Neurologic and Neurosurgical Emergencies

JULIO CRUZ, M.D., Ph.D.

Adjunct Professor of Neurosurgery
Allegheny University of the Health Sciences
Philadelphia, Pennsylvania, USA

Director, The Comprehensive International Center for Neuroemergencies
São Paulo, Brazil

Former Assistant Professor of Neurosurgery
University of Pennsylvania Medical Center
Philadelphia, Pennsylvania, USA

Former Visiting Assistant Professor of Neurosurgery
The University of Texas Medical School at Houston
Houston, Texas, USA

Neurologic and Neurosurgical Emergencies

W.B. SAUNDERS COMPANY
A Division of Harcourt Brace & Company
Philadelphia London Toronto Montreal Sydney Tokyo

W.B. SAUNDERS COMPANY
A Division of Harcourt Brace & Company

The Curtis Center
Independence Square West
Philadelphia, Pennsylvania 19106

Library of Congress Cataloging-in-Publication Data

Neurologic and neurosurgical emergencies / [edited by] Julio Cruz.—1st ed.

p. cm.

ISBN 0–7216–6105–X

1. Central nervous system—Diseases. 2. Medical emergencies.
3. Neurological intensive care. I. Cruz, Julio.
[DNLM: 1. Nervous System Diseases—therapy. 2. Nervous System Diseases—diagnosis. 3. Emergencies. 4. Emergency Treatment. WL 140 N49155 1998]

RC361.N46 1998 616.8′0425—dc21

DNLM/DLC 98–7038

NEUROLOGIC AND NEUROSURGICAL EMERGENCIES ISBN 0–7216–6105–X

Printed in the United States of America.

Last digit is the print number: 9 8 7 6 5 4 3 2 1

This book is dedicated to my father
Julio Adamor Cruz *(in memoriam),*
for his daily demonstrations on the value of hard work and humanitarian help to human beings;

and to my Neurosurgical Instructor
Vittorio Rolando Boccaletti, M.D. *(in memoriam),*
for his superb teaching of Neurosurgery and Humanitarian Medicine at Hospital São Paulo, Escola Paulista de Medicina, Federal University of São Paulo, São Paulo, Brazil

Contributors

Anthony L. Alcantara, M.D.

Assistant Professor (Clinical), FTA, Diagnostic Radiology, Wayne State University School of Medicine; Vice Chief, Diagnostic Radiology, Detroit Receiving Hospital, Detroit, Michigan

Initial Evaluation and Management of Neuroemergencies

Ann Marie Angelucci, M.S.N., R.N., C.C.R.N.

Staff Nurse, University of Pennsylvania Health System, Philadelphia, Pennsylvania

Neuroemergency Nursing

Thomas P. Bleck, M.D.

Professor of Neurology, Neurological Surgery and Internal Medicine, The Louise Nerancy Professor in Neurology; Director, Nerancy Neurologic Intensive Care Unit, University of Virginia, Charlottesville, Virginia

Cardiovascular Disorders Related to Neuroemergencies; Acute Stroke Management

Derek A. Bruce, M.B., Ch.B.

Clinical Associate Professor, Department of Neurosurgery, University of Texas Southwestern Health Sciences Center; Director, Pediatric Neurosurgery, Columbia Children's Hospital, Dallas, Texas

Pediatric Neuroemergencies With Intracranial Hypertension

Werther B. de Carvalho, M.D.

Adjunct Professor of Pediatrics and Chief, Pediatric Intensive Care Unit, Hospital São Paulo, Escola Paulista de Medicina, Federal University of São Paulo, São Paulo, Brazil

Severe Acute Brain Trauma

Peter B. Crino, M.D., Ph.D.

University of Pennsylvania School of Medicine and University of Pennsylvania Medical Center, Philadelphia, Pennsylvania

Acute Seizure Disorders

Julio Cruz, M.D., Ph.D.

Adjunct Professor of Neurosurgery, Allegheny University of the Health Sciences, Philadelphia, Pennsylvania, USA; Director, The Comprehensive International Center for Neuroemergencies, São Paulo, Brazil; Former Assistant Professor of Neurosurgery, University of Pennsylvania Medical Center, Philadelphia, Pennsylvania, USA; Former Visiting Assistant Professor of Neurosurgery, The University of Texas Medical School at Houston, Houston, Texas, USA

Severe Acute Brain Trauma

Eugene S. Flamm, M.D.

Charles Harrison Frazier Professor and Chairman, Department of Neurosurgery, University of Pennsylvania School of Medicine, Philadelphia, Pennsylvania

Parasurgical Management of Aneurysmal Subarachnoid Hemorrhage; Surgical Management of Spontaneous Intracranial Hemorrhage

Gwendolyn F. Ford-Lynch, M.D.

Assistant Professor of Neurology, Rush University; Assistant Attending Physician, Director, Neurologic Critical Care Program, Rush–Presbyterian–St. Luke's Medical Center, Chicago, Illinois

Acute Stroke Management

Alberto A. Gabbai, M.D.

Professor of Neurology, Chair, Department of Neurology, Escola Paulista de Medicina, Federal University of São Paulo, São Paulo, Brazil

Acute Neuromuscular Diseases

Steven L. Galetta, M.D.

Professor of Neurology, University of Pennsylvania School of Medicine; Professor of Neurology and secondary appointment in Ophthalmology, University of Pennsylvania School of Medicine, Philadelphia, Pennsylvania

Neuroemergencies During Pregnancy; Neuro-Ophthalmologic Emergencies

Thomas A. Gennarelli, M.D.

Professor and Chairman, Department of Neurosurgery, Allegheny University of the Health Sciences, Philadelphia, Pennsylvania

Pituitary Emergencies

Gary Goldberg, M.D.

Associate Professor, Department of Physical Medicine and Rehabilitation, Temple University School of Medicine; Attending Psychiatrist, Drucker Brain Injury Center; Co-Director, Electrodiagnostic Center, Moss Rehabilitation Hospital, Philadelphia, Pennsylvania

Neurorehabilitation

Virginia Graziani, M.D.

Assistant Professor, Department of Rehabilitation Medicine, Jefferson Medical College; Assistant Professor, Department of Rehabilitation Medicine, Thomas Jefferson University Hospital, Magee Rehabilitation Hospital, Philadelphia, Pennsylvania

Neurorehabilitation

C. William Hanson III, M.D.

Assistant Professor of Anesthesiology, Surgery and Internal Medicine, and Medical Director, Surgical Intensive Care Unit, University of Pennsylvania Medical Center, Philadelphia, Pennsylvania

Acute Respiratory Failure in Neuroemergencies

Robin Haskell, M.S.N., R.N., C.R.N.P., C.C.R.N.

Nurse Practitioner, University of Pennsylvania Health System, Philadelphia, Pennsylvania

Neuroemergency Nursing

Robert W. Hurst, M.D.

Associate Professor of Radiology, Neurosurgery, and Neurology, University of Pennsylvania, Philadelphia, Pennsylvania

Cervicocerebral Interventional Neuroradiology

Kevin D. Judy, M.D.

Assistant Professor of Neurosurgery, Hospital of the University of Pennsylvania, Philadelphia, Pennsylvania

Intracranial Tumor Emergencies

Scott E. Kasner, M.D.

Assistant Professor of Neurology, University of Pennsylvania School of Medicine; Co-director, Comprehensive Stroke Center, University of Pennsylvania Medical Center, Philadelphia, Pennsylvania

Neuroemergencies During Pregnancy

Rosemary Kennedy, B.S.N., R.N., C.C.R.N.

Staff Nurse, University of Pennsylvania Health System, Philadelphia, Pennsylvania

Neuroemergency Nursing

Dennis L. Kolson, M.D., Ph.D.

Assistant Professor of Neurology, Department of Neurology, Hospital of the University of Pennsylvania, Philadelphia, Pennsylvania

Infectious and Parasitic Emergencies of the Central Nervous System

David J. Langer, M.D.

Chief Resident, Neurosurgery, Department of Neurosurgery, Hospital of the University of Pennsylvania, Philadelphia, Pennsylvania

Parasurgical Management of Aneursymal Subarachnoid Hemorrhage

Daniel T. Laskowitz, M.D.

Associate in Neurology, Department of Medicine (Division of Neurology), Duke University Medical Center, Durham, North Carolina

Infections and Parasitic Emergencies of the Central Nervous System; Neuro-Ophthalmologic Emergencies

Suzana M. F. Malheiros, M.D.

Attending Neurologist, Escola Paulista de Medicina, Federal University of São Paulo, São Paulo, Brazil

Acute Neuromuscular Diseases

Eileen Maloney-Wilensky, B.S.N., R.N., C.C.R.N., C.N.R.N.

Assistant Nurse Manager, University of Pennsylvania Health System, Philadelphia, Pennsylvania

Neuroemergency Nursing

Paul J. Marcotte, B.Sc., M.D.

Assistant Professor of Neurosurgery, University of Pennsylvania, Philadelphia, Pennsylvania

Acute Spinal Disorders

Etienne Marguinaud, M.D.

Attending Physician for Anesthesiology and Critical Care, Service de Neurochirurgie, Centre Hospitalier Universitaire de Bordeaux, Bordeaux, France

Severe Acute Brain Trauma

Ayrton R. Massaro, M.D.

Attending Neurologist, Hospital das Clínicas, University of São Paulo, São Paulo, Brazil

Acute Neuromuscular Diseases

Riccardo Massei, M.D.

Professor of Anesthesiology, University of Milano, and Chief, Servizio di Anestesia e Rianimazione, Ospedale di Lecco, Lecco, Italy

Severe Acute Brain Trauma

Cristina Mattioli, M.D.

Attending Physician in Neuro Intensive Care, Ospedale San Raffaele, University of Milano, Milano, Italy

Severe Acute Brain Trauma

Daniel B. Michael, M.D., Ph.D.

Assistant Professor of Neurological Surgery, Adjunct Assistant Professor of Anatomy and Cell Biology, Wayne State University School of Medicine; Chief of Neurosurgery and Surgical Director of the Neurologic Intensive Care Unit, Detroit Receiving Hospital, Detroit, Michigan

Initial Evaluation and Management of Neuroemergencies

Linda J. Michaud, M.D.

Associate Professor of Clinical Physical Medicine and Rehabilitation and Clinical Pediatrics, University of Cincinnati College of Medicine; Director of Pediatric Rehabilitation, Children's Hospital Medical Center, Cincinnati, Ohio

Neurorehabilitation

Giulio Minoja, M.D.

Assistant Professor of Anesthesiology and Intensive Care, University of Pavia–Varese; Associate Chief of Anesthesia and Intensive Care, Ospedale di Circolo–Fondazione Macchi, Varese, Italy

Severe Acute Brain Trauma

Kazuo Okuchi, M.D.

Director of Neurosurgery, Nara Prefectural Emergency and Critical Care Center, and Lecturer, Nara Medical University, Nara, Japan

Severe Acute Brain Trauma

Acary S. B. Oliveira, M.D.

Attending Neurologist, Escola Paulista de Medicina, Federal University of São Paulo, São Paulo, Brazil

Acute Neuromuscular Diseases

Brian J. O'Neil, M.D.

Associate Professor, Department of Emergency Medicine, Wayne State University School of Medicine; Research Director, Department of Emergency Medicine, Grace Hospital, Detroit, Michigan

Initial Evaluation and Management of Neuroemergencies

Götz Penkert, M.D.

Associate Professor, Consultant Neurosurgeon, Nordstadt Hospital, Hannover, Germany

Traumatic Disorders of the Peripheral Nervous System

Patti L. Peterson, M.D.

Associate Professor of Neurology and Emergency Medicine, Wayne State University School of Medicine; Chief of Neurology, Detroit Receiving Hospital, Detroit, Michigan

Initial Evaluation and Management of Neuroemergencies

Marie-Edith Petitjean, M.D.

Attending Physician and Lecturer, Departement des Urgences, Centre Hospitalier Universitaire de Bordeaux, Bordeaux, France

Severe Acute Brain Trauma

Matthew F. Philips, M.D.

Clinical Instructor in Neurosurgery, Resident in Neurosurgery, Hospital of the University of Pennsylvania, Philadelphia, Pennsylvania

Intracranial Tumor Emergencies

Marguerite Phillips, B.S.N., R.N.

Staff Nurse, University of Pennsylvania Medical Center, Philadelphia, Pennsylvania

Neuroemergency Nursing

J. Javier Provencio, M.D.

Senior Resident in Neurology and Internal Medicine, University of Virginia, Charlottesville, Virginia

Cardiovascular Disorders Related to Neuroemergencies

Kathy Paulik Ramson, M.S.N., R.N., C.C.R.N.

Staff Nurse, University of Pennsylvania Health System, Philadelphia, Pennsylvania

Neuroemergency Nursing

Eric C. Raps, M.D.

William N. Kelley Professor of Neurology, Associate Professor of Neurology and Neurosurgery, University of Pennsylvania School of Medicine; Director of Stroke and Neurointensive Care, Medical Director, Neuroscience Acute Care Unit, University of Pennsylvania Medical Center, Department of Neurology, Philadelphia, Pennsylvania

Neuroemergencies During Pregnancy; Neuro-Ophthalmologic Emergencies

Keith M. Robinson, M.D.

Assistant Professor, Department of Rehabilitation Medicine, University of Pennsylvania Medical Center, Philadelphia, Pennsylvania

Neurorehabilitation

Kristin M. Sagedy, B.S.N., R.N., C.C.R.N.

Staff Nurse, University of Pennsylvania Health System, Philadelphia, Pennsylvania

Neuroemergency Nursing

Madjid Samii, M.D.

Professor, Hannover Medical School; Director of Neurosurgical Clinic at Nordstadt Hospital and Hannover Medical School, Nordstadt Hospital, Hannover, Germany

Traumatic Disorders of the Peripheral Nervous System

M. Elizabeth Sandel, M.D.

Medical Director, Kaiser Foundation Rehabilitation Center; Chief, Rehabilitation Medicine, Kaiser Foundation Hospital, Vallejo, California

Neurorehabilitation

Diane Schretzman, M.S.N., R.N., C.N.R.N.

Staff Nurse, University of Pennsylvania Medical Center, Philadelphia, Pennsylvania

Neuroemergency Nursing

Ellen G. Shaver, M.D.

Medical College of Georgia, Augusta, Georgia; Eisenhower Army Medical Center, Fort Gordon, Georgia

Acute Spinal Disorders

Mark M. Stecker, M.D., Ph.D.

Assistant Professor, Department of Neurology, University of Pennsylvania; Assistant Professor of Neurology, Hospital of the University of Pennsylvania, Philadelphia, Pennsylvania

Acute Seizure Disorders

John R. Vender, M.D.

Assistant Professor of Neurosurgery, Medical College of Georgia, Augusta, Georgia

Pituitary Emergencies

Robert J. Weil, M.D.

Resident in Neurosurgery, Hospital of the University of Pennsylvania, Philadelphia, Pennsylvania

Acute Spinal Disorders

Eric L. Zager, M.D.

Associate Professor of Neurosurgery, University of Pennsylvania; Attending Neurosurgeon, Hospital of the University of Pennsylvania, Children's Hospital of Philadelphia, Philadelphia Veterans Administration Medical Center, Graduate Hospital, and Presbyterian Hospital, Philadelphia, Pennsylvania

Parasurgical Management of Aneurysmal Subarachnoid Hemorrhage; Surgical Management of Spontaneous Intracranial Hemorrhage

Preface

The International Society for Neuroemergencies (ISONEUREM) was founded with the aim of converging nonsurgical (neurologic) and neurosurgical emergencies into a single body of scientific information, heavily based on clinical experience (without extrapolation from animal experimentation). The first ISONEUREM symposium (NEUROEMERGENCY '96), held in July 1996 in Freeport, Bahamas, was a very friendly, unbiased, and productive event, where all neuroemergency professionals could exchange clinically relevant information from the initial event through the emergency room and all phases of hospitalization, up to neurorehabilitation.

This book represents an original effort to concentrate in a single volume the roots of ISONEUREM, namely, to address unbiased, updated information regarding adult and pediatric neuroemergency issues in a most comprehensive fashion.

Up until now, the term *neuroemergency* has not yet been defined in medical dictionaries. According to the ISONEUREM standards, however, neuroemergency issues are expected to be covered in a combined and multidisciplinary fashion, rather than in isolated islands of pertinent medical information.

At the second ISONEUREM symposium (NEUROEMERGENCY '99), to be held in Italy, the above-described philosophy will be further enhanced, and all future ISONEUREM events will highlight the merit of addressing unbiased, strongly scientific and clinically relevant information on the diagnosis, pathophysiology, and management of acute insults to the nervous system.

It is therefore believed that this book will provide the reader with truly useful information on this rather complex topic, beyond previously published books or journal papers addressing questionable information regarding neurologic and neurosurgical emergencies, and neuro intensive care medicine.

JULIO CRUZ, M.D., PH.D.

Acknowledgments

Incentive and support are frankly appreciated from my family members in the cities of Rio de Janeiro, São Paulo, and Guarujá, in Brazil.

Educational support is acknowledged from my teachers at Externato São Paulo and Instituto Estadual de Educação Prof. Alberto Levy, for my pre-graduate studies in the city of São Paulo, Brazil.

Pre-graduate medical educational support from my teachers at Curso Objetivo in the city of São Paulo, Brazil, is also frankly appreciated.

Graduate medical teaching is also strongly appreciated from my professors at Faculdade de Medicina do ABC, in Santo André, São Paulo, Brazil.

Following medical graduation, I strongly acknowledge the support of my neurosurgical professors at Escola Paulista de Medicina, Federal University of São Paulo, São Paulo, Brazil, and the University of Pennsylvania School of Medicine, Philadelphia, Pennsylvania, USA.

As a faculty member, I heavily thank the physicians, nurses, scientists, and technicians from the University of Texas Medical School at Houston, Texas, USA, the University of Pennsylvania Medical Center, Philadelphia, Pennsylvania, USA, and the Allegheny University of the Health Sciences, Philadelphia, Pennsylvania, USA.

My 1980–81 experience as a Post-Graduate Fellowship Award recipient, sponsored by The Rotary Foundation of Rotary International, was rather gratifying and unforgettable.

JULIO CRUZ, M.D., PH.D.

Contents

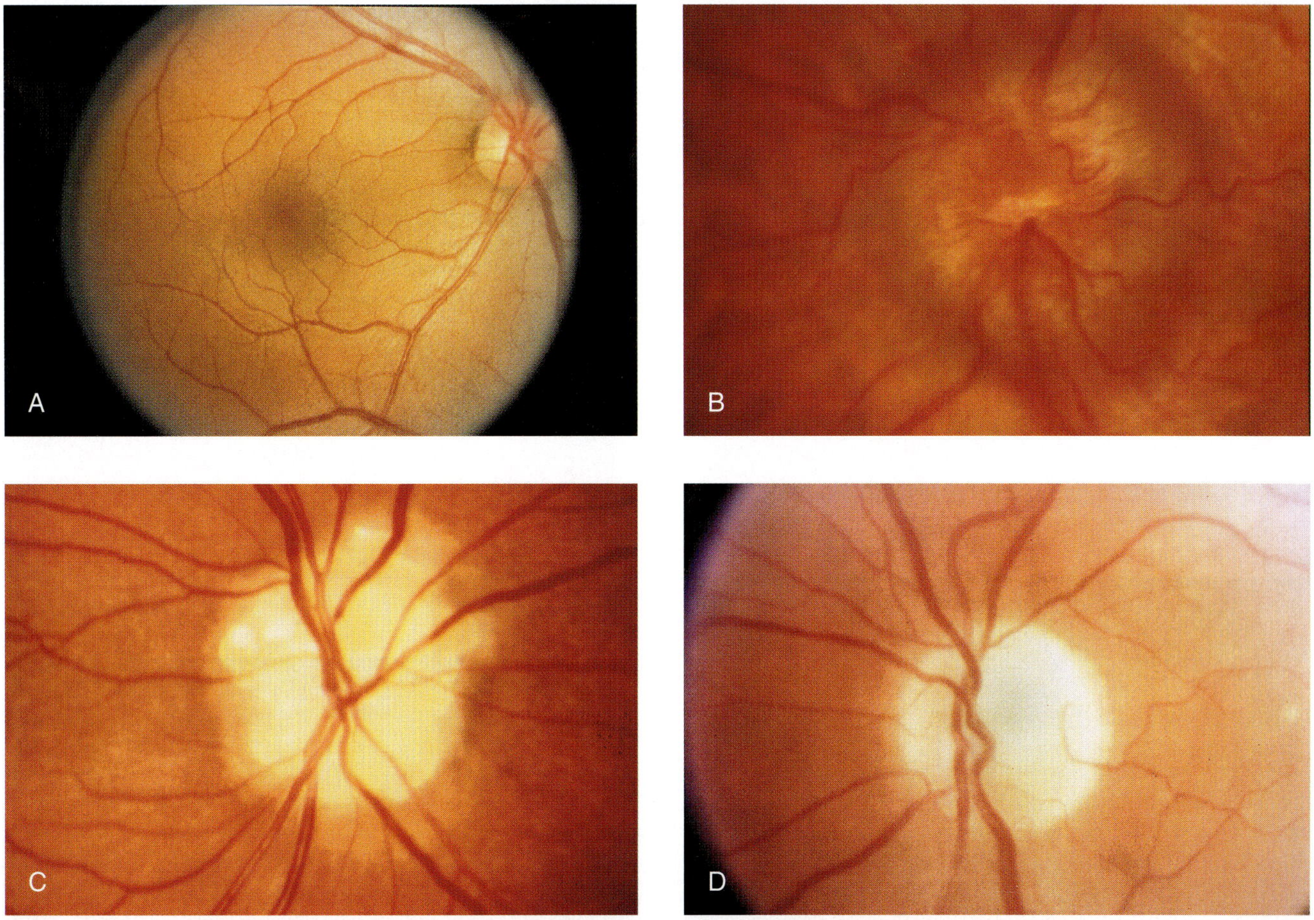

FIGURE 7–1 • *A*, Normal optic disc. *B*, Fully developed papilledema, demonstrating disc swelling, hyperemia, venous distention, and hemorrhages. *C*, Disc drusen (pseudopapilledema): note central origination of vessels and absence of peripapillary nerve fiber layer swelling. *D*, Segmental atrophy secondary to anterior ischemic optic neuropathy.

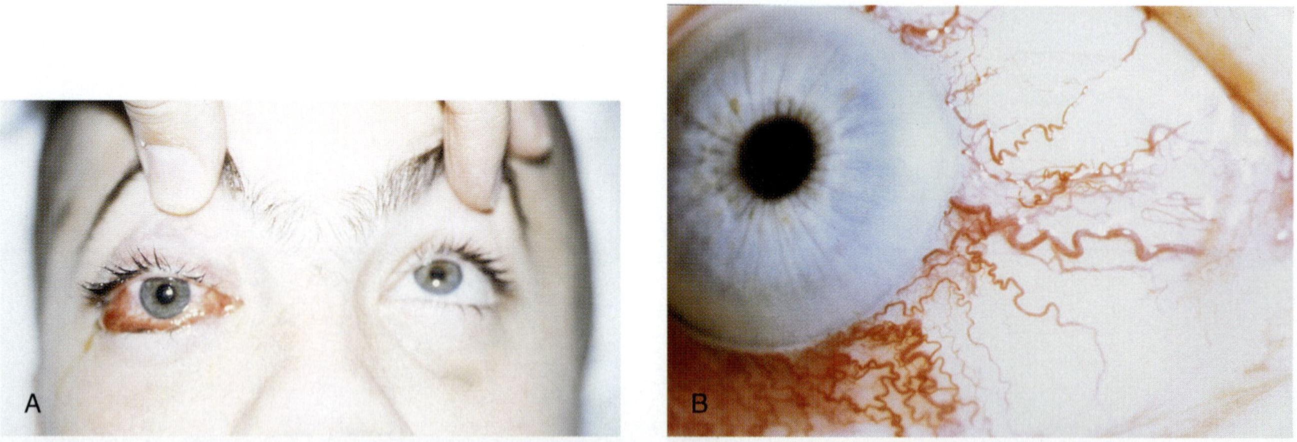

FIGURE 7–6 • *A*, Arterialized conjunctival and scleral vessels, exophthalmos, and chemosis due to orbital congestion from carotid-cavernous fistula. Impaired eye elevation may be from muscle and nerve dysfunction. *B*, Close up of arterialized conjunctival vessels.

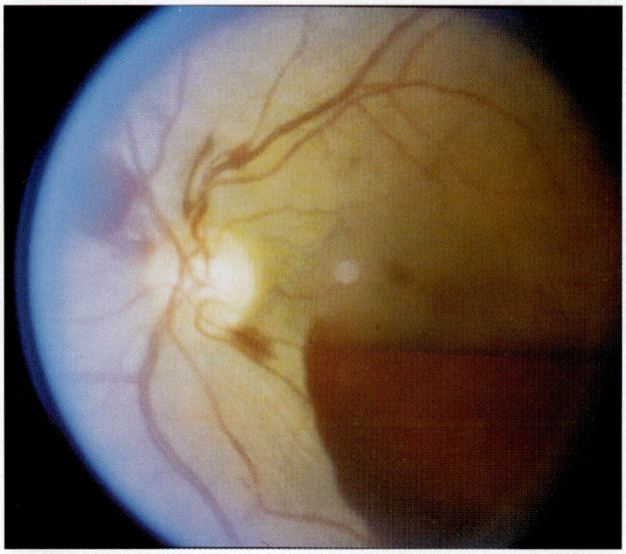

FIGURE 7–8 • Terson's syndrome: subhyaloid "boat-shaped" hemorrhage secondary to rupture of anterior communicating artery aneurysm.

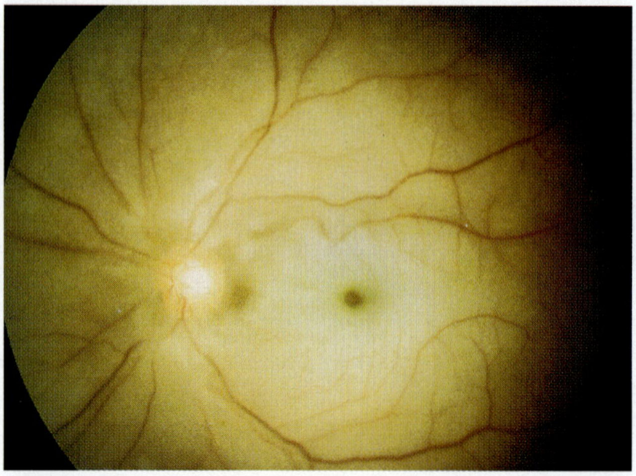

FIGURE 7–9 • Central retinal artery occlusion. Note pale retina, with attenuation of vessels.

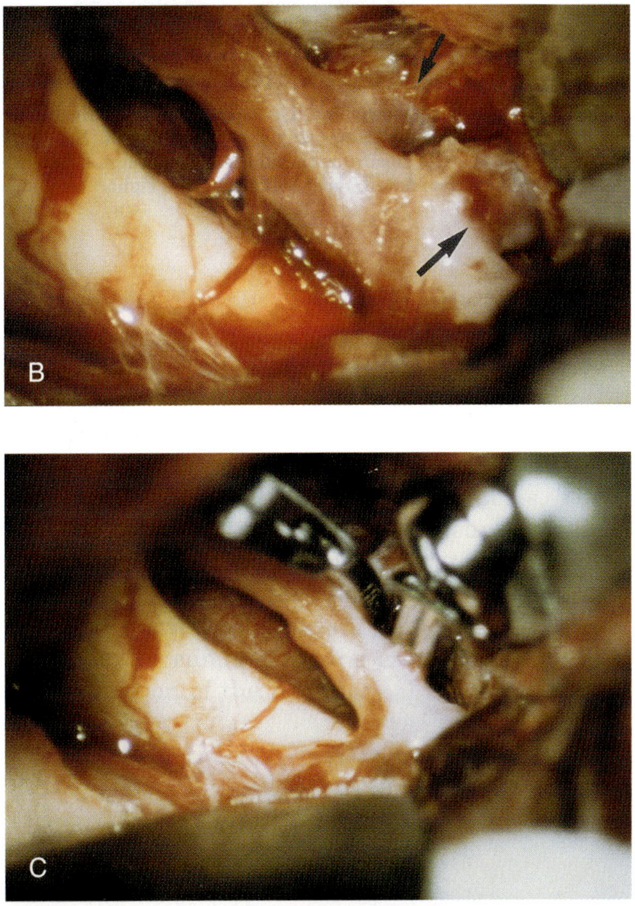

FIGURE 10-16 • *B*, Intraoperative photomicrograph showing both aneurysms (PComA aneurysm—small arrow; AChA aneurysm—large arrow). *C*, Following clip obliteration of both aneurysms.

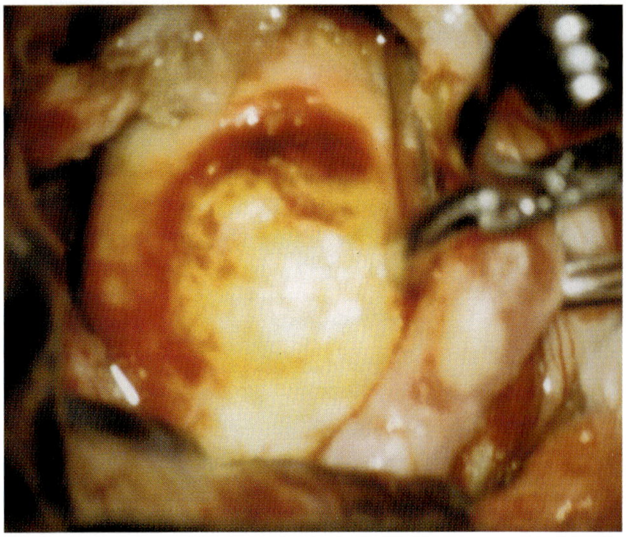

FIGURE 10-30*B* • Intraoperative photomicrograph showing the heavily calcified, atherosclerotic aneurysm dome, which was repaired with an angled fenestrated clip.

opiate overdose or hypoglycemia and the appropriate equipment is available (e.g., Dextrostix, glucometer, naloxone [Narcan], glucose, and restraints), therapy may be initiated prior to hospital arrival.

Initial Emergency Department Evaluation and Management

Resuscitation

In all neurologic and neurosurgical emergencies, the initial evaluation and stabilization of the patient are of paramount importance to eventual neurologic outcome. It is well documented that hypotension, hypoxemia, seizures, hyperthermia, and other factors clearly increase secondary injury.[11–13]

The goals of resuscitation are to stabilize vital functions (airway, breathing, and circulation: the ABCs, vital signs and oxygenation) and perform a systematic evaluation of the patient in order to determine what emergent interventions are necessary. In all patients, the cervical spine (c-spine) should be assessed and stabilized and overt hemorrhage immediately controlled.

AIRWAY

The airway must be patent. A number of airway adjuncts exist and include the chin lift and establishment of nasopharyngeal or oropharyngeal airways; all improve airway patency. It must be stressed that these are only temporizing techniques and if oxygenation does not improve, a definitive airway technique (i.e., intubation of the trachea) is necessary.

BREATHING

The patient's respiration must be of adequate rate and tidal volume in order to avoid hypoxia and hypercapnia. Supplemental oxygen should be administered to patients who are severely traumatized or hypoxic as indicated by pulse oximetry. Oxygenation should be actively facilitated either with a bag-valve mask (if the patient is spontaneously breathing, it is best to assist ventilation during inspiration) or by use of 100% oxygen via a nonrebreather mask. The Sellick maneuver (application of cricoid pressure) reduces insufflation of the stomach during active oxygenation or during rapid-sequence induction. Rapid-sequence induction refers to the technique of rapidly preparing a patient for intubation while reducing the risk of pulmonary aspiration.[14]

Patients who are either comatose (Glasgow Coma Scale[15] score < 9 [Table 1–1]), hypotensive and refractory to volume replacement, unable to maintain adequate oxygen saturation despite the use of 100% oxygen, or unable to protect their airway should be intubated. Prior to intubation, preoxygenation can be achieved either actively with a bag-valve mask or by letting the patient breathe 100% oxygen via a non-rebreather mask, as previously described.

TABLE 1–1 **GLASGOW COMA SCALE**

Eye Opening			
	Opens	Spontaneously	4
		To verbal commands	3
		To pain	2
	No Response		1
Best Motor Response			
	To verbal command	Obeys	6
	To pain stimulus	Localizes pain	5
		Flexion withdrawal	4
		Flexion abnormal	3
		Extension abnormal	2
	No response		1
Best Verbal Response			
	Oriented and converses		5
	Disoriented and converses		4
	Verbalizes		3
	Vocalizes		2
	No response		1
Glasgow Coma Score (GCS) =	**TOTAL**		**3-15**

All patients should be presumed to have a full stomach at the time of presentation to the emergency department. The neurohormonal response to trauma predisposes these patients to aspiration. This is especially true in the case of shock and head injury. The coexistence of multiple trauma and head injury alters the approach to airway management. Cerebral blood flow (CBF), intracranial pressure (ICP), volume status, and cardiovascular function must be considered simultaneously so that no single factor is compromised.[16] Laryngoscopy and intubation may result in bradycardia, tachycardia, hypertension, and increased ICP.[17]

Intubation Techniques

Numerous intubation techniques and pharmacologic regimens for tracheal intubation currently exist, and the subject of airway management in the acutely ill patient is a controversial subject. For the sake of brevity, the most common intubation techniques and pharmacologic therapies will be reviewed and recommendations made.

Orotracheal intubation with rapid-sequence induction is becoming the procedure of choice for traumatic airway management. Blind nasotracheal intubation has long been advocated as the procedure of choice in patients with suspected c-spine injury. This procedure requires spontaneous breathing and that the intubator can clearly recognize the patient's inspiration and expiration. In order to perform this procedure optimally, the nasal mucosa must be premedicated with an anesthetic and a vasoconstrictor (i.e., 4% lidocaine and 1% Neo-Synephrine). The effect of these medications is not immediate, and even after appropriate premedication, epistaxis can still occur. This may increase the patient's chance of aspiration and further complicate orotracheal intubation attempts.[18] Nasotracheal intubation causes intense cardiovascular stimulation that may cause a deleterious increase in ICP.[19] If nasotracheal intubation is performed, the patient should be adequately sedated, receive IV lidocaine (which may ameliorate some of the sympathetic circulatory effects), the c-spine should be immobilized, Sellick's maneuver should be performed, and the patient should be adequately oxygenated.

Despite the high success rate associated with orotracheal and nasotracheal intubation, it may be necessary to establish a surgical airway (cricothyroidotomy), if the nonsurgical procedures have failed or the patient has sustained massive facial and/or upper airway injuries.

Lidocaine (1.5–2 mg/kg/intravenous push [IVP] 2–3 minutes prior to intubation) attenuates much of the hemodynamic and cough reflex and rise in ICP during intubation.[20–22] The mechanism by which lidocaine accomplishes this is currently unclear. Etomidate (Amidate) is a nonbarbiturate, non-narcotic hypnotic agent that reliably facilitates induction in less than 1 minute, with a duration of action of 4–6 minutes.[23] Etomidate, when given in the above induction dose, has little effect on heart rate and cardiac output when compared with equipotent doses of thiopental.[24] Etomidate also has much less respiratory depressant effects than the barbiturates traditionally used in rapid-sequence induction, although transient apnea can occur if etomidate is given too rapidly.[25] Similar to the barbiturates, etomidate results in a reduction of ICP in a dose-dependent manner by decreasing CBF and cerebral metabolic rate.[26, 27] The aforementioned therapeutic attributes make etomidate an ideal induction agent in the setting of multiple trauma, head injury, and the potentially difficult airway.

Succinylcholine (1 mg/kg/IVP) provides rapid onset (<1 minute) and short duration of action (4–6 minutes) and makes it the paralytic of choice during rapid-sequence induction. The side effects of succinylcholine are fasciculations, hyperkalemia, and transient rise in intracranial, intragastric, and intraocular pressures. The fasciculations and increased intracranial, intragastric, and intraocular pressures all can be blocked by administration of a defasciculating dose of a nondepolarizing agent (e.g., 0.01 mg/kg/IVP of vecuronium [Norcuron]) 2–3 minutes prior to succinylcholine administration.[28] If a defasciculating agent is used, the dose of succinylcholine should be increased to 1.5–2 mg/kg/IVP in order to ensure rapid onset of action. A small number of individuals may develop vagally mediated bradycardia, histamine-induced hypotension, or malignant hyperthermia; unfortunately, there is no way to predict which patients will respond in this manner.

The recommended procedure for rapid-sequence induction is as follows:

1. Preoxygenation with 100% oxygen and use of the Sellick maneuver during active oxygenation.
2. Administration of lidocaine 1.5–2 mg/kg/IVP and vecuronium 0.01 mg/kg/IVP.
3. Slow administration of etomidate 0.3 mg/kg/IVP. The dosage should be reduced to 0.1–0.2 mg/kg/IVP if the patient becomes hypotensive.
4. Administration of succinylcholine 1.5–2 mg/kg/IVP.
5. Performance of the Sellick maneuver and orotracheal intubation of the trachea. The cuff should be inflated, breath sounds verified, tube placement confirmed, and the Sellick maneuver released.
6. Neuromuscular paralysis should be maintained, if indicated, with vecuronium 0.1 mg/kg/IVP.
7. End-tidal carbon dioxide detectors can be used to discriminate tracheal from esophageal intubation.

CIRCULATION

Circulation can be assessed according to the patient's vital signs and assessment of end-organ perfusion. All hypotensive patients (systolic blood pressure < 90 mm Hg) and those with signs of end-organ hypoperfusion (oliguria, poor capillary refill, confusion) should receive aggressive volume resuscitation with crystalloids, colloids, or packed red blood cells. Hypotension should never be attributed to head injury until an exhaustive search for other causes has been carried out. Hypotension secondary to intracranial injury occurs only as a terminal event resulting from failure of the medullary centers. Hypotension, however, can occur due to hemorrhage from scalp lacerations and also from high cervical cord injuries. It is also important to recall that vital signs alone are a poor indicator of shock states, as blood pressure drops only after loss of 30% of the blood volume. Intravenous access should be obtained and appropriate laboratory studies drawn.

Bedside glucometry and screening laboratory studies should be performed. Screening laboratory tests should include complete blood count, electrolytes, blood glucose, blood urea nitrogen and creatinine, prothrombin time and partial thromboplastin time, blood type and screen (in the trauma patient), and arterial blood gases. If the patient has a nonfocal neurologic examination, urine and several tubes of blood should be saved in order to obtain serum and urine drug screens; liver enzymes; calcium, ammonia, carboxyhemoglobin and cyanide levels; serum osmolality; and anticonvulsant or other drug levels as indicated by the clinical presentation. The initial evaluation should also include an electrocardiogram (to rule out myocardial infarction or arrhythmia) and x-rays (to rule out lung, abdomen, and vascular abnormalities).

Rectal temperature, heart rate, blood pressure, respiratory rate, pulse oximetry, and cardiac rhythm should be closely monitored throughout the evaluation. In comatose patients, a urinary catheter and nasogastric tube should be carefully inserted if no contraindications exist (i.e., possible basilar skull fracture or urethral injury) while the appropriate invasive monitoring (e.g., central venous line, arterial line, ICP monitor) is placed.

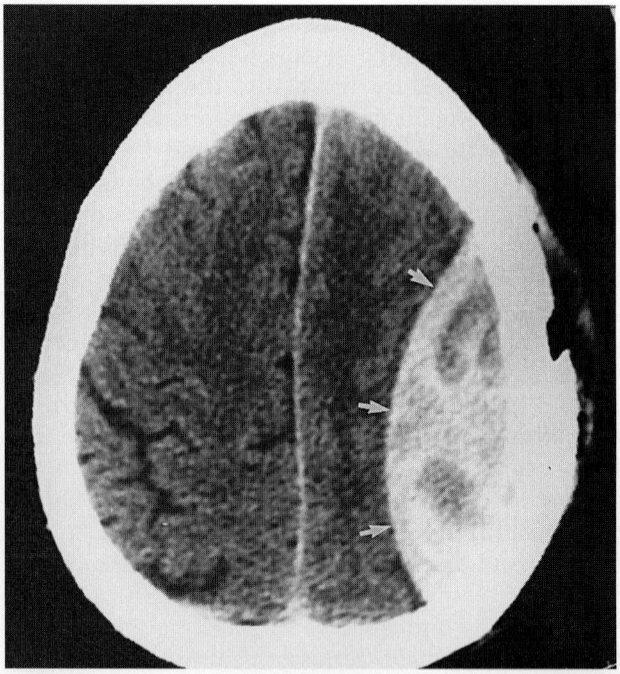

FIGURE 1-1 • A depressed skull fracture in the left parietal region is associated with a large epidural hematoma.

Initial Clinical Examination

The purpose of the initial clinical evaluation is to assess the patient's injuries/clinical disorder and prioritize further management. After the patient has been initially stabilized, a clinical evaluation should be performed in order to rapidly identify neurologic signs that indicate the need for immediate intervention (e.g., drainage of an epidural hematoma [Fig. 1–1]). The patient's level of consciousness should be assessed and examination of the pupils and oculomotor function performed.

A postresuscitation Glasgow Coma Scale (GCS) score and serial GCS evaluations should be performed in order to identify early signs of neurologic deterioration. The advantages of the GCS are its simplicity and high inter-rater reliability. The disadvantages are that the score is unreliable in patients who have sustained significant facial trauma (those whose eyes are swollen shut); are pharmacologically paralyzed, intubated, or dysphasic; in patients who are hypotensive; or in those who have suffered a spinal cord injury.

Initial Emergency Management

If bedside glucometry reveals a low glucose level, glucose should be administered (25–50 g/IVP). In suspected nutritionally deficient patients, e.g., alcoholics or chemotherapy patients, 100 mg of thiamine (1–2 mg/kg/IVP) should be administered prior to the administration of glucose. Thiamine is given to promote carbohydrate metabolism and to prevent the acute onset of Wernicke's disease (see later section). The newer formulations of thiamine do not cause anaphylactoid reactions when intravenously administered.

Naloxone (Narcan) should be administered (2 mg/IVP in adults) and repeated when indicated if narcotic intoxication is a consideration. If precipitation of opiate withdrawal is a concern, smaller doses (0.01 mg/kg/IVP) should be given and repeated if necessary. Naloxone is an effective antagonist of opiates and synthetic narcotics (e.g., propoxyphene), although with propoxyphene, larger doses may be needed to reverse the endorphin effects. Patients who are emerging from opiate overdose can become confused or combative and should be appropriately restrained prior to naloxone administration. If poisoning is a possibility, it may be necessary to lavage the stomach; emesis should be induced only in the alert adult patient (ipecac 30 mL orally). Evacuation of the stomach has been shown to be effective only after acute ingestion (<2 hours) unless drugs that decrease gastric motility (i.e., anticholinergics) have been ingested.

Elevations in systemic arterial pressure should not be treated, particularly in those patients who have sustained a cerebral infarction, intracerebral hemorrhage, or post-traumatic hemorrhage, unless (1) the systolic blood pressure exceeds 220 mm Hg or the diastolic blood pressure exceeds 120 mm Hg on three repeated measurements at 15-minute intervals; or (2) cardiac failure or aortic dissection is identified. The blood pressure usually decreases by 10% over the first 24 hours of the stroke, and aggressive use of calcium channel blockers and other antihypertensive drugs can lead to further decrease in cerebral perfusion.[29]

Situations that necessitate immediate therapeutic intervention include severe central nervous system (CNS) trauma (Fig. 1–2), status epilepticus, toxic and metabolic disorders, and meningitis. If these conditions are not expeditiously managed (as described in later sections and other chapters), neurologic outcome will be significantly compromised. If there is evidence of herniation (see later section) or seizure activity, immediate diagnostic/therapeutic intervention should be initiated. Hyperventilation, with a goal to initially maintain the arterial P_{CO_2} between 28 and 32 torr (kPa value between 3.7 and 4.3), may provide a rapid decrease in ICP (if there is evidence of herniation). Administration of mannitol (0.5 g/kg bolus) may also provide valuable time to initiate definitive, surgical therapy; as well as to exert a synergistic effect with hyperventilation. This latter effect simultaneously decreases abnormally high ICP and improves cerebrovenous oxygenation (by increasing cerebral blood flow).

Neuroimaging

After the neurologically impaired patient has been resuscitated and stabilized, an initial clinical evalu-

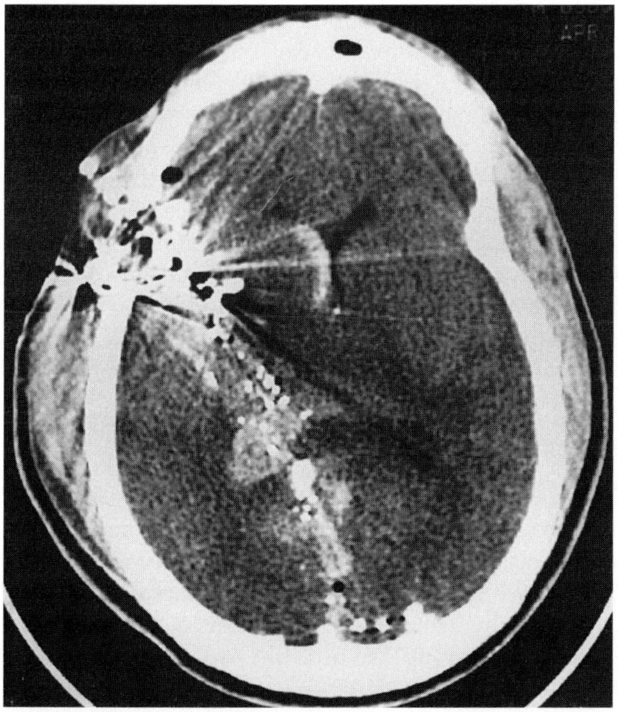

FIGURE 1-2 • Gunshot wound. Bullet and bone fragments are scattered through the brain parenchyma from a close range gunshot to the right temporal region.

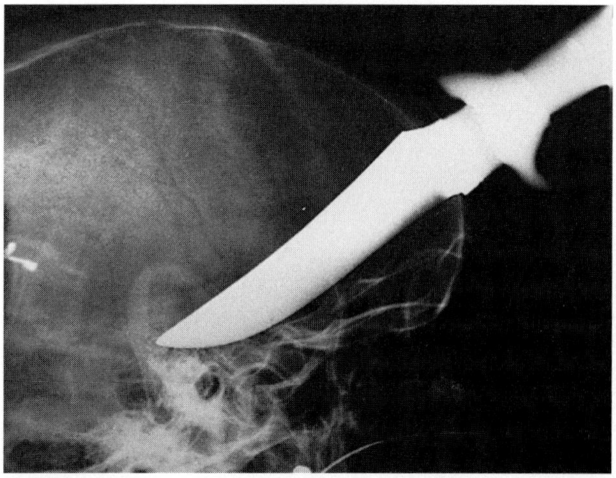

FIGURE 1-3 • Acute penetrating trauma. A Bowie knife was impaled through the frontal bone to the level of the clivus.

ation has been performed, screening laboratory studies have been sent for analysis, and initial emergency management has been provided, appropriate neuroimaging studies (e.g., computed tomography [CT] scan of the head, cervical spine radiography) and other radiologic studies can be performed.

All comatose patients and those who have suffered trauma (especially above the clavicles) should be suspected to have a c-spine injury, immobilized in a rigid cervical collar in the neutral position, and stabilized on a back board until a c-spine injury can be ruled out. The physical examination alone does not reliably predict c-spine injury.[30] Lateral c-spine radiography can miss up to 30% of c-spine injuries (most of which are ligamentous in nature),[31] and even a complete c-spine series does not exclude cervical injury if a concomitant neurologic and musculoskeletal examination cannot be performed. In cases in which the diagnosis is apparent (Fig. 1–3), appropriate neuroimaging studies can guide further immediate management.

Clinical Examination

The clinical evaluation of the neurologically compromised, particularly the comatose patient, may be a difficult diagnostic and management dilemma. It is extremely important that the clinician's approach to the patient is systematic so that no critical factors are overlooked.

History

In some patients, the cause of neurologic impairment may appear obvious (witnessed cardiac arrest, generalized seizure, or trauma [Fig. 1–4]); however, it is important to systematically review whether there are any additional contributing factors that

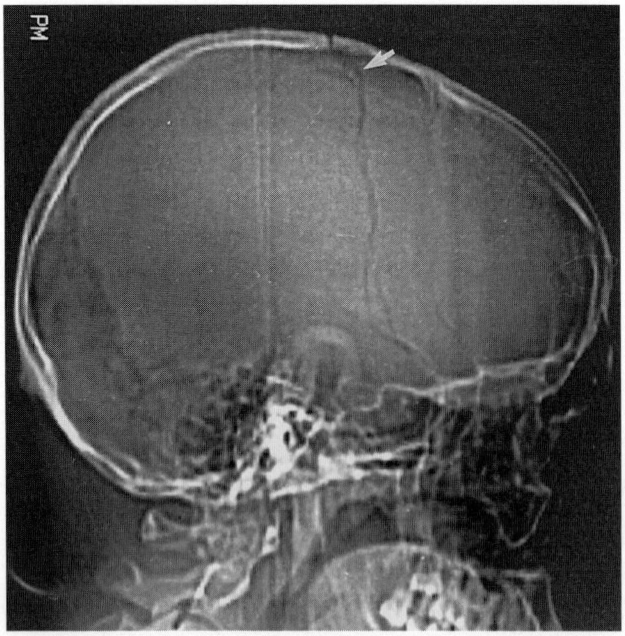

FIGURE 1-4 • Linear skull fracture. A vertically oriented linear fracture in the right parietal region is well seen on the lateral tomogram (arrows).

may compromise the patient's neurologic outcome. Causes of focal signs and symptoms should be sought, such as seizures, trauma, infection, illicit drug use, or hypoglycemia.

A description of the onset of neurologic impairment or prior occurrence is invaluable; unfortunately, however, such description is frequently not available. The EMS, emergency department (including transfer records from another hospital), and intensive care unit (ICU) records should be carefully reviewed (particularly any details regarding the onset of neurologic deterioration, repeated vital signs, focal neurologic complaints, headache, and prior medications). When available, those accompanying the patient to the emergency department (EMS, family or friends) should be carefully questioned. Prior medical and psychiatric health status of the patient, medication history, circumstances surrounding the illness or accident, deterioration of neurologic status, how the patient was found, and recent stressful events should be documented.

Physical Examination

The patient's vital signs including heart rate, blood pressure, respiratory rate, rectal temperature, pulse oximetry, and the GCS should be serially monitored while in the emergency department. Bradycardia, systolic hypertension, and respiratory irregularity (Cushing's triad) may indicate increased ICP.

The physical appearance of the patient should be noted and may be helpful when the patient is nonresponsive and there is no available history. Cachexia may be seen in advanced cancer, HIV infection, or chronic malnutrition. Poor hygiene may suggest underlying dementia, a problem with substance abuse, or a psychiatric disorder. Skin color may provide important diagnostic clues (e.g., cyanosis of the lips or nailbeds [hypoxia], jaundice [hepatic failure], pallor [hypotension], sallow color [pituitary hypofunction], or "cherry red" color [carbon monoxide poisoning]). Diaphoresis may occur in hypotension, or the skin may be dry as in diabetic ketoacidosis or uremia; dry skin and high fever may indicate heat stroke or poisoning with anticholinergics. Telangiectasia and spider angiomas suggest a chronic alcohol abuse history. The presence of compression blisters indicates the patient has been in one position for a prolonged period of time and may be helpful in determining the length of time the patient has been unconscious.

The patient's breath may have the characteristic odor of alcohol, acetone, or fetor hepaticus. Evidence of urinary or fecal incontinence or bruising or laceration of the tongue is suggestive of the occurrence of a generalized seizure. Resistance to passive, forward flexion of the neck may suggest intracranial infection, hemorrhage, or herniation. The greater the compromise of consciousness, the less reliable meningismus is as a diagnostic sign. In elderly patients, degenerative joint disease (DJD) may result in what appears as meningismus; however, in the presence of DJD, lateral motion of the neck is typically also restricted.

Evaluation of the fundi may reveal evidence of hypertensive retinopathy, Roth's spots, diabetic retinopathy, retinal ischemia, subhyaloid hemorrhage, optic atrophy, or papilledema.

The remainder of the physical examination may provide useful information regarding the patient's prior health/surgical status; evidence of multisystem trauma, such as tenderness, bruising (Battle's sign [Fig. 1–5]) or raccoon eyes, lacerations, swollen or deformed limbs; or pertinent additional findings (e.g., otorrhea, dysrhythmia, neck bruits).

Neurologic Examination of the Comatose Patient

The neurologic examination of the neurologically impaired subject is of critical importance in determining how to further evaluate and manage the patient while in the emergency department.[32–34] In patients who are comatose, the neurologic examination can provide invaluable information as to whether the cause of coma is structural or due to a toxic or metabolic disorder. Structural disorders cause coma by affecting the function of the reticular activating system (RAS) either directly or indirectly.

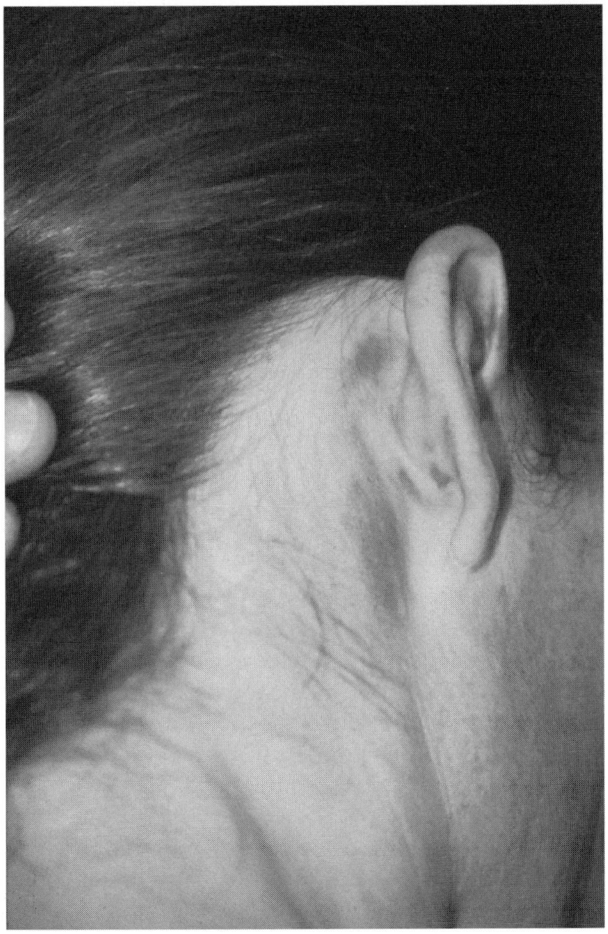

FIGURE 1–5 • Battle's sign. Postauricular ecchymosis subsequent to an acute assault with a baseball bat.

The RAS is a polysynaptic collection of neurons primarily located in the core of the medulla, pons, and midbrain.[35, 36] Metabolic disorders may result in coma by affecting neuronal energy metabolism, by disrupting neuronal membrane activity, or may be multifactorial. The most common etiologies of coma are summarized in Table 1–2.

The neurologic examination of the comatose patient consists of an assessment of the respiratory pattern, spontaneous movements, evaluation of the cranial nerves, and motor response to stimuli.[37]

TABLE 1–2 **ETIOLOGY OF COMA**

Structural Disorders

Damage to the reticular activating system (RAS)
- Direct (hemorrhage, infarction, trauma, tumor, infection)
- Indirect (herniation)

Metabolic Disorders

Disorders affecting energy metabolism (ischemia, anoxia/hypoxia, hypoglycemia, hyper/hypothermia)

Disorders affecting neuronal membrane activity (electrolyte imbalance, acid-base disorders, hyper/hypo-osmolar states, generalized seizure, concussion)

Disorders that are multifactorial
- Organ failure (hepatic, renal, pulmonary, pancreatic)
- Poisonings, intoxications
- Infections

RESPIRATORY PATTERNS

The pattern of respiration can be useful in localizing the lesion responsible for the patient's altered level of consciousness. The most frequently encountered abnormal respiratory pattern of pathologic significance is Cheyne-Stokes respiration and is characterized by a crescendo-decrescendo rate and depth of respiration followed by an apneic period. It is typically seen with deep, midline, bihemispheric lesions or diffuse cortical impairment.[38, 39] Central neurogenic hyperventilation, which is not commonly seen, is characterized by rapid, rhythmic hyperventilation and is associated with midbrain lesions.[40] Apneustic respiration and ataxic breathing are infrequently identified, as the patient is typically recognized to be in respiratory distress and quickly intubated. Apneustic breathing is characterized by a postinspiratory pause and is associated with structural lesions of the lateral tegmentum of the midcaudal pons.[41] In ataxic breathing (Biot's breathing), respirations are irregularly cycled and there is associated medullary dysfunction.

SPONTANEOUS MOVEMENTS

It is very useful to observe the patient at rest. Observation may reveal purposeful, spontaneous movements such as postural changes or manipulation of the bedclothes. Abnormal movements such as twitching, myoclonus, or tremor should be noted and may indicate seizure activity or a toxic/metabolic disorder. Spontaneous movements or posture that is asymmetric, such as an externally rotated lower extremity, may indicate a focal motor deficit. The brain stem component of the RAS is presumed to be intact when spontaneous chewing, blinking, or yawning is seen and helps to localize the cause of coma to the cerebral hemispheres.

CRANIAL NERVE EXAMINATION

The cranial nerve examination of the patient may reveal asymmetries suggestive of a structural lesion. In general, the comatose patient with normal brain stem reflexes most likely has diffuse cortical impairment of a metabolic etiology.

Examination of symmetry, size, shape, and direct and consensual pupillary light response is very useful. Disparity in pupil size can be caused by a number of nonemergent pathologic causes such as previous eye surgery or trauma, a glass eye, or topical cycloplegics (such as in accidental instillation of

Neo-Synephrine during procedures such as nasotracheal intubation). Only instillation of topical cycloplegics is unresponsive to topical constrictors like pilocarpine. The single most helpful factor in determining if the cause of the coma is toxic/metabolic is the pupillary response to light, because the light reflex is highly resistant to toxic/metabolic disorders.

Toxicologic causes of miosis include cholinergic and antiadrenergic agents (e.g., acetylcholine, monoamine oxidase inhibitors). Toxicologic mydriasis can be caused by anticholinergic agents (i.e., antidepressants) and adrenergic agents (i.e., cocaine). Anisocoria—unequal size and reactivity of the pupils—is not necessarily indicative of an acute structural lesion. Ptosis, miosis, and anhidrosis may be seen, and their evolution may be the first evidence of an ipsilateral, supratentorial mass effect due to compression of the hypothalamus. Horner's syndrome, with miosis, ptosis, and anhidrosis, is seen with ipsilateral, lateral pontine, medullary, and ventrolateral cervical cord lesions. Unilateral mydriasis is usually due to supratentorial compression of the oculomotor nerve as occurs in herniation. Mydriasis occurs prior to dysfunction of the motor component of the third nerve because the parasympathetic sphincter fibers, on the exterior of the nerve, are initially impaired. Since the sympathetic fibers are unopposed, the pupil becomes widely dilated.

Oval pupils may be seen when there is patchy involvement of the fibers innervating the sphincter and may be seen in herniation. Bilaterally dilated and unreactive pupils are seen with severe midbrain damage or with anticholinergic poisoning. Lesions of the midbrain tegmentum may be associated with pear-shaped pupils due to irregular constriction of the sphincter of the iris or with displacement of the pupil to one side (corectopia). Lesions of the tectum of the midbrain are associated with spontaneous oscillations in the size of the pupil and are referred to as hippus. Pinpoint and reactive pupils are characteristic of pontine lesions and are due to interruption of the descending sympathetic fibers.

Corneal reflexes should be elicited and any asymmetries in response noted. If the upper pons and midbrain are intact, stimulation of the cornea will cause the eyes to deviate upward (Bell's phenomenon).

Evaluation of eye movements in coma is invaluable in the identification of a structural etiology, as the RAS, nuclei, and tracts subserving eye movements are closely intercalated within the substance of the brain stem. The third, fourth, and sixth cranial nerve nuclei; and the descending sympathetic fibers are situated directly within the neuronal network of the RAS. Damage to these nuclei and tracts is associated with abnormalities of eye movements and the pupils and provides clinical information that the etiology of the coma is structural in nature.

The patient's resting lid tone may be evaluated by raising the eyelids and noting the rate and completeness of eyelid closure. The deeper the coma, the slower and more incomplete eyelid closure. The position of the eyes and spontaneous movements should be noted. In the drowsy patient, it is normal for the eyes to appear divergent in the horizontal plane. When the patient awakens, the eyes become conjugate. Abduction of one eye at rest, associated with pupillary dilatation, indicates third cranial nerve compression. Adduction may be due to damage to the sixth cranial nerve or may be a false localizing sign due to increased ICP. Skew deviation (resting dysconjugate vertical gaze) may be seen with damage or dysfunction at various levels of the brain stem and cerebellum.

There are a number of spontaneous eye movements that are helpful in localizing lesions in the comatose patient. If the brain stem is intact, the eyes may be seen to drift slowly from side to side (roving eye movements). Horizontal eye movements are preserved and damage to the caudal portion of the pons has been described in association with ocular bobbing. Ocular bobbing is associated with a fast downward phase and a slow return to the resting position. Ocular dipping is associated with a slow downward phase followed by a rapid return to the resting position and occurs with diffuse anoxic insults. Acute thalamic lesions may cause sustained deviation of the eyes down and in.

Barbiturates, diphenylhydantoin (Dilantin), diazepam (Valium), tricyclic antidepressants, and ethanol intoxication may suppress reflex ocular movements; however, the pupillary response to light remains intact. Ping-pong gaze, in which the eyes rove from side to side in a cyclical fashion, is seen with bilateral cerebral damage. Repetitive conjugate deviation may be seen in focal motor seizures involving the frontal eye fields. Conjugate horizontal deviation of the eyes may be seen in destructive, hemispheric frontal lesions, in which case the eyes deviate toward the lesion. The deviation may be overcome with either the oculocephalic or oculovestibular (caloric) maneuvers. In deep cerebral lesions, the eyes may deviate away from the side of the lesion (wrong way eyes). In lesions affecting the tegmentum of the pons, the eyes deviate away from the side of the lesion (toward the hemiparesis) and cannot be overcome with maneuvers. Damage to the tegmental region of the midbrain may abolish vertical gaze.

Eye movements can be assessed in the comatose patient by performing the oculocephalic maneuver (doll's eyes). This should never be performed in a patient who may have sustained a cervical spine injury. As a rule, cerebral gaze palsies can be overcome with the doll's eye maneuver whereas palsies due to brain stem damage cannot be overcome. If the response is absent, it is necessary to use a stronger stimulus and caloric stimulation should be performed.

The oculovestibular reflex or caloric testing is ideally performed with the patient supine and the head flexed at 30 degrees (if the c-spine has not been cleared, the test is still very accurate without head flexion). The patient should not be hypothermic or pharmacologically paralyzed. The tympanic membrane (TM) should be visualized, and if TM perforation is present caloric testing should not be performed, although hemotympanum is not a contraindication to this procedure. In the adult subject, 50mL of ice cold water should be instilled into the external auditory canal with either a plastic angiocatheter or, preferably, tubing from a butterfly catheter. If both eyes deviate opposite the instilled ear and nystagmus occurs, the cause of coma is likely to be metabolic. If both eyes deviate toward the cold water without nystagmus, the cause of coma is likely to be structural in nature. If there are no eye movements despite adequate stimulation to both ear canals, the prognosis for functional recovery is poor.

MOTOR SYSTEM

A progressive increase in intensity and type of stimulation can be used to assess the depth of coma. Verbal stimuli, such as calling the patient's name or shouting, followed by light superficial tactile stimulation to the nasal mucosa with a cotton swab, the face, or the limbs are effective. If these stimuli produce no response, deep pain may be produced by compression of the nailbeds or the supraorbital nerves. The depth of coma can be estimated by the type of stimulation necessary to arouse the patient and the length of time the patient maintains arousal.

The specific motor response to noxious stimuli is also helpful in evaluating patients. The noxious stimulus is administered and the motor response observed. The patient may withdraw appropriately or may assume a reflexive position such as decorticate or decerebrate posturing. Either decorticate or decerebrate posturing may be seen with toxic/metabolic disorders (hypoglycemia, liver failure) and in structural causes of coma; however, focal motor deficits are usually indicative of structural damage.

Decorticate posturing is characterized by adduction of the shoulder and arm, flexion at the elbow, and pronation and flexion at the wrist. The lower extremity remains extended at the hip and knee. In decerebrate posturing, there are extension and pronation of the upper extremities and forcible plantar flexion of the feet. Decerebrate posturing is associated with transection at the collicular level below the red nuclei that leaves the pontine reticular formation and vestibular nuclei intact and removes the normal supratentorial inhibition.

Abnormal, adventitious movements such as tremor, asterixis, and myoclonus are most commonly seen in toxic/metabolic disorders. The tremor seen in metabolic encephalopathies is coarse and irregular and ranges from 8 to 10 cycles per second. Asterixis is a sudden, brief loss of postural tone that is translated into a flapping movement when the hand is held in dorsiflexion at the wrist and the fingers are extended and abducted. Asterixis can be seen in virtually any body part that has the capacity for voluntary movement. Multifocal myoclonus is a sudden, nonrhythmic twitching most commonly seen in the facial and proximal limb musculature in uremic and hyperosmolar-hyperglycemic encephalopathy, as well as in carbon dioxide narcosis. Generalized myoclonus, which predominantly involves the axial musculature, occurs most commonly after severe anoxic damage.

SUMMARY

In summary, the neurologic evaluation of the comatose patient, including assessment of respiratory patterns, spontaneous movements, cranial nerves, and motor system examination, can be very helpful in determining whether the etiology of the coma is structural or metabolic.

When the patient is awake enough to participate in the examination, considerably more information can be obtained regarding the status of the patient's nervous system.

HERNIATION SYNDROMES

It is imperative that the clinician in the emergency department be able to identify incipient herniation. Once identified, it is possible to intervene in the process of herniation by administering mannitol and/or hyperventilating the patient until further diagnostic and management steps can be taken.

In herniation, cerebral tissue is displaced from one intracranial location to another, typically by a mass effect. The bony constraints of the skull also contribute to this displacement. This usually involves the movement of tissue by a rigid septum such as the falx or the tentorium cerebelli with subsequent compression and dysfunction of neuronal tissue. The most common type of herniation, transfalcial, involves the herniation of the cingulate gyrus under the falx and may result in infarction of the anterior cerebral artery and additional mass effect as infarction and edema evolve.

Supratentorial, or transtentorial, herniation includes uncal and central herniation and involves the passage of tissue below the tentorium. Uncal herniation occurs as a result of a laterally placed mass lesion (e.g., subdural or epidural hematoma, large middle cerebral artery infarction, temporal lobe tumor) and may be associated with stepwise, progressive compression and dysfunction of adjacent anatomic structures. Initially, the oculomotor nerve is compressed as the inferomedial portion of the temporal lobe herniates over the tentorium. This results in dilatation of the pupil ipsilateral to the mass lesion. The patient may have contralateral hemiparesis or, more rarely, an ipsilateral hemiparesis (Kernohan's phenomenon). The posterior cerebral artery may become compressed and infarct. As the mass effect evolves, increasing midline shift of structures occurs, the midbrain is compressed, hemorrhage occurs, the ascending portion of the RAS is compromised and the patient's level of consciousness progressively deteriorates.

In central transtentorial herniation, a centrally located, supratentorial mass lesion (e.g., thalamic hemorrhage) exerts a downward mass effect upon the brain stem and diencephalon. Progressive, rostrocaudal deterioration of brain stem function may occur. Diffuse (symmetric) and severe traumatic brain swelling may also lead to transtentorial herniation.

The most common causes of supratentorial mass lesions are vascular (large middle cerebral or internal carotid artery infarction or hemorrhage, basal ganglia or intraventricular hemorrhage); post-traumatic with extra or intradural or intraparenchymal collection of blood (subdural, epidural, cerebral contusion, or intraparenchymal collection); neoplastic (primary or metastatic); or an infectious etiology (abscess, granuloma, or empyema). Hemispheral (asymmetric) traumatic brain swelling may also result in uncal herniation.

Herniation from infratentorial mass lesions also may occur. Mass lesions within the posterior fossa (e.g., cerebellar hemorrhage) may cause the contents of the posterior fossa to herniate upward and compress the midbrain, or there may be herniation of the cerebellar tonsils down through the foramen magnum. In the latter situation, the compromise of consciousness is due to anoxic/ischemic encephalopathy as the cerebellar tonsils compress the medulla and result in sudden apnea and cardiac arrest.

The remainder of the chapter will discuss specific, neurologic disorders that are commonly encountered in the emergency department.

METABOLIC DISORDERS

Despite the fact that the human brain accounts for only 2% of the total body weight, it has a very high rate of oxygen consumption. The brain requires a constant supply of oxygen and glucose to support oxidative metabolism. This requires a high rate of CBF in order to meet the metabolic needs. Blood glucose is the primary, though not the sole, source of energy for the brain, and greater than one third of the total blood glucose delivered to the brain is extracted. When stressed, the brain has the capacity to oxidize ketone bodies, amino acids, and free fatty acids. One half of the energy consumed by the brain is used to support the ATP-driven Na^+-K^+ plasma membrane pump in order to re-establish the membrane potential and render the cell electrically excitable. Other important energy-dependent needs of the brain include support of neurotransmitter metabolism, blood-brain barrier transport, protein synthesis, and axonal transport.[42, 43]

When there is not enough ATP available, the ionic homeostasis of the cell cannot be maintained and neural injury occurs. In the excitotoxic hypothesis of neural injury, there is insufficient ATP to support reuptake of excitatory amino acids (particularly glutamate). The neurotransmitter remains active at the synapse, and the cell is unable to regulate the intracellular concentration of electrolytes, particularly calcium. Intracellular calcium concentration rises, and degradative enzymes (i.e., phospholipases, proteases, and endonucleases) are activated. The enzymes digest the cellular structure. Currently, considerable research is being conducted to explore various pharmacologic interventions that will prevent or ameliorate the cellular damage that results from activation of the degradative cascade, as previously discussed.

A patient's level of consciousness will become impaired when neuronal oxidative phosphorylation is compromised. This may occur when there is an inadequate amount of the substrates oxygen and glucose delivered to the brain (i.e., hypoxia, hypoglycemia) or when there is a decrease in cerebral blood flow resulting in cerebral ischemia. There normally is a very delicate balance between the delivery of substrates to the brain and its metabolism. The normal mean cerebral blood flow is 50 mL/100 g/minute, and it is considered to be critically reduced when it falls below 18 mL/100 g/minute. The latter is true for a conscious subject, whose cerebral oxygen consumption is normal (unlike comatose patients). If there is a cessation of cerebral blood flow, consciousness is lost within 10 seconds, spontaneous electrical activity stops in 15 seconds, and structural damage occurs in approximately 5 minutes. Cardiac arrest is the most common cause of global ischemia,[44, 45] while other causes that may result in clinically significant cerebral ischemia include impaired cardiac function, a fall in peripheral vascular resistance, increased cerebral vascular resistance, and disseminated small vessel vascular occlusion.

Hypoglycemia is a commonly encountered cause of neurologic impairment in the emergency department and is arbitrarily defined as a blood glucose concentration of less than 50 mg/dL (2.8 mmol/L).[46] Most of the initial signs and symptoms of hypoglycemia are the result of a sympathetic response that results in tachycardia, diaphoresis, and anxiety. Additionally, it significantly increases cerebral blood flow. The patient frequently initially complains of headache, dizziness, and loss of fine motor skills followed later by confusion, behavioral abnormalities, seizures, and coma. In the normal individual, acutely dropping the blood glucose to 50 mg/dL will result in clinical symptoms.[47] Patients with preexisting systemic disease (e.g., diabetes, cardio- or cerebrovascular disease) are more likely to become symptomatic at higher blood glucose levels.[48] The normal response to hypoglycemia is an increase in cerebral blood flow, which also may be impaired in patients with vascular disease. The most commonly encountered cause of hypoglycemia in the emergency department is excessive administration of insulin in the diabetic patient. It is important to recall that hypoglycemia alone may result in focal neurologic deficits. Fortunately, the clinical outcome of patients with hypoglycemia is significantly better than in hypoxia/anoxia or cerebral ischemia.

Hypoxia may also compromise brain function. Significant hypoxia can occur when there is inadequate delivery of oxygen to the brain as occurs with anemia; when there is pulmonary compromise; or during acute exposure to high altitudes. Altered levels of consciousness may occur when the $Pa{O_2}$ is 25–40 torr (3.3–5.3 kPa). The severity depends on the degree and duration of hypoxia. As in hypoglycemia, the cerebral blood flow increases to compensate for the decrease in arterial oxygen content, which has the effect of increasing the supply of oxygen and glucose to the tissue. Arterial oxygen tension becomes the limiting factor for oxidative metabolism at 45–50 torr (6.0–6.6 kPa), which is the point at which cerebral dysfunction occurs. Since the synthesis and metabolism of norepinephrine, dopamine, and serotonin are dependent upon an adequate supply of oxygen, neurotransmitter dysfunction occurs early in hypoxemia.[43]

Electrolyte and acid-base disorders and hypo- and hyperosmolar (<260 or >330 mOsm/L) states may also impair neurologic function by affecting neuronal membrane activity and impairing neuronal metabolism. Shifts in serum sodium affect the brain by altering serum osmolality and intracellular water content. Hyponatremia leads to intracellular edema, which usually does not occur until the serum sodium concentration falls below 125 mEq/L. Hypernatremia and hyperglycemia can lead to intracellular dehydration and dysfunction. Hyper- and hypocalcemia can also cause altered mental status. With all electrolyte abnormalities, it is not only the degree of change but also the rapidity of change that causes the eventual effects.

Systemic organ failure (e.g., hepatic, renal failure) is a recognized cause of neurologic impairment. Rapid elevations in ammonia lead to altered mental status; these patients also are prone to hypoglycemia secondary to decreased glycogen stores. Neurologic dysfunction from hepatic failure is thought to result from toxins that are not filtered from the circulation. The altered mental status is due to a number of factors: rapid elevations in ammonia, false neurotransmitters that compete with normal neurotransmitters, and fatty acid metabolism and sodium-potassium ATPase pump abnormalities.[49] Ammonia is known to interfere with oxidative metabolism and protein synthesis. The longer the period of time the brain has been exposed to the effects of ammonia, the smaller the rise in ammonia level required to result in clinical compromise.[50–52]

Uremic encephalopathy occurs when the glomerular filtration rate falls below 10% of the normal rate and is thought to be due to retention of urea, proteins, phosphates, and a number of ill-defined compounds. Uremic coma is associated with changes in serum osmolality as the blood urea nitrogen (BUN) rises. Cerebral water will adjust to gradual changes in BUN, but coma may develop with a rapid rise in nitrogenous wastes.[53, 54]

Neuronal oxidative metabolism may also be compromised by a deficiency of enzymatic cofactors. The most commonly encountered deficiency is thiamine deficiency.[55] Thiamine deficiency results in impaired activity of key enzymes in oxidative phosphorylation. Clinically, the patient presents with mental status changes and the classic clinical triad of Wernicke's disease, which includes encephalopathy, ataxia, and oculomotor abnormalities.

CENTRAL NERVOUS SYSTEM TRAUMA

The emergency department evaluation of the patient who has suffered central nervous system trauma is a common occurrence, particularly in Level 1 trauma centers, and has been summarized in several articles.[56–59] The goals of initial management are to stabilize the vital signs; minimize secondary brain injury by avoiding hypotension, hypoxia, hypoglycemia, and hyperthermia[11–13]; and prioritize management of the patient's injuries.

Head Injury

In the United States, it has been estimated that nearly 7 million people sustain some form of a head injury annually, though the great majority do not seek medical treatment.[60] Of this population, approximately 500,000 traumatic brain injured patients per year are hospitalized[60] at a societal cost estimated between 48 and 83.5 billion dollars per year.[61] Of those patients who are seen in the emergency department, as many as 50% are intoxicated or have used illicit drugs.[62] The majority of individuals are young (15–29 years of age) and male.[63]

Traumatic brain injury (TBI) can be classified according to the GCS score, the mechanism of injury (motor vehicle accident, assault, fall, gunshot wound, etc.), or the results of neuroimaging. TBI is classified using the GCS scores into mild (GCS 13–15), moderate (GCS 9–12), and severe (GCS 3–8) injuries. Fortunately, the majority of patients seen in the emergency department have suffered a mild degree of injury (approximately 80%).

Neuroimaging is also a useful means of classification, and the results of a nonenhanced CT scan of the head, skull x-rays, or, in some cases, magnetic resonance imaging help to clarify the intracranial pathology. The most common abnormalities encountered are diffuse or hemispheral brain swelling, traumatic subarachnoid hemorrhage, pneumocephalus, intracerebral contusion, intraparenchymal hemorrhage, diffuse axonal injury, subdural hemorrhage, and epidural hemorrhage. Figures 1–1 through 1–4 and 1–6 through 1–9 are illustrative examples.

As previously mentioned, the most common head injury encountered in the emergency population is mild TBI. The difficult decision for the clinician is whether to obtain neuroimaging (typically a nonenhanced CT scan of the head) and whether the patient is safe to be discharged from the emergency department. Those patients who did not have a loss of consciousness, or significant post-traumatic amnesia, and have a normal neurologic examination may not require a CT scan of the head. Patients who are intoxicated, elderly, have focal neurologic signs on clinical examination, are at high risk for intracranial hemorrhage (e.g., anticoagulant use), or have suffered a mechanism of injury that is associated with intracranial hemorrhage (e.g., fall from a height, assault with a blunt object) may need to be scanned. Skull x-rays are useful if the mechanism of injury (e.g., penetrating injury) or clinical examination suggests the study is indicated (see Fig. 1–4). Those patients with a normal CT scan of the head may be discharged home unless they experience persistent vomiting or neurologic deterioration. Ibuprofen (Motrin) 400–800 mg at 6-hour intervals is very effective for post-traumatic headaches.

Patients with an abnormal CT scan or a moderate/severe degree of head injury should receive immediate neurosurgical consultation. Once the patient is appropriately resuscitated, further management depends on the specific clinical situation. Once again, it is imperative to adequately manage conditions that have the potential to exacerbate secondary injury, as previously described. The decision to treat intracranial hypertension, place an ICP monitoring device in the emergency department, or determine whether the patient should be transferred immediately to the operating room or the intensive care unit is the prerogative of the neurosurgeon. The management of patients with severe traumatic brain injury is discussed in Chapter 16.

Spinal Cord Injury

In comparison to traumatic brain injury, spinal cord injury fortunately is relatively uncommon. In the United States, approximately 10,000 new cases occur each year[64] and the majority are the result of motor vehicle accidents, although sporting injuries, falls, and gunshot wounds are also frequently reported.[65]

Spinal cord injury is typically classified by the level of injury (the lowest level with both normal motor and sensory function is the neurologic level of injury), and by whether the injury is complete or incomplete. The presence of "sacral sparing" (rectal

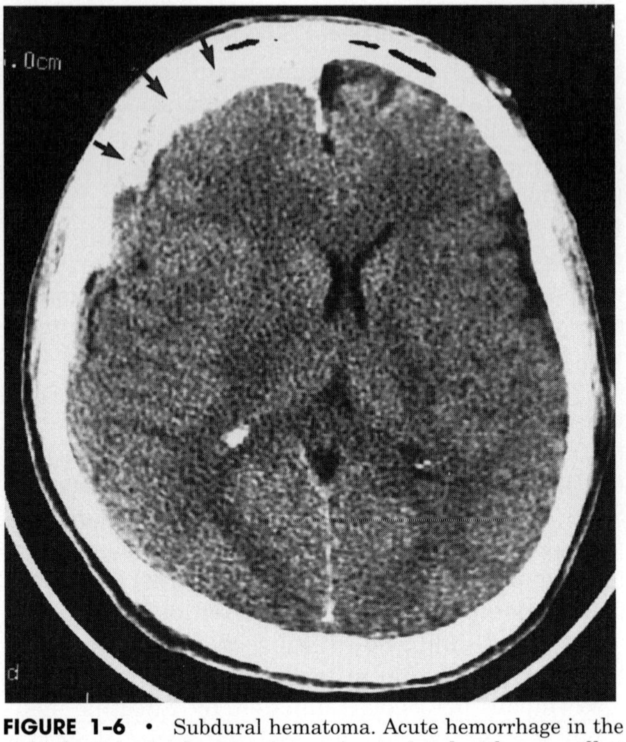

FIGURE 1–6 • Subdural hematoma. Acute hemorrhage in the right frontoparietal region (arrows) associated with mass effect and midline shift.

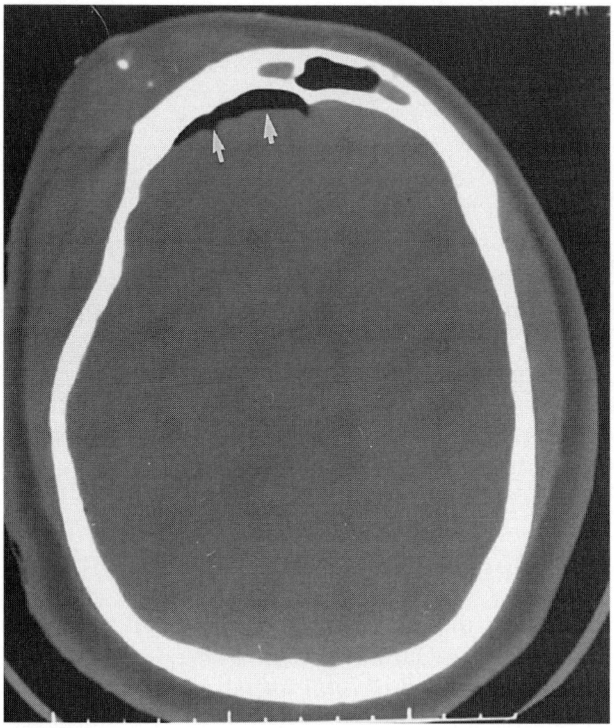

FIGURE 1-7 • Pneumocephalus. Subdural air is seen in the right frontal region (arrows), secondary to open skull fracture.

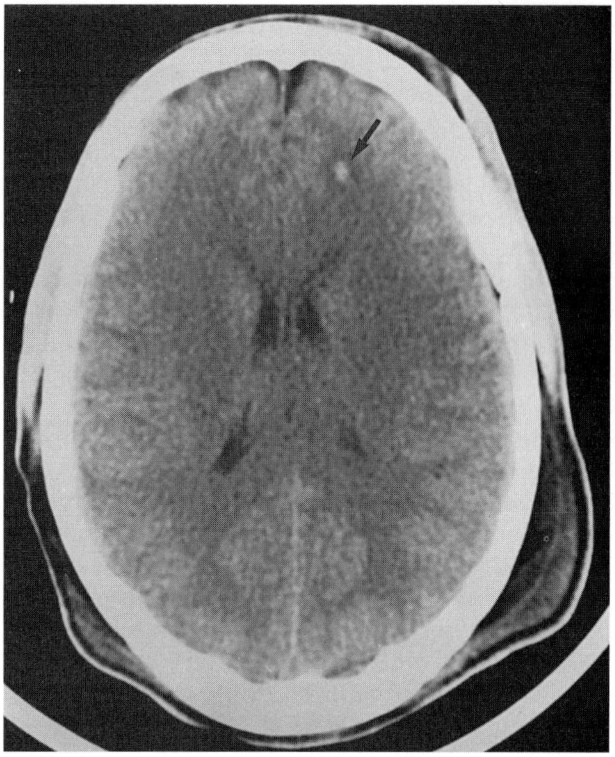

FIGURE 1-8 • Diffuse axonal injury. Hyperdense focus in the vertex of the brain (arrow) indicates a small shearing injury.

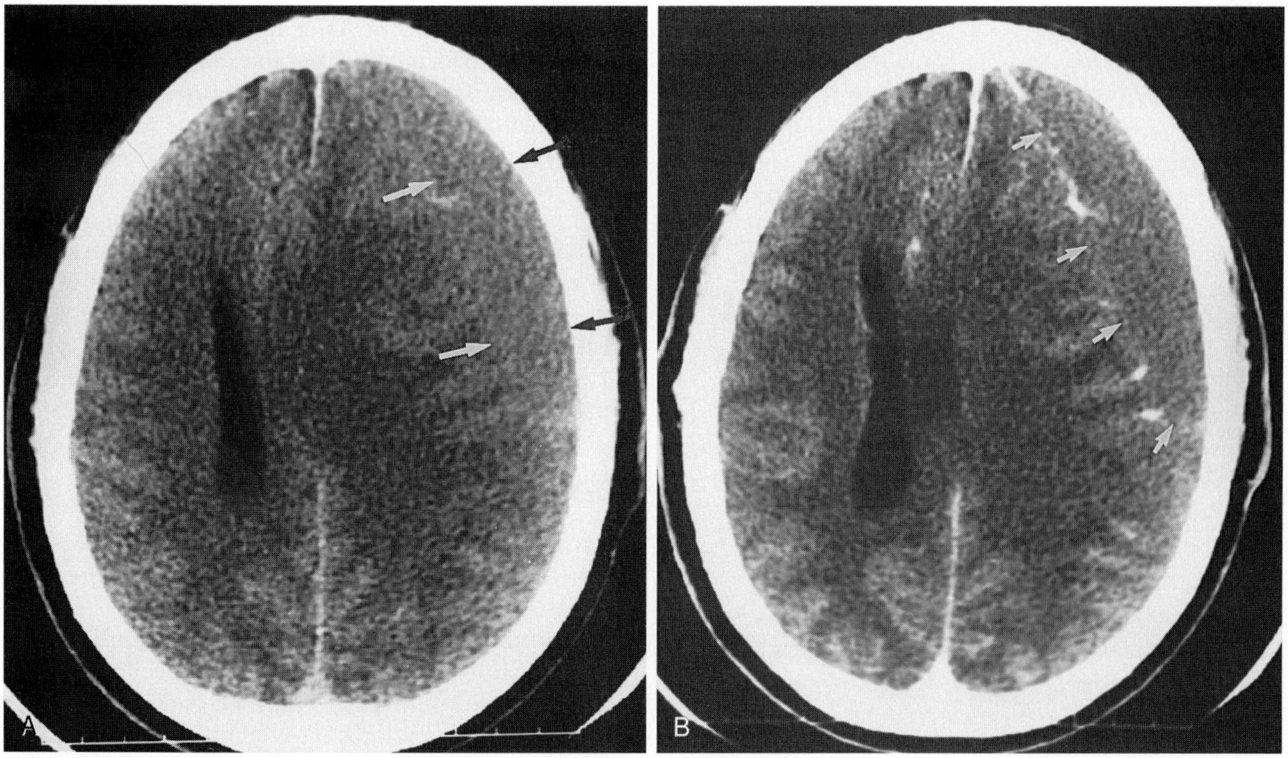

FIGURE 1-9 • Chronic subdural hematoma. *A,* Subdural hemorrhage in the left frontoparietal region has become isodense to the gray matter (arrows). *B,* Identification of the hematoma is clearly facilitated by contrast enhancement.

tone or the presence of perianal sensation) carries a better prognosis.[66–68]

In the emergency department, it is important to always have a high index of suspicion of spinal cord injury, particularly in patients involved in motor vehicle accidents and falls, and to ensure that the spinal column is adequately immobilized and stabilized. The airway should be secured. If a simple chin lift does not establish adequate airway, the patient should be intubated, preferably by nasotracheal intubation, as hyperextension of the neck is not required. If there are no spontaneous respirations, careful laryngoscopically guided orotracheal intubation should be performed. Once the airway has been secured and the patient adequately ventilated, the circulatory status should be assessed.

Hypotension is a frequent problem in spinal cord injury and may be due to hypovolemic or neurogenic shock, or a combination of the two. Neurogenic shock is typically seen in severe cervical or upper thoracic spinal cord injuries and results from sympathetic nervous system dysfunction with a loss of peripheral sympathetic drive and subsequent decreased peripheral vascular resistance.[69] Clinically, these patients are usually bradycardiac despite their hypotension, and this provides an important clinical clue to the possibility of a spinal cord injury. If volume expansion fails to increase the blood pressure, 0.5–1.0 mg IV atropine or 0.1 mg IV glycopyrrolate should be administered in the adult subject. Patients should be vigorously fluid resuscitated, and it may be necessary to use vasopressor drugs (i.e., dopamine, Neo-Synephrine) if the patient remains hypotensive. The blood pressure should be carefully monitored using an arterial line. It is particularly important to place a nasogastric tube and urinary catheter in patients with spinal cord injury,

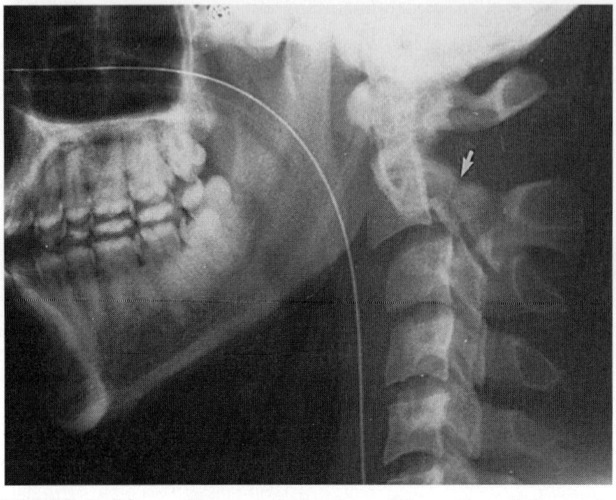

FIGURE 1-10 • Hangman's fracture. Disruption of the posterior arch of C2 (arrow) is present with anterior subluxation of C2 on C3.

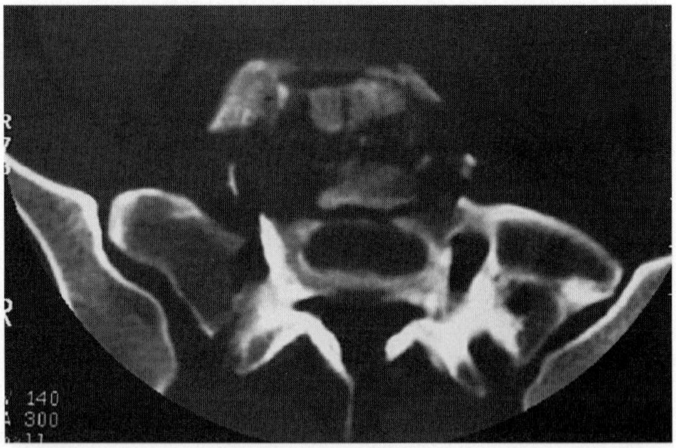

FIGURE 1-11 • Lumbar spine fracture. Comminuted fracture of the L5 vertebral body is seen on CT scan.

as gastric atony and bladder distention may occur. Systemic intravascular volume titration is better achieved by monitoring with either a central venous line or a Swan-Ganz catheter.

If the diagnosis is established within 8 hours of the injury, methylprednisolone should be administered as an intravenous bolus of 30 mg/kg followed in 1 hour by a continuous infusion of 5.4 mg/kg/hour for the ensuing 23 hours.[70, 71] After the patient has been resuscitated and the initial dose of methylprednisolone has been administered, appropriate radiologic evaluation should be performed (Figs. 1–10 and 1–11). A lateral cervical spine radiograph should be obtained to T1, and anteroposterior and lateral views of the thoracic and lumbar spine should be performed. If these studies are unremarkable, oblique views should be obtained. If the initial films indicate the patient should be immobilized, this should be done. In cervical spine injuries, this is usually accomplished with Gardner-Wells tongs. Computed tomography is invaluable in imaging the spinal column and should be performed if the initial studies do not reveal a suspected fracture. Magnetic resonance imaging is the diagnostic study of choice for intra-axial spinal cord lesions.

A complete discussion of this topic can be found in Chapter 15.

CEREBROVASCULAR DISORDERS

Stroke is a major cause of death in acute care hospitals and the leading cause of brain damage in adults. Despite the decreasing mortality, there are approximately 500,000 new strokes annually in the United States.[6] The term "stroke" encompasses all cerebrovascular disease whether it is ischemic or hemorrhagic in nature. Transient ischemic attacks (TIAs) are focal neurologic complaints that resolve within a 24-hour period. Ischemic cerebrovascular disease is due to thrombosis of a vessel or embolism to a particular vascular territory. These patients tend to have characteristic clinical presentation depending on which vascular territory is affected. Hemorrhagic cerebrovascular disease occurs less frequently than ischemic disease and includes cerebral hemorrhage[72] and subarachnoid hemorrhage (SAH) (Fig. 1–12). Patients with cerebral hemorrhage (Fig. 1–13) and SAH tend to present to the emergency department earlier in their course of illness than those with ischemic disease and are more likely to have an altered level of consciousness. Patients with SAH may present with only a complaint of severe headache, and emergency room clinicians should have a high index of this diagnostic suspicion, particularly if there is meningismus.

The majority of patients with stroke will not present as a medical code and will not require resuscitation. It is important that the neurologic or neurosurgical consultant be informed of the patient's presence as soon as possible. The patient should be stabilized and airway, breathing, and circulation appropriately assessed. Intravenous access should be obtained. Blood pressure should be controlled as previously described. Hypertension should not be aggressively treated in the absence of specific indications such as myocardial infarction, arterial dissection, or systolic blood pressure ≥ 220 mm Hg or ≥ 120 mm Hg diastolic on repeated measurements over 30 to 60 minutes.[29, 73]

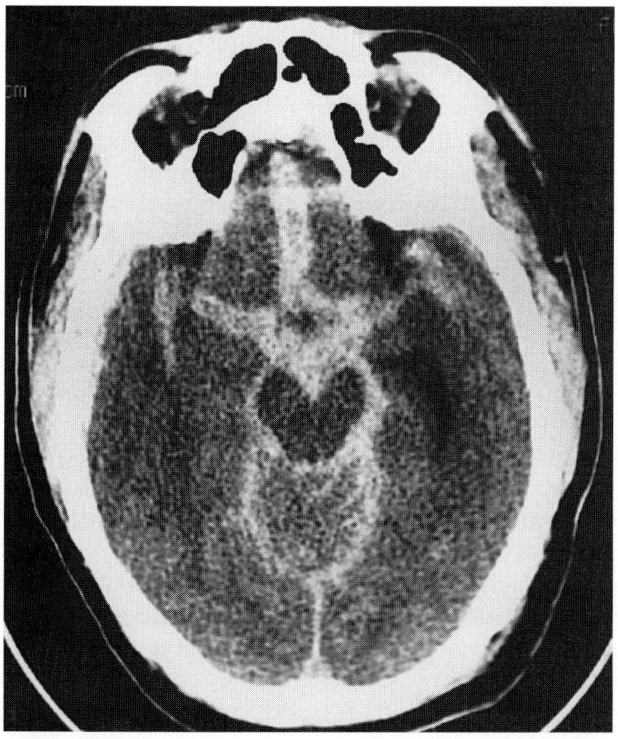

FIGURE 1–12 • Subarachnoid hemorrhage. Hyperdense acute hemorrhage is present in the suprasellar cistern and surrounding the brain stem after rupture of an aneurysm.

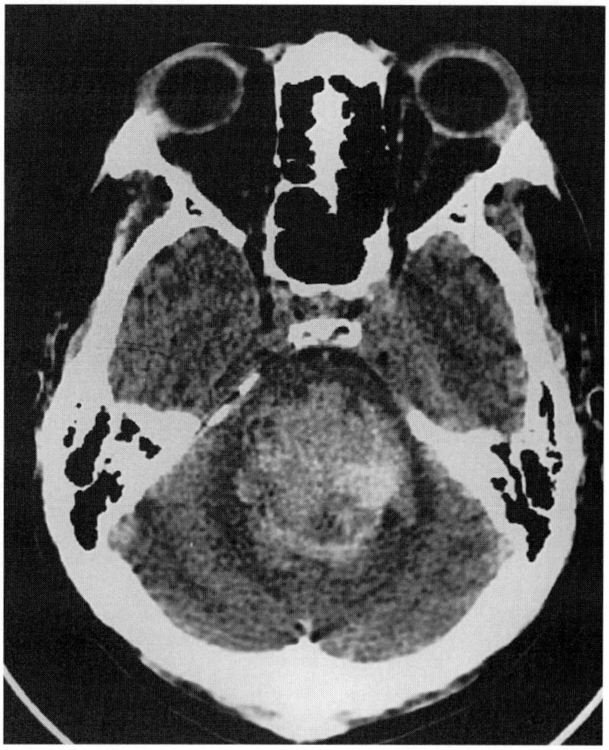

FIGURE 1–13 • Pontine hemorrhage. A large brain stem hemorrhage obliterates the pons.

Most patients are conscious and able to provide a history of the time and mode of onset of their stroke. A history of seizure disorder, trauma, infection, and illicit drug use (particularly cocaine) is important to elicit, as these can mimic stroke. A thorough general examination should be performed with attention to signs of trauma, infection, and meningismus. The heart should be examined for dysrhythmia or murmurs, and the peripheral pulses should be palpated. The neck should be auscultated for bruits.[74, 75]

Blood studies should be obtained and include, as a minimum, complete blood count (CBC), differential, electrolytes, creatinine, platelets, prothrombin time, partial thromboplastin time, and blood glucose. An electrocardiogram and a chest x-ray should be obtained.

The type of stroke can usually be determined based on history, neurologic examination, and results of neuroimaging. In the emergency department, most patients will receive a noncontrast CT scan due to its reliability in distinguishing ischemic from hemorrhagic disease. It is important to recall that the CT scan may appear normal despite the occurrence of acute infarction during the first 12–24 hours (Fig. 1–14). Patients with atypical presentations should have a contrasted CT scan performed.[76] Additional studies such as emergent angiography (e.g., in the SAH patient) should be performed as soon as possible.

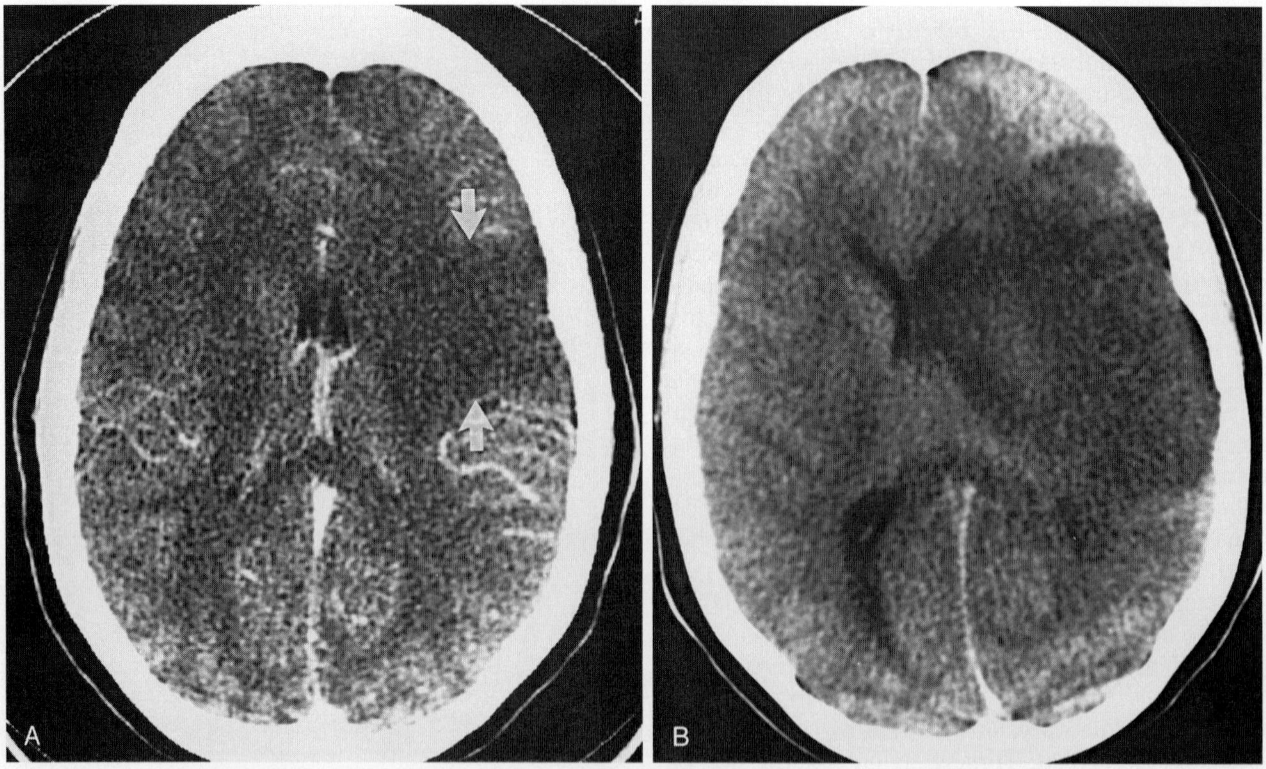

FIGURE 1–14 • Acute infarction. *A,* Initial CT scan with contrast demonstrates a subtle area of low attenuation with decreased perfusion (between arrows). *B,* Follow-up CT scan shows a large area of ischemia and edema in the left middle cerebral artery distribution with midline shift.

The earlier that evaluation and treatment of stroke is initiated, the better the outcome.[77] Unfortunately, there is a tendency for patients to delay in seeking medical treatment and also a lack of urgency on the part of health care providers in recognizing stroke as an emergency. Earlier recognition and a sense of "urgency" will become more imperative as new therapies are developed. New pharmacotherapies that are neuroprotective, agents that lyse clots, thrombolytics (urokinase, streptokinase), new heparinoid agents, defibrinating agents, and calcium channel blockers all show promise in future therapy. For additional information on acute cerebrovascular disorders, see also Chapters 8 through 11.

SEIZURE DISORDERS

New-Onset Seizures

New-onset seizures frequently occur in the emergency department and, in the majority of the urban population, may result from sleep deprivation, metabolic disturbances, or intracranial infections. They may also be related to the use of illicit substances, particularly cocaine, or alcohol withdrawal seizures. Other risk factors for the occurrence of new-onset seizures include a family history of seizure disorder and prior traumatic brain injury. The recurrence rate after a single seizure is estimated to be between 26% and 71%.

It is important to obtain as much relevant information as possible, including that from family and friends. Laboratory studies should include a CBC with differential; electrolytes, including magnesium and calcium; indices of liver and renal function; blood glucose; arterial blood gases (or pulse oximetry); and a serum and urine drug screen. A lumbar puncture should be performed if indicated. In older patients and those whose neurologic examination is focal, both a noncontrast and contrast CT scan of the head should be performed (Fig. 1–15). The decision to admit the patient is dependent upon the clinical situation,[78] as is the appropriate anticonvulsant for newly diagnosed adult epilepsy.[79] Monotherapy is superior to polytherapy in the majority of patients. Antiepileptic therapy should be initiated only when the diagnosis of epilepsy can be established. In the typical situation, once the diagnosis of epilepsy is established, the patient should be treated for a period of 2 years and re-evaluated.

Status Epilepticus

In the United States, convulsive status epilepticus is a neurologic emergency that affects over 50,000 patients per year[80] with a high morbidity and mortality. Early appropriate therapy is critical to neurologic outcome. Status epilepticus is defined as more than 30 minutes of continuous seizure activity or two or more seizures without full recovery of consciousness between seizures.[81] The most common causes of status epilepticus in adults are an acute cerebrovascular event (Fig. 1–16), anticonvulsant medication change, anoxia, and substance abuse.[81]

The immediate management of the patient in status epilepticus is adequate resuscitation and stabilization according to the ABCs of emergency management. Monitoring of vital signs and skilled vigilant nursing care are imperative. The first priority is to stop the convulsive movements, which is ideally accomplished with the use of a benzodiazepine (lorazepam [Ativan] 0.1 mg/kg at 1–2 mg/minute to 10 mg, or diazepam [Valium] 0.2 mg/kg at 2 mg/minute to 20 mg); however, if convulsive activity and intubation is delayed, a short-acting neuromuscular blocker (e.g., vecuronium [Norcuron]) can be administered. It is important to note that neuromuscular blockade merely stops the clinically evident convulsive movements while the seizure activity in the brain persists. Benzodiazepines, also, are not definitive therapy because their half-life is short lived.[81–83]

Definitive therapy consists of intravenous phenytoin (Dilantin) 20 mg/kg (<50 mg/minute). The dose should be decreased in the elderly (15 mg/kg). The drug is incompatible with glucose-containing solutions and should be administered with normal saline.

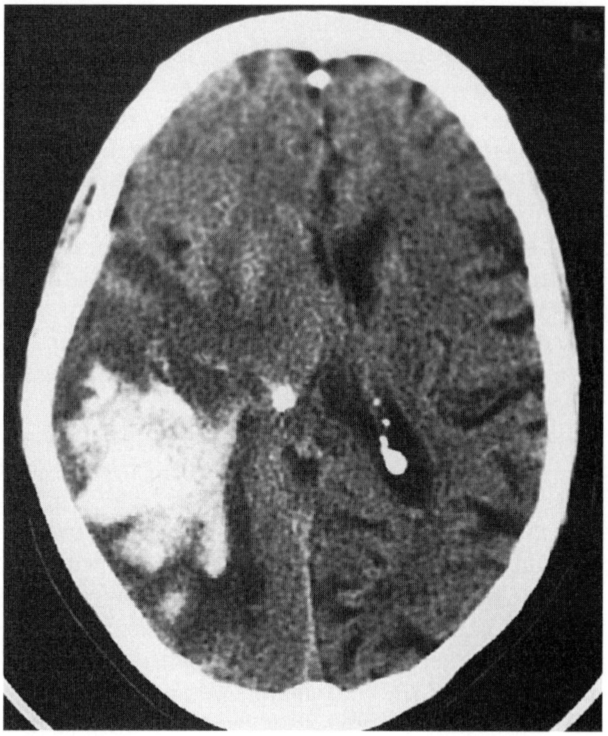

FIGURE 1-16 • Hypertensive hemorrhage. Extensive acute hemorrhage has occurred in the right temporo-occipital region with surrounding edema and mass effect.

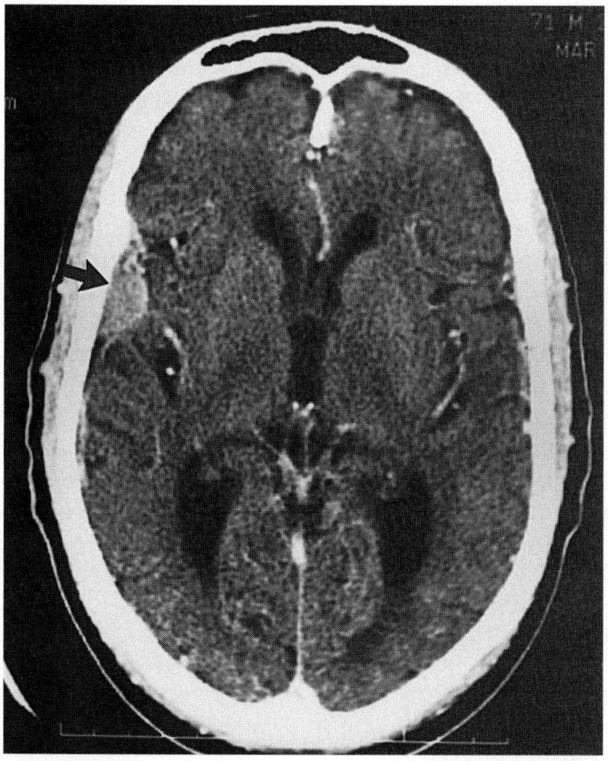

FIGURE 1-15 • Metastases. Contrast-enhanced CT scan demonstrates a dural-based mass in the right temporal region (arrow) in a patient with advanced prostate cancer.

If status persists, an additional bolus of intravenous phenytoin 5–10 mg/kg should be given. If seizures continue, intravenous phenobarbital 20 mg/kg (<100 mg/minute) can be given and increased to anesthetizing doses (boluses of 5–10 mg/kg at 20-minute intervals) until the seizures stop or the patient becomes significantly hypotensive. Pentobarbital coma is an alternative and can be administered in a loading dose of 5 mg/kg followed by an infusion of 0.5–3 mg/kg per hour until the seizures stop. Anesthetic doses of phenobarbital and pentobarbital are frequently associated with significant hypotension requiring vasopressor therapy and increased morbidity with continued use. Propofol has also proven to be efficacious in certain situations.[84] Continuous electroencephalographic (EEG) monitoring is ideal but usually not available.[85] An EEG should be obtained as soon as possible. For a more complete description of status epilepticus, the reader is referred to Chapter 4.

TOXICOLOGY

Neurologically impaired or comatose patients may present to the emergency department after inhalation, ingestion, or administration of a toxic substance or toxic amounts of a drug. Rapid identification of the intoxicant facilitates appropriate management. As in other neurologic emergencies, the patient is first resuscitated and stabilized with attention to the ABCs of emergency management. As previously recommended, adult patients with an altered mental status should receive naloxone (Narcan) 2 mg IVP, thiamine 100 mg IV, and glucose 1–2 ampules of 50% dextrose IVP. In patients suspected of chronic opiate abuse, it is advised to titrate the dose of naloxone administered (0.4 mg) to avoid abrupt withdrawal.

Table 1–3 summarizes clinical signs and symptoms that are characteristic of particular classes of drugs. If the patient is alert enough to give a history, this can be invaluable. It is important to keep in mind that suicidal patients may not willingly provide this information. Routine laboratory studies allow the calculation of the anion gap and osmolar gap and are useful in conjunction with the clinical presentation of the patient in identifying the toxic agent. Serum and urine drug screens are helpful in identifying the more common drugs of abuse.

Acute intoxications are managed by preventing further absorption of the intoxicant by decontaminating the skin and gut. The gut can be decontaminated by inducing emesis using syrup of ipecac, gastric lavage, activated charcoal, and whole bowel irrigation using, for example, GoLYTELY. Measures used to enhance elimination include hemodialysis, hemoperfusion, and serial activated charcoal. Hyperbaric oxygen, alkalization of the urine, and specific antidotes are also available.

Toxic ingestions of drugs and other chemicals are the leading cause of altered mental status. Cyanide disrupts oxidative phosphorylation and carbon monoxide displaces oxygen from hemoglobin, both of which alter mental status and produce clinical hypoxia. Lithium influences the CNS by affecting the monoaminergic neurotransmitters and neuronal membrane potentials.[86]

TABLE 1–3 **SIGNS AND SYMPTOMS OF DRUG INTOXICATION**

Opioids	**Sympathomimetics**
Hypothermia	Hypertension, tachycardia
Hypotension, hypoventilation	Mydriasis
Miosis	Hyperthermia
	Diaphoresis, tremor

Anticholinergics	**Cholinergics**
Hypertension, tachycardia	Hypothermia
Hyperthermia	Diaphoresis
Dry, flushed skin	Salivation, fasciculations
Mydriasis	Miosis
Urinary retention	Increased urination
Decreased bowel sounds	Increased bowel activity

INFECTIOUS DISORDERS

In the United States, even in large, busy emergency departments, it is not common to encounter a patient with bacterial meningitis. However, the topic will be briefly mentioned due to the importance of rapid, accurate diagnosis and treatment.

The typical patient with bacterial meningitis presents with complaints of headache, stiff neck, and irritability. Seizures, cranial nerve palsies, and focal neurologic signs may be present. Kernig's and Brudzinski's signs may be present and indicate meningeal irritation. High-grade fever is usually present but may be absent in the very young and very old. Consciousness is clouded in most cases. A maculopapular rash suggests meningitis caused by *Streptococcus pneumoniae* or *Staphylococcus aureus,* whereas subconjunctival hemorrhages, petechial hemorrhages, and purpura are associated with meningococcal meningitis.

A lumbar puncture (LP) is indicated when the diagnosis is suspected. The only absolute contraindication to performing an LP is infection at the proposed site of the LP. If it is possible to obtain a CT scan of the head prior to the LP, this is desirous, particularly if there is papilledema or a focal neurologic examination.[87] The opening pressure should be recorded and is considered elevated when it is greater than 200 mm H_2O. Analysis of the cerebrospinal fluid (CSF) typically reveals a pleocytosis (200–10,000 white blood cells/mm^3) that is predominantly polymorphonuclear. CSF protein is elevated in excess of 100 mg/mL, and the CSF/blood glucose ratio is less than two thirds. In contrast, in viral meningitis, the clinical complaints are much milder and CSF examination reveals 25–300 white blood cells/mm^3, which are predominantly lymphocytic or mononuclear. In the majority of cases, Gram stain of the CSF will reveal the bacteria. Counterimmunoelectrophoresis for bacterial capsular antigens is routinely available for the most common causes of meningitis. Blood cultures should be drawn.

The patient should be vigorously fluid resuscitated if in shock and should be kept well hydrated. The appropriate antibiotic therapy depends on the age of the patient and risk factors. Empiric therapy to produce rapid sterilization of the CSF is recommended and includes a third-generation cephalosporin (cefotaxime 2 g IV every 4 hours, ceftazidine 2 g IV every 6 hours, or ceftriaxone 2 g every 12 hours) in addition to ampicillin 2 g IV every 4 hours in adults.[88] For additional information on infectious emergencies of the CNS, the reader should refer to Chapter 5.

BRAIN DEATH

Brain death, according to the American Academy of Neurology, is the irreversible loss of the clinical function of the brain, including the brain stem. The determination of brain death is not typically a concern in the emergency department; however, in some cases (e.g., severe CNS trauma), it may be indicated.

The clinical diagnosis of brain death may be made when the cause of coma is known and irreversible and the patient is comatose with absent brain stem reflexes and apneic. The procedural guidelines for determination of brain death vary with individual states and hospitals. In those cases in which the diagnosis of brain death cannot be made by clinical criteria (e.g., severe facial trauma, patient is too hemodynamically unstable for apnea testing), confirmatory tests may be performed. These include cerebral angiography, electroencephalography, transcranial Doppler ultrasonography, technetium-99m hexamethylpropyleneamineoxime brain scan, and somatosensory evoked potentials.[89]

References

1. Young W: Role of calcium in central nervous system injuries. J Neurotrauma 1992;9:Suppl 1:s9–s25.
2. Choi D, Hartley D: Calcium and glutamate-induced cortical neuronal death. In Waxman S (ed): Molecular and Cellular Approaches to the Treatment of Neurological Disease, p 23. New York, Raven Press, 1993.
3. Siesjo B: Pathophysiology and treatment of focal cerebral ischemia. Part I: Pathophysiology. J Neurosurg 1992;77:169–184.
4. Siesjo B: Pathophysiology and treatment of focal cerebral ischemia. Part II: Mechanisms of damage and treatment. J Neurosurg 1992;77:337–354.
5. Siesjo B: The role of calcium in cell death. In Price D, Thoenen H, Aguayo A (eds): Neurodegenerative Disorders: Mechanisms and Prospects for Therapy, p 35. Chichester, UK, John Wiley and Sons, 1993.
6. Chang C, Bleck T: Drug therapy for cerebral protection. Pharm Therap 1995;155:129–135.
7. Stein D, Sabel B: Pharmacologic Approaches to the Treatment of Brain and Spinal Cord Injury. New York, Plenum Press, 1988.
8. McIntosh T: Pharmacologic strategies in the treatment of experimental brain injury. J Neurotrauma 1992;9:201–209.
9. Faden A, Salzman S: Pharmacological strategies in CNS trauma. Trends Pharm Sci 1992;13:29–35.
10. Peterson P, Phillis J: Novel Therapies for CNS Injuries. Rationales and Results. Boca Raton, FL, CRC Press, 1996.
11. Chesnut R, Marshall L: Analysis of the role of secondary brain injury in determining the outcome from severe head injury. J Neurosurg 1992;72:360A.
12. Chesnut R: Secondary brain insults after head injury: Clinical perspectives. New Horizons 1995;3:366–375.
13. Doberstein C, Hovda D, Becker D: Clinical considerations in the reduction of secondary brain injury. Ann Emerg Med 1993;22:993–997.
14. Walls R: Rapid sequence intubation in head trauma. Ann Emerg Med 1993;22:1008–1013.
15. Teasdale G, Jennett B: Assessment of coma and impaired consciousness. A practical scale. Lancet 1974;ii:81–84.
16. Walls R: Airway management. Emerg Med Clin North Am 1993;11:53–60.
17. Shribman A, Smith G, Achola J: Cardiovascular and catecholamine responses to laryngoscopy with and without tracheal intubation. Br J Anesth 1987;50:295–299.
18. Young W, McCormick P: Perioperative management of intracranial catastrophes. Crit Care Clin 1989;5:821–824.
19. Donegan M, Bedford R: Intravenously administered lidocaine prevents intracranial hypertension during endotracheal suctioning. Anesthesiology 1980;52:516–518.
20. Hamil J, Bedford R, Weaver D, et al: Lidocaine before endotracheal intubation: Intravenous or laryngotracheal? Anesthesiology 1981;55:578–581.
21. Bedford R, Persing J, Pobereskin L, et al: Lidocaine or thiopental for rapid control of intracranial hypertension. Anesth Analg 1980;59:435–437.
22. Yukioka H, Hayashi M, Terai T, et al: Intravenous lidocaine as a suppressant of coughing during endotracheal intubation in the elderly. Anesth Analg 1993;77:309–312.
23. Stoelting R: Nonbarbiturate induction agents. In Stoelting R (ed): Pharmacology in Anesthetic Practice, 2nd ed, p 134. Philadelphia, JB Lippincott, 1991.
24. Kissin I, Motomura S, Aultman B, et al: Inotropic and anesthetic potencies of etomidate and thiopental in dogs. Anesth Analg 1983;62:961–965.
25. Choi S, Spaulding B, Gross J, et al: Comparison of the ventilatory effects of etomidate and methohexital. Anesthesiology 1985;62:442–447.
26. Dearden N, McDowall D: Comparison of etomidate and althesin in the reduction of increased intracranial pressure after head injury. Br J Anesth 1985;57:361–368.
27. Modica P, Tempelhoff R: Intracranial pressure during induction of anesthesia and tracheal intubation with etomidate-induced EEG burst suppression. Can J Anesth 1992;39:236–241.
28. Minton M, Grosslight K, Stirt J, et al: Increases in intracranial pressure from succinylcholine: Prevention by prior non-depolarizing blockade. Anesthesiology 1986;65:165–169.
29. Broderick J, Brott T, Barsan W, et al: Blood pressure during the first hours of acute focal cerebral ischemia. Neurology 1990;40:145.
30. McCabe J, Angelos M: Injury to the head and face in patients with cervical spine injury. Am J Emerg Med 1984;2:333–335.
31. Sinclair D, Schwartz M, Gruss J: A retrospective review of the relationship between facial fractures, head injuries and cervical spine injuries. J Emerg Med 1988;6:109–112.
32. Caronna J, Simon R: The comatose patient: A diagnostic approach and treatment. Int Anesthiol Clin 1979;17:3–18.
33. Fisher C: Neurological examination of the comatose patient. Acta Neurol Scand 1969;45:1–56.
34. Brazis P, Masden J, Biller J: Localization in Clinical Neurology. Boston, Little, Brown, 1990.
35. Moruzzi G, Magoun H: Brain stem reticular formation and activation of the EEG. Electroenceph Clin Neurophys 1949;1:455.
36. Pappas C, Carrion C: Altered levels of consciousness and the reticular activating system. BNI Quarterly 1989:5:2–8.
37. Plum F, Posner J: The Diagnosis of Stupor and Coma, 3rd ed. Philadelphia, FA Davis, 1988.
38. Brown H, Plum F: The neurologic basis of Cheyne-Stokes respiration. Am J Med 1961;30:849–860.
39. Cherniak N, Longobardo G: Cheyne-Stokes breathing. An instability in physiologic control. Am J Med 1973;288:952–957.
40. Plum F, Swenson A: Central neurogenic hyperventilation in man. Arch Neurol Psych 1959;81:535–549.
41. Plum F, Alvorn E: Apneustic breathing in man. Arch Neurol 1961;10:101–112.
42. Arieff A, Griggs R: Metabolic Dysfunction in Systemic Disorders. Boston, Little, Brown, 1992.
43. McCandless D: Cerebral Energy Metabolism and Metabolic Encephalopathy. New York, Plenum Press, 1985.
44. Safar P: Cerebral resuscitation after cardiac arrest: A review. Circulation 1986;74:138–153.
45. White B, Grossman L, Krause G: Brain injury by global ischemia and reperfusion: A theoretical perspective on membrane damage and repair. Neurology 1993;43:1656–1665.
46. Sieber F, Traystman R: Special issues: Glucose and the brain. Crit Care Med 1992;20:104–114.
47. Malouf R, Brust J: Hypoglycemia: Causes, neurological manifestations and outcome. Ann Neurol 1985;17:421–430.

48. Boyle P, Schwartz N, Shah S, et al: Plasma glucose concentrations at the onset of hypoglycemia symptoms with poorly controlled diabetes and non diabetes. N Engl J Med 1988;318:1487–1492.
49. Fraser C, Arieff A: Hepatic encephalopathy. N Engl J Med 1985;313:865–873.
50. Cooper A, Plum F: Biochemistry and physiology of brain ammonia. Physiol Rev 1987;67:440–519.
51. Zieve L: Pathogenesis of hepatic encephalopathy. Metab Brain Dis 1987;2:147–165.
52. Mullen K, Gacad R: Pathogenetic mechanisms of acute hepatic encephalopathy. New Horizons 1994;2:505–511.
53. Fraser C, Arieff A: Nervous system complications in uremia. Ann Intern Med 1988;109:143–153.
54. Fraser C, Arieff A: Metabolic encephalopathy as a complication of renal failure: Mechanisms and mediators. New Horizons 1994;2:518–526.
55. Blass J, Gibson G: Abnormality of a thiamine-requiring enzyme in patients with Wernicke-Korsakoff syndrome. N Engl J Med 1977;297:1367–1370.
56. Narayan R: Emergency room management of the head-injured patient. In Becker D, Gudeman S (eds): Textbook of Head Injury, pp 23–66. Philadelphia, WB Saunders, 1989.
57. Miller JD: Assessing patients with head injury. Br J Surg 1990;77:241–242.
58. Stein S, Ross S: Moderate head injury: A guide to initial management. J Neurosurg 1992;77:562–564.
59. Marion DW: Acute head injuries in adults. In Rakel RE (ed): Conn's Current Therapy 1998, pp 959–963. Philadelphia, WB Saunders, 1998.
60. Graves E: Detailed diagnoses and procedures. National Hospital Discharge Survey 1991;13:1–239.
61. Lewin I: The cost of disorders of the brain. The National Foundation for Brain Research Survey, 1992.
62. Dacey R, Alves W, Rimel R, et al: Neurosurgical complications after apparently minor head injury. J Neurosurg 1986;65:203–210.
63. Kraus J, Black M, Hessol N, et al: The incidence of acute traumatic brain injury and serious impairment in a defined population. Am J Epidemiol 1984;119:186–201.
64. DeVivo M: National Spinal Cord Injury Statistical Center Fact Sheet, University of Alabama, Birmingham, 1994.
65. Jellinger K: Neuropathology of cord injuries. In Errico T, Bauer R, Waugh R (eds): Spinal Cord Injury, Chap 4. Amsterdam, North Holland Publishing, 1976.
66. Ditunno J: Standards for Neurological and Functional Classification of Spinal Cord Injury. Chicago, American Spinal Injury Association, 1992.
67. Stauffer E: Diagnosis and prognosis of acute cervical spinal cord injury. In Urist M (ed): Trauma to the Spinal Cord. Philadelphia, JB Lippincott, 1975.
68. Walters R, Adins R, Yakura J: Definition of complete spinal injury. Paraplegia 1991;29:573–581.
69. Pasarin G, Green B: Emergency room assessment and stabilization of spinal injury. In Greenberg J (ed): Handbook of Head and Spine Trauma, p 413. New York, Marcel Dekker, 1993.
70. Bracken M, Shepard M, Collins W, et al: A randomized, controlled trial of methylprednisolone or naloxone in the treatment of acute spinal cord injury. N Engl J Med 1990;322:1405–1411.
71. Bracken M, Shepard M, Collins W, et al: Methylprednisolone or naloxone treatment after acute spinal cord injury: 1-year follow-up data. J Neurosurg 1992;76:23–31.
72. Diringer M: Intracerebral hemorrhage: Pathophysiology and management. Crit Care Med 1993;21:1591–1603.
73. Lisk D, Grotta J, Lamki L, et al: Should hypertension be treated after acute stroke? A randomized controlled trial using single photon emission computed tomography. Arch Neurol 1993;50:855–862.
74. National Stroke Association Consensus Statement: Stroke: The first six hours. Emergency evaluation and treatment. NSA 1993;3–7.
75. Grotta J: Acute stroke management: Diagnosis (Part 1). Stroke Clin Updates 1993;5:17–21.
76. Libman R, Wirkowski E, Alvir J, et al: Conditions that mimic stroke in the emergency department. Implications for acute stroke trials. Arch Neurol 1995;52:1119–1122.
77. Rosen D: New directions for acute stroke therapy. Med J Austral 1993;158:78–80.
78. Henneman P: Determining the need for admission in patients with new onset seizures. Am Emerg Med 1994;24:1108–1114.
79. Heller A, Chesterman P, Elwes R, et al: Phenobarbitone, phenytoin, carbamazepine or sodium valproate for newly diagnosed adult epilepsy: A randomized monotherapy trial. J Neurol Neurosurg Psych 1995;58:44–50.
80. Hauser W: Status epilepticus: Epidemiologic considerations. Neurology 1990;40:9–13.
81. Treatment of convulsive status epilepticus. Recommendations of the Epilepsy Foundation of the American Working Group on Status Epilepticus. JAMA 1993;270:854–859.
82. Shepherd S: Management of status epilepticus. Emerg Med Clin North Am 1994;12:941–961.
83. DeLorenzo R, Towne A, Pellock J et al: Status epilepticus in children, adults and the elderly. Epilepsia 1992;33:15–25.
84. Merigian K, Browning R, Leeper K: Successful treatment of amoxapine-induced refractory status epilepticus with propofol (Diprivan). Acad Emerg Med 1995;2:128–133.
85. Jordan K: Status epilepticus. A perspective from the neuroscience intensive care unit. Neurosurg Clin North Am 1994;5:671–686.
86. Whinchester J: Lithium. In Haddad L, Winchester J (eds): Clinical Management of Poisoning and Drug Overdose, p 656. Philadelphia, WB Saunders, 1990.
87. Archer B: Computed tomography before lumbar puncture in acute meningitis: A review of the risks and benefits. Can Med Assoc 1993;148:961–965.
88. Talan D, Hoffman J, Yoshikawa T: Role of empiric parenteral antibiotics prior to lumbar puncture in suspected bacterial meningitis: State of the art. Rev Infect Dis 1988;10:365–376.
89. Report of the Quality Standards Subcommittee of the AAN. Neurology 1994;44:1537–1540.

2

Acute Respiratory Failure in Neuroemergencies

C. William Hanson III, M.D.

The brain receives about 15% of the resting cardiac output, accounts for 20% of the resting oxygen consumption, and has essentially no reserve: total cessation of blood flow to the brain results in unconsciousness within 5–10 seconds. The brain works with what might be called a just-in-time oxygen supply, using today's jargon. Because of the high metabolic rate of neurons and the lack of glycogen or oxygen stores in the brain, it is uniquely sensitive to interruptions in blood flow and oxygen delivery. It is presumably for this reason that cerebral autoregulation of blood flow, and therefore regional oxygen delivery, is so exquisite. Conversely, the brain adjusts the rate of alveolar ventilation to maintain the arterial partial pressure of oxygen and carbon dioxide within very narrow limits.

The interdependence of respiration and the brain is nowhere more apparent than in the intensive care unit (ICU). The prognosis of head-injured and neurosurgical patients has improved dramatically in the past 30 years owing, in part, to advances in ventilatory technology. Patients with diseases of the peripheral nerves, such as acute inflammatory demyelinating disease and myasthenia gravis, routinely undergo mechanical ventilation for periods of weeks to months with every expectation of survival.

At the same time that ICUs have improved the outlook for neurologically compromised patients, new diseases have arisen as a consequence of the interventions employed in the ICU. Multiple organ dysfunction syndrome (MODS) is a disease entity created, in a sense, by modern intensive care that involves both the brain and the lungs and is the most common cause of death in the modern ICU. Similarly, critical illness polyneuropathy[1, 2] is a poorly understood, newly recognized disease entity found in patients with MODS, predominantly involving the distal extremities, causing atrophy, weakness, and absent reflexes with sensory sparing.

Neuromuscular blocking agents (NMBs), which are used to paralyze patients with respiratory failure, have permitted intensivists to manage one disease while creating another. NMBs are implicated in several syndromes of persistent weakness in the intensive care patient. Vecuronium is typically thought to be a short-acting nondepolarizing muscle relaxant, but an active, renally excreted metabolite (3-desacetyl vecuronium) has been demonstrated to cause prolonged weakness in a cohort of critically ill patients with renal failure.[3, 4] A second entity attributed to neuromuscular blocking agents is an acute myopathy, characterized by a rapidly evolving quadriparesis.[5] Finally, prolonged use of nondepolarizing agents causes up-regulation of nicotinic acetylcholine receptors, which may account for the prolonged muscle paralysis seen in some patients.[6]

The modern era of respiratory failure and its treatment began, appropriately, with efforts to treat the complications of polio. In 1930, a negative-pressure ventilator designed by the Drinker brothers was used to treat a student with polio and respiratory failure who subsequently recovered. The Drinker "iron lung" was designed with financial support from New York's Consolidated Gas Company because of the significant incidence of respiratory failure in employees exposed to smoke and gas.

Iron lungs were used for the management of respiratory failure over the next quarter century but were attended by problems with patient isolation, skin breakdown, and nursing care. Positive-pressure ventilation had been used experimentally as early as the sixteenth and seventeenth century by Vesalius and Hooke, but the development of barotrauma with the primitive apparatus of the time derailed further experimentation until the 1950s, when positive-pressure ventilators developed by Engström, Lundia, and Bang were used in the management of patients in the Danish polio epidemic of 1952. Two thousand seven hundred and twenty-two polio patients were admitted to the Hospital for Communicable Diseases in Copenhagen from July 24th to December 3, over three hundred of whom required respiratory support. Twenty-seven of the first thirty-one patients with respiratory failure died. As with many other medical advances (such as war and trauma surgery), the large numbers and potential scope of the tragedy resulted in ingenious solutions.

Aspiration en route to the hospital, which led to the death of many patients early in the epidemic, was eliminated by sending expert medical care to the patient's home, where suctioning, ventilation, and even tracheostomy were initiated for transport. This presaged the development of critical care transport teams.

Tracheostomy was employed routinely to secure the airway, and hand ventilation performed by rotating teams of medical students, nurses, and technicians. Chest physical therapy, postural drainage, the application of sighs to prevent atelectasis, aspiration of secretions from the airway, humidification of inspired gas, and administration of blended gases (oxygen with nitrogen to avoid oxygen toxicity) were all developed during this period and continue to be used to this day. The use of these measures reduced mortality from 90% to less than 30%.[7] The same measures were applied in American polio epidemics in the mid to late 1950s. By 1960, mass immunization with the Salk and Sabin vaccines had effectively eradicated polio, but by this time the unquestioned success of intensive respiratory therapy had led to the development of the first wards dedicated to the management of patients with respiratory failure.

Further impetus for creation of ICUs came from the recognition of new disease entities, the success of cardiac care units, and advances in surgery and anesthesia. Although earlier descriptions exist,[8, 9] Ashbaugh is widely credited with identifying the entity that has subsequently been called adult respiratory distress syndrome[10] (ARDS) and, more recently, acute lung injury (ALI), which is generally acknowledged to have been an important impetus for the development of ICU's. Cardiac care units were the first to demonstrate the efficacy of intensive care in reducing mortality.[11] Concurrent advances in neurosurgery and neuroanesthesia have led to the development of specialized units (or portions of units) dedicated to the management of acutely ill neurologic and neurosurgical patients.

PULMONARY PHYSIOLOGY

The lung rests at functional residual capacity (FRC), which is an essential reference point for any discussion of pulmonary pathophysiology: any process that decreases FRC results in diminished respiratory reserve. Advancing age, obesity, changes in body position, and smoking all lessen FRC, which is the lung volume at the end of passive exhalation, and the point at which several forces are balanced. At the end of normal exhalation, the actions of gravity, the elastic recoil of the lung, and surface tension in the alveoli, which favor collapse of the lung, are balanced by the forces of the muscles of respiration and ribs, negative intrapleural pressure, elastic recoil of the lung, surfactant, intra-alveolar nitrogen, and physiologic positive end-expiratory pressure.

The ribs normally provide an elastic, expandable infrastructure to which the muscles of respiration are attached, although with age and certain disease, elasticity diminishes. On inspiration, the external intercostal muscles contract, causing the ribs to move upward and forward, expanding the anteroposterior and lateral dimensions of the chest cavity. This has been likened to the motion of a bucket handle. Other muscles employed during quiet inspiration are the diaphragm, which flattens from its usual domed configuration during contraction, increasing the volume of the thorax, and the muscles that support the upper airway, maintaining a patent channel for gas flow. Additional muscles can be recruited during periods of stress or exercise for hyperventilation, such as the scalenes, alae nasi, and sternomastoid: the accessory muscles of respiration.

Expiration is usually passive but becomes active during exercise, voluntary hyperventilation, and with certain diseases (chronic obstructive pulmonary disease, asthma), when the internal intercostal, muscles rectus abdominis, internal and external obliques, and the transversus abdominis are recruited.

Movements of the chest wall and muscles of respiration are translated to the lungs via the pleural space, which normally contains only a few milliliters of fluid and is at subatmospheric pressure (-2.5 to -10 cm H_2O), permitting apposition of the serosal surface of the lung to the pleura. When the pleural space is violated, however, as with a puncture or rib fracture, intrapleural pressure equilibrates with the atmosphere, the serosa is no longer apposed to the pleura, and the forces of the chest wall are no longer transmitted to the lung, resulting in a pneumothorax.

Elastic recoil results from elastin and collagen in the pulmonary parenchyma. It acts locally to collapse a given segment of lung but, in so doing, expands distant segments. This paradoxic concept is termed *interdependence* and is a function of the large number of interconnecting units in the lung.[12, 13] Elastic recoil is increased in lung fibrosis, acute lung injury, and interstitial edema, increasing the tendency toward atelectasis.

Surfactant is a detergent-like molecule that reduces surface tension in the alveolus. It is secreted by alveolar pneumocytes and becomes more effective in reducing surface tension as the alveolus becomes smaller, thereby counteracting alveolar collapse. Processes that deplete surfactant or injure alveolar pneumocytes, such as inhalation injury, aspiration of gastric contents, and mediator activation, invariably lead to atelectasis.

The role of intra-alveolar nitrogen in maintaining alveolar expansion is generally ignored in discussions of lung mechanics, but its importance cannot be overemphasized. Nitrogen is poorly absorbed and amounts to almost 80% of atmospheric gas. It acts to maintain alveolar patency in units with poor gas exchange by remaining behind after all of the oxygen has been absorbed. As the fraction of inspired oxygen is increased, the concentration of nitrogen in inhaled gas decreases, and lung units that exchange gas poorly with atmosphere (due to secretions or bronchial constriction) collapse.

Finally, physiologic positive end-expiratory pressure results from turbulent gas flow during exhalation through the vocal cords and upper airway and resulting back pressure on the alveoli. This is lost with endotracheal intubation with a large-bore tube.

CONTROL OF RESPIRATION

The muscles of respiration are controlled by the pons and medulla, which act as the seat of the "central pattern generator," which is a term describing a physiologic function rather than an anatomic location. The central pattern generator (CPG) is not well understood but appears to represent interactions among several separate areas in the brain including the pontine pneumotaxic center, which appears to participate fine control;[14] the apneustic center, which acts as an inspiratory cut-off switch;[15] the dorsal (DRG) and ventral (VRG) respiratory groups in the medulla; and perhaps a gasping center in the rostral medulla (which is normally suppressed but may become active with severe stress or diffuse brain stem injury). The resting respiratory pattern results from cross-talk between the DRG, which has primarily inspiratory units, and the VRG, which has a mix of inspiratory and expiratory units. Our current understanding of neural control of respiration derives from early experiments in which selective portions of the (cat) brain stem were transected,[16–18] revealing characteristic patterns of abnormal breathing.

Normal breathing (eupnea), as paced by the CPG, is modulated by feedback from various receptors located in (1) the brain stem itself; (2) the carotid and aortic bodies; (3) the airways; and (4) the lung. The pH-sensitive receptors on the surface of the medulla respond to changes in CO_2 that diffuses into cerebrospinal fluid (CSF) from the bloodstream.[19] The carotid and aortic bodies respond to hypoxia, hypercapnia, and pH, as well as blood pressure changes and sympathetic activity. When chemically or mechanically stimulated, the airways of the nose and pharynx can trigger sneezing, apnea, or bradycardia, while laryngeal and tracheal receptors evoke coughing, slow deep breathing, or apnea. Pulmonary receptors can be categorized as stretch receptors, irritant receptors, or J receptors. Stretch receptors are activated by distention of the lungs and participate in the Hering-Breuer reflex, which inhibits inspiration. Irritant receptors are activated by chemical and mechanical irritants[20] and elicit bronchoconstriction and hyperpnea. The J or juxtapulmonary capillary receptor responds to capillary interstitial pressure and produces the pulmonary chemoreflex, which is characterized by apnea, bradycardia, and hypotension.

Many of the abnormal respiratory patterns seen with acute lesions of the central nervous system (CNS) can be understood with a working knowledge of the respiratory circuit as diagrammed in Fig. 2–1, as can the responses to peripheral lesions. The archetypal abnormal respiratory pattern is Cheyne-Stokes breathing,[21] characterized by a cyclical rise and fall in the rate of ventilation with periods of apnea, which, while more typically central in character, can also be obstructive.[22] Cheyne-Stokes breathing was first noted in cardiac and neurologic disease but has subsequently been described with the administration of sedatives or opiates, as well as in normal subjects at high altitude. This respiratory pattern results from processes that affect normal feedback control of the CPG, such as increased circuit length (prolonged circulation time), increased controller gain (as in the response to hypoxia at high altitudes), or decreased damping (sedatives, opiates).

There are several other characteristic respiratory patterns indicative of abnormalities in the central respiratory control (Fig. 2–2).[23, 24] *Central neurogenic hyperventilation* occurs during the acute and convalescent phases of injuries to the high pons. It is very difficult to control and often results in a sustained respiratory alkalosis. With *apneustic* or *ratchet breathing*, inspiration occurs in a series of steps and indicates injury to the mid pontine area

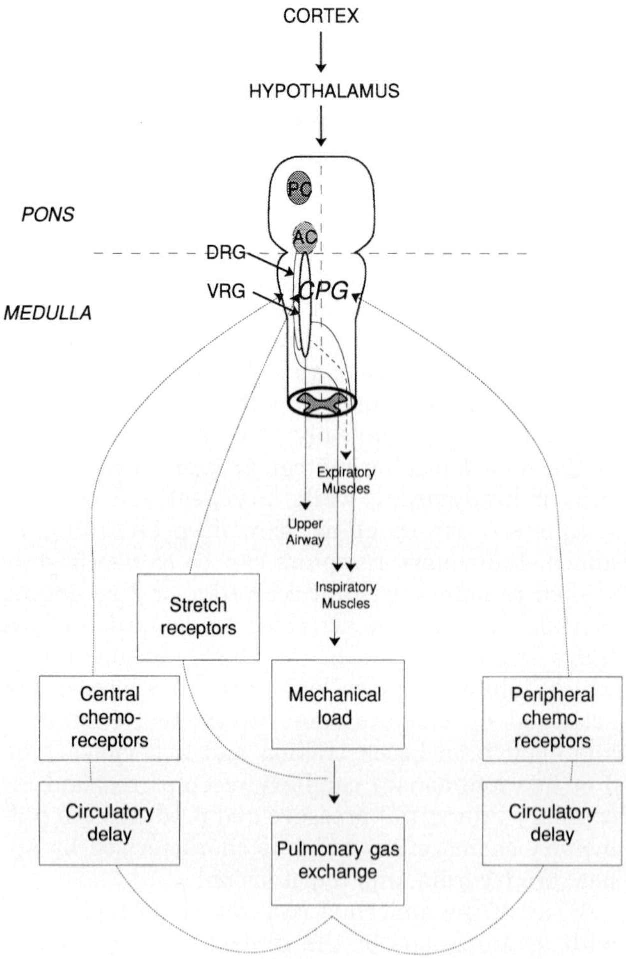

FIGURE 2–1 • The respiratory control circuit with central contribution from the cortex and hypothalamus, the pneumotaxic center (PC), the apneustic center (AC), the dorsal respiratory group (DRG), and the ventral respiratory group (VRG), which contribute to the central pattern generator (CPG). These nuclei project crossed (expiratory and inspiratory muscles) and uncrossed (upper airway) neurons to the effector muscles. Respiratory control is modulated by feedback from central and peripheral chemoreceptors as well as stretch receptors.

(where the apneustic center is speculated to exist). *Cluster breathing* is seen with low pontine lesions and encephalitis. *Ataxic breathing*, which occurs with injury to the low pons and the medulla, is the least coordinated and probably indicative of the most profound injury. *Hiccups* may result from an injury to the nucleus tractus solitarii, appear to be potentiated by hypocapnia, and may be relieved by CO_2 rebreathing or vagal stimuli. *Ondine's curse* is named for a water nymph in German mythology who, when jilted by her mortal husband, took from him all automatic functions, thereby requiring him to breathe volitionally.[25] Ondine's curse probably represents one end of a continuum of abnormalities associated with sleep apnea wherein central apnea predominates and there is a flat CO_2/ventilation response curve. This is also found, to some extent, with chronic poliomyelitis and the pickwickian syndrome.

Sleep apnea has many similarities to Cheyne-Stokes breathing, and while central obstructive episodes can be attributed to abnormal feedback control, obstructive episodes may be due to dysynchronous activation of the thoracic cage muscles and the muscles of the upper airway, with contraction of the first during relaxation of the latter. Alternatively, out-of-phase oscillations in activity of chest wall muscles and upper airway muscles could explain both obstructive and central apneas (Fig. 2–3).

Anomalous respiration also results from abnormalities of the peripheral nervous system that are manifested by irregular mechanics rather than patterns of breathing. When the phrenic, intercostal, and cranial nerves fail to act synchronously, several forms of paradoxic respiration result, in which the chest and the abdomen do not rise and fall together. These include obstructive apnea as described above, as well as the breathing pattern associated with cervical cord injuries, in which the phrenic nerve is

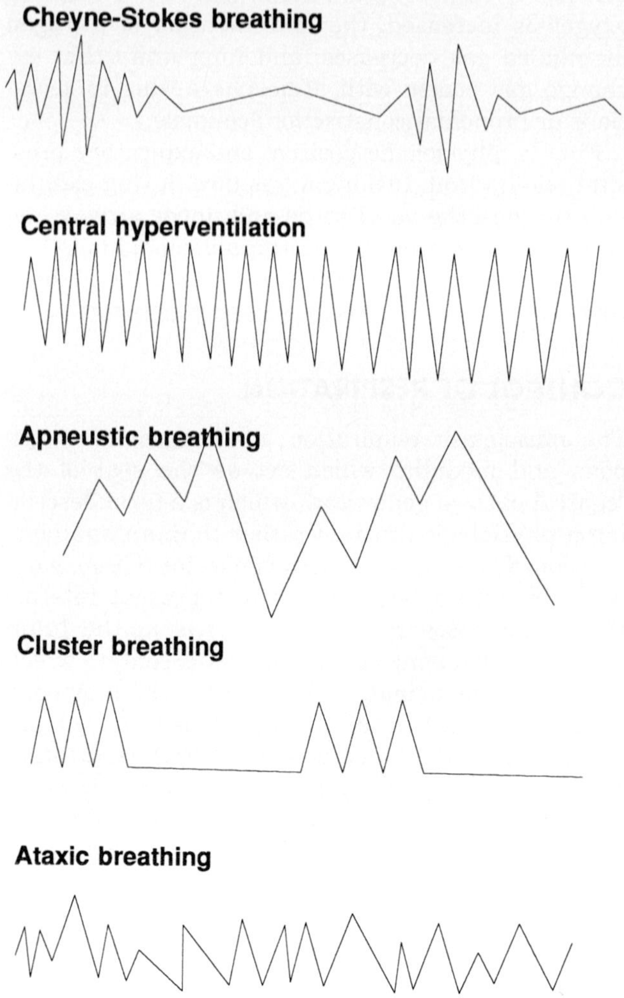

FIGURE 2–2 • Characteristic respiratory patterns indicative of disorders in central respiratory control.

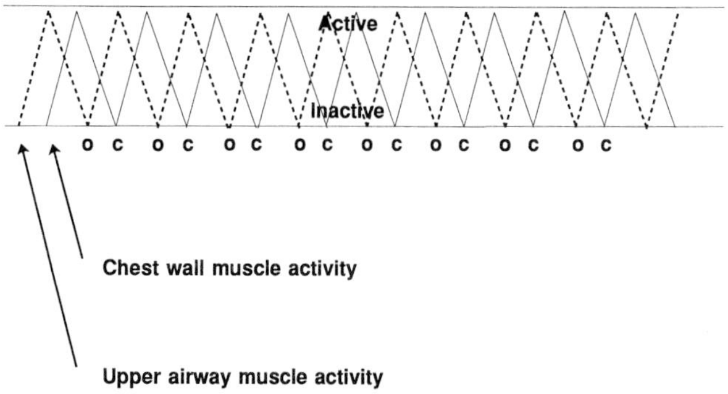

FIGURE 2-3 • Hypothetical explanation for sleep apnea, wherein oscillations of the upper airway are out of phase with those of the chest wall. Obstructive apneas (O) occur when there is activity of the chest wall with absence of activity in the upper airway, while central apneas (C) occur with absence of chest wall activity.

intact and chest wall innervation is interrupted, and the breathing pattern seen with bilateral phrenic nerve injury, in which the intercostal muscles function, but the diaphragm is flaccid. With cervical cord injuries and the resulting loss of intercostal innervation, the chest wall retracts on inspiration when the diaphragm descends. Conversely, with phrenic nerve injury and loss of diaphragmatic innervation, the chest wall rises on inspiration while the abdomen descends. Careful physical examination permits ready differentiation among these lesions (Fig. 2–4). Paradoxic respiration also occurs with expiratory obstruction as with asthma or chronic obstructive pulmonary disease (COPD), wherein expiration becomes an active process, and the abdominal recti and the internal intercostal muscles contract during exhalation, causing the chest to appear to rise while the abdomen contracts.

Finally, it is clear that abdominal surgery and thoracotomy, as well as injury to the chest or abdomen, can lead to reflex inhibition of the diaphragm and intercostal muscles.[26–28] Pasteur was the first to observe that postoperative atelectasis was caused by "paralysis of the muscles that are the direct extenders of the lung—the diaphragm and the intercostals."[29] This reflex may be mediated by the vagus or splanchnic nerve[30, 31] and results in substantial loss of functional residual capacity (FRC). Several studies have shown that the use of regional analgesia in the postoperative period, as with epidural analgesia or intercostal nerve blocks, attenuates the loss of FRC (Fig. 2–5).[32–34]

RESPIRATORY PRINCIPLES IN NEUROLOGIC AND NEUROSURGICAL EMERGENCIES

The dynamic interplay between dysfunction of the nervous system and respiratory failure is illustrated in Fig. 2–6. Central nervous system injury can lead to aspiration of gastric contents that exacerbates the CNS injury. Peripheral nervous system lesions can cause aspiration, hypoxia, and resultant CNS injury. CNS injury can cause neurogenic pulmonary edema or dysfunction. The management of concomitant CNS and pulmonary dysfunction is complicated by the degree to which the manage-

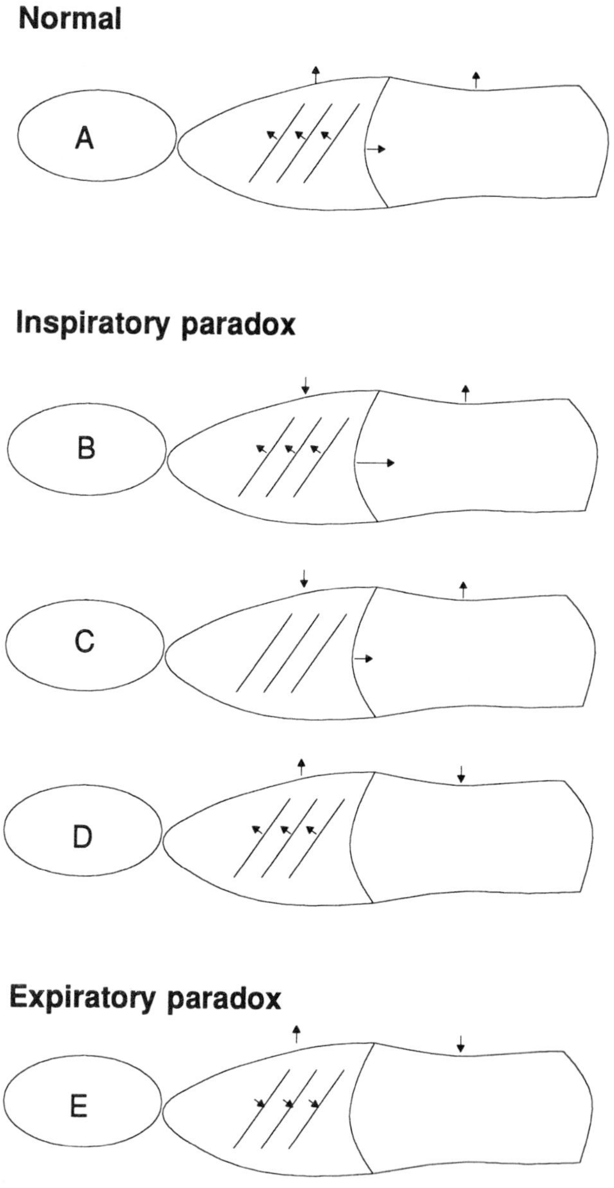

FIGURE 2-4 • Contrast normal respiration *(A)*, in which the chest and abdomen rise simultaneously, with several paradoxic patterns. Inspiratory paradox can occur with upper airway obstruction *(B)*, where the diaphragm and the intercostal both contract simultaneously, but the diaphragm "wins," pulling the chest down. Alternatively, with spinal cord lesions *(C)*, the diaphragm may function, but the intercostals do not. Several different processes, including phrenic nerve injury and diaphragmatic fatigue, allow the intercostals to work more effectively than the diaphragm *(D)*. Expiratory paradox *(E)* occurs when the abdominal rectus muscles contract forcibly, as do the obliques, to assist alveolar emptying.

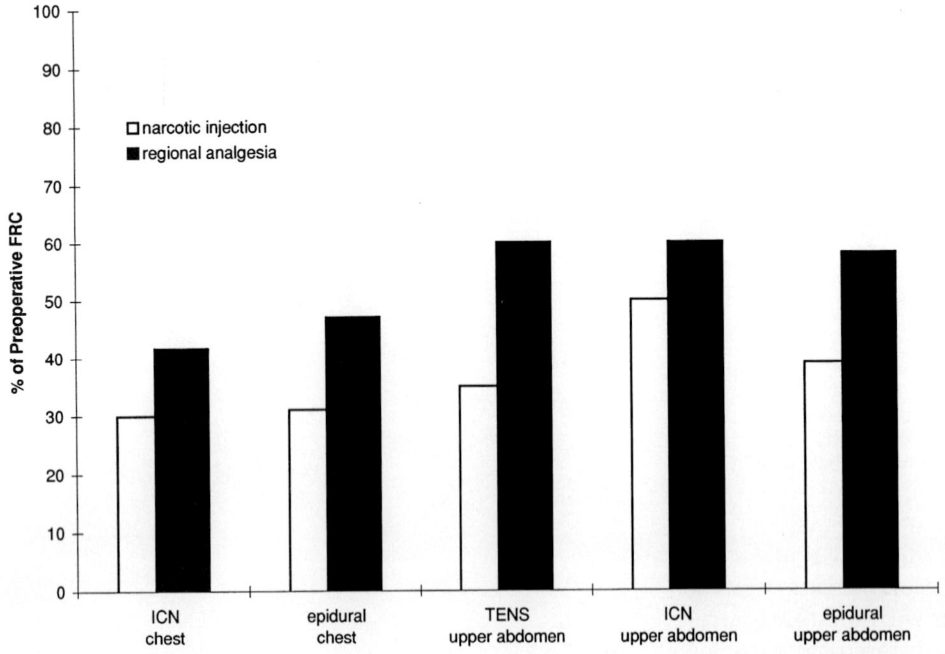

FIGURE 2-5 • The graphic shows the difference in postoperative functional residual capacity (FRC) as a percentage of preoperative values, when standard pain therapy (intravenous morphine as needed) is contrasted with regional analgesia. Procedures involving the thorax (with intercostal nerve blocks [ICN] and epidural analgesia) are contrasted with those involving the upper abdomen (transepidermal nerve stimulator [TENS], ICN, and epidural).

ment of the former affects the management of the latter.

CNS Injury

Injury to the central nervous system, whether it be surgical or traumatic, is often accompanied by respiratory failure.

Upper Airway Obstruction

The upper airway often functions ineffectively in patients with decreased level of consciousness, with resulting obstruction, desaturation, and hypoventilation. Normal respiration requires coordinated activity of a number of muscles, including those of the nasopharynx and the oropharynx, the larynx, the intercostals, and the diaphragm. When stressed, a number of secondary, "accessory" muscles are brought into play, including the sternocleidomastoid muscles and the abdominal muscles.

During normal inspiration, contraction of the diaphragm and the external intercostal muscles results in expansion of the thoracic cavity, development of subatmospheric pressure in the chest and pharynx, and air flow into the lungs. The subatmospheric pressure in the pharynx tends to pull the tongue backward (as does gravity when in the supine position) with resulting upper airway obstruction. This tendency is counteracted by the intrinsic muscles of the tongue, those that control the position of the mandible and the hyoid bone, and the oropharyngeal dilator muscles, of which the genioglossus is the most important. Patency of the nasopharynx is additionally maintained by the tensor velum palatini, palatoglossus, and palatopharyngeus muscles.

Factors that predispose to upper airway obstruction are anatomic or neurologic. Examples of the former include excess soft tissue in the tongue or around the pharynx. This is characteristic of the obese patient but may also be seen with edema of the tongue or tissues around the airway (after trauma), or in certain anaphylactoid reactions, such as the tongue swelling occasionally seen with angiotensin-converting enzyme inhibitors. The genioglossus muscle demonstrates both tonic and phasic inspiratory activity on electromyography.[35, 36] The onset of activity of upper airway activation slightly precedes contraction of the diaphragm. Activity of the upper airway musculature increases with hypercapnia, hypoxia, certain stimulatory chemicals such as nicotine, and arousal. Conversely, hypocapnia, sedatives such as alcohol and anesthetics, and CNS depression during sleep (and in particular REM sleep) are accompanied by significant reductions in upper airway tone. Upper airway obstruction with head injury is presumably due to both the loss of static CNS output and asynchronous activation of the airway muscles.

While the innervation of the larynx is quite complex, upper airway obstruction is infrequently caused by laryngeal processes, although laryngospasm can certainly occur at light levels of anesthesia in the neurosurgical patient.

The patient with upper airway obstruction and CNS injury is at particular risk because of the potential for exacerbation of the primary CNS injury due to hypoxemia and ischemia, as well as for increased cerebral blood flow and intracranial pressure due to hypercapnia and hypoxemia. Prompt restoration of adequate oxygenation and ventilation is essential.

Upper airway obstruction can be relieved transiently in some patients by arousal using vocal or physical stimuli. Painful stimuli are effective but should be avoided in patients with intracranial hypertension to avoid dangerous increases in intracranial pressure. CNS depressants, such as narcotics or benzodiazepines, can be reversed using pharmacologic antagonists. Maneuvers to open the airway are often successful. The "sniffing position" (Fig. 2–7), in which the neck is flexed forward and the head extended, relieves obstruction in many cases, as do oral or nasopharyngeal airways. This maneuver is obviously inappropriate when cervical spine injury is suspected. The application of continuous positive airway pressure by mask ("mask CPAP"), which was originally developed to treat obstructive sleep apnea, has gained increasing acceptance in the intensive care environment as a short-term measure to treat upper airway obstruction. Mask CPAP relieves obstruction by distending the oropharynx. The "jaw thrust" maneuver, in which anterior displacement of the mandible is achieved by pressure on the angle of the jaw, relieves obstruction by several mechanisms, including periosteal pain with CNS arousal and elevation of the tongue. In many instances, the upper airway obstruction is expected to be of sufficient duration that oral intubation of the trachea is required.

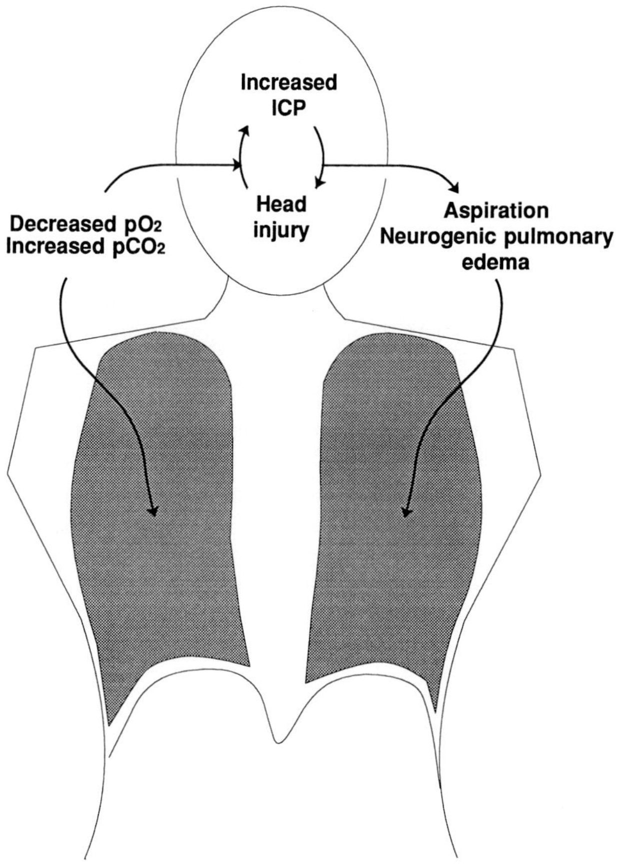

FIGURE 2–6 • The inter-relationship between head injury and lung disease. ICP, intracranial pressure.

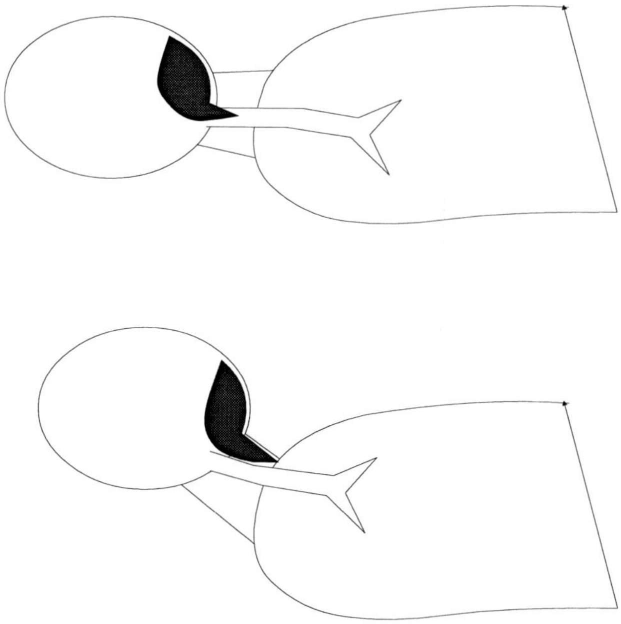

FIGURE 2–7 • The "sniffing position" tends to open the retropharynx by displacing the tongue forward (bottom).

Aspiration of Gastric Contents

Aspiration is more likely to occur in the setting of trauma or an acute CNS event than in the elective neurosurgical patient, and it significantly complicates management of the primary disease.

Traumatic injuries, strokes, or CNS bleeds usually occur within a few hours of the most recent oral intake. Factors that contribute to the degree of lung injury sustained after aspiration are the volume, the nature, and the acidity of the gastric contents. Smaller, well-digested material tends to lodge in the distal bronchi, causing lobar obstruction, atelectasis, and pneumonia, while larger material lodges in the trachea. The most common site of proximal obstruction is the vocal cords, which are the narrowest portion of the adult airway.

Depending on the degree of digestion, gastric contents range from predominantly liquid to solid. With greater time since ingestion, acidity and the enzymatic activity increase. Wynne et al. studied the relative contributions of acidity and particulate matter to lung injury in a mouse model[37] and found that food particles, gastric enzymes, and pH act synergistically to injure the airway. The most severe and durable injuries were sustained when the combination was instilled in the airway. Other studies indicate that aspirated contents with pH below 2.5 and volume greater than 0.5 cc/kg are most likely to cause damage in humans. The damage is manifested by loss of ciliated cells in the trachea, destruction of alveolar pneumocytes, surfactant depletion, and increased vascular permeability.

The anatomy of the normal lung often leads to localization of the aspirated material in the right lower lobe of the lung (because the right mainstem bronchus is straighter than the left) (Fig. 2–8), although body position at the time of injury determines the location in most instances. When the aspiration is of sufficient magnitude, ARDS typically results. Aspiration is one of the two most common risk factors for the development of ARDS.[38]

The diagnosis of aspiration, when not witnessed, is dependent on the appropriate setting, clinical course, and radiographic studies. Unless the aspiration is massive, there are often no signs of pulmonary distress immediately following the event, but over the succeeding 1–3 hours bronchospasm, dyspnea, and tachypnea develop coincident with the appearance of infiltrates on chest x-ray. Intubation, mechanical ventilation, and inotropic support are necessary to support cardiopulmonary function in severe cases.

When particulate matter is suspected to play a significant role in aspiration, bronchoscopic evaluation and, when appropriate, removal of foreign bodies should be undertaken. Rigid bronchoscopy is necessary to remove large foreign bodies, whereas fiberoptic lavage can be used with smaller-sized particles. Routine lavage with large volumes of saline solution should not be performed because of the likelihood of dispersing small particles into the lung, which would otherwise be eliminated by normal protective reflexes.

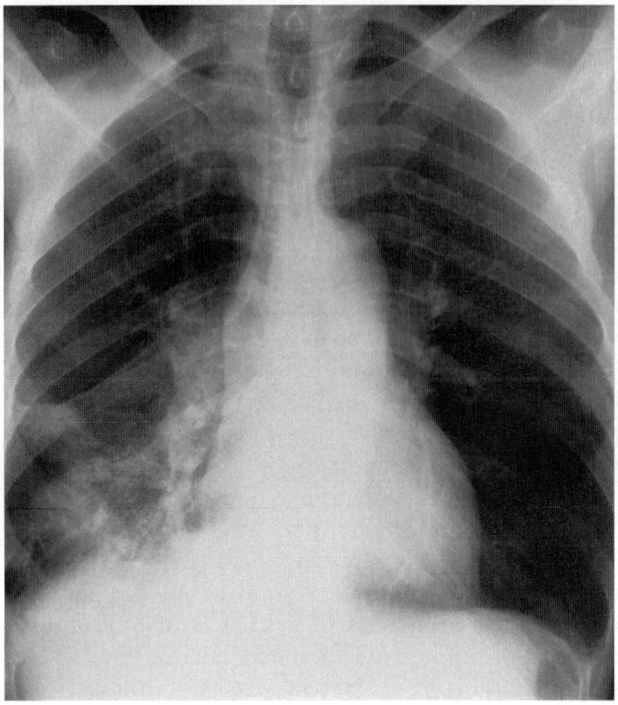

FIGURE 2-8 • Roentgenogram of aspiration pneumonia involving the right lower lobe.

Massive aspirations result in volume shifts into the alveoli and interstitial edema with attendant hypotension and hemoconcentration. Volume resuscitation should be performed cautiously in order to prevent exacerbation of the lung injury by increasing pulmonary artery and pulmonary artery wedge pressures. The use of a pulmonary artery catheter to guide fluid administration is essential. The inevitable debate about the appropriate fluid for volume resuscitation can be answered only by stating that no therapeutic benefit has ever been demonstrated with colloid over crystalloid. Bronchoalveolar lavage fluid shows the same concentration of albumin as in plasma with severe aspiration injuries, suggesting that large portions of the alveolar barrier have become ineffective in preventing transudation of albumin.[39] Similarly, colloid is more effective neither in restoring intravascular volume nor in altering the course of the injury.[40]

The use of empiric antibiotics is controversial when aspiration is presumed or witnessed. Clinical practice is varied, and although experimental evidence clearly supports the use of antibiotics only in culture proven bacterial infections,[41] many practitioners routinely prescribe antibiotics with any aspiration. A second area of controversy is the use of steroids for the empiric treatment of aspiration. Several studies, however, have definitively demonstrated an increased rate of complications when steroids are used.[42–44]

Neurogenic Pulmonary Edema

Neurogenic pulmonary edema (NPE) is characterized by pulmonary congestion occurring in the setting of head injury, grand mal seizures[45] or electroconvulsive therapy,[46] subarachnoid hemorrhage, brain tumor, vertebral artery ligation[47] or cervical cord injury,[48] and in the absence of aspiration. Histology demonstrates flooding of the alveoli with proteinaceous, hemorrhagic fluid. Radiographically, NPE is indistinguishable from cardiogenic pulmonary edema (Fig. 2–9). It is characteristically seen with severe head injury or subarachnoid hemorrhage and has a poor prognosis.

There are several theories as to the etiology of this process (Fig. 2–10) that can be roughly separated into hemodynamic phenomena and changes in capillary permeability.

Intense sympathetic activity, mediated by the hy-

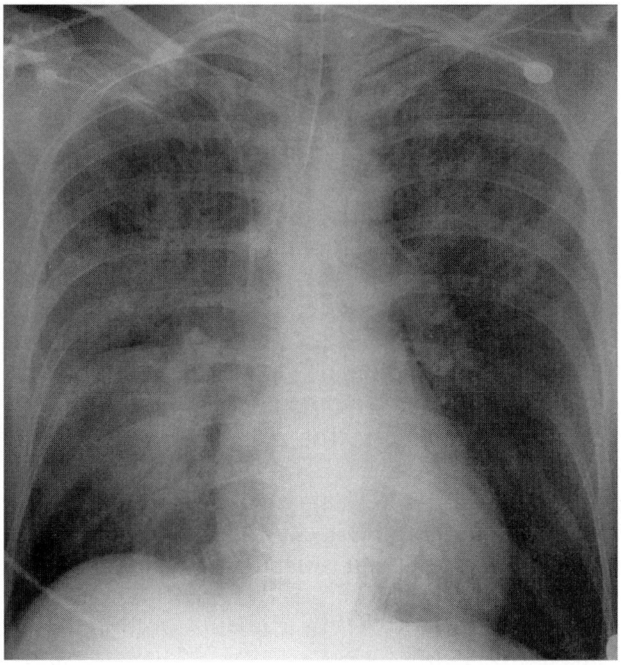

FIGURE 2-9 • Roentgenogram of neurogenic pulmonary edema.

pothalamus,[49–51] occurs shortly after CNS injury. This results in peripheral vasoconstriction, increased cardiac output, tachycardia, and vasoconstriction. The increase in afterload applied to the heart may result in left ventricular failure, elevated pulmonary capillary wedge pressure, and transudation of fluid into the alveoli.[52, 53] Another explanation for the left ventricular failure is excessive venous return due to venoconstriction, although this is probably not of major importance.[54] The left ventricle might fail because of reduced diastolic relaxation time,[55] although this is, again, probably not significant.[56] There is even evidence that left ventricular function can be directly affected (by an unknown mechanism) when the CNS is injured.[57]

An alternative hemodynamically based theory attributes the same effects to direct sympathetic activity on the pulmonary vasculature rather than failure of the left ventricle.[58, 59] The experimental evidence supporting this theory indicates that patients can develop significant hypoxemia and infiltrates in the absence of elevations in left atrial pressure.[60]

A second body of research suggests that NPE results from primary pulmonary capillary leak, and that pulmonary hypertension is not a necessary cocontributor.[61–63] Extravascular lung water has been shown to increase markedly during intracerebral hemorrhage despite normal pulmonary artery pressure, pulmonary capillary wedge pressure, and cardiac output.[64] In another study, in which intracranial pressure was gradually increased in laboratory animals, there was a threefold increase in pulmonary vascular permeability to protein,[65] while increasing venous pressures to extremely high levels had minimal effects on permeability.[66]

Yet another school of thought attributes NPE to constriction of the lymphatics due to sympathetic activation.[67] This theoretically causes decreased lymphatic flow, filling of the interstitial space and, eventually, the alveoli.

The neural pathways that participate in the development of NPE are uncertain. The medulla, the vasomotor center of the brain, contains two clusters of neurons capable of mediating responses like NPE: area A1, in the ventrolateral medulla, and A5, in the upper medulla. Ablation of the A1 area causes hypertension, bradycardia, and NPE.[68] Fibers for spinal sympathetic outflow project from area A5,[69] which responds to electrical stimulation with responses similar to those evoked by ablation of A1. Sectioning the cervical spinal cord prevents NPE. The nuclei of the solitary tract and the area postrema also have potential roles in the development of NPE.

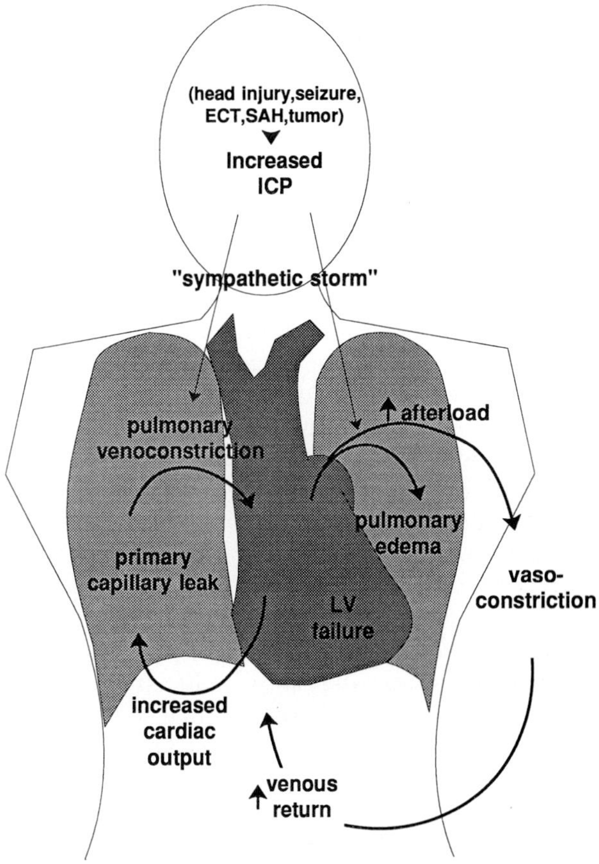

FIGURE 2-10 • This figure demonstrates the various etiologies that may account for the development of neurogenic pulmonary edema, including (1) left ventricular (LV) failure due to increased afterload and venous return, (2) pulmonary venoconstriction and increased cardiac output, and (3) primary pulmonary capillary leak. ECT, electroconvulsive therapy; SAH, subarachnoid hemorrhage; ICP, intracranial pressure.

One method of reconciling the several theories is known as the "blast theory,"[70–72] which suggests that CNS injury leads to a transient increase in systemic vascular tone with translocation of blood into the pulmonary circulation. The sudden increase in pulmonary vascular volume causes increased pulmonary capillary hydrostatic pressure with resulting injury to the capillaries. Despite the subsequent resolution of the hemodynamic abnormalities, the capillaries remain damaged and leaky.

It is unclear whether neurogenic pulmonary dysfunction (NPD) represents a separate entity or a mild form of NPE. It is clear that pulmonary dysfunction characterized by hypoxemia and a normal or near-normal chest x-ray can occur in the hours to days following head injury. Possible alternative explanations include disruption of normal ventilation-perfusion relationships,[73] microatelectasis, and retained secretions. Colice has speculated that NPE and NPD represent the dichotomous presentation of the same entity,[74] while others argue that the two are separate entities.[75]

The variety of clinical presentations categorized under the aegis of NPE and the absence of a universally accepted explanation for its etiology confound any discussion of management approaches, but, as with ARDS, supportive care is the cornerstone of therapy.

Spinal Cord Injury

Depending on the level of the injury, spinal cord injury ranges from negligible to catastrophic impact on the respiratory system. Injuries of most significance can be divided into the high cervical (C1 and C2) and mid to low cervical injuries (C3–C8). Injuries above the C3 level produce paralysis of the respiratory musculature, apnea, and immediate death unless respiratory support is initiated.

Phrenic nerve outflow originates in the C3 through C5 roots, and injury at this level produces immediate and substantial diminishment in inspiratory and expiratory flow rates, and pulmonary function tests consistent with a restrictive process.[76]

Injuries below C5 primarily affect the intercostal muscles, while sparing the diaphragm. Patients with low cervical and thoracic spinal cord injuries breathe paradoxically, as described above, because the muscles of the chest wall do not function. On inspiration, the diaphragm descends and the chest is paradoxically pulled inward. There is also substantial phasic inspiratory activity of the sternocleidomastoid, trapezius, platysma, myohyoid, and sternohyoid muscles,[77] which results in upward movement of the superior sternum during inspiration. Expiratory reserve is preserved to some extent if innervation of the upper pectoralis major muscle is preserved, as it often is in lower cervical cord injuries.[78] Lobar atelectasis is a common complication with injuries at this level, partly because of the loss of the "bucket-handle" action of the chest wall usually provided by the intercostal muscles, as well as the lack of an effective cough to clear secretions. In quadriplegic patients, the character of the bronchial mucus changes in about 20% of patients, becoming thicker and more tenacious, possibly under the influence of neural mechanisms.[79]

Another characteristic of spinal injury patients is the atypical way in which they respond to changes in position. Normal individuals have a diminished vital capacity when in the recumbent position, because of the pressure on the diaphragm from the abdominal contents. The pressure and resulting change in diaphragmatic curvature are actually advantageous to the quadriplegic, in whom it permits greater excursion of the diaphragm. The erect position is disadvantageous and results in loss of vital capacity in cord-injured patients. The use of an abdominal binder reverses the loss of vital capacity inherent in the upright position.

Neuromuscular, Degenerative, and Hereditary Diseases

This group of diseases involve the muscles of respiration either primarily or secondarily, including the intercostals, diaphragm, and those of the upper airway, and put the patient at risk for hypercapneic respiratory failure. Diseases falling under this category include the primary myopathic disorders, amyotrophic lateral sclerosis, myasthenia gravis, multiple sclerosis, Guillain-Barré syndrome, and Parkinson's disease.

The muscular dystrophies that most characteristically result in respiratory failure are myotonic dystrophy and Duchenne's muscular dystrophy. A variety of other congenital and acquired myopathies can cause some degree of respiratory embarrassment, including congenital myopathy, metabolic myopathies, periodic paralysis, and the inflammatory myopathies. In this group of patients, however, vital capacity is typically reduced only by 10%–15% due to decreased residual volumes.[80]

Myotonic dystrophy is an autosomal dominant disorder characterized by delayed muscular relaxation, weakness, cardiac and endocrine defects, and cataracts. Patients with this disease are susceptible to a number of respiratory disorders, including weakness and myotonia of the respiratory muscles, dysfunction of pharyngoesophageal musculature,[81] central hypoventilation with an altered response to hypoxia and hypercapnia,[82] and sleep-related problems. Complications include dyspnea, aspiration, extreme susceptibility to anesthesia, and excessive daytime somnolence.

Duchenne's dystrophy is an X-linked recessive muscle-wasting disorder, which presents in early childhood with difficulty in running and jumping due to proximal muscle weakness and progresses to wheelchair dependence, respiratory failure, and death by age 20 in many cases. Duchenne's patients develop progressive scoliosis, which, when combined with muscle weakness, leads to loss of vital capacity, tachypnea, hypercapnia, and pulmonary infections. Spinal fixation has been employed as a means of preventing respiratory deterioration,[83] but is not clearly efficacious.[84] Tracheostomy and ventilator dependency are the inevitable outcome of Duchenne's.

Amyotrophic lateral sclerosis (ALS) is a neurodegenerative disease of the voluntary motor system, affecting upper and lower motor neurons, which eventually progresses to respiratory deterioration and death. While ALS can present with primary respiratory dysfunction due to phrenic nerve involvement,[85, 86] it more characteristically appears with weakness of the intercostal muscles and diaphragm in the setting of bulbar muscle weakness. ALS patients develop daytime alveolar hypoventilation, which worsens with sleep. Aminophylline and theophylline have been shown to produce a modest increase in vital capacity and inspiratory flow rates in ALS patients,[87] while oxygen therapy is used to prevent nocturnal oxygen desaturation. Impaired swallowing, due to bulbar involvement, substantially increases the risk of aspiration, and gastrostomy is often performed to permit safe enteral feeding. Nocturnal nasal positive-pressure or negative-pressure ventilation (with a cuirass or poncho ventilator) interrupts the inevitable respiratory decline by providing periods of rest.[88, 89] Refractory respiratory failure eventually supervenes, and tracheostomy and permanent ventilatory support inevitably become necessary.

Myasthenia gravis is an acquired disease of the neuromuscular junction caused by antibodies to the acetylcholine receptor, which is manifested by fatigue and weakness worsened by exercise. Neuromuscular transmission is impaired by "drop-out" of acetylcholine receptors.

Myasthenia affects both inspiratory and expiratory muscles. While the most sensitive indicators of early respiratory muscle weakness are the maximal inspiratory and expiratory pressures,[90, 91] the vital capacity is generally used to follow patients with imminent respiratory failure. An abnormal fall in vital capacity when the patient assumes the supine position is indicative of severe muscle weakness, as is a vital capacity less than 10–15 cc/kg. Endotracheal intubation and mechanical ventilation are indicated when these parameters are reached, both to support ventilation and to prevent aspiration in patients with bulbar muscle weakness. The prognosis of myasthenic patients who require intubation is excellent: in a Mayo Clinic study of 22 patients with respiratory failure over a 2-year interval, 21 were successfully weaned from mechanical ventilation.[92] Maximal inspiratory force (MIF < -20 cm H_2O) and vital capacity (VC $>$ 15 cc/kg) are used to predict successful weaning from mechanical ventilation.[93]

Multiple sclerosis (MS) is a demyelinating disease involving the central nervous system white matter. The etiology is obscure; however, there is evidence for both genetic and environmental contributions to its development. Although there is no characteristic course, patients generally deteriorate over the long term. While respiratory failure is not a typical cause of death in most series,[94, 95] Smeltzer and colleagues have conducted a series of studies demonstrating that respiratory muscle dysfunction proceeds in parallel with neurologic impairment.[96, 97] Bedridden patients were shown to have abnormal inspiratory and expiratory pressures, reduced maximal voluntary ventilation, difficulty clearing secretions, and weak cough. In another study,[98] respiratory muscle weakness was demonstrated in a majority of evaluated patients, who were also shown to have bulbar dysfunction, abnormalities of respiratory control, paroxysmal hyperventilation, and obstructive sleep apnea. From these data, the authors developed a rating score for pulmonary dysfunction in MS.

The specific manifestation of respiratory failure is dependent on the site of involvement of the CNS.[99] Lesions in the corticospinal tracts, brain stem, or upper cervical cord result in an inability to voluntarily increase tidal volume or rate, while automatic breathing is intact. Conversely, lesions of the medulla, nucleus ambiguus, and medial lemniscus result in apnea during sleep, as in Ondine's curse. Diaphragmatic paralysis can be unilateral or bilateral and results from lesions of the upper cervical cord. Brain stem involvement causes a variety of abnormal respiratory patterns, including hyperventilation and apneustic respirations. Neurogenic pulmonary edema has been reported in cases with involvement of the medulla in the region of the nucleus tractus solitarius.[100]

While acute respiratory failure occurs rarely in MS patients, the scale developed by Smeltzer and colleagues, which includes a careful history and physical examination, can be used as an indicator of impending respiratory dysfunction.[101]

Guillain-Barré syndrome (GBS), also known as acute inflammatory demyelinating polyneuropathy, is an autoimmune disease that symmetrically involves the peripheral nervous system and is characterized by weakness and decreased tendon reflexes. Often preceded by a viral illness, other infectious processes,[102] cancer,[103] and surgery[104] can also act as immune system activators in GBS.

Respiratory involvement occurs in approximately one third of patients,[105] and GBS is the peripheral neuropathy most likely to cause respiratory failure. GBS affects central respiratory drive, upper airway protection, and respiratory muscle strength. GBS patients demonstrate an abnormal response to CO_2 rebreathing,[106] possibly due to central adaptation to chronic neuromuscular failure.[107] Aspiration of saliva and positional obstruction of the upper airway result from denervation of the bulbar musculature. Respiratory muscle weakness causes poor cough, decreased vital capacity and tidal volume, and atelectasis, which results in shunting and hypoxia.

Mortality rates in GBS patients requiring mechanical ventilation may exceed 15% and often result from pulmonary complications.[108, 109] Typical complications include atelectasis (40%), pneumonia (25%–40%), and (rarely) pulmonary embolism (2%).

When the diagnosis of GBS is made, extreme vigilance must be exercised in monitoring the patient's respiratory performance. Vital capacity should be determined every 4–6 hours, and when it falls below 15–20 cc/kg (Table 2–1), elective intubation of the trachea should be performed. Similarly, a maximal inspiratory force less than 20–30 cm H_2O presages imminent respiratory failure.

Because of the susceptibility to pulmonary complications and dysautonomia, GBS patients must be managed impeccably throughout the period of frank respiratory failure. Chest physiotherapy and suctioning are appropriate modalities, although patients with severe dysautonomia can develop cardiovascular collapse during therapy.[110] Intubation of the GBS patient should be performed with extreme care. Sedative agents, such as barbiturates and benzodiazepines, can provoke hypotension, and succinylcholine, a depolarizing muscle relaxant, can cause severe hyperkalemia when administered to these patients. In GBS, denervation of the neuromuscular junction results in a compensatory increase in acetylcholine receptor population. Administration of succinylcholine activates the abnormally large number of receptors and causes excessive potassium release, which can cause cardiac arrhythmias and death.[111, 112] Early performance of a tracheostomy is appropriate in GBS patients who are likely to require prolonged mechanical ventilation and effective pulmonary suctioning. Since one third of GBS patients will not require ventilatory support after 2 weeks,[113] it is reasonable to make a decision at that landmark.

Management of mechanical ventilation with GBS is not substantially different from that of any intubated patient. No modality or scheme has definitively been shown to be superior to any other.

The indications that neuromuscular performance has improved to the point that weaning and extubation should be entertained are similar to those of other chronic respiratory processes. Maximal inspiratory force less than −20 cm H_2O, forced vital capacity greater than 20 cc/kg,[114] and maximal CO_2 stimulated ventilation greater than 20 L/minute[115] have all been shown in association with successful weaning.

Parkinson's disease and syndrome include primary parkinsonism, Shy-Drager syndrome, olivopontocerebellar degeneration, and multiple system atrophy. Respiratory abnormalities that include disorders in breathing during sleep,[116] dyspnea,[117] reduction in maximal voluntary ventilation,[118] increase in airway resistance,[119] and upper airway obstruction[120] have been found in parkinsonian patients. L-Dopa, which is used to treat Parkinson's disease, has also been reported to cause apnea, dyspnea, and tachypnea. This has been attributed to respiratory dyskinesia by several investigators.[121, 122]

TABLE 2-1 **VITAL CAPACITY, RESPIRATORY PATHOPHYSIOLOGY, AND INTERVENTIONS IN GUILLAIN-BARRÉ SYNDROME**

VITAL CAPACITY (cc/kg)	PATHOPHYSIOLOGY	MANAGEMENT
>30	Normal	No intervention
20–30	Poor cough, accumulated secretions, atelectasis	Respiratory therapy: chest physiotherapy, incentive spirometry
<20	Hypoxemia, hypercapnia	Elective endotracheal intubation

Cerebral Ischemia

While focal seizures or stimulation of areas of the cortex has clearly been shown to cause apnea,[123, 124] cortical strokes typically have minimal respiratory effects. Bilateral hemispheric strokes, however, are associated with Cheyne-Stokes breathing,[125] as are single hemispheric lesions in patients with concomitant pulmonary or cardiac dysfunction.[126] Injuries to specific areas of the brain stem depend on the level of the injury and location of the lesion. The dorsolateral portion of the medulla contains most of the essential respiratory control neurons, and lesions to this area are usually fatal.[127] Conversely, an extensive injury to the brain stem that spares the dorsolateral medulla is compatible with prolonged survival.[128]

A lesion of the autonomic respiratory pathway elicits Ondine's curse, which is characteristically seen with injury to the lateral medulla (often seen with occlusion of the distal vertebral artery), in which there is impairment or absence of automatic respiration. The opposite condition, in which the patient is unable to voluntarily alter breathing pattern or rate but has preserved automatic respiration, can be seen with a midpontine lesion.[129]

Seizure Disorders

Generalized seizures are often accompanied by upper airway obstruction and abnormal diaphragmatic movements.[130] While the respiratory manifestations of grand mal seizures are typically self-limited, the effects of combined respiratory acidosis, from the increase in CO_2 production and decrease in elimination, and metabolic acidosis can cause dangerous metabolic derangements. Serum potassium levels can rise to dangerous levels, precipitating cardiac arrhythmias. Aspiration of gastric contents and neurogenic pulmonary edema are other potential complications of generalized seizures.

A distinctly more unusual complication, in which acute respiratory failure occurred in the absence of motor activity, was observed in a patient with a known seizure disorder and presumed to be due to "propagation of seizure discharges leading to dysfunction of brain stem respiratory centers."[131]

Acute generalized seizures rarely require intervention to protect the airway or to provide ventilation and are typically managed by maneuvers to open the airway with or without supplemental oxygen. Because permanent brain damage has been reported with seizures persisting for periods of 30 minutes,[132] the management of status epilepticus requires support of airway and breathing and often requires intubation and mechanical ventilation.

Respiratory Failure and Mechanical Ventilation

When patients with neurologic disease require ventilatory assistance, the clinician must determine the urgency of intervention based upon the security of the airway and blood supply to the brain. Because of the dependence of the brain on a continuous supply of oxygen, and its lack of reserve, endotracheal intubation and mechanical ventilation with supplemental oxygen should be employed early in patients with suspected brain injury. Even a brief period of hypoxia can result in extension of the primary injury.

A number of methods for providing long-term mechanical ventilation outside of the hospital setting or in chronic care facilities have become available in the past several years. These include negative-pressure ventilators, such as the cuirass and poncho ventilators. These are typically used at night to provide a period of rest for the patient with COPD or neuromuscular diseases. Noninvasive ventilation, as with nasal biPAP (wherein the pressure applied to a tightly fitting nasal mask is alternated from high to low), is gaining in popularity and is often used with sleep apnea patients. Many patients with chronic respiratory failure undergo positive-pressure ventilation through a tracheostomy. Each mode has associated financial costs and requires understanding and competence by the patient or family in its application.

Aspiration of gastric contents and the development of aspiration pneumonitis represent a potentially catastrophic complication to the neurologically impaired patient. Similarly, the combination of hypoxia and hypercapnia, with the resulting increase in cerebral blood flow, can be lethal to the patient with increased intracranial pressure. The strategies and modalities applied to the respiratory care of patients with neurologic disease are generally not significantly different from those employed in caring for any patient requiring mechanical ventilation, with the exception of those patients with increased intracranial pressure.

The management of mechanical ventilation in patients with intracranial hypertension is quite complex because of the interplay between injuries to the brain and secondary or concomitant lung pathology described in the foregoing paragraphs, as well as the effects of mechanical ventilation on venous return to the thorax and therefore to venous drainage from the head (Fig. 2–11). Some authors recommend the use of continuous jugular bulb oxygen saturation monitoring to determine the best balance of therapies available to the brain-injured patient.[133–135]

Positive-pressure ventilation and positive end-expiratory pressure (PEEP), while frequently necessary for the care of patients with intracranial hypertension, can increase intracranial pressure by several mechanisms. Increased intrathoracic pressure impairs venous return from the brain primarily. Engorgement of epidural veins, resulting from transmitted positive intrathoracic pressure, can compress the subarachnoid space and translocate cerebrospinal fluid to the intracranial vault. In some patients, the application of positive pressure to the intrathoracic space results in decreased venous return to the right and left side of the heart and diminished cardiac output, blood pressure, and cerebral perfusion.

Although the application of PEEP warrants caution for the aforementioned reasons, it is clear that

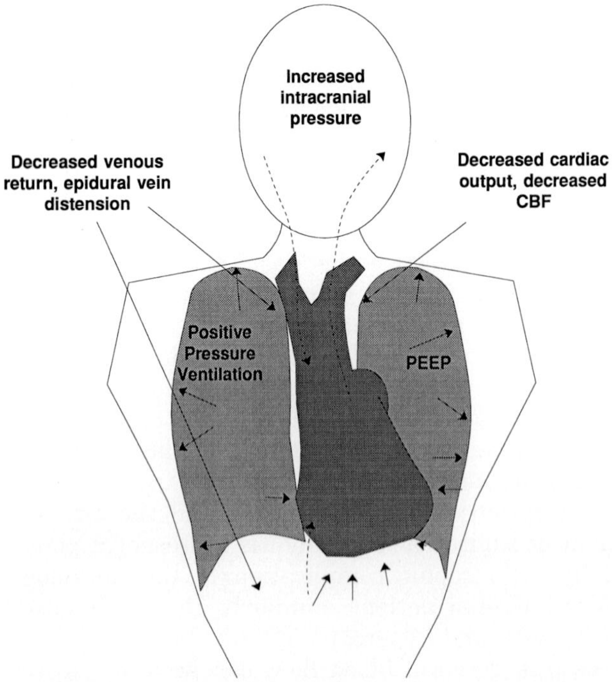

FIGURE 2-11 • The effect of positive-pressure ventilation and positive end-expiratory pressure (PEEP) on intracranial pressure. CBF, cerebral blood flow.

moderate degrees of PEEP (≤15 cm H_2O) can safely be used in the management of patients with poor intracranial compliance,[136] particularly when pulmonary compliance is poor. Less positive pressure is transmitted to the mediastinum when the lungs are stiff, which providentially is the circumstance in which PEEP is most likely to be effective. PEEP should be applied in small increments and titrated to the minimal level consistent with the desired clinical effect (i.e., adequate oxygenation on nontoxic levels of inspired oxygen). Concurrent repletion of intravascular volume deficits diminishes the effect of PEEP on cardiac output.

The mortality rate for ARDS has not changed substantially in the last 25 years, despite trials of extracorporeal membrane oxygenation, high-dose steroids, supraphysiologic PEEP, nonsteroidal anti-inflammatory agents, and exogenous surfactant. Current recommendations for the management of ARDS, while not yet supported by large, randomized, prospective studies, can be extrapolated from smaller studies and animal data. The terms *volutrauma* and *barotrauma* have come into general acceptance and refer to the fact that animals undergoing mechanical ventilation with large tidal volumes for short periods develop lung pathology indistinguishable from ARDS.[137, 138] Overdistention, with fracture of the basement membrane of the healthy alveolus, is the likely culprit. Hickling et al. reported a mortality rate of 16% in 50 patients with severe ARDS,[139] and a predicted mortality rate of 40% using a ventilator strategy designed to minimize mean airway pressure and alveolar distention. A large, multicenter prospective study is currently under way to test differences between "low-stretch" and "high-stretch" ventilation. Liposome encapsulated prostaglandin E_1 was shown to improve oxygenation and reduce dependence on mechanical ventilation in a phase 2 study,[140] and partial liquid ventilation with a perfluorocarbon solution has shown promise in adult[141] and pediatric[142] patients. Other potentially promising agents include ketoconazole[143] and steroids in the fibroproliferative phase of ARDS.[144]

CONCLUSION

As recently as 15–20 years ago, coexistent neurologic and respiratory failure resulted in a uniformly fatal outcome. Advances on a number of fronts, including the field management of head-injured patients (definitive airway intervention in the field), the evolution of intensive care units and nurses dedicated to the management of patients with neurologic diseases (spinal cord units, head injury centers), the therapy of increased intracranial pressure, and respiratory therapy (allowing prolonged periods of mechanical ventilation), have dramatically improved outcomes in this patient population.

References

1. Bolton CF, Gilbert JJ, Hahn AF, et al: Polyneuropathy in critically ill patients. J Neurol Neurosurg Psychiatr 1984;47:1223–1231.
2. Bolton CF, Laverty DA, Brown JD, et al: Critically ill polyneuropathy: Electrophysiological studies and differentiation from Guillain-Barré syndrome. J Neurol Neurosurg Psychiatr 1986;49:563–573.
3. Segredo V, Caldwell JE, Matthay MA, et al: Persistent paralysis in critically ill patients after long-term administration of vecuronium. N Engl J Med 1992;327:524–528.
4. Segredo V, Matthay MA, Sharma ML, et al: Prolonged neuromuscular blockade after long-term administration of vecuronium in two critically ill patients. Anesthesiology 1990;72:566–570.
5. MacFarlane IA, Rosenthal AD: Severe myopathy after status asthmaticus. Lancet 1977;ii:615.
6. Dodson BA, Kelly BJ, Braswell, LM, et al: Changes in acetylcholine receptor number in muscle from critically ill patients receiving muscle relaxants: An investigation of the molecular mechanism of prolonged paralysis. Crit Care Med 1995;23:815–821.
7. Mörch ET: History of mechanical ventilation. In Kirby RR, Banner MJ, Downs JB (eds): Clinical Applications of Ventilatory Support, pp 1–61. New York, Churchill Livingstone, 1990.
8. Burford TH, Burbank B: Traumatic wet lung. J Thorac Surg 1945;14:415–424.
9. Moon VH: Pathological features following shock with delayed death. Am J Pathol 1936;12:788–791.
10. Ashbaugh DG, Bigelow OB, Petty TL, et al: Acute respiratory distress in adults. Lancet 1967;ii:319–323.
11. Hilberman M: The evolution of intensive care units. Crit Care Med 1975;3:159–165.
12. Mead J: Mechanical properties of lungs. Physiol Rev 1961;41:281–330.

13. West JB: Respiratory Physiology: The Essentials, 3rd ed. Baltimore, Williams and Wilkins, 1985.
14. Gautier H, Bertrand F: Respiratory effects of pneumotaxic center lesions and subsequent vagotomy in chronic cats. Respir Physiol 1975;23:71–85.
15. Berger AJ, Mitchell RA, Herbert DA: Properties of apneustic respiration. Fed Proc 1976;35:633–653.
16. Lumsden T: Observation on the respiratory centers in the cat. J Physiol Lond 1923;57:153–160.
17. Lumsden T: Observations on the respiratory centers. J Physiol Lond 1923;57:354–367.
18. Lumsden T: The regulation of respiration I. J Physiol Lond 1923;58:81–91.
19. Bruce EN, Cherniack NS: Central chemoreceptors. J Appl Physiol 1987;62:389–402.
20. Sampson SR, Vidruk EH: Properties of irritant receptors in canine lung. Resp Physiol 1975;25:9–22.
21. Lange RL, Hecht HH: The mechanism of Cheyne-Stokes respiration. J Clin Invest 1962;41:42–52.
22. Lyons HA, Burno, Stone RW: Pulmonary compliance in patients with periodic breathing. Circulation 1958;17:1056–1061.
23. Bolton CF: Assessment of respiratory function in the intensive care unit. Can J Neurol Sci 1994;21:S28–S34.
24. Loh L: Neurological and neuromuscular disease. Br J Anaesth 1986;58:190–200.
25. Nunn JF: Control of breathing. In Nunn JF: Nunn's Applied Physiology, 4th ed, p 94. Oxford, Butterworth-Heinemann, 1994.
26. Beecher HK: Effect of laparotomy on lung volume: Demonstration of a new type of pulmonary collapse. J Clin Invest 1932;12:651–658.
27. Craig DB: Postoperative recovery of pulmonary function. Anesth Analg 1981;60:46–52.
28. Meyers JR, Lembeck L, O'Kane H, et al: Changes in functional residual capacity of the lung after operation. Arch Surg 1975;110:576–582.
29. Pasteur W: Massive collapse of the lung. Lancet 1908;ii:1351.
30. Reeve EB, Nanson EM, Rundle RF: Observations on inhibitory respiratory reflexes during abdominal surgery. Clin Sci 1951;10:65–87.
31. De Troyer A, Rosso J: Reflex inhibition of the diaphragm by afferents. Neurosci Lett 1982;30:43–46.
32. Ullman DA, Wimpy RE, Fortune JB, et al: The treatment of patients with rib fractures using continuous thoracic epidural narcotic infusion. Reg Anaesth 1989;14:43–47.
33. Yeager MP, Glass DD, Neff RK: Epidural anesthesia and analgesia in high-risk surgical patients. Anesthesiology 1987;66:729–736.
34. Rutberg H, Hakanson E, Anderberg B, et al: Effects of the extradural administration of morphine or bupivacaine on the endocrine response to upper abdominal surgery. Br J Anaesth 1984;56:233–237.
35. Remmers JE, deGroot WJ, Sauerland EK, et al: Pathogenesis of upper airway occlusion during sleep. J Appl Physiol 1978;44:931–938.
36. Sauerland EK, Sauerland BAT, Orr WC, et al: Noninvasive electromyography of human genioglossal (tongue) activity. Electromyogr Clin Neurophysiol 1981;21:279–286.
37. Wynne JW, Ramphal R, Hood CI, et al: Tracheal mucosal damage after aspiration: A scanning electron microscope study. Am Rev Respir Dis 1981;124:728–732.
38. Fowler AA, Hamman RD, Good JT, et al: Adult respiratory distress syndrome: risk with common predisposition. Ann Intern Med 1983;98:593–597.
39. Peitzman AB, Shires GT, Illner H, et al: The effect of intravenous steroids on alveolar capillary membrane permeability in pulmonary acid injury. J Trauma 1982;22:347–352.
40. Peitzman AB, Shires GT, Illner H, et al: Pulmonary acid injury: Effects of positive end-expiratory pressure and crystalloid versus colloid fluid resuscitation. Arch Surg 1982;117:662–668.
41. Lewis RT, Burgess JH, Hampson LG: Cardiorespiratory studies in critical illness: Changes in aspiration pneumonitis. Arch Surg 1971;103:335–340.
42. Buchman SR, Sugerman HJ, Tatum JL: Failure of methylprednisolone, ibuprofen or prostacyclin to reduce HCl induced pulmonary albumin leak in dogs. Surgery 1984;92:163–170.
43. Gates S, Huang T, Cheney FW: Effects of methylprednisolone on resolution of acid aspiration pneumonitis. Arch Surg 1983;118:1262–1265.
44. Wynne JW, Demarco FJ, Hood CI: Physiological effects of corticosteroids in food-stuff aspiration. Arch Surg 1981;116:46–49.
45. Archibald RB, Armstrong JD Jr: Recurrent postictal pulmonary edema. Postgrad Med 1978;63:210–213.
46. Buisseret P: Acute pulmonary oedema following grand mal epilepsy and as a complication of electric shock therapy. Br J Dis Chest 1982;76:194–195.
47. Waters HR, Gooding MR: Pulmonary oedema following vertebral artery ligation. Anesthesia 1972;27:450–453.
48. Poe RH, Reisman JL, Rodenhouse TG: Pulmonary edema in cervical spinal cord injury. J Trauma 1978;18:71–73.
49. Graf CJ, Rossi NP: Catecholamine response to intracranial hypertension. J Neurosurg 1978;49:862–868.
50. Moss I, Lisbon A, Levine JF, et al: The effects of increased intracranial pressure on respiratory functions. In Lundberg N, Ponten U, Brock M (eds): Intracranial Pressure II, p 315. Berlin, Springer-Verlag, 1975.
51. Clifton GL, Ziegler MG, Grossman RG: Circulating catecholamines and sympathetic activity after head injury. Neurosurgery 1981;8:10–14.
52. Chen HI, Chai CY: Pulmonary edema and hemorrhage as a consequence of a systemic vasoconstriction. Am J Physiol 1974;227:144–151.
53. Ducker TB, Simmons RL: Increased intracranial pressure and pulmonary edema. Part 2. The hemodynamic response of dogs and monkeys to increased intracranial pressure. J Neurosurg 1968;128:118–123.
54. Brashear RE, Ross JC: Hemodynamic effects of elevated cerebrospinal fluid pressure: Alterations with adrenergic blockade. J Clin Invest 1970;49:1324–1333.
55. Luisada AA: Mechanism of neurogenic pulmonary edema: Ann Cardiol 1967;20:66–68.
56. Glantz SA, Parmley WW: Factors which affect the diastolic pressure volume curve. Circ Res Vol 1978;42:171–180.
57. Colice GL, Matthay MA, Bass E: Neurogenic pulmonary edema. Am Rev Respir Dis 1984;130:941–948.
58. Minnear FL, Barrie PS, Malik AB: Effects of epinephrine and norepinephrine infusion on lung fluid balance in sheep. J Appl Physiol 1981;50:1353–1357.
59. Malik AB, Minnear FL, Popp AJ: Catecholamine induced pulmonary edema. Gen Pharmacol 1983;14:55–60.
60. Popp AJ, Gottlieb ME, Paloski WH, et al: Cardiopulmonary hemodynamics in patients with serious head injury. J Surg Res 1982;32:416–421.
61. Garcia-Uria J, Hoff JT, Miranda S: Experimental neurogenic pulmonary edema. Part 2: The role of cardiopulmonary pressure change. J Neurosurg 1981;54:632–636.
62. Hoff JT, Nisimura M, Garcia-Uria J: Experimental neurogenic pulmonary edema. Part 1: The role of systemic hypertension. J Neurosurg 1981;54:627–631.
63. Millen JE, Glauser FL: Low levels of concussive brain trauma and pulmonary edema. J Appl Physiol 1983;54:666–670.
64. Touho H, Karasawa J, Shishido H, et al: Hypoxemia in the acute stage of intracerebral hemorrhage with special reference to increased extravascular lung water (in Japanese). Neurol Med Chir (Tokyo) 1989;29:724–727.
65. McClellan MD, Dauber IM, Weil JV: Elevated intracranial pressure increases pulmonary vascular permeability to protein. J Appl Physiol 1989;67:1185–1191.
66. Maron MB: Effect of elevated vascular pressure transients on protein permeability in the lung. J Appl Physiol 1989;67:305–310.
67. McHale NG, Roddie IC: Peripheral lymph flow during

intravenous noradrenaline infusion in sheep (abstract). J Physiol (Lond) 1983;334:50P.
68. Blessing WW, West MJ, Chalmers J: Hypertension, bradycardia and pulmonary edema in the conscious rat after brainstem lesions coinciding with the A1 group of catechol neurons. Circ Res 1981;49:959–970.
69. Loewy AD, McKellar S: The neuroanatomical basis of central cardiovascular control. Fed Proc 1980;39:2495–2503.
70. Ducker TB, Simmons RL: Increased intracranial pressure and pulmonary edema. Part II. The hemodynamic response of dogs and monkeys to increased intracranial pressure. J Neurosurg 1968;28:118–123.
71. Carlson RW, Schaeffer RC, Michaels SG: Pulmonary edema following intracranial hemorrhage. Chest 1979;75:731–734.
72. Theodore J, Robin ED: Speculations on neurogenic pulmonary edema (NPE). Am Rev Respir Dis 1976;113:405–411.
73. Schumacker P, Rhodes GB, Newell JC: Ventilation-perfusion imbalance after head trauma. Am Rev Respir Dis 1979;119:33–43.
74. Colice GL: Neurogenic pulmonary edema. Clin Chest Med 1985;6:473–489.
75. Popp AJ, Shah DM, Berman RA, et al: Delayed pulmonary dysfunction in head injured patients. J Neurosurg 1982;57:784–790.
76. Huldtgren AC, Fuglemeyer AR, Jonasson E, et al: Ventilatory dysfunction and respiratory rehabilitation in post-traumatic quadraplegia. Eur J Respir Dis 1980;61:347–356.
77. De Troyer A, Estenne M, Vincken W: Rib cage motion and muscle use in high tetraplegics. Am Rev Resp Dis 1986;133:115–119.
78. Estenne M, Knoop C, Vanvaerenbergh J, et al: Effect of pectoralis muscle training in tetraplegic subjects. Am Rev Respir Dis 1989;139:1218–1222.
79. Bhaskar KR, Brown R, O'Sullivan DD, et al: Bronchial mucous hypersecretion in acute quadriplegia. Am Rev Res Dis 1991;143:640–648.
80. Rideau Y, Jankowski LW, Grellet J: Respiratory function in the muscular dystrophies. Muscle Nerve 1981;4:155–164.
81. Swick HM, Werlin SL, Dodds WJ, et al: Pharyngoesophageal motor dysfunction in patients with myotonic dystrophy. Ann Neurol 1981;10:454–457.
82. Hansotia P, Frens D: Hypersomnia associated with alveolar hypoventilation in myotonic dystrophy. Neurology 1981;31:1336–1337.
83. Kurz LT, Mubarak SJ, Schultz P, et al: Correlation of scoliosis and pulmonary function in Duchenne muscular dystrophy. J Pediatr Orthop 1983;3:347–353.
84. Miller RG, Chalmers AC, Dao H, et al: The effect of spine fusion on respiratory function in Duchenne muscular dystrophy. Neurology 1991;41:38–40.
85. Daras M, Spiro AJ, Swerdlow M: Respiratory failure in amyotrophic lateral sclerosis: N Y State J Med 1984;84:570–572.
86. Fromm GB, Wisdom PJ, Block AJ: Amyotrophic lateral sclerosis presenting with respiratory failure. Chest 1977;71:612–614.
87. Schiffman PL, Belsh JM: Effect of inspiratory resistance and theophylline on respiratory muscle strength in patients with amyotrophic lateral sclerosis. Am Rev Resp Dis 1989;139:1418–1423.
88. Bach JR, Alba AS: Management of chronic alveolar hypoventilation by nasal ventilation. Chest 1990;97:52–57.
89. Braun SR, Sufit RL, Giovannoni R, et al: Intermittent negative pressure ventilation in the treatment of respiratory failure in progressive neuromuscular disease. Neurology 1987;37:1874–1875.
90. Ringqvist I, Ringqvist T: Respiratory mechanics in untreated myasthenia gravis with special reference to the respiratory forces. Acta Med Scand 1971;190:499–508.
91. Mier-Jedrzejowicz AK, Brophy C, Green M: Respiratory muscle function in myasthenia gravis. Am Rev Respir Dis 1988;138:867–873.
92. Gracey DR, Divertie MB, Howard FM: Mechanical ventilation for respiratory failure in myasthenia gravis: Two year experience with 22 patients. Mayo Clin Proc 1983;58:597–602.
93. Borel CO, Tilford C, Nichols DG, et al: Diaphragmatic performance during acute ventilatory failure in Guillain-Barré syndrome and myasthenia gravis. Chest 1991;99:444–451.
94. McAlpine D, Compston N: Some aspects of the natural history of disseminated sclerosis. Q J Med 1952;21:135–168.
95. Carter S, Sciarra D, Merritt HH: The course of multiple sclerosis as determined by autopsy proven cases. Research Publications, Association for Research in Nervous and Mental Disease 1950;28:471.
96. Smeltzer SC, Utell MJ, Rudick RA, et al: Pulmonary function and dysfunction in multiple sclerosis. Arch Neurol 1988;45:1245–1249.
97. Smeltzer SC, Skurnick JH, Troiano R, et al: Respiratory function in multiple sclerosis: Utility of clinical assessment of respiratory muscle function. Chest 1992;101:479–484.
98. Howard RS, Wiles CM, Hirsch NP, et al: Respiratory involvement in multiple sclerosis. Brain 1992;115:479–494.
99. Carter JL, Noseworthy JH: Ventilatory dysfunction in multiple sclerosis. Clin Chest Med 1994;15:693–703.
100. Simon RP, Gean-Marton AD, Sander JE: Medullary lesion inducing pulmonary edema. A magnetic resonance imaging study. Ann Neurol 1991;30:727–730.
101. Smeltzer SC, Skurnick JH, Troiano R, et al: Respiratory dysfunction in multiple sclerosis: Utility of clinical assessment of respiratory muscle function. Chest 1992;101:479–494.
102. Kleyweg RP, van der Meche FGA, Banffer JRJ: Campylobacter infection in the Guillain-Barré syndrome. J Neurol 1988;235(suppl):23.
103. Lisak RP, Mitchell M, Zweiman B, et al: Guillain-Barré syndrome and Hodgkin's disease: Three cases and immunological studies. Ann Neurol 1977;1:72–78.
104. Arnason BG, Asbury AK: Idiopathic polyneuritis after surgery. Arch Neurol 1968;18:500–507.
105. Moore P, James O: Guillain-Barré syndrome: Incidence, management and outcome of major complications. Crit Care Med 1981;9:549–550.
106. Borel CO, Teitelbaum JS, Hanley DF: Ventilatory drive and CO_2-response in ventilatory failure due to myasthenia gravis and Guillain-Barré. Crit Care Med 1993;21:1717–1726.
107. Bigland-Ritchie B: Muscle fatigue and the influence of changing neural drive. Clin Chest Med 1984;5:21–34.
108. Sunderrajan EV, Davenport J: The Guillain-Barré syndrome: Pulmonary neurologic correlations. Medicine 1985;64:33–41.
109. Gracey DR, McMichan JC, Divertie MB, et al: Respiratory failure in Guillain-Barré syndrome: A 6-year experience. Mayo Clin Proc 1982;57:742–746.
110. Dalos NP, Borel C, Hanley DF: Cardiovascular autonomic dysfunction in the Guillain-Barré syndrome. Therapeutic implications of Swan-Ganz monitoring. Arch Neurol 1988;45:115–117.
111. Beach TP, Stone WA, Hamelburg W: Circulatory collapse following succinylcholine: Report of a patient with diffuse lower motor neuron disease. Anesth Analg 1971;50:431–437.
112. Fergusson RJ, Wright DJ, Willey RF, et al: Suxamethonium is dangerous in polyneuropathy. Br Med J Clin Res Ed 1981;282:298–29.
113. Ropper AH, Kehne SM: Guillain-Barré syndrome: Management of respiratory failure. Neurology 1985;35:1662–1665.
114. Chevrolet JC, Deleamont P: Repeated vital capacity measurements as predictive parameters for mechanical

ventilation need and weaning success in Guillain-Barré syndrome. Am Rev Respir Dis 1991;144:814–818.
115. Borel CO, Tilford C, Nichols DG, et al: Diaphragmatic performance during recovery from acute ventilatory failure in Guillain-Barré syndrome and myasthenia gravis. Chest 1991;99:444–451.
116. Apps MCP, Sheaff PC, Ingram DA, et al: Respiration and sleep in Parkinson's disease. J Neurol Neurosurg Psychiatr 1985;48:1240–1245.
117. Nugent CA, Harris HW, Cohn J, et al: Dyspnea as a symptom in Parkinson's syndrome. Am Rev Tuberc 1958;78:682.
118. Neu HC, Connolly JJ Jr, Schwertley FW, et al: Obstructive respiratory dysfunction in parkinsonian patients. Am Rev Respir Dis 1967;95:33–47.
119. Obenour WH, Stevens PM, Cohen AA, et al: The causes of abnormal pulmonary function in Parkinson's disease. Am Rev Respir Dis 1972;105:382–387.
120. Vincken WG, Gauthier SG, Dollfuss RE, et al: Involvement of upper-airway muscles in extrapyramidal disorders. A cause of airflow limitation. N Engl J Med 1984;311:438–442.
121. Granerus AK, Jagenburg R, Nisson NJ, et al: Respiratory disturbance during L-dopa treatment of Parkinson's syndrome. Acta Med Scand 1974;195:39–43.
122. Zupnick HM, Brown LK, Miler A, et al: Respiratory dysfunction due to L-dopa therapy for parkinsonism: Diagnosis using serial pulmonary function tests and respiratory inductive plethysmography. Am J Med 1990;89:109–114.
123. Coulter DL: Partial seizures with apnea and bradycardia. Arch Neurol 1984;41:173–174.
124. Nelson DA, Ray CD: Respiratory arrest from seizure discharges in limbic system. Arch Neurol 1968;19:199–207.
125. Heyman A, Birchfield RI, Sieker HO: Effects of bilateral cerebral infarction on respiratory center sensitivity. Neurology 1958;8:694–700.
126. Lee MC, Klassen AC, Resch JA: Respiratory pattern disturbances in ischemic cerebral vascular disease. Stroke 1974;5:612–616.
127. Devereaux MW, Keane JR, Davis RL: Automatic respiratory failure associated with infarction in the medulla. Arch Neurol 1973;29:46–52.
128. Feldman MH: Physiological observations in a chronic case of "locked-in" syndrome. Neurology 1971;21:459–478.
129. Munschauer FE, Mador MJ, Ahuja A, et al: Selective paralysis of voluntary but not limbically influenced automatic respiration. Arch Neurol 1991;48:1190–1192.
130. Walton NY: Systemic effects of generalized convulsive status epilepticus. Epilepsia 1993;34:S54–S58.
131. Malatinsky J, Prochazka M, Samel M: Respiratory failure as a seizure phenomenon. Br J Anaesth 1975;47:1019–1022.
132. Browne TR, Mikati M: Status epilepticus. In Ropper AH, Kennedy SF (eds): Neurological and Neurosurgical Intensive Care, pp 269–284. Rockville, MD, Aspen, 1987.
133. Cruz J, Raps EC, Hoffstad OJ, et al: Cerebral oxygenation monitoring. Crit Care Med 1993;21:1242–1246.
134. Cruz J: On-line monitoring of global cerebral hypoxia in acute brain injury. Relationship to intracranial hypertension. J Neurosurg 1993;79:228–233.
135. Cruz J, Jaggi JL, Hoffstad OJ: Cerebral blood flow, vascular resistance, and oxygen metabolism in acute brain trauma. Redefining the role of cerebral perfusion pressure? Crit Care Med 1995;23:1412–1417.
136. Cooper KR, Boswell PA, Choi SC: Safe use of PEEP in patients with severe head injury. J Neurosurg 1985;63:552–555.
137. Dreyfuss D, Basset G, Soler P, et al: Intermittent positive pressure hyperventilation with high inflation pressures produces pulmonary microvascular injury in rats. Am Rev Respir Dis 1985;132:880–884.
138. Parker JC, Hernandez LA, Peevy KJ. Mechanisms of ventilator induced lung injury. Crit Care Med 1993;21:131–143.
139. Hickling KG, Walsh J, Henderson S, et al: How mortality using low volume pressure limited ventilation with permissive hypercapnia in ARDS: A prospective study. Crit Care Med 1994;22:1568–1578.
140. Abraham E, Park YC, Covington P, et al: Liposomal prostaglandin E1 in acute respiratory distress syndrome: A placebo-controlled, randomized, double-blind, multicenter clinical trial. Crit Care Med 1996;24:10–15.
141. Hirschl RB, Overbeck MC, Parent A, et al: Liquid ventilation provides uniform distribution of perfluorocarbon in the setting of respiratory failure. Surgery 1994;116:159–168.
142. Gauger PG, Pranikoff T, Schreiner RJ, et al: Initial experience with partial liquid ventilation in pediatric patients with acute respiratory distress syndrome. Crit Care Med 1996;24:16–22.
143. Yu M, Tomasa G: A double-blind, prospective, randomized trial of ketoconazole, a thromboxane synthetase inhibitor, in the prophylaxis of the adult respiratory distress syndrome. Crit Care Med 1993;21:1635–1642.
144. Meduri GU, Chinn AJ, Leeper KV, et al: Corticosteroid rescue treatment of progressive fibroproliferation in late ARDS: Patterns of response and predictors of outcome. Chest 1994;105:1516–1527.

3

Cardiovascular Disorders Related to Neuroemergencies

J. Javier Provencio, M.D. • Thomas P. Bleck, M.D.

Acute changes in cardiovascular function can have profound impact on morbidity and mortality in acute neurologic injury. More than 90% of acute stroke patients have measurable cardiovascular sequelae.[1] They can range from transient moderate hypertension to shock. Patients with stroke, subarachnoid hemorrhage (SAH), seizure, intracerebral hemorrhage (ICH), tumor, abscess, and acute trauma have all been shown to be susceptible to cardiovascular complications. In some cases, these complications resulted in death. For these reasons, a thorough understanding of the physiology and pathophysiology of cardiovascular complications is essential to appropriate treatment in the acute setting.

Cardiovascular sequelae of acute injury to the brain have been often overlooked in formal discussions of treatment. The combination of cardiologic and neurologic complications do not lend themselves to study by neuroscientists or cardiac physiologists. Advances in emergency room monitoring of blood pressure and electrocardiogram and the development of neurologic intensive care units have made awareness and study of these fields more feasible. This has resulted in the rapid rate of advances in diagnosis and treatment over the last decade.

It has long been known that blood pressure is in part controlled by the brain. The understanding that blood pressure is modulated by "medullary centers" in the brain stem was investigated initially by Dittmar in 1870.[2] Work performed by Alexander in 1945[3] and Bard in 1960[4] established the concept of the "vasomotor center," which regulates systemic blood pressure.

Wallace and Levy systematically addressed the relationship of increased blood pressure and stroke in humans.[5] They showed that in patients in whom initial increase in blood pressure was seen, the majority resolved within 24 hours. Moreover, they showed that bed rest and pharmacologic treatment were similarly effective. This cast doubt on the necessity of treating hypertension in the acute setting.

Doba and Reis,[6] and Blessing, West, and Chalmers[7] showed that elevation in blood pressure could be experimentally induced by lesioning noradrenergic neurons in the brain stems of rodents. Since then, many workers have searched for the neurologic pathways that are affected in increased blood pressure after neurologic injury. Many researchers are now looking for more precise localization of the structures in the brain stem responsible for increased blood pressure in acute injury. Oppenheimer[8] has proposed the insular cortex as a possible site for elevated blood pressure.

The observation that patients with neurologic lesions can experience cardiac electrical complications as well as myocardial abnormalities is more recent. Arrhythmias associated with SAH were first noted in 1938 by Aschenbrenner and Bodechtel.[9] Abnormalities including atrial fibrillation, ventricular tachycardia, and elongation of the QT interval leading to torsades de pointes have been documented in humans. Animal studies conducted by Satinsky et al.[10] to investigate the cause of these arrhythmias found that stimulation of the midbrain in dogs causes vasospasm of the coronary vessels that leads to ventricular tachycardia. This, and related work, brought to the forefront clinical observations[11] that SAH can cause electrographic findings indistinguishable from myocardial ischemia. Related work has been centered around the causes of acute pulmonary edema in neurologically injured patients.[12]

All of these findings lead to a unifying hypothesis of how the brain interacts with the cardiovascular system through the sympathetic pathways. With the exception of neurogenic shock, which is caused by a decrease in sympathetic tone, the complications mentioned above have excessive catecholamine release implicated as the mechanism of injury. In fact, the subdivisions of this chapter are artificial, because all of the complications mentioned above can occur concurrently. Some patients seem to preferentially have some complications, and not others. A patient with an SAH may develop hypertension and pulmonary edema but not cardiac arrhythmias. Why this occurs is unclear. It may be that there are pathological or genetic differences in certain patients' end organs (i.e., heart, lungs, vasculature, etc.) that predispose them to certain complications. It may be that different patients' neuroanatomy or physiology differ, which may change their response to certain stressors.

Samuels proposes a hypothesis of sympathetic overload precipitating myocardial damage and arrhythmias.[13] He postulates that neurologic injuries and stress can cause the release of catecholamines both in the blood (a lesser effect) and in the sympathetic nerve terminals. This in turn causes activation of catecholamine-responsive Ca^{++} channels, which cause prolonged contraction of myofibrils resulting in electrocardiographic changes. If the catecholamine excess continues and/or there is a period of ischemia (caused by prolonged contraction of the myocardium) followed by reperfusion, there is free radical release that leads to cell death (Fig. 3–1).

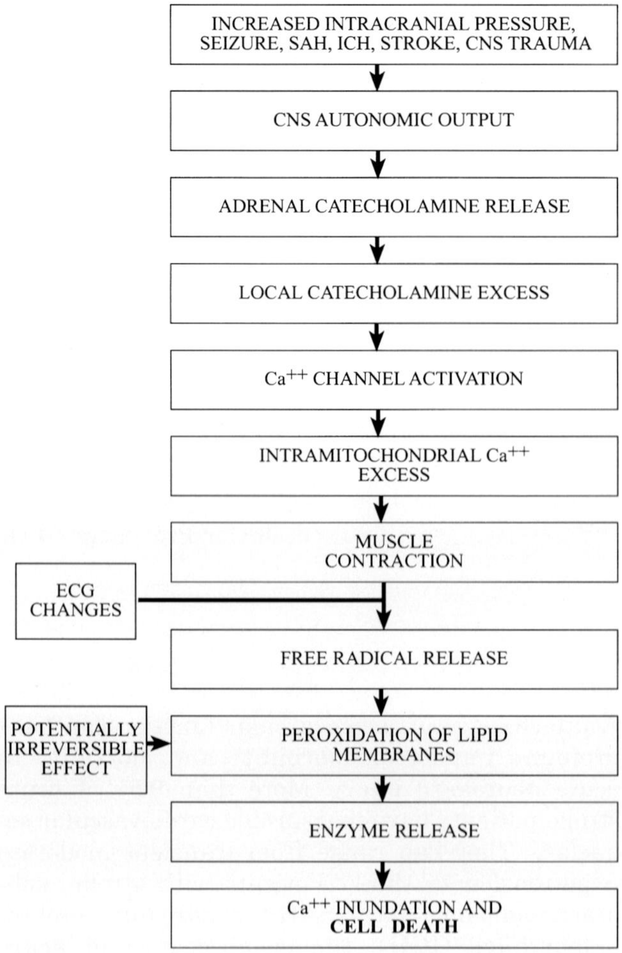

FIGURE 3–1 • Events leading to cardiac cell death due to neurologic injury. SAH, subarachnoid hemorrhage; ICH, intracerebral hemorrhage; CNS, central nervous system; ECG, electrocardiogram. (Adapted from Samuels MA: Cardiopulmonary aspects of acute neurologic diseases. In Ropper AH [ed]: Neurological and Neurosurgical Intensive Care, 3rd ed, pp 103–119. New York, Raven Press, 1993.)

HYPERTENSION

Hypertension in patients with stroke and SAH is difficult to manage in the acute setting. In a study by Wallace and Levy,[5] 80% of patients with acute stroke had increased systemic blood pressure. The standard of practice has fluctuated from aggressive normalization of blood pressure to tolerance of high blood pressures up to the point at which there is evidence of end-organ damage. Over the last 10 years, attempts have been made to reach consensus about the best management of hypertension to optimize brain perfusion in the setting of neurologic injuries.[14]

In the emergency room, as well as the critical care setting, it is often difficult to determine the right parameters or time course for treatment with antihypertensive medications. Some neurologic injuries may have unique requirements for blood pressure management that do not have optimal perfusion as the final end point. The best example of this is in SAH, of which a large subset is caused by rupture of aneurysms. In this setting, prior to clipping or obliteration of the aneurysm, decreasing the amount of bleeding is as important or more important as optimal blood flow. Common practice is to keep blood pressure within the standard normal ranges.

Regulation of Blood Pressure

Regulation of arterial blood pressure is a dynamic process that involves both nervous system control and local effects. The primary chemical regulator of pressure is the sympathetic system. Norepinephrine and epinephrine acting on alpha and beta receptors change the smooth muscle tone in the arterial and arteriolar vessel walls. In addition, the sympathetic and parasympathetic systems regulate cardiac rate and contractibility. It is the combination of these effects that causes immediate changes in systemic blood pressure that allow the body to ensure perfusion to vital organs.

Cerebral extraction of oxygen from the blood differs from that in the rest of the body. The brain more efficiently extracts oxygen from the blood than do other tissues. The brain is uniquely dependent on adequate perfusion for oxygen delivery, and its vasculature is adapted to control cerebral perfusion in a unique way.

The vasculature of the brain vasodilates and vasoconstricts in response to local pH, P_{CO_2}, and possibly potassium fluxes. This process of active regulation is called metabolic autoregulation. Increases in P_{CO_2} cause vasodilation of the cerebral vessels, whereas decreased P_{CO_2} causes vasoconstriction. In addition, pressure autoregulation acts to keep the blood flow to the brain relatively constant over a wide range of systemic blood pressures. In normal individuals, between the mean arterial blood pressures of 60 and 160 mm Hg, cerebral blood flow remains constant. This ensures that hypertension and hypotension do not remarkably change the amount of blood received by the brain.

When the brain experiences ischemia due to infarction or bleeding, the cerebral vessels in the area of compromise lose their ability to autoregulate. The brain becomes dependent on systemic blood pressure to get adequate blood flow. The medullary response is to release catecholamines, thus increasing cerebral perfusion pressure. This, in turn, increases systemic blood pressure. Therefore, increases in systemic blood pressure in the acute setting may be adaptive.

Complications

Increases in systemic blood pressure fail to be adaptive when the systemic blood pressure reaches such a level as to cause end-organ damage, so-called malignant hypertension. The final common pathway for damage is the development of generalized arteriolar fibrinoid necrosis. The most commonly compromised tissues are those of the brain, the kidneys, and the retinas.

Hypertensive encephalopathy results from extravasation of blood out of the cerebral vasculature as the pressure (hydrostatic and oncotic) in the vessels exceeds the oncotic and hydrostatic pressure in the interstitium of the brain. Also, necrosis of arterioles in the brain can cause small hemorrhages. This process can lead to increased intracranial pressure that can compromise cerebral blood flow, which in a severe form can cause strokes. Increased intracranial pressure can cause herniation of the brain stem through the foramen magnum if allowed to progress.

Retinal changes include papilledema and retinal hemorrhages. Papilledema occurs when increased pressure in the optic nerve ending impedes venous return through the optic nerve, causing stasis of blood in the nerve head, which results in poor perfusion and can lead to optic nerve ischemia and infarction. Permanent damage to vision occurs if the intracranial pressure elevation is not resolved prior to optic nerve infarction. Impeded venous drainage can occur because of increased intracranial pressure or because of increased pressure in the retinal arterioles. Retinal hemorrhages due to hypertension are caused by rupture of arterioles in the outermost layer of the retina due to fibrinoid necrosis. This causes infarctions of the retina with permanent visual loss in the corresponding field of vision.

Treatment

Debate about when to treat hypertension in the acute setting continues. Hypertension after acute stroke usually resolves to premorbid levels with or without medication in about 7 days in the majority of patients, and bed rest seems to be as effective as pharmacologic agents.[5] The risk of hypotension and increased brain ischemia is greater with pharmacologic agents and has caused some clinicians to propose that seldom is pharmacologic intervention warranted in the acute setting of stroke.[15]

To further complicate the issue, studies in animals have shown that in the chronically hypertensive subject, the autoregulatory curve is shifted to higher mean arterial blood pressures, so that reduction of blood pressure to a level that is considered "normal" compromises cerebral blood flow.[16]

In the case of SAH and ICH, the danger of hypertension is more acute. Because the majority of SAH is caused by ruptured cerebral aneurysms, increased pressure can cause the rupture site to remain open, leading to further bleeding. The same argument is proposed for ICH, in which the etiology is rupture of a smaller cerebral vessel. In these cases, there is an apparent benefit to lowering blood pressure, despite the risk of compromising cerebral blood flow. The rational for tightly controlling blood pressure in SAH and ICH is that further bleeding would increase intracranial pressure by the volume of the blood in the extravascular space and by increased cerebral edema. The benefit of the increased cerebral perfusion with hypertension may be outweighed by the risk of continued bleeding.

The most accepted treatment rationale in patients with acute stroke is to examine the patient frequently with bed rest as the only treatment for systemic hypertension. Arbitrary treatment parameters of systolic blood pressures of greater than 210 mm Hg have been set by some investigators and may have some utility for routine orders given to nurses if close medical monitoring cannot be achieved. If close monitoring is available, evidence of malignant changes such as proteinuria, papilledema, or encephalopathy should be the guide to treatment.

Once the decision to treat is made, the choice of antihypertensive agents is important. Dihydropyridine calcium channel blockers (such as nifedipine) and alpha-adrenergic blockers tend to precipitously drop systemic blood pressure on initial administration; angiotensin-converting enzyme inhibitors (with the exception of enalaprilat) work too slowly to be effective; and nitroprusside, although titratable and fast acting, causes cerebral venodilation preferentially, which can increase intracranial pressure. Diuretics can be used in very specific circumstances but are usually not good choices because they cause decreased intravascular volume, which may lead to precipitous fluctuations in mean arterial pressure. Since hypotension may increase the area of ischemia and cause areas that are recoverably hypoperfused to become irreversibly hypoperfused, vasodilators such as labetalol and hydralazine, which do not appear to affect the intracranial vessels, are first-line agents. Both are intravenous preparations, which is beneficial in the acute setting. Administration of small doses repeated at constant intervals until blood pressure is out of the dangerous range is the best way to minimize the risk of hypotension (see also Chapter 8).

CARDIAC ARRHYTHMIAS

Cardiac arrhythmias are seen in several types of neurologic pathology. In one study, 90% of patients with SAH had abnormalities on the electrocardiogram (ECG) at the time of admission. Arrhythmias accounted for a significant proportion of the abnormalities.[1] In stroke, the presence of arrhythmias has been long known but more difficult to implicate in neurologic disease due to the high incidence of coincident atherosclerotic heart disease. Other neurologic problems such as mass lesions causing increased intracranial pressure and epilepsy have been reported to cause sudden death due to arrhythmia.

A clinical study conducted by Norris[17] showed that in acute stroke and cerebral hemorrhage, the incidence of cardiac abnormalities was similar. The most common finding was arrhythmias, which accounted for 48% of the total. Second was ectopic depolarizations, which comprised 30%. Atrial fibrillation was about half as common as ectopic depolarizations, and a category called "miscellaneous" accounted for the rest. Critics of this study claim that the data do not point to cerebral ischemia as the causal agent. Some investigators have interpreted similar data as evidence of underlying cardiovascular disease in patients predisposed to stroke and hemorrhage; experimental data suggest otherwise. Andreoli et al.[18] showed that in patients with SAH followed by a Holter monitor, 91% had some arrhythmia compared with only 28% in controls without pre-existing heart disease. Only 4% of patients in that study[18] had life-threatening arrhythmias, and the arrhythmias subsided within 24 hours.

Work by Oppenheimer and colleagues[19] showed that stimulation of the insular cortex of human patients undergoing temporal lobectomy for epilepsy caused increased heart rate and blood pressure if stimulations occurred on the right side, and bradycardia if stimulations occurred on the left. Lane et al.[20] have reported that patients with right hemispheric stroke are more likely to have supraventricular tachycardia. They also found that there is a tendency for patients with left hemispheric stroke to have more severe ventricular arrhythmias (the results were not significant). These are the first studies that address the cortical control of sympathetic influence on the cardiac conduction system. The lateralization that was seen in both of these studies suggests that there may be different risks associated with strokes or SAH that occur on the left versus the right side. More work needs to be done before risk assessment can be accomplished.

Classification and Treatment

The abnormalities seen in neurologic disease include increased number of ventricular premature depolarizations (VPDs), atrial abnormalities such as atrial fibrillation and flutter, ventricular tachycardia and ventricular fibrillation, prolongation of the QT interval, and torsades de pointes, as well as signs of ischemia (discussed later). The frequencies of these particular abnormalities are shown in Table 3–1. Among the disturbances in heart rhythm (VPDs, atrial fibrillation and flutter, ventricular fibrillation, torsades de pointes, etc.), VPDs are the most common. Although the latter are in themselves not usually fatal, they may presage ventricular tachycardia. Premature complexes that differ from complex to complex are called polymorphic VPDs. The significance of these polymorphic complexes is not known, but their popular name, "multifocal VPDs," implies multiple foci and more serious disease, although this has not been conclusively shown. In typical patients, the frequency of VPDs increases rapidly after the onset of neurologic symptoms and signs and reaches a peak as intracranial pressure increases. If the increased intra-

TABLE 3-1 **FREQUENCY OF ELECTROCARDIOGRAM (ECG) ABNORMALITIES IN 120 PATIENTS WITH SUBARACHNOID HEMORRHAGE**

ELECTROGRAPHIC FINDINGS	NO. OF PATIENTS	%
T wave abnormalities	15	12
ST segment changes	44	37
PR interval > 0.20 seconds	1	0.8
Interventricular conduction delay	4	3
Atrial fibrillation	1	0.8
Ventricular premature depolarizations	5	4
Total abnormal ECG	*81*	*67*

Adapted from Pinelli G, Andreoli A, Manini G, et al: Holter detection of cardiac arrhythmias in intracranial subarachnoid hemorrhage. Am J Cardiol 1987;59:596–600. With permission from Excerpta Medica, Inc.

cranial pressure is controlled, the frequency decreases to a less frequent (although not always baseline) state for several days. If intracranial pressure is not controlled, the VPDs become more frequent and can lead to more serious arrhythmias.

Pharmacologic treatment of VPDs is seldomly warranted if increased intracranial pressure can be managed promptly. The appearance of couplets and triplets makes close monitoring essential because they may predict subsequent ventricular tachycardia. In cases in which intracranial pressure cannot be managed quickly, intravenous lidocaine is the drug of choice in the acute setting. Other agents that can be tried include procainamide, beta blockers, and amiodarone (a class 1C antiarrhythmic). Special care needs to be taken in treatment decisions for patients with increased frequency of premature contractions. Because of the large comorbidity of heart disease in many of these patients, it is imperative that cardiac causes of abnormal conduction be investigated. Unfortunately, there are no characteristics of premature complexes due to cardiac disease that help differentiate them from those caused by neurologic injury.

Ventricular tachycardia and atrial fibrillation are the most common serious arrhythmias found in this setting (Fig. 3–2). The definition of ventricular tachycardia is more than three VPDs in a row. A distinction is made by most authors between nonsustained and sustained ventricular tachycardia. The amount of depolarizations or time necessary to delineate one from the other is a question of semantics. The longer the abnormal ventricular focus is the dominant rhythm, the more likely the patient will experience hypotension or have the rhythm degenerate to ventricular fibrillation. Ventricular fibrillation is disorganized ventricular activity that in itself always causes hypotension and also can lead to asystole (lack of ventricular electrical and mechanical activity).

The diagnosis of ventricular tachycardia can be confused with other types of arrhythmias, especially atrial fibrillation with aberrant conduction of atrial impulses through an accessory conduction pathway. The distinction is important from a pharmacologic standpoint. The points that distinguish the two are (1) atrial fibrillation will most always be irregular in rhythm, whereas ventricular tachycardia is oftentimes regular; and (2) ventricular tachycardia usually has some evolution from a low frequency to a higher frequency and, although atrial fibrillation can do this, it is less common.

The treatment of ventricular tachycardia is dependent on the duration of the arrhythmia and the stability of the patient. Nonsustained rhythms often need not be treated, while sustained ventricular arrhythmias are always treated. The decision to use DC electrocardioversion versus pharmacologic treatment is based on the stability of the patient. If there is significant hypotension or if the patient has angina or loses consciousness, DC cardioversion is preferred for its speed. If the patient is stable, pharmacologic treatment is preferred. Lidocaine and procainamide are the first-line drugs used in most acute care settings. An initial dose of each with continuation of the agent that works best is standard practice. Quinine can be tried if the other two agents are unsuccessful. Usually, it is recommended that failure of lidocaine and procainamide lead to electrical cardioversion. Very low doses of DC electricity are oftentimes successful in converting the aberrant rhythm back to a sinus rhythm. Sequentially increasing settings of DC electricity are used until the rhythm is converted to another rhythm.

Torsades de pointes is a special case of ventricular tachycardia that is very refractory to treatment. The arrhythmia is multifocal ventricular tachycardia characterized by waves of changing amplitude that form a sinusoidal pattern around the isoelectric baseline. Torsades de pointes is thought to be precipitated by prolongation of the QT interval. In this syndrome, the T wave from the previous ventricular depolarization is superimposed on the Q wave of the subsequent ventricular complex. In animal studies, it has been shown that acute brain injury and increased intracranial pressure can cause prolongation of the QT interval.

Treatment of torsades de pointes is very difficult. Since deficits of magnesium can cause the torsades de pointes, infusion of magnesium sulfate has been tried to stop the arrhythmia. Other causes of torsades de pointes include medications such as amiodarone and quinidine. If such medicines are being used at the time of the arrhythmia, they should be stopped. Class 1B antiarrhythmic agents such as lidocaine and phenytoin can also be tried. Other classes of antiarrhythmics have little effect usually.

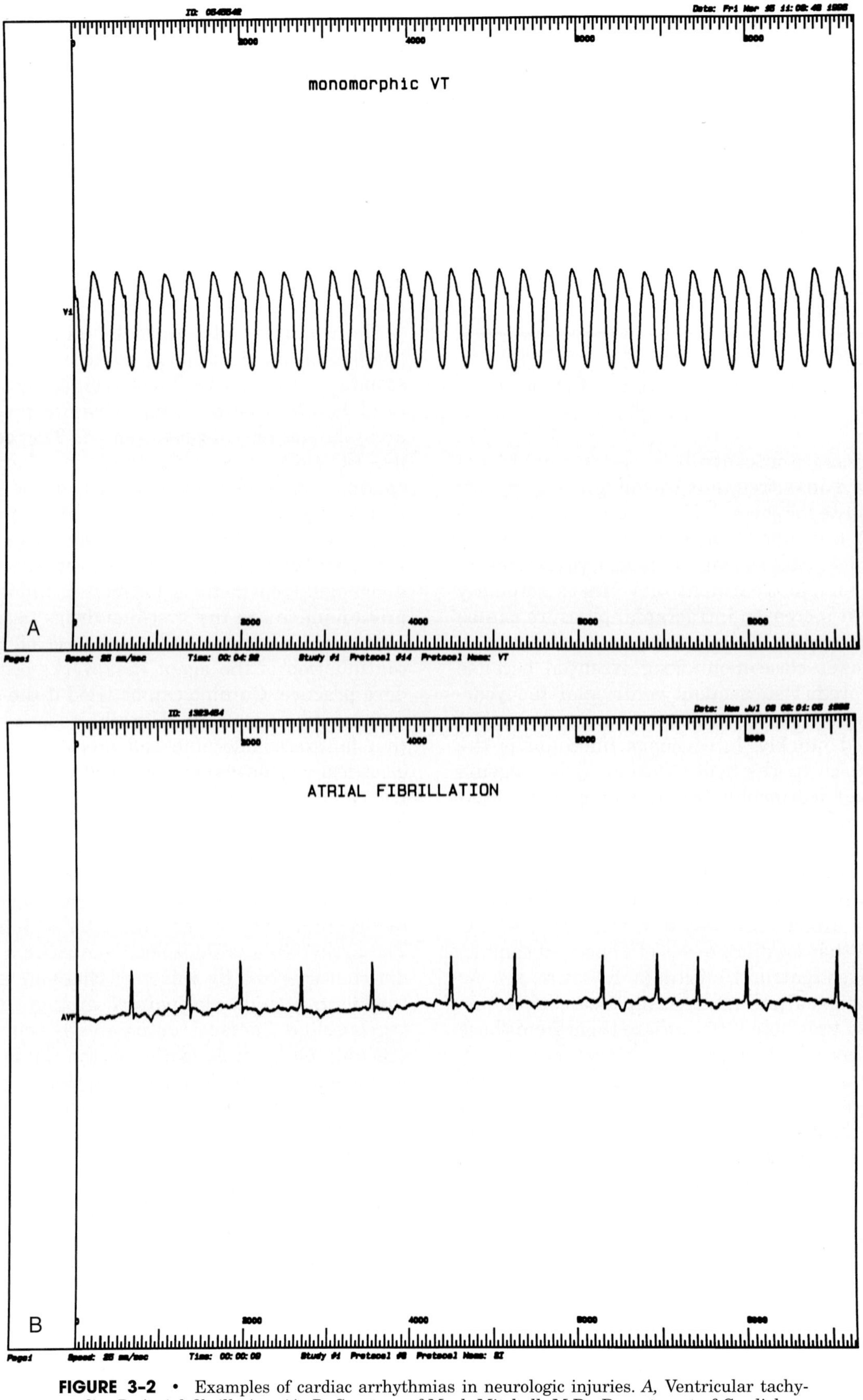

FIGURE 3–2 • Examples of cardiac arrhythmias in neurologic injuries. *A,* Ventricular tachycardia. *B,* Atrial fibrillation. (*A, B,* Courtesy of Mark Mitchell, M.D., Department of Cardiology, University of Virginia.)

Temporary pacing has also been successful in controlling the arrhythmia.

Supraventricular arrhythmias are seen less commonly in the setting of acute neurologic injury. Atrial fibrillation, which is the most common, when seen in acute stroke, must be considered as an etiology as well as a consequence. It is characterized by dyssynchronous electrical activity in the atrial conduction system that leads to fibrillation of the atria. On standard ECG, there is a typical irregularly irregular rhythm. Conduction to the ventricle can be through the atrioventricular (AV) node or through accessory pathways. If the conduction is not through the AV node, wide ventricular complexes can be seen, which can be confused with ventricular tachycardia. Atrial flutter is characterized by rapid rate of atrial electrical activity that can exceed the limitations of the refractory period of AV node and cause intermittent blocking of conduction to the ventricles. The typical ECG pattern is multiple, saw-toothed P waves interposed between normal QRS complexes that are triggered by the preceding p wave. Other supraventricular arrhythmias are seen less frequently in acute neurologic events and will not be addressed here.

Atrial fibrillation is oftentimes seen concurrently with neurologic injury. Clot formation and embolization in atrial fibrillation are a common cause of stroke. In other brain injuries such as SAH and traumatic injury, atrial fibrillation occurs more frequently than in non–brain-injured patients. It has not been conclusively shown that sympathetic mechanisms are directly responsible. Decreased myocardial contractility can increase pressure in the right atrium and cause distention of the atrial wall (a phenomenon known to precipitate atrial fibrillation).

Treatment of atrial fibrillation hinges on the duration of the rhythm. If the rhythm can reliably be determined to be new (<2 days) in a stable patient, pharmacologic therapy with procainamide is appropriate. If the patient becomes unstable or the pharmacologic treatment fails, electrical cardioversion with low-power synchronous DC shock is preferred. This often does not need to be administered on an emergent basis.

In patients who become hypotensive or experience heart failure or angina, electrical cardioversion is mandatory treatment. On the other hand, if it cannot be determined that the onset of atrial fibrillation is within 2 days and the patient remains stable, a course of warfarin anticoagulation for a period of 6 weeks to 2 months is recommended prior to electrical or mechanical cardioversion to allow time for possible atrial clots to dissolve.[21]

CARDIAC ISCHEMIC CHANGES

ECG changes after acute neurologic injuries were one of the earliest cardiovascular manifestations noted in the scientific literature. As early as the 1940s and 1950s, there were reports of peaked T waves and depression of ST segments on ECG (Fig. 3–3). Burch et al.[22] popularized the term "cerebral T waves" from his study of patients with SAH. In 1960, Cropp and Manning[23] described a series of patients with SAH who had ECG findings of myocardial ischemia. In their series of 15 patients, four died and were reported to have normal-appearing hearts both grossly and microscopically. Later autopsy studies using more sensitive techniques showed evidence of subendocardial ischemia in patients who had ECG changes.[24]

The incidence of ECG changes of ischemia in patients with brain insults is not known. In studies conducted exclusively on SAH patients, the incidence ranges from 50% to 90%.[23] The most frequent finding is of peaked T waves followed by ST depression then ST elevation. The mortality of patients who exhibit these changes has been found to be higher than in patients who do not.[25]

Since the early studies that failed to show changes microscopically in hearts of patients with ECG abnormalities, there have been considerable

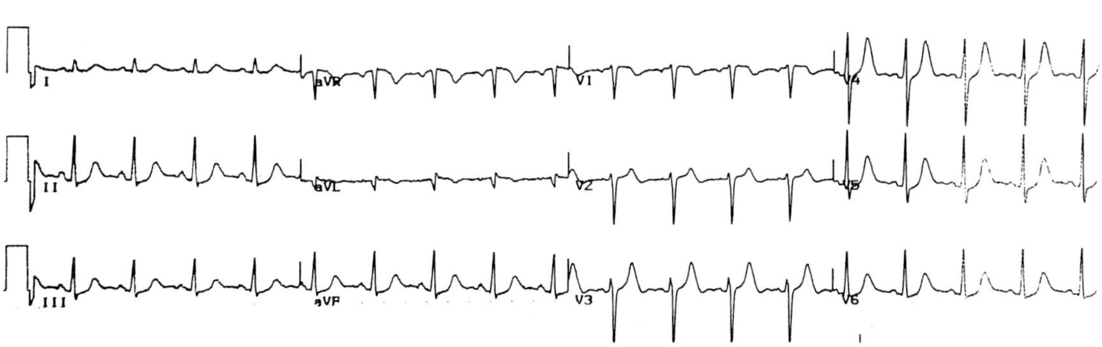

FIGURE 3–3 • Example of cerebral T waves in a 47-year-old woman who presented with subarachnoid hemorrhage. Twenty-six hours after onset of symptoms, high-peaked T waves are seen with mild ST depression in leads aVF and V_5.

advances that now make it possible to see specific changes in the myocardium that are thought to be due to release of catecholamines. Hearts of affected patients exhibit *contraction band necrosis,* a nonischemic lesion of individual myofibrils (Fig. 3–4). This has also been seen in the setting of pheochromocytoma with elevated levels of circulating catecholamines. In the most severe cases, patients can exhibit hypokinesia of the anterior wall of the heart and decreased ejection fraction of blood as seen by echocardiogram.

Chemical testing of patients with ECG abnormalities shows increased levels of creatine kinase MB fraction in most patients. Levels of the MB fraction are similar to the levels seen in acute myocardial infarctions. The BB fraction (the isozyme of creatine kinase that is found mostly in the brain) can also be elevated, which is likely due to injury to the brain. Lactate dehydrogenase levels and serum glutamic-oxaloacetic transaminase (SGOT) levels increase in a time frame compatible with acute myocardial infarction. To date, there have been no novel elevations of testable blood chemistries that reliably detect myocardial contraction band necrosis.

Experimental models in animals have successfully induced contraction band necrosis with infusion of supraphysiologic doses of catecholamines. In these studies, animals exhibited changes in ECG similar to those of humans and had elevated levels of myocardial enzymes. Infusion of beta blockers and other sympatholytics have been shown to block these changes.[26] No studies have been conducted in humans that investigate the survival of patients after beta-blocker therapy.

Treatment

The treatment of patients with ECG changes after neurologic injury is complicated. The mortality of patients with ECG abnormalities (ischemic changes and arrhythmias) is higher than that of patients who do not exibit changes. No studies have looked at whether patients with ischemic ECG changes in neurologic injuries suffer long-term cardiac sequelae. The most effective treatment to correct ECG changes is to correct the neurologic injury. Some researchers have proposed treatment with beta blockers to make the heart less sensitive to catecholamine surges.[26] Since the mortality in patients with ECG changes is higher than in other patients, there is a great interest in finding new treatments.

With injuries such as SAH and acute stroke, there is a large comorbidity with ischemic heart disease; in fact, in stroke, myocardial ischemia can be the primary pathology. It is difficult at times to decide whether to treat the changes as true myocardial ischemia or the sequelae of the neurologic injury. The pathological basis for ECG changes in contraction band necrosis and atherosclerotic heart disease is ischemia of the heart muscle. It is therefore impossible to differentiate between the two entities on the basis of ECG.

The most prudent course of action in patients who present with injuries to the brain and ECG changes is to look closely at the patient's medical history, family history, risk factors for myocardial ischemic disease, and the clinical situation. Given these factors, one can decide whether it is more likely that the changes represent the neurologic injury or true ischemic heart disease. If the patient has appropriate risk factors and the clinical situation is plausible for acute myocardial ischemia, the patient should be treated with standard therapy for acute myocardial infarction. If the situation is not suggestive of acute myocardial infarction, a course of beta blockers may be tried but the strategy should be one of watchful waiting. If myocardial compromise is apparent, Swan-Ganz catheterization and echocardiogram may be helpful in acutely managing the patient. In some cases, cardiac angiography may be necessary to differentiate true atherosclerotic myocardial damage and catecholamine-induced contraction band necrosis.

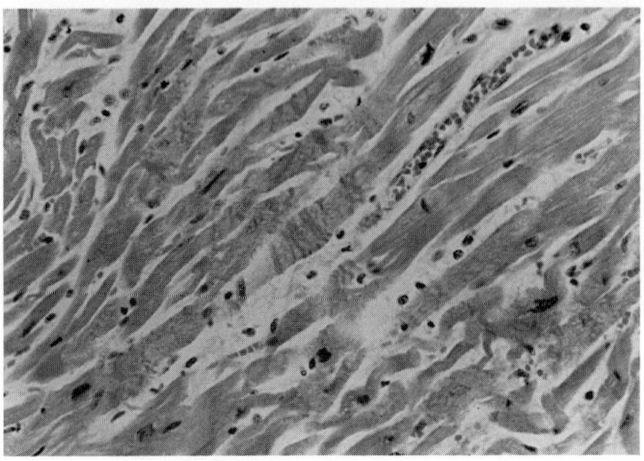

FIGURE 3–4 • Photomicrograph of contraction band necrosis of the heart. The banded pattern of the muscle fibers and fiber necrosis is seen. (Courtesy of William Glass, M.D., Ph.D., Department of Pathology, University of Virginia.)

NEUROGENIC PULMONARY EDEMA

Neurogenic pulmonary edema (NPE) is a phenomenon of pulmonary edema after neurologic insult that seems likely to be caused directly by the injury to the brain and not by a secondary route from cardiac or blood pressure changes discussed above. The phenomenon has been reported for many years, although skepticism about the primary neurologic mechanism has been prominent until recently. Animal studies have shown that both the onset time and chemical composition of the pleural exudate make it less likely to be a strictly cardiac and hypertensive entity.[27]

The classic description of NPE is a rapidly occurring pulmonary edema that has been noted to occur after SAH, brain trauma, seizure, stroke, and other insults to the nervous system. Although work has attempted to determine which patients are at risk for developing NPE, it is still unclear why this rare phenomenon occurs. In animal studies, it has been shown that the exudated fluid from NPE is higher in protein than pulmonary exudates that are seen in left-sided heart failure and hypertension.[28] This has led to questions about the mechanism of fluid extravasation.

In the normal functioning lung, fluid balance is sustained by the interplay between interstitial fluid oncotic pressure and interstitial fluid hydrostatic pressure with the vascular fluid oncotic pressure and the vascular fluid hydrostatic pressure (Fig. 3–5). This relationship is made possible by tight junctions between the endothelial cells that do not allow large fluxes of fluid in any direction. In the case of left-sided heart failure, the vascular fluid hydrostatic pressure increases as a result of poor forward flow of blood out of the left ventricle. This shifts the balance of fluids, causing fluid to extravasate out of the blood vessels and into the lung interstitium. In low-protein states such as malnutrition (another cause of pulmonary edema), the interstitial fluid oncotic pressure decreases, causing fluid to extravasate out of the blood vessels and into the interstitium of the lung. In cases of lung infection or chemical irritation, the tight junctions that separate the interstitium from the vessel lumens are damaged, allowing fluid and protein to extravasate out into the interstitial space.

In the case of NPE, the extravasation of fluid occurs quickly, causing "flash pulmonary edema." In animal studies, it has been shown that the protein content of the fluid is higher than what would be expected in simple extravasation of fluid across the basal membrane. This implies that the tight junction mechanism is compromised during this process.[27]

Mechanism

The innervation of the lungs is from the sympathetic and parasympathetic nervous systems. The parasympathetic innervation is supplied by the vagus nerve; the sympathetic innervation is supplied by nerves that exit the spinal cord in the thoracic area. There is clear evidence that both systems act on the vascular smooth muscles in the lung to dilate and constrict them. There is also good evidence that the sympathetic system acts on the respiratory smooth muscles to constrict and dilate the respiratory bronchioles. Clinical evidence that NPE is autonomically mediated comes largely from the fact that patients who have complete cervical spinal cord interruption are protected from the phenomenon.

The reasonable theory of the autonomic influence is that the autonomic system causes a compromise of the tight junction endothelial lining of the vascular-interstitial interface that allows the extravasation of proteinaceous fluid into the interstitium. This does not preclude the possibility that the cardiac and hypertensive effects discussed above are partially responsible for the fluid component of the interstitial fluid.

Treatment

The treatment of NPE is largely symptomatic. Despite the fact that the fluid is different in composi-

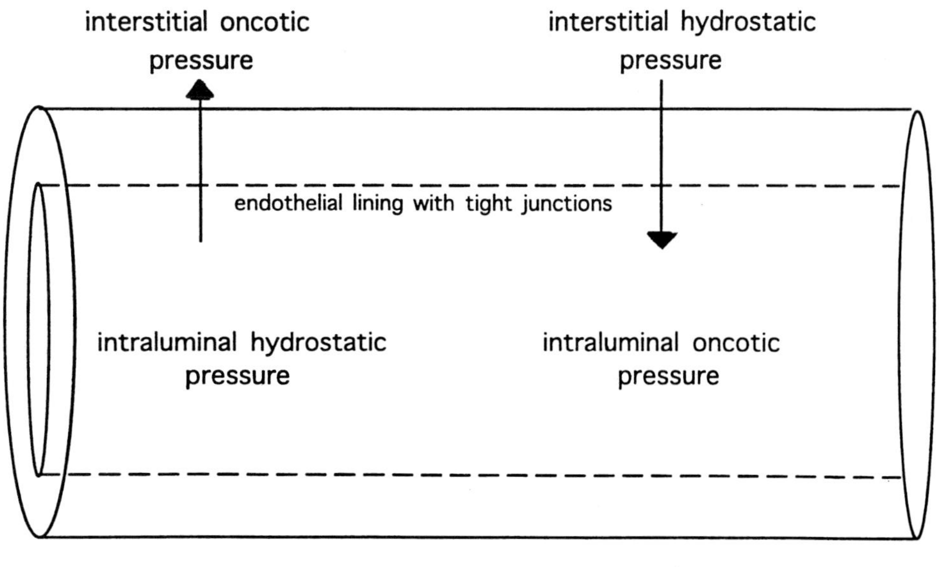

FIGURE 3–5 • Forces acting on diffusion of fluid from intravascular space to interstitial space and vice versa. Due to the capillary endothelium tight junctions, protein molecules do not pass readily from one compartment to the other.

tion than that of cardiogenic pulmonary edema, the initial treatment strategy is the same. The two hallmarks of treatment are to decrease interstitial fluid and maximize oxygenation. Increased fluid in the lungs will cause decreased oxygen transport, which can be treated with supplemental oxygen. This can be done with nasal prong/facemask oxygen if the patient is spontaneously breathing or by increased fraction of inspired oxygen on ventilator settings if the patient is intubated.

The removal of fluid from the lungs is difficult in the clinical setting of acute neurologic injury. In cases in which increased intracranial pressure is a concern or where cerebral perfusion pressure may be compromised, treatment with diuretics can be detrimental to the patient. Judicious use of loop diuretics is the treatment of choice for decreasing interstitial fluid with close monitoring of the cerebral perfusion pressure. Some investigators have recommended the use of albumin and other oncotic agents to help increase the vascular fluid oncotic pressure. This strategy only transiently increases the vascular fluid oncotic pressure and may actually allow increased available protein to extravasate into the lung interstitium causing a larger shift of fluid into the interstitium. Some researchers have also recommended surgical techniques for decreasing intracranial pressure such as decompressive craniotomy or ventriculostomy. Although these procedures make the management of the pulmonary edema easier, it is unclear whether the risk of a surgical procedure in someone with compromised oxygenation outweighs the benefit of simplifying the management of pulmonary edema. This may be an optimal choice in selected patients but will probably never be considered a universal treatment.

The use of morphine to decrease sympathetic vasoconstriction and reduce anxiety is the mainstay of treatment for acute cardiogenic pulmonary edema. The pitfall of this therapy for neurologic patients is that obtundation due to morphine can compromise the ability to follow the neurologic examination. Theophylline has been used in some cases to increase renal blood flow and to dilate the bronchioles, thus making oxygenation easier. Its usefulness in cardiogenic pulmonary edema has been questioned, but it is untested in neurologic injuries.

Although the treatment of pulmonary edema is more complicated in patients with neurologic diseases, treatment strategies should be based on assessment of the whole patient and prioritization of needs. If the patient is at risk from pulmonary edema, all of the therapies above must be used regardless of the effect on the cerebral perfusion pressure. If pulmonary edema is manageable with increased oxygen therapy and judicious use of diuretics, considerations of cerebral perfusion pressure and increased intracranial pressure should dominate.

Early intubation of the patient with NPE is recommended. This is the best way to ensure adequate oxygenation of the brain and will allow for the control of increased intracranial pressure. It may also be preferable to paralyze the patient after intubation. Although this compromises the ability to follow the neurologic examination, it will reduce the systemic oxygen demand allowing more available oxygen to the brain. Ventilation is made easier by decreasing intercostal muscle tone and thereby increasing compliance. Patients who are paralyzed should have paralytics reversed periodically to evaluate neurologic status. In patients whose intracranial pressure is a concern, monitoring is advisable to detect sudden increases in intracranial pressure, which could signal a cerebral bleed or herniation.

SHOCK

In neurologic circles, the term "shock" is used in two different ways. The term "neurogenic shock" is used to signify systemic hypotension causing hypoperfusion of vital organs due to neurologic disease. The term "spinal shock" is used to signify the state of depressed upper motor neuron findings in patients with damage to the corticospinal tracts acutely after injury. Here we will address only neurogenic shock.

Arterial blood pressure is maintained by the combination of cardiac output and systemic vascular resistance. Cardiac output depends in turn on stroke volume of the cardiac ventricles and heart rate:

$$\text{Cardiac output} = \text{stroke volume} \times \text{heart rate}$$

Systemic vascular resistance is directly dependent on the viscosity of the blood and the vessel length and inversely proportional to the fourth power of the luminal diameter of the vessels. The neural control of these processes is mediated through the sympathetic and parasympathetic nervous systems. The sympathetic system is responsible for the vascular tone in the arterial system. In addition, the sympathetic endocrine system of epinephrine and norepinephrine affects the rate of the myocardial pacemakers.

Release of sympathetic mediators causes the heart rate to increase. With the absence of these mediators at baseline levels, the heart rate decreases to the intrinsic rate of the cardiac pacemaker. The parasympathetic system, when activated, can slow the heart rate by direct effect of the vagus nerve on the cardiac pacemaker. The parasympathetic system, when activated, causes dilation of the venous system, which leads to pooling of blood in the venules, decreasing cardiac preload.

Diseases of the brain can acutely change systemic vascular resistance, heart rate, and heart contractility. Spinal cord injuries are the most common cause of neurogenic shock. The sympathetic fibers that exit the thoracic spinal cord are responsible for the sympathetic tone of the blood vessels, especially the arterioles of the systemic circulation. Because the most important variable in the equation of systemic vascular resistance is the luminal diameter, small changes in the sympathetic tone of the smooth muscles in the walls of the arterioles can make large differences in the systemic vascular resistance. Injuries to the sympathetic fibers that innervate these arteriolar walls can lead to profound hypotension. The lack of chronotropic effect of sympathetic innervation to the heart causes the heart rate to fall to the baseline rate of the pacemaker cells. What is seen clinically is a patient with profound hypotension and bradycardia. On electrophysiologic monitoring, one sees a moderate bradycardia that may be accompanied by multiple VPDs.

The other mechanisms that can cause shock due to neurologic disease include herniation involving the brain stem. When intracranial pressure increases and causes herniation, it initially causes increased blood pressure (Cushing's response), but later, as the sympathetic fibers become interrupted, hypotension ensues. Autonomic seizures have been reported to cause hypotension, although shock has not been reported. Finally, the consequences of neurodegenerative diseases can exaggerate hypotension in the face of a systemic insult. In patients with Shy-Drager syndrome, advanced Parkinson's disease, and other neurodegenerative disorders, bacterial infections can cause hypoperfusion of vital organs more quickly due to decreased autonomic reserve.

Treatment

Hypotension in patients with shock due to spinal cord lesions responds well to the addition of sympathomimetic agents. Patients are often very sensitive to very low doses of dopamine intravenously. Dopamine increases the heart rate and contributes to vascular tone (of note, in these patients, dopamine can cause increase in arrhythmias). Other important therapies include lower extremity compression to prevent vascular pooling and supine positioning of the patient to decrease the effect of gravity. Eventually, despite lack of sympathetic outflow, patients develop some self-regulation of systemic vascular resistance. Eventually, they become independent of dopamine and with only lower extremity compression they can sit up. Throughout the acute phase of injury, they continue to have periods of hypotension that are thought to be due to arrhythmias.

CONCLUSION

Neurologic diseases can have profound effects on the cardiovascular system. Unfortunately, there are very little data about the morbidity and mortality of these complications. Although it may simply be that patients with more severe neurologic disease are more prone to cardiovascular insults, it seems unlikely. Questions remain about the mechanism of injury to the heart and vasculature. A great deal of work is left to understand the mechanism by which the brain brings about cardiac, pulmonary, and vascular changes. Work is currently being performed on elucidating the mechanism of injury and finding effective therapies. Sympatholytic medication has been proposed as a possible therapy, as have free radical scavengers.[12] Studies and clinical trials are ongoing, but much work is necessary before these or any other therapies are approved for use as treatment.

References

1. Dimant J, Grob D: Electrocardiographic changes and myocardial damage in patients with acute cerebrovascular accidents. Stroke 1997;8:448–455.
2. Dittmar C: Ein Neuer beweis fur die reizbarkeit der centripetalen fesern des rickemmarks. Ber sachs ges (akad) wiss 1870;22:18–48.
3. Alexander R: The effects of blood flow and anoxia on spinal cardiovascular centers. Am J Physiol 1945;143:698–708.
4. Bard P: Anatomical organization of the central nervous system in relation to control of the heart and blood vessels. Physiol Rev 1960;40(Suppl 4):3–26.
5. Wallace J, Levy L: Blood pressure after stroke. JAMA 1981;246:2177–2180.
6. Doba N, Reis D: Acute fulminating neurogenic hypertension produced by brain stem lesions in the rat. Circ Res 1981;32:584–593.
7. Blessing W, West M, Chalmers J: Hypertension, bradycardia, and pulmonary edema in the conscious rabbit after brain stem lesions coinciding with the A1 group of catecholamine neurons. Circ Res 1981;49:949–958.
8. Oppenheimer S: Neurologic cardiac effects of cerebrovascular disease. Curr Opin Neurol 1994;7:20–24.
9. Aschenbrenner R, Bodechtel G: Uber EKG-veranderungen bei hirntumorkranken. Clin Wochenschr 1938;17:298–302.
10. Satinsky J, Kosowsky B, Lown B: Ventricular fibrillation induced by hypothalamic stimulation during coronary occlusion (abstract). Circulation 1971;44(Suppl II):60.
11. Beard E, Robertson J, Robertson R: Spontaneous subarachnoid hemorrhage simulating acute myocardial infarction. Am Heart J 1951;58:755–759.
12. Samuels MA: Cardiopulmonary aspects of acute neurologic diseases. In Ropper AH (ed): Neurologic and Neurosurgical Intensive Care, 3rd ed, pp 103–119. New York, Raven Press, 1993.
13. Samuels MA: Neurogenic heart disease: A unifying hypothesis. Am J Cardiol 1987;60:15J–19J.
14. Adams H, Brott T, Crowell R, et al: Guidelines for the management of patients with acute ischemic stroke. Stroke 1994;25:1901–1914.

ated along the axon. Approximately 1 msec after the action potential generation, Na^+ channels close and prohibit further entry of Na^+. As Na^+ channels are inactivated, K^+ channels open to permit K^+ to rapidly exit the intracellular space. The K^+ efflux and coincident Cl^- influx result in membrane hyperpolarization and the termination of electrical activity at that point along the cell membrane.[5]

As the action potential reaches the axon terminal, voltage-dependent Ca^{++} channels open, permitting entry of Ca^{++} ions into the terminal. The subsequent influx of Ca^{++} ions into the presynaptic terminal triggers a chain of molecular events that results in neurotransmitter release. The maintenance of membrane potential and transient changes in ion flux that culminate in the generation of an action potential is entirely dependent on the tight regulation of ion permeability into neurons. Thus, changes or abnormalities at any point along this electrical cascade could have a dramatic impact on the excitability and epileptogenicity of individual neurons.[6]

Because virtually all neurons have the ability to fire in a rapid, repetitive fashion, it is clear that generating a recurrent cycle of membrane depolarizations and action potentials may be critical in the initiation and propagation of an ictal discharge. Furthermore, many neocortical and hippocampal neurons normally exhibit intrinsic bursting activity in which populations of cells fire in a rhythmic, repetitive manner.[7] This property may be dependent on a complex array of ionic conductances that operate in addition to those that regulate action potential generation. Specifically, high-threshold inward Ca^{++} currents; low-threshold, slowly inactivating Na^+ and Ca^{++} currents; a hyperpolarization associated with low-threshold Ca^{++} current; and several K^+ currents with distinct activation thresholds contribute to burst firing in intrinsically rhythmic neurons in neocortex and hippocampus.[4] Moreover, many cells with the ability to fire rapid action potential bursts require a depolarizing Ca^{++}-dependent after-potential to sustain repetitive volleys of action potentials.[8]

The effects of neuronal activity are mediated via synaptic connections between neocortical, thalamocortical, and corticothalamic projections. Excitatory impulse volleys pass continuously between the thalamus and cortex, with each subset of neurons entraining their efferent targets. Impulses culminate in either excitatory, depolarizing postsynaptic potentials (EPSPs) or hyperpolarizing inhibitory postsynaptic potentials (IPSPs). Excitatory inputs are mediated primarily by neurotransmitters such as glutamate and aspartate (see below), while inhibitory inputs are transmitted via gamma-aminobutyric acid (GABA, see below). Other neurotransmitters and neuromodulators such as acetylcholine, norepinephrine, serotonin, and neuropeptides also contribute to excitatory and inhibitory synaptic connectivity.

Seizure propagation may be especially likely in cells with intrinsic bursting abilities if the balance between excessive excitatory or inadequate inhibitory inputs is altered. In the absence of appropriate inhibitory regulation (loss of IPSPs), populations of neurons may begin to fire synchronously leading to a seizure. Indeed, in the many clinical settings in which refractory seizures may develop, it is likely that both local and widespread disruption of ionic conductances and regulation of ionic concentrations result in ictal discharges. It is quite plausible, for example, that in epileptogenic regions of cortex adjacent to brain tumors or within ischemically injured brain tissue, K^+ or Ca^{++} metabolism is altered, so that appropriate hyperpolarization and cessation of nerve impulses are diminished. This would result in impaired ability to terminate overactive spontaneous bursting (Fig. 4–1).

Neurochemistry

Because the action potentials described above are the result of the action of neurotransmitters released by presynaptic terminals on postsynaptic receptors, an understanding of the basic pharmacology of these neurotransmitters and receptors is essential groundwork for establishing a rational basis on the use of anticonvulsants in SE.

Several neurotransmitters have been implicated in the generation of seizures. Gamma-aminobutyric acid (GABA) is likely a critical inhibitory modulator of neuronal activity in the brain.[9] GABAergic neurons are primarily smooth, sparsely spinous interneurons in cortex and may be identified by their immunoreactivity for glutamic acid decarboxylase (GAD), the primary synthetic enzyme for GABA. In the hippocampus, GABAergic cells are mostly basket cells within the dentate gyrus, which synapse with the pyramidal neurons. GABA mediates synaptic inhibition in the hippocampus by generation of IPSPs, which counterbalance excitatory inputs from other brain regions. Of the two primary GABA receptor subtypes—GABA A and GABA B—the GABA A receptor is believed to be more intimately involved in the neurochemical features of epilepsy. The GABA A receptor is believed to be a pentameric complex composed of two alpha, two beta, and one gamma subunit, which organize as a holoprotein to form a chloride channel through which chloride ions can flow into the postsynaptic region.[10]

When GABA binds to the GABA A–chloride channel complex, there is an influx of chloride ions through the chloride channel, which results in an inhibitory postsynaptic potential and, hence, hyper-

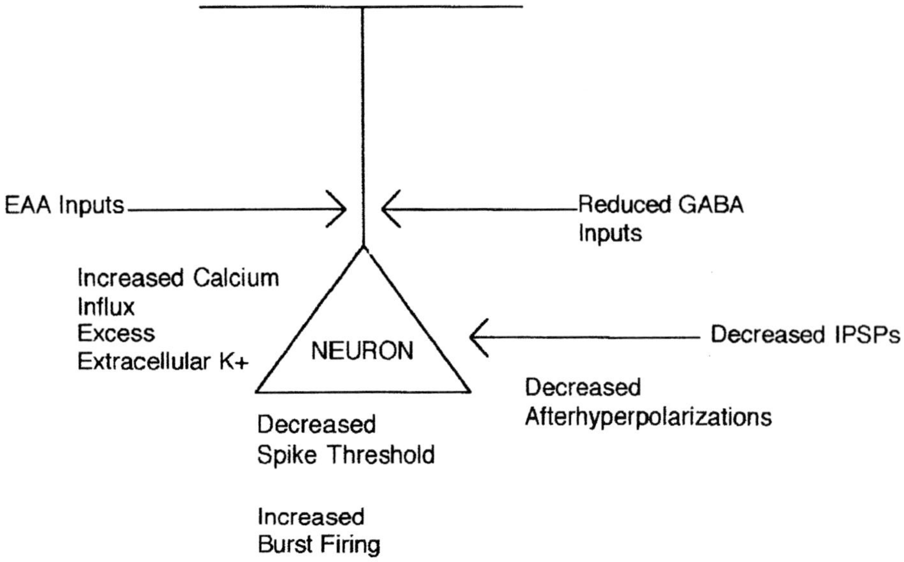

FIGURE 4–1 • Basic neurophysiologic factors that may contribute to status epilepticus (see text).

polarization (inhibition) of postsynaptic neurons. Two classes of anticonvulsant compounds—benzodiazepines and barbiturates—are modulators of GABA neurotransmission and are believed to act by binding directly to a site on the GABA A receptor–chloride channel complex, thereby facilitating chloride entrance into the cell. Thus, by increasing the generation of IPSPs and maintaining a hyperpolarized state, these drugs may inhibit seizure initiation and propagation.

A large body of evidence suggests that disruption of GABAergic function may be central to the molecular pathophysiology of epilepsy.[2] Interruption of integrated GABA-mediated inhibition in cortex could compromise a primary mechanism for inhibition of neuronal firing and, theoretically, result in a lowered threshold for ictal discharges. Evidence for this mechanism comes from animal models, which show that GABA A antagonists may provoke seizures, while GABA agonists (such as benzodiazepines) prevent seizures. Similarly, compounds that raise endogenous levels of GABA tend to have anticonvulsant properties, while those that inhibit GABA synthesis can cause seizures. Finally, in the face of recurrent rapid experimental electrical stimulation, many cortical GABAergic synapses exhibit tetanic and post-tetanic depression.[11] This results in impaired inhibitory synaptic transmission during rapid repetitive firing, similar to what occurs during seizures. Thus, the protective inhibitory role of GABA may be lost during prolonged seizures and may contribute to the pathogenesis of SE.

In contrast to GABA, glutamate is the primary excitatory amino acid (EAA) neurotransmitter used in the brain, particularly by corticocortical, corticofugal, and commissural projection neurons. Glutamate and aspartate, other putative EAA transmitters, act by binding to a variety of EAA receptors. These receptors may be broadly subdivided into metabotropic and ionotropic classes, based on their pharmacologic and molecular biologic properties.[12] The ionotropic receptors are postsynaptic cation permeable channels and include the AMPA (amino-3-hydroxy-5-methyl-4-isoxazole-propionate), NMDA (*N*-methyl-D-aspartate), and kainic acid–binding sites. The metabotropic receptors may be located pre- or postsynaptically and act via second-messenger systems such as inositol triphosphate and adenylate cyclase. Both receptor subtypes have been identified on glia as well as neurons and exhibit a heterogeneous though ubiquitous pattern of distribution in various brain regions.

Virtually all neurons express some type of glutamate receptor. The actions of glutamate are terminated when glutamate is removed from synapses by a sodium-dependent glutamate uptake site on neurons and glia. Thus, the effects of glutamate on neurons are likely to be widespread and ideally suited to propagate excitatory neuronal activity over large regions of cortex. While normal functioning of the EAA system is essential to processes such as learning and memory, overactivity of the EAA pathways in the brain can lead to neuronal damage and death. EAA agonist compounds such as kainic acid induce profound regional neuronal death when injected into neocortex and hippocampus,[13] which is similar to that observed following prolonged seizures.[14] Furthermore, recurrent seizures frequently resulted from kainic acid injection.

It is widely believed that the neurotoxic effects of EAA compounds stem, in part, from alterations in Ca^{++} permeability through EAA receptor channel complexes, which results in an increase in intracellular Ca^{++} levels.[15] Dramatic changes in Ca^{++} concentrations may induce a cascade of Ca^{++}-dependent intracellular events, such as activation of proteases and lipases, influx of other cations such as Na^{+}, and osmotic swelling of neurons that culminates in cell death. Under circumstances in which repetitive EAA neurotransmission is in effect, such as in prolonged seizures, these cellular pathways are almost certainly induced.

The role of EAA in epilepsy is being more fully defined, although clearly, glutamate and aspartate contribute to the initiation, spread, and maintenance of epileptic activity in cortex.[3] Furthermore, glutamate antagonists can attenuate the spread of seizure activity. In animal models of epilepsy, such as the EL (epilepsy-like) strain, release of glutamate in response to calcium influx is enhanced. In kindling, an experimental model of epileptogenesis, there is increased release of EAA transmitters and alterations in AMPA and NMDA receptor populations.[16] Similarly, activation of excitatory amino acid receptors may also be involved because antagonists block high K^{+}-induced seizures.

EAA antagonists can attenuate or suppress the kindling process. Indeed, in general, EAA antagonist compounds function as anticonvulsants while EAA agonists serve as proconvulsants. In human epilepsy patients, increased levels of EAA compounds such as aspartate have been identified using microdialysis catheters immediately prior to the onset of seizure activity.[17] Similarly, increased numbers of NMDA and kainate receptor levels have been identified autoradiographically in resected temporal lobe specimens from patients with refractory complex seizures.[18] Increased numbers of AMPA and kainate receptors have also been identified in the dentate gyrus as well. It remains to be shown whether EAA compounds such as glutamate play a central role in the pathogenesis of epilepsy. If so, excessive EAA activity during seizures could account for some of the neuropathologic changes observed following prolonged ictal discharges such as SE.

One interesting study demonstrated that an increased level of mRNA for the connexin family of proteins is elevated in patients with refractory epilepsy.[19] These proteins combine as oligomers to form gap junctions between neurons. The latter would allow electrotonic—i.e., nonsynaptic—coupling between neurons and facilitate rapid simultaneous changes in ions, such as calcium, in large numbers of neurons at once. If electrotonic coupling between neurons is enhanced in patients with epilepsy, this would provide a novel mechanism through which synchronization of depolarizing or hyperpolarizing ion fluxes could occur simultaneously in many cells, and thus facilitate the spread of an ictal discharge.

At the cellular and molecular biologic levels, several changes have been observed that reflect dynamic alterations in the phenotype of neurons in response to seizures.[20] In addition to classic neurotransmitters such as GABA and glutamate, neuropeptides such as neuropeptide Y (NPY), somatostatin, enkephalins, and cholecystokinin (CCK) may be affected by prolonged seizures in experimental models of epilepsy. For example, seizures induced by ablation of the dentate gyrus within the hippocampus or by intracerebroventricular injection of kainic acid alter the expression of dynorphin, preproenkephalin, enkephalin, CCK, and NPY within hippocampal neurons.

Furthermore, changes in the levels of mRNA that encode these compounds, or the synthetic enzymes necessary for their generation, may also be noted using in situ hybridization. Alterations in mRNA suggest that prolonged seizures may induce changes in gene expression within individual populations of neurons. Most recently, it has been shown that the expression of certain immediate early genes including the proto-oncogenes *c-fos* and *c-jun*[21] may be altered by seizures. These transcription factors are critical messages within cells, which are necessary for gene expression, and thus serve as on-off switches. The latter regulate which genes are transcribed in response to a variety of stimuli.

Perhaps most interesting has been the demonstration that growth factors, including nerve growth factor (NGF), brain-derived neurotrophic factor (BDNF), and neurotrophin-3 (NT-3), may also be affected by seizures within the hippocampus.[21–23] These compounds play a central role in the maintenance and possible outgrowth of neurons. Thus, increased levels of growth factor mRNA following several seizure paradigms suggest that some of the pathologic changes, including mossy fiber sprouting within the dentate gyrus following prolonged seizures, may result in the expression of transcription factors, such as *c-fos*. This would permit or facilitate gene expression and growth factors, which may induce morphologic changes.

Neural Networks

Since seizures are transient abnormal electrical events in which there is synchronous and repetitive firing of groups of neurons within the cerebral cortex,[6] it is important to understand how the single-cell events described above are part of the larger neural network. While synchronous firing may not occur continuously, neurons within an epileptogenic focus are believed to be electrically hyperexcitable and, therefore, may have a propensity for rapid development of synchronous firing. From an electrophysiologic perspective, the initiation and propagation of an ictal discharge likely result from aberrant regulation of the ionic and neurochemical messengers, which mediate action potential generation and termination. It is hypothesized that a population of neurons within an epileptic focus in cortex undergo paroxysmal synchronous depolarization termed a *paroxysmal depolarizing shift (PDS),*[23] which results in an abnormal burst of action potentials that continue in synchronous volleys without appropriate inhibition.

The PDS, in animal models of epilepsy, is reflected in the EEG as an interictal spike. The PDS likely stems from a giant EPSP, although the exact mechanisms of generation remain unknown. Following the PDS, neurons exhibit after-hyperpolarization and are briefly but dramatically inhibited.[24] In the transition from PDS to seizure, several mechanisms may be responsible. For example, with a repetitive PDS, the characteristic after-hyperpolarizing potential becomes smaller and eventually is replaced by an after-depolarization.[24] With recurrent PDS, repetitive after-depolarizations merge and result in high-frequency action potential generation. Synchronous depolarization may then spread rapidly to other brain regions and entrain other neurons, the output of which produce additional volleys of firing. Among other things, this can be caused by a fundamental disregulation of intracellular or extracellular Na^+, K^+, Cl^-, or Ca^{++} ion permeability. This hypothesis is supported by the fact that phenytoin and carbamazepine, which putatively inhibit rapid firing in Na^+ channels, are potent anticonvulsant medications.

Experimental analysis on how synchronization of recurrently firing neurons culminates in an ictal or epileptic discharge suggests that certain neurons, such as pyramidal cells in neocortex and hippocampus, have a lower threshold for seizures than other cell types. Whether ictal discharges in these neurons result from a loss of inhibition or excessive excitation is unclear. Several experimental animal models have been used to study the development and propagation of ictal discharges. For example, repetitive electrical stimulation of small cortical regions (kindling) can alter the neuronal network so that it will generate spontaneous seizures. Systemic administration of drugs such as penicillin or pentylenetetrazol, and local ablation by freezing, electrolysis, or excitotoxic compounds such as kainic acid,[6, 26] can reliably induce seizures in experimental animals.

Seizure-like electrical events have been identified in vitro in slices of rat hippocampus, by altering the ionic concentration of the incubation media. For example, exposure of hippocampal neurons to high extracellular K^+ facilitates the appearance of ictal discharges within CA1 pyramidal neurons in rodent hippocampal brain slices.[27] Similarly, elevated K^+ levels have been identified in cat cortex during and after seizures. Although elevated extracellular K^+ may induce seizures, the appearance of seizures is also dependent on intact synaptic inputs from the CA3 to CA1 regions, which appear to facilitate the transition from normal to ictal cell firing. At the single-channel and molecular level of analysis, it is not clear how elevated K^+ could favor the initiation of seizure activity. Traynelis and Dingledine[27] have postulated that high extracellular K^+ produces a positive shift in the reversal potential of K^+, which partially depolarizes neuronal cell membranes.

Partial depolarization moves the overall membrane potential closer to the threshold for initiation of an action potential.[6] Moreover, pyramidal neurons normally generate an after-hyperpolarization following a prolonged burst discharge that limits recurrent firing. With an elevated K^+, this afterpotential is diminished, thereby reducing a control mechanism that, under normal circumstances, inhibits recurrent depolarization. Over time, repetitive firing of CA1 pyramidal cells further increases extracellular K^+ levels, which, in turn, fosters the repetitive generation of action potentials. As these bursts of depolarization become synchronized by a yet unknown mechanism, a seizure is generated.

A particularly cogent insight into the ways in which the basic cellular mechanisms act to generate seizures comes from the work of Traub et al.,[28, 29] who generated mathematical simulations of the behavior of "real" neurons. In this model, the following components are required in order to generate large-scale synchronized behavior of the type seen during seizures: (1) there are neurons with an intrinsic capability for generating bursts of high-frequency discharges; (2) there is a sufficient number of excitatory connections that each neuron can excite at least one other neuron; and (3) there is after-hyperpolarization of the firing neurons, as a result of either intrinsic properties or the convergence of IPSPs onto the firing neuron. Chemical or structural factors affecting these properties of neural networks will have predictable effects on the appearance of large-scale synchronized firing of model neurons, just as in actual neurons described above.

CLINICAL SCIENCE

Definition of Status Epilepticus

The first step in recognizing SE is to appropriately define it. There are many definitions of SE. Perhaps the most often used is as follows: the occurrence of two or more seizures so closely together in time that the patient does not recover to baseline between seizures, or continuous seizure activity persisting more than 30 minutes. This definition presents some limitations: one limitation is that, when encountering a patient for the first time, it is often difficult to determine whether there has been recovery to baseline between seizures or not. The major limitation of the above definition, however, is that many patients with chronic epilepsy regularly have clusters of seizures. It is not uncommon for these patients to have one seizure followed by a prolonged postictal state and another seizure. It is clear that this latter situation is quite different from that of a patient who experiences a new seizure pattern manifested by complex partial seizures occurring every few minutes. Thus, the treatment of a patient cannot be based solely on whether or not he or she meets the above definition of SE.

Perhaps a more appropriate modification of the above definition of status addressing these issues would be *(1) the occurrence of two or more seizures in a pattern that is atypical for the individual patient, so closely together in time that the patient does not recover to baseline between episodes (or does not recover to normal, if information about the patient's baseline is not available); or (2) continuous seizure activity persisting either more than 30 minutes or much longer than the patient's typical seizure.* Even this definition does not remove all ambiguities from the term "status epilepticus," since it may be difficult for a clinician to know what a typical or atypical pattern of seizure activity is for a new patient. However, in the absence of a premorbid history, it would be reasonable to assume as atypical any seizure in which the patient experienced signs of significant systemic instability, such as physical injury, or obvious respiratory compromise with oxygen desaturation. We will employ this latter definition in this review, although the reader must be wary about treating patients purely on the basis of whether or not they fit any definition for SE.

Diagnosis of Status Epilepticus

After a preliminary definition of SE, it becomes important to determine when a patient actually presents with status. The main tool in making this diagnosis is the clinical neurologic examination, although in complex situations other testing including EEG, SPECT, and MRI can be of considerable importance.

Adequate neurologic examination is critical in the evaluation of a patient with suspected SE. The first step in the neurologic examination is to observe for spontaneous movements. Movements associated with SE may take many forms, but the crucial factor distinguishing them from movements seen in other neurologic disorders is evolution in frequency, amplitude, or location over time (Table 4–1). In particular, myoclonus, although typically arrhythmic, can occasionally be associated with somewhat rhythmic movements; however, these movements often have a sudden onset and cessation not typical of seizure-related movements. In addition, the movements associated with tremor or myoclonus are generally position-dependent, whereas epileptic movements generally are not. Major exceptions to this rule are the focal seizures associated with hyperglycemia, which are often stimulus-sensitive.[30] It is important to remember as well that the movements may be extremely subtle, especially in patients who have received some anticonvulsant treatment, or patients who have had long durations of status.[2, 31] These movements may be seen only in restricted regions even if the electrical seizure activity involves both hemispheres.[32] Thus, it is important to be certain that there are no abnormal movements involving the eyes, the tongue, the mouth, the neck, and abdomen, as well as the hands or legs.

TABLE 4–1 **CHARACTERISTICS OF THE MOVEMENTS SEEN IN PATIENTS WITH MYOCLONUS, TREMOR, SEIZURES, AND PSEUDOSEIZURES**

MOVEMENT TYPE	STIMULUS-SENSITIVE	EVOLUTION	POST-DEPENDENT	MULTIFOCAL (GENERALIZED)	RESPONDS TO BENZODIAZEPINES
Myoclonus	Yes	No	Yes	Usually	Yes
Tremor	No	No	Yes	Yes	Yes
Seizures	Rarely Photic sensitivity in primary generalized Sensory stimulus Sensitive with hyperglycemia	Yes	No	Yes When movements are generalized, they are usually correlated in the extremities	Yes
Pseudoseizure	Yes	Atypical changes in movements are often abrupt rather than gradual as in epileptic seizures	No	Occasionally	Occasionally

Because the movements seen in SE can often be subtle, it is important to accumulate evidence that will help corroborate an initial diagnosis of status. The most helpful corroborative information is whether or not the patient responds in any meaningful way to stimuli. If the patient has complex and purposeful responses in the face of bilateral movements, SE would be unlikely. Exceptions to this rule occur in the case of frontal lobe complex partial seizures and the myoclonus seen in the primary generalized epilepsies. It is also important to realize that in the early stages of status, in which the patient experiences frequent discrete seizures, purposeful responses to external stimuli may be seen in the postictal phase. One must also be aware that "primitive" responses such as posturing or triple flexion may be preserved during status. Despite these caveats, response to stimulation can be helpful in distinguishing patients with nonepileptic from those with true epileptic movements, although no factor in and of itself is diagnostic.

A general neurologic examination is important, especially when focal findings suggest a neurologic lesion that might hold a cause-and-effect relationship with SE. Papilledema may point to increased intracranial pressure and, hence, a structural lesion as the possible etiology of the patient's seizures. In some cases, disruption of the pupillary light reflex may be the sole sign of neurologic dysfunction. Early in the course of SE, there may be pupillary constriction followed subsequently by dilation. Asymmetries may occur, but, in general, the pupillary light reflex should be preserved. A unilateral unreactive pupil may provide a clue to impending tentorial herniation. In addition, careful observation of spontaneous eye movements is important. In the setting of a hemispheric structural lesion, the eyes normally deviate toward the side of the lesion; however, during seizures, eye deviation will often be contralateral to the hemispheric seizure focus. Although ipsilateral deviation may occur, contralateral eye deviation without evidence of a brain stem lesion will lower the examiner's threshold in making the diagnosis of ongoing seizure activity.

Much of the time, the neurologic examination is sufficient to make a reasonable determination of SE. If the examiner is uncertain, the immediate options are to (1) continue observation without treatment; (2) continue observation during treatment with less sedating anticonvulsants such as phenytoin; (3) continue observation during treatment with more sedating anticonvulsants such as the benzodiazepines; or (4) withhold further treatment pending the results of an emergency EEG. In scenarios 1–3, the examiner will generally obtain an EEG as well, unless the patient has substantially recovered to baseline prior to the time that the EEG can be performed.

There are five patterns that may be seen in the EEG of a patient with SE (Table 4–2). First, as illustrated in Figure 4–2, the EEG may show discrete seizures of focal onset with a clear beginning, evolution, and end. As noted by Treiman et al.,[31] this pattern is often seen at the beginning of SE. However, as SE continues, often the EEG will demonstrate continuous ictal activity as illustrated in Figure 4–3. Often this pattern is difficult to recognize, but its hallmark is the presence of continuous evolution with a pattern that changes from moment to moment and is not sensitive to external stimuli, such as painful stimulation or passive eye opening and eye closure. Even more difficult to interpret are EEG patterns in patients showing periodic complexes because, under certain circumstances, similar patterns recorded at the scalp are clearly interictal (Fig. 4–4*A*), and in other circumstances they are clearly an ictal pattern (Fig. 4–4*B*).

Reiher et al.[33] has attempted to classify these periodic discharges into PLEDS (periodic lateralized epileptiform discharges) and PLEDS-PLUS according to whether there are bursts of fast activity accompanying the periodic discharges. Figure 4–5 is a segment of the EEG of a patient demonstrating PLEDS over the left hemisphere, and independently occurring PLEDS-PLUS over the right hemisphere. The PLEDS-PLUS pattern was found commonly after SE, whereas the PLEDS pattern was much less specific. In particular, Reiher et al. showed that there was a 50% chance of recording a clear electrographic seizure within 17 minutes of the time that an EEG showed the PLEDS-PLUS pattern, while when an EEG showed only PLEDS the probability was only 6%. Reiher et al.[33] and Grand'Maison et al.[34] however, could not determine whether the PLEDS-PLUS pattern was ictal. This problem remains an important issue for future study. In patients with either spike wave stupor or a primary generalized epilepsy, the EEG may show bursts of generalized spike and wave activity (Fig. 4–6). Finally, it is also possible that an EEG obtained in a patient with SE may show no ictal activity, if the EEG is of short duration and is per-

Text continued on page 63

TABLE 4–2 **EEG PATTERNS DURING STATUS EPILEPTICUS**

Partial Epilepsy or Acute Brain Injury
- Discrete seizure activity (see Fig. 4–2)
- Continuous seizure activity (see Fig. 4–3)
- Periodic complexes (see Fig. 4–4)
- Interictal (see Fig. 4–5)

Generalized Epilepsy or Spike Wave Stupor
- Generalized spike and wave activity (see Fig. 4–6)

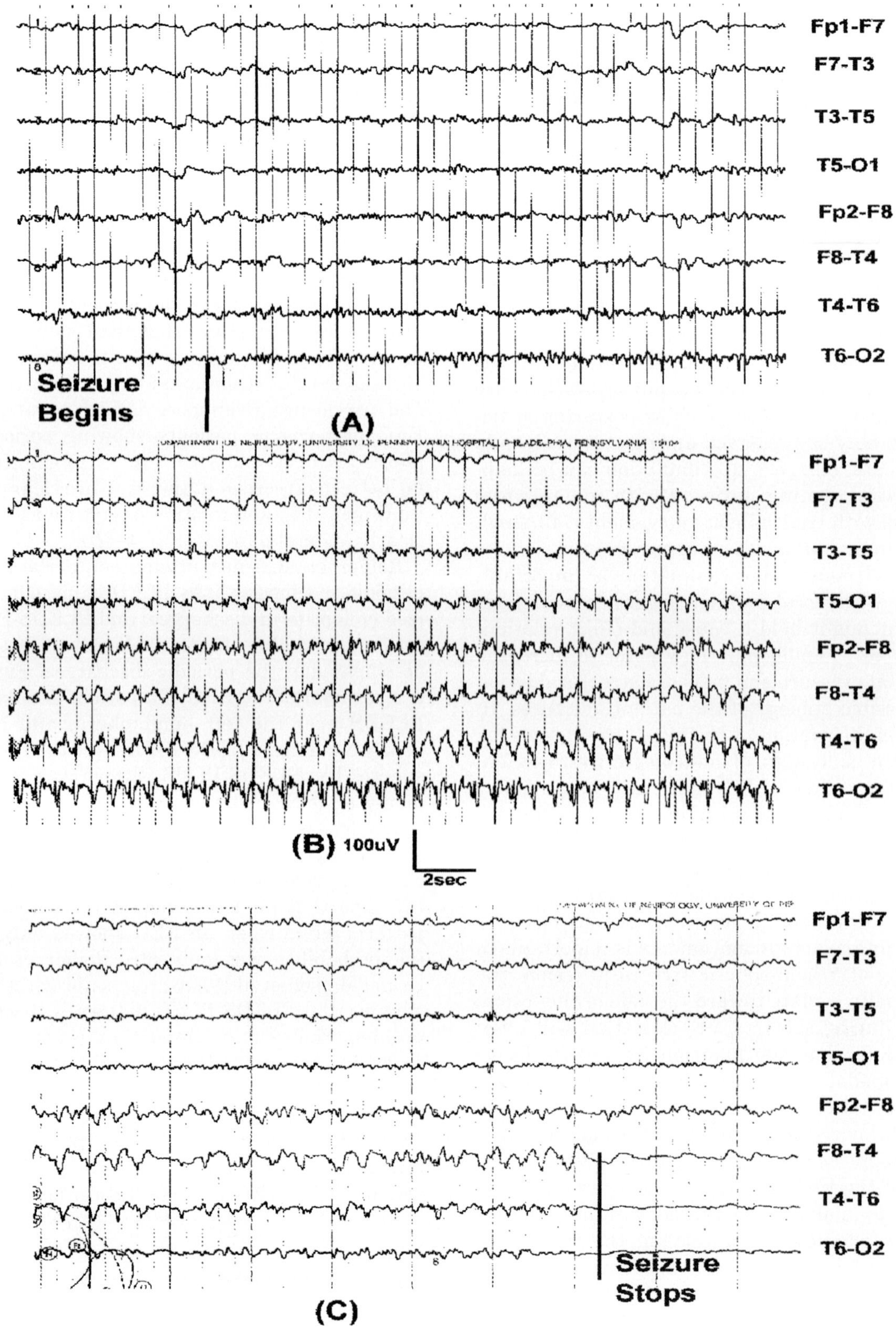

FIGURE 4–2 • A focal onset electrographic seizure in a patient with status epilepticus. *A,* Seizure onset in the right posterior regions with increased fast activity. *B,* Seizure continues with the build-up of higher amplitude slower activity over the right posterior regions. *C,* Seizure stops with subsequent postictal flattening of the EEG, especially in the right posterior regions.

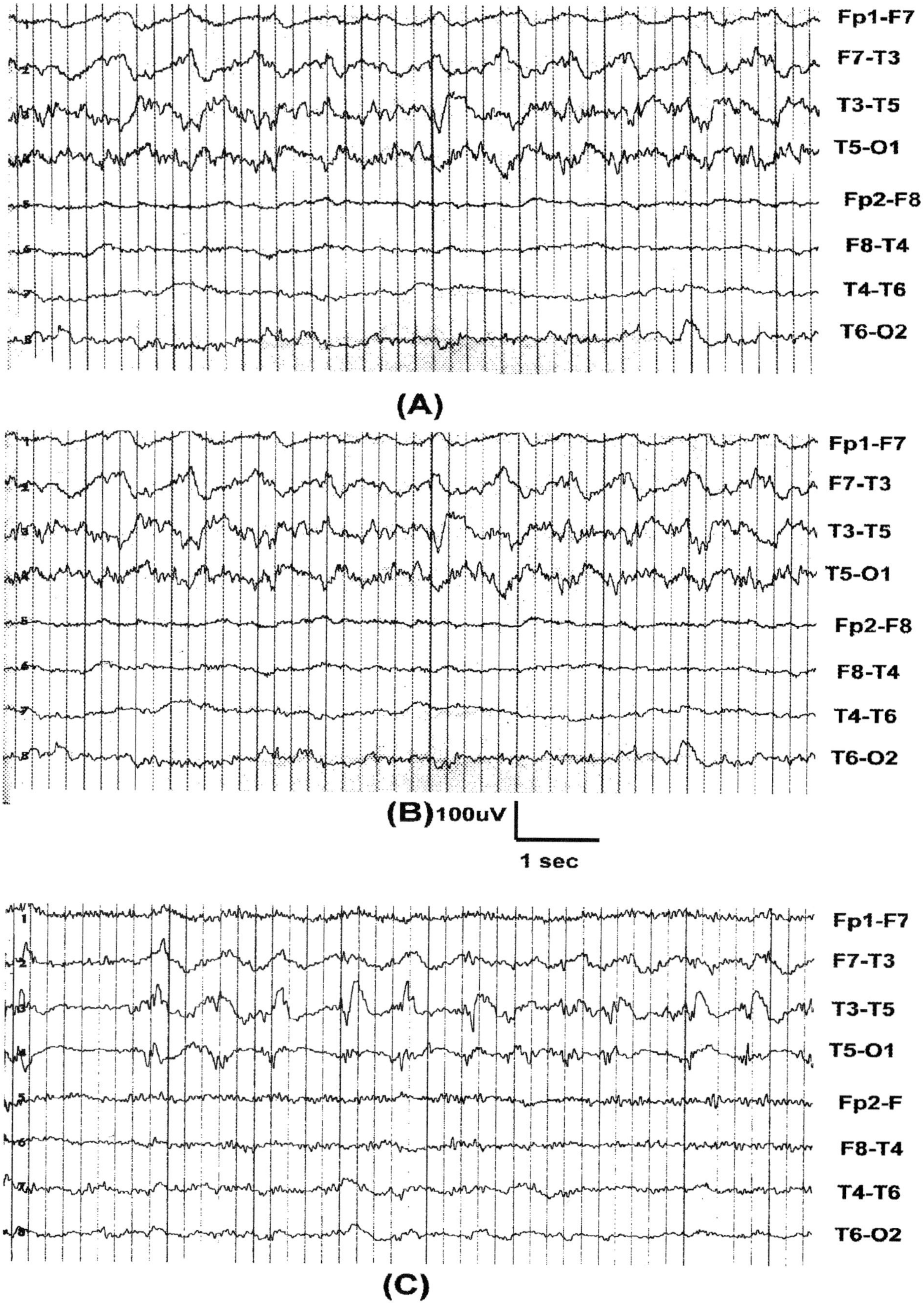

FIGURE 4-3 • Continuous electrographic ictal activity over the left posterior regions. The three segments of this figure *(A–C)* illustrate the variation in electric activity from moment to moment that is the hallmark of continuous electrographic status.

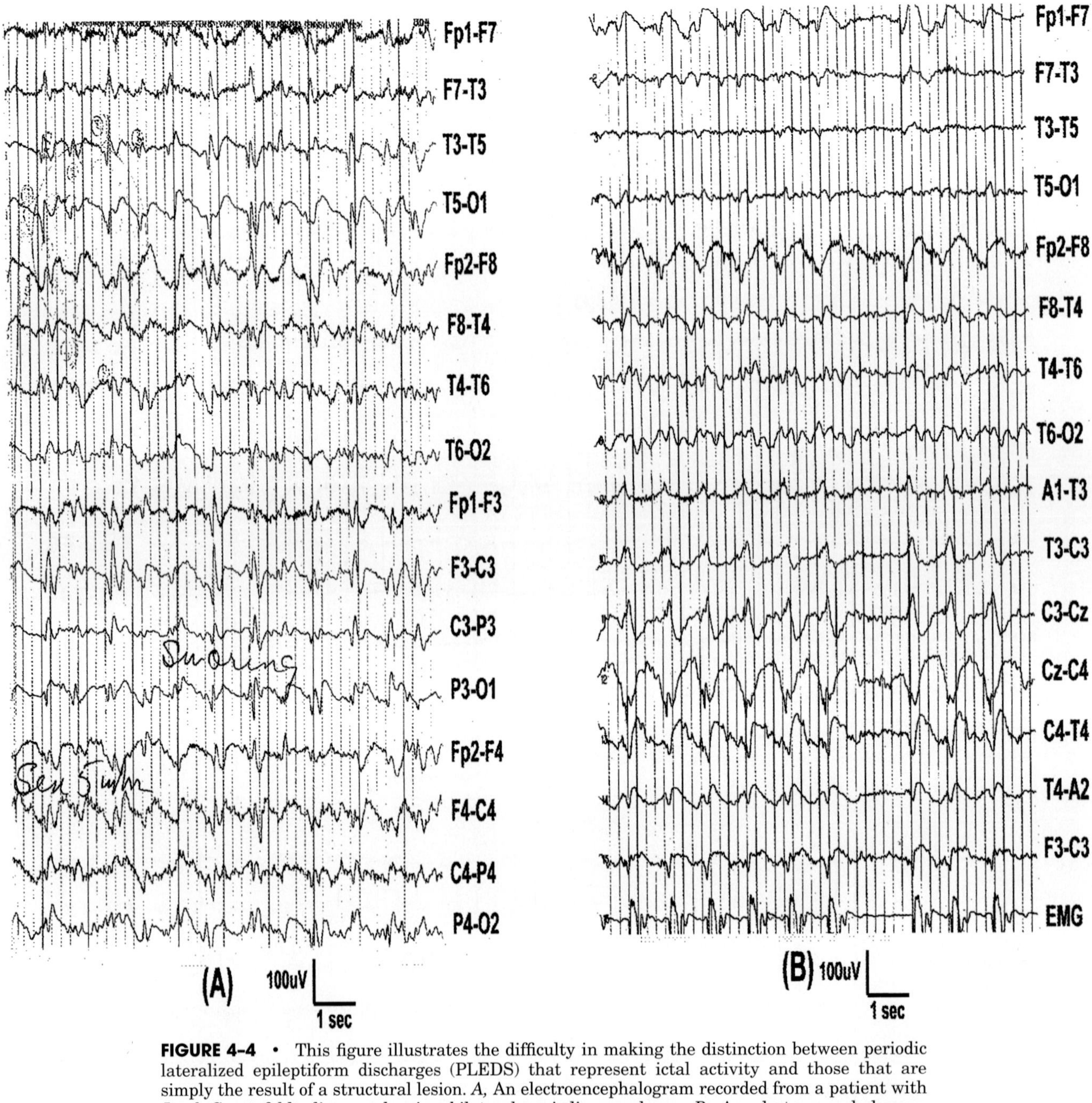

FIGURE 4–4 • This figure illustrates the difficulty in making the distinction between periodic lateralized epileptiform discharges (PLEDS) that represent ictal activity and those that are simply the result of a structural lesion. *A*, An electroencephalogram recorded from a patient with Jacob-Creutzfeldt disease showing bilateral periodic complexes. *B*, An electroencephalogram recorded from a patient experiencing intermittent seizures manifested by altered responsiveness and intermittent twitching. This recording also demonstrates periodic complexes that can be seen bilaterally (with maximum amplitude at the vertex) but are present only during the patient's clinical seizures.

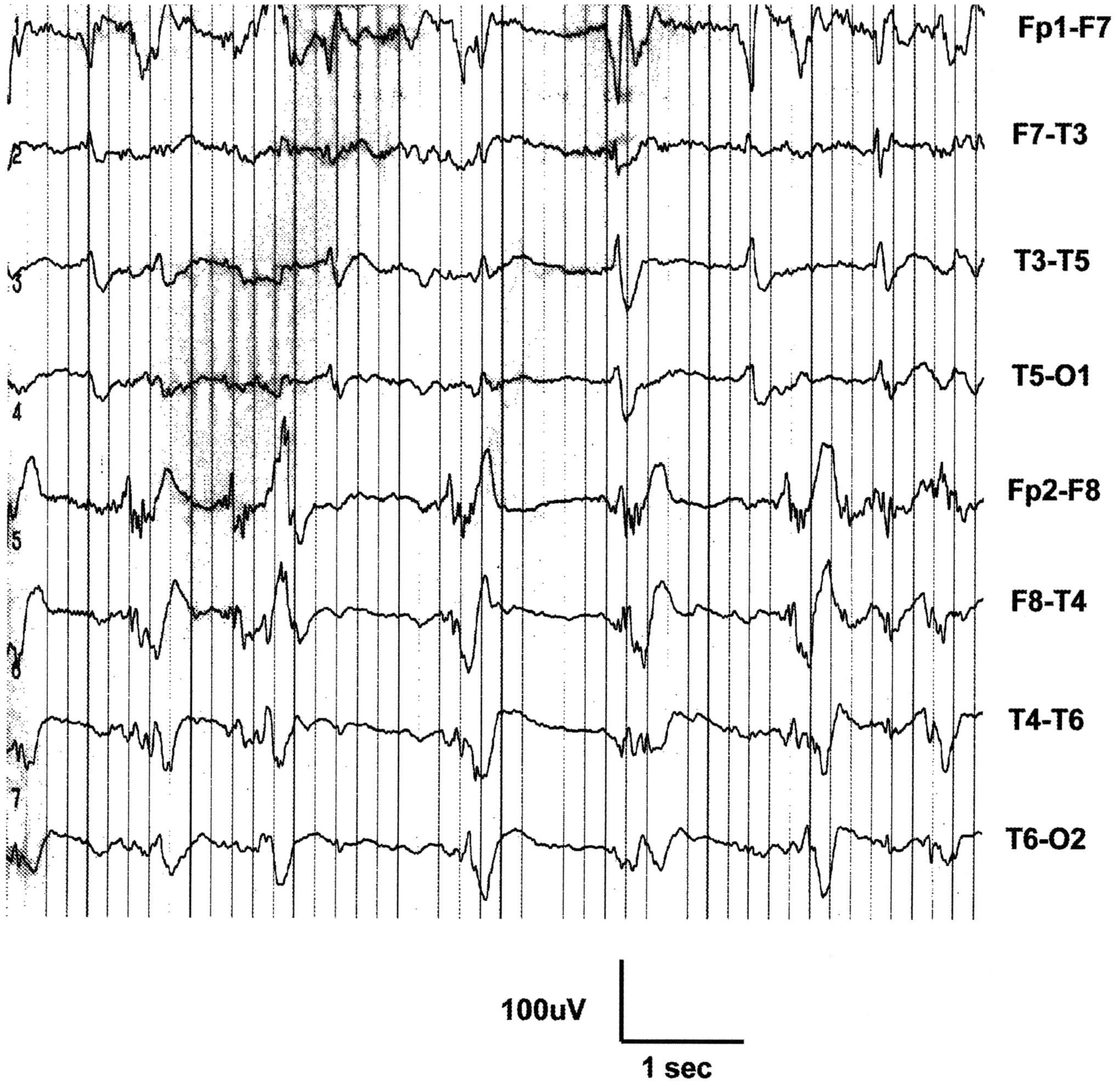

FIGURE 4–5 • The difference between PLEDS and PLEDS PLUS. The electroencephalogram over the left hemisphere demonstrated PLEDS and, over the right hemisphere, PLEDS PLUS. The major difference is the fact that the PLEDS PLUS are accompanied by short bursts of faster activity.

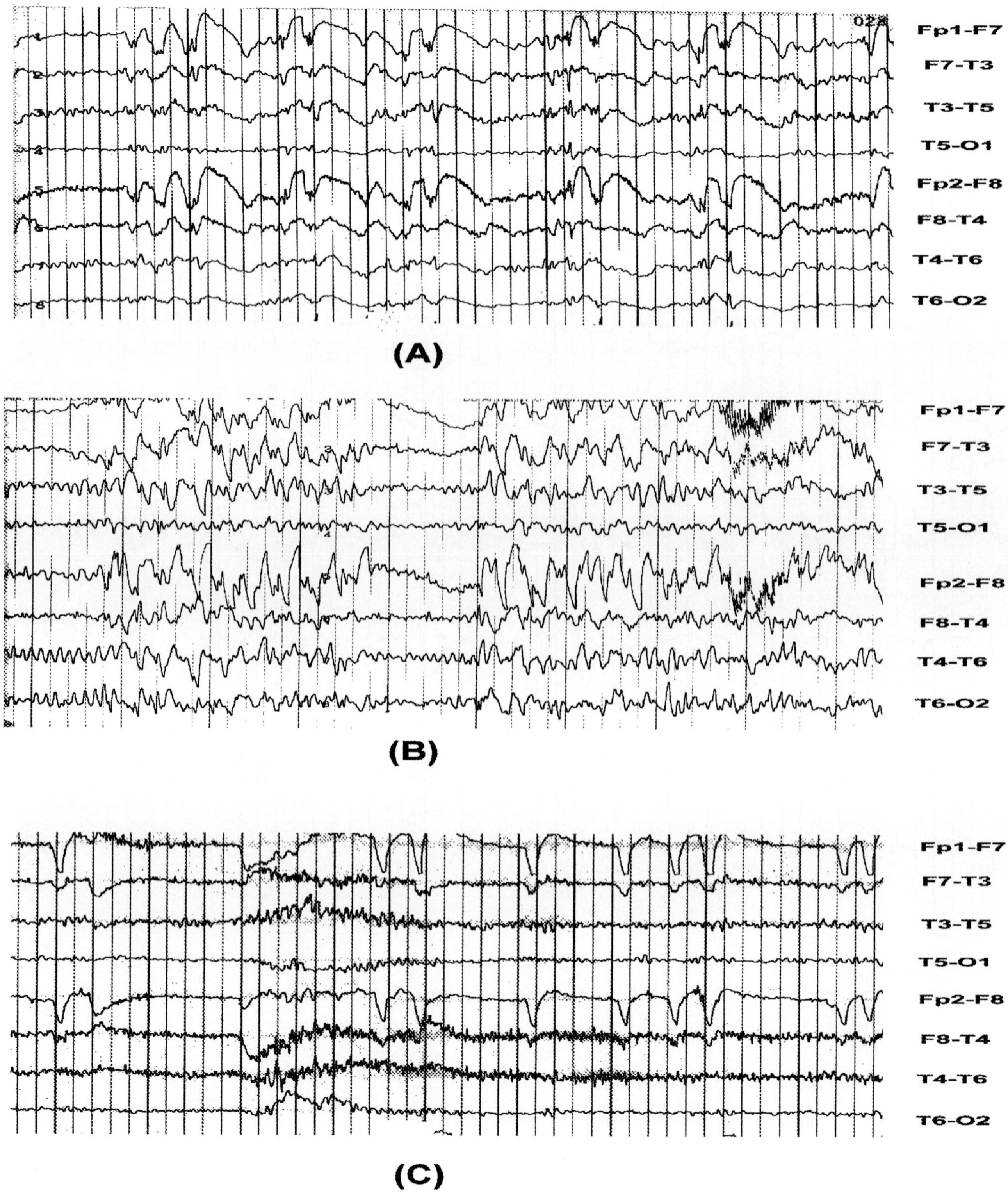

FIGURE 4-6 • *A, B,* Bursts of spike and wave activity occurring during spike-wave status in a patient with altered mental status. Note that the morphology of the spike and wave activity is not as well defined as is often seen interictally. *C,* The EEG of this patient after treatment with benzodiazepines for comparison.

formed between seizures. It is thus important, if status is suspected, that the EEG be carried out for a prolonged period of time if no ictal abnormalities are seen at the outset of the record.

Because of the difficulties in interpreting the EEG in the presence of continuous subclinical seizure activity, it is occasionally important to use other testing to help confirm a diagnosis of SE. In particular, Tatum et al.[35] demonstrated that SPECT with technetium-hexamethylpropyleneamineoxime (Tc-HMPAO) shows areas of focal hyperperfusion in patients with partial SE, but not in patients with other neurologic conditions being evaluated for the possibility of SE, even when the electrographic abnormalities were difficult to interpret. However, it is well known that after SE, areas of focal hyperperfusion can persist for weeks.[36] Thus, SPECT can detect patients who currently have or have recently had focal SE, but cannot necessarily be used to determine whether a patient is in status at the time the study is performed.

Figure 4–7*A* illustrates an example of a Tc-HMPAO SPECT scan performed during focal SE in a patient having episodes of aphasia, demonstrating a region of increased regional blood flow in the left temporal region. Figure 4–7*B* illustrates a Tc-HMPAO SPECT scan for the same patient after status had ended. In interpreting these SPECT studies, it is important to correlate the areas of focal hyperperfusion with the results of other imaging studies because, for instance, new infarcts and tumors may be associated with areas of breakdown in the blood-brain barrier and cause a localized increase in the uptake of Tc-HMPAO. Serial SPECT studies can sometimes be used to answer the question of whether focal areas of hyperperfusion are due to continuing ictal activity or are the residua of terminated ictal activity. This is because gradual diminution in hyperperfusion over time indicates that status has terminated.

Although positron emission computed tomography (PET) is a powerful tool in the evaluation of the metabolic activity and blood flow during seizures, its use as an adjunct in helping to establish

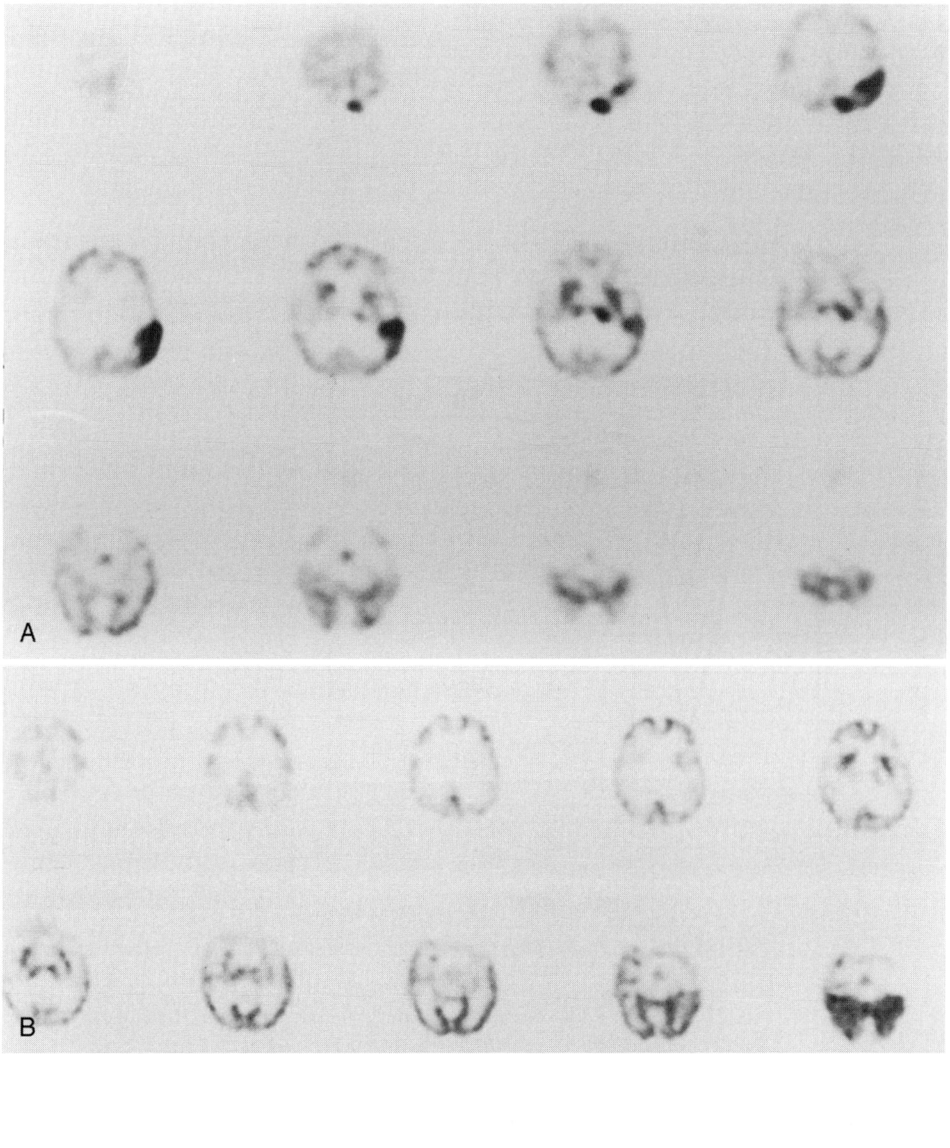

FIGURE 4–7 • *A,* Tc-HMPAO SPECT scan of patient in nonconvulsive status epilepticus showing greatly increased blood flow in the left occipital, parietal, and temporal regions. *B,* Repeat SPECT scan on the same patient days after status had ended demonstrating a much smaller degree of asymmetry of blood flow between the right and left hemispheres.

the diagnosis of SE will be likely limited, at least in the near future, because of the logistic difficulties in obtaining images at short notice.

MRI also may have a role in helping to elucidate the diagnosis of SE, in addition to its role in detecting lesions that could be responsible for SE, such as stroke, hemorrhage, tumor, etc. In particular, Henry and colleagues[37] have demonstrated localized changes in the intensity of T2-weighted images during seizures on routine MRI studies. Warach et al.[38] have demonstrated hyperperfusion in a patient with SE using the gadolinium bolus tracking method. Figure 4–8*A* illustrates the typical finding of more rapid change in signal intensity over the area from which the seizures originated, in comparison with a homologous region located in the opposite hemisphere. Figure 4–8*B* shows the regions from which the data from Figure 4–8*A* are derived. Righini and associates[39] have elucidated changes in the apparent diffusion coefficient using MRI in animal models of SE. Jackson and coworkers[40] have demonstrated that BOLD (brain oxygen level–dependent) or "functional" MRI images, which are sensitive to the relative regional abundance of oxy- and deoxyhemoglobin, can be used to provide images of regional changes during seizures.

Magnetic resonance spectroscopy may in the future become an important tool in evaluating patients with suspected SE by virtue of its ability to yield direct information on the metabolic state of regions of the brain.[46] In particular, Younkin et al.,[41] using ^{31}P NMR spectroscopy, demonstrated that the ratio of phosphocreatine (P_{cr}) to inorganic phosphate (P_i) declined during seizures, and that P_{cr}/P_i ratios less than .8 were associated with a poor neurologic prognosis. They also demonstrated a dramatic effect of anticonvulsant treatment in quickly increasing this ratio toward normal levels. Petroff and colleagues[42] have demonstrated this effect in bicuculline-induced SE in animals. ^{1}H NMR spectroscopy has been used to demonstrate elevated lactate during seizures,[44] as well as to determine that there are increased free fatty acids in the brain after electroconvulsive therapy.[45] ^{1}H NMR spectroscopy has been reported to measure GABA and glutamine levels in the brain and show their alterations by vigabatrin.[47]

There is much less utility of imaging techniques in patients with suspected primary generalized SE, since EEG abnormalities are always prominent and the focal abnormalities that are easily distinguished on imaging studies are absent.

Etiology of Status Epilepticus

Once a diagnosis of SE is made, a consideration of potential causes (Table 4–3) is essential in order to develop a rational treatment plan.

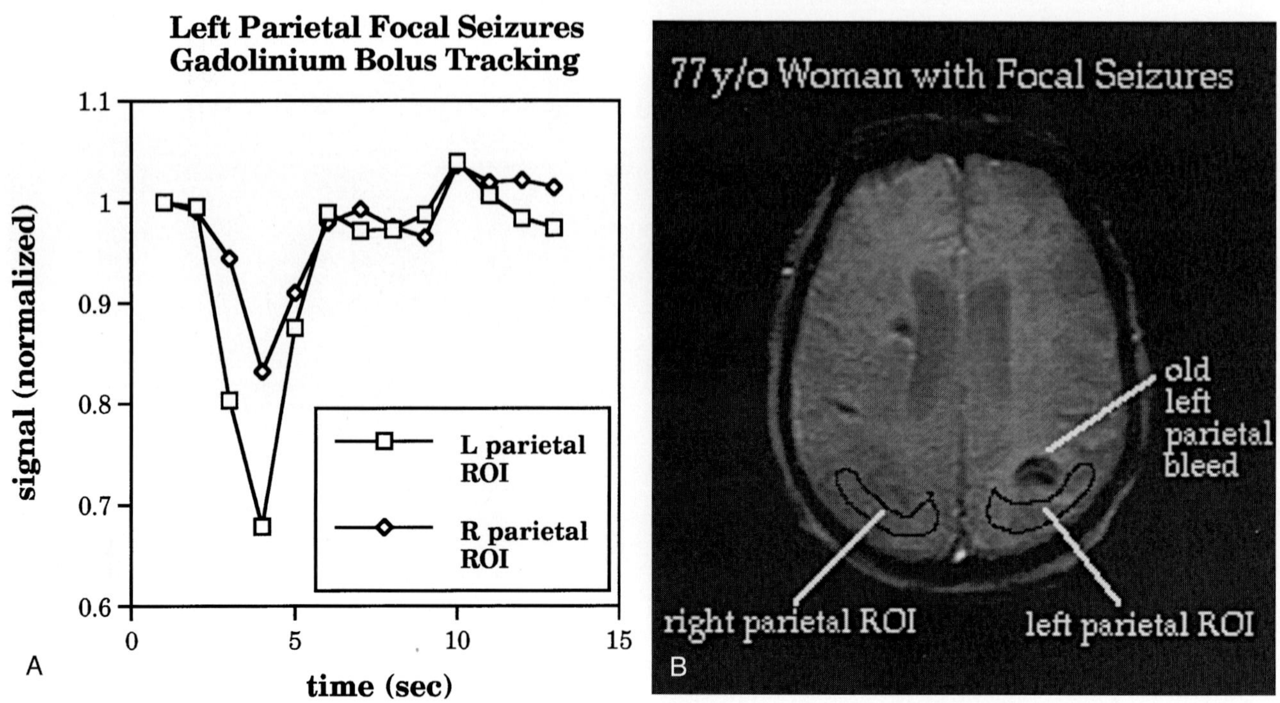

FIGURE 4–8 • *A,* Normalized time course of signal intensity after injection of gadolinium as a function of time, showing greater change over the left parietal region of interest (ROI) than over the right parietal region of interest. The seizure focus was in the left parietal region. *B,* Illustration of regions of interest on the patient's MRI. (Courtesy of Dr. J. Detre, Department of Neurology, Hospital of the University of Pennsylvania.)

TABLE 4–3 **ETIOLOGIES OF STATUS EPILEPTICUS**

Mass lesions	Congenital anomalies
Brain tumors	Tuberous sclerosis
Arteriovenous malformations	Sturge-Weber syndrome
Epidural hematoma	Cortical dysplasia (hemimegalencephaly, polymicrogyria, lissencephaly)
Subdural hematoma	Metabolic
Carcinomatous meningitis	Hypoglycemia
Paraneoplastic syndromes	Hyponatremia
Infectious	Hypocalcemia
Bacterial abscess	Hypoxemia
Tuberculosis	Renal failure
Cryptococcosis	Hepatic failure
Toxoplasmosis	Drug intoxications
Bacterial meningitis	Ethanol
Viral encephalitis (especially herpes)	Methanol
Vascular	Cocaine
Cerebral infarction (especially embolic)	Amphetamine
Vasculitis	Tricyclic antidepressants
Intracerebral hemorrhage	Lithium
Subarachnoid hemorrhage	Cyclosporine
Arteriovenous malformations	Isoniazid
	Theophylline

Most etiologic studies tend to focus on convulsive SE, and estimates are that from 60,000 to 200,000 individuals in the United States will suffer SE within any given year.[48] Of the patients presenting to emergency rooms with SE, in one third it reflects their first seizure. Nonconvulsive SE, which includes complex partial, tonic, myoclonic, and absence SE, also occurs, but in only approximately 14% of all cases.[49] Among all patients with epilepsy, some type of SE is likely to occur in 1%–16% of patients.[48] The risk of SE is highest among children and adults over the age of 60 years.

Although there are many possible etiologies for SE, patients can be broadly divided into two categories: those with an acute central nervous system insult, i.e., structural, infectious, or toxic-metabolic; and those without a de novo brain injury.[50] In particular, Aminoff and Simon[32] noted that 52% of patients in their study of SE had previous seizures, and those were overwhelmingly classified into the second of these categories.

One frequent precipitant of SE in patients with known epilepsy is anticonvulsant drug (ACD) withdrawal. In fact, this was the etiology in 57% of patients with known epilepsy,[32] and approximately 28% of all cases of SE, although Scholtes et al.[49] cite this as a cause in only 6% of their patients with SE. Anticonvulsant withdrawal seizures are a greater problem with the benzodiazepines and barbiturates than the other anticonvulsants but can occur with any anticonvulsant.[51]

In adults, common structural brain lesions that cause SE include stroke in 8% of all cases of generalized tonic-clonic status,[49] intracranial hemorrhage (2%, Scholtes[49]), head injury (8.9%, Scholtes[49]; 4%, Aminoff and Simon[32]), chronic static encephalopathy (35%, Scholtes[49]), and brain tumor (5%, Aminoff and Simon[32]); however, the estimates of the relative frequency of these conditions is highly variable from study to study. Infectious etiologies (5%, Aminoff and Simon[32]; 3%, Scholtes[49]) include bacterial or fungal meningitis, brain abscess, and encephalitis especially as a result of herpesvirus infection.

Another important cause of SE in patients both with and without previous seizures is ethanol abuse. Aminoff and Simon[32] implicate this as the etiology of SE in 15% of cases, whereas Lowenstein and Alldredge[52] cite a figure of 25% in the years 1980–1990, and Scholtes[49] uses 2.5%. Ng[53] indicates that the majority of alcohol withdrawal seizures occurred between 7 and 72 hours after cessation of drinking, although he did not find an increased probability of seizures in the 12–24 hour period after cessation of drinking, as suggested by Victor.[54] Ng also indicated that risk of seizures was present only in patients taking 50 g of absolute alcohol a day or more, and that the risk of seizures tripled for every additional 100 g daily intake of alcohol above this point up to 300 g daily.

Drug intoxication from tricyclic compounds, isoniazid, cocaine, amphetamines, cyclosporine, and theophylline may induce prolonged seizures. These types of intoxication are important to diagnose as soon as possible, since treatment with pyridoxine will be useful in managing seizures from isoniazid, and treatment with physostigmine (0.25–1 mg IV) may have some value in managing seizures occurring as a result of tricyclic overdose.[55] In theophylline and cyclosporine intoxication, it is important to discontinue the medication as soon as possible, or at least hold dosing until levels are in the low therapeutic range. Similarly, acute withdrawal of sedative-hypnotic compounds such as barbiturates and benzodiazepines, especially clonazepam, may precipitate SE.

Metabolic derangements such as anoxia, hypoxia-ischemia, hypo- or hyperglycemia, hyponatremia, hypocalcemia, and hypomagnesemia may precipitate SE in many individuals, especially hospitalized patients (8%, Aminoff and Simon[32]). SE may occur in patients with uremic and, less commonly, hepatic encephalopathy. Acute Wernicke's encephalopathy may also present as SE.

Endocrinologic dysfunction such as hyper- or hypothyroidism, Addison's disease, or hyperparathyroidism may be rare causes of SE. Rare iatrogenic causes of SE include metrizamide myelography[60] and cerebral angiography.[61] Treatment with high-dose intravenous penicillin G, lidocaine, or imipenem can also cause seizures as well as treatment with the quinolone antibiotics. Electroconvulsive therapy[56, 57] has also rarely been reported to cause SE.

Morbidity and Mortality

There are two types of complications from SE: those related to central nervous system effects, and those related to systemic effects. In order to understand the prognosis of patients, it is important to first have a rough idea about the general statistical studies on the outcome of status, as a function of etiology and type of SE. However, as the group of patients with SE is heterogeneous, it is important to understand more fully the CNS and systemic effects of status, so that the neurologist can make better estimates of the prognosis for each patient.

General Statistics

Several studies have attempted to identify immediate and long-term medical, neurologic, and neuropsychologic consequences of SE[58] in both adults and children. SE may account for up to 8% of all hospital admissions[58]; however, this number is highly variable and depends greatly on the patient population served by any given hospital. Thus, the statistics we summarize below will function primarily as a rough guideline regarding outcome in SE.

The major morbidity and mortality of SE are related to several factors, the most prominent of which are the duration of seizures and underlying neurologic or medical illnesses. In one series of 98 patients, serious or fatal complications occurred in 28 individuals,[32] 10 of which were related only to the occurrence of SE and not to an underlying illness. Two of these patients (2.5%) died. Further support for a specific effect of SE on outcome is offered in a series of 42 patients with SE studied by Rowan and Scott.[59] In this study, the mean duration of status was 1.5 hours in the group of patients with no subsequent neurologic deterioration, and 12 hours in the group of patients that either died or experienced neurologic deterioration as a result of status. Scholtes et al.[49] examined the effect of duration of status on morbidity and mortality of patients with status. They concluded that, in cases in which the underlying etiology of status was directly considered as the outcome determinant, the duration of status had no effect on outcome. However, in the other cases in that series, when the duration of status exceeded 4 hours, morbidity and mortality increased from approximately 1%–2% to 50%–60%. Lowenstein and Alldredge[52] found significant correlations between outcome and duration of status only for patients with alcohol-related SE and patients with CNS infections. In patients with anticonvulsant withdrawal or drug toxicity, there was a statistically insignificant trend to poorer outcome with longer duration of status.

In addition to the duration of status, the outcome in SE depends greatly on the type of treatment required to control it. In particular, as shown in Table 4–4, mortality of SE in general ranged from

TABLE 4–4 **COMPARISON OF THE MORTALITY OF ALL PATIENTS WITH STATUS WITH PATIENTS REQUIRING BARBITURATE COMA FOR TREATMENT**

ALL PATIENTS		BARBITURATE COMA	
Investigator	**Mortality (%)**	**Investigator**	**Mortality (%)**
Oxbury and Whitty[69]	8.3	Yaffe and Lowenstein[110]	53
Aminoff and Simon[32]	2.5	Rashkin et al.[113]	77
Lowenstein and Alldredge[52]	14.5	Osorio and Reed[111]	16
Rowan and Scott[59]	21	Van Ness[109]	42
Scholtes et al.[49]	11		

The effect on outcome of treatment required to stop status epilepticus. Barbiturate coma is considered one of the most aggressive treatments, needed only in difficult to control cases of status. The mortality associated with this treatment is significantly greater than that of the entire group of patients with status epilepticus. This is more likely a reflection of the seizures in patients requiring barbiturate coma, rather than a specific effect of the treatment.

TABLE 4–5 **EFFECT OF ETIOLOGY OF STATUS EPILEPTICUS ON MORTALITY**

	LOWENSTEIN/ALLDREDGE[52]	CELESIA ET AL.[135]	OXBURY/WHITTY[69]	SCHOLTES ET AL.[49]
Alcohol related	10%	—	—	0%
Head trauma	0%	—	—	10%
CNS infection	35%	—	11%	50%
Cardiac arrest/anoxia	80%	69%	—	80%
Cerebrovascular	70%	—	0%	50%
Tumor	40%	—	20%	16%
Chronic epilepsy	20%	—	0%	7%
Anticonvulsant withdrawal	10%	—	—	—

Outcome as a function of etiology of status. Lowenstein and Alldredge used poor outcome as their measure instead of mortality. This included both patients who died and patients left with a severe neurologic disability requiring full supportive care. Note that the above statistics, especially for the Oxbury and Whitty study, were based on small numbers of patients in each group and, hence, are quite variable.

2% to 21%, whereas in patients requiring treatment with barbiturate coma, mortality ranged from 16% to 77%.

In addition to the effects of treatment and duration of status, etiology has a powerful effect on outcome. As shown in Table 4–5, patients with status in the setting of anoxia/cardiac arrest had a dismal prognosis, while patients with status as a result of alcohol use or anticonvulsant withdrawal had a much better prognosis.

Neural Damage As a Consequence of Status Epilepticus

One central question that remains to be answered is whether recurrent seizure activity can cause neuronal injury. In several animal models of SE, histopathologic evidence of neuronal damage was identified within the CA1 and CA3 sectors of the hippocampus; layers 3, 5, and 6 of neocortex; Purkinje cells within the cerebellum; the thalamus; and amygdala following more than 60 minutes of seizures.[14] However, it was not clear whether the observed neuronal injury resulted from the excessive electrical activity characteristic of recurrent seizures or from metabolic derangements such as hypoxemia, metabolic acidosis, and hyperpyrexia. These latter changes also occur during prolonged seizures and could have independent detrimental effects on brain function distinct from the effects of continuous seizures.

For example, one worrisome consequence of SE is hypoxemia. During generalized tonic-clonic seizures, there can be inactivity of the diaphragm with subsequent respiratory arrest. Blood oxygen tension and oxygen saturation may fall to dangerously low levels, putting certain neurons at risk for hypoxic injury. Interestingly, neurons injured by hypoxia were similar to those damaged by prolonged seizures, i.e., pyramidal neurons within the CA1 and CA3 hippocampal sectors, Purkinje cells in the cerebellum, and cortical pyramidal cells in layers 3, 5, and 6. Thus, the question remained as to whether neuronal injury identified following SE resulted form ictal activity or hypoxia. In experimental models of SE in which primates were given mechanical ventilation and neuromuscular blockade, continuous seizures resulted in neuronal damage restricted primarily to hippocampus and cortex if seizures continued for 60 minutes or more.[14, 62, 63] Thus, independent of hypoxia and systemic acidosis, localized cell death may occur with prolonged seizures. It has been hypothesized that neuronal injury results, in large part, from excessive EAA compounds such as glutamate and aspartate released during prolonged seizures. Through interaction with postsynaptic EAA receptors, glutamate and aspartate cause excessive intracellular calcium increases,[64] which activate a variety of neuronal proteases and cause cell death.[15] Indeed, when EAA agonists such as kainic acid are injected into the brain, similar types of damage may be detected.[65]

The extent to which neurocognitive abnormalities can be identified in human survivors of SE[66] is a complex problem. Most analyses have been retrospective studies performed on children. Few have used formal neuropsychologic testing protocols. In addition, it has often been difficult to determine whether cognitive deficits following SE result from prolonged seizures, from the underlying neurologic disease that induced SE, or are secondary to the systemic changes seen in status. In several clinical series of patients with SE, a variety of neurocognitive deficits were observed following prolonged seizures, although formal neuropsychologic assessment was not performed.[32, 67–69] A general trend was that longer seizure duration was associated with more extensive neurocognitive deficits.

In three prospective studies, formal IQ testing (Wechsler scales for adults and children) was performed on patients with epilepsy who subsequently suffered SE. In two studies that analyzed children,[70, 71] no clear difference in IQ was identified. In the third study, which studied adults, a mild decrement in formal IQ test results was noted in patients with an episode of SE.[66] In summary, there is a suggestion that SE may diminish neurocognitive abilities, although the extent of these deficits needs to be further assessed using formal neuropsychologic testing.

Systemic Effects of Status Epilepticus

Besides the effects of SE on the brain, its systemic effects (Table 4–6) are also important in determining the type and rapidity of treatment. Some of the systemic effects of SE are a direct result of continued muscle contractions, such as rhabdomyolysis, systemic acidosis, and increased temperature. Generally, rhabdomyolysis does not occur with convulsions lasting shorter than 7 minutes or so, unless the patient falls and directly injures muscles.

Blood pH values less than 7.2 are uncommon, unless the duration of a convulsion is greater than 7 minutes or there is significant respiratory dysfunction. In the study of Aminoff and Simon,[32] approximately 50% of patients presented with pH values less than 7.3. Some of them had a primary metabolic acidosis, while others had a primary respiratory acidosis. Wijdicks and Hubmayr[72] studied the arterial blood gas results of patients with status arriving at the emergency room, prior to mechanical ventilation and other treatments. In this study, 42% of patients had respiratory acidosis, 37% had metabolic acidosis with an associated elevated anion gap, and 21% had respiratory alkalosis. Wijdicks also determined that patients with respiratory acidosis were not statistically more likely to have evidence of aspiration on chest x-ray than other patients.

Aminoff and Simon[32] noted that approximately 50% of patients with status had temperatures greater than 38.1° C, although only 3% of patients had evidence of infection. One patient had temperatures up to 41.6° C after convulsive status lasting 9 hours without evidence of underlying infection.

Other systemic consequences of SE, such as tachycardia and pulmonary edema, can occur purely in the absence of motor activity, although extreme motor activity can worsen these consequences. Dramatic increases in circulating catecholamine levels occur early in SE even in the presence of neuromuscular blockade.[73] These changes are associated with arterial hypertension, hyperglycemia, and tachycardia. However, as the duration of status increases, the magnitude of this effect diminishes and the patient can develop arterial hypotension and hypoglycemia. In the studies on sheep performed by Benowitz et al.,[73] plasma epinephrine levels rose from 124 pg/mL to 49,000 pg/mL for the first 60 minutes after the onset of status, then began to slowly decline over the next 2 hours, with concomitant decreases in systemic arterial pressure. These changes were similar to those seen in humans by Simon et al.[74]

Both in cerebrospinal fluid (CSF) and peripheral blood, leucocytosis can occur in status, with peripheral white blood cell (WBC) counts as high as 28,000 WBC/mm^3, even in the absence of infection. Simon[75] states that this phenomenon is largely due to demargination of WBCs. In fact, it is rare to see bands in the differential of patients with status who do not have an intercurrent infection. CSF pleocytosis to 80 WBC/mm^3 has been noted after status[76] but is transient and seen in only 2% of patients when CSF is drawn within 72 hours of the seizure.

Increased intracranial pressure (ICP) may also be a manifestation of SE, which occurs even in the absence of the excessive Valsalva maneuvering or arterial hypertension during a convulsion.[77, 78] In particular, White et al.[77] studied 21 paralyzed patients undergoing seizures induced by pentylenetetrazol and demonstrated an ICP increase to the range of 40 mm Hg during the seizure. For the otherwise neurologically normal individual, increased ICP may be mildly problematic. However, for patients in whom elevated ICP already presents a threat to neurologic function, such as those with brain trauma, subarachnoid hemorrhage, brain tumor, meningitis, hepatic encephalopathy, Reye's syndrome, intracerebral hemorrhage, or stroke, prolonged seizures may make the effective management of increased ICP intractable and put the patient at risk for neurologic deterioration.

TABLE 4–6 **SYSTEMIC EFFECTS OF STATUS EPILEPTICUS**

FACTOR	EFFECT
Body temperature	Increased with prolonged motor seizures
Heart rate	Increased
Blood pressure	Increased—initially Decreased—in later stages
Respiratory drive	Minimally decreased—initially Decreased—in later stages
Aspiration pneumonia	Occasionally
Pulmonary edema	Rarely
Rhabdomyolysis	With prolonged motor activity
Acute tubular necrosis	Secondary to rhabdomyolysis
pH (blood)	Decreased
Lactate (blood)	Increased
Creatine kinase (blood)	Increased
Glucose (blood)	Increased—initially Decreased—in later stages
White blood cell count	Increased—up to 28,000/mm^3 in patients without infection

Clinical Pharmacology of Status Epilepticus

Once the diagnosis of SE has been made, it is important to quickly devise and then act on a rational plan of treatment whether SE occurs in the hospital ward, at home, or in the emergency room. Before this, it is important that one understand the pharmacology of the various medications that can be used in treating SE. Thus, we will digress to explore the pharmacology of these drugs in detail before returning to a detailed discussion of the actual treatment of SE.

It is also crucial to understand that, as the etiology of SE is heterogenous, and the treatment of status requires rapid action (often with many different medications), all studies on treatment are difficult to perform and difficult to compare. In particular, this means a study showing that a drug is effective on a certain small group of patients with status does not indicate that it will be effective in other groups.

Benzodiazepines

As mentioned earlier, benzodiazepines are a family of drugs with sedative-hypnotic and anxiolytic properties, which are believed to interact with the GABA A receptor–chloride channel complex and, thus, potentiate the inhibitory effects of GABA on neurons.[79] Benzodiazepines increase chloride channel opening at static GABA levels and, thus, increase the magnitude of inhibitory postsynaptic potentials at GABAergic synapses. Because these compounds are quite sedating and because patients readily develop tolerance to their antiepileptic effects, these drugs have had limited usefulness as long-term anticonvulsants. However, diazepam and lorazepam are extremely effective initial agents to terminate SE.

In several animal models of epilepsy, such as seizures induced by pentylenetetrazol and maximal electroshock, benzodiazepines have proven to be effective anticonvulsant compounds. Both torazepam and diazepam can be administered intravenously and, because of their lipophilicity, pass easily through the blood-brain barrier. In direct comparison studies of diazepam versus lorazepam, both agents appear to be equally effective in terminating SE, with lorazepam possibly being somewhat more potent.[80] Therapeutic brain levels of benzodiazepines may be achieved rapidly following intravenous administration. Because both diazepam and lorazepam are potent CNS depressants, they share similar side effect profiles, such as respiratory depression, respiratory arrest, and hypotension. Indeed, when benzodiazepines are administered with other CNS depressants, such as barbiturates or in the presence of ethanol, their toxic effects may be potentiated.

Diazepam (Valium) was first used to treat seizures in 1965[81] and remains a standard first-line agent for the treatment of SE. It is effective in providing lasting control of SE in 48%–100% of patients.[82] It may be administered intravenously, orally, intramuscularly, and rectally with varying efficacy. High serum and brain levels may be attained within 0.5–3 hours by oral and rectal routes, but within 10–15 seconds intravenously. Suppression of ictal activity has been observed within 10–15 seconds following intravenous diazepam administration,[82] but peak brain levels are seen only approximately 8 minutes later.

Diazepam is 90%–95% bound to plasma proteins but, as a lipophilic compound, it readily enters the brain and adipose tissue.[83] Diazepam exhibits dual-phase pharmacokinetics. Initially, its serum half-life is related to drug distribution to body and CNS compartments. The second phase is a function of its metabolism and excretion. Diazepam is metabolized in the liver to two centrally active compounds—nordiazepam and oxazepam—which may achieve levels similar to diazepam. Diazepam and diazepam metabolites are excreted in the urine with an elimination half-life of 1–2 days.[83] Despite the long elimination half-life of diazepam, its effective or therapeutic half-life is approximately 15 minutes when used to control seizures. This is most likely the result of its large volume of distribution (.3–2.0 L/kg for diazepam and 1.0–1.6 L/kg for lorazepam[82]), making it possible for diazepam to redistribute more easily than other benzodiazepines. For the treatment of SE, usual doses of diazepam in adults are 0.25 mg/kg body weight. Thus, for the 70-kg adult, approximately 10–20 mg should be given intravenously at a rate of less than 5 mg/minute, as a single bolus dose. The effective serum concentration is approximately 500 ng/mL.

Lorazepam (Ativan) is also a sedative/anxiolytic agent, which is useful in the management of SE. In several studies summarized by Treiman,[82] lorazepam has been effective in 63%–100% of patients with SE. Leppik et al.[80] conducted a double-blinded study of patients with SE treated with a solution of either 5 mg/mL diazepam or 2 mg/mL torazepam. Two milliliters of the solution was administered immediately, and an additional 2 mL was administered by the physician if seizures continued or recurred. No difference was shown in the ability of diazepam and lorazepam to control status.

Like diazepam, lorazepam is extensively (85%–93%) protein bound but, in contrast, it is glucuronidated in the liver to inactive metabolites, which are excreted in the urine. The effective elimination half-life of lorazepam is 8–25 hours.[82] Unlike diazepam, lorazepam has a smaller volume of distribution and, thus, higher sustained plasma levels may be attained for longer duration. It enters the brain within approximately 2–3 minutes and peaks within 30 minutes.[82] Its effective serum concentration is approximately 30–100 ng/mL. For SE, a total dose of lorazepam is typically administered of between 0.05 and 0.2 mg/kg. A reasonable initial lorazepam dose for a 70-kg adult in convulsive SE is 0.1 mg/kg infused at a rate of 2 mg/minute or less.[82] If the patient is not in convulsive status, it should be recalled that lorazepam takes longer to distribute into the brain than diazepam. It is thus important to give a dose of lorazepam some time (approximately 1 minute) to show an effect, before giving additional doses, in order to avoid the possibility of respiratory depression resulting when too much lorazepam is administered.

Intravenous infusions of clonazepam[82, 84] have also been used to treat SE and have an efficacy similar to that of diazepam or lorazepam. However, intravenous clonazepam is not available in the United States.

Another benzodiazepine agent that has been identified as having some benefit in treating SE is midazolam (Versed).[85–87] This short-acting benzodiazepine penetrates the CNS rapidly and has an elimination half-life of 1.5–3 hours. In one study of patients with refractory generalized tonic-clonic SE, midazolam was effective in terminating seizures in four patients, when given as an initial intravenous loading dose of 200 μg/kg, followed by a continuous infusion of 0.75–10 μg/kg/minute until cessation of seizures was noted on continuous EEG monitoring.[87]

Phenytoin

Since its development and clinical institution in 1938, phenytoin (Dilantin) has proven to be an extremely useful agent in the treatment of epilepsy. Because it is so effective in the termination of generalized tonic-clonic seizures and because it can be administered intravenously, phenytoin has been used extensively in treatment of SE.

The neuropharmacologic effects of phenytoin on neurons still remain to be completely elucidated. However, it is widely believed that the primary action of phenytoin is to prevent the spread of ictal discharges from a hyperexcitable epileptic focus within the brain.[88] Experimentally, phenytoin likely inhibits the activity of voltage-dependent sodium channels and, thus, the passage of sodium ions intracellularly, especially within regions in which neurons are exhibiting high-frequency sustained repetitive firing.[89] In addition, phenytoin may facilitate the flux of potassium ions from the intracellular to extracellular space, as well as movement of chloride ions intracellularly. Finally, phenytoin also diminishes voltage-dependent intracellular calcium flow, thus decreasing neurotransmitter release from the presynaptic terminal. The net effect of these actions is to maintain and stabilize neurons closer to the resting membrane potential, or even in a somewhat hyperpolarized state, thereby reducing the likelihood of cellular depolarization.

Phenytoin is 70%–95% plasma protein bound. Metabolism occurs via the hepatic P-450 mixed oxidase system with zero-order kinetics. These metabolites are excreted in the bile and then reabsorbed through the gut and excreted in the urine. It has a relatively long elimination half-life (range 7–42 hours, mean 22 hours[90]) and a relatively smaller volume of distribution (0.78 L/kg[90]), than diazepam or lorazepam.

Phenytoin remains an important drug in the management of SE.[91] In animal studies, phenytoin suppresses seizures within minutes of administration.[92] It rapidly penetrates the blood-brain barrier, reaching peak levels in the brain in approximately 15 minutes,[90] and is effective at terminating seizures in up to 90% of patients with status.[93] Treiman et al.[94] compared the efficiency of .1 mg/kg lorazepam versus 18 mg/kg of intravenous phenytoin in terminating nonconvulsive SE within a 15-minute time period. Lorazepam controlled seizures as the first drug in 77% and phenytoin as the first drug in 55%, although when phenytoin was used as a second drug, it controlled five of six seizures that were refractory to lorazepam. In addition, with proper dosing and administration, phenytoin does not cause the same degree of respiratory depression and sedation caused by benzodiazepines and barbiturates. Administration should be via oral or intravenous routes.

For the treatment of SE, phenytoin should be administered intravenously mixed in normal saline solution and should not be mixed with other medications. Admixture with dextrose-containing solutions or with other medications may cause precipitation of the drug. Because of the long half-life of phenytoin, a substantial loading dose is required to obtain therapeutic levels in a short period of time. The typical loading dose for phenytoin in SE is 18–20 mg/kg, given no faster than 50 mg/minute. Thus, a full loading dose will take approximately 20–30 minutes to be completely infused. Typical blood levels of phenytoin after such an infusion are 10–13 mg/L; thus, if seizures continue after a loading dose, an additional 5–10 mg/kg may be given.

When given too rapidly, phenytoin has been associated with severe arterial hypotension, although Wilder and colleagues[95] did not note hypotension at infusion rates of even 93 mg/minute. Cranford et al.[93] noted that hypotension was more frequent in the elderly patient. Shaner and coworkers[96] did not note a significant difference in the occurrence of hypotension or arrhythmias in patients treated with phenobarbital or phenytoin and diazepam. Louis et al.[96] demonstrated that propylene glycol, in which the intravenous form of phenytoin is dissolved when administered intravenously, can produce arterial hypotension and bradycardia, as well as arrhythmias that are actually reduced by premedication with phenytoin. These authors also demonstrated that intravenous administration of phenytoin in cats in nonglycol solutions produced a mild drop in blood pressure but no ECG changes, bradycardia, or arrhythmia. They suggested that the glycol diluent played a major role in the cardiac side effects attributed to intravenous phenytoin infusions. This is supported by the work of Wyte and Berk,[98] in which 57 patients with oral phenytoin overdose (levels > 40 mg/L) were studied. These patients did not demonstrate any evidence of change in heart rate or ECG and did not experience any phenytoin-related arrhythmias.

Whatever the etiology of cardiac side effects from intravenous infusion of phenytoin, significant arrhythmias have rarely been seen during this infusion in humans. These include bradycardia, heart block, and asystole.[99–102] Earnest et al.[103] studied the complications of intravenous phenytoin infusion in 200 patients. In this series, they noted only 3 cases (1.5%) with arterial hypotension and bradycardia, which were only minimally symptomatic and resolved with halting the phenytoin infusion. Two patients (1%) in that study experienced "premature contractions" and two experienced sinoatrial nodal block, both of which were transient. Despite the low frequency of cardiac complications from intravenous phenytoin infusion, continuous ECG monitoring should be ongoing during intravenous phenytoin loading. Bradycardia, widening of the QT interval, or arterial hypotension is an indication to slow or stop phenytoin infusion. If needed, coincident administration of low-dose intravenous dopamine may be helpful in maintaining blood pressure during intravenous phenytoin infusion.

Barbiturates

Phenobarbital is a safe, inexpensive drug that may be administered orally, intravenously, or intramuscularly. From a neuropharmacologic perspective, phenobarbital acts on the GABA A receptor–chloride channel complex. Its primary action is to potentiate the effects of GABA in inducing inhibitory postsynaptic potentials.

Phenobarbital is 40%–60% protein bound. Its volume of distribution is similar to that of phenytoin (0.6–0.7 L/kg[104]), but its half-life of 87–100 hours[104] is much longer than that of phenytoin. Phenobarbital is hydroxylated and glucuronidated in the liver. Both phenobarbital and its metabolites are excreted in the urine. Approximately 40% of an administered dose of phenobarbital is excreted unchanged, while the remainder is excreted as inactive metabolites. Peak serum concentrations are achieved within 6–8 hours after oral administration. However, after intravenous administration, brain concentrations can become significant in less than 5 minutes[105] and reach peak levels within 30 minutes. Shaner et al.[96] reported a response latency for treatment with phenytoin and diazepam to be approximately 15 minutes, whereas the response latency for treatment with intravenous phenobarbital was only 5 minutes, supporting the fact that phenobarbital may rapidly cross the blood-brain barrier.

For the treatment of SE, phenobarbital is typically administered after adequate dosages of benzodiazepines and phenytoin have failed to terminate seizures either clinically or electrographically. Shaner and associates,[96] however, indicate that the use of only a phenobarbital infusion can be quite effective in rapidly terminating seizures. A 20 mg/kg loading dose of phenobarbital is typically given in SE by rapid infusion at a rate less than 100 mg/minute. This rapid infusion is stopped or slowed if the seizures terminate during the infusion. If hypotension occurs with intravenous administration, it may be ameliorated by slowing the infusion rate. If seizures persist and hypotension occurs during phenobarbital infusion, the infusion should be continued and a pressor such as dopamine should be administered at low dose. The patient should not be volume depleted.

Most patients who require intravenous phenobarbital as a second-line agent for the treatment of SE will require ventilatory support, since respiratory depression is a significant side effect of phenobarbital. This is especially true when other sedating medications, such as benzodiazepines, have already been administered. One of the drawbacks of using phenobarbital is that its long half-life often mandates that patients remain intubated for prolonged periods, thus increasing respiratory complications and morbidity, as well as prolonging stay in the intensive care unit.

In addition to phenobarbital, other barbiturates are useful in the management of seizures. Walker et al.[106] surveyed intensive care specialists in England and found that approximately 10% of respondents used phenobarbital and 10% used thiopental infusions early in treatment of status refractory to Dilantin and diazepam; 80% indicated that thiopental was their drug of choice for SE that continued despite all other measures. Pentobarbital was chosen by only 1% of respondents in this study, although the use of pentobarbital is more popular in the United States.

Pentobarbital has a half-life of 11–50 hours and

has no active metabolites, whereas thiopental has a somewhat longer half-life and saturable kinetics and has pentobarbital as one of its metabolites. Thiopental has also been shown to be associated with a greater degree of cardiac toxicity than pentobarbital.[107] In particular, Roesch et al.[107] demonstrated more ventricular arrhythmias in animals treated with thiopental than animals treated with pentobarbital at doses less than those required to cause a flat EEG. At higher doses than those required to produce a flat EEG, only 2 of 7 dogs treated with thiopental survived while all 17 dogs treated with pentobarbital survived. In this regard, it is well known that pentobarbital causes dose-dependent decreases in systemic blood pressure[107] as well as a negative inotropic effect on the heart that is responsive to dobutamine.[108] Thus, we prefer pentobarbital over thiopental when treatment with phenytoin, lorazepam, and phenobarbital is unsuccessful at stopping seizures.

A number of studies have investigated the role of high-dose pentobarbital infusions in order to stop seizures refractory to lorazepam, phenobarbital, and phenytoin.[109–116] All studies indicate a high mortality (16%–77%) of patients with refractory status requiring high-dose pentobarbital infusions, likely due to the underlying nature of the neurologic injury associated with refractory seizures. Our usual protocol for such infusions involves administration of pentobarbital at a rate of less than 100 mg/minute until seizures stop. This usually occurs at a total dose of 10–20 mg/kg pentobarbital, although a rare patient has required significantly more than this to stop seizures. Once the seizures stop, a continuous infusion of 1–4 mg/kg/hour is instituted and titrated to keep the EEG in a burst-suppression pattern for 24 hours. The pentobarbital infusion is then tapered off over the next 24 hours. If seizures recur, pentobarbital infusion is reinstituted for another 48 hours and then discontinued slowly over the following 24 hours.

Propofol

Propofol (2,6 di-isopropylphenol) is an alkylphenol that has been used as a general anesthetic. It has been demonstrated that propofol increases chloride conductances into neurons and thus facilitates synaptic inhibitory effects of GABA.[117] A number of authors have reported its use in treating SE.[118–120] Propofol has a number of potential advantages in the treatment of refractory SE over the barbiturates, in that it has an extremely large volume of distribution of 10–12 L/kg and, after administration, quickly partitions into body lipid with a half-life of 2–4 minutes.

In our experience, a loading dose of 2 mg/kg given over 10 minutes can be effective in eliminating refractory seizures. However, because of the short half-life of propofol, continuous electrographic monitoring must be available in order to determine the rate of continuous infusion needed to maintain the EEG in a burst-suppression pattern. The rate of maintenance infusion is usually between 1 and 12 mg/kg/hour. It is of extreme importance that the propofol infusion not be stopped suddenly, as this will often produce seizures. Our usual protocol is to continue the propofol infusion to maintain EEG burst-suppression for 24 hours and then taper the infusion by 5% of the initial rate each hour until it is discontinued.

The advantages of propofol include the ability to rapidly treat seizures and to rapidly leave the CNS after treatment, thus potentially reducing the recovery time for patients. There are, however, a number of potential problems. Propofol infusions do significantly reduce the arterial blood pressure, especially in patients who are volume depleted. Pressors must be available during the infusion and are almost always required. Propofol is a powerful respiratory suppressant, and thus the patient must be intubated prior to or at the time of treatment. Because of its short half-life, continuous electrographic monitoring must be available and be interpreted in real time in order to control the dosing of the propofol.

Propofol should be considered a promising agent for the treatment of status, but additional studies will be required to fully define the dosing and its effectiveness relative to high-dose barbiturate therapy.

Paraldehyde

Paraldehyde was one of the mainstays in the treatment of SE. In the review of Rowan and Scott,[59] describing patients seen in the years 1948–1968, this treatment was used in 42 of 50 episodes of SE. In adults, paraldehyde is best administered in established status as a continuous infusion of 50–100 mL/hour of a 4%–5% solution dissolved in 5% dextrose in water. Extreme caution must be taken because paraldehyde reacts with rubber and plastics, is locally toxic if given too rapidly, and decomposes rapidly.[121] It may be associated with a lesser degree of hypotension than other agents, but carries with it the risk of pulmonary hemorrhage, pulmonary edema, as well as some degree of arterial hypotension and renal or hepatic failure.[122] Paraldehyde is not available in intravenous form in the United States.

Chloral Hydrate

Lampl et al.[123] noted the chemical similarities between chloral hydrate and paraldehyde and observed the effects of administering chloral hydrate to five patients with status in whom treatment had failed with 20 mg of intravenous diazepam and a 20 mg/kg load of intravenous phenytoin. Chloral hydrate administration was begun within 30–50 minutes of the onset of status. All patients received a rectal dose of 30 mg/kg and all experienced cessation of seizures within 5–12 minutes, although two of five patients experienced recurrent seizures 8–21 hours after administration of chloral hydrate. No patient experienced a significant complication of treatment that was directly attributable to the drug.

Because of the minimal information available on the use of chloral hydrate in this situation, its use should be reserved for those cases in which more standard treatments have failed, such as treatment with high-dose barbiturates.

Chlormethiazole

Chlormethiazole is related to the thiazole moiety of thiamine[124] and is thought to act by potentiation of GABA at the GABA A receptor.[125] It is often used in the United Kingdom to treat SE, but its use in the United States is rare. Walker and colleagues[106] reported that approximately 12% of intensivists treating SE in the United Kingdom considered this their first-line agent for status refractory to phenytoin and lorazepam. Harvey et al.[126] studied the effect of chlormethiazole in nine patients with status refractory to treatment with diazepam and/or thiopental. Seizures stopped in all patients with an infusion rate of 500–1000 mg/hour (as a .8 g/100 mL solution), although seizures returned in two patients on this treatment. No patient experienced arterial hypotension or other significant side effects from the drug in this study.[126] Noreng and coworkers[127] confirmed this experience in the treatment of a single child with SE.

One positive aspect of treatment with this agent is its relatively short half-life of 5.3 hours.[124] Drawbacks include the potential for saturation kinetics,[121] especially when an infusion is continued for longer than 12 hours. Local thrombophlebitis, arterial hypotension, fluid overload, adsorption of the drug to PVC tubing, and electrolyte imbalances are other potential complications of its use. This agent is considered investigational in the United States but appears very promising.

Lidocaine

Lidocaine is occasionally suggested in the treatment of refractory seizures.[91] Pascual et al.[128] studied the effect of lidocaine in the treatment of SE in 36 patients who suffered a total of 42 episodes of status. Fourteen patients received diazepam and phenytoin prior to lidocaine infusion, and 22 received phenytoin and then lidocaine prior to infusion of diazepam. In this experience, 74% of episodes of status were considered responsive to an initial dose of 1.5–2 mg/kg given over 2 minutes; however, in 60% of the patients responding to lidocaine, seizures recurred between 3 and 30 minutes after the initial bolus. Many of the patients that experienced seizure recurrence after the initial lidocaine bolus responded to a second bolus and then to a continuous infusion of 3–5 mg/kg/hour. In particular, 3 out of 7 patients treated with this continuous infusion experienced cessation of seizures while the infusion was continued. The other 4 patients experienced either no or transient responses to the infusion.

Our own limited experience with the use of lidocaine has not been very favorable, and so we would recommend that treatment of SE with lidocaine be reserved to those patients who do not respond or cannot tolerate more standard therapies.

Valproate

Vajda et al.[129] administered 200–800 mg of sodium valproate in lipid-based suppositories every 6 hours to patients with an average of 12 seizures per day. Valproic acid levels greater than 50 μg/mL were obtained 24–48 hours after initiation of treatment. With this regimen, the frequency of seizures diminished gradually and eventually complete control was obtained in five of six patients studied. Although therapeutic concentrations of valproic acid can be obtained rectally, the slow time course over which therapeutic levels are attained and seizures are controlled makes this a poor choice for patients with ongoing seizures, although patients with intermittent discrete seizures may benefit.

Anesthetics

General anesthesia with inhalational anesthetics has been suggested in the treatment of refractory SE. Among the various available agents, Ropper et al.[130] suggest that isoflurane may be more effective than either nitrous oxide or halothane and does not have the systemic side effects of halothane. A number of investigators have reported on the use of isoflurane in managing refractory status.[130–133] Their experience has been that, in general, this treatment is very effective in doses of .5–2%. However, seizures often recur after treatment. Kofke et al.[132] noted that in 8 of 11 patients treated with isoflurane, seizures recurred immediately after treatment. Arterial hypotension is also common during treatment. It is clear that, although this treatment is effective in the short term, seizure recurrence and the necessity of using an operating room with continuous EEG monitoring during treatment suggest that this treatment be used mainly as a temporary measure, while the etiology of the patient's seizures is investigated, and while other anticonvulsants are brought up to therapeutic levels.

Treatment of Status Epilepticus

Although there is a bewildering array of medical treatments for SE, the most important rules in successfully treating status are, in order of importance:

1. DON'T PANIC![134]
2. Ensure that the patient is stable from the pulmonary and cardiac standpoints.
3. Do not expect that timely treatment will occur without a neurologist being physically present.
4. Use a medication regimen with which you are familiar. Do not use a new regimen just because it is the subject of a number of recent papers.
5. Do not forget to seek an etiology and assess overall prognosis.

With these cautionary statements aside, we will now outline a protocol for treating patients with SE, which is graphically illustrated, in part, in Figures 4–9 through 4–11.

Hyperacute Management (Time 0–40 Minutes)

INITIAL ASSESSMENT

As in other emergency situations, the initial management of a patient with SE should consist of the ABCs: airway, breathing, and circulation. Respiratory compromise may become a problem in the patient with SE for several reasons. First, aspiration of food, gastric contents, or oral secretions can predispose the individual to pneumonia or the acute respiratory distress syndrome. In addition, these secretions may partially occlude the airway, making effective air exchange difficult. Although patients with seizures do not "swallow their tongue," the tongue can certainly occlude the airway in the unconscious patient. Thus, inspection of the oropharynx should routinely be performed if possible, and a nasal airway inserted if possible. It is generally counterproductive to place anything in the mouth, as this can cause damage to the patient's teeth and may potentially force objects in the mouth into the patient's trachea.

Continuous monitoring of oxygen saturation using pulse oximetry is a valuable addition to the clinical examination in determining when there is significant respiratory compromise. However, it must be noted that oxygen saturation will be only a later indicator of respiratory compromise, and intermittent assessment of respiratory rate or arterial CO_2 concentrations is important as well. An arterial blood gas measurement should be obtained at some point early in the patient's course, as further documentation of the patient's respiratory status. Each patient with SE should have supplemental oxygen delivered by means of either nasal canula or facemask. The head and neck should be placed in a position that will help minimize the possibility of aspiration. In most individuals, placement of an endotracheal tube can be avoided, although if high-dose barbiturates are infused, virtually all patients will require intubation.

Assessment and subsequent monitoring of heart rate and rhythm should be initiated immediately by examination and telemetry. The blood pressure should be measured immediately by cuff and monitored intermittently.

At least one intravenous line should be established at this time, with a larger (16–18) gauge being better than a smaller (22) gauge catheter.

At the same time that treatment is commencing, it is important to obtain relevant and important elements of the patient's history. In the emergency department setting, where little information may be available about a patient who arrives in SE, a quick search for a Medic-Alert bracelet or necklace may be useful in identifying a patient with epilepsy or another important chronic medical condition that may be useful in discovering the etiology of seizures (such as a diabetic who may be suffering from hypoglycemia following an insulin overdosage). In addition, any available relatives, friends, or Emergency Medical Teams may provide critical pieces of the patient's medical and medication history. Important questions to ask include whether there is a history of epilepsy, prior brain injury or tumor, toxic ingestion, or substance abuse. It is also important to ascertain whether the patient is taking any medications. In the emergency room, valuable information about the onset of the event may be available from the ambulance or fire rescue team that brought the patient to the hospital. In particular, evidence that the patient's seizures were preceded by an anoxic event caused by a primary cardiac or respiratory event should be aggressively sought. In the hospital setting, similar information may be obtained from a quick chart and medication list review.

INITIAL MEDICAL TREATMENT

As the patient's intravenous line is inserted, blood is drawn for a complete blood count, electrolytes, calcium, magnesium, blood urea nitrogen and creatinine, liver function studies, and serum anticonvulsant levels of phenytoin, carbamazepine, phenobarbital, and valproate, if the patient's anticonvulsant medication history is unknown. A serum and urine

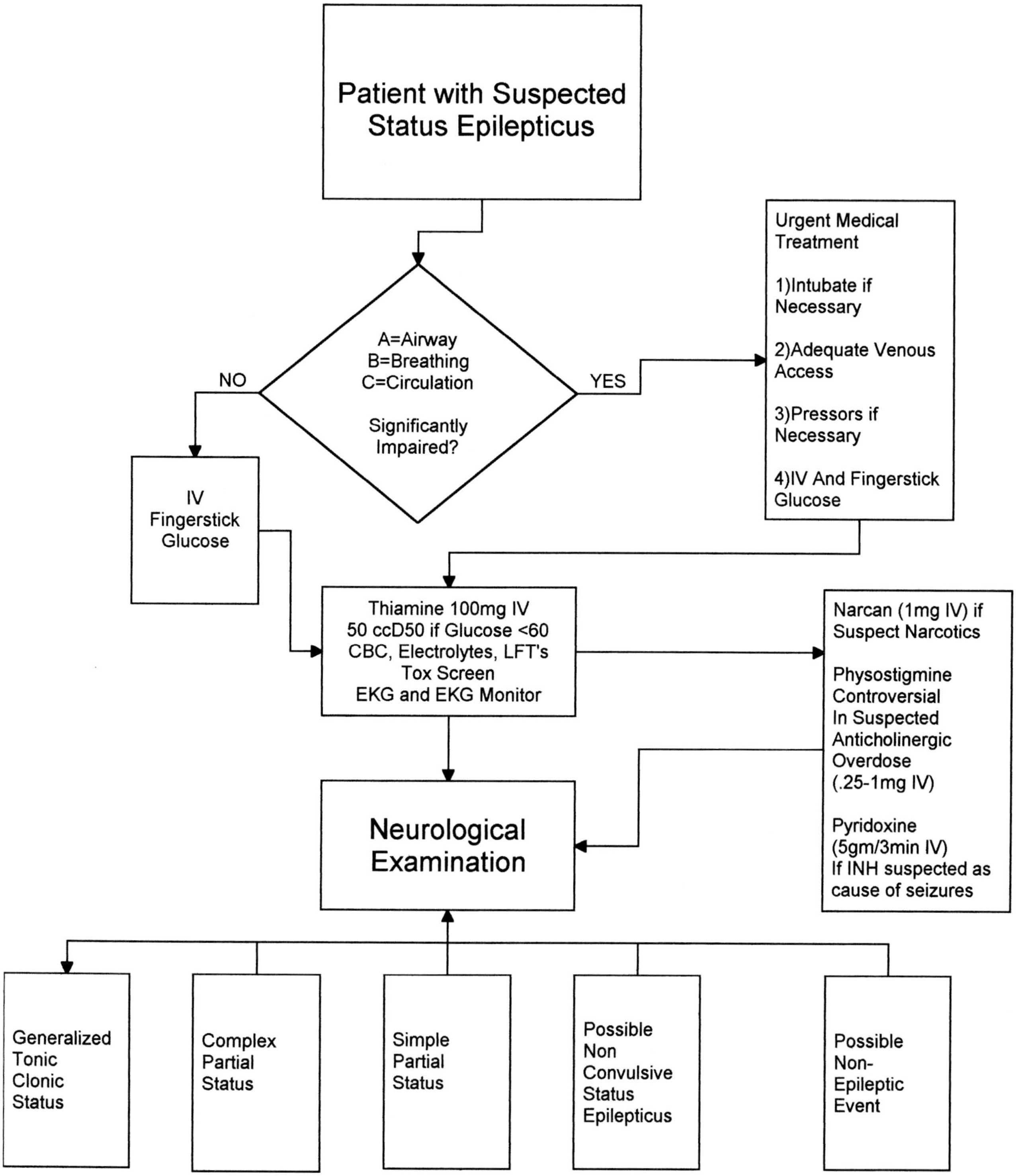

FIGURE 4-9 • Flow chart illustrating an approach to managing patients with suspected status epilepticus. IV, intravenous; D50, 50% dextrose; CBC, cell blood count; LFT's, liver function tests; Tox, toxicologic; EKG, electrocardiogram; INH, isonicotine hydrazine (used for preparations of isoniazid).

screen for ingestion of toxic substances such as cocaine, amphetamines, narcotics, barbiturates, tricyclic antidepressants, and benzodiazepines should be sent if the etiology for status is not clearly evident. A blood alcohol level (ethanol and methanol) is also important, since acute ethanol or methanol intoxication or ethanol withdrawal can precipitate seizures. Because a potential cause of seizures is hypoglycemia, even in patients who do not take oral hypoglycemic agents or insulin, a fingerstick glu-

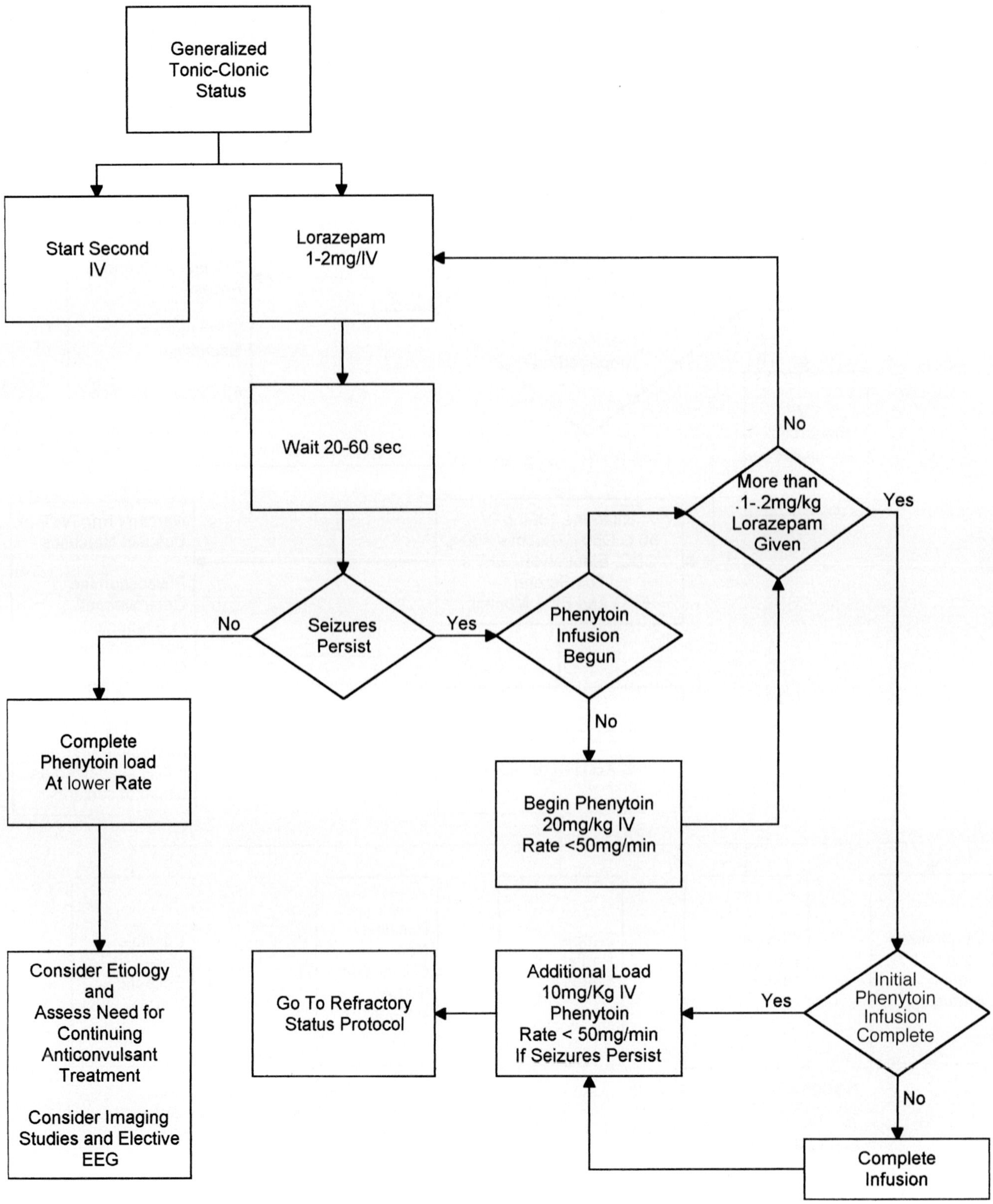

FIGURE 4–10 • Flow chart illustrating the initial phases of management of patients with generalized tonic-clonic or complex partial status. IV, intravenous; EEG, electroencephalogram.

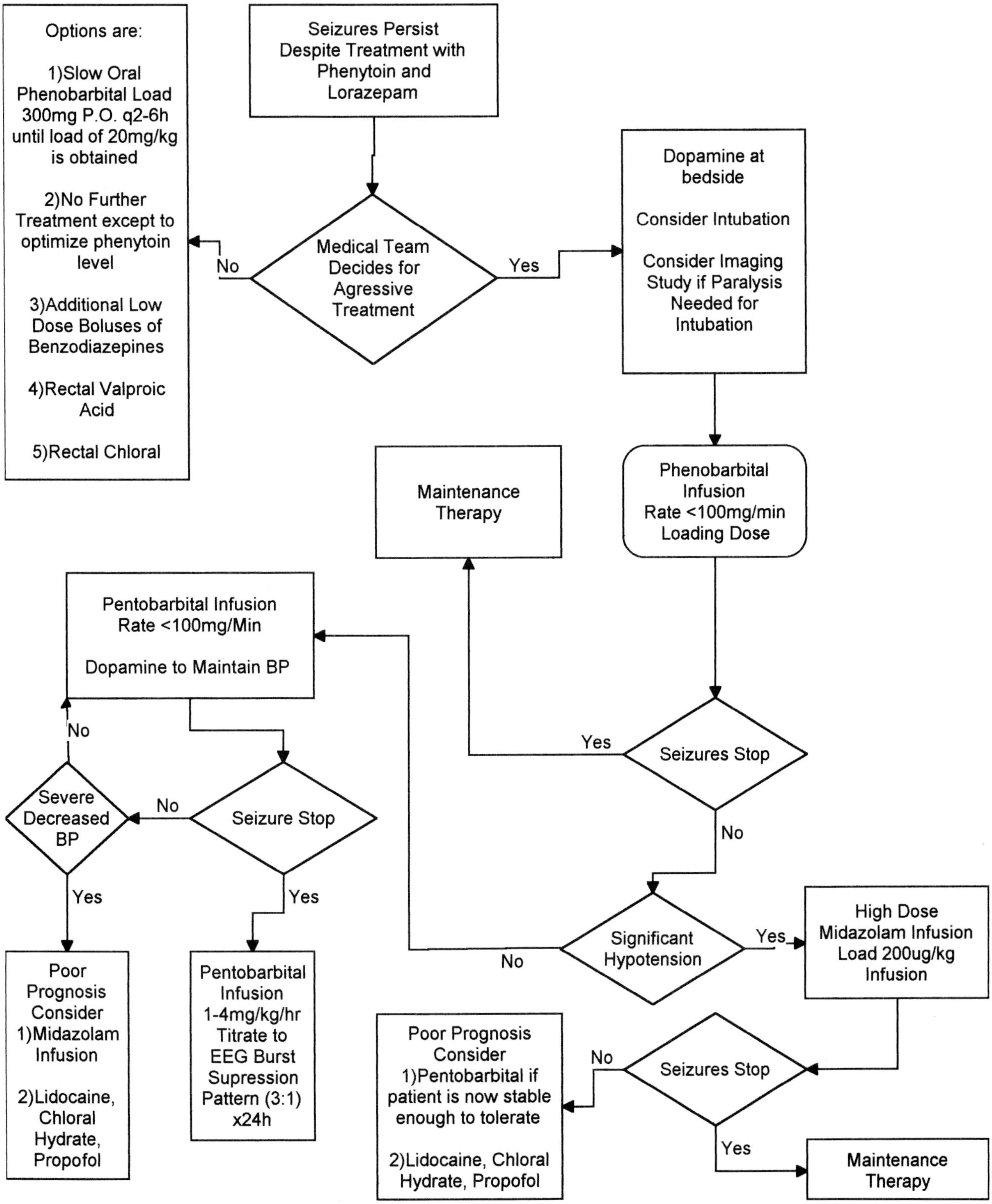

FIGURE 4-11 • Flow chart illustrating the treatment of patients with refractory status epilepticus. P.O., per oral route; q 2-6h, every 2 to 6 hours; BP, blood pressure; EEG, electroencephalogram; ×24h, over 24-hour period.

cose measure should be obtained early in the patient's course prior to the administration of anticonvulsant drugs. In the adult patient, if the fingerstick glucose concentration is less than 60 mg/dL or a fingerstick glucose cannot be obtained, a single bolus of 50 mL of 50% dextrose should be administered until the results of the laboratory glucose measurement are available. Before administration of glucose, 100 mg of intravenous thiamine should be given.

INITIAL NEUROLOGIC ASSESSMENT

Once all of the steps have been performed, it is appropriate to conduct a brief neurologic assessment as discussed above. The goal of this assessment is to determine whether there is a high likelihood of SE and what type of status there is. The initial categorization should include whether the patient is likely to have generalized tonic-clonic status, simple partial status, or nonconvulsive SE. The remainder of the protocol outlined below will be for generalized tonic-clonic status. Later we discuss the differences between the treatment of generalized tonic-clonic status, simple partial status, and nonconvulsive status.

INITIAL PHARMACOLOGIC TREATMENT

At this point, it is usually 5–7 minutes after the patient's seizures have come to medical attention. In the adult patient, pharmacologic treatment begins usually with 1–2 mg of intravenous lorazepam given over 60 seconds. We use this in preference to 5–7 mg of diazepam because of the longer duration of action in seizure suppression of lorazepam. In older patients, it is often wise to start with as little as 1 mg IV and, in younger patients or known alcohol abusers, with 2 mg IV. If convulsions continue and the patient remains stable from the cardiac and pulmonary standpoints in the next 60 seconds, another 1–2 mg is infused over another 60 seconds with careful monitoring of respiration and blood pressure. At this time, another intravenous line should be inserted so that a longer acting agent such as phenytoin can be infused. Phenytoin should not be infused through the same tubing as the lorazepam, unless it has been flushed vigorously. This is because there is a high risk of precipitating the phenytoin if traces of lorazepam or diazepam remain in the tubing. This could occlude the intravenous line and render it useless.

If seizures persist at this point, an intravenous infusion of phenytoin should be begun at a rate of 50 mg/minute and should target a loading dose of 20 mg/kg through the second intravenous line. This infusion will take approximately 20 minutes to complete. During this period of time, as long as the patient remains stable, additional doses of lorazepam 1–2 mg IV can be given up to a typical dose of 0.1–0.15 mg/kg (although, in some circumstances, we have successfully used up to 0.25 mg/kg). It is important to know that it can take 30–60 seconds for lorazepam to have its maximal effect, and so one should wait at least this long between additional doses in order to fully assess its effect.

Acute Management (40–80 Minutes)

If seizures persist after treatment with a loading dose of 20 mg/kg of phenytoin and up to 0.15 mg/kg lorazepam, another 10 mg/kg loading dose of phenytoin can be administered again at a rate of up to 50 mg/minute. If this is unsuccessful, the next level of treatment involves the use of barbiturates. At this point, it is important to be aware of a number of issues before proceeding.

First, patients may experience an "electromechanical dissociation" after treatment, in that clinically evident SE may stop while the EEG reveals continuous ictal activity. Thus, it is appropriate if the patient has stopped having clinical seizure activity, but does not begin to become more responsive over time, to obtain an EEG in order to rule out nonconvulsive status.

Second, if the patient has not already been intubated at this point, this is a good time to intubate. Most patients will be at a high risk of aspiration if seizures continue at this point, and in addition, the risk of significant respiratory depression when barbiturates and benzodiazepines are combined is high. If continuous EEG monitoring is not available at this point, it is important to use only short-acting neuromuscular blocking agents, such as vecuronium or atracurium, in order to facilitate the intubation. Long-term neuromuscular blockade will make it impossible to determine clinically whether the patient is still in status without the help of the EEG.

Third, if EEG monitoring is not already in place and there is a high suspicion for a structural lesion, it may be appropriate at this point to obtain an imaging study such as CT or MRI, after adequate positioning of the endotracheal tube is confirmed. This is true because it will be difficult to assess the patient while he or she is paralyzed and, hence, the effect of additional treatment for status cannot be assessed. This is also an appropriate time for an imaging study, not only because the patient will not be moving due to the paralytic agents, but also because the patient will be more stable from a cardiovascular standpoint than after treatment with high-dose barbiturates.

Fourth, because the use of barbiturates after phenytoin and lorazepam will likely be associated with a prolonged intubation and ICU stay, issues of prognosis must be addressed at this stage. For example, in a patient with end-stage metastatic cancer, it may be more appropriate to consider alternative treatments depending on the wishes of the patient and family. These might include treatment with lidocaine or propofol. Another option that we have used often is a slow oral load of phenobarbital (described below under simple partial status), which can be effective in patients who would be expected to be at high risk if they required intubation.

Once the decision is made to continue aggressive treatment, the patient is intubated, the decision has been made as to whether or not to obtain an imaging study, and there is evidence that seizures are continuing either clinically or by EEG, a dopamine infusion is placed at bedside. Once this is done, infusion of phenobarbital at a rate of less than 100 mg/minute to a total dose of 10–25 mg/kg is infused. If seizures stop during this infusion, the smaller dose can be given; but if seizures persist, the larger dose can be administered. This can be done either by continuous intravenous infusion or by intermittent bolus infusion. In any case, it is important to very carefully monitor blood pressure during this time. Usually the neurologist, in conjunction with the medical team, sets a well-defined level of blood pressure parameters at this stage. As a general guideline, if the patient's blood pressure drops below 90 mm Hg systolic in a young person, or more than 25 mm Hg below the usual blood pressure for a patient with suspected cerebrovascular disease, the dopamine infusion is started and titrated to keep the pressure within a predefined range. The phenobarbital infusion may be slowed somewhat but should not be discontinued unless severe arterial hypotension develops. It is important to make sure that the patient is not volume depleted, and infusions of normal saline or albumin may be of great value in maintaining the patient's blood pressure in addition to the dopamine. Close attention to the electrocardiogram may indicate signs of cardiac ischemia due to arterial hypotension.

Management of Refractory Status

If seizures persist despite treatment with phenytoin, lorazepam, and phenobarbital, one next step is to begin treatment with pentobarbital. General anesthesia with inhalational agents is another possibility but involves moving an unstable patient from the ICU to the operating room and is associated with a significant risk of seizure recurrence. Thus, this is not the favored choice under most circumstances. Propofol may be useful in this situation, but its use under these circumstances has been studied less than that of pentobarbital and, more importantly, neurologists are less familiar with propofol than pentobarbital. Thus, pentobarbital infusion would be favored at this point, unless the patient is at high risk of complications of long-term sedation and an anesthesiologist is available to assist with management.

Another alternative at this point is a high-dose midazolam infusion and, although good success has been noted with this treatment, it is still less well studied than pentobarbital in this situation. Midazolam infusion, however, becomes the treatment of choice when the patient experiences severe hypotension from barbiturates, since midazolam is generally associated with less arterial hypotension than pentobarbital infusion.[86] It may also be better to use midazolam in patients with multiorgan failure, as Yaffe and Lowenstein[110] have indicated that this group of patients is at an extremely high risk if receiving pentobarbital infusions. Labar et al.[136] have also suggested that an intravenous lorazepam infusion may be of value for the same reasons.

Before the pentobarbital infusion begins, it is extremely helpful to have continuous EEG monitoring to guide treatment. Pentobarbital infusion is begun at a rate of less than 100 mg/minute and continues until seizures stop or until significant arterial hypotension ensues. By this period, it will be evident how the patient's blood pressure responds to barbiturates, and so the infusion can be tailored to a rate that is appropriate to the individual. Although the typical loading dose is approximately 10 mg/kg, occasionally significantly higher doses need to be administered in order to stop the seizures. In rare circumstances, certain patients have required up to 60 mg/kg of pentobarbital in order to stop seizures! If seizures are controlled, or arterial hypotension ensues before their control, a continuous infusion of 1–4 mg/kg/hour can be instituted while other therapies are attempted. Our choice in this situation would be a midazolam infusion begun with a bolus of 200 μg/kg and continued at a rate of 1–20 μg/kg/minute. If this is not successful, other treatments such as lidocaine or chloral hydrate could be attempted. However, if seizures persist at this point, the likelihood of neurologic survival is very small.

Maintenance Therapy

Once seizures stop, the pentobarbital infusion is titrated in the range of 0.5–6 mg/kg/hour (although typically 1–4 mg/kg/hour is required) to keep the EEG in a burst-suppression pattern. The burst-suppression pattern is chosen primarily because it is easy to identify visually, so housestaff and nurses can titrate the infusion without the assistance of an electroencephalographer. Usually the target is to have three times as much suppression as burst in the record (3:1) if the patient's blood pressure will tolerate this.

During this period of time, it is important to realize that the patient will have a complete ileus and, hence, must receive all nutrition parenterally. The patient will also likely lose all reflexes, even pupillary reflexes, and so must be turned on a regular basis to prevent decubitus ulcers. A Foley catheter is also necessary, as bladder contractility will be diminished. Because the patient will not have cough and gag reflexes, good pulmonary toilet is important as well.

After 24 hours of pentobarbital infusion titrated to burst-suppression, maintenance anticonvulsant levels are checked and maintained in the high therapeutic range. This usually includes phenytoin levels of 20–25 mg/L and phenobarbital levels of 30–40 mg/L. Clinically, one can decide either to continue both phenytoin and phenobarbital as maintenance anticonvulsants or to continue only the phenobarbital. In our experience, there is not much difference between these alternatives, although this has not been studied formally. The pentobarbital infusion is then tapered off over a period of 12–24 hours, with intermittent EEG monitoring to observe for seizure recurrence. If seizures recur during this taper, a small bolus of pentobarbital is given to stop the seizures, and the continuous infusion is again begun at a rate that will be sufficient to regain seizure control and produce a burst-suppression pattern on the EEG. The pentobarbital infusion is then continued for another 48–60 hours and is tapered over 24 hours with maintenance anticonvulsant levels of at least 45 mg/L for phenobarbital and 22–26 mg/L for phenytoin.

If seizures recur in this setting, the prognosis is extremely poor and, in only exceptional cases, do we reinstitute barbiturate coma. Exceptions occur when another factor is found that can be ameliorated, such as a severe worsening CNS infection, severe hyponatremia, etc. It must be remembered, however, that patients may experience some myoclonus during recovery from barbiturate coma, and that the EEG can display periodic complexes during this time. Therefore, one should take great care in diagnosing recurrent seizures. Consideration may be given to rectal valproic acid or rectal carbamazepine at this point, although the therapeutic value of such treatment will be low.

Simple Partial Status

The treatment of simple partial SE is different from that of generalized tonic-clonic status, since there is less of a risk of systemic injury from seizures that are localized than seizures that are generalized. In addition, as the patient with simple partial status is awake by definition, it is likely that the risk of aspiration will be low. In this situation, the cardinal rule is to not cause more problems with treatment than the seizure itself would cause.

The first step is to consider the results of a fingerstick glucose. If the patient's fingerstick glucose level is high and there is no other evidence of a neurologic abnormality, the major treatment is based on lowering the glucose levels. With this approach, seizures will usually stop without additional anticonvulsants. If a fingerstick glucose concentration is not available or is not greater than approximately 300 mg/dL, small amounts of intravenous lorazepam (0.5–1 mg) can be given slowly intravenously and then repeated in 2–5 minutes. The rapidity and aggressiveness of treatment depend on how severe the simple partial seizures are. If there is just minor twitching in, for example, a hand muscle, treatment should progress gradually and slowly in order to avoid side effects of medication treatment. If, however, there are violent movements of an entire arm or language is significantly affected, it is generally best to be more aggressive in order to prevent injury and rhabdomyolysis. If small amounts of lorazepam are not effective in controlling the seizures, a loading dose of phenytoin can be administered. If the patient is stable and able to swallow, this can often be accomplished orally, in order to avoid the side effects of intravenous phenytoin. Oral phenytoin dosage in these circumstances is 300 mg every 2–6 hours until 20 mg/kg is administered. This purely oral phenytoin load is often too prolonged for some patients, and in this situation, a partial (5–10 mg/kg) intravenous load may be given at a rate of 10–20 mg/minute, followed by 10–15 mg/kg oral load. The phenytoin level should be checked within a few hours of starting the loading dose, with a target of obtaining levels up to 25 mg/L if seizures persist. If phenytoin is not successful, oral phenobarbital or oral carbamazepine (Tegretol) can be useful in the treatment of these patients.

Hepatic and Renal Failure

In tertiary care settings, a relatively large number of patients with status may have severe hepatic or renal failure. It is important to know how to treat these patients appropriately for SE. In general, the acute management of these patients is EXACTLY THE SAME as that of any other patient, although there are a number of minor points that are important to realize when treating such patients. These patients may be more heavily sedated for longer periods than other patients from the medication treatment, but the major immediate concern of seizure control outweighs this factor in the short term. Accordingly, the following considerations would apply to managing these patients:

1. Lorazepam would be preferred over diazepam for treatment of seizures in renal or hepatic failure. Lorazepam does not have significant active metabolites, whereas diazepam does. Therefore, the elimination of metabolites may be reduced in either hepatic or renal failure, and the effect of renal or hepatic failure will be greater on diazepam.
2. Phenytoin loading doses are the same as in patients without renal or hepatic failure. This is true despite the fact that, in patients with renal failure, the amount of bound phenytoin is lower than in normals. This effect tends to increase free phenytoin levels and, thus, increase the effect seen with a given total level of phenytoin. However, since the rule in the urgent treatment of status is to treat on the basis of clinical response to medications, this effect is of only minor importance. Such an effect is more important in determining the appropriate maintenance doses of phenytoin to be administered.
3. If the patient is being dialyzed, it is important to know that only a small amount of phenytoin will be removed from the system, because it is highly protein bound. However, a relatively larger amount of phenobarbital or pentobarbital will be removed during dialysis, because these latter agents are less protein bound than phenytoin. In this situation, it is important to obtain pre- and postdialysis anticonvulsant levels and to give additional barbiturate doses as necessary during dialysis.

CLINICAL CASES

Because of the heterogeneity of patients with SE, it would be incorrect to consider any of the above treatment guidelines as hard-and-fast rules. It is, thus, as important to know the times when the above guidelines are useful, as when they break down. Accordingly, discussion of a number of difficult clinical scenarios can be of great importance, as follows:

Illustrative Case 1

A 25-year-old asthmatic patient suffered a respiratory and subsequent cardiac arrest. The time between arrest and initiation of cardiopulmonary resuscitation (CPR) was 10 minutes. Another 5 minutes of CPR were required before a spontaneous cardiac rhythm and blood pressure could be obtained. On arrival in the emergency room, her initial pH was 6.80 with an arterial P_{CO_2} of 55 torr and P_{O_2} of 30 torr. Her initial neurologic examination revealed intact pupillary responses but otherwise absent brain stem reflexes, and no response to painful stimulation. She was intubated and brought to the medical intensive care unit. A few hours later, it was noted that her brain stem reflexes had been recovered, including corneals and oculocephalics, but there was now focal twitching of the left hand. An EEG was ordered and revealed continuous ictal activity beginning over the right hemisphere and occasionally spreading to the left. An intravenous injection of lorazepam (2 mg) was administered without effect, and a phenytoin load of 20 mg/kg at a rate of 50 mg/minute was begun. Additional boluses of lorazepam to a total dose of 10 mg were given, which did not stop the underlying ictal activity even after the phenytoin infusion had ended and the patient's blood pressure had decreased by 40 mm Hg (to 80/50 mm Hg).

This is a difficult situation but, unfortunately, one that is all too common. The options are to continue to pursue aggressive treatment of status or to reduce the level of treatment based on the overall prognosis. At this point, our preference is to perform a CT scan of the head. This is because the neurologic prognosis is extremely poor, and it would be important to rule out a structural lesion (hemorrhage, etc.), and then to discuss the options with the family. We would encourage treatment with 2–4 mg additional lorazepam and an additional bolus of phenytoin 10 mg/kg (if the patient's blood pressure will tolerate it), but if no response is noted, we would suggest discontinuing EEG monitoring and simply maintaining a phenytoin level in the range of 20–25 mg/L. We would discourage the use of barbiturates because of the poor prognosis of postanoxic SE; however, we would inform the family of this option and that we believe that further treatment would be unlikely (though not impossible) to allow the patient to recover neurologically. We would abide by the family's decisions in this matter.

Illustrative Case 2

A 64-year-old woman with a history of a previous right middle cerebral artery infarct was admitted to the emergency room because of twitching in the left hand that began 8–12 hours earlier. The episodes of twitching lasted 40–60 seconds and involved primarily the abductor pollicis brevis initially, but spread to involve the abductor digiti minimi in the same hand. They recurred every 2–3 minutes. The twitching was not stimulus-sensitive and did not resolve with changing position of the hand. No twitching was noted in other muscle groups. The patient did not seem to be in distress and was not bothered by the twitching. Her fingerstick glucose level was normal, as were the rest of her electrolytes and blood cell count. Initially, 1 mg of intravenous lorazepam was infused without effect on the twitching, although the patient became somewhat lethargic. At this point, an EEG was obtained and demonstrated continuous slowing over the right hemisphere, with frequent spikes over the right frontal regions. No electrographic seizures were seen during episodes of twitching.

The fact that the EEG showed no seizures did not mean that the patient's twitching was not ictal, since the EEG does not always reveal ictal changes during simple partial seizures. It does, however, help to rule out the possibility of complex partial status, which would require more aggressive treatment. At this point, we planned to load the patient orally with 300 mg of phenytoin every 2 hours for four doses. Serum phenytoin level was checked every 6 hours after the phenytoin was begun. This level was 12 mg/L, and an additional 300 mg of oral phenytoin was administered in addition to the doses already planned. On the next day, the twitching persisted, phenytoin blood levels were 25 mg/L, and the patient was slightly lethargic.

One could argue that it would be reasonable to just continue the treatment with phenytoin at this point, as long as the seizure activity did not cause the patient any discomfort. Our belief was that, as long as the patient was doing well without any systemic complications, we should try to continue treating this focal motor seizure. It is hoped that shortening the duration of seizure activity would allow for the potential of additional neuronal recovery. At this point, one could use lorazepam 1 mg IV again, but as this patient previously became lethargic with lorazepam, and this drug would only be a temporizing measure in any case, our preference would be to use a slow oral phenobarbital load. In this case, we would suggest administering 200 mg phenobarbital orally every 6–8 hours until a loading dose of 20 mg/kg is attained. We would slow down the rate of administration if the patient became too lethargic to swallow safely. We would also be certain to obtain vital signs just before and 1 hour after each oral dose of phenobarbital. Aspiration precautions should be taken as well in this situation.

Illustrative Case 3

A 63-year-old right-handed woman presented at the emergency department with a 3-day history of confusion, slurred speech, and falling. She had been neurologically normal until 3 days prior to admission, when dysarthria and confusion were noted. On several occasions, she fell to the ground and was noted to have a right facial asymmetry. On neurologic examination, she appeared somnolent and she was moderately dysarthric. She could state her name and was oriented to year but not date. She could not perform serial sevens but could follow one-step commands. At times she became unresponsive, and a right facial twitch was noted. After approximately 2–3 minutes, she became more arousable again. There was a mild pronator drift on the right, and the right plantar response was extensor.

The initial clinical differential diagnosis included a left hemispheric stroke, recurrent transient ischemic attacks, and recurrent complex partial seizures. A CT scan revealed a 2 × 2 cm left hemispheric meningioma along the sylvian fissure, but no evidence of infarction. EEG revealed focal sharp waves and spikes of maximum amplitude over the left frontotemporal region. During periods of unresponsiveness, electrographic seizures were seen beginning with sharply contoured theta activity in the left frontotemporal region. Following the seizure, there was a brief attenuation of the background activity, with mild left hemispheric slowing.

The clinical picture of this patient was initially suggestive of transient and possibly crescendo ischemic attacks with aphasia versus complex partial SE. The patient had identifiable risks for cerebrovascular disease, such as hypertension, but little in the clinical history to suggest seizures. However, the intermittent twitching and the alternating mental status suggested possible seizures, and this was confirmed by the EEG.

During the EEG, the patient then suffered a generalized tonic-clonic seizure, which was briefly slowed with 4 mg of intravenous lorazepam but which subsequently returned. The patient was loaded with 18 mg/kg of phenytoin without effect. An additional 5 mg/kg of phenytoin was given, and a post-phenytoin bolus level was 28 mg/dL. In the face of ongoing convulsions, the patient was intubated and given intravenous phenobarbital until a burst-suppression pattern was achieved. She remained in the intensive care unit, in burst-suppression for 6 days without further seizures. Intravenous phenobarbital was slowly tapered and switched to oral phenobarbital. She was ultimately discharged from the hospital on phenytoin and phenobarbital, with no obvious neurologic sequelae.

This case underscores several important clinical points regarding the diagnosis of SE. First, in any patient with episodic and transient neurologic dysfunction, or a waxing-and-waning mental status, the diagnosis of recurrent seizures or complex partial SE must be considered. Although in this patient the initial diagnosis was believed to be transient ischemic attacks with aphasia and facial weakness, continuous EEG monitoring in the emergency department was critical in making the diagnosis of SE. Second, even in patients with no history of epilepsy or neurologic disease, SE may be the presenting seizure. Third, neuroimaging plays a central role in the assessment of many neurologic diseases including seizures. In this patient, despite no history of neurologic impairment, she had a meningioma, which likely caused changes in the perisylvian cortex and, thus, was the cause of her seizures. The CT scan ruled out a stroke or intracerebral hemorrhage.

Finally, although this patient initially presented in complex partial SE, she suddenly developed convulsive seizures. It is important when managing patients with SE to be mindful of the possibility of nonconvulsive seizures, so that quick, effective steps may be taken to terminate seizure activity. As discussed earlier, perhaps the single most important indicator of clinical outcome in patients with SE is the duration of seizures prior to termination. In this patient, despite adequate doses of benzodiazepines and phenytoin, phenobarbital was required to control the seizures. However, despite the need for intensive care monitoring and ventilatory support, she ultimately left the hospital without sequelae.

Note that in this patient an intravenous phenobarbital infusion was administered rather than an intravenous pentobarbital infusion. Although both treatment modalities will cause burst-suppression and will likely have similiar anticonvulsant effects, pentobarbital will have a shorter half-life and, hence, reduce the time the patient might have spent in the ICU in burst-suppression.

Illustrative Case 4

A 57-year-old woman was noted in the hospital to have nearly continuous left face, arm, and leg twitching, as well as leftward eye deviation. She had been admitted to the intensive care unit for worsening hepatic failure, aspiration pneumonia requiring ventilatory support, dehydration, mild rhabdomyolisis, and possible sepsis in the setting of chronic alcohol abuse and acute intoxication. There was a history of two prior generalized tonic-clonic seizures related to alcohol withdrawal several years previously, although she was not maintained on anticonvulsants. Within the 48 hours prior to the onset of her left-hemibody twitching, she had developed progressive renal failure with rapidly rising blood urea nitrogen (BUN) and creatinine, complicated by hypotension requiring intravenous pressor agents, and fever.

On neurologic examination, she was comatose with only decerebrate posturing to deep pain stimuli. The pupils were 5 mm in diameter and sluggishly reactive to light, while weak oculocephalic reflexes persisted. Reflexes were brisk in the arms and legs and 4^+ at the ankles with clonus. Plantar responses were extensor bilaterally. She was observed to have episodes of twitching approximately every 3 minutes during which the left face, then arm and leg exhibited rhythmic jerking followed by tonic leftward eye deviation. These episodes lasted approximately 3 minutes, after which the patient became motionless until the next episode. Laboratory values were remarkable for a serum sodium of 122 mEq/L, BUN/creatinine of 80/4.4 mg/dL, elevated liver function tests (transaminases and bilirubin), a peripheral white blood cell count of 17,000/mm^3, and a platelet count of 90,000/mm^3. A CT scan of the head performed on the day prior to worsening mental status showed only cerebral cortical atrophy.

Bedside EEG monitoring revealed generalized slowing with mixed low-amplitude theta and delta activity. However, immediately prior to episodes of twitching, there was a rhythmic build-up of generalized low-voltage fast activity evolving to generalized high-amplitude spike wave discharges lasting approximately 2.5 minutes, which correlated with left-sided twitching and eye deviation. Upon termination of seizure activity, the EEG showed periodic lateralized epileptiform discharges for approximately 2 minutes, which were then replaced by diffuse slowing.

The patient was given lorazepam (0.15 mg/kg) in two divided doses without effect. An intravenous phenytoin load (18 mg/kg) was attempted at a rate of 50 mg/minute, but hypotension (systolic blood pressure < 70 mm Hg) and bradycardia (heart rate < 40 beats per minute) were noted. Despite slowing the infusion rate, fluid challenges, and increasing the infusion rate of pressors already being administered, hypotension remained. Phenytoin was discontinued, and the patient's blood pressure began to return to baseline. Intravenous phenobarbital was begun until a burst-suppression pattern was obtained. Over the next 48 hours, the patient remained in a burst-suppression pattern without clinical or electrographic seizures. However, she expired, likely secondary to overwhelming sepsis and respiratory failure.

Management of complicated cases involving SE superimposed on multiple serious medical problems can prove to be a real challenge for the neurologist. However, this case illustrates that, despite numerous potential contributing factors and etiologies encountered, the essential algorithm for treatment of SE remains the same in virtually all patients. Indeed, it is important to stress that, even in spite of multisystem organ failure, the clinician treating SE should maintain the same goal of quickly and effectively terminating seizures. In this patient, multiple possible etiologies could have caused SE. Both hepatic and renal failure are associated with SE, as is hyponatremia. In the patient with alcohol abuse, status may be seen in the withdrawal phase and acutely intoxicated state as well. In addition, moderate head trauma may be a common though often unnoticed occurrence in alcoholic individuals and may cause enough brain injury to provide an anatomic substrate for seizures. This patient had a history of two prior seizures, which should make the clinician sensitive to the possibility of recurrent seizure activity. Finally, in all patients with a history of alcohol abuse, prophylac-

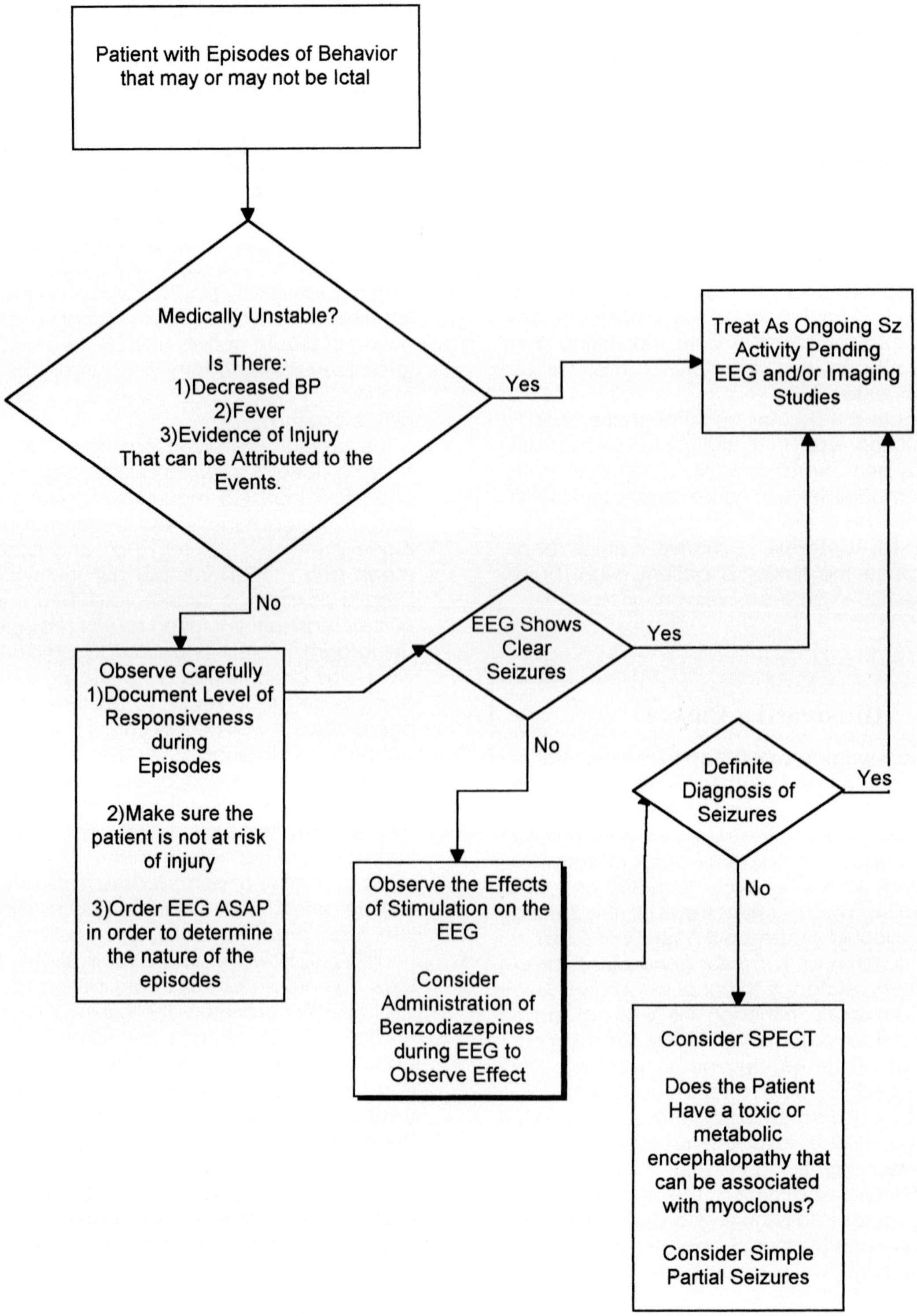

FIGURE 4–12 • Flow chart illustrating an approach to patients with possible nonepileptic events. BP, blood pressure; EEG, electroencephalogram; ASAP, as soon as possible; Sz, seizure; SPECT, single photon emission computed tomography.

tic therapy should be instituted with multivitamins and thiamine (100 mg/day), to prevent or ameliorate Wernicke's encephalopathy.

Although in many patients with acute renal or hepatic failure, the pharmacokinetic metabolism and clearance of anticonvulsants may be altered, in treating SE it is essential that full loading doses be administered. Achieving a high or even toxic phenytoin or phenobarbital level that stops status is far better than inadequately dosing the medication and failing to terminate seizures. However, our patient proved challenging in that, despite multiple methods, she exhibited significant hypotension with the phenytoin infusion and required a more rapid use of phenobarbital. It was difficult to determine whether her hypotension stemmed only from the phenytoin infusion (although this effect is more likely due to the glycol diluent, see above) or also was worsened by her intravascular dehydration and sepsis. Regardless, fluid resuscitation, slowing of the phenytoin infusion, and intravenous pressor agents such as dopamine may aid in completing a full phenytoin loading dose in the setting of infusion-related hypotension.

Illustrative Case 5

A 27-year-old male with a history of seizures in childhood began to have tonic-clonic movements postoperatively, after a urologic procedure. He was unresponsive to verbal stimulation and to painful stimulation. The tonic-clonic movements would be generalized and last from 1–3 minutes, followed by a postictal period of lethargy. These movements persisted despite 6 mg of lorazepam administered intravenously and a loading dose of phenytoin of 20 mg/kg. In preparation for treatment with high-dose barbiturates, an emergency EEG was ordered. The EEG revealed only generalized beta activity and a small amount of diffuse slowing even during the patient's tonic-clonic movements. At this point, nursing staff and medical staff left the bedside and the patient woke up spontaneously. It is important to realize that, occasionally, one will encounter nonepileptic seizures that look outwardly very much like generalized tonic-clonic convulsions. In this particular case, the patient would have been intubated and received high-dose barbiturates without the information provided by the EEG. See Figure 4–12 for an outline of the approach to patients with suspected nonepileptic events.

References

1. Walsh GO, Delgado-Escueta AV: Status epilepticus. Neurol Clin North Am 1993;11:835–856.
2. Lothman E: The biochemical basis and pathophysiology of status epilepticus. Neurology 1990;40(Suppl 2):13–23.
3. Meldrum B: The role of glutamate in epilepsy and other CNS disorders. Neurology 1994;44(Suppl 8):S14–S23.
4. Selzer ME, Dichter MA: Cellular pathophysiology and pharmacology of epilepsy. In Asbury AK, McKhann GM, McDonald WI (eds): Diseases of the Nervous System: Clinical Neurobiology, pp 916–935. Philadelphia, WB Saunders, 1992.
5. Hille B: Ion Channels of Excitable Membranes, pp 1–426. Sunderland, MA, Sinauer Associates, 1984.
6. McNamara JO: Cellular and molecular basis of epilepsy. J Neurosci 1994;14:3413–3425.
7. Connors BW, Gutnick MJ: Intrinsic firing patterns of diverse neocortical neurons. Trends Neurosci 1990;13:99–104.
8. Wong RK, Prince DA: Afterpotential generation in hippocampal pyramidal cells. J Neurophysiol 1981;45:86–97.
9. Gale K: GABA and epilepsy: Basic concepts from preclinical research. Epilepsia 1992;33(Suppl 5):S3–S12.
10. Barnard EA, Darlison MG, Fujita N, et al: Molecular biology of the GABA A receptor. Adv Exp Med Biol 1988;236:31–45.
11. Dichter MA: Modulation of inhibition and the transition to seizures. In Dichter MA (ed): Mechanisms of Epileptogenesis: The Transition to Seizure, pp 169–181. New York, Plenum Publishing, 1988.
12. Greenamyre JT, Porter RH: Anatomy and physiology of glutamate in the CNS. Neurology 1994;44(Suppl 8):S1–S7.
13. Lothman EW, Collins RC: Kainic acid induced limbic seizures: Metabolic, behavioral, electroencephalographic, and neuropathologic correlates. Brain Res 1981;218:299–319.
14. Meldrum BS, Brierly JB: Prolonged epileptic seizures in primates: Ischemic cell change and its relation to ictal physiologic events. Arch Neurol 1973;28:10–17.
15. Rothman SM, Olney JW: Excitotoxicity and the NMDA receptor. Trends Neurosci 1987;10:299–304.
16. Flavin HJ, Wieraszko A, Seyfried TN: Enhanced aspartate release from hippocampal slices of epileptic (EL) mice. J Neurochem 1991;56:1007–1011.
17. During MJ, Spencer DD: Extracellular hippocampal glutamate and spontaneous seizure in the conscious human brain. Lancet 1993;341:1607–1610.
18. McDonald JW, Garofalo EA, Hood T: Altered excitatory and inhibitory amino acid receptor binding in hippocampus of patients with temporal lobe epilepsy. Ann Neurol 1991;29:529–541.
19. Naus CC, Bechberger JF, Paul DL: Gap junction gene expression in human seizure disorder. Exp Neurol 1991;111:198–203.
20. Gall C, Lauterborn J, Isaackson P, et al: Seizures, neuropeptide regulation and mRNA expression in the hippocampus. Prog Brain Res 1990;83:371–390.
21. Labiner DM, Butler LS, Cao Z, et al: Induction of c-fos mRNA by kindled seizures: Complex relationship with neuronal burst firing. J Neurosci 1993;13:744–751.
22. Gall C, Lauterborn J: The dentate gyrus: A model system for studies of neurotrophin regulation. Epilepsy Res 1992;7(Suppl):171–185.
23. Goldensohn ES, Purpura DP: Intracellular potentials of cortical neurons during focal epileptogenic discharges. Science 1963;139:840–842.
24. Dichter MA, Spencer WA: Penicillin-induced interictal discharges from the cat hippocampus. II. Mechanisms underlying origin and restriction. J Neurophysiol 1969;32:662–687.
25. Schwartzkroin P: Basic mechanisms of epileptogenesis. In Wyllie E (ed): The Treatment of Epilepsy. Philadelphia, Lea and Febiger, 1993.
26. Rutecki PA, Lebeda FJ, Johnston D: Epileptiform activity induced by changes in extracellular potassium in the hippocampus. J Neurophysiol 1985;54:1363–1374.
27. Traynelis SF, Dingledine R: Potassium-induced spontaneous electrographic seizures in the rat hippocampus slice. J Neurophysiol 1988;59:259–276.
28. Traub RD, Miles R, Wong RK, et al: Models of synchro-

nized hippocampal bursts in the presence of inhibition. II. Ongoing spontaneous population events. J Neurophysiol 1987;58:752–764.
29. Traub RD, Wong RK: Cellular mechanism of neuronal synchronization in epilepsy. Science 1982;216:745–747.
30. Brick JF, Gutrecht JA, Ringel RA: Reflex epilepsy and non-ketotic hyperglycemia in the elderly. Neurology 1989;39:394–399.
31. Treiman DW, Walton NY, Wickboldt C, et al: Predictable sequence of EEG changes during generalized convulsive status epilepticus in man and three experimental models of status epilepticus in the rat. Neurology 1987;34:244–245.
32. Aminoff MJ, Simon RP: Status epilepticus: Causes, clinical features, and consequences in 98 patients. Am J Med 1980;69:657–666.
33. Reiher J, Rivest J, Grand'Maison F, et al: Periodic lateralized epileptiform discharges with transitional rhythmic discharges: Association with seizures. Electroenceph Clin Neurophys 1991;78:12–17.
34. Grand'Maison F, Reiher J, Leduc CP: Retrospective inventory of EEG abnormalities in partial status epilepticus. Electroenceph Clin Neurophys 1991;79:264–270.
35. Tatum WO, Alavi A, Stecker MM: Technetium-99m-HMPAO SPECT in partial status epilepticus. J Nucl Med 1994;35:1087–1094.
36. VanLandingham KE, Lothman EW: Self-sustaining limbic status epilepticus. I. Acute and chronic cerebral metabolic studies: Limbic hypermetabolism and neocortical hypometabolism. Neurology 1991;41:1942–1949.
37. Henry TR, Drury I, Brunberg JA, et al: Focal cerebral magnetic resonance changes associated with partial status epilepticus. Epilepsia 1994;35:35–41.
38. Warach S, Levin JM, Schomer DL, et al: Hyperperfusion of ictal seizure focus demonstrated by MR perfusion imaging. AJNR 1994;15:965–968.
39. Righini A, Pierpaoli C, Alger J, et al: Brain parenchyma apparent diffusion coefficient alteration associated with experimental complex partial status epilepticus. Magn Reson Imaging 1994;12:865–871.
40. Jackson GD, Connelly A, Cross JH, et al: Functional magnetic resonance imaging of focal seizures. Neurology 1994;44:850–856.
41. Younkin DP, Delivoria-Papadopoulos M, Maris J, et al: Cerebral metabolic effects of neonatal seizures measured with in vivo ^{31}P NMR spectroscopy. Ann Neurol 1986;20:513–519.
42. Petroff OAC, Prichard JW, Behar KL, et al: In vivo phosphorus nuclear magnetic resonance spectroscopy in status epilepticus. Ann Neurol 1984;16:169–177.
43. See reference 42.
44. Matthews PM, Andermann F, Arnold DL: A proton magnetic resonance spectroscopy study of focal epilepsy in humans. Neurology 1990;40:985–989.
45. Woods BT, Chiu TM: Induced and spontaneous seizures in man produce increases in regional brain lipid detected by in vivo proton magnetic resonance spectroscopy. Adv Exp Med Biol 1992;318;267–274.
46. Prichard JW: Nuclear magnetic resonance spectroscopy of seizure states. Epilepsia 1994;35(Suppl 6):S14–S20.
47. Petroff OAC, Rothman D, Behar K, et al: The effect of vigabatrin on GABA, glutamate, and glutamine levels in human brain measured in vivo with ^{1}H NMR spectroscopy. Soc Magn Res Med Abstr 1993;12:434.
48. Hauser WA: Status epilepticus: Etiology and neurologic sequelae. Adv Neurol 1983;34:3–14.
49. Scholtes FB, Renier WO, Meinardi H: Generalized convulsive status epilepticus: Causes, therapy, and outcome in 346 patients. Epilepsia 1994;35:1104–1112.
50. Engel J: Seizures and Epilepsy. Philadelphia, FA Davis, 1989.
51. Dean JC, Penry JK: General principles: Discontinuation of antiepileptic drugs. In Levy RH, et al (eds): Antiepileptic Drugs, 3rd ed, pp 133–142. New York, Raven Press, 1989.
52. Lowenstein DH, Alldredge BK: Status epilepticus at an urban public hospital in the 1980's. Neurology 1993;43:483–488.
53. Ng SKC: Alcohol related seizures: A diversity of mechanisms? In Porter RJ, et al (eds): Alcohol and Seizures, pp 162–178. Philadelphia, FA Davis, 1990.
54. Victor M: Alcohol withdrawal seizures: An overview. In Porter RJ, et al (eds): Alcohol and Seizures, pp 148–161. Philadelphia, FA Davis, 1990.
55. Kunisaki TA, Augenstein WL: Drug and toxin induced seizures. Emerg Med Clin North Am 1994;12:1027–1055.
56. Kaufman KR, Finstead BA, Kaufman ER: Status epilepticus following electroconvulsive therapy. Mt Sinai J Med 1986;53:119–122.
57. Scott AIF, Riddle W: Status epilepticus after electroconvulsive therapy. Br J Psych 1989;155:119–121.
58. Hauser WA: Status epilepticus: Epidemiologic considerations. Neurology 1990;40(Suppl 2):9–13.
59. Rowan AJ, Scott DF: Major status epilepticus: A series of 42 patients. Acta Neurol Scand 1970;46:573–584.
60. Russel D, et al: Complex partial status epilepticus following myelography with metrizamide. Ann Neurol 1980;8:325–327.
61. Vickrey BG, Bahls FH: Nonconvulsive status epilepticus following cerebral angiography. Ann Neurol 1989;25:199–201.
62. Meldrum BS, Vigaroux RA, Brierly JB: Systemic factors and epileptic brain damage: Prolonged seizures in paralyzed, artificially ventilated baboons. Arch Neurol 1973;29:82–87.
63. Menini C, Meldrum BS, Riche D, et al: Sustained limbic seizures induced by intra-amygdaloid kainic acid in the baboon: Symptomatology and neuropathological consequences. Ann Neurol 1980;8:501–509.
64. Meldrum BS: Cell damage in epilepsy and the role of calcium in cytotoxicity. Adv Neurol 1986;44:849–853.
65. Nadler JV, Perry BW, Cotman CW: Intraventricular kainic acid preferentially destroys hippocampal pyramidal cells. Nature 1978;271:676–677.
66. Dodrill CB, Wilensky AJ: Intellectual impairment as an outcome of status epilepticus. Neurology 1990;40(Suppl 2):23–27.
67. Aicardie J, Chevrie JJ: Convulsive status epilepticus in infants and children: A study of 239 cases. Epilepsia 1970;11:187–197.
68. Dodrill CB: Correlates of generalized tonic-clonic seizures with intellectual, neuropsychological, emotional, and social functioning in patients with epilepsy. Epilepsia 1986;27:399–411.
69. Oxbury JM, Whitty CWM: Causes and consequences of status epilepticus in adults. Brain 1971;94:733–744.
70. Ellenberg JH, Nelson KB: Febrile seizures and later intellectual performance. Arch Neurol 1978;35:17–21.
71. Ellenberg JH, Hirtz DG, Nelson KB: Do seizures in children cause intellectual deterioration? N Engl J Med 1986;314:1085–1088.
72. Wijdicks EFM, Hubmayr RD: Acute acid-base disorders associated with status epilepticus. Mayo Clin Proc 1994;69:1044–1046.
73. Benowitz NL, Simon RP, Copeland JR: Status epilepticus: Divergence of sympathetic activity and cardiovascular response. Ann Neurol 1986;19:197–199.
74. Simon RP, Aminoff MJ, Benowitz N: Changes in plasma catecholamines after tonic-clonic seizures in man: Possible role in sudden death during seizures. Neurology 1984;34:255–257.
75. Simon RP: Physiologic consequences of status epilepticus. Epilepsia 1985;26(Suppl 1):S58–S66.
76. Schmidley JW, Simon RP: Postictal pleocytosis. Ann Neurol 1981;9:81–84.
77. White PT, Grant P, Mosier J, et al: Changes in cerebral dynamics associated with seizures. Neurology 1961;11:354–361.
78. Gabor AJ, Brooks AG, Scobey RP, et al: Intracranial pressure during epileptic seizures. Electroenceph Clin Neurophys 1984;57:497–506.

79. Haefely W: Benzodiazepines: Mechanisms of action. In Levy RH, et al (eds): Antiepileptic Drugs, 3rd ed, pp 133–142. New York, Raven Press, 1989.
80. Leppik IE, Derivan AT, Homan RW, et al: Double blind study of lorazepam and diazepam in status epilepticus. JAMA 1983;249:1452–1454.
81. Gastaut H, Naquet R, Poire R, et al: Treatment of status epilepticus with diazepam. Epilepsia 1965;6:167–182.
82. Treiman DM: Pharmacokinetics and clinical use of benzodiazepines in the management of status epilepticus. Epilepsia 1989;30(Suppl 2):S4–S10.
83. Schmidt D: Benzodiazepines: Diazepam. In Levy RH, et al (eds): Antiepileptic Drugs, 3rd ed, pp 735–764. New York, Raven Press, 1989.
84. Sato S: Benzodiazepines: Clonazepam. In Levy RH, et al (eds): Antiepileptic Drugs, 3rd ed, pp 765–784. New York, Raven Press, 1989.
85. Kumar A, Bleck TP: Intravenous midazolam for the treatment of refractory status epilepticus. Crit Care Med 1992;20:483–488.
86. Rivera R, Segnini M, Batodano A, et al: Midazolam in the treatment of status epilepticus in children. Crit Care Med 1993;21:991–994.
87. Parent JM, Lowenstein DH: Treatment of refractory generalized status epilepticus with continuous infusion of midazolam. Neurology 1994;44:1837–1840.
88. Delgado-Escueta AV, Horan MP: Phenytoin: Biochemical membrane studies. Adv Neurol 1980;27:377–398.
89. McLean MJ, MacDonald RL: Multiple actions of phenytoin on mouse spinal cord neurons in culture. J Pharmacol Exp Ther 1983;227:779–789.
90. Woodbury DM: Phenytoin: Absorption, distribution, and excretion. In Levy RH, et al (eds): Antiepileptic Drugs, 3rd ed, pp 177–195. New York, Raven Press, 1989.
91. Delgado-Escueta AV, Wasterlain C, Trieman DM, et al: Management of status epilepticus. N Engl J Med 1982;306:1337–1340.
92. Leppik IE, Sherwin AL: Intravenous phenytoin and phenobarbital anticonvulsant action, brain content, and plasma binding in rats. Epilepsia 1979;20:201–207.
93. Cranford RE, Patrick B, Anderson CB, et al: Intravenous phenytoin: Clinical and pharmacokinetic aspects. Neurology 1978;28:874–880.
94. Treiman DM, DeGiorgio E, Ben-Menachem D, et al: Lorazepam versus phenytoin in the treatment of generalized convulsive status epilepticus: Report of an ongoing study. Neurology 1985;35(Suppl 1):284.
95. Wilder BJ, Ramsay RE, Willmore LJ, et al: Efficacy of intravenous phenytoin in the treatment of status epilepticus: Kinetics of central nervous system penetration. Ann Neurol 1977;1:511–518.
96. Shaner DM, McCurdy SA, Herring MO, et al: Treatment of status epilepticus: A prospective comparison of diazepam and phenytoin versus phenobarbital and optional phenytoin. Neurology 1988;38:202–207.
97. Louis S, Kutt H, McDowell F: The cardiocirculatory changes caused by intravenous Dilantin and its solvent. Am Heart J 1967;74:523–529.
98. Wyte CD, Berk WA: Severe oral phenytoin overdose does not cause cardiovascular morbidity. Ann Emerg Med 1991;20:508–512.
99. Zoneraich S, Zoneraich O, Siegel J: Sudden death following intravenous sodium diphenylhydantoin. Am Heart J 1976;91:375–377.
100. York RC, Coleridge ST: Cardiopulmonary arrest following intravenous phenytoin loading. Am J Emerg Med 1988;6:255–259.
101. Unger AH, Sklaroff HJ: Fatalities following intravenous use of sodium diphenylhydantoin for cardiac arrhythmias. JAMA 1967;200:335–336.
102. Gellerman GL, Martinez C: Fatal ventricular fibrillation following intravenous sodium diphenylhydantoin therapy. JAMA 1967;200:337–338.
103. Earnest MP, Marx JA, Drury LR: Complications of intravenous phenytoin for acute treatment of seizures. JAMA 1983;249:762–765.
104. Rust RS, Dodson WE: Phenobarbital: Absorption, distribution and excretion. In Levy RH et al (eds): Antiepileptic Drugs, 3rd ed, pp 293–304. New York, Raven Press, 1989.
105. Simon RP, Copeland JR, Benowitz N, et al: Brain phenobarbital uptake during prolonged status epilepticus. J Cereb Blood Flow Metab 1987;7:783–788.
106. Walker MC, Smith SJM, Shorvon SD: The intensive care treatment of convulsive status epilepticus in the UK. Anaesthesia 1995;50:130–135.
107. Roesch C, Haselby KA, Paradise RR, et al: Comparison of cardiovascular effects of thiopental and pentobarbital at equivalent levels of CNS depression. Anesth Analg 1983;62:749–753.
108. Segel LD, Rendig SV: Sodium pentobarbital effects on cardiac function and response to dobutamine. J Cardiovasc Pharmacol 1986;8:392–397.
109. VanNess PC: Pentobarbital and EEG burst suppression in treatment of status epilepticus refractory to benzodiazepines and phenytoin. Epilepsia 1990;31:61–67.
110. Yaffe K, Lowenstein DH: Prognostic factors of pentobarbital therapy for refractory generalized status epilepticus. Neurology 1993;43:895–900.
111. Osorio I, Reed RC: Treatment of refractory generalized tonic-clonic status epilepticus with pentobarbital anesthesia after high dose phenytoin. Epilepsia 1989;30:464–471.
112. Orlowski JP, Erenberg G, Lueders H, et al: Hypothermia and barbiturate coma for refractory status epilepticus. Crit Care Med 1984;12:367–372.
113. Rashkin MC, Youngs C, Penovich P: Pentobarbital treatment of refractory status epilepticus. Neurology 1987;37:500–503.
114. Partinen M, Kovanen J, Nilsson E: Status epilepticus treated by barbiturate anesthesia with continuous monitoring of cerebral function. Br Med J 1981;282:520–521.
115. Young GB, Blume WT, Bolton CF, et al: Anesthetic barbiturates in refractory status epilepticus. Can J Neurol Sci 1980;7:291–292.
116. Lowenstein DH, Aminoff MJ, Simon RP: Barbiturate anesthesia in the treatment of status epilepticus. Neurology 1988;38:395–400.
117. Orser BA, Wang LY, Pennefather PS, et al: Propofol modulates activation and desensitization of GABA A receptors in cultured murine hippocampal neurons. J Neurosci 1994;14:7747–776.
118. Borgeat A, Wilder-Smith OHG, Jallon P, et al: Propofol in the management of refractory status epilepticus: A case report. Int Care Med 1994;20:148–149.
119. Pitt-Miller P, Elcock B, Maharaj M: The management of status epilepticus with a continuous propofol infusion. Anesth Analg 1994;78:1193–1194.
120. Mackenzie SJ, Kapadia F, Grant IS: Propofol infusion for control of status epilepticus. Anaesthesia 1990;45:1043–1045.
121. Shorvon S: Tonic clonic status epilepticus. J Neurol Neurosurg Psychiatry 1993;56:125–134.
122. Sheperd SM: Management of status epilepticus. Emerg Med Clin North Am 1994;12:941–961.
123. Lampl Y, Eshel Y, Gilad R, et al: Chloral hydrate in intractable status epilepticus. Ann Emerg Med 1990;19:674–676.
124. Fulton B, Park GR: Intravenous chlormethiazole. Br J Hosp Med 1992;48:742–746.
125. Hales TG, Lambert JJ: Modulation of GABA A and glycine receptors by chlormethiazole. Eur J Pharm 1992;210:239–246.
126. Harvey PKP, Higenbottam TW, Loh L: Chlormethiazole in treatment of status epilepticus. Br Med J 1975;2:603–605.
127. Noreng MF, Christensen PA, Theissen P, et al: Chlormethiazole treatment in a child with status epilepticus. Acta Paediatr Scand 1987;76:839–840.
128. Pascual J, Ciudad J, Berciano J: Role of lidocaine in managing status epilepticus. J Neurol Neurosurg Psychiatry 1992;55:49–51.
129. Vajda FJE, Mihaly GW, Miles JL, et al: Rectal administration of sodium valproate in status epilepticus. Neurology 1978;28:897–899.

130. Ropper AH, Kofke A, Bromfield EB, et al: Comparison of isoflurane, halothane, and nitrous oxide in status epilepticus. Ann Neurol 1986;19:98–99.
131. Meeke RI, Soifer BE, Gelb AW: Isoflurane for the management of status epilepticus. DICP Ann Pharmacol 1989;23:579–581.
132. Kofke WA, Young RSK, Davis P, et al: Isoflurane for refractory status epilepticus: A clinical series. Anesthesiology 1989;71:653–659.
133. Hilz MJ, Bauer J, Claus D, et al: Isoflurane anaesthesia in the treatment of convulsive status epilepticus. J Neurol 1992;239:135–137.
134. Adams D: The Hitchhiker's Guide to the Galaxy. New York, Harmony Books, 1980.
135. Celesia GG, Grigg MM, Ross E: Generalized status myoclonicus in acute anoxia and in toxic-metabolic encephalopathies. Arch Neurol 1988;45:781–784.
136. Labar DR, Ali A, Root J: High-dose intravenous lorazepam for treatment of refractory status epilepticus. Neurology 1994;44:1400–1403.

5

Infectious and Parasitic Emergencies of the Central Nervous System

Dennis L. Kolson, M.D., Ph.D. • Daniel T. Laskowitz, M.D.

An enormous number of infectious and parasitic agents invade the central nervous system (CNS) and may establish acute, subacute, and indolent neurologic syndromes. This chapter is directed toward pathogens affecting significant numbers of patients worldwide in clinical syndromes considered to be neurologic and/or neurosurgical emergencies. It covers selected bacterial, parasitic, and viral agents. Certain topics dealing with less acute clinical presentation (e.g., human immunodeficiency virus [HIV] encephalopathy) are not covered in this review despite their profound clinical impact on large numbers of patients worldwide. In some emergent conditions (e.g., viral encephalitides), curative treatments are not yet established but nonetheless are likely on the horizon.

BACTERIAL MENINGITIS

The overall incidence of bacterial meningitis in the United States is 0.1–10 cases/100,000 per year, with the highest incidence in the late fall through early spring. In general, meningitis does not present as a neurosurgical emergency except in rare instances of associated masses (abscess, tuberculoma; see under Brain Abscesses) or cerebrospinal fluid (CSF) outflow obstruction. In many cases of abscess, drainage is the treatment of choice; in the case of outflow obstruction, ventricular shunting may be used. Meningitis and meningoencephalitis may be clinically indistinguishable under certain circumstances, so recognition and empiric treatment of meningitis is essential for the practicing clinician.

Pathophysiology. Bacterial meningitis occurs when invading pathogens overcome host defense mechanisms and reach the subarachnoid space, where replication is associated with release of proinflammatory cytokines and other cellular toxins.[1–4] The most important determinant of pathogenicity is the bacterial capsule *(Haemophilus influenzae* type b, *Neisseria meningitidis, Streptococcus pneumoniae).* Nasopharyngeal colonization is necessary to establish local invasion through the nasopharyngeal epithelium in persons without neutralizing antibodies that block adhesion.[5] This invasion results in a bacteremia that allows adherence to the epithelium of the choroid plexus, followed by meningeal infection, and seeding of the subarachnoid space. *H. influenzae* infection in particular may result in ventriculitis with subsequent thrombosis of pial veins, cortical arterioles, and venous sinuses with formation of subdural effusions.[6] In general, death from bacterial meningitis occurs from increased intracranial pressure (ICP) from cerebral edema, which may result from vasogenic edema secondary to increased blood-brain barrier permeability, cytotoxic swelling and lysis of cells from toxins released from polymorphonuclear cells and bacteria, and obstructive hydrocephalus.[7] Treatment of bacterial meningitis is directed toward inhibition of replication of the invading pathogens, prevention of cerebral edema, and in some cases prevention of secondary effects of proinflammatory cytokine release within the subarachnoid space.

Clinical Presentation. The clinical presentation of bacterial meningitis typically involves headache, photophobia, and meningismus in 80% of cases,

TABLE 5–1 **BACTERIAL PREVALENCE IN MENINGITIS IN ADULTS**

PATHOGEN	PREVALENCE
Haemophilus influenzae	1%–3%
Streptococcus pneumoniae	30%–50%
Neisseria meningitidis	10%–35%
Staphylococci	5%–15%
Gram-negative bacilli	1%–10%
Group B *Streptococcus* (*S. agalactiae*)	5%
Listeria monocytogenes	5%

Adapted from Roos KL, et al: Acute bacterial meningitis in children and adults. In Scheld WM, et al (eds), Infections of the Central Nervous System, pp 335–409. New York, Raven Press, 1991.

along with fever (85%), malaise, and vomiting. The "classic" Kernig's sign (resistance to leg extension when the examiner flexes the patient's thigh on the abdomen and passively extends the leg) and Brudzinski's sign (passive flexion of the neck causing flexion of the knees and hips) are present in only 50% of cases of adults and thus are not reliable diagnostic tools.[5]

Focal neurologic signs are generally not helpful in making the diagnosis, although cranial nerve deficits, especially VIII, may be prominent in each of the three major bacterial meningitides.[6, 8, 9] In addition, *H. influenzae* meningitis may present with acute mania[3] after a several-day prodrome of fever, otitis media, and pharyngitis.[6] Pneumococcal meningitis should be suspected in patients with defective splenic function (sickle cell disease, post splenectomy) and previous head injury with or without skull fracture.[8] CNS syndromes with *Listeria monocytogenes* are notoriously clinically varied and include the following: (1) diffuse encephalitis (especially in renal transplant patients); (2) localized abscesses in the hemispheres, thalamus, and brain stem; (3) cerebritis with focal neurologic deficits; and (4) brain stem encephalitis (see under Brain Stem Encephalitis).[10] Tuberculous meningitis often presents with multiple cranial nerve deficits because of its predilection for the basilar meninges, and it may have an insidious clinical course.[11] In cases of suspected tuberculous meningitis, one must be alert to the possible presence of tuberculomas of the brain and spinal cord (see under Intraparenchymal Abscess and Figs. 5–10, 5–11, 5–12, and 5–13). Finally, meningitis from *N. meningitidis* may be associated with meningococcemia, from which a rapidly developing petechial-purpuric rash may develop within hours (50% of patients).[4] Once recognized, the presence of this rash demands immediate institution of antibiotic therapy without any further diagnostic delays.[4, 9] Of note, a purpuric rash sometimes occurs in *H. influenza* and *S. pneumoniae* meningitis, though rarely.[9]

Microorganisms. The microorganisms responsible for most cases of bacterial meningitis are listed in Table 5–1. *S. pneumoniae* is the most common bacterial cause of meningitis in adults, and *H. influenza* is the most common cause in children, although effective vaccination against *H. influenza* type b may alter the prevalence in children.[3, 4, 12] However, there is a distinct age predilection for specific pathogens, as indicated in Table 5–2. For example, group B *Streptococcus* and *Listeria* are major pathogens in neonates; *Listeria* is also preva-

TABLE 5–2 **AGE SUSCEPTIBILITY AND EMPIRIC ANTIBIOTIC CHOICES FOR MENINGITIS**

AGE RANGE	MOST COMMON PATHOGENS	EMPIRIC ANTIBIOTIC CHOICE*
< 1 mo	Group B *Streptococcus*, *Listeria monocytogenes*, *Escherichia coli*	Cefotaxime + ampicillin Gentamicin + ampicillin
1 mo to 5 yrs	*Haemophilus influenzae* type b (95% are type b; others are types a–f)	Ceftriaxone + ampicillin Chloramphenicol + ampicillin + dexamethasone
5–29 yrs	*Neisseria meningitidis*	Ceftriaxone + ampicillin + dexamethasone
> 29 yrs	*Streptococcus pneumoniae*	Ceftriaxone + ampicillin + dexamethasone

*Recommended antibiotic doses are as follows:

Ampicillin	*< 1 mo old:* 100–200 mg/kg/day IV *Children:* 300–400 mg/kg/day *Adults:* 2 g IV every 6 hrs
Ceftriaxone	*Children:* 75 mg/kg initial dose, then 100 mg/kg every 12 hrs IV (not to exceed 4 gm/day) *Adults:* 2 g IV every 12 hrs
Cefotaxime	0–7 days: 100 mg/kg/day IV every 12 hrs > 7 days: 150 mg/kg/day IV every 8 hrs (not to exceed 12 gm/day)
Chloramphenicol	*Children:* 100 mg/kg/day IV *Adults:* 0.5 g every 6 hrs IV or PO
Gentamicin	*Children:* 5 mg/kg/day IV *Adults:* Load 2 mg/kg, then 5 mg/kg/day
Dexamethasone	0.15 mg/kg IV every 6 hrs × 4 days, started within 30 minutes of antibiotics

IV, intravenous; PO, per os (oral); mo, month; yrs, years.
Data are summarized from Sanford JP, Gilbert DN, Sande MA, Geberding JE (eds): The Sanford Guide to Antimicrobial Therapy, pp 4, 5, 113–115. Dallas, Antimicrobial Therapy, 1997; and from Wenger JD, Broome CV: Bacterial meningitis: Epidemiology. In Lambert HP (ed), Infections of the Central Nervous System, p 19. Philadelphia, BC Decker, 1991.

lent in elderly and immunocompromised patients. Adults are more likely to have *N. meningitidis* or *S. pneumoniae* meningitis.[4, 13]

Radiographic Diagnosis. Brain imaging results are generally normal except in cases of global cerebral edema or abscess formation, as discussed under Brain Abscesses. Exceptions to this general rule are demonstrated in following sections discussing tuberculous meningitis (see Fig. 5–14), where basilar enhancement may be seen, or in cases of *Listeria* brain stem encephalitis (see Fig. 5–18). Occasionally, *H. influenza* meningitis results in the formation of subdural effusions.[6]

Laboratory Diagnosis. Suspicion of bacterial meningitis requires immediate examination of the CSF by lumbar puncture in all cases except: (1) clinically important cardiovascular compromise in a neonate; (2) clinical signs of increased ICP; and (3) infection in the areas where the needle would transverse. The Gram stain is the most sensitive diagnostic tool in the diagnosis of meningitis and is about 90% sensitive for *S. pneumoniae* meningitis and somewhat less sensitive for *H. influenzae* and *N. meningitidis.*[8] For antigen detection in the CSF, latex agglutination kits have replaced the counterimmunoelectrophoresis techniques, because they are generally more rapid, requiring less than an hour for results.[14]

Typical CSF findings in acute bacterial meningitis include the following: (1) opening pressure of 200–300 mm H_2O; (2) white blood cell count of 1000–5000 × 10^6/L; (3) greater than or equal to 80% neutrophils; (4) protein level 100–500 mg/dL; (5) glucose level less than or equal to 40 mg/dL; (6) Gram stain positive in 60%–90% (highest for *S. pneumoniae);* and (7) culture positive in 70%–85%.[5] Spanos et al.[15] determined a 99% predictive value for CSF parameters that included a glucose level less than 1.9 mmol/L, a CSF/blood glucose ratio less than 0.33, a protein level greater than 2.2 g/L, a leukocyte level of more than 2000 × 10^6/L, or a neutrophil level of more than 1180 × 10^6/L.

Treatment of Bacterial Meningitis. Because third-generation cephalosporins such as ceftriaxone have broad-spectrum coverage over all of these pathogens except *Listeria,* they are generally combined with ampicillin (for *Listeria* coverage) as empiric treatment for suspected meningitis in all ages of patients (except neonates up to 3 weeks of age) until organisms are identified.[5, 13, 16] In neonates up to 3 weeks old, cefotaxime is the third-generation cephalosporin of choice because of its effects on bilirubin metabolism in this age group.[5] Alternatively, in neonates, ampicillin plus an aminoglycoside may be used.[17] After identification of the infecting organism, antibiotic therapy may be modified, based on sensitivities of the bacterium. For example, methicillin-sensitive *Staphylococcus aureus* may be treated with nafcillin or oxacillin, whereas methicillin-resistant organisms should be treated with vancomycin.[16] The duration of treatment is 10–14 days, except in the case of *Listeria,* wherein at least 3 weeks of treatment is recommended.[10]

The use of dexamethasone has been recommended in cases of *H. influenza* meningitis because it decreases the likelihood of hearing loss due to eighth-nerve damage in children.[1, 6] It has been proposed to decrease the effects of proinflammatory cytokines and metabolites released in the subarachnoid space, which are thought to contribute to complications of bacterial meningitis.[1, 18] Some evidence suggests a possible beneficial effect in *N. meningitidis* encephalitis as well, although the data are less convincing.[19] It is also unknown whether it has a beneficial effect on the outcome of *S. pneumoniae* meningitis, and some authors have recommended its use.[20] It should be noted that the use of dexamethasone in acute bacterial meningitis is nonetheless controversial, and routine use is not recommended by other authors.[21] Dexamethasone is given at a dose of 0.15 mg/kg every 6 hours for a total of 4 days, and it should be started immediately before or within 30 minutes of the institution of antibiotics.[16] In tuberculous meningitis, dexamethasone improves outcome in patients presenting in stupor or with intracranial tuberculomas.[11]

Neurosurgical Treatment and Other Adjunctive Therapy. Neurosurgical intervention is generally limited to drainage of subdural empyemas or intraparenchymal abscesses that may complicate bacterial meningitis. A communicating hydrocephalus due to impaired arachnoid villi reabsorption of CSF may require shunting, and such a decision must be based on the overall condition of the patient. Patients who are stuporous or comatose, precluding clinical assessment of neurologic status, may benefit from ICP monitoring, with treatment aimed at maintaining ICP at less than 20 mm Hg.[2, 5, 22, 23] ICP may be reduced by the following measures[5]: (1) elevation of the head of the bed to 30 degrees to maximize venous drainage while minimizing decreases in cerebral blood flow; (2) hyperventilation (maintaining arterial P_{CO_2} between 25 and 30 torr [3.3–4 kPa]), which causes cerebral vasoconstriction; (3) use of hyperosmolar agents such as mannitol (0.25 to 0.50 g/kg every 4 to 8 hours as necessary; (4) free-water restriction to 1000 mL normal saline per square meter of body surface area per day; and (5) CSF drainage through intracranial ventricular shunts.

BRAIN ABSCESSES

Intraparenchymal Abscesses

Bacterial

In the United States, the frequency of brain abscess is 1.1/100,000, and two-thirds of all cases are diagnosed at autopsy.[24] Organisms gain entrance into the CNS most commonly through infection within the sinuses and ears (50%) but also via hematogenous spread (20%) from the mouth, lung, skin, gastrointestinal tract, and heart. Approximately 10% of brain abscesses result from penetrating injuries to the skull.[24] Brain abscesses may occur intraparenchymally or as subdural or epidural empyemas. Epidural abscesses are more likely to form from mastoid infection, and the dura may provide an effective barrier that walls off the infection. Subdural abscesses form over the hemispheric convexities as a result of sinusitis, and parenchymal abscesses may result from sinus infection, hematogenous seeding, traumatic injury, and direct infection through the cribriform plate.

Clinical Presentation. The clinical presentation of brain abscesses may be insidious, often with nonspecific symptoms. Headaches that are worse with exertion are common (~50%) as are altered mental status (~40%), fever (~40%), seizures (~33%), and meningismus (~20%).[25] Depending on the location of the abscess, one may experience local pain around the sinuses or suffer a stroke syndrome secondary to cortical thrombophlebitis and ischemic infarction of the brain.[25] In a recent series of 44 infants and children with brain abscesses Ersahin et al.[26] found the following presenting signs: papilledema (~45%), hemiparesis (~34%), coma (~34%), cranial nerve palsies (~27%), and nuchal rigidity (~17%).

Microorganisms. The microorganisms responsible for formation of most brain abscesses include aerobic and anaerobic bacteria, *Mycobacterium tuberculosis*, fungi, and parasites, including *Echinococcus, Toxoplasmosis,* and *Cysticercosis*. Approximately 40% of brain abscesses contain *Streptococci* (including anaerobes) and about 30% contain *Bacteroides* in addition to aerobes.[24] The bacterial flora varies, depending on the route of inoculation into the CNS. Abscesses resulting from infection within the ear usually contain gram-negative organisms, especially *Proteus,* whereas sinus infections seed *Streptococcus* and *Pneumococcus.* Penetrating skull injuries often result in *Staphylococcus pyogenes* abscesses, whereas hematogenously seeded abscesses contain mixed flora. The route of inoculation also determines the likely location of the abscess. The frontal lobes are seeded via the frontal, ethmoid, and sphenoid sinuses; the temporal lobes are seeded via the sphenoid and maxillary sinuses; and the cerebellum is seeded via the mastoid air cells. Predisposing factors for brain abscess include immunosuppression, congenital heart disease, or pulmonary arteriovenous malformations with right-to-left shunt.

Radiographic Diagnosis. The diagnosis of brain abscess depends on imaging with either contrasted head computed tomography (CT) or magnetic resonance imaging (MRI), and appearances may vary. Scans may reveal an isodense ring representing enhancement of the capsule of the abscess (Fig. 5–1). This enhancement is thought to be due to breakdown of the blood-brain barrier with increased capillary permeability with the inflammation around the abscess and increased vascularity.[24, 27] This capsular rim, 1 to 3 mm thick, is the cardinal feature of abscesses, differentiating them generally from tumors and granulomas. There may also be surrounding edema, which contributes to mass effect. In addition, abscesses due to tuberculomas or fungal infection may appear as focal areas of low attenuation that may show either homogeneous enhancement or thick enhancing rims with central cavities (reviewed in reference 24). Although CT and MRI appear to be equally suitable for detection of abscesses, CT is preferably for detection of subdural empyemas.[27] As Figure 5–2 shows, one may see a hypodense area parallel to the calvarium or falx with enhancing margins.

Complication of Brain Abscesses. The overall fatality rate for abscesses is approximately 10%, but this varies widely with the age of the patient and time to diagnosis.[24] Cortical thrombophlebitis (which can result in focal neurologic deficits) is common following subdural empyema but may also occur with intraparenchymal abscesses. Rupture of an abscess into the subarachnoid space or a ventricle may result in meningitis and ventriculitis, which may be fatal. Finally, increased ICP from mass effect is a major factor in mortality.[25]

Treatment of Brain Abscesses. The treatment of choice for abscesses is drainage of pus from the intracranial compartment. This may be performed by aspiration through a burr hole or open craniotomy. CT-guided or even ultrasound-guided approach biopsy[28] is the preferred technique. The abscess must be cultured for aerobes, anaerobes, fungus, and *M. tuberculosis,* and it is important to note that 20% of drained abscesses are "sterile" either as a result of previous antibiotic treatment or because of the fastidious growth requirements of some organ-

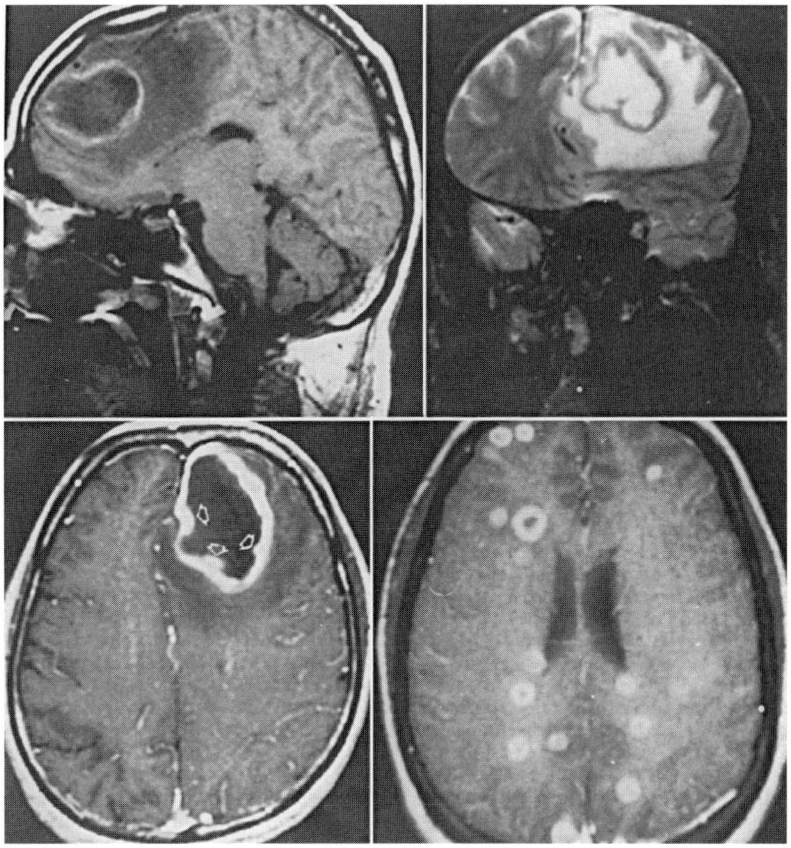

FIGURE 5-1 • MRI of brain abscesses. *Upper left,* Unenhanced T1-weighted sagittal image demonstrating frontal lobe high-intensity ring with low intensity surrounding the *Streptococcal* abscess. *Upper right,* T2-weighted coronal image revealing surrounding vasogenic edema. *Lower left,* T1-weighted image showing ring-enhancement with nodular inner face and smoother outer face, characteristic of abscesses. *Lower right,* Multiple peptostreptococcal abscesses. (From Grossman RI, Yousem DM: Infectious and noninfectious inflammatory diseases of the brain. In Farrell RJ [ed]: Neuroradiology: The Requisites, p 179. St. Louis, Mosby–Year Book, 1994.)

isms.[24] The appropriate antibiotic coverage until culture results dictate treatment should include at the least a combination of penicillin and metronidazole (Table 5–3). In adult patients, typical intravenous doses are penicillin, 4 million units every 6 hours; metronidazole, 7.5 mg/kg IV every 6 hours. If the abscess is a result of traumatic brain injury, a penicillinase-resistant penicillin is used in addition (flucloxacillin, nafcillin, oxacillin, cloxacillin, dicloxacillin). A third-generation cephalosporin (cefotaxime) should be added when an otogenic source is suspected.[16] A recent study used a combination of cefotaxime and metronidazole alone in 15 consecutive patients with good results.[29] Both of these show good CNS abscess penetration and may provide an acceptable alternative for patients with penicillin allergies.

Amebic Abscesses

NAEGLERIA AND *ACANTHAMOEBA*

Of particular interest are amebic brain abscesses due to *Naegleria* and *Acanthamoeba,* which are responsible for most amebic CNS infections.[30, 31] In addition, *Entamoeba histolytica* is responsible for brain abscesses in areas where intestinal amebiasis is endemic. *Naegleria* causes meningoencephalitis, and all amebic CNS infections carry high rates of morbidity and mortality.[32]

Naegleria amoebae are found primarily in soil and fresh water, and a flagellated form of the larvae can survive in chlorinated swimming pools, fresh water lakes, thermal springs, and human throat and nasal cavities.[33] Infection usually occurs during either swimming or bathing; cases have been reported from Australia, Belgium, Western Europe, India, New Zealand, Puerto Rico, Uganda, and Venezuela, and in the United States in Virginia, Florida, Texas, Nevada, and New York. The *Naegleria fowleri* amoeba invades the olfactory neuroepithelium and follows the unmyelinated nerves to the subarachnoid space, from which it spreads to other parts of the CNS.[30] *Acanthamoeba* may enter the CNS via hematogenous spread, and primary infection is thought to occur either through skin lesions or through the lower respiratory tract.[32, 34]

Clinical Presentation. Amebic meningoencephalitis due to *N. fowleri* may present as *acute amebic meningoencephalitis* (AAM), whereas *Acanthamoeba* may cause subacute or chronic meningoencephalitis, which is called *granulomatous amebic encephalitis* (GAE).[33] In AAM, one sees a rapid and fulminant course resembling bacterial meningitis: unremitting headache, fever, nausea, vomiting, photophobia, seizures, and coma are common. One may experience ageusia or parosmia, because the olfac-

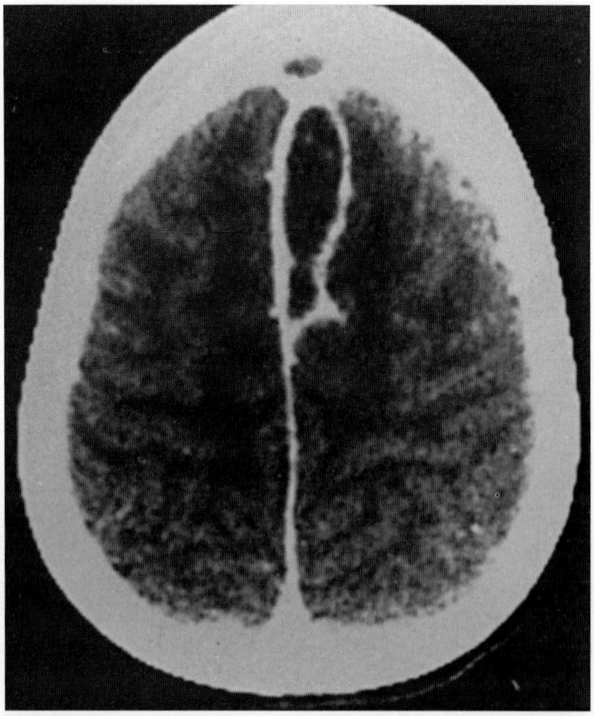

FIGURE 5-2 • Contrasted computed tomography (CT) of a subdural empyema. This scan shows a low-attentuation collection in the extra-axial space within the interhemispheric fissure. The morphologic features on CT are similar to those of brain abscesses on magnetic resonance imaging (see Fig. 5–1, upper left). (From Jungreis CA, Grossman RI: Intracranial infections and inflammatory diseases. In Latchaw RE [ed]: MR and CT Imaging of the Head, Neck, and Spine, p 307. St. Louis, Mosby–Year Book, 1991.)

tory tracts are affected early.[33] Signs include nuchal rigidity, cranial nerve palsies with signs of increased ICP, and herniation. There may be associated myocarditis, and in most cases death occurs within a week.[30] The major differential diagnoses of AAM are acute bacterial meningitis and herpes simplex meningoencephalitis. CSF examination is critical to demonstrate the absence of bacteria on stain and culture. Furthermore, the characteristic electroencephalographic pattern of focal spikes or periodic (2–3 second intervals) sharp wave complexes or periodic lateralized epileptiform discharges (PLEDS) over the temporal lobe characteristic of herpes simplex encephalitis is not seen with AAM.[33]

GAE due to *Acanthamoeba* is most common in debilitated or immunosuppressed patients and presents similarly to brain abscesses (see earlier) with an insidious course. It occurs occasionally in acquired immunodeficiency syndrome (AIDS) patients.[32, 35] It tends to present with a variable clinical picture, which may include focal or diffuse neurologic signs: hemiparesis, cranial nerve palsies, diplopia, drowsiness, personality changes, and seizures with a low-grade fever. Signs of meningitis may be absent, and the disease is almost invariably fatal because of cerebral edema and intracranial herniation.[33]

Laboratory Diagnosis of Amebic Infection. In AAM, CSF leukocytosis is typical with greater than 90% neutrophils.[33] CSF pressure is almost always elevated (300–650 mm H_20), as is the protein level.[32] Glucose is usually low, often less than 10 mg/dL. For identification of free-living amoebae, a modified trichrome stain is useful for fresh CSF specimens for detection of the trophozoites (Table 5–4), which are from 10 to 35 μm in diameter.[30, 32] Amoebae on trichrome stain or Wright's smear are often mistaken for mononuclear cells. Figure 5–3*A* illustrates a *Naegleria* trophozoite with a large eccentric nucleus in a trichrome stain in CSF, compared with a smaller leukocyte. Figure 5–3*B* illustrates a Wright's-stained cytospin preparation of CSF with a degenerating amoeba surrounded by lymphocytes and polymorphonuclear cells.

Cultures for free-living amoebae are positive within 24–48 hours, and trophozoites may be identified in culture medium. Figure 5–4 shows both mononuclear and binuclear organisms, and multinu-

TABLE 5–3 **EMPIRIC TREATMENT FOR BRAIN ABSCESSES**

MODIFYING CIRCUMSTANCES	ETIOLOGIES	REGIMEN
Otogenic (temporal, parietal, cerebellar) or unknown	*Streptococcus viridans,* anaerobic *Streptococcus, Bacteroides,* Enterobacteriacaea	Penicillin, 4 million U every 6 hrs + metronidazole + cephalosporin (third-generation)
Primary paranasal sinuses (frontal)	Anaerobes, *Streptococcus* species, *Streptococcus pneumoniae, Haemophilus influenzae*	Penicillin, 4 million U every 6 hrs + metronidazole
Young adult	*Staphylococcus aureus*	Penicillinase-resistant penicillin + metronidazole
Postsurgical, traumatic	*Staphylococcus aureus,* Enterobacteriacaea	Penicillinase-resistant penicillin + cephalosporin (third-generation) + rifampin
HIV-1 infected (AIDS)	*Toxoplasma gondii*	Pyrimethamine and sulfadiazine, or clindamycin

Data are summarized from Sanford JP, Gilbert DN, Sande MA, Geberding JE (eds): The Sanford Guide to Antimicrobial Therapy, p 4. Dallas, Antimicrobial Therapy, 1997.

TABLE 5–4 WHEATLEY TRICHROME STAIN FOR FREE-LIVING AMEBAE (MODIFIED SHORT VERSION)

Materials: Schaudinn's fixative, 70% ethyl alcohol plus iodine, 70% ethyl alcohol, Trichrome stain (Scientific Products or Meridian Diagnostics, Cincinnati; or Renel, Lenexa, KS), 90% alcohol acidified, 95% ethyl alcohol, 100% ethyl alcohol, xylene, Permount (Fisher Scientific, Norcross, GA), No. 1 coverslip.

Set up 10 coplin jars. Fill in jars with above reagents in order.

Staining procedure:

Prepare thin smear. Immediately proceed to the following:

(1) Schaudinn's fixative: 1 hr (room temperature)/5 min (50° C)
(2) 70% ethyl alcohol plus iodine: 1 min*
(3) 70% ethyl alcohol: 1 min
(4) 70% ethyl alcohol: 1 min
(5) Trichrome stain: 4 min
(6) 90% ethyl alcohol acidified: 1 dip†
(7) 95% ethyl alcohol: 1 dip
(8) 95% ethyl alcohol: 1 dip
(9) Carbol xylene: 3 min
(10) Xylene: 3 min
(11) Permount: 1 or 2 drops

Cover with No. 1 coverslip. Let dry. Examine with oil-immersion lens.

Interpretation:

Trophozoite: Cytoplasm green with a tinge of purple, depending on age; karyosome red.

Cyst: Wall green; cytoplasm purplish green.

*Add iodine crystals to 70% ethyl alcohol until the color looks like port wine.

†Use 947.4 mL of 95% ethanol and bring up to 1000 mL with glass-distilled water; add 4.5 mL glacial acetic acid.

From Ma P, Visvesvara GS, Martinez AJ, et al: Naegleria and acanthamoeba infections: Review Infect Dis 1990;12:509–510. University of Chicago, publisher.

cleated forms are not uncommon. Free-living amoebae as etiologic agents should be suspected in every case of purulent meningitis wherein bacteria are not identified by smear, culture, counterimmunoelectrophoresis, or latex agglutination.[32] Table 5–4 describes the technique for trichrome staining for amoebae.

Serological testing in AAM is generally not useful because of the rapid progression of disease. In GAE, CSF usually reveals modest pleocytosis (mononuclear cells) with mildly elevated protein levels and a normal to low-normal glucose level; amoebae are usually neither seen nor cultured.[33] Brain biopsy for identification of *Acanthamoeba* is necessary for definitive diagnosis. The *Acanthamoeba* cyst is 10–25 μm in diameter and is double-walled, with the outer wall somewhat irregular (Fig. 5–5*A*), whereas *Naegleria* displays a single wall (see Fig. 5–5*B*).

Radiographic Diagnosis. In AAM, the radiographic findings may include basal arachnoiditis with enhancement of the sulci and adjacent gray matter reflecting inflammation, but the findings are generally nonspecific.[30] In GAE, multiple abscesses may be seen, both enhancing and nonenhancing with surrounding edema on CT (Fig. 5–6).[36]

Treatment. In AAM, intravenous amphotericin B (1 mg/kg daily) is the treatment of choice.[16, 37] Because CNS penetration of amphotericin B is poor, it may be given in addition through an Ommaya reservoir at lower doses (0.1 mg/kg daily).[30] Experimental evidence suggests that adjunctive therapy with rifampin, tetracycline, or minocycline may have synergistic or additive effects against *N. fowleri.*[33] However, despite marked in vitro sensitivity

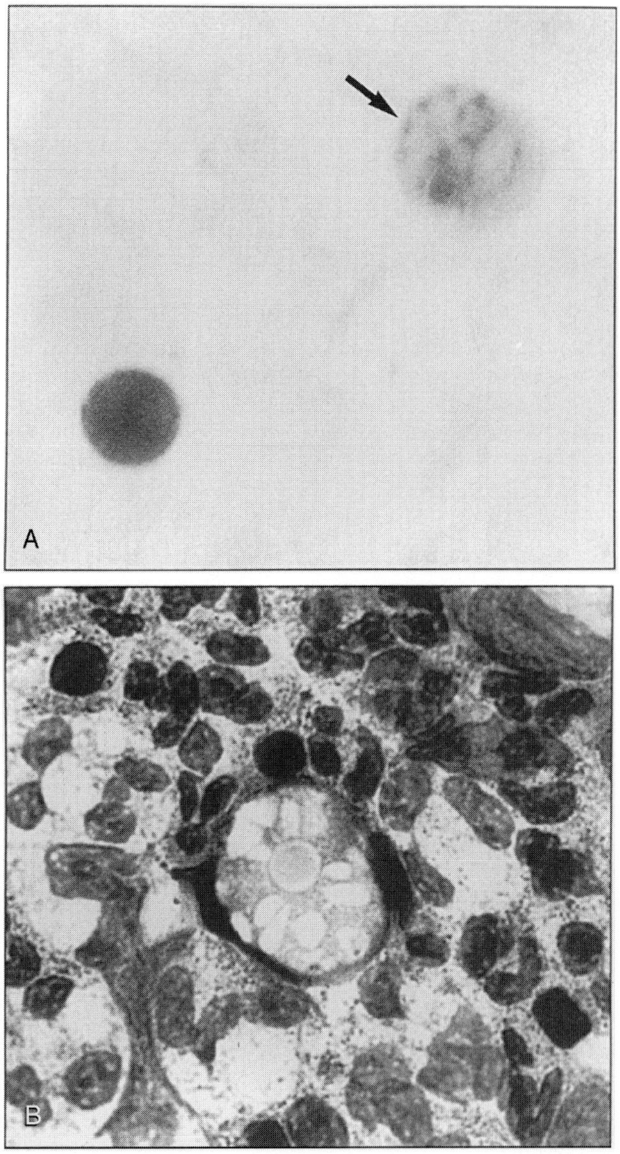

FIGURE 5–3 • *Naegleria fowleri* trophozoites. *A*, This is a trichrome-stained smear of human cerebrospinal fluid, illustrating a large nucleated trophozoite (arrow) with an eccentric nucleus. A smaller leukocyte is present in the lower left portion of the field. Organisms seen in cerebrospinal fluid and tissues are typically smaller than the trophozoites seen in culture. *B,* This is a Wright-stained cytospin preparation of cerebrospinal fluid showing a degenerating amoeba surrounded by lymphocytes and polymorphonuclear leukocytes. This organism has a large central nucleus. (From Ash LR, Griebel TC: Atlas of Human Parasitology, p 67. Chicago, American Society of Clinical Pathologists, 1990.)

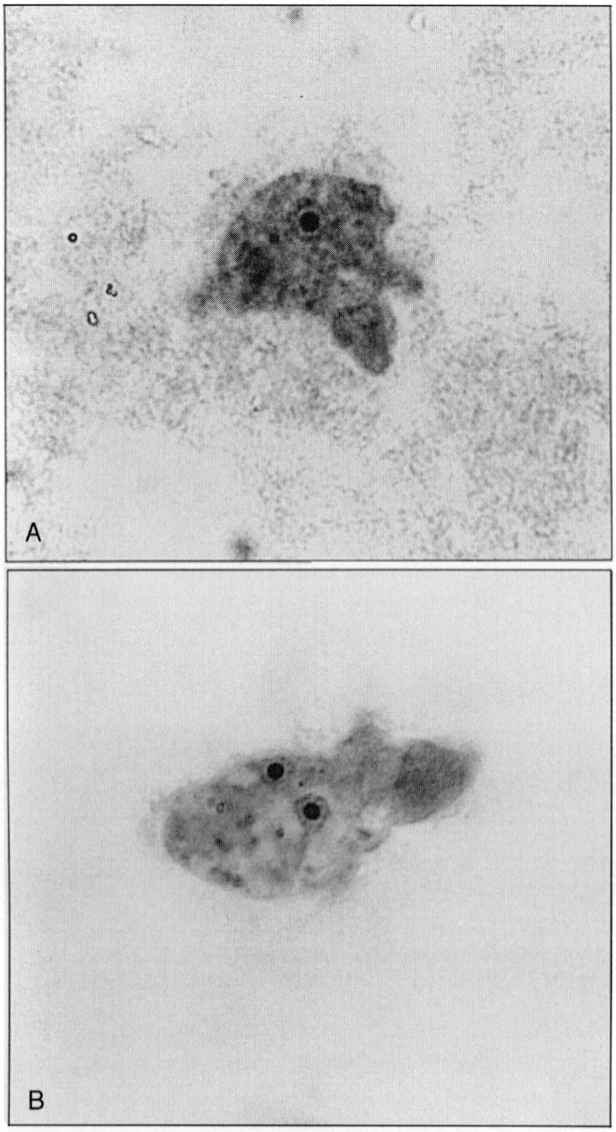

FIGURE 5-4 • *Naegleria fowleri* trophozoites in culture medium. Trichrome-stained trophozoites with one (*A*) and two (*B*) nuclei. In culture, it is not uncommon to find organisms with multiple nuclei. (From Ash LR, Griebel TC: Atlas of Human Parasitology, p 67. Chicago, American Society of Clinical Pathologists, 1990.)

of *N. fowleri* to amphotericin B, few patients survive AAM, and death occurs within 5–10 days.[32]

No effective chemotherapy has been developed for CNS *Acanthamoeba* infection, although excision of focal lesions may be attempted.[38] Agents that have been used include fluconazole, ketoconazole, 5-fluorocytosine, paromomycin, neomycin, and rifampin.[39, 40]

ENTAMOEBA

Epidemiology. Unlike *Naegleria* and *Acanthamoeba, E. histolytica* is an obligate parasite. Up to 10% of the world population is infected, and the annual mortality rate is up to 100,000 deaths/year worldwide.[30, 41] Most infections do not produce symptoms, but approximately 10% of infected patients suffer mild to moderate gastrointestinal symptoms, including abdominal pain, fever, tenesmus, and bloody diarrhea.[42] Brain abscess due to *E. histolytica* is a relatively rare complication of systemic infection (0.6%–8% of patients with hepatic *E. histolytica* abscesses) and occurs generally only in patients with hepatic abscesses.[43] Infection spreads by the fecal-oral route via contaminated water or through sexual transmission.[42]

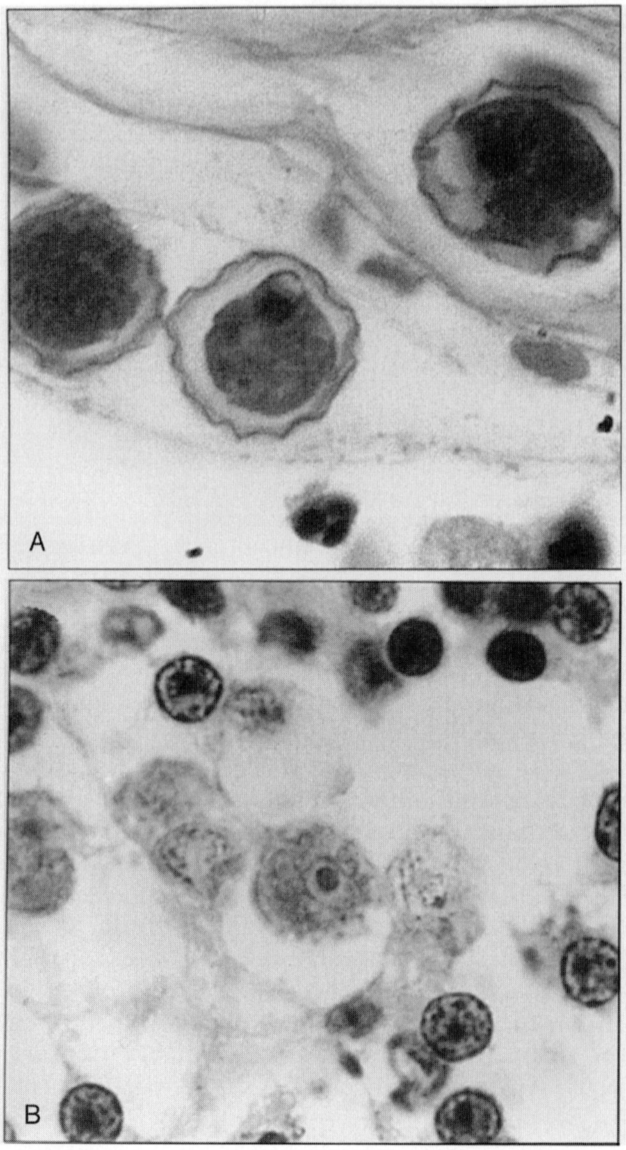

FIGURE 5-5 • *Acanthamoeba* and *Naegleria* organisms in human brain tissue. *A,* Three cysts of *Acanthamoeba* within the wall of a vein in this section of human brain stained with hematoxylin and eosin. The wrinkled appearance of the cyst wall is clearly evident. *B,* The *Naegleria* amoeba within this section of human brain stained with hematoxylin and eosin demonstrates a smooth single cell wall and prominent nucleus. (From Ash LR, Griebel TC: Atlas of Human Parasitology, p 71. Chicago, American Society of Clinical Pathologists, 1990.)

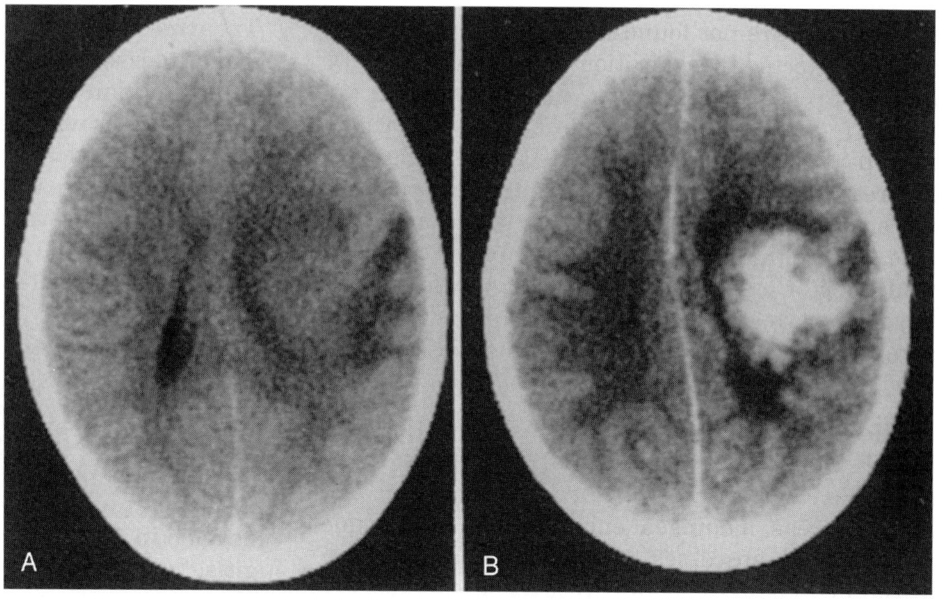

FIGURE 5–6 • Computed tomography of a 7-year-old female patient with *Acanthamoeba*-induced granuloma of left parietal lobe, presenting as right upper-extremity weakness. After surgical excision, the patient's symptoms resolved, and a 1-year follow-up scan showed no evidence of recurrence. *A,* Noncontrasted scan. *B,* Post-metrizamide scan. (From Ofori-Kwakye SK, Sidebottom DG, Herbert J, et al: Granulomatous brain tumor caused by Acanthamoeba: Case report. J Neurosurg 1986; 64:506.)

Pathophysiology. *E. histolytica* has at least two morphologically identifiable forms, one of which is pathogenic.[41] After the host ingests the cyst, trophozoites escape and invade the intestinal epithelium and disseminate to extrahepatic sites, most frequently the right lobe of the liver.[41] This may result in intestinal ulcerations and perforation, secondary bacterial infections, liver abscesses, and dissemination of infection to the lungs, pericardium, skin, and brain.

Clinical Presentation. Patients with noninvasive *Entamoeba* infection may exhibit nonspecific gastrointestinal symptoms, including abdominal pain and loose stools, whereas invasive infection may result in more severe abdominal pain, diarrhea, and occult blood in the stools. Approximately one-third of patients have fever. When abscesses occur in the brain, the clinical symptoms are essentially those of other brain abscesses as described earlier in the setting of symptoms of chronic systemic infection. Occasionally, patients present with meningeal signs.[44]

Laboratory Diagnosis. *Entamoeba* trophozoites or cysts are found in the stool in less than one-third of adults with systemic disease and in up to 60% of children.[30] Fig. 5–7 shows a trichrome stain of *Entamoeba* trophozoites from a fecal smear. They may also be found in hepatic aspirate samples. Al-

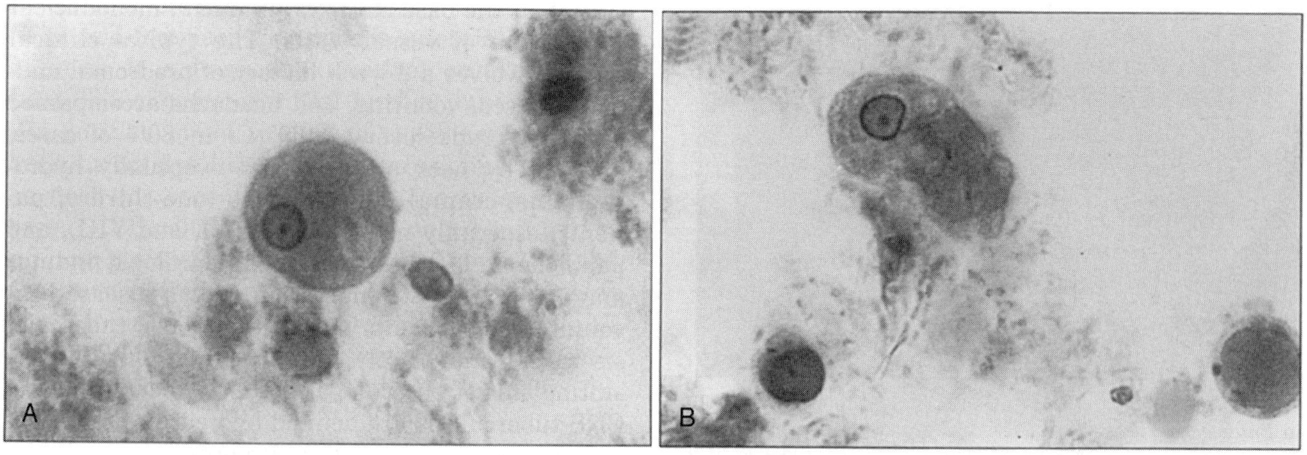

FIGURE 5–7 • *Entamoeba histolytica* trophozoites. This represents two typical appearances of the trophozoites. In trichrome-stained fecal smears trophozoites may have a green to purple appearance and a round (*A*) or elongated (*B*) shape. The cytoplasm typically is finely granular and does not contain debris, although red blood cells may be ingested in amebic dysentery. Vacuolization of the cytoplasm may be apparent in preparations that are left standing for hours prior to fixation. (From Ash LR, Griebel TC: Atlas of Human Parasitology, p 33. Chicago, American Society of Clinical Pathologists, 1990.)

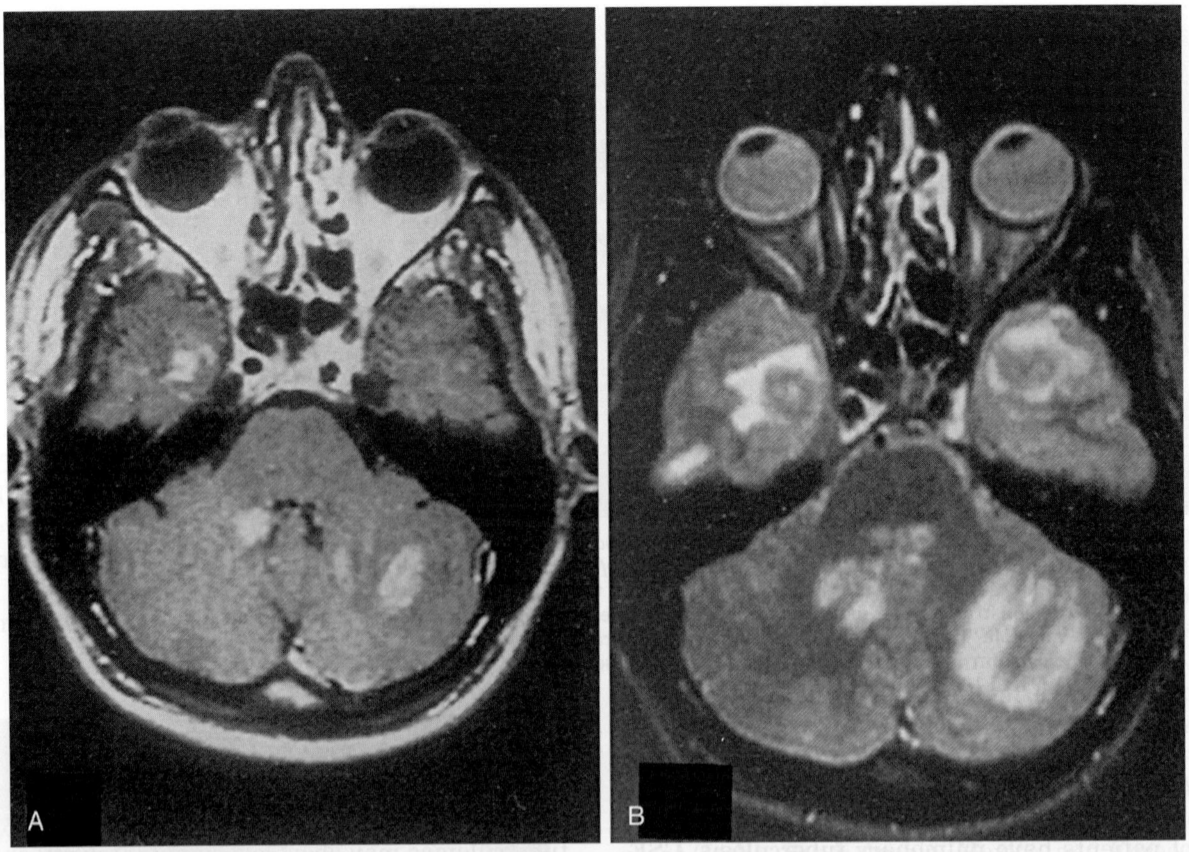

FIGURE 5–11 • Multiple intracranial tuberculomas in a 40-year-old man seropositive for HIV. *A,* Axial contrast-enhanced T1-weighted MRI revealing enhancing lesions within the right temporal lobe and both cerebellar hemispheres. *B,* Axial T2-weighted MRI revealing multiple lesions with isointense central core surrounded by a high-intensity rim. (From Kioumehr F, Dadsetan MR, Rooholamini SA, et al: Central nervous system tuberculosis: MRI. Neuroradiology 1994; 36:95.)

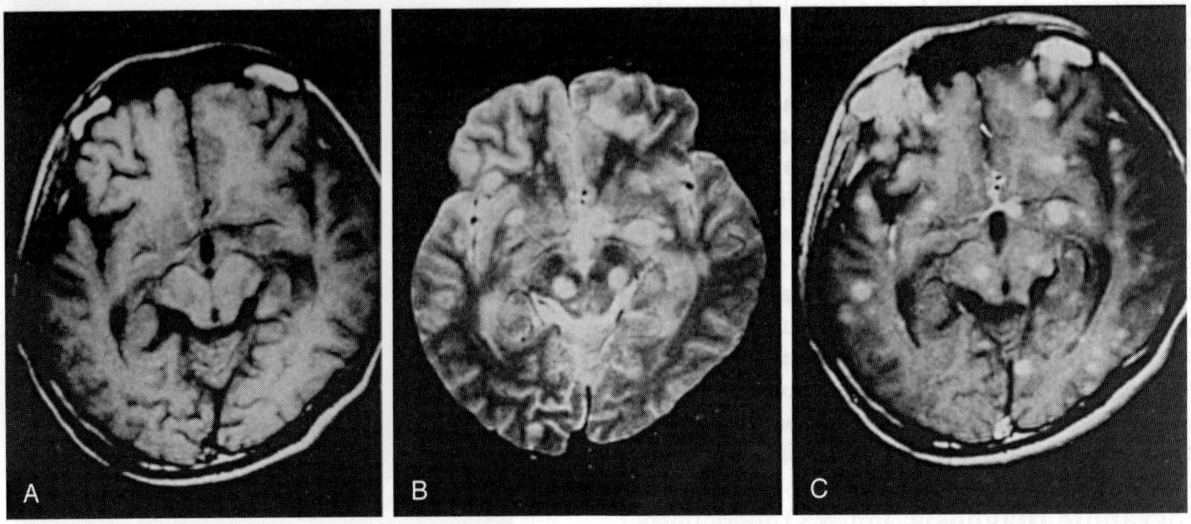

FIGURE 5–12 • Multiple intracranial tuberculomas in a 30-year-old man with miliary tuberculosis and sudden onset of fever and leg weakness. *A,* Axial T1-weighted MRI with isointense lesions within the brain that were visualized on T2-weighted images. *B,* Axial T2-weighted images revealing multiple lesions within the cerebral hemispheres and brain stem. *C,* Contrast-enhanced T1-weighted image revealing enhancement of the nodules. (From Shen W-C, Cheng T-Y, Ho Y-J, et al: Disseminated tuberculomas in spinal cord and brain demonstrated by MRI with gadolinium-DTPA. Neuroradiology 1993;35:214.)

lar enhancement[48] (Fig. 5–11). Although tuberculous meningitis cannot be differentiated from other meningitides by MRI, the characteristic T2 shortening of intraparenchymal tuberculomas is not found on most other space-occupying lesions[48] (see Fig. 5–11*B*). Immature tuberculomas appear as scattered areas of varied intensity (Fig. 5–12), whereas mature tuberculomas may appear as space-occupying lesions with a central area of low signal and surrounding edema (see Fig. 5–11).[49] Calcification is rare, and about one-third of tuberculomas are multiple.[50] As many as half may attach to the dura and resemble meningiomas. Intramedullary spinal cord tuberculomas are rare (~1%–5% of all CNS tuberculomas) and may appear primarily as single lesions in the thoracic area as hyperintense T2 signals with marked gadolinium enhancement (Fig. 5–13).[51] Most intramedullary cord tuberculomas resolve with adequate chemotherapy.[51, 52]

The development of symptoms of increased ICP, seizures, or focal neurologic signs in treated cases of CNS tuberculosis should raise suspicion of paroxysmal enlargement of intracranial tuberculomas.[46, 53] Suspicious lesions on CT or MRI require biopsy for definitive diagnosis in view of a high rate of false-positive radiographic findings that may mimic gliomas, cysticercosis, fungal granulomas, and metastases.[49] The positive predictive value for CT diagnosis is only about 33%.[49, 54]

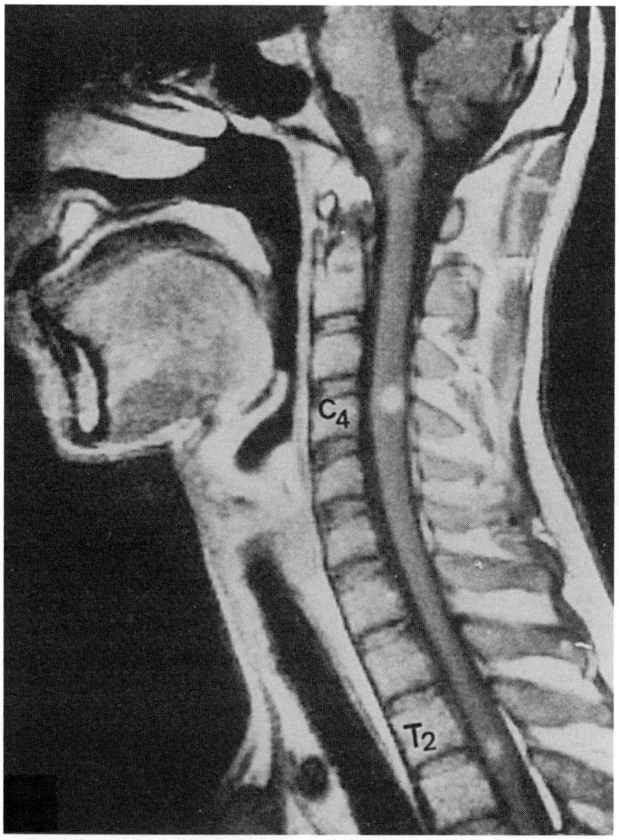

FIGURE 5–13 • Intramedullary cervical cord tuberculoma in same patient as in Figure 5–12. Contrast-enhanced T1-weighted MRI revealing enhancing tuberculomas in spinal cord. (From Shen W-C, Cheng T-Y, Ho Y-J, et al: Disseminated tuberculomas in spinal cord and brain demonstrated by MRI with gadolinium-DTPA. Neuroradiology 1993;35:214.)

TABLE 5–5 **TUBERCULOSIS THERAPY FOR ADULTS AND CHILDREN**

DRUG	DAILY DOSE	
	Adults	**Children**
Isoniazid	5 mg/kg PO or IM	10–20 mg/kg PO or IM
Rifampin	10 mg/kg PO or IV	10–20 mg/kg PO or IV
Pyrazinimide	15–30 mg/kg PO	15–30 mg/kg PO
Ethambutol	15–25 mg/kg PO	15–25 mg/kg PO
Streptomycin	15 mg/kg IM	20–40 mg/kg IM

PO, oral; IV, intravenous; IM, intramuscular.
Adapted from Preheim LC: Tuberculosis and other mycobacterial infections. In Carlson RW, Geheb MA (eds): Principles and Practice of Medical Intensive Care, p 425. Philadelphia, WB Saunders, 1993.

Treatment. Tuberculomas generally respond to medical treatment for tuberculosis. The currently recommended regimen for tuberculosis for children and adults is a combination of isoniazid, rifampin, and pyrazinamide (Table 5–5), and therapy should last 6 months or longer, depending on isolate sensitivity and clinical response.[55]

When clinical deterioration (to stage III) or an increase in lesion size is demonstrated, corticosteroids are recommended (dexamethasone 0.2–0.4 mg/kg every 6 hours) in addition to continued antituberculosis medications for up to 6 months.[46] Surgical intervention should be considered for patients in whom this medical regimen fails.

Epidural Abscesses

Epidemiology. Although not frequently encountered, infections of the epidural space are important by virtue of their nonspecific clinical presentation and high level of associated morbidity if not promptly identified and treated. Hematogenous spread is responsible for 25%–50% of cases, and patients with pre-existing back trauma or degenerative joint disease are at particular risk for metastatic seeding.[56, 57] These cases often result from the transient bacteremia associated with intravenous drug use, skin, dental, urinary tract, or upper respiratory infections.[57, 58] Alternatively, infection may be caused by direct invasion of the epidural space by surgery, by vertebral osteomyelitis, by paraspinal abscess, by penetrating trauma, or rarely after lumbar puncture or epidural anesthesia.[59, 60] Elderly, immunocompromised, and dialysis-dependent patients appear to be at the greatest risk for infection. In a relatively recent study performed at a large urban tertiary care hospital, the incidence of admission for epidural abscess was 2.8 cases per 10,000 admissions.[61] This is a significant increase from earlier studies, which may reflect the aging population and higher incidence of hematogenous spread from intravenous drug use in the community served. Although it may occur at any age, several studies suggest that epidural abscess is most common in the fifth decade of life and is distinctly uncommon in childhood.[61]

In descending order of frequency, epidural abscesses occur in the thoracic, lumbar, and cervical spine. Infection usually tracks along the posterior epidural space, because the dura of the anterior aspect of the spinal cord is tightly adherent to the vertebral bodies. Involvement of the anterior compartment is more likely to be associated with infection of the cervical or lumbar cord, where the epidural space widens.[57] Infection of the anterior epidural space is also more likely to result in meningitis due to invasion of the subarachnoid space.

Clinical Presentation. The clinical presentation of epidural abscess has been classically divided into four stages.[62] The patient may initially present with spinal ache, often accompanied by local tenderness and fever. As the syndrome progresses, the patient may experience true radicular pain, often associated with long tract signs and segmental reflex loss. Nuchal rigidity and headache are not uncommon. As the infection evolves, the patient may experience progressive weakness, bowel or bladder dysfunction, and an ascending sensory level. Prompt recognition of progressive spinal cord compression is essential, because weakness may herald precipitous deterioration, and irreversible paralysis may follow within hours.[61] Progressive neurologic deficit may be due either to direct compression of the spinal cord or to secondary ischemia resulting from venous inflammation and thrombosis.

The tempo of symptom progression from epidural abscess may vary widely. Acute epidural abscess (usually defined as symptom duration of less than 2 weeks) is most often caused by hematogenous seeding and is more apt to be associated with acute signs of systemic infection, such as fever, chills, and leukocytosis. A history of often trivial pyogenic skin, dental, upper respiratory, or urinary tract infection may be elicited. Chronic abscesses are more likely to arise from pre-existing osteomyelitis or extension of adjacent infection. Unfortunately, these patients often do not appear to be acutely ill, and the diagnosis may be missed.[57] Thus, a high index of suspicion should be entertained, especially in the patient with unexplained back pain who is immunocompromised or aged.

Many other disease processes may mimic the symptoms of epidural abscess (Table 5–6). Common problems such as disc herniation may cause similar radicular and myelopathic symptoms. Lymphoma and metastatic prostate, lung, or breast cancer may cause a syndrome of subacute cord compression that may be hard to differentiate from epidural abscess. Uncomplicated vertebral osteomyelitis may also be difficult to distinguish from epidural abscess, especially when vertebral collapse causes progressive myelopathy. Even when the diagnosis of uncomplicated vertebral osteomyelitis is correctly made, these patients should be followed closely, because 20% eventually develop chronic epidural abscess.[57] Transverse myelitis, epidural hematoma, psoas abscess, or intra-abdominal processes such as pyelonephritis, pancreatitis, or peptic ulcer should also be considered in the differential diagnosis of unexplained back pain. The rare entity of epidural lipo-

TABLE 5–6 **DIFFERENTIAL DIAGNOSIS OF EPIDURAL ABSCESS**

DIFFERENTIAL DIAGNOSIS	ASSOCIATED SIGNS, SYMPTOMS, AND HISTORY	ANCILLARY DIAGNOSTIC TESTS
Metastatic disease	Prior history of lung, breast, or prostate cancer or lymphoma	MRI, plain films, CSF for cytology
Intrinsic tumor or syrinx	Subacute progression of dull, poorly localized back pain over weeks or months; multiple segments often involved. Suspended, disassociated sensory level over arms and trunk may be present	MRI
Transverse myelitis	Prior history of multiple sclerosis or optic neuritis; recent viral infection	CSF may show mild pleocytosis, oligoclonal bands; MRI evidence of demyelinating lesions in brain or spinal cord
Abdominal, retroperitoneal infection	Prior history of genitourinary, pelvic infection; elevated amylase, lipase	Leukocytosis, abdominal/spine imaging
Epidural hematoma	Acute onset of pain, myelopathic symptoms in the setting of bleeding diathesis, anticoagulation, trauma	MRI, consider angiography if arteriovenous malformation suspected
Ischemia	Acute onset of anterior cord syndrome (loss of pain and temperature sensation, paralysis, with preservation of vibration, proprioception); vascular risk factors (smoking, diabetes mellitus, peripheral vascular disease)	Absence of structural lesion on MRI

CSF, cerebrospinal fluid; MRI, magnetic resonance imaging.

matosis may cause a syndrome of radicular pain and subacute myelopathy and should be considered in the patient with a history of chronic steroid use.

Laboratory Diagnosis. When present, nonspecific evidence of systemic response to infection, including an elevated sedimentation rate and leukocytosis, may be helpful in suggesting occult infection. These findings are not invariable, however, and may be absent in patients who are elderly, are immunocompromised, and have chronic infection. Blood cultures are positive in two-thirds of cases and have a high correlation with organisms cultured at surgical exploration.[61] *Staphylococcus aureus* is the most common pathogen, and *Staphylococcus* bacteremia in the setting of unexplained back pain should raise the index of suspicion for epidural abscess.[63] *Streptococcus* species are the second most common pathogens. Several recent studies have suggested an increased incidence of gram-negative organisms, especially in intravenous drug users.[56, 58] The possibility of atypical pathogens, including *Aspergillus,* should be considered in immunocompromised or transplant patients.[64]

It is usually recommended that lumbar puncture not be routinely performed because of the risk of seeding the subarachnoid space. If CSF is obtained, the glucose is usually normal and the protein is markedly elevated, especially if complete spinal block is present. Mild pleocytosis of polynuclear and mononuclear cells is common. Although chronic epidurals may have fewer than 40 cells/mm^3, a completely normal CSF formulation is distinctly unusual and should suggest an alternative diagnosis.[65]

Radiographic Diagnosis. Because MRI is noninvasive and provides excellent anatomic detail of the paraspinal structures, it has supplanted myelography at many institutions as the initial procedure of choice in patients suspected of harboring epidural infection.[66] A typical enhancing epidural abscess in the cervical spine is demonstrated in Figure 5–14. MRI is also sensitive at identifying associated osteomyelitis and most other lesions that may cause a syndrome of subacute spinal cord compression. Occasionally, MRI is nondiagnostic, especially in the setting of coexistent meningitis. In this situation or when MRI is not readily available, myelography remains the mainstay of diagnosis and usually demonstrates partial or complete obstruction of CSF flow. Spinal CT is not adequate to exclude the diagnosis of nontuberculous epidural abscess, although it may be helpful when used in conjunction with myelography. A postcontrast MRI, however, remains the preferred test (Fig. 5–15). Plain films may demonstrate evidence of osteomyelitis but are not sensitive in making the diagnosis of epidural abscess. Radionucleotide studies are sufficiently nonspecific that they rarely provide additional useful information.

Treatment. Most authors agree that surgical drainage and decompression is a crucial step in the management of nontuberculous epidural abscess. Certainly, progressive neurologic deterioration mandates emergent surgical intervention. The administration of glucocorticoids in the setting of progressive neurologic deficit remains controversial. In a recent study, the use of steroids was associated with poor outcome, although the patients who received steroids had more severe neurologic deficits prior to their administration.[61] The possibility of exacerbating infection remains at least a theoretical concern, although this complication has not been well documented in this setting. Intravenous antibiotics should be started immediately, and empirical treatment should provide adequate antistaphylococcal coverage. The optimal length of treatment has not been well established. Osteomyelitis is present in up to one-half of patients with chronic epidural abscess and in 15% of patients with acute infection; it should be treated with an extended course of antibiotics.[67] There is some indication that patients who are HIV-1 positive may also not respond adequately to standard treatment and should receive a prolonged course of antibiotic therapy.[68]

There is good evidence that neurologic outcome is directly related to the patient's neurologic status at the time of surgical intervention.[61] In general, patients with abscess involving the anterior paraspinal space tend to have more complete recovery. Overall, approximately one-half of patients recover completely, one-quarter are left with significant neurologic deficit, and 10% are left paralyzed.[61] The mortality rate ranges from 14% to 32% in different series.[56, 58, 61]

OTHER PARASITIC INFECTIONS

Echinococcus

Epidemiology. Two species of echinococcus tapeworm infest the human CNS, *Echinococcus granulosus* and *Echinococcus multilocularis,* with the former being more common in hot climates (middle East, South America, Australia, and India) in areas where sheep are raised, and the latter being more common in cooler climates (Wales, western England, former Soviet Union, United States, Germany, and China). The brain is infected in approximately 2% of all cases of *Echinococcus granulosus* infection, although brain infection is as high as 8% among children in Mediterranean countries.[69] Hydatid cyst disease refers to formation of walled cysts con-

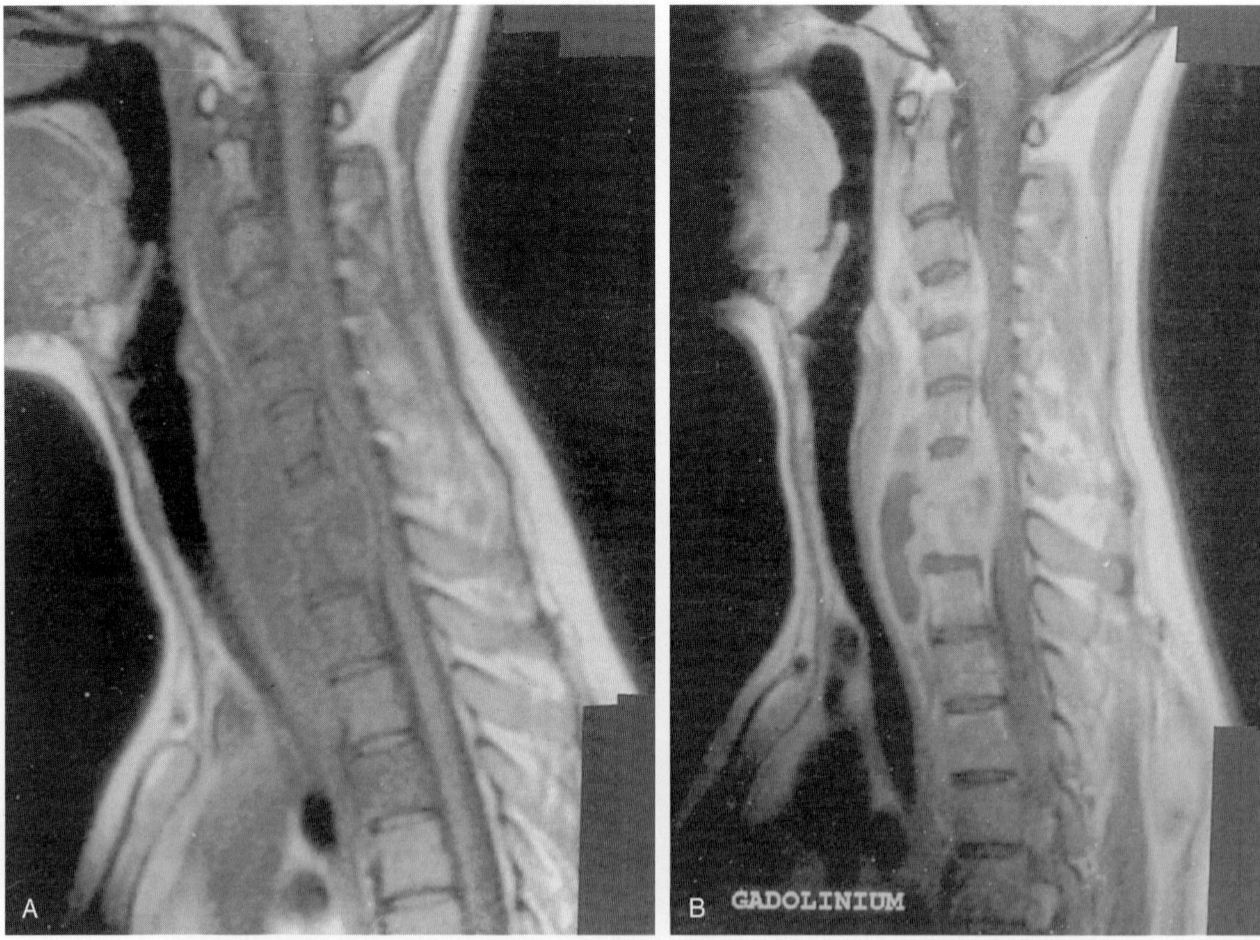

FIGURE 5-14 • MRI of epidural abscesses. These are cervical spinal cord MRI images in a 20-year-old Asian woman presenting with gradual onset of pain and stiffness in her neck and paresthesias in her left arm. *A,* T1-weighted sagittal image of the cervical cord before contrast. *B,* Postcontrast imaging revealing an irregularly enhancing anterior spinal mass causing cord compression associated with bone and disc abnormalities. Note the presence of a mass also in the posterior soft tissues at the upper thoracic level. (From Lang IM, Hughes DG, Jenkins JPR, et al: MR imaging appearances of cervical epidural abscess. Clin Radiol 1995;50:469.)

taining larvae, which may appear in the liver, lung, and brain, with brain involvement more common in children than adults.[70]

Pathogenesis. *Echinococcus* eggs passed in the feces of infected dogs and foxes that have fed on the carcasses of the primary host (sheep) are ingested by humans, who become intermediate hosts.[71] Once swallowed, embryos are liberated from the eggs and invade the bloodstream, passing via the portal vein to the liver, where larvae become entrapped and form cysts (60%–70%) or proceed further to form cysts within the lung (10%–15%) or brain.[43, 45, 71, 72] Although 80% of cysts are solitary,[45] once established within the brain, a single mother cyst may rupture and seed multiple secondary cysts by spilling of the scolices.[73] Hydatid cysts may form within the brain parenchyma, skull bones, epidural space, and intraventricular space.[69, 71, 74]

Clinical Presentation. Symptoms of increased ICP are prominent and include headache and vomiting in a majority of patients, followed in frequency by seizures in 50%,[75] visual disturbances, and focal weakness.[71] Fifty percent to 75% of intracranial hydatid cysts occur in children[75]; in a series of 19 children undergoing surgical excision of intracranial cysts, Ersahin et al.[71] documented papilledema in 16 (84%) and hemiparesis in 10 (55%). Children may present with a marked expansion of the cranium due to cyst enlargement in the epidural space or diploe.[71, 74]

Laboratory Diagnosis. Eosinophilia in the peripheral blood is an inconstant feature. ELISAs for detection of genus-specific antigens isolated from unilocular hydatid cyst fluid are being developed.[42]

Radiographic Diagnosis. CT reveals cystic lesions containing fluid isodense with CSF and possibly grape-like clusters of scolices, often with ring enhancement with contrast dye, with or without surrounding edema (Fig. 5–16). MRI may reveal a heterogeneous low-signal mass or masses on T1 weighting, whereas T2 weighting may reveal significant edema.[76] The cysts are most commonly found in the parietal lobes and only rarely in the posterior fossa and ventricles; they may enlarge at a rate of several centimeters per year.[69, 73] Plain skull films sometimes reveal erosion of bone and linear calcifications at the cystic edges.[70, 74, 77] Identification of intracranial cysts demands a thorough examination of the rest of the viscera, because infection is most common in the liver (60%) and lungs (25%).[45]

Treatment. The treatment of choice for cerebral hydatid cysts is surgical excision, although oral mebendazole and albendazole (10 mg/kg every 12 hours during 3 months) have been shown to be effective in some cases of systemic hydatid cysts.[16, 72, 78] The cysts should be removed without rupture because of the immediate risk of anaphylaxis (in response to hydatid fluid), meningitis, and subsequent recurrence due to seeding of larvae.[70, 79] Surgical approaches include puncture and aspiration of cystic fluid, wide excision, and "birthing" of the cyst by irrigation of the cyst/brain interface to gently dislodge the cyst, which unlike hepatic cysts, have well-defined margins without adhesions.[69, 73, 76] Some authors recommend prophylactic use of mebendazole after surgery when either multiple cysts are found or rupture occurs, to delay or prevent recurrence of cysts.[71] Perioperative mortality rates range from 8% to 25%.

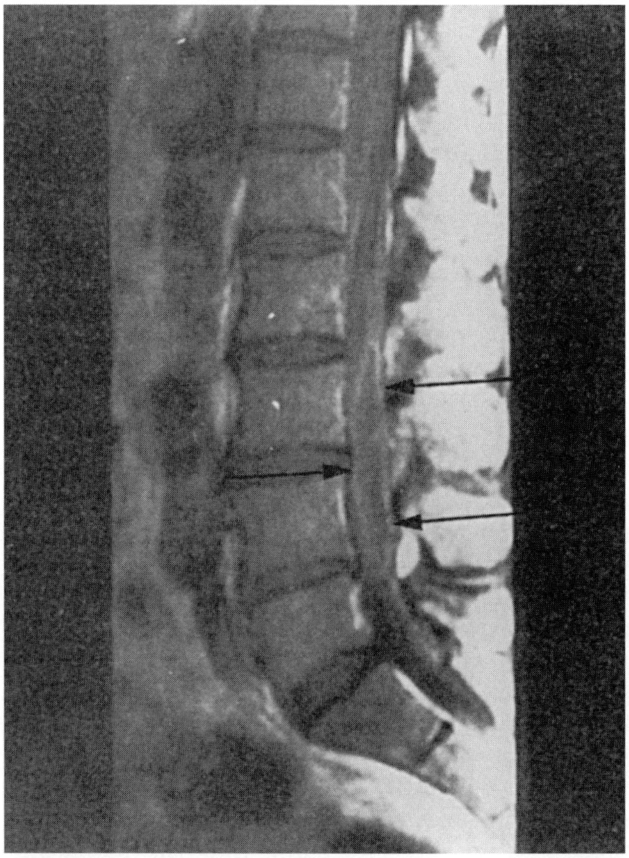

FIGURE 5-15 • MRI of lumbosacral epidural abscess. This is a postcontrast T1-weighted sagittal image of the lumbosacral spine of a 64-year-old man taken 3 days after receiving an epidural anesthetic procedure for angioplasty of his femoral arteries. The abscess is apparent in the dorsal epidural space and demonstrates a thin margin of high signal enhancement at its periphery (arrows). (From Mamourian AC, Dickman CA, Drayer BP, et al: Spinal epidural abscess: Three cases following spinal epidural injection demonstrated by magnetic resonance imaging. Anesthesiology 1994;78:206.)

Neurocysticercosis

Epidemiology. Neurocysticercosis is caused by infection of the larval stage *(Cysticercus cellulosa)* of the pig tapeworm *Taenia solium,* which is the most common helminth to produce CNS infection in man.[42] Infection is endemic in all continents except in Australia; it is common in Latin America, especially Mexico, where cysticercosis is found in up to 4% of autopsies.[80] Neurocysticercosis is becoming more frequent in the United States as a result of immigration of people from endemic areas. It is the most common parasitic infection of the CNS[81] in the world, including the United States.[82]

Pathogenesis. Humans acquire the pork tapeworm by eating undercooked pork carrying the larval stage of *T. solium,* which results in the attachment and growth of a single tapeworm in the human host. Human cysticercosis arises when eggs, rather than larvae, are ingested in food or water contaminated with human feces. The egg wall is dissolved, and the resultant oncospheres (released primary larvae) penetrate the intestinal mucosa and enter the lymphatics and mesenteric vessels. From there they enter skeletal muscles, other tissues, and the CNS. Within 2–3 months cysticerci (secondary larvae) develop and evoke a local reaction, including capsule formation, fibrosis, and infiltration by neutrophils and eosinophils.[83] These space-occupying cysts may persist for decades and eventually become calcified.[84] Patients may autoinfect themselves through inadvertent ingestion of their own fecal material.[43]

Clinical Presentation. Signs and symptoms result from meningeal inflammation, mass effects of the cysts, and intense inflammatory responses due to death of the cysticerci.[81] Symptoms occur anywhere from 2 months to 30 years after infection, and systemic symptoms of subcutaneous nodule for-

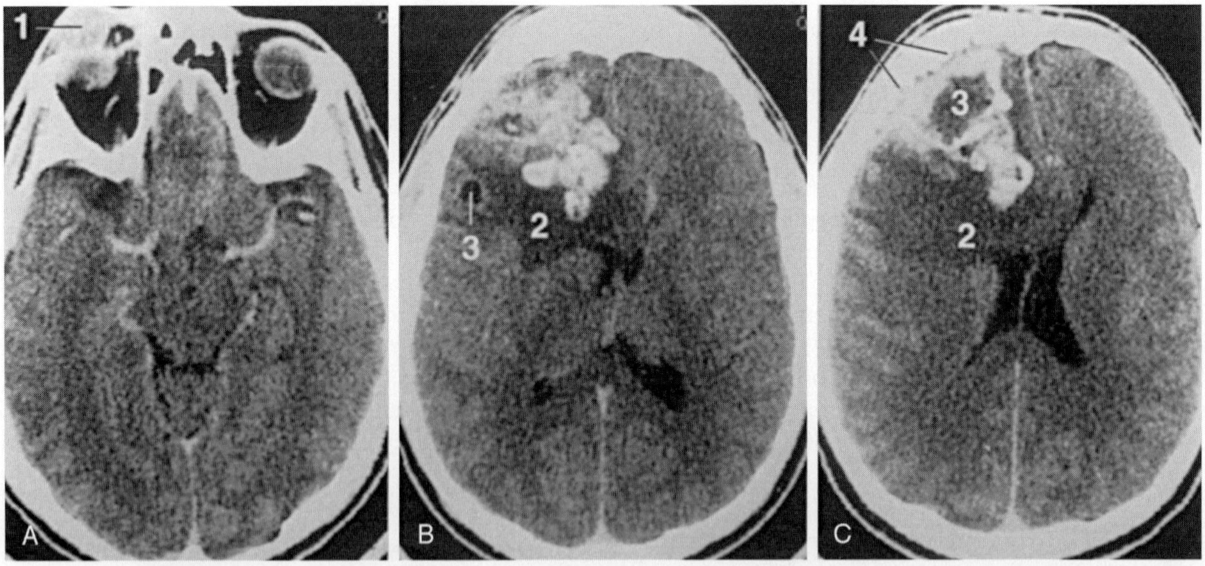

FIGURE 5–16 • Contrast-enhanced computed tomography in a 48-year-old French farmer with headaches and a prior history of pulmonary alveolar hydatid cyst. *A,* A rounded palpebral mass [1]. *B,* There is also a large right frontal mass, with posterior displacement of the corpus callosum, which contains nodular and ring cacification, partial contrast enhancement, and surrounding edema [2]. A nonenhancing, noncalcified parasitic cyst [3]. *C,* Anterior to the mass, the inner table of the skull is irregular [4]. (From Bensaid AH, Dietemann JL, Filippi de la Palavesa MM, et al: Intracranial alveolar echinococcosis: CT and MRI. Neuroradiology 1994;36:289.)

mation and myositis are common. Approximately 50% of patients develop CNS symptoms, the most common of which are: seizures (50%), hydrocephalus with increased ICP (30%), and stroke (4%–12%) (Table 5–7).[42, 85, 86] Signs and symptoms may be attributed to the anatomic location of the cyst:

1. Parenchymal cysts may result in seizures, focal abnormalities, and increased ICP secondary to obstructive hydrocephalus.
2. Meningeal cysts are often in the basal meninges and can cause meningitis, hydrocephalus, and stroke.
3. Ventricular cysts commonly infect the fourth ventricle and may cause obstructive hydrocephalus, which may be intermittent.
4. Spinal cord cysts are the least common but may result in arachnoiditis with transverse myelitis or local spinal cord syndrome.

TABLE 5–7 **PRESENTING SIGNS AND SYMPTOMS IN NEUROCYSTICERCOSIS**

SIGNS AND SYMPTOMS	FREQUENCY
Seizures	53%
Headaches	43%
Papilledema	28%
Vomiting	27%
Pyramidal tract signs	21%
Altered mentation	16%
Others:	1%–10%
ataxia, visual loss, optic atrophy, psychosis, diplopia, vertigo, tremor, and cranial nerve palsies	

Adapted from Sotelo J, Guerrero V, Rubio F: Neurocysticercosis: A new classification based on active and inactive forms: A study of 753 cases. Arch Intern Med 145:443. Copyright 1985, American Medical Association.

The most common causes of death are status epilepticus and herniation due to increased ICP. Table 5–7 lists signs and symptoms in order of decreasing frequency in a series of 700 patients from Mexico City.[42]

Laboratory Diagnosis. Approximately 50% of patients with neurocysticercosis have subcutaneous nodules containing cysticercal cysts.[45] CSF pressure may be elevated, and other abnormalities depend on the location of the cysts. There may be pleocytosis of 5 to 500 cells with an eosinophil or lymphocyte preponderance. Total protein and IgG may be elevated, and the glucose may be low.[42] An ELISA for CSF has recently shown promising results in neurocysticercosis.[87] In this study, Chang-Yuan et al. used a monoclonal antibody–based ELISA to detect antigen in 95 of 116 patients (82%) diagnosed by a combination of CT, physical examination, and serology. In active cysticercosis, one may find IgG or IgM antibodies in the serum or CSF using ELISA, complement fixation, or hemagglutination inhibition[42, 86]; some authors claim that the diagnostic yield of the CSF ELISA may be as high as 93%.[87]

Radiographic Diagnosis. Both CT and MRI are useful in diagnosis. Acute lesions may show edema and postcontrast enhancement, and they are described as well circumscribed when the larvae are living[88] (Fig. 5–17). These cystic lesions may be single or multiple. Pedunculated larvae may be identified within cystic lesions by T1-weighted MRI.[42] In two-thirds of adult patients, one may see small punctate calcifications in the parenchyma, which are thought to represent cysts in which the larvae have died.[88]

Treatment. Albendazole is considered the drug of choice of neurocysticercosis. This includes intraparenchymal cysts and subarachnoid cysts.[84, 89, 90] For fourth ventricular cysts, spinal lesions, or large mass lesions that result in mass effects, surgical excision is the treatment of choice. In a comparison between albendazole and praziquantel therapy for neurocysticercosis, Takayanagui and Jardim[90] compared 21 patients treated with praziquantel with 21 patients treated with albendazole. Albendazole was more effective in decreasing the total number of cysts according to CT, and the cysts completely disappeared in 55% of patients treated with albendazole and in 15% of patients treated with praziquantel. Typical doses are 15 mg/kg per day orally for 8 days of albendazole or praziquantel 20 mg/kg three times daily orally for 14 days.

Concomitant use of dexamethasone is controversial but directed toward decreasing acute inflammatory responses of the death of the cysticerci during the first few days of therapy.[16, 42, 82] It is specifically recommended in patients (especially children) who develop seizures, headache, or vomiting for a period of 72 hours after initiating cysticidal therapy.[82, 89] In addition, it is recommended when subarachnoid cysts are present, and it should be administered before, during, and for several days after the course of anti-cysticercal drug treatment to avoid possible occlusive endarteritis due to destruction of subarachnoid cysticerci.[89] Dexamethasone may increase the plasma level of albendazole while decreasing the plasma praziquantel.[16] Overall, one may expect destruction of 60%–70% of parenchymal brain cysts by praziquantel, whereas albendazole destroys 75%–90% of such lesions.[89] In addition, albendazole has better penetration into the subarachnoid space, allowing treatment of meningeal cysticerci.

Anti-cysticerci drugs should be used with caution in patients with cysticercotic encephalitis, because these drugs may exacerbate intracranial hypertension. Furthermore, when hydrocephalus accompanies parenchymal brain cysts, the drug should be used after ventricular shunting to avoid further increases in ICP as a result of drug therapy. And finally, patients with calcifications alone but with no cysts need not receive brain therapy because these lesions contain dead parasites.

Because epilepsy is the most frequent clinical manifestation of neurocysticercosis, concurrent anti-epileptic therapy has been recommended.[91, 92] In a series of 40 patients with treated neurocysticercosis,[91] a relapse seizure rate of 50% after drug withdrawal was found within 3 to 4 months after initiation of therapy. Seizure recurrence was associated with edema appearing around calcifications left after drug treatment. This suggests that many patients require long-term anti-epileptic medica-

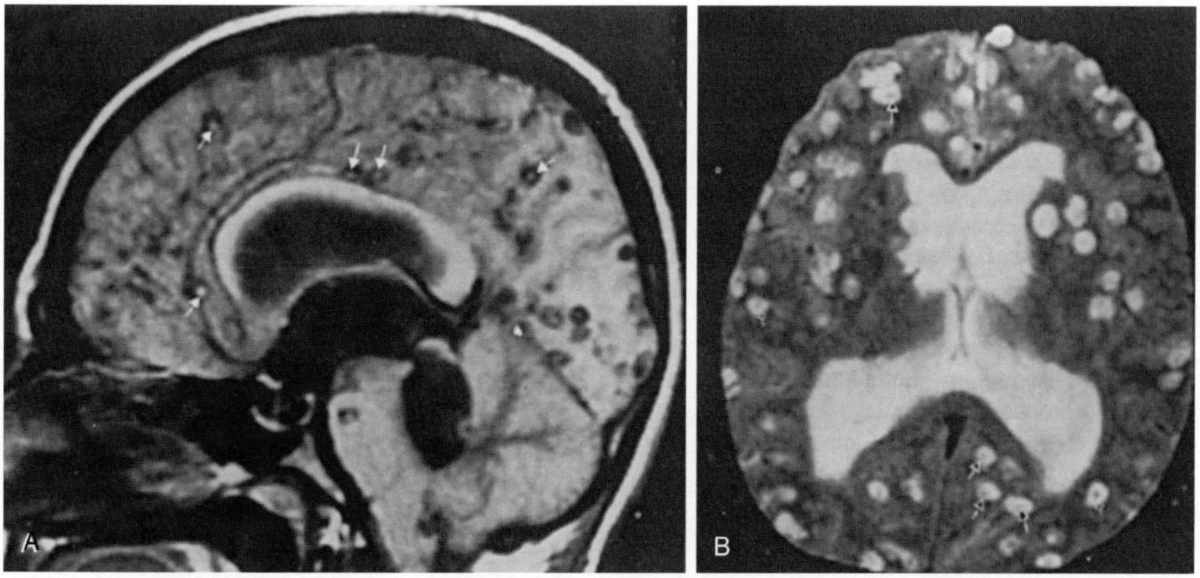

FIGURE 5–17 • MRI of neurocysticercosis. *A,* Sagittal T1-weighted MRI demonstrating numerous cystic lesions with arrows indicating intracystic scolices (larvae). *B,* T2-weighted image again indicating intracystic scolices (arrows) and demonstrating that the vesicular fluid is isointense with cerebrospinal fluid on both T1- and T2-weighted images. (From Grossman RI, Yousem DM: Infectious and noninfectious inflammatory diseases of the brain. In Farrell RJ [ed]: Neuroradiology: The Requisites, p 195. St. Louis, Mosby–Year Book, 1994.)

tions, especially those with parenchymal brain calcifications and multiple cysts.

Malaria

Epidemiology. Malaria affects as many as 300 million humans in the world per year and contributes to the deaths of more than 1 million persons annually in tropical Africa alone.[42] Malaria is endemic in most of Africa, Asia, and Latin America. It is imported occasionally into the United States by immigrants, military personnel, and visitors. Cerebral malaria is the most common pediatric encephalopathy in Africa with a mortality rate of 10%–40% and a 10% rate of severe neurologic sequelae including hemiparesis, blindness, epilepsy, and aphasia.[93]

Pathogenesis. Malaria is a protozoan disease transmitted to humans by the bite of Anopheles mosquitos that transmit the genus *Plasmodium.* There are four *Plasmodia* species known to infect humans, including *P. vivax, P. ovale, P. malariae,* and *P. falciparum.*[43] *P. falciparum's* infection has the highest mortality and drug resistance and is the cause of cerebral malaria.[93–96] After the mosquito bite and inoculation of sporozoites, the organisms infect hepatocytes where they multiply to form merozoites which, after 1–6 weeks, infect red blood cells and become intracellular parasites. Within 48 hours, the cell ruptures and releases infectious organisms capable of reinfecting red cells. Some cells are parasitized by sexual forms (gametocytes) that do not lyse the cells but remain dormant unless ingested by a mosquito vector.

The erythrocyte phase of infection is accompanied by chills, fevers, headaches, and myalgias in association with hepatomegaly, icterus, splenomegaly, and gastrointestinal symptoms. Untreated, anemia may occur, and subsequent renal failure, liver failure, and visceral ischemia may occur because of capillary blockage by infected erythrocytes. Cerebral malaria is also a complication. The sequelae of cerebral infection is thought to result from sequestration of infected erythrocytes altering tissue perfusion and oxygenation. This may be secondary to widespread blockage of small vessels by parasitized erythrocytes.[93, 94] Histologic examination of tissues from fatal *P. falciparum* malaria has shown accumulation of parasitized red blood cells in the brain, heart, lungs, and gut.[94]

Clinical Presentation. The incubation period is 6–16 days and heralded by a prodrome that begins with vague constitutional symptoms, including headaches, malaise, abdominal pain, or myalgias.[42] Paroxysms of chills and fever 40° C or higher occur at varying intervals interspersed with periods of few symptoms.

Cerebral malaria may present as disturbances of consciousness, acute organic mental syndromes, movement disorders, focal neurologic signs, and acute personality changes. CNS involvement often begins abruptly with generalized seizures and alterations of consciousness. The movement disorders include flexor or extensor posturing, severe chorea and myoclonus, and focal neurologic signs, including hemiparesis, monoparesis, or cranial nerve palsies. Retinal hemorrhages may occur in 15% of cases but in adults are not usually accompanied by signs of increased ICP, including papilledema.[42] Such increases in ICP, however, may be more common in childhood cerebral malaria.[93, 95] Most neurologic symptoms persist for 24–72 hours and then proceed to death or to complete recovery.[42]

Laboratory Diagnosis. Perhaps the most useful diagnostic test is identification of parasitized red blood cells in the peripheral blood smear.[42] Serial blood samples should be taken, because parasites may be absent early in the course of infection. In addition, serologic diagnosis using ELISAs are useful[97] but again may be negative early in infection. Nucleic acid hybridization techniques are highly sensitive.[98, 99] Laboratory findings may vary according to the severity of the illness with anemia, elevation of hepatic transaminase levels, mild hyponatremia (125–135 mEq/L), hypoglycemia, or thrombocytopenia.

CSF is usually normal, although modest elevation of protein and cell counts have been noted; elevated cell counts should suggest diagnoses other than cerebral malaria, however.[42, 43]

Radiographic Diagnosis. CT of the head is usually normal but may show diffuse swelling, especially in children.[93]

Treatment. Treatment of cerebral malaria depends on whether chloroquine resistance is significant in the geographic area where infection occurred (Table 5–8). Areas with chloroquine-resistant strains of *P. falciparum* include: sub-Saharan Africa, Asia, North and South America, New Guinea, and the Indian subcontinent. Where chloroquine resistance is a problem and the adult patient is able to take oral medications, recommended antibiotics are oral quinine sulfate plus doxycycline 100 mg every 12 hours for 7 days, or clindamycin or the combination of sulfadoxine and pyrimethamine (Fansidar) (if malaria is not acquired in Southeast Asia or the Congo Basin).[16] Where the organism is chloroquine-sensitive, recommended treatment is oral chloroquine phosphate (1 g loading dose, then 0.5 g in

TABLE 5–8 **DRUG TREATMENT OF CEREBRAL MALARIA *(P. falciparum)***

MENTAL STATUS	CHLOROQUINE-SENSITIVE	CHLOROQUINE-RESISTANT
Patient arousable	*Adult:* Chloroquine phosphate 1 g (600 mg base) PO, then 0.5 g in 6 hrs, then 0.5 g every day for 2 days (total 2.5 g) *Child:* Chloroquine phosphate 10 mg base/kg (max. 600 mg base) PO, then 5 mg base/kg in 6 hrs, then 5 mg base/kg every day for 2 days	*Adult:* Quinine sulfate 600 mg (500 mg base) PO every 8 hrs for 3–7 days *plus* Doxycycline 100 mg PO every 12 hrs for 7 days *or* Clindamycin 450 mg PO every 6 hrs for 3 days *or* Pyrimethamine sulfdoxine (Fansidar), 3 tablets PO single dose *Child:* Quinine sulfate 25 mg/kg divided 3 times daily for 3 days *plus* Pyrimethamine sulfdoxine: *< 1 yr:* ¼ tablet *1–3 yrs:* ½ tablet *4–8 yrs:* 1 tablet *9–14 yrs:* 2 tablets, single dose
Patient unarousable or unable to take oral medication	*Adult:* Quinidine gluconate 10 mg/kg IV loading dose (max. 600 mg) over 1 hr, then 0.02 mg/kg constant infusion until oral therapy with chloroquine is tolerated *Child:* Same as adult dose	Qunindine gluconate IV (same regimen as for chloroquine-sensitive strains, except that quinine sulfate in combination with pyrimethamine sulfdoxine or mefloquine is used for oral therapy)

IV, intravenous; PO, per os (orally); yrs, years; hr, hour.
Data are summarized from Bale JF: Parasitic and rickettsial infections of the nervous system; Tyler KL, Martin JB (eds): Infectious Diseases of the Central Nervous System, p 272. Philadelphia, FA Davis, 1993; and from Sanford JP, Gilbert DN, Sande MA, Geberding JE (eds): The Sanford Guide to Antimicrobial Therapy, pp 77–80. Dallas, Antimicrobial Therapy, 1994.

6 hours and then 0.5 g daily for 2 days, or a total dose of 2.5 g).[16] Drug treatments for cerebral malaria are summarized in Table 5–8, for both adults and children.

VIRAL ENCEPHALITIS

Viral encephalitis most commonly involves the cerebral hemispheres but may preferentially affect the brain stem instead. In this section, the common viral encephalitides are discussed first, followed by a discussion of brain stem encephalitis as a separate diagnostic entity.

Epidemiology. Most primary forms of encephalitis are caused by viruses, where direct cellular damage is less commonly significant than delayed hypersensitivity, because most viruses are recognized as foreign to their host and in many cases result in antibody formation. The clinical manifestations are diverse in severity, onset, and progression, but they generally share the features of fever, headache, and malaise followed by alteration of mentation. Although the diagnosis always requires a high degree of clinical suspicion, a careful history, including seasonal predominance and geography, and neurologic examination along with appropriate diagnostic tests can often identify the specific etiologic agent and sometimes suggest specific treatment. Nonetheless, of all cases of infectious encephalitis in the United States reported to the Centers for Disease Control and Prevention in 1977, 72.9% were of undetermined etiology, 10.7% were associated with arboviruses, 5.9% were associated with exanthem viruses, 3.3% were associated with mumps, and 7.3% were associated with other viruses.[100]

Clinical Presentation. Fever, headache, neck stiffness, and altered sensorium are nearly universal, though nonspecific. In such a clinical setting, focal neurologic signs such as aphasia, focal seizures, and cranial nerve deficits strongly indicate infectious encephalitis and can even suggest specific viral agents. Evaluation must be directed by geographic and seasonal considerations (*summertime* arboviruses, *sporadic* herpes and parainfectious sources) and requires examination of CSF and appropriate specific serum or CSF antibody titers, usually IgM.[101] Virus isolation is possible in a few cases.

Increased ICP is indicated by the absence of spontaneous venous pulsations in the optic disc and often precedes papilledema and diffuse brain swelling. Such findings are common in Eastern equine and Herpes simplex encephalitis. Facial hemiparesis (cranial nerve VII) should alert one to Eastern equine, St. Louis, Venezuelan, Japanese B, and herpes simplex. Cutaneous vesicles in the distribution of the trigeminal nerve, especially V_1, or in the ear canal suggest varicella-zoster (zoster ophthalmicus, Ramsay Hunt syndrome, respectively). Multiple cranial nerve palsies indicating brain stem encephalitis are common in varicella-zoster, rabies, and

St. Louis encephalitis. Hemiparesis suggests herpes simplex, Eastern equine, and varicella-zoster. Tetraparesis suggests Eastern equine and rabies; rabies also shows hyporeflexia.

With the exception of AIDS-associated encephalitis, which is a subacutely developing clinical entity, the more common clinical viral encephalitides are discussed with reference to epidemiology, pathology, symptoms and diagnostic studies, and treatment. They are grouped as *endemic* (herpes simplex, varicella-zoster, and rabies); *epidemic arboviral* (Eastern equine, Western equine, St. Louis, Venezuelan equine, Japanese B, and La Crosse); *epidemic nonarboviral* (influenza, enterovirus, and mumps); and *parainfectious* (measles).

TABLE 5–9 **SYMPTOMS AND SIGNS IN PATIENTS WITH BRAIN-CULTURE POSITIVE HERPES SIMPLEX ENCEPHALITIS**

Altered consciousness	97%
Fever	90%
Headache	81%
Dysphasia	76%
Personality change	71%
Seizures	67%
Vomiting	47%
Ataxia	40%
Hemiparesis	33%
Cranial nerve deficits	32%
Memory loss	24%
Visual field loss	14%
Papilledema	14%

These data are from the National Institute of Allergy and Infectious Disease (NIAID) Collaboratove Antiviral Study Group, summarized in Goldsmith SM, Whitley RJ: Herpes simplex encephalitis. In Lambert HP (ed). Infections of the Central Nervous System, p 286. Philadelphia, BC Decker, 1991. They summarize clinical findings in 112 patients in whom the diagnosis of herpes simplex encephalitis was confirmed by virus culture from the brain. Ages ranged from 6 months to > 60 years, with equal distribution by decade. Males and females were equally represented; whites constituted 86% of patients.

Endemic Encephalitis

Herpes Simplex Encephalitis (HSE)

Epidemiology. Encephalitis due to infection by herpes simplex type 1 virus is the most common sporadic viral encephalitis in adults, estimated to occur in 2%–10% of all encephalitis cases.[102] There is no seasonal or geographic predominance, and males and females are equally affected. Only one-third of cases are preceded by a history of gingivostomatitis.[103] Untreated, HSE has a mortality rate of 70%–90%, with only 2.5% of patients surviving without neurologic sequelae.[104]

Clinical Presentation. In HSE, one typically sees that a 4 to 10 day prodromal period of fever and malaise is followed by a characteristic clinical presentation: alteration in consciousness (97%), fever (90%), headache (81%), and personality changes (71%)[105] (Table 5–9). Focal motor seizures affecting the face and upper extremities are common, indicating the predilection of herpes simplex for the temporal and frontal lobes.[105] Other focal neurologic signs, including hemiparesis and aphasia, are more common with HSE than with other viral encephalitides.

Laboratory Diagnosis. Definitive diagnosis can now be made not only by brain biopsy but also by recently developed polymerase chain reaction (PCR) techniques that are highly sensitive and specific.[106–109] Brain biopsy should be directed by neuroimaging studies to areas of suspected involvement or to the nondominant temporal lobe. With immunofluorescence staining for viral antigens (sensitivity 80%, specificity 95%), a positive result can be obtained in 2–3 hours. Viral culture from the brain tissue usually requires 48 hours. Electron microscopy is about 98% specific but only about 48% sensitive and therefore not routinely used.

A recent publication from the National Institute of Allergy and Infectious Diseases Collaborative Antiviral Study Group recommends PCR detection of herpes simplex virus DNA as the standard for diagnosis of HSE.[106] Using CSF and brain tissue from 54 patients with biopsy-proven HSE, these authors demonstrated a sensitivity of 98%, specificity of 94%, positive predictive value of 95%, and negative predictive value of 98% for PCR in the CSF of patients. Furthermore, this 98% sensitivity estimate applied to specimens collected from patients up to 7 days after initiation of antiviral therapy, after which sensitivity dramatically decreased (47% during days 8–14 of treatment). PCR assay may confirm the diagnosis as early as the first day of neurologic signs and symptoms.[110]

The CSF typically shows lymphocytosis of 10–400 cells/mm^3 (though 20% of CSF specimens are normal in the first few days), along with increased protein (80–1000 mg/dL) and up to 1000 red blood cells/mm^3 (median ~130), indicating hemorrhagic necrosis.[102] Glucose is normal or decreased.

Radiographic Diagnosis. CT with intravenous contrast shows gyral enhancement, temporal lobe lucencies, or mass effect in up to 65% of biopsy-proved cases by day 5 or later of clinical signs and symptoms,[111] whereas MRI scanning may be more sensitive, especially earlier, and may allow monitoring of response to acyclovir therapy.[112, 113] Figure 5–18 shows a typical T2-weighted MRI scan on a patient with HSE, revealing increased signal intensity within the right temporal lobe. The electroencephalogram (EEG) is often helpful, showing PLEDS unilaterally or bilaterally in the temporal

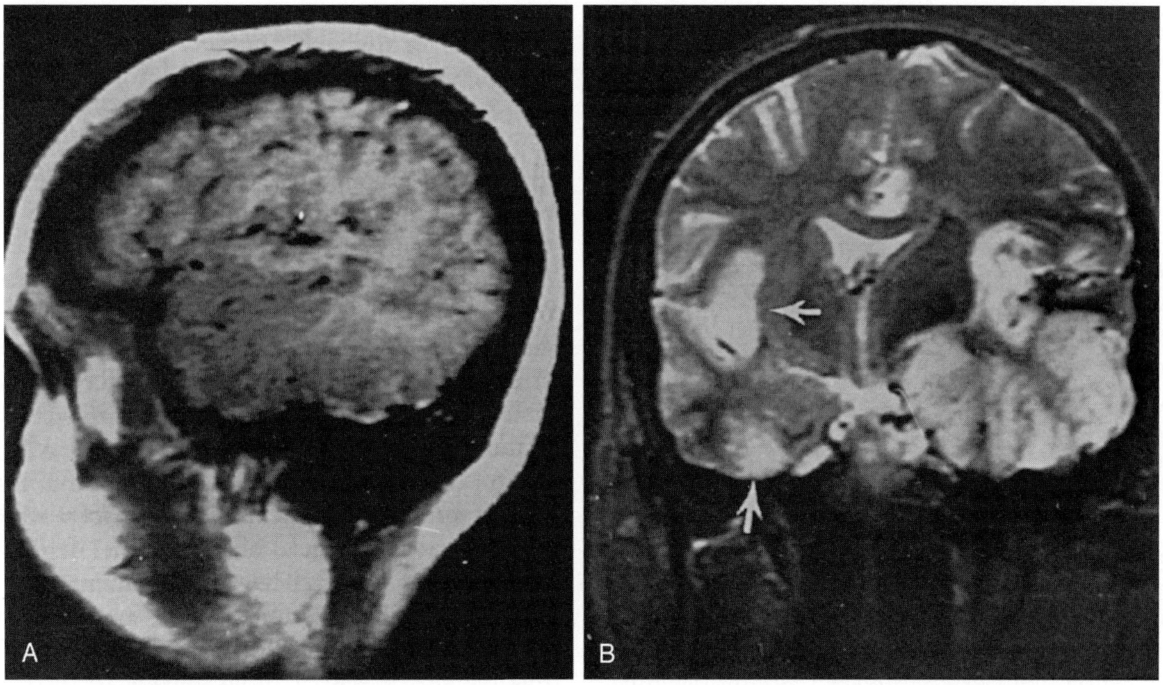

FIGURE 5–18 • MRI of herpes simplex encephalitis. *A,* Sagittal T1-weighted image with low intensity in the swollen temporal lobe. *B,* T2-weighted image demonstrating high signal intensity diffusely in the left temporal lobe, along with asymmetrical high signal intensity in the right temporal lobe (arrows). (From Grossman RI, Yousem DM: Infectious and noninfectious inflammatory diseases of the brain. In Farrell RJ [ed]: Neuroradiology: The Requisites, p 183. St. Louis, Mosby–Year Book, 1994.)

regions as early as 2 days into the course, and is localizing in up to 81% of patients.[114]

Treatment. Treatment of HSE potentially involves the management of increased ICP and seizures, in addition to antiviral therapy as follows:

I. Management of increased ICP should include:
   A. Elevation of the head of the bed to about 30 degrees
   B. Restriction of free water to 1000 mL normal saline solution per square meter of body surface per day
   C. Hyperventilation to maintain arterial P_{CO_2} at 25–30 torr (3.3–4 kPa). This decreases cerebral blood volume and decreases ICP.
   D. Use of hyperosmolar agents (e.g., intravenous mannitol 0.25–0.50 g/kg every 4–8 hours as necessary). Steroids are not recommended in viral encephalitis.
   E. (Optional): Placement of an intraventricular CSF pressure monitor may be used to keep ICP below 20–25 mm Hg by drainage. This depends on the lack of clinical response to hyperosmolar agents and the severity of the mass effect as determined by neuroimaging studies.

II. *Seizures* can be managed by slow intravenous push of phenytoin (Dilantin) at a dose of 18 mg/kg in normal saline solution at a rate of less than 50 mg/min. Maintenance doses of about 300–400 mg daily in three divided doses are used to keep the serum level between 10 and 20 μg/mL in adults. Alternatively, phenobarbital may be loaded at a dose of 10 mg/kg. Divided daily doses of about 60–120 mg are used to maintain serum levels at 20–40 μg/mL in adults. This may depress the sensorium. Valproate syrup (250 mg per 5 mL) can be administered via clamped rectal tube in a total volume of 30 mL with water at a dose of 250–500 mg every 6–8 hours to maintain blood levels of 50–100 μg/mL in adults. This may lead to elevated blood ammonia levels and liver enzymes.

III. *Antiviral treatment.* Acyclovir (acycloguanosine) reduces the mortality rate to about 19%, if administered early, with up to 38% of survivors showing no significant sequelae.[104, 115] It is administered at an intravenous dose of 10 mg/kg every 8 hours for 10 days. Side effects include reversible elevation in serum creatinine (10%), local phlebitis (4%), and nausea (2%). A review of acyclovir neurotoxicity suggested that tremors, myoclonus, confusion, and lethargy secondary to acyclovir infusion occur very rarely.[116] Alternatively, ara-A may be used at an intravenous dose of 15 mg/kg in at least 25 mL of 5% dextrose in normal saline solution given over 12 hours. Estimates of a 28% mortality rate with about 19% of survivors being normal are published.[115]

Varicella-Zoster Encephalitis (VZE)

Epidemiology. VZE, like HSE, shows no seasonal or geographic predilection. Varicella-zoster infects nearly 100% of the population in temperate parts of the world.[117] VZE occurs in about 0.05% of childhood chickenpox cases, appearing typically 5–6 days after the rash[118] or up to 5 weeks later.[119] It is heralded by fever, headache, and obtundation or delirium and must be distinguished from the more common acute cerebellar ataxia, which develops 1 week after infection, with nystagmus, dysarthria, and ataxia.[120]

VZE is more common in adults after the age of 40, with an incidence of 0.5% after cutaneous zoster eruption.[121] Approximately 35%–45% of patients have an antecedent cranial nerve (usually trigeminal) or mixed cranial-cervical nerve zoster dermatomal lesion, and the average time to occurrence of CNS signs and symptoms is 9 days but as long as 53 days.[119] The average duration of signs and symptoms is 16–24 days, and the average mortality rate is about 20% but is much higher in the immunosuppressed.[119]

Clinical Presentation. Symptoms and signs include fever, headache, stiff neck, obtundation, delirium, or personality changes following zoster skin eruptions, especially in immunocompromised patients with Hodgkin's disease and chronic lymphocytic leukemia.[119] Seizures are uncommon. An important association with necrotizing myelitis has been reported in isolated cases.[122] A clinical stroke picture of hemiparesis may develop secondary to varicella-induced vasculitis ipsilateral to ophthalmic involvement of the trigeminal nerve.[123] Although varicella infection of the CNS is not a common complication of AIDS (~2%–4%), VZE may occur in AIDS patients in the absence of cutaneous skin eruptions, especially late in their course.[124] Ventriculitis and necrotizing myelitis are also rare but well-recognized complications of varicella-zoster virus infection in AIDS.[124, 125]

Varicella-zoster involving cranial nerve VII may be associated with facial paralysis and vesicles in the external auditory meatus and eardrum (Ramsay-Hunt syndrome). This may progress to focal brain stem encephalitis involving cranial nerves V, VI, VIII, IX, and X.[126, 127]

Laboratory Diagnosis. The CSF usually shows less than 500 white blood cells per cubic millimeter, but protein levels can vary widely.[119, 128] Glucose may be low. Jemsek et al.[119] reported detection of specific antibody to varicella-zoster membrane antigen (FAMA) in the CSF from 7 of 7 patients showing clinical encephalitis after zoster infection. In another series of 16 patients with zoster-associated encephalitis, 94% had elevated (>1:2) titers in the CSF, whereas none of 25 controls with other CNS pathology had positive CSF titers.[129] Using an antibody-capture ELISA technique, van Loon et al.[130] demonstrated varicella-zoster virus–specific IgG, IgM, and IgA in CSF from patients with zoster encephalitis.

Radiographic and Electrophysiologic Diagnosis. In diagnosis of VZE, head MRI and CT are not generally helpful. The EEG shows diffuse slowing in nearly all cases.

Treatment. No controlled clinical trials of antiviral treatment for VZE are reported. Controlled trials of intravenous acyclovir in cutaneous zoster infection have demonstrated its efficacy in halting cutaneous dissemination and development of visceral zoster in immunocompromised patients.[131, 132] Reports of improvement of VZE in several patients over several days of treatment with intravenous acyclovir suggest efficacy.[133] An intravenous treatment dosage similar to that used in immunocompromised patients (acyclovir, 1500 mg/m^2 per day) has been suggested, pending further studies.[126] The usefulness of steroids in VZE has not been demonstrated.

Rabies Encephalitis

Epidemiology. Rabies virus causes acute encephalomyelitis following centripetal movement of the virus from peripheral nerve motor end plates to the spinal cord and eventually brain. All warm-blooded mammals, as well as birds, are susceptible to the virus, and the disease is present on all continents except Australia and Antarctica. Up to 50,000 rabies-induced deaths per year occur in India, and other countries with a high incidence of human rabies include Pakistan, Bangladesh, Sri Lanka, the Philippines, Thailand, Indonesia, Brazil, Colombia, El Salvador, Peru, Ecuador, Mexico, and China.[134] In the United States in 1988, approximately 12% of the total cases were in domestic animals, cats (35%) most commonly for the first time, followed by cattle (31%) and dogs (23%). Among wild animals, skunks (38%), raccoons (31%), and bats (14%) account for most cases.[135] Other important animal reservoirs include foxes in the Arctic; mongooses in Granada and Puerto Rico; vampire bats in Trinidad, Mexico, and South America; wolves, jackals, and small carnivores in

Africa and Asia; and foxes, wolves, raccoon dogs, and insectivorous bats in Europe.[134] The risk of developing rabies from the bite of an affected animal is 5%–15%[135]; higher risk is associated with bites on the head and face.

Pathogenesis. The virus gains access to the CNS after entry into peripheral nerves either (1) at a wound site, through mucous membranes, or via aerosolization (laboratory animals and bats) or (2) via transplanted corneas.[136] Typically, nerve entry is heralded by paresthesias at the wound site; virus enters myocytes where cytoplasmic replication is followed by extracellular shedding and entry into nerves. Retrograde movement through the axoplasm occurs at an estimated rate of 3 mm/hour to the spinal cord and then to the brain, where extensive viral replication occurs in neurons, especially in the limbic system. The clinical manifestations are thought to follow virus replication in neurons, after which virus moves along axoplasmic routes to salivary glands and other tissues. There is no hematogenous spread.

Clinical Presentation. Antemortem diagnosis depends on recognition of the clinical syndromes following exposure, which is difficult in the absence of a history of a recent animal bite. Typically, an incubation period lasts from 30 to 90 days (ranging from 7 days to a year or more),[137] leading to a 2 to 7 day prodrome of fever, headache, myalgia, cough, sore throat, and malaise. An important warning sign is paresthesias around the wound site, present in 44%–50% of cases.[138] Within days of this nonspecific prodrome, one sees either of two clinical courses. More commonly (80%) restlessness, delirium, intolerance to sensory stimuli, and 1 to 5 minute attacks of frenzy alternating with lucid intervals. Pharyngeal spasms may be precipitated by attempts to drink or by fanning the face. Approximately 20% of patients experience a rapidly progressive, ascending paralysis resembling Guillain-Barré syndrome. In either case, progression to stupor, coma, and death occurs in 3–7 days. Once clinically established, rabies encephalomyelitis is nearly uniformly fatal, though several cases of survival have been reported.[138, 139]

Laboratory Diagnosis. The white blood cell count is often elevated (10,000–20,000 cells/mm^3) with elevated polymorphonuclear neutrophils, and the CSF typically shows less than 125 mononuclear cells/mm^3, although cell counts are normal in 40% of patients in the first week of illness.[134] CSF protein may be mildly elevated, whereas glucose is normal. The most reliable serologic test is detection of serum antibody in unvaccinated subjects.

In a retrospective study of 22 patients, Anderson and associates[140] found that 100% developed positive titers between days 6 and 15 of clinical illness, with mean titers increasing from 1:8 (day 6) to 1:288 (day 15). Virus isolation from either throat swab or saliva was the test found likeliest to yield positive results early in the illness, as early as 2 days in four of four confirmed cases. Rapid antemortem diagnosis can also be made by immunofluorescent staining for virus antigen in corneal scrape specimens or neck skin biopsy,[141] though these are diagnostic in only about 50% of early cases. Virus can be isolated in neuroblastoma cells in 2–4 days.[134]

Radiographic and Electrophysiologic Diagnosis. Head CT results are normal, and EEGs are diffusely slow.[142]

Treatment. A decision for treatment must be made before the development of clinical disease. Immediate cleansing of the wound with soap and water, 1%–2% benzalkonium chloride, or 40%–70% alcohol is recommended. A decision for postexposure prophylaxis should be based on the animal type, disposition, and geographic area (Table 5–10). If prophylaxis is required, human rabies immune globulin (HRIG) at a dose of 20 IU/kg body weight is used, if the patient has not been previously vaccinated. One-half of the dose is infiltrated around the wound; the remainder is administered intramuscularly in the gluteus (Table 5–11) or another area away from the subsequent of vaccine injection. In nonvaccinated patients, 1.0 mL of either human diploid cell vaccine (HDCV) or adsorbed rabies vaccine (RVA) is given intramuscularly in the deltoid (never gluteus) on days 0, 3, 7, 14, and 28. In previously vaccinated persons, this dose is given only on days 0 and 3, after initial wound cleansing. If HRIG was not given prior to the vaccination, it *can* be administered through the seventh day after the first dose of vaccine. Concomitant use of steroids, immunosuppressants, or antimalarials is contraindicated, because they can interfere with active immunity after vaccination.

Reactions after vaccination with HDCV and RVA are much less common than with prior vaccines. These include local pain, erythema, swelling around the injection site in 30%–74% of patients, and headache, nausea, vomiting, and myalgias in 5%–40%. Several cases of a reversible Guillain-Barré–like illness have been reported. HRIG has not been associated with significant complications.

Once clinical rabies encephalomyelitis is established, supportive care is all that can be offered. Respiratory disturbances occur in all cases, requiring intubation for management of secretions as well

TABLE 5–10 **RABIES POSTEXPOSURE PROPHYLAXIS GUIDE, UNITED STATES, 1991**

ANIMAL TYPE	EVALUATION AND DISPOSITIONS OF ANIMAL	POSTEXPOSURE PROPHYLAXIS RECOMMENDATIONS
Dogs and cats	Healthy and available for 10 days of observation	Should not begin prophylaxis unless animal develops symptoms of rabies*
	Rabid or suspected rabid	Immediate vaccination
	Unknown (escaped)	Consult public health officials
Skunks, raccoons, bats, foxes, and most other carnivores; woodchucks	Regarded as rabid unless geographic area is known to be free of rabies or until animal proven negative by laboratory tests†	Immediate vaccination
Livestock rodents, and lagomorphs (rabbits and hares)	Consider individually	Consult public health officials. Bites of squirrels, hamsters, guinea pigs, gerbils, chipmunks, rats, mice, other rodents, rabbits, and hares almost never require antirabies treatment

*During the 10-day holding period, begin treatment with HRIG and HDCV or RVA (see text) at first sign of rabies in a dog or cat that has bitten someone. The symptomatic animal should be killed immediately and tested.
†The animal should be killed and tested as soon as possible. Holding for observation is not recommended. Discontinue vaccine if immunofluorescence test results of the animal are negative.
From Centers for Disease Control: Rabies prevention—United States, 1991.
Recommendations of the Immunization Practices Advisory Committee (ACIP). MMWR 1991;40:1.

as respiratory distress and increased ICP. Seizures can be expected in two-thirds of cases, and cardiac arrhythmias occur almost invariably. Other CNS dysfunctions include thermal dysregulation, diabetes insipidus, and autonomic dysfunction.

Epidemic Encephalitis

Arbovirus Encephalitis

Epidemiology. Most epidemic encephalitides throughout the United States are caused by the arboviruses (arthropod-borne viruses), with the mosquito as the major vector. These viruses include three major groups: (1) the Togaviridae *Alphavirus* group, which causes Eastern equine encephalitis (EEE), Western equine encephalitis (WEE), and Venezuelan equine encephalitis (VEE); (2) the Togaviridae *Flavivirus* group, which causes St. Louis encephalitis (SLE) and Japanese B encephalitis (JBE), among others; and (3) the Bunyaviridae California serogroup, which causes La Crosse encephalitis.

Unlike sporadic encephalitides, arboviral encephalitides show a clear seasonal and geographic pattern of expression. Cases appear in May and peak in July and August, followed by a dramatic decrease by the late fall (November), corresponding to peaks in the mosquito population. Generally, subclinical infection is widespread, with few persons showing disease. Of the six major types listed, EEE is the least frequent but most deadly, whereas SLE accounts for most arboviral cases of encephalitis in the United States.

During 1993, 78 cases of arboviral encephalitis

TABLE 5–11 **RABIES POSTEXPOSURE PROPHYLAXIS SCHEDULE, UNITED STATES, 1991**

VACCINATION STATUS	TREATMENT	REGIMEN*
Not previously vaccinated	Local wound cleansing	All postexposure treatment should begin with immediate thorough cleansing of all wounds with soap and water.
	HRIG	20 IU/kg body weight. If anatomically feasible, up to one-half the dose should be infiltrated around the wound(s), and the rest should be administered IM in the gluteal area. HRIG should not be administered in the same syringe or into the same anatomic site as vaccine. Because HRIG may partially suppress active production of antibody, no more than the recommended dose should be given.
	Vaccine	HDCV or RVA, 1.0 mL, IM (deltoid area†), one each on days 0, 3, 7, 14, and 28.
Previously vaccinated‡	Local wound cleansing	All postexposure treatment should begin with immediate thorough cleansing of all wounds with soap and water.
	HRIG	HRIG should not be administered.
	Vaccine	HDCV or RVA, 1.0 mL, IM (deltoid area†), one each on days 0 and 3.

IU, international units; IM, intramuscular; HRIG, human rabies immune globulin; HDCV, human diploid cell vaccine; RVA, adsorbed rabies vaccine.
*These regimens are applicable for all age groups, including children.
†The deltoid area is the only acceptable site of vaccination for adults and older children. For younger children, the outer aspect of the thigh may be used. Vaccine should never be administered in the gluteal area.
‡Any person with a history of pre-exposure vaccination with HDCV or RVA, prior postexposure prophylaxis with HDCV or RVA, or previous vaccination with any other type of rabies vaccine and a documented history of antibody response to the prior vaccination.
From Centers for Disease Control: Rabies prevention—United States, 1991.
Recommendations of the Immunization Practices Advisory Committee (ACIP). MMWR 1991;40:1.

were reported to the Centers for Disease Control and Prevention, of which 55% were California serogroup, 23% St. Louis, 16% Western equine, and 6% Eastern equine.[144]

ST. LOUIS ENCEPHALITIS (SLE)

Epidemiology. First described in 1933, outbreaks of SLE occur in approximately 5- to 15-year intervals (last in 1990), peaking in August and September primarily in the Ohio-Mississippi Valley, eastern Texas, Florida, Kansas, Colorado, and California. In certain endemic areas, seroprevalence is about 3.6%, and up to 6% in epidemics, with an estimated ratio of inapparent to apparent infection of 800:1 in children to 80:1 in the elderly. Attack rates are estimated at 1–800 per 100,000 population.[145] The clinical presentation of encephalitis in an endemic area during the months of July or August should alert one to the diagnosis.

Clinical Presentation. Clinical manifestations appear on average 4–12 days after exposure, and are most common in patients over 60 years of age.[145] Sudden onset of fever (100%), headache (95%), nausea and vomiting (61%), stiff neck (37%), and myalgias is typical, followed in 1–4 days by confusion, irritability, disorientation, or apathy. Brain stem and cerebellar findings, such as a lower motor neuron VII deficit (20%), tremors (50%), ataxia, nystagmus, and myoclonus, may appear.[146] Unusual associated symptoms of urinary urgency, frequency, and incontinence were reported in 25% of patients in one series, as well as syndrome of inappropriate antidiuretic hormone secretion.[146, 147] The mortality rate has been estimated at 10%, and 80% of deaths occur in the first 2 weeks. Residual complaints of fatigue may persist for several years in 20% of patients, with no long-term cognitive sequelae.

Laboratory Diagnosis. The rapid, early diagnosis of SLE is best achieved with an IgM-capture ELISA on acute and convalescent sera.[148] IgM antibodies are detectable in 71% of cases between days 0 and 3 of illness, 94% between days 4 and 21, with gradual decline after the first 10 days of illness, being generally undetectable at 4 months. There is limited cross-reactivity with related flaviviruses (e.g., Japanese B), making this the best serodiagnostic test, replacing the standard hemagglutination inhibition (HI), complement fixation (CF), and neutralizing antibody (Nt) tests formerly used.

The CSF shows pleocytosis (average ~100 cells/mm^3) on initial lumbar puncture, with early neutrophil predominance in up to 94% of patients and elevated protein (average 78 mg/dL) in over 80%.[146] By the second week of illness, 75% of the cells are lymphocytes.[147]

Radiographic and Electrophysiologic Diagnosis. CT is generally not helpful. In the series of Brinker et al.,[146] the EEG showed diffuse abnormalities in all cases, though the severity of the disease did not correlate with the severity of the EEG abnormalities.

Treatment. No effective antiviral treatment is currently available; supportive care is the rule. Particular attention must be paid to the fluid management (free water restriction) when syndrome of inappropriate antidiuretic hormone secretion develops.

EASTERN EQUINE ENCEPHALITIS (EEE)

Epidemiology. EEE is the deadliest arboviral encephalitis, with a mortality rate of 50%–80%, highest in adults, with most cases occurring in the Atlantic and Gulf coast states, upper New York, and western Michigan. Epidemics typically occur in late summer/early fall following a period of heavy rainfall. Of the four major arboviral encephalitides in the United States, EEE has the lowest ratio of inapparent to apparent infection, ranging from 8:1 in infants to 50:1 in young adults.[149] The human infection rate during epidemics is low, estimated at 2.3%.

Assessments of morbidity and mortality suggest a complete recovery rate of only 3%. Severe neurologic sequelae, primarily mental retardation but also hemiparesis and aphasia, occur in up to two-thirds of patients, usually children.[150] Infection in adults more often results in death, with fewer patients showing permanent sequelae. Evidence suggests that longer prodromal periods are associated with lower morbidity and mortality.[151]

Clinical Presentation. EEE is a fulminant disease characterized by the onset of signs and symptoms 1–4 days after infection. These include high fever (39°–40° C), lethargy (92%), convulsions (74%), stiff neck (62%), and vomiting (52%), leading to stupor, coma, and death in as little as 24 hours and up to 5 days.[151] Cranial nerve palsies and hemiparesis sometimes occur (resembling HSE), and seizures occur in about 75% of patients, usually children. In adults, a febrile prodrome may precede the clinical encephalitis by as much as 11 days; in children this is not generally the case.

Laboratory Diagnosis. As with SLE, rapid and early diagnosis of EEE can be made with an IgM-capture ELISA antibody test on serum.[152] In a retrospective series of 20 confirmed cases, all patients had positive titers, one as early as 1 day after clinical disease onset, with maximum titers at 1–2 weeks. There was no cross-reactivity with sera from either WEE or VEE patients.[153] This test is replacing the standard HI, CF, and Nt serologic tests used to diagnose the equine encephalitides. The diagnosis has also been made by electron microscopic identification of virus particles in a brain biopsy specimen from an infant.[154] In two series of patients,[155, 156] the initial CSF nearly always showed an increased opening pressure and protein (45–100 mg/dL in 62%) with an average white blood cell count of 900–1000 cells/mm^3 (60% neutrophils) within 48 hours of the onset of signs and symptoms. Notably, xanthochromia was present in the CSF of over half of the patients, again resembling HSE.

A recent study using in-situ hybridization techniques demonstrated EEE viral DNA in paraffin-embedded tissues from infected horses as well as infected cells in culture using in-situ hybridization.[157]

Radiographic and Electrophysiologic Diagnosis. Although head CT usually shows generalized swelling, focal lesions may be seen on both CT and MRI.[158] The EEG shows generalized slowing, though PLEDS, resembling those seen in HSE, sometimes occur.[114]

Treatment. No clinically useful pharmacologic therapy is available.[159] Supportive care must be directed toward the control of brain swelling, as described earlier.

WESTERN EQUINE ENCEPHALITIS (WEE)

Epidemiology. WEE is generally a mild disease, clinically difficult to distinguish from SLE, but nearly always found west of the Mississippi River, particularly the San Joaquin Valley of California, Texas, and Colorado.[126] WEE and SLE epidemics peak slightly earlier in the summer (July/August) than do those of EEE (August/September).[160] The ratio of inapparent to apparent infection is estimated at 60:1 in children and 1100:1 in adults, with increased severity of disease in infants less than 1 year of age. Between 25% and 30% of WEE cases occur in children less than 1 year of age, and 50% of these have severe neurologic sequelae, including mental retardation, spasticity, and seizures, due to structural damage to the developing brain.[161, 162] Adults have a less than 5% risk of neurologic sequelae. The overall mortality rate is 2%–3%, but it is 10%–23% in adults over the age of 55.[160] Interestingly, the incidence rate in males is twice that of females by age 5–9 years, presumably because of increased exposure during outdoor activities.[163] A recent report demonstrated vertical transmission of WEE virus in mosquitoes, which allows the virus to persist in endemic regions between transmission seasons.[164]

Clinical Presentation. As with each of the equine encephalitides, one must be alert for cases in mid and late summer; WEE particularly occurs in infants less than 1 year of age. The incubation period appears to be about 2 weeks, followed by a sudden onset of mild headache, fever, nausea, vomiting, and malaise, often with photophobia and vertigo. After several days, the headache progresses in severity, and the patient becomes lethargic or even comatose (~15%). In mild cases, these symptoms persist for about 10 days, then subside; in severe cases the fever may reach 40°–41° C, and the lethargy may progress to stupor, coma, and death in 4–7 days. Seizures occur in up to 90% of infants and in 40% of children between ages 1 and 4 years, but rarely in adults.[165] Physical examination usually reveals stiff neck and commonly hyporeflexia and weakness. Cranial nerves are spared. Children often exhibit muscular rigidity, involuntary movements, and paralysis.[163]

Laboratory Diagnosis. Again, as for EEE and SLE, rapid and early diagnosis is possible with an IgM-capture ELISA antibody test, though in WEE there is more cross-reactivity with several other, geographically isolated viruses.[152] Fourteen of 17 (84%) patients previously confirmed with WEE by acute and convalescent HI, CF, and Nt antibody titers had specific IgM antibody titers, several within the first 2 days of illness.[153] As for EEE, this single determination test was more sensitive and specific for *recent* infection than the standard HI, CF, and Nt titers. However, as for EEE, the serodiagnosis can be made by confirmation of a fourfold rise in the standard acute and convalescent titers.

Unlike in EEE, the CSF typically shows a normal opening pressure and protein and fewer than 200 cells/mm^3, with a mononuclear predominance developing in the first 2 days.

Radiographic and Electrophysiologic Diagnosis. CT and EEG are generally not helpful in the diagnosis of WEE.

Treatment. There is no specific antiviral treatment; however, aggressive supportive care in these patients can often result in complete recovery.

JAPANESE B ENCEPHALITIS (JBE)

Epidemiology. JBE has affected more people and accounts for more morbidity and mortality than any other form of arboviral encephalitis, resulting in 10,000 annual cases in China with several thousand deaths. The virus is distributed throughout Asia, southeastern Russia, and China to India on the west and the Philippines to the east, and it may affect travelers to those areas, especially servicemen.[166] Swine are an important source of infection for those species of mosquito that transmit JBE virus to humans.[167] In nonvaccinated populations, children less than 15 years of age have the highest incidence of disease.[168] The ratio of inapparent to apparent infection may be as high as 500:1.[168] In the 1980s, the use of inactivated JBE viral vaccine dramatically decreased the morbidity and mortality rates of JBE (estimated at 20%–50%).[169] Both the mortality rate and the neurologic sequelae rate (3%–32%) are greatest in children; such sequelae include psychosis, intellectual impairment, spasticity, and paresis.[126] Rapid appearance of antibodies in the CSF is a predictor of less severe disease.[170, 171]

Clinical Presentation. Prodromal symptoms are not common. The 4 to 20 day incubation period is followed by a rapid onset of fever (100%), headache (80%), and nuchal rigidity (100%), with altered sensorium, which may range from lethargy to agitation. Interesting features in some cases include masked-like facies resembling Parkinsonism; ocular tremors and coarse tremors of the face, lips, and hands; and occasionally a lower motor neuron facial (nerve VII) paresis.[166] In fatal cases, death usually occurs on the fifth to ninth day.

Laboratory Diagnosis. The most useful early test is the IgM-capture ELISA antibody titer in the CSF. This has confirmed the diagnosis in 68% (day 1) and 100% (day 7) of cases eventually diagnosed by conventional HI assays.[171] Standard CF antibody tests are consistently positive only after weeks of infection. Virus can be cultured from the CSF but it requires more time than the IgM test.[170]

The CSF shows approximately 20–400 mixed polymorphonuclear cells and lymphocytes per cubic millimeter in 90% of cases up to day 4, with conversion completely to lymphocytes by day 7.[166] These cell counts may remain elevated for months, though they steadily decline. Protein levels and opening pressure are minimally elevated.

Radiographic and Electrophysiologic Diagnosis. Isolated case reports suggest no specific findings on head CT or EEGs.

Treatment. There is no effective antiviral treatment. Purified Japanese encephalitis vaccine made from whole virus derived from mouse is estimated to be 91% effective at preventing disease in children.[169]

VENEZUELAN EQUINE ENCEPHALITIS (VEE)

Epidemiology. VEE in man is generally a benign disease in adults. It is most common in Central and South America and in the southern United States, where a major epidemic occurred in 1971.[172] That year, over 16,000 cases occurred in Mexico, and 75% of the deaths occurred in children under 5 years of age and only 5% in adults over the age of 45 years. Overall, a death rate of 0.2%–0.6% is estimated. The majority of infections are believed to lead to systemic disease, though only a fraction suffer encephalitis. VEE virus is highly infectious by the aerosol route and poses a risk to laboratory personnel.

Clinical Presentation. Disease due to infection with VEE virus can be categorized into three forms: (1) *influenzal* (most common in adults), manifested by constitutional symptoms including nausea, vomiting, myalgias, and pharyngitis, with a febrile course of 1–4 days; (2) *fulminant* (most common in children), characterized by several days of fever followed by shock, coma (2%), and convulsions (6%), and leading to sequelae; and (3) *encephalitic* (~20%, more common in children), characterized by a diphasic febrile course of over 2 weeks, with CNS manifestations of confusion, drowsiness, hallucinations, or ataxia during the second phase.[165, 172, 173] Of all patients acutely ill with VEE virus, 100% show fever, 43% lethargy, and 22% pharyngitis.

Laboratory Diagnosis. HI antibody titers in acute and convalescent sera remain the standard serologic diagnostic tool,[163] though the IgM-capture ELISA assay shows specificity in the limited number of cases tested.[163] Virus can be isolated from sera during the first 48 hours of illness, as well as from throat swabs by injection into suckling mice.[163] In a small number of cases, the CSF has been reported to contain 300+ lymphocytes/mm^3 by day 3 of disease, with protein levels of 50 mg/dL. Leukopenia occurs in 75% of patients, unlike the case with WEE, SLE, and EEE.

Treatment. Although no effective antiviral therapy is as yet known, polyinosinic-polycytidylic acid has shown some effectiveness in murine and primate models.[159]

LA CROSSE ENCEPHALITIS

Epidemiology. Since the 1970s, La Crosse encephalitis has been second only to SLE in the number of arboviral cases in the United states (~5% of all viral CNS infections).[174] The majority of cases (~100/year) occur in Ohio, Wisconsin, Minnesota, New York, and Indiana, and over 90% occur in children less than 15 years of age, with a peak incidence between ages 4 and 10 years. Most cases occur in August and September. The ratio of inapparent to apparent infection is estimated at 26:1, and exposure to woodland mosquitoes is a consistent historical risk factor.[175] Fatalities are rare (0.5%), and seizures may persist in up to 19% of patients.[175–177]

Clinical Presentation. The most common presentation is a 2 to 3 day period of fever, headache (90%), malaise, abdominal pain, nausea, and vomiting, followed by signs of meningitis, all of which resolve in approximately 1 week. Less common is a picture more typical of equine encephalitis: abrupt onset of fever (100%), disorientation (90%), nuchal rigidity (38%), seizures (50%), tremors (20%), papilledema, and coma, from which most patients recover over a 2-week period.[126, 177] The peripheral blood shows leukocytosis, and CSF shows fewer than 300 lymphocytes per cubic millimeter in 97% of patients.[175, 178]

Laboratory Diagnosis. An IgM-capture ELISA has been developed to diagnose infection in acute serum. In one series of 29 patients, specific IgM was detected in 83% by day 3 after the onset of clinical symptoms.[179] This test is replacing the standard HI, CF, and Nt tests formerly used on paired sera to make the diagnosis.[180]

Radiographic and Electrophysiologic Diagnosis. EEGs are nearly uniformly abnormal, showing generalized or focal slow waves.[181] Head CT is not diagnostic.

Treatment. There is no effective antiviral treatment. Long-term seizure prophylaxis has been recommended for persons having seizures during the acute illness.[177]

Non-arboviral Epidemic Encephalitis

INFLUENZA ENCEPHALITIS AND REYE'S SYNDROME

Epidemiology. Although the frequency of CNS complications with influenza is low, varied clinical syndromes may result: acute encephalitis, acute paralysis, and parainfectious processes—encephalomyelitis, acute hemorrhagic leukoencephalopathy, transverse myelitis, acute ataxia of childhood, and Reye's syndrome (influenza B). A small number of encephalitis cases due to influenza A occur at 2- to 3-year intervals during epidemics and worldwide pandemics every 10–15 years. Complete recovery is the rule, although influenza A has been proposed as the etiologic agent responsible for von Economo's encephalitis, which may result in Parkinsonism.[182]

Clinical Presentation. Diagnosis is difficult and case reports are few. Neurologic signs such as depression of consciousness, disorientation, stupor, coma, and seizures in the setting of fever occurring 2–7 days after constitutional symptoms of headache, dry cough, and myalgias are typical.[183, 184] Acute psychoses following influenza symptoms are also reported, with recovery occurring for all these symptoms over 4 weeks. Myoclonus has been described as a possible postinfectious syndrome following influenza-like illnesses, but an etiologic link between influenza strains and myoclonus has not been established.[185]

Reye's syndrome (encephalopathy with fatty degeneration of the liver) may follow influenza B, influenza A, or varicella-zoster infection in children less than 14 years of age (90% of cases) and rarely in adults. It is heralded by recurrent vomiting followed by lethargy, with markedly elevated serum transaminases, ammonia levels, and prothrombin time in the setting of a normal bilirubin, and by absence of signs of CNS infection or focal neurologic deficits.

Laboratory Diagnosis. A fourfold rise in serum HI or CF antibody titers in acute and convalescent (day 14–21) sera, or virus isolation from throat swabs is presumptive evidence for acute infection. Alternately a single rapid hemolysis test for detection of antibody to influenza virus hemagglutinin may allow more rapid early serologic diagnosis.[186]

Radiographic Diagnosis. MRI may show high signal intensity with T2 weighting in cases of influenza encephalitis, though few cases are described.[182]

Treatment. Amantadine hydrochloride has demonstrated effectiveness in the treatment of influenza A infections, but its use in the treatment of CNS complications has not been studied. Although not tested in clinical trials for influenza encephalitis, aerosolized ribavirin protected mice intracerebrally injected with influenza A from encephalitis and reached levels sufficient to inhibit virus replication.

One successful management protocol for the treatment of Reye's syndrome is as follows[187]:

1. Placement of an intraventricular CSF pressure monitor

2. Mechanical ventilation to maintain arterial P_{CO_2} at 23–25 torr (3–3.3 kPa)
3. Phenobarbital maintenance of blood levels at 30–40 μg/mL
4. Intravenous mannitol boluses of 0.25–1.0 g/kg to keep ICP below 20–25 mm Hg
5. CSF drainage if mannitol boluses fail

ENTEROVIRUS ENCEPHALITIS

Epidemiology. The enterovirus group include the polioviruses, Cocksackie A and B, echoviruses, enteroviruses, and hepatitis A, all of which infect the human alimentary tract. Of those patients with a clinical presentation, aseptic meningitis is the most frequent neurologic manifestation (35%), followed by encephalitis (11%) and paralysis (1%). Most cases of meningitis or encephalitis occur in July through September, primarily in the 10 to 29 year age group.[188] Outcome of enteroviral encephalitis is usually benign, though a mortality rate of 2.5% is reported.

Clinical Presentation. The clinical picture of the meningoencephalitis is nonspecific. Enterovirus-70, for example, often heralds infection with self-limiting acute hemorrhagic conjunctivitis within 1–10 days of infection.[126] In a small number of cases it is followed in 1–5 weeks by radicular pain with asymmetric flaccid paralysis, which may be permanent. Cocksackie viruses may cause aseptic meningitis associated with herpangina, pleurodynia, pericarditis, and rashes. Enterovirus-71 more commonly causes aseptic meningitis and encephalitis.

Laboratory Diagnosis. Routine serologic screening of most enteroviral infections is impractical, requiring antibody titering against specific viruses, because of lack of group specific antigens. Therefore, emphasis is on viral isolation from throat swabs, stool, blood, and CSF (which was demonstrated in 41% of 111 pediatric cases of meningitis or meningoencephalitis in one report[189]). During specific outbreaks, however, a fourfold antibody rise against the specific virus is diagnostic.

Radiographic and Electrophysiologic Diagnosis. CT and EEG are generally not helpful in the diagnosis of enteroviral infections of the CNS.

Treatment. No specific antiviral therapies are available.

Parainfectious Encephalitis

Parainfectious encephalomyelitis is a term describing presumed immune-mediated damage to the CNS arising in temporal relation to overt CNS infection (measles/subacute sclerosing panencephalitis; chicken pox/acute disseminated encephalomyelitis), and others, or post vaccination (rabies, smallpox, and others).

Measles Encephalitis

Epidemiology. Measles infection peaks in the 5 to 9 year old age group, and 99% of subjects by age 20 years have been exposed. Measles encephalitis is most common in the winter and spring seasons; the incidence may reach as high as 16/100,000 in the very young (< 2 years old), decreasing dramatically by age 15 years.[190]

Clinical Presentation. Typically, 10–11 days after exposure comes a 2 to 4 day prodromal phase of fever, malaise, cough, rhinitis, and conjunctivitis with the characteristic Koplik's spots on the buccal mucosa, which fade in 2–4 days. A distinctive maculopapular rash follows the prodrome, first on the head and face, moving centrifugally in 3–4 days to cover the body. Encephalitis following measles infection is rare and includes any one of three syndromes:

1. Subacute measles encephalitis (SME) occurs in immunosuppressed patients, typically leukemic children undergoing radiation therapy. Incubation ranges from 5 weeks to 6 months, followed by focal myoclonic seizures, hemiplegia, stupor, coma, and death after a course of weeks or a few months.[191, 192] In a review of 33 cases, Mustafa et al.[191] documented the following clinical characteristics of SME: altered consciousness (100%), seizures (97%), hemiparesis/hemiplegia (36%), ataxia/weakness (24%), aphasia/slurred speech (21%), and visual symptoms/cortical blindness (15%).
2. Acute measles postinfectious encephalitis occurs in about 1/1000–5000 measles cases within 8 days of onset of measles, with a 15% mortality rate. It is characterized by resurgent fever, headache, seizures, cerebellar ataxia, and coma. Approximately 20%–40% of those who recover have permanent neurologic deficits, including retardation, seizures, and hemiparesis.
3. Subacute sclerosing panencephalitis (SSPE) affects 1 in 1 million measles cases approximately 6–8 years after acute infection. The initial measles attack occurs before the age of 2 years in approximately 50% of patients. Generalized intellectual deterioration, psychologic or personality disturbances, and hallucinations lasting weeks or months are followed by dyspraxia, extrapyramidal movement disorders, myoclonus,

aphasia, and convulsions. In 75% of cases viral chorioretinitis occurs, which can lead to blindness. Overall, the course of SSPE varies, and spontaneous remissions occur in only 5% of cases.[193] Death occurs in 1–3 years in 70%–90% of cases. It is thought to result from either slow replication of structurally defective virus in neurons and oligodendrocytes or immune attack upon these cells.

Laboratory Diagnosis. Diagnosis of SSPE can be made in the appropriate clinical setting with demonstration of oligoclonal IgG antibody in the CSF. ELISAs for IgM measles specific antibody in acute and convalescent serum can confirm the diagnosis of measles during the initial illness. HI testing is also commonly used. PCR detection of measles virus has been used in brain biopsy specimens to make the diagnosis in biopsy-proved SSPE.[191]

Radiographic and Electrophysiologic Diagnosis. The EEG often shows a characteristic burst suppression pattern of high-amplitude slow wave complexes occurring at a rate of one every 4–20 seconds. CT may show cortical atrophy and focal or multifocal lucencies in the white matter. MRI studies may show high-signal T2 intensities in the gray matter.[194]

Treatment. Immunosuppressed patients infected with measles viruses should receive human anti-measles gamma globulin 0.25–0.5 mL/kg within the first 3 days after exposure. It is ineffective if given 6 or more days after exposure.[195]

In general, medical therapy for SSPE is symptomatic, although antiviral agents have been used successfully in isolated cases. Myoclonus can be treated with benzodiazepines or valproate; seizures can be treated with standard anticonvulsants. The antiviral agent isoprinosine (Inosoprex) at a dose of 100 mg/kg of body weight in divided doses every 4 hours by mouth for the course of the disease has been shown to markedly improve long-term survival and diminish neurologic disability in several nonrandomized trials.[193, 196] In a case report of an AIDS patient with disseminated measles infection, a treatment regimen consisting of intravenous ribavirin at a dose of 15 mg/kg per day in divided doses every 8 hours for 6 days, followed by intravenous gamma globulin at a dose of 400 mg/kg per day, resulted in marked improvement in encephalopathy and systemic manifestations.[197]

For SME, ribavirin has been used with varying success. In a pediatric case report and review of the literature, Mustafa et al.[191] reported clinical and radiographic (brain MRI) improvement in an immunocompromised patient treated with 20 mg/kg for several weeks. Additional scattered case reports suggest possible benefit of ribavirin, though no randomized placebo-controlled study has been published to date.[191]

Mumps Encephalitis

Epidemiology. Before the widespread vaccination for mumps began in 1967, mumps encephalitis affected 400 patients per year in the United States, or about 0.3% of all mumps patients; the total number of encephalitis cases dropped to 26 in 1978, with a concomitant tenfold decrease in the total number of nonencephalitic mumps cases.[126] Other estimates put the frequency of mumps meningitis with or without signs of encephalitis as high as 11% of mumps cases.[198] As many as one-third of mumps infections are asymptomatic, whereas as many as half of all clinical mumps cases have CSF pleocytosis, irrespective of the presence of neurologic symptoms. The peak incidence in the United States occurs in March and April and is highest in the 5 to 9 year age range, and approximately 92% of children acquire mumps antibody by age 15. Although mumps affects males and females equally, males are more susceptible to the development of encephalitis (3:1).[199] Although 0.5%–2.3% of all mumps encephalitis cases are fatal, most patients show marked clinical improvement within 2–4 days and recover fully.[198]

Clinical Presentation. In general, the incubation period from exposure to the clinical signs of mumps is 18 days. In those patients developing CNS signs and symptoms, the distinction between meningitis and encephalitis is blurred.[200] Signs of fever, headache, vomiting, neck stiffness, and lethargy develop in 5 days following the onset of parotitis; of these patients, 20%–30% have seizures with or without focal neurologic signs. However, only about 50% of encephalitis cases have antecedent parotitis, which occurs in 95% of all mumps patients. Occasionally, encephalitis even precedes parotitis.[201] Mumps encephalitis is extremely rare in adults, although a cerebellar encephalitis syndrome can occur.[202]

Laboratory Diagnosis. CSF pleocytosis is present in nearly all encephalitis cases, even in 40%–50% of all cases without CNS symptoms. Mononuclear cells predominate from the onset of CNS disease, and peak counts occur around day 3 of CNS symptoms (averaging 250 cells/mm^3 but as high as 1000 or more).[201] This declines over weeks. Protein is markedly elevated in 60%–70% of cases, and low CSF glucose levels may occur on average in one-fourth of cases.

Virus can be cultured from the CSF,[203] throat swabs, and testes, and they can be identified by electron-microscopic analysis of ependymal cells in the CSF.[204]

An IgM-capture ELISA has been developed for detection of mumps virus in serum and CSF; positive titers were found in 100% of confirmed cases in at least one series.[205] This will probably prove to be the most sensitive early diagnostic test for CNS infection. Similar results were found for IgM ELISAs on acute phase sera, and these IgM tests appear more reliable for early detection than conventional HI, CF, or Nt assays.[206–208]

Radiographic Diagnosis. Radiographic studies are generally not helpful in the diagnosis of mumps encephalitis, although one report has suggested detection of asymptomatic optic neuritis by MRI in a pediatric case of mumps encephalitis.[209]

Treatment. No specific antiviral therapy has been proved efficacious for mumps meningoencephalitis; however, ribavirin shows in-vitro activity against mumps virus.[210]

Brain Stem Encephalitis

Brain stem encephalitis is clinically manifested by progressive alteration of level of consciousness and bulbar dysfunction, often with prominent neuro-ophthalmologic signs. A diverse range of infectious and inflammatory processes may cause this clinical pattern (Table 5–12).[211–213] Prompt recognition of the etiology of progressive brain stem dysfunction is important for both management and prognosis.

Listeria monocytogenes is a relatively common cause of meningitis in the elderly and immunocompromised. Rarely, it causes brain stem encephalitis (rhombencephalitis). In a review, Armstrong and Fung described the clinical progression of *Listeria* rhombencephalitis.[214] Neurologic signs and symptoms are usually preceded by several days of nonspecific constitutional symptoms, including headache, nausea, vomiting, and malaise. Neurologic signs and symptoms may develop precipitously and often include asymmetric cranial nerve deficits, ataxia, hemiparesis, or hemisensory loss. The early diagnosis of *Listeria* rhombencephalitis may be elusive, because only one-half of patients show evidence of meningeal irritation or change in mental status upon initial presentation. The CSF may also look surprisingly benign, and approximately one-quarter of these patients have fewer than four white blood cells per cubic millimeter (mononuclear predominant). The CSF glucose level is often normal, although there is usually a modest elevation in protein. Initial CT of the head is unrevealing in almost

TABLE 5–12 **DIFFERENTIAL DIAGNOSIS OF BRAIN STEM ENCEPHALITIS**

DIFFERENTIAL DIAGNOSIS	ASSOCIATED HISTORY, SIGNS, AND SYMPTOMS	ANCILLARY DIAGNOSTIC TESTS
Viral encephalitis		Lumbar puncture; acute and convalescent serologies; viral cultures
Listeria rhombencephalitis	2 to 4 day prodrome of constitutional symptoms (malaise, nausea, vomiting, headache); abrubt onset of asymmetrical cranial nerve deficits, ataxia, long tract signs	Lumbar puncture
Acute disseminated encephalomyelitis	Recent viral infection, vaccination	Multiple areas consistent with demyelination on MRI; lumbar puncture (mild leukocytosis, elevated protein)
Bickerstaff's encephalitis	Preceding viral illness; ophthalmoparesis, ataxia; long tract signs may be present	MRI
Miller-Fisher variant of Guillain-Barré syndrome	Preceding gastrointestinal or upper respiratory illness; areflexia, ataxia, extremity weakness may be present	Lumbar puncture (albuminocytologic dissociation); electrodiagnostic studies
Central pontine myelinolysis	Recent history of rapid electrolyte fluctuations (rapid correction of hyponatremia)	MRI
Wernicke's encephalopathy	History of alcohol abuse or malnutrition; nystagmus, ataxia, a confusional state; physical stigmata of long-term alcohol abuse may be present	Improvement with thiamine
Behçet's disease	Oral or vaginal apthous ulcers, uveitis, conjunctivitis, arthritis, thrombophlebitis, skin lesions (erythema nodosum, acneiform rash); fever, subacute progression of of brain stem signs	ESR, CBC (mild anemia and leukocytosis); lumbar puncture (mild pleocytosis, elevated protein)
Brain stem stroke	History of cardiac arrhythmia, vascular disease, diabetes mellitus; bilateral long tract signs and skew deviation may be present	MRI
Paraneoplastic syndrome	Sensory neuronopathy, limbic encephalitis; most commonly associated with small cell carcinoma of the lung	Work-up for occult malignancy; type 1 antineuronal nuclear antibody

MRI, magnetic resonance imaging; ESC, erythrocyte sedimentation rate; CBC, cell blood count.

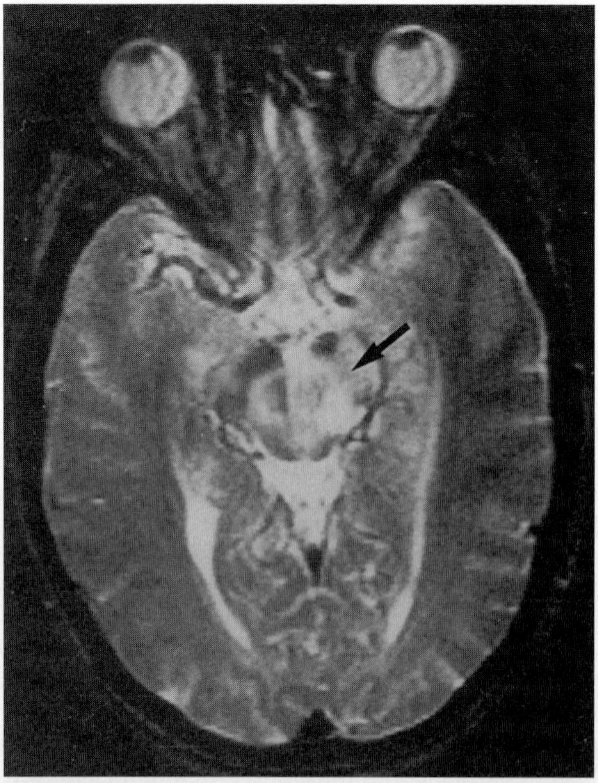

FIGURE 5–19 • *Listeria monocytogenes* brain stem encephalitis. A 48-year-old man presented with a 12-day history of right facial numbness, weakness, diplopia, clumsiness, and a tendency to fall toward the right. Ten days later, this magnetic resonance image demonstrated high-signal abnormality in the left cerebral peduncle and the dorsolateral aspect of the midbrain, as shown (arrow). (From Faidas A, Shepard DL, Lim J, et al: Magnetic resonance imaging in Listerial brain stem encephalitis. Clin Infect Dis 1993;16:187. University of Chicago, publisher.)

half of cases, although MRI is much more sensitive.[214] Figure 5–19 demonstrates MRI findings in a case of *Listeria* brain stem encephalitis from a 48-year-old man who presented with facial numbness, diplopia, confusion, and falling to the right. His MRI results revealed high-signal lesions in the left cerebral peduncle and cerebellar peduncles, and he improved with ceftriaxone and ampicillin.[215] Prompt recognition of this condition is essential, because the timely administration of appropriate antibiotic therapy (usually ampicillin) greatly improves prognosis.

Viral infections may also cause brain stem encephalitis. Herpes infections usually involve the temporal lobes, but cases of herpetic brain stem encephalitis have been reported.[211, 216] St. Louis encephalitis may also cause focal brain stem findings.[217] Patients usually present with typical features of nuchal rigidity, fever, and confusion. A high index of suspicion should be maintained for this entity in the summer and early autumn, especially in endemic areas. Rarely, focal brain stem findings result from other viral infections, including EEE and Japanese encephalitis.[218, 219]

In some cases, it is unclear whether brain stem inflammation is caused by direct viral infection or an immune-mediated postinfectious process. In 1951, Bickerstaff and Cloake described a series of patients who presented with ataxia and ophthalmoparesis.[220] Bickerstaff's encephalitis has since been used to describe the clinical syndrome of external ophthalmoparesis, ptosis, and ataxia. This syndrome is often preceded by viral infection, and associations have been made with cytomegalovirus and herpesviruses.[221, 222] Its etiology is unclear, but the syndrome is believed to be a postinfectious autoimmune-mediated process. Although the clinical presentation of progressive bulbar dysfunction is ominous, Bickerstaff's encephalitis generally has a benign prognosis.[223] The clinical presentation of ophthalmoplegia and ataxia bears a striking similarity to Miller-Fisher syndrome, and there has been some controversy over the relationship of these two entities. Miller-Fisher syndrome is generally believed to be due to demyelinating peripheral neuritis, whereas Bickerstaff's encephalitis may be associated with mild hemiparesis, extensor plantar responses, and other signs and symptoms suggesting CNS involvement. Despite these apparent differences, a recent report identified an antigen that was common to both these disorders, anti-GQ_{1b}, which raises the possibility that both of these entities share a common pathogenesis.[224]

References

1. Lebel MH, Freij BJ, Syrogiannopoulos GA, et al: Dexamethasone therapy for bacterial meningitis. N Engl J Med 1988;319:964–971.
2. Roos KL, Scheld WM: The management of fulminant meningitis in the intensive care unit. Crit Care Clin 1988;4:375–392.
3. Lambert HP: Meningitis. J Neurol Neurosurg Psychiatry 1994;57:405–415.
4. Martin JB, Tyler KL, Scheld WM: Bacterial meningitis. In Tyler KL, Martin JB (eds): Infectious Diseases of the Central Nervous System, pp 176–187. Philadelphia, FA Davis, 1993.
5. Tunkel AR, Scheld WM: Bacterial meningitis. In Carlson RW, Geheb MA (eds): Principles & Practice of Medical Intensive Care, pp 454–466. Philadelphia, WB Saunders, 1993.
6. Dobson SRM, Moxon ER: *Haemophilus influenzae:* Syndromes and treatment. In Lambert HP (ed): Infections of the Central Nervous System, pp 105–116. Philadelphia, BC Decker, 1991.
7. Tunkel AR, Scheld WM: Bacterial meningitis: Pathogenic and pathophysiologic mechanisms. In Lambert HP (ed): Infections of the Central Nervous System, pp 1–15. Philadephia, BC Decker, 1991.
8. Conway SP: Pneumococcal and other gram-positive coccal meningitides. In Lambert HP (ed): Infections of the Central Nervous System, pp 125–149. Philadelphia, BC Decker, 1991.
9. Lambert HP: Meningitis: Diagnostic problems. In Lambert HP (ed): Infections of the Central Nervous System, pp 32–39. Philadelphia, BC Decker, 1991.
10. Farrar WE, Reboli AC: Meningitis due to *Listeria monocytogenes* and other gram-positive bacilli. In Lambert HP

(ed): Infections of the Central Nervous System, pp 175–188. Philadelphia, BC Decker, 1991.

11. Teoh R, Humphries M: Tuberculous meningitis. In Lambert HP (ed): Infections of the Central Nervous System, pp 189–207. Philadelphia, BC Decker, 1991.
12. Moxon ER, Kroll JS, Kayhty MH: *Haemophilus infuenzae* type B meningitis: Pathogenesis and immunology. In Lambert HP (ed): Infections of the Central Nervous System, pp 99–104. Philadelphia, BC Decker, 1991.
13. Bell WE, McGuinness GA: Antibacterial and antifungal therapy for CNS infections. In Tyler KL, Martin JB (eds): Infectious Diseases of the Central Nervous System, pp 305–353. Philadelphia, FA Davis, 1993.
14. McGowan KL: The Report on Pediatric Infectious Diseases 1992;2:29–32.
15. Spanos A, Harrell FE, Durack DT: Differential diagnosis of acute meningitis. JAMA 1989;262:2700–2707.
16. Sanford JP: The Sanford Guide to Antimicrobial Therapy. Dallas, Antimicrobial Therapy, 1997.
17. de Louvois J: Neonatal meningitis. In Lambert HP (ed): Infections of the Central Nervous System, pp 161–174. Philadelphia, BC Decker, 1991.
18. Tauber MG, Khayam-Bashi H, Sande MA: Effects of ampicillin and corticosteroids on brain water content, cerebrospinal fluid pressure, and cerebrospinal fluid lactate levels in experimental pneumococcal meningitis. J Infect Dis 1985;151:528–534.
19. Milligan NM, Newcombe R, Compson DA: A double-blind controlled trial of high dose methylprednisolone in patients with multiple sclerosis: 1. Clinical effects. J Neurol Neurosurg Psychiatry 1987;50:511–516.
20. Jensen K, Ranek L, Rosdahl N: Bacterial meningitis. Scand J Infect Dis 1969;1:21–30.
21. Prasad K, Haines T: Dexamethasone treatment for acute bacterial meningitis: How strong is the evidence for routine use? J Neurol Neurosurg Psychiatry 1995;59:31–37.
22. Tang L-M: Ventriculoperitoneal shunt in cryptococcal meningitis with hydrocephalus. Surg Neurol 1990;33:314–319.
23. Eddy VA, Vitsky JL, Rutherford EJ, Morris JA: Aggressive use of ICP monitoring is sage and alters patient care. Am Surg 1995;61:24–29.
24. Bell BA, Britton JA: Brain abscess. In Lambert HP (ed): Infections of the Central Nervous System, pp 361–373. Philadelphia, BC Decker, 1991.
25. Seydoux C, Francioli P: Bacterial brain abscesses: Factors influencing mortality and sequelae. Clin Infect Dis 1992;15:394–401.
26. Ersahin Y, Mutluer S, Guzelbag E: Brain abscess in infants and children. Child's Nerv Syst 1994;10:185–189.
27. Tsuchiya K, Makita K, Furui S, et al: Contrast-enhanced magnetic resonance imaging of sub- and epidural empyemas. Neuroradiology 1992;34:494–496.
28. Lunardi P, Acqui M, Maleci A, et al: Ultrasound-guided brain biopsy: A personal experinece with emphasis on its indication. Surg Neurol 1993;39:148–151.
29. Sjolin J, Lilja A, Eriksson N, et al: Treatment of brain abscess with cefotaxime and metronidazole: Prospective study on 15 consecutive patients. Clin Infect Dis 1993;17:857–863.
30. Campbell S: Amebic brain abscess and meningoencephalitis. Semin Neurol 1993;13:153–160.
31. Schmidtmayer J, Jacobsen C, Miksch G, Sievers J: Blood monocytes and spleen macrophages differentiate into microglia-like cells on monolayers of astrocytes: Membrane currents. Glia 1994;12:259–267.
32. Ma P, Visvesvara GS, Martinez AJ, et al: Naegleria and Acanthamoeba infections: Review. Rev Infect Dis 1990;12:490–513.
33. Duma RJ: Primary amebic meningoencephalitis: Infection by free-living amebae. In Lambert HP (ed): Infections of the Central Nervous System. Philadelphia, BC Decker, 1991;253–263.
34. Lawande RV, Abraham SN, John I, Egler LJ: Recovery of soil amebas from the nasal passages of children during the dusty harmattan period in Zaria. Am J Clin Pathol 1979;71:201–203.
35. Wiley CA, Safrin RE, David CE, et al: Acanthamoeba meningoencephalitis in a patient with AIDS. J Infect Dis 1987;155:130–133.
36. Dietz R, Schanen G, Kramann B, Erpelding J: Intracranial amebic abscesses: CT and MR findings. J Comp Asst Tom 1991;15:168–170.
37. Stevens AR, Shulman ST, Lansen TA, et al: Primary amoebic meningoencephalitis: A report of two cases and antibiotic and immunologic status. J Infect Dis 1981;143:193–199.
38. Ofori-Kwakye SK, Sidebottom DG, Herbert J, et al: Granulomatous brain tumor caused by *Acanthamoeba.* Case report. J Neurosurg 1986;64:505–509.
39. Das SR, Asiri S, El-Scofi A, Baer HP: Protective and curative effects of rifampicin in *Acanthamoeba* meningitis of the mouse. J Infect Dis 1991;163:916–917.
40. Martinez AJ: Infection of the central nervous system due to *Acanthamoeba.* Rev Infect Dis 1991;13:S399–S402.
41. Bruckner DA: Amebiasis. Clin Microbiol Rev 1992;5:356–369.
42. Bale JF: Parasitic and rickettsial infections of the nervous system. In Tyler KL, Martin JB (eds): Infectious Diseases of the Central Nervous System, pp 259–304. Philadelphia, FA Davis, 1993.
43. Bia FJ, Barry M: Parasitic infections of the central nervous system. In Booss J, Thornton GF (eds): Neurologic Clinics: Infectious Diseases of the Central Nervous System, pp 171–207. Philadelphia, WB Saunders, 1986.
44. Lombardo L, Alonso P, Saenz-Arroyo L, et al: Cerebral amebiasis. J Neurosurg 1964;215:704–708.
45. Cook GC: Protozoan and helminthic infections. In Lambert HP (ed): Infections of the Central Nervous System, pp 264–282. Philadelphia, BC Decker, 1991.
46. Afghani BN, Leiberman JM: Paradoxical enlargement or development of intracranial tuberculomas during therapy: Case report and review. Clin Infect Dis 1994;19:1092–1099.
47. Berenguer J, Moreno S, Laguna F, et al: Tuberculous meningitis in patients infected with the human immunodeficiency virus. N Engl J Med 1992;326:668–672.
48. Levine DP: Infections in intravenous drug abusers. In Carlson RW, Geheb MA (eds): Principles & Practice of Medical Intensive Care. Philadelphia, WB Saunders, 1993.
49. Selvapandian S, Rajshekhar V, Chandy MJ, Idikula J: Predictive value of computed tomography–based diagnosis of intracranial tuberculomas. Neurosurgery 1994;35:845–850.
50. Garner CV, Baker AS: Upper respiratory tract infections. In Carlson RW, Geheb MA (eds): Principles & Practice of Medical Intensive Care, pp 474–480. Philadelphia, WB Saunders, 1993.
51. Shen W-C, Cheng T-Y, Ho Y-J, Lee K-R: Disseminated tuberculomas in spinal cord and brain demonstrated by MRI with gadolinium-DTPA. Neuroradiology 1993;35:213–215.
52. Eide FF, Gean AD, So YT: Clinical and radiographic findings in disseminated tuberculosis of the brain. Neurology 1993;43:1427–1429.
53. Silman JB, Peters JI, Levine SM, Jenkinson SG: Development of intracranial tuberculomas while receiving therapy for pulmonary fibrosis. Am J Respir Crit Care Med 1994;150:1439–1440.
54. Gupta RK, Pandey R, Khan EM, et al: Intracranial tuberculomas: MRI signal intensity correlation with histopathology and localised proton spectroscopy. Mag Res Imaging 1993;11:443–449.
55. Preheim LC: Tuberculosis and other mycobacterial infections. In Carlson RW, Geheb MA (eds): Principles & Practice of Medical Intensive Care, pp 422–433. Philadelphia, WB Saunders, 1993.
56. Kaufman DM, Kaplan JG, Litman N: Infectious agents in epidural abscesses. Neurology 1980;30:844–850.
57. Verner EF, Musher DM: Spinal epidural abscess. Med Clin North Am 1985;69:375–384.
58. Baker AS, Ojemann RG, Swartz MN, et al: Spinal epidural abscess. N Engl J Med 1975;293:463–468.

59. Schemtzhard E, Aichner F, Dierck RA: New perspectives in acute spinal epidural abscess. Neurochirurgica 1986;80:105–108.
60. Bergman I, Wald ER, Meyer JD, et al: Epidural abscess and vertebral osteomyelitis following serial lumbar punctures. Pediatrics 1983;72:476–480.
61. Danner RL, Hartman BJ: Update on spinal epidural abscess: Thirty five cases and a review of the literature. Rev Infect Dis 1987;9:265–274.
62. Heusner AP: Nontuberculous spinal epidural infections. N Engl J Med 1948;239:845–854.
63. Schulman JA, Blumberg HM: Paraspinal and spinal infections. In Lambert HP (ed): Infections of the Central Nervous System, pp 374–390. Philadelphia, BC Decker, 1991.
64. Byrd BF, Weiner MH, McGee ZA: Aspergillus spinal epidural abscess. JAMA 1982;248:3138–3139.
65. DiNubile MJ: Spinal epidural abscess. In Schlossberg D (ed): Infection of the Nervous System, pp 171–178. New York, Springer-Verlag, 1990.
66. Bertino RE, Porter BA, Stimak GK, et al: Imaging spinal osteomyelitis and epidural abscess with short T1 inversion recovery. Am J Neuroradiol 1988;9:563–564.
67. Sapico FL, Montgomerie JZ: Pyogenic vertebral osteomyelitis: Report of nine cases and review of the literature. Rev Infect Dis 1979;1:754–776.
68. Koppel BS, Tuchman AJ, Mangiardi JR: Epidural spinal infection in intravenous drug users. Arch Neurol 1988;45:1331–1337.
69. Lunardi P, Missori P, DiLorenzo N, Fortuna A: Cerebral hydatidosis in childhood: A retrospective survey with emphasis on long-term follow-up. Neurosurgery 1991;29:515–518.
70. Kaya U, Ozden B, Turker K, Tarcan B: Intracranial hydatid cysts: A study of 17 cases. J Neurosurg 1975;42:580–584.
71. Ersahin Y, Mutluer S, Guzelbag E: Intracranial hydatid cysts in children. Neurosurgery 1993;33:219–225.
72. Sayek I, Cakmakci M: The effect of prophylactic mebendazole in experimental peritoneal hydatidosis. Surg Gynecol Obstet 1986;163:351–353.
73. Bilge T, Barut S, Bilge S, et al: Primary multiple hydatid cysts of the brain: Case report. Surg Neurol 1993;39:377–379.
74. Saminy E, Ali Zadeh F: Cranial and intracranial hydatidosis with special reference to roentgen-ray diagnosis. J Neurosurg 1965;22:425–433.
75. Pearl M, Kotsilimbos DG, Leher HZ, et al: Cerebral echinococcosis, a pediatric disease: Report of two cases with one successful five-year follow-up. Pediatrics 1978;61:915–920.
76. Bensaid AH, Dietemann JL, Filippi de la Palavesa MM, et al: Intracranial alveolar echinococcosis: CT and MRI. Neuroradiology 1994;36:289–291.
77. Carcassonne M, Aubrespy P, Dor V, Choux M: Hydatid cysts in childhood. Prog Pediatr Surg 1973;5:1–35.
78. Todorov T, Vutova K, Petkov D, Balkanski G: Albendazole treatment of multiple cerebral hydatid cysts: Case report. Trans R Soc Trop Med Hyg 1988;82:150–152.
79. Hamza R, Toubi S, Jamoussi M, et al: Intracranial and orbital hydatid cysts. Neuroradiology 1982;22:211–214.
80. Feuerstein N, Chan PK, Mond JJ: Identification of numatrin, the nuclear matrix protein associated with induction of mitogenesis, as the nucleolar protein B23. J Biol Chem 1988;263:10608–10612.
81. Hirsch MS, Schooley RT: Drug therapy. Treatment of herpesvirus infections. N Engl J Med 1983;309:963, 1034.
82. St.Geme JW, Maldonado YA, Enzmann D, et al: Consensus: Diagnosis and management of neurocysticercosis in children. Pediatr Infect Dis J 1993;12:455–461.
83. Jackson A, Dobson MJ, Cooper PN: The Swiss cheese brain. Br J Radiol 1992;65:1042–1044.
84. Del Brutto OH, Sotelo J, Aguirre R, et al: Albendazole therapy for giant subarachnoid cysticerci. Arch Neurol 1992;49:535–538.
85. Alarcon F, Hidalgo F, Moncayo J, et al: Cerebral cysticercosis and stroke. Stroke 1992;23:224–228.
86. Garcia HH, Gilman R, Martinez M, et al: Cysticercosis as a major cause of epilepsy in Peru. Lancet 1993;341:197–200.
87. Chang-Yuan W, Hong-Hua Z, Ling-Yun G: A Mab-based ELISA for detecting circulating antigen in CSF of patients with neurocysticercosis. Hybridoma 1992;11:825–827.
88. Carpio A, Placencia M, Santillan F, Escobar A: A proposal for classification of neurocysticercosis. Can J Neurol Sci 1994;21:43–47.
89. Del Brutto OH: Medical treatment of cysticercosis-effective. Arch Neurol 1995;52:102–104.
90. Takayanagui OM, Jardim E: Therapy for neurocysticercosis. Arch Neurol 1992;49:290–294.
91. Del Brutto OH: Prognostic factors for seizure recurrence after withdrawal of antiepileptic drugs in patients with neurocysticercosis. Neurology 1994;44:1706–1709.
92. Rajshekhar V: Albendazole therapy for persistent, solitary cysticercus granulomas in patients with seizures. Neurology 1993;43:1238–1240.
93. Newton CRJC, Peshu N, Kendall B, et al: Brain swelling and ischaemia in Kenyans with cerebral malaria. Arch Dis Child 1994;70:281–287.
94. Turner GDH, Morrison H, Jones M, et al: An immunohistochemical study of the pathology of fatal malaria: Evidence for widespread endothelial activation and a potential role for intercellular adhesion molecule-1 in cerebral sequestration. Am J Pathol 1994;145:1057–1069.
95. Waller D, Crawley J, Nosten F, et al: Intracranial pressure in childhood malaria. Trans R Soc Trop Med Hyg 1991;85:362–364.
96. Clark IA, MacMicking JD, Gray KM, et al: Malaria mimicry with tumor necrosis factor: Contrasts between species of murine malaria and Plasmodium falciparum. Am J Pathol 1992;140:325–336.
97. Facer CA, Bentley A, Withers M, Kataaha PK: Malaria and ELISA HTLV-III antibody reactivity. Trans R Soc Trop Med Hyg 1986;80:351–352.
98. Bruce-Chwatt LJ: From Laveran's discovery to DNA probes: New trends in diagnosis of malaria. Lancet 1987;1509–1511.
99. Malaria Action Programme World Health Organization: The use of DNA probes for malaria diagnosis: Memorandum from a WHO meeting. Bull WHO 1986;64:641–652.
100. Downs AG: Arboviruses. In Evans AS (ed): Viral Infections of Humans: Epidemiology and Control, p 114. New York, Plenum, 1989.
101. Reiber H, Lange P: Quantification of virus specific antibodies in cerebrospinal fluid and serum: Sensitive and specific detection of antibody synthesis in brain. Clin Chem 1991;37:1153–1160.
102. Koskiniemi M, Vaheri A, Taskinen E: Cerebrospinal fluid alterations in herpes simplex virus encephalitis. Rev Infect Dis 1984;6:608.
103. Longson M: Herpes simplex. In Zuckerman AJ, Banatvala JE, Pattison JR (eds): Principles and Practice of Clinical Virology, 2nd ed, p 2. West Sussex, England, John Wiley & Sons, 1990.
104. Whitley RJ, Soong SJ, Hirsch MS, et al: Herpes simplex encephalitis: Vidarabine therapy and diagnostic problems. N Engl J Med 1981;304:313–318.
105. Whitley RJ, Soong SJ, Linneman C Jr, et al: Herpes simplex encephalitis: Clinical assessment. JAMA 1982;247:317–320.
106. Lakeman FC, Whitley RJ, the National Institue of Allergy and Infectious Diseases Collaborative Antiviral Study Group: Diagnosis of Herpes simplex encephalitis: Application of polymerase chain reaction to cerebrospinal fluid from brain-biopsied patients and correlation with disease. J Infect Dis 1995;171:857–863.
107. Shoji H, Koga M, Kusuhara T, et al: Differentiation of herpes simplex virus 1 and 2 in cerebrospinal fluid of patients with HSV encephalitis and meningitis by stringent hybridization of PCR-amplified DNAs. J Neurol 1994;241:526–530.
108. Dennett C, Klapper PE, Cleator GM, Lewis AG: CSF pretreatment and the diagnosis of herpes encephalitis using

the polymerase chain reaction. J Virol Methods 1991;34:101–104.
109. Soong S-J, Watson NE, Caddell GR, et al: Use of brain biopsy for diagnositic evaluation of patients with suspected herpes simplex encephalitis: A statistical model and its clinical applications. J Infect Dis 1991;163:17–22.
110. Aurelius D, Johansson B, Skoldenberg B, et al: Rapid diagnosis of herpes simplex encephalitis by nested polymerase chain reaction assay of cerebrospinal fluid. Lancet 1991;337:189.
111. Davis JM, Davis KR, Kleinman GM, et al: Computed tomography of herpes simplex encephalitis, with clinicopathological correlation. Radiology 1978;129:409.
112. Schroth G, Gawehn J, Thron A, et al: Early diagnosis of herpes simplex encephalitis by MRI. Neurology 1987;37:179–183.
113. Lester JW, Carter MP, Reynolds TL: Herpes encephalitis: MR monitoring of response to acyclovir therapy. J Comp Asst Tom 1988;12:941–943.
114. Aminoff MJ: Electroencephalography: General principles and clinical applications. In Aminoff MJ (ed): Electrodiagnosis in Clinical Neurology, 2nd ed, p 21. New York, Churchill Livingstone, 1986.
115. Whitley RJ: Herpes simplex virus infections of the central nervous system: A review. Am J Med 1988;85:61–67.
116. Adair JC, Gold M, Bond RE: Acyclovir neurotoxicity: Clinical experience and review of the literature. South Med J 1994;87:1227–1231.
117. Schimdbauer M, Budka H, Pilz P, et al: Presence, distribution and spread of productive varicella zoster virus infectrion in nervous tissues. Brain 1992;115:383–398.
118. Tensor RB: Herpes simplex and herpes zoster: Nervous system involvement. In Johnson KP (ed): Neurologic Clinics: Symposium on Neurovirology, pp 215–239. Philadelphia, WB Saunders, 1984.
119. Jemsek J, Greenberg SB, Taber L, et al: Herpes zoster–associated encephalitis: Clinicopathologic report of 12 cases and review of the literature. Medicine 1983;62:81–97.
120. Ho DD, Hirsch MS: Acute viral encephalitis. Med Clin North Am 1985;69:415.
121. Ragozzino MW, Melton LJ III, Kurland LT, et al: Population-based study of herpes zoster and its sequelae. Medicine 1982;61:310–316.
122. Hogan EL, Krigman MR: Herpes zoster myelitis. Arch Neurol 1973;29:309.
123. Elliot KJ: Other neurological complications of herpes zoster and their management. Ann Neurol 1994;35:S57–S61.
124. Gray F, Belec L, Lescs C, et al: Varicella-zoster virus infection of the central nervous system in the acquired immune deficiency syndrome. Brain 1994;117:987–999.
125. Chretien F, Gray F, Lescs MC, et al: Acute varicella-zoster virus ventriculitis and meningo-myelo-radiculitis in acquired immunodeficiency syndrome. Acta Neuropathol 1993;86:659–665.
126. Booss J, Esiri ME: Viral Encephalitis: Pathology, Diagnosis, and Management. Boston, Blackwell Scientific, 1986.
127. Aviel A, Marshak C: Ramsay Hunt syndrome: A cranial polyneuropathy. Am J Otolaryngol 1982;3:61–66.
128. McKendall RR, Klawans HI: Varicella zoster virus complications. In Vinken PJ, Bruyn GW (eds): Handbook of Clinical Neurology, vol 34, Infections in the Nervous System, p 161. New York, North Holland, 1978.
129. Gershon A, Steinberg S, Greenberg S, Taber L: Varicella zoster–associated encephalitis: Detection of specific antibody in cerebrospinal fluid. J Clin Microbiol 1980;12:764–767.
130. van Loon AM, van der Logt JTM, Heessen FWA, et al: Antibody-capture enzyme-linked immunosorbent assays that use enzyme-labelled antigen for detection of virus-specific immunoglobulin M, A and G in patients with varicella or herpes zoster. Epidemiol Infect 1992;108:165–174.
131. Balfour HH, Bean B, Laskin O, et al: Acyclovir halts progression of herpes zoster in immunocompromised patients. N Engl J Med 1983;308:1448.
132. Shepp DH, Dandliker PS, Meyers JD: Treatment of varicella-zoster infection in severely immunocompromised patients. N Engl J Med 1986;314:208.
133. Steele RW, Keeney RE, Bradsher RW, et al: Treatment of varicella-zoster meningoencephalitis with acyclovir—Demonstration of virus in cerebrospinal fluid by electron microscopy. Am J Clin Pathol 1983;80:57.
134. Warrell DA, Warrell MJ: Rabies. In Lambert HP (ed): Infections of the Central Nervous System, pp 317–328. Philadelphia, BC Decker, 1991.
135. Eng TR, Hamaker TA, Dobbins JG: Rabies surveillance, United States. MMWR 1988;38:1.
136. Houff SA, Burton RC, Wilson RW, et al: Human-to-human transmission of rabies virus by corneal transplant. N Engl J Med 1979;300:603.
137. Chopra JS, Banerjee AK, Murthy JMK, et al: Paralytic rabies: A clinicopathological study. Brain 1980;103:789.
138. Bernard KW, Fishbein DB: Rabies virus. In Mandell GL, Doylous RG, Bennett JE (eds): Principles and Practice of Infectious Diseases, 3rd ed, p 1291. New York, John Wiley & Sons, 1990.
139. Whitley RJ, Soong S-J, Dolin R, et al: Adenosine arabinoside therapy of biopsy-proved herpes simplex encephalitis. N Engl J Med 1977;297:289–294.
140. Anderson LJ, Karl G, Nicholson MB, et al: Human rabies in the United States, 1960 to 1979: Epidemiology, diagnosis, and prevention. Ann Intern Med 1984;100:728.
141. Bryceson AD, Greenwood BM, Warrell DA, et al: Demonstration during life of rabies antigen in humans. J Infect Dis 1975;131:71.
142. Maton PN, Pollard JD, Newsom Davis J. Human rabies encephalomyelitis. BMJ 1976;1:1038.
143. Kastrukoff LF, Lau AS, Kim SU: Multifocal CNS demyelination following peripheral inoculation with herpes simplex virus type 1. Ann Neurol 1987;22:52–59.
144. CDC: Arbovirus disease—United States, 1993. JAMA 1994;272:262–264.
145. Monath TP: Flaviviruses. In Fields BN, Knipe DM, Chanock RM, et al (eds): Virology, 2nd ed, pp 763–814. New York, Raven Press, 1990.
146. Brinker KR, Paulson G, Monath T, et al: St. Louis encephalitis in Ohio, September 1975. Arch Intern Med 1974;139:561–566.
147. Quick DT, Thompson JM, Bond JO: The 1962 epidemic of St. Louis encephalitis in Florida. IV: Clinical features of cases occurring in the Tampa Bay area. Am J Epidemiol 1965;81:415–427.
148. Monath TP, Nystrom RR, Bailey RE, et al: Immunoglobulin M antibody capture enzyme-linked immunosorben assay for diagnosis of St. Louis encephalitis. J Clin Microbiol 1984;20:784–790.
149. Johnson RT: Viral Infections of the Nervous System. New York, Raven Press, 1982.
150. Aryes JC, Feemster RF: The sequelae of eastern equine encephalomyelitis. N Engl J Med 1949;240:960.
151. Feemster RF: Equine encephalitis in Massachusetts. N Engl J Med 1957;257:701–704.
152. Calisher CH, el-Kafrawi AO, Al-Deen Mahmud MI, et al: Complex-specific immunoglobulin M antibody patterns in humans infected with alphaviruses. J Clin Microbiol 1986;23:155–159.
153. Calisher CH, Berardi VP, Muth DJ, Buff EE: Specificity of immunoglobulin M and G antibody responses in humans infected with eastern and western equine encephalitis viruses: Application to rapid serodiagnosis. J Clin Microbiol 1986;23:369–372.
154. Kim JH, Booss J, Manuelidis EE, Duncan CC: Human eastern equine encephalitis. Electron microscopic study of a brain biopsy. Am J Clin Pathol 1985;84:223–227.
155. Farber S, Connerly ML, Dingle JH: Encephalitis in infants and children. JAMA 1940;114:1725–1731.
156. Prezelomski MM, O'Rourke E, Grady GF, et al: Eastern equine encephalitis in Massachusetts: A report of 16 cases, 1970–1984. Neurology 1988;38:736.
157. Schmidt P, Meyer H, Hubert P, et al: In-situ hybridization for demonstration of equine herpesvirus type 1 DNA in paraffin wax–embedded tissues and its use in horses with

disseminated necrotizing myeloencephalitis. J Comp Pathol 1994;110:215–225.
158. Piliero PJ, Brody J, Zamani A, Deresiewicz RL: Eastern equine encephalitis presenting as focal neuroradiographic abnormalities: Case report and review. Clin Infect Dis 1994;18:985–988.
159. Huggins JW: RNA viruses that cause hemorrhagic, encephalitic, and febrile disease. In Galasso GJ, Whitley RJ, Merigan TC (eds): Antiviral Agents and Viral Diseases of Man, 3rd ed, p 691. New York, Raven Press, 1990.
160. McGowan JE, Bryan JA, Gregg MB: Surveillance of arboviral encephalitis in the United States, 1955–1971. Am J Epidemiol 1973;97:199–207.
161. Finley KH, Fitzgerald LH, Richter RW, et al: Western encephalitis and cerebral ontogenesis. Arch Neurol 1967;16:140–164.
162. Earnest MP, Goolishian HA, Calverley JR, et al: Neurologic, intellectual, and psychologic sequelae following western encephalitis. Neurology 1971;21:969–974.
163. Peters CJ, Dalrymple JM: Alphaviruses. In Fields BN, Knipe DM, Chanock RM, et al (eds): Virology, 2nd ed, pp 713–761. New York, Raven Press, 1990.
164. Fulhorst CF, Hardy JL, Eldridge BF, et al: Natural vertical transmission of western equine encephalomyelitis virus in mosquitoes. Science 1994;263:676–678.
165. Ho M: Acute viral encephalitis. In Vinken PJ, Bruyn GW (eds): Handbook of Clinical Neurology, vol 34, Infections in the Nervous System, p 63. New York, North Holland, 1978.
166. Dickerson RB, Newton JR, Hansen JE: Diagnosis and immediate prognosis of Japanese B encephalitis. Am J Med 1952;12:277.
167. Rosen L: The natural history of Japanese encephalitis virus. Annu Rev Microbiol 1986;40:395.
168. Umenai T, Krzysko R, Bektimirov A, et al: Japanese encephalitis: Current worldwide status. Bull WHO 1985;65:625.
169. Hoke CH, Nisalak A, Sangwhipa N, et al: Protection against Japanese encephalitis by inactivated vaccines. N Engl J Med 1988;319:608.
170. Burke DS, Nisalak A, Ussery MA, et al: Kinetics of IgM and IgG responses to Japanese encephalitis virus in human serum and cerebrospinal fluid. J Infect Dis 1985;151:1093.
171. Burke DS, Lorsomrudee W, Leake CJ, et al: Fatal outcome in Japanese encephalitis. Am J Trop Med Hyg 1985;34:1203.
172. Ehrenkranz NJ, Ventura AK: Venezuelan equine encephalitis in man. Annu Rev Med 1974;25:9.
173. Bowen GS, Fashinell TR, Dean PB, Gregg MB: Clinical aspects of human Venezuelan equine encephalitis in Texas. Bull Pan Am Health Organ 1976;10:46–57.
174. Porterfield JS: Alphaviruses, flaviviruses and Bunyaviridae. In Zuckerman AJ, Banatvala JE, Pattison JR (eds): Principles and Practice of Clinical Virology, 2nd ed, p 435. New York, John Wiley & Sons, 1990.
175. Gundersen CB, Brown KL: Clinical aspects of La Crosse encephalitis: Preliminary report. In Calisher CH, Thompson WH (eds): California Serogroup Viruses, p 169. New York, Alan R. Liss, 1983.
176. Gonzalez-Scarano F, Nathanson N: Bunyaviruses. In Fields BN, Knipe DM, Chanock RM, et al (eds): Virology, 2nd ed, pp 1195–1228. New York, Raven Press, 1990.
177. Deering WM: Neurologic aspects and treatment of La Crosse encephalitis. In Calisher CH, Thompson WH (eds): California Serogroup Viruses, p 187. New York, Alan R. Liss, 1983.
178. Chun RWM, Thompson WH, Grabow JD, et al: California arbovirus infection in children. Neurology 1968;18:369.
179. Jamnback TL, Beaty BJ, Hildreth SW, et al: Capture immunoglobulin M system for rapid diagnosis of La Crosse (California encephalitis) virus infections. J Clin Microbiol 1982;16:577–580.
180. Beaty GJ, Jamnback TL, Hildreth SW, et al: Rapid diagnosis of La Crosse virus infections: Evaluation of serologic and antigen detection techniques for the clinically relevant diagnosis of La Crosse encephalitis. In Calisher CH, Thompson WH (eds): California Serogroup Viruses, p 293. New York, Alan R. Liss, 1983.
181. Chun RWM: Clinical aspects of La Crosse encephalitis: Neurological and psychological sequelae. In Calisher CH, Thompson WH (eds): California Serogroup Viruses, p 193. New York, Alan R. Liss, 1983.
182. Sievers J, Parwaresch R, Wottge H-U: Blood monocytes and spleen macrophages differentiate into microglia-like cells on monolayers of astrocytes: Morphology. Glia 1994;12:245–258.
183. Sulkava R, Rissanen A, Pyhala R: Post-influenzal encephalitis during the influenza A outbreak in 1979/1980. J Neurol Neurosurg Psychiatry 1982;44:161.
184. Potter CW: Influenza. In Zuckerman AJ, Banatvala JE, Pattison JR (eds): Principles and Practice of Clinical Virology, p 214. New York, John Wiley & Sons, 1990.
185. Kleppner SR, Robinson KA, Trojanowski JQ, Lee VM-Y: Transplanted human neurons derived from a teratocarcinoma cell line (NTera-2) mature, integrate, and survive for over 1 year in the nude mouse brain. J Comp Neurol 1995;357:618–632.
186. Schild GC, Pereira MS, Chakraverty P: Single-radial-hemolysis is a new method for the assay of antibody to influenza hemagglutinin. Bull WHO 1975;52:42.
187. Shaywitz BA, Rothstein P, Venes JL: Monitoring and management of increased intracranial pressure in Reye's syndrome: Results in 29 children. Pediatrics 1980;66:198.
188. Moore M: Enteroviral diseases in the United States. J Infect Dis 1982;146:103.
189. Chonmaitree T, Menegus MA, Powell KR: The clinical relevance of "CSF viral culture." JAMA 1982;247:1843–1847.
190. Koskiniemi M, Rautonen J, Lehtokoski-Lehtinieme E, Vaheri A: Epidemiology of encephalitis in children: A 20-year survey. Ann Neurol 1991;29:492–497.
191. Mustafa MM, Weitman SD, Winick NJ, et al: Subacute measles encephalitis in the young immunocompromised host: Report of two cases diagnosed by polymerase chain reaction and treated with ribavirin and review of the literature. Clin Infect Dis 1993;16:654–660.
192. Chen RE, Chir B, Ramsay DA, et al: Immunosuppressive measles encephalitis. Pediatr Neurol 1994;10:325–327.
193. Durant RH, Dyken PR, Swift AV: The influence of inosiplex treatment on the neurological disability of patients with subacute sclerosing panencephalitis. J Pediatr 1982;101:288.
194. Carpentier MAB, Billard C, Maheut J, et al: Acute measles encephalitis of the delayed type: Neuroradiological and immunological findings. Eur Neurol 1992;32:235–237.
195. Carter MJ, Ter Meulen V: Measles. In Zuckerman AJ, Banatvala JE, Pattison JR (eds): Principles and Practice of Clinical Virology, 2nd ed, p 314. New York, John Wiley & Sons, 1990.
196. Jones CE, Dyken PR, Huttenlocher PR, et al: Inosiplex therapy in subacute sclerosing panencephalitis. A multicentre, non-randomised study in 98 patients. Lancet 1982;i:1034.
197. Ross LA, Kim KS, Mason WH, Gomperts E: Successful treatment of disseminated measles in a patient with acquired immunodeficiency syndrome: Consideration of antiviral and passive immunotherapy. Am J Med 1990;88:313–314.
198. Wolinsky JS, Waxham MN: Mumps virus. In Fields BN, Knipe DM, Chanock RM (eds): Virology, 2nd ed, p 989. New York, Raven Press, 1990.
199. Reuler JB, Chang MK: Herpes zoster: Epidemiology, clinical features, and management. South Med J 1984;77:1149–1156.
200. Wood MJ: Current experience with antiviral therapy for acute herpes zoster. Ann Neurol 1994;35:S65–S68.
201. Adour KK: Otological complications of herpes zoster. Ann Neurol 1994;35:S62–S64.
202. Alfaro A: Cerebellar encephalitis in adults. J Neurol 1993;240:505–508.
203. Bistrian B, Phillips CA, Kaye IS: Fatal mumps meningoencephalitis. JAMA 1972;222:478.

204. Herndon RM, Johnson RT, Davis LE, et al: Ependymitis in mumps virus meningitis: Electron microscopical studies of cerebrospinal fluid. Arch Neurol 1974;30:475.
205. Glinkmann G, Pederson M, Mordhorst CH: Detection of specific immunoglobulin M to mumps virus in serum and cerebrospinal fluid samples from patients with acute mumps infection, using an antibody-capture enzyme immunoassay. Acta Pathol Microbiol Immunol Scan 1986;94:145.
206. Morishima T, Miyazu M, Ozaki T, et al: Local immunity in mumps meningitis. Am J Dis Child 1980;134:1060–1064.
207. Gnann JW: New antivirals with activity against varicella-zoster virus. Ann Neurol 1994;35:S69–S72.
208. Ukkonen P, Vaisanen O, Penttinen K: Enzyme-linked immunosorbent assay for mumps and parainfluenza type 1 immunoglobulin G and immunoglobulin M antibodies. J Clin Microbiol 1980;11:319.
209. Ando SM, Minamitani K, Miyamoto H, Niimi H: Magnetic resonance imaging: A case of mumps postinfectious encephalitis with asymptomatic optic neuritis. Eur J Pediatr 1991;150:773–775.
210. Kirsi JJ, McKernan PA, Burns NJ, et al: Broad-spectrum synergistic antiviral activity of selenazofurin and ribavirin. Antimicrob Agents Chemother 1984;26:466–475.
211. Kindley AD, Harris F: Herpes simplex infection presenting as brainstem encephalitis. Lancet 1978;i:212–213.
212. Kuroiwa Y, Tohgi H, Kanayama H: Neurobechet's disease with alternating hemiparesis. Neuroradiology 1986;28:284.
213. Mortomura S, Tabira T, Kuroiwa Y: A clinical comparative study of multiple and neuro-Behçet's syndrome. J Neurol Neurosurg Psychiatry 1980;210–213.
214. Armstrong WA, Fung PC: Brainstem encephalitis (rhombencephalitis) due to *Listeria monocytogenes:* Case report and review. Clin Infect Dis 1993;16:689–702.
215. Faidas A, Shepard DL, Lim J, et al: Magnetic resonance imaging in Listerial brain stem encephalitis. Clin Infect Dis 1993;16:186–187.
216. Roman-Campos G, Toro G: Herpetic brainstem encephalitis. Neurology 1980;30:981–985.
217. Feit H, Luby JP, Mollenrich S: Brainstem encephalitis with serological evidence of St. Louis encephalitis. J Neurol Neurosurg Psychiatry 1981;44:368.
218. Johnson RT, Burke DS, Elwell M: Japanese encephalitis: Immunocytochemical studies of viral antigen and inflammatory cells in fatal cases. Ann Neurol 1985;18:567–573.
219. Bastian FO, Wende RD, Singer DB, et al: Eastern equine encephalitis: Histopathological and ultrastructural changes with isolation of the virus in a human case. Am J Clin Pathol 1975;64:10–13.
220. Bickerstaff ER, Cloake PC: Mesencephalitis and rhombencephalitis. BMJ 1957;2:1384–1387.
221. Kanzaki A, Yabuki S, Yuki N: Bickerstaff's brainstem encephalitis associated with cytomegalovirus infection. J Neurol Neurosurg Psychiatry 1995;58:260–261.
222. Maran AG: Bickerstaff's encephalitis. J Laryngol 1980;66:520–523.
223. Yaqub BA, Al-Deeb SM, Daif AK, et al: Bickerstaff's brainstem encephalitis: A grave non-demyelinating disease with benign prognosis. J Neurol Sci 1990;96:29–40.
224. Yuki N, Sato S, Tsuji S, et al: An immunologic abnormality common to Bickerstaff's brainstem encephalitis and Fisher's syndrome. J Neurol Sci 1993;118:83–87.

6

Neuroemergencies During Pregnancy

Scott E. Kasner, M.D. • Eric C. Raps, M.D. • Steven L. Galetta, M.D.

The neurologic and neurosurgical management of the pregnant woman is unique by necessity, because efforts must be directed toward the simultaneous care of two patients, mother and fetus. Alterations in maternal-fetal physiology are associated with an increased incidence of several pathological phenomena (Table 6–1). Some disorders, such as preeclampsia and eclampsia, occur exclusively in the setting of pregnancy. Others, including stroke and cerebral venous thrombosis, occur more frequently among pregnant women. Myasthenia gravis has an increased tendency to flare in the puerperium. Guillain-Barré syndrome is no more common during pregnancy than at other times, but it can significantly complicate an otherwise normal pregnancy. In every case, both mother and child are vulnerable to the potential toxicity and teratogenicity of our diagnostic and therapeutic endeavors (Table 6–2). Over 20% of maternal mortality is attributed to neurologic disease,[1, 2] and a multi-disciplinary approach of obstetric, medical, and neurologic critical care is required for maximally effective management.

MATERNAL-FETAL PHYSIOLOGY

Mother

Major adjustments in the pulmonary, cardiovascular, endocrine, renal, and neurologic systems occur as pregnancy progresses, and these play important roles in the pathophysiology of maternal disease. Oxygen consumption increases by 15% during the second and third trimesters in order to meet increased demands of the fetus, but total lung capacity and vital capacity are reduced by 5%.[1] To compensate, tidal volume must increase 30%–40%. Mild respiratory alkalosis results and is symptomatically experienced by the gravid patient as dyspnea and decreased exercise tolerance. Cardiac output increases 30%–50% in association with a 40%–55% expansion of the circulating blood volume, and the heart rate increases 15%–20%.[1] The heart becomes

TABLE 6–1 **TIMETABLE OF NEUROEMERGENCIES DURING PREGNANCY AND THE PUERPERIUM**

	1st TRIMESTER	2nd TRIMESTER	3rd TRIMESTER	LABOR AND DELIVERY	1st WEEK POSTPARTUM	2nd TO 6th WEEKS POSTPARTUM
Stroke	+	+	+ + +	+ +	+ + +	+ +
Cerebral venous thrombosis					+	+ + +
AVM-SAH	+ +	+ + +	+ +	+ +	+	+
Aneurysm-SAH	+	+ +	+ + +	+	+	+
Eclampsia		+	+ + +	+ + +	+ + +	+
Wernicke's encephalopathy	+ + +	+				
Central pontine myelinolysis	+ + +	+				
Hepatic encephalopathy/AFLP		+	+ + +	+		
Myasthenia gravis					+ + +	+ + +

AVM, arteriovenous malformation; SAH, subarachnoid hemorrhage; AFLP, acute fatty liver of pregnancy.

TABLE 6–2 **POTENTIAL ADVERSE EFFECTS OF MEDICATIONS DURING PREGNANCY**

MEDICATION	MATERNAL TOXICITY	FETAL TOXICITY
Aspirin	Peripartum hemorrhage, prolongation of labor	Premature closure of ductus arteriosus
Warfarin	Peripartum hemorrhage	Teratogenic, optic atrophy, mental retardation, fetal demise
Heparin	Peripartum hemorrhage, osteopenia, thrombocytopenia	
Thrombolytic agents	Massive hemorrhage	
Nimodipine		(Teratogenic and embryotoxic in animals)
Mannitol	Hypotension	Profound fetal dehydration
Phenytoin	Hypotension	Teratogenic
Phenobarbital	Hypotension	Teratogenic
Carbamazepine		Teratogenic
Valproic acid		Teratogenic
Benzodiazepines		Neonatal respiratory depression
Magnesium sulfate	Respiratory depression	Neonatal hypermagnesemia: hypotonia, weak suck, respiratory depression
Hydralazine	Hypotension, reflex tachycardia	
Diazoxide	Hypotension, tocolytic prolongation of labor	Hyperglycemia
Labetalol		(?Low birth weight)
Sodium nitroprusside	Thiocyanate toxicity, elevated intracranial pressure	Thiocyanate toxicity
Corticosteroids		Cleft lip and palate
Antimetabolites (azathioprine, cyclophosphamide)		Teratogenic
Intravenous immunoglobulin		Neonatal neutropenia

hyperdynamic and is displaced upward within the thorax. Systemic vascular resistance falls by 25% in response to the vasodilatory effects of progesterone. Blood pressure, however, is not significantly altered. A relative hypercoagulable state is established in pregnancy because of increased levels of fibrinogen and factors V, VII, VIII, IX, X, and XII, along with decreased levels of protein S, antithrombin III, and tissue plasminogen activator.[3, 4] Platelet aggregability is also augmented, but platelet number does not change. Although these alterations reach their extremes in the middle of the third trimester, they may persist for several weeks into the postpartum period.[1, 5]

Fetus

The uterine arteries are the sole blood supply to the fetus. As pregnancy progresses, perfusion increases from 50 mL/min at 10 weeks' gestation to about 600 mL/min, or almost 20% of maternal cardiac output, near term.[6] These vessels lack autoregulation, so uteroplacental blood flow depends entirely on maternal mean arterial pressure, blood viscosity, and intrauterine pressure. This system provides some margin of safety in that fetal hypoxia does not occur until oxygen delivery falls by 30%–50%.[6, 7]

Fetal ischemia may occur in the setting of normal maternal vital signs and requires a more direct assessment. However, the available techniques for antepartum evaluation of fetal hemodynamics are neither direct nor specific. Fetal heart monitoring may detect tachycardia, bradycardia, abnormal heart rate variability, or decelerations as signs of fetal distress. Fetal ultrasonography may demonstrate gross cardiac or other anatomic malformations that may affect fetal circulation. Because of the limitations of these methods, fetal injury may be clinically silent and remain undetected until delivery or later.

STROKE

Pregnancy may be a risk factor for cerebral ischemia and infarction in young women. Stroke has long been held to occur up to 13 times more often in pregnant women than in nonpregnant women of the same age,[8–12] although this contention has been recently challenged.[13] Conversely, approximately one-third of strokes in women of child-bearing age occur during pregnancy.[9] Cerebral infarction is due to arterial occlusion in 60%–80% of patients; the remainder are a result of cerebral venous thrombosis.[8, 11] Often additional cerebrovascular risk factors can be identified in pregnant women with stroke. Pre-existing or gestationally acquired diabetes mellitus, hypertension, cardiac abnormalities, hyperlipidemia, hypercoagulable states, and smoking are frequently implicated simultaneously. Alternatively, venous disease appears to be a more direct consequence of altered maternal physiology and hypercoagulability. Cerebral infarction can occur at any time during gestation, yet 25% occur during the first week after delivery, and an additional 17% occur during postpartum weeks 2 through 5.[8]

Diagnosis

The majority of strokes during pregnancy are characterized by large arterial occlusion, most often involving the middle cerebral artery or the internal carotid artery. Involvement of the posterior circulation is uncommon. The presenting symptoms depend on the site of infarction, and the clinical diagnosis and localization of cerebral infarction is usually not difficult. The etiologic differential diagnosis is extensive, however, and despite the temptation to label the event as a complication of pregnancy alone, full investigation of cerebral infarction in a young person should be considered. A thorough history, including a review of familial diseases, may suggest the underlying etiology. General physical examination may reveal evidence of systemic disease or stigmata of cardioembolic disease. Laboratory studies should include a screening panel consisting of a complete blood count, coagulation profile, erythrocyte sedimentation rate, syphilis serology, and an antinuclear antibody profile. Further laboratory diagnostic testing should be directed by the clinical scenario and the results of the screening studies.

In pursuit of the etiology of stroke, a number of imaging studies must be performed. Computerized tomography (CT) scan of the head is relatively safe in pregnancy and is the appropriate initial diagnostic study to exclude intracranial hemorrhage. With abdominal shielding, the radiation dose to the fetus is less than 1 mrad and of no consequence to the developing fetus.[14] Intravenous iodinated contrast crosses the placenta and should be avoided if possible, although no untoward effects on the fetus have been observed.[14] Carotid and transcranial ultrasound studies as well as echocardiography can be performed safely in pregnancy.[15] Conventional cerebral angiography may ultimately be required for definitive examination of the vasculature. This procedure is not contraindicated in pregnancy, but the abdomen should be thoroughly shielded as soon as the catheter is advanced into the thorax. Fetal monitoring should also be considered during the procedure.[5]

Magnetic resonance imaging (MRI) can also be used to examine the infarcted territory, and magnetic resonance angiography (MRA) can assist in visualization of the blood vessels. The safety of MRI and MRA in pregnancy has been generally accepted; therefore, they serve as useful screening tools in this setting.[14, 16] Gadolinium injection should be avoided in routine studies if possible, because this agent also crosses the placenta. However, no significant adverse effects have been demonstrated.[14, 16]

Cardioembolic Stroke

The majority of cerebral infarctions in pregnant women result from cardioembolic events. Congenital and acquired abnormalities, such as intracardiac right-to-left shunt, valvular disease, and arrhythmia, are not rare among pregnant women with stroke.

Paradoxical embolization may occur in patients with a patent foramen ovale (PFO). This abnormality is present in 5%–20% of the general population and usually remains asymptomatic throughout life.[17, 18] Because the pressure in the left atrium is normally higher than that in the right atrium, the foramen remains physiologically closed. However, in conditions that increase right-sided pressure, such as the Valsalva maneuver, blood may flow from right to left.[18, 19] This has been demonstrated to occur asymptomatically in 20% of normal volunteers with PFO and can be evaluated with microbubble contrast echocardiography and transesophageal echocardiography.[19] In studies of young (nonpregnant) patients who suffered cerebral infarction, the prevalence of PFO was nearly 50%.[18, 20] In pregnancy, the incidence of thrombophlebitis in the lower extremities is dramatically increased; it becomes maximal during the first several weeks post partum and is further increased after cesarean section or forceps delivery.[1] Other potential sources of paradoxical emboli include amniotic fluid embolism after parturition and air embolism after surgical delivery or abortion.[5] Thus, the pregnant woman with a PFO may be at increased risk for paradoxical embolus, although the incidence of such an event is as yet undetermined.

Pregnant women with valvular disease have an increased incidence of cardioembolic stroke. Patients with prosthetic valves are at particularly high risk for formation and embolization of a valvular thrombus. In pregnant patients with artificial valves, 25% had systemic emboli while on aspirin alone, whereas those on heparin had an embolic rate of only 4%.[21] As is discussed later, warfarin (Coumadin) is contraindicated during pregnancy. Mitral valve prolapse (MVP), found in 6% of healthy young women,[22] may also be associated with a mildly elevated risk of cardioembolic stroke.[23] Stroke related to MVP in pregnancy is rare, and anticoagulation is not generally recommended for primary prevention.

Infectious endocarditis is rare in patients with normal native cardiac valves. However, transient bacteremia follows 5% of vaginal deliveries and is more frequent after instrumented delivery or cesarean section.[24] The role of antibiotic prophylaxis at the time of delivery is controversial in patients with normal valves but is widely recommended in those with valvular abnormalities.[24] The most common organisms are *Streptococcus viridans* and *Staphylococcus aureus*.[25] In addition, *Enterococcus* (e.g., *Streptococcus faecalis*) is a prevalent cause of endocarditis after cesarean section.[26] Embolic cerebral infarction occurs in about 21% of patients with bacterial endocarditis[25] and may be the first clinical manifestation.[8] Antibiotic therapy must be directed at the specific pathogen. Anticoagulation is not indicated.[24, 25]

Peripartum cardiomyopathy (PPCM) is an unusual complication of pregnancy. Multiparous black women appear to be at greatest risk. PPCM is characterized by congestive heart failure during the last month of pregnancy or the first 5 months after delivery that occurs in the absence of a pre-existing or coexisting cause of heart failure.[27] Development of a mural thrombus with subsequent systemic embolization is a frequent complication, occurring in 25% of patients.[27] Further, cardiac arrhythmias including atrial fibrillation may further complicate the clinical picture. Hypotension due to systolic dysfunction or acute blood loss at delivery can result in infarction in the watershed zones.[27, 28] Management of PPCM usually requires bed rest, diuresis, and anticoagulation with heparin.[11] Only half of patients with PPCM return to normal within 6 months, whereas approximately 85% of patients with persistent cardiomegaly die of heart failure within 5 years,[24] unless heart transplantation is performed. Patients with a history of PPCM are often advised to consider sterilization because of the high recurrence rate in subsequent pregnancies.[24]

Atrial fibrillation in pregnancy often accompanies decompensated valvular disease or cardiomyopathy. The risk of systemic embolic events ranges from 10% to 23%, and approximately half of these events present as cerebral infarction.[8, 29] Chronic atrial fibrillation and rheumatic heart disease are associated with a maternal mortality rate of 19% and a fetal mortality rate of 58%.[29] Treatment should include anticoagulation with heparin. In cases of new-onset atrial fibrillation, attempts at electrocardioversion are considered safe and appropriate during pregnancy.[29]

Arterial Thrombotic Stroke

Atherosclerosis is responsible for up to 25% of cerebral infarctions in pregnancy.[8] As in the population at large, stroke risk is associated with cigarette smoking, diabetes mellitus, hypertension, hyperlipidemia, family history, and advancing age.[5] The hypercoagulable state induced by pregnancy may further contribute to the formation of intra-arterial thrombus.

Other structural arterial abnormalities may predispose the pregnant woman to cerebral ischemia. Carotid and vertebral artery dissection has been reported after labor and delivery, presumably due to violent neck injury.[30] Moya-Moya disease[31] and Takayasu's arteritis[32] may be exacerbated during pregnancy, although case reports are rare. Idiopathic pregnancy–induced reversible intimal hyperplasia or reversible cerebral segmental vasoconstriction has been reported to cause cerebral ischemia and death during pregnancy as well.[33–35]

Stroke and Hematologic Disorders

Pregnant women with sickle cell anemia are at especially high risk for cerebrovascular disease. About half of these patients experience at least one sickle cell crisis during pregnancy, which may result in cerebral infarction, cerebral vein thrombosis, or subarachnoid hemorrhage.[5, 36] Sickle cell trait also poses a mildly increased risk of cerebrovascular disease during pregnancy. The pathophysiology is related in part to microvascular occlusion by aggregated sickled cells but more importantly may be due to intimal proliferation after ischemic injury to the walls of large arteries with subsequent thrombosis.[36] Plasma exchange and transfusion used early in sickle cell crisis has reduced maternal and fetal mortality[36] and may prevent cerebral infarction.

Antiphospholipid antibodies (aPLa), including the lupus anticoagulant and anticardiolipin antibodies, are associated with an adverse outcome in pregnancy. They are present in approximately 2% of women of reproductive age.[37] Among women with recurrent spontaneous abortion, fetal demise, intrauterine growth retardation, placental abruption, and early preeclampsia, the prevalence of aPLa is dramatically higher, approaching 40% in some series.[38, 39] The presence of aPLa may be an isolated abnormality or may accompany systemic lupus erythematosus (SLE) and other collagen vascular disorders.[37] Many authors do not recommend screening all pregnant women for aPLa, although this remains controversial.[37, 39, 40] Patients with a history of potentially aPLa-associated complications of prior pregnancy, SLE, deep venous thrombosis, or stroke should be tested. In addition, routine prenatal VDRL or rapid plasma reagin testing and partial thromboplastin time may be falsely abnormal because of the presence of aPLa[37, 40] and may promote further investigation. Patients may have a negative test result for aPLa when they are not pregnant but then demonstrate a positive result during pregnancy during the second and third trimesters.[37] The mechanism by which aPLa may cause thrombosis is uncertain: aPLa appear to cause intra-arterial fibrin deposition, platelet aggregation, prostacyclin inhibition, and reduction of antithrombin III activity.[37] Arterial and venous thrombosis and thrombocytopenia are the most common nonobstetric consequences of the syndrome. The treatment for patients with the aPLa syndrome is intensely debated, and successful pregnancy without thrombosis has been reported with various combinations of corticosteroids, aspirin, heparin, dipyridamole, and immunosuppressive agents.[37, 39–41] However, no randomized controlled trials are available so far.

Thrombotic thrombocytopenic purpura (TTP) is characterized by fever, thrombocytopenia, microangiopathic hemolytic anemia, renal abnormalities, and neurologic deficits. Although rare in the general population, TTP occurs three times as often in pregnant woman compared with other women of similar age. Untreated, it carries a mortality rate of 80%–90%.[24, 42] Consumptive coagulopathy develops in the microvasculature, resulting in transient ischemic attacks, subcortical and cortical cerebral infarctions, seizures, or diffuse ischemic encephalopathy.[8, 43] TTP presents late in pregnancy and may be difficult to distinguish from preeclampsia/eclampsia on the basis of both clinical and laboratory findings.[42–44] Often the diagnosis is made by therapeutic responsiveness. Preeclampsia/eclampsia should improve after delivery of the fetus. If the fetus is not yet viable or the patient does not rapidly improve with delivery, empiric plasmapheresis should be initiated.[24, 44] Plasmapheresis and transfusion therapy are effective in the majority of patients.[42]

Other rare hematologic disorders, including polycythemia vera, essential thrombocythemia, paroxysmal nocturnal hemoglobinuria, and deficiencies of antithrombin III and proteins C and S, may cause cerebrovascular disease in young women as well. They do not appear to occur with increased frequency during pregnancy. These are discussed elsewhere in this text.

Management and Prognosis

Treatment of cerebral infarction consists largely of the prevention of progression and recurrence. Therapy must be directed at the specific cause, if one can be identified. The choice of therapeutic agents is further constrained by the potential effects on the fetus.

Aspirin antiplatelet therapy is recommended in patients with atherosclerotic disease and idiopathic stroke. Some authors also recommend aspirin for patients with aPLa without a history of thrombotic or embolic events.[3] Aspirin has no known teratogenic effect.[45] However, chronic aspirin use can prolong labor and has been associated with intrauterine growth retardation and maternal and fetal hemorrhage.[45] Aspirin inhibits prostaglandin synthesis and may cause premature closure of the ductus arteriosus in utero.[46] Low-dose aspirin (80 mg daily) has no demonstrable untoward effects on the fetus and can be used as prophylaxis against stroke during pregnancy.[11, 46]

Anticoagulation is indicated as prophylaxis for patients with atrial fibrillation and artificial cardiac valves.[3, 5, 8] It is also generally used to prevent recurrent cardioembolic events in patients with paradoxical embolus and cardiomyopathy, arterial thrombotic events due to dissection, and some hypercoagulable states.[3] Anticoagulation has also been recommended for severe atherosclerotic disease that is not amenable to surgery, recurrent idiopathic cerebral infarction, and for stroke-in-evolution.[5, 11]

Oral anticoagulation with warfarin has been associated with multiple fetal abnormalities and fetal wastage.[3] It readily crosses the placenta and is a known teratogen during the first trimester. Even beyond this period, optic atrophy and mental retardation may occur.[45, 46] Women who become pregnant while taking warfarin should undergo extensive and frequent obstetric evaluations to exclude fetal malformation.[3] Maternal and fetal hemorrhages may further complicate pregnancy, most significantly at the time of labor and delivery.[3, 45] Warfarin is therefore recommended only for those patients who cannot tolerate heparin because of thrombocytopenia or who continue to have recurrent thromboembolic events while on heparin.

Heparin does not cross the placental barrier and is safe for the fetus.[3, 45] However, it requires a parenteral route of administration, and long-term use can be difficult to sustain. More importantly, chronic heparin use is associated with maternal bleeding, thrombocytopenia, and osteopenia.[3] Bone demineralization depends on both the dose and duration of heparin use and may be reversible when the drug is stopped.[45, 46] Heparin-induced thrombocytopenia is a consequence of the formation of heparin-dependent antibodies and requires immediate discontinuation.[47] Low-molecular-weight (LMW) heparin also does not cross the placenta, affords effective anticoagulation, and possesses several advantages over conventional heparin.[48] LMW heparin has a longer half-life and may be administered via a single daily subcutaneous injection. LMW heparin also carries a reduced risk of osteopenia.[48] The widespread use of LMW heparin is not advocated at this time, because studies are ongoing to determine optimal dosage and efficacy during pregnancy.

Thrombolysis with intravenous tissue plasminogen activator was found to be effective for acute ischemic stroke in recent trials. Although pregnant women were excluded from these studies, the use of these agents during pregnancy is not unprecedented. Intravenous streptokinase has been used successfully in the management of a pregnant woman with prosthetic mitral valve thrombosis[49] and in another with massive pulmonary embolus.[50] Because of the profound fibrinolytic action of these medications, however, the risk of severe hemorrhage from the placenta will likely preclude their systemic use during pregnancy in all but the most devastated patients. Trials of intra-arterial administration of thrombolytic agents are also underway and may carry a lower risk of systemic bleeding.

Acute surgical intervention in the form of carotid endarterectomy has not been evaluated in pregnancy. However, carotid artery thrombectomy was performed in a patient with cardioembolic stroke within 4 hours of the onset of postpartum hemiplegia, and her symptoms resolved.[51] Until further investigation, no clear recommendations can be made regarding surgical management of occlusive cerebrovascular disease during pregnancy.

Specific treatments are important in several disease entities, but these may be restricted during pregnancy. In patients with stroke due to cerebral vasculitis, corticosteroids and immunosuppressive drugs may be required. These agents may cause fetal malformation, and close monitoring of fetal development is suggested. Appropriately chosen antibiotics are indicated for infectious endocarditis. Cardiac surgery with cardiopulmonary bypass may be necessary for patients with deteriorating valvular function. This surgery is associated with a maternal mortality rate of less than 2%, but the fetal mortality rate of 17%[52] mandates that it be performed only when maximal medical therapy has failed or, if possible, after the fetus becomes viable and is delivered. Plasma exchange for sickle cell anemia and plasmapheresis for TTP are safe and effective during pregnancy,[36, 44] although fluctuations in blood pressure should be avoided.

Further medical management of acute stroke is directed at providing maximal cerebral perfusion and oxygen delivery while avoiding elevation of intracranial pressure. The management of elevated intracranial pressure may pose a risk to the fetus. Intravenous mannitol may cause severe fetal dehydration with profound systemic and neurologic injury and should therefore be avoided. Hyperventilation, on the other hand, appears to cause no additional harm to the fetus.[11]

The prognosis for stroke during pregnancy and the puerperium is relatively good. Women who have a stroke during this period without an identified cause seldom have recurrent events during subsequent pregnancies. Furthermore, in the absence of other systemic disease, the young stroke patient can be expected to recover a major proportion of lost function quickly, typically within 1–2 months.[11]

CEREBRAL VENOUS THROMBOSIS

Cerebral venous thrombosis (CVT) is an important cause of morbidity in young women. Although both infectious and noninfectious processes may cause CVT, septic phlebitis is most common in children with infections of the head and neck. In adults, more than half of the cases of aseptic CVT are associated with pregnancy and the puerperium.[53] Oral contraceptive agents have also been implicated as risk factors. Infrequent etiologies include severe dehydration, sickle cell anemia, malignancy, hypercoagulable states, and myeloproliferative disorders. CVT occurs in the puerperium in approximately 95% of cases, with 60%–80% presenting in the second to fifth postpartum week.[8, 53] This is in marked contradistinction to the majority of arterial strokes, which occur either during pregnancy or the first week postpartum.

The incidence of puerperal CVT is estimated to be one to two cases per 10,000 childbirths.[8, 9] Risk factors for the development of CVT are uncertain. Neither maternal age nor parity is associated. The features of the pregnancy, labor, and delivery also seem unrelated. Dehydration after childbirth may increase the risk of CVT.[11]

Diagnosis

The clinical appearance of CVT may be diverse, depending on the specific cerebral venous spaces involved. The cerebral cortical veins are most commonly thrombosed during the puerperium, with frequent extension into the superior sagittal sinus.[53] The lateral sinuses are less often implicated as the primary site, and cavernous sinus thrombosis is not associated with pregnancy.[11] Severe headache accompanied by nausea and vomiting are general features of CVT. Headache is believed to be a consequence of venous distention and inflammation. Papilledema, when present, may be the only objective clinical abnormality on examination during the early phases of the disease. Some patients have clinical evidence of venous thrombosis elsewhere, particularly in the pelvis and lower extremities. When the cortical veins are primarily affected, fluctuating focal neurologic deficits, such as unilateral weakness or numbness, aphasia, and seizures, may appear. These signs often accompany the peak in severity of headache symptoms and may coincide with cerebral infarction or hemorrhage due to venous hypertension.[8, 11] As thrombus spreads into adjacent venous spaces, clinical deficits worsen, seizures may evolve into generalized status epilepticus, and the level of consciousness can deteriorate.

CVT in pregnancy typically has a more acute onset than thrombosis in the general population.[53] CVT is often not recognized until the condition of the patient begins to decline, because an otherwise nonspecific headache is common during the puerperium. Other early diagnostic confounders include migraine,[54] pseudotumor cerebri, late postpartum preeclampsia/eclampsia, herpes encephalitis, and meningitis. In some cases of CVT, the finding of fever and an elevated white blood cell count lead to further investigation.[55, 56] Lumbar puncture may reveal normal cerebrospinal fluid (CSF) or increased pressure,[53] but the finding of red cells, elevated protein, or xanthochromia suggests that venous infarction or hemorrhage has already occurred.[11]

Radiologic diagnosis of CVT may be made with CT. An initial noncontrast study is used to determine if acute hemorrhage or mass effect is present. A subsequent study with contrast may demonstrate the "empty delta sign" in the posterior sagittal sinus in one-third of patients,[53] which is a result of dural enhancement around the clot in the sinus. However, MRI (Fig. 6–1) and magnetic resonance venogram are superior in defining the anatomy of the cerebral venous system and have better sensitivity for detection of CVT.[53, 54, 57, 58] Digital subtraction angiography or conventional cerebral angiography (Fig. 6–2) is required in some cases to fully evaluate the venous anatomy and clot burden. Because CVT is largely a postpartum phenomenon, the issues regarding fetal exposure to radiation and iodinated contrast are irrelevant.

Management and Prognosis

The role of anticoagulation in the treatment of CVT is rooted in a long history of controversy and remains unresolved. In patients with hemorrhagic venous infarction due to CVT, anticoagulation may cause further intracerebral bleeding and mass effect with herniation.[11, 59] It may also promote excessive bleeding from the postpartum endometrium. Alternatively, anticoagulation can prevent further thrombus formation and thereby prevent the development of venous infarctions, both bland and hemorrhagic. Many authors favor anticoagulation with heparin only in patients without radiologic and CSF evidence of hemorrhage, or for those patients with coexisting hypercoagulable states.[11, 55, 60] Other authors favor a more aggressive stance and recommend heparin even in patients with documented hemorrhagic infarctions.[56, 61] Initiation of intravenous heparin without an initial bolus dose may reduce the risk of bleeding. Anticoagulants are used for 1–3 months[11, 55, 56, 61]; patients are then re-evaluated, usually with magnetic resonance venography, to determine if flow is re-established. Prolonged anticoagulation therapy may be required for refractory cases.

Systemic thrombolytic therapy for CVT has been of value in a few case series,[62, 63] but data are insufficient and the risks of systemic bleeding complications are high. Local urokinase infusion into a dural sinus thrombosis has been reported to be successful in several patients and may be associated with less risk of significant hemorrhage.[64, 65] Additional medical management of CVT should be directed toward

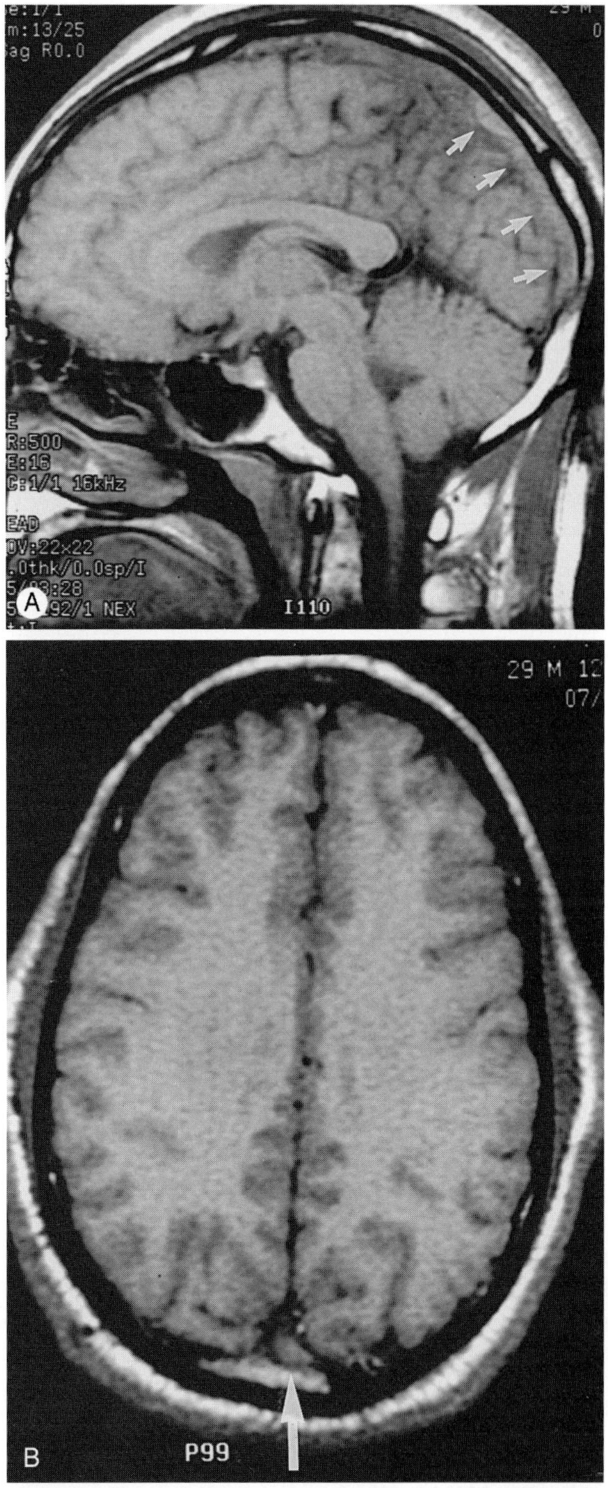

FIGURE 6–1 • Cerebral venous thrombosis. The patient presented with severe headache, left hemianopsia, and left hemisensory deficit. *A,* Sagittal T1-weighted magnetic resonance imaging (MRI) demonstrates clot in the posterior portion of the superior sagittal sinus (arrows). *B,* The MRI delta sign is shown on the axial T1-weighted MRI (arrow).

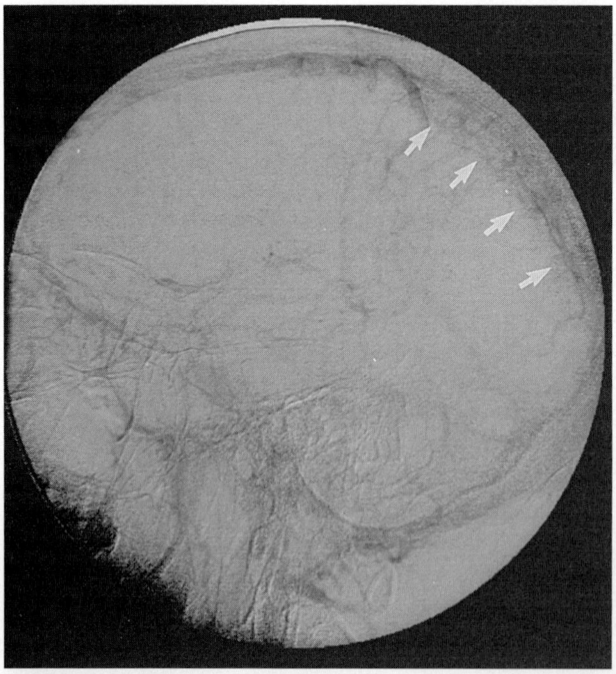

FIGURE 6-2 • Cerebral venous thrombosis. Conventional angiography (performed on the patient from Fig. 6–1) demonstrated poor flow due to obstruction of the posterior portion of the superior sagittal sinus (arrows) as well as the transverse sinuses bilaterally. Small collateral veins are engorged near the obstructed sinuses.

treatment of seizures, metabolic derangements, and elevated intracranial pressure, as dictated by the clinical situation.

The mortality rate from CVT in the United States is estimated to be 5%–30%,[11, 53, 66] although older studies suggest much higher rates. Prolonged coma and status epilepticus are associated with the poorest outcome. Most patients, however, have a good prognosis and are left with less residual deficit than are patients with a comparable arterial stroke.[9, 55, 56] Furthermore, pregnant women with CVT have a better prognosis than patients with CVT due to other causes.[53] Recovery may be aided by the presence of an intact arterial supply of oxygenated blood when thrombosis occurs in the venous circulation. There appears to be a mild risk for recurrence with subsequent pregnancies.[55, 56]

INTRACRANIAL HEMORRHAGE

Subarachnoid hemorrhage (SAH) complicates one to five of every 10,000 pregnancies,[67, 68] is associated with a fatality rate of 30%–40%, and causes approximately 10% of maternal mortality.[68–70] Nontraumatic SAH is the third most common cause of indirect obstetric death.[70, 71] The majority of SAH during pregnancy is due to rupture of an intracranial aneurysm or arteriovenous malformation (AVM). Other etiologies of spontaneous intracranial hemorrhage during pregnancy include eclampsia, metastatic choriocarcinoma, endocarditis, CVT, pituitary apoplexy, hematologic disorders, vasculitis, and cocaine abuse.

Pregnancy may be a risk factor for SAH, although this is controversial. The physiologic changes during pregnancy, as described earlier, may play a role. Expanded blood volume, increased cardiac output, and Valsalva maneuvers during active labor are hypothesized as hemodynamic factors contributing to SAH; high levels of circulating estrogens may dilate and alter abnormal vascular structures.[11]

Diagnosis

The clinical presentation of SAH in pregnant women is no different from its appearance in the general population and depends on the site and severity of the hemorrhage. The common symptoms and signs include headache of sudden onset accompanied by nausea, vomiting, photophobia, meningismus, seizures, focal weakness, and declining level of consciousness. Often a history of sentinel or warning headache is elicited at the time of presentation with a major SAH.[72] In a pregnant or postpartum woman, eclampsia may present similarly and is an important alternative in the differential diagnosis.[67] The two disorders may be difficult to distinguish, although findings of profound proteinuria, hemolytic anemia, elevated transaminases, and low platelet count support the diagnosis of eclampsia.

Diagnosis of SAH can be made in 90% of patients with CT. Lumbar puncture reveals xanthochromia and blood after SAH. Four-vessel conventional angiography (with abdominal shielding) is mandatory prior to surgical intervention, because multiple aneurysms may be present, and an AVM may be supplied by several vessels. MRI can detect angiographically occult vascular malformations. All of the procedures can be performed safely in pregnancy, as previously discussed. The diagnostic evaluation of SAH is described more extensively elsewhere in this text.

Multidisciplinary Considerations

The treatment of AVMs and aneurysms during pregnancy requires some compromise between obstetric and neurosurgical concerns. Often the acuteness of the situation for the mother and the viability of the fetus are the most important factors. Several important differences further distinguish the approaches to AVMs and aneurysmal hemorrhages. Other potential causes of cerebral hemorrhage during pregnancy need to be recognized in order to direct specific therapy toward the underlying disease process. Moreover, the care of the pregnant woman in the neurosurgical suite must be amended to provide an appropriate margin of safety for the fetus.

Arteriovenous Malformations

In pregnancy, AVMs are most likely to present with the symptoms and signs of SAH, whereas in the general population they more often initially present with seizures.[73] AVMs are responsible for 25%–50% of SAHs during pregnancy. Women who bleed from AVMs tend to be younger than those with aneurysmal hemorrhage. SAH due to AVM also appears to be more common in primigravidas than in multiparous women, possibly reflecting an increased tendency for these congenital lesions to rupture during pregnancy,[73] although this contention has been recently challenged.[68]

Hemorrhage from an AVM is most common during the second trimester and during delivery but may occur at any time during pregnancy and the puerperium.[11, 74] Bleeding during the second trimester may be related to engorgement of vessels. During labor, SAH may be due in part to the hemodynamics of bearing-down. The Valsalva maneuver is associated with a marked increase in intrathoracic, intra-abdominal, and intracranial pressure in association with a transient fall and then rise in systemic blood pressure that may result in SAH. The breathing methods taught to pregnant women aim to prevent bearing-down by maintaining an open glottis during uterine contractions.[11]

Women with AVMs face an important decision regarding pregnancy. Several small series have demonstrated a markedly increased risk of hemorrhage from an AVM during pregnancy.[73, 75] However, in a recent study of 451 women with an AVM, the risk of first hemorrhage during pregnancy was 3.5%, not significantly different from that of age-matched nonpregnant controls.[71] Women with a history of hemorrhage due to an AVM before becoming pregnant were found to have an elevated (5.8%) risk of bleeding during pregnancy.[71] Furthermore, once an AVM bleeds during pregnancy, the risk of recurrent bleeding during the same pregnancy is about 27%.[75] The mortality rate of SAH from AVM during pregnancy approaches 28%, which is higher than it is in nonpregnant patients.[68] Because of these risks and uncertainties, some women with known AVMs may elect to undergo treatment for the malformation prior to contemplating pregnancy.

The neurosurgical approach to AVMs during pregnancy varies considerably and depends on the site of the malformation, the vascular supply, and the clot burden. Although excision can be performed successfully in pregnant women, the efficacy of such a procedure during pregnancy is of uncertain benefit. Dias and Sekhar showed that maternal and fetal mortality were not significantly different in surgically treated and nonoperatively treated groups.[68] Many advocate postponement of surgical excision of AVMs until after childbirth, unless neurosurgical intervention is acutely required[68, 71, 75] or if hemorrhage occurs during labor. SAH during active labor is an indication for emergent delivery by cesarean section with possible subsequent surgical excision of the AVM.[11] If the patient is not in active labor at the time of SAH, she should be managed according to neurosurgical considerations as if she were not pregnant,[68, 74] although attention to choice of medications and other exposures is necessary to ensure fetal well-being. Thus, a large hematoma with mass effect or a ventricular clot with obstructive hydrocephalus would require urgent evacuation or ventriculostomy.[74] Neurosurgery may be less technically difficult if it can be delayed until the end of the puerperium when the hematologic and hemodynamic changes of pregnancy have abated.[75] The safety of the fetus would also no longer be a consideration with regard to anesthetic and surgical manipulations (see later).

Because labor and delivery appear to be associated with high risk of SAH from AVM, some authors favor performing elective cesarean section at 34–38 weeks' gestation in order to prevent the onset of labor completely.[66, 75, 76] This is then followed by conventional angiography and further treatment of the AVM. No conclusive data support this practice, however. Other authors argue that in women with uncomplicated AVMs, the method of delivery should be dictated strictly by obstetric criteria, because the maternal and fetal mortality rates for vaginal and surgical delivery are not significantly different.[68]

AVMs can also be treated with embolization or radiosurgery in some cases. These techniques have not been sufficiently evaluated during pregnancy to recommend their widespread use.

Aneurysms

Intracranial aneurysms are found in approximately 1% of women of child-bearing age. Although previously believed to cause the vast majority of SAH during pregnancy, more recent data suggest that aneurysms and AVMs cause SAH in about equal proportions. Aneurysms occur at the same sites in pregnancy as in the general population, most often at branch points within the circle of Willis.[77] They occur with the same epidemiologic risk factors, including family history, smoking, Ehlers-Danlos syndrome, fibromuscular dysplasia, polycystic kidney disease, and Marfan's syndrome.[67] The risk of aneurysmal rupture increases with age in pregnant and nonpregnant patients, and pregnant women with aneurysmal SAH are usually older than women with hemorrhage from AVMs. The risk of bleeding also increases with the duration of pregnancy and extends into the early puerperium, with the majority of ruptures occurring during the third trimester.[68, 73] Again, the alterations in maternal hemodynamic and endocrine physiology may play a role in this temporal pattern. Surprisingly, aneurysmal rupture is relatively rare during labor and delivery despite the dramatic but transient hemodynamic fluctuations observed during this time.[73]

The management of aneurysmal hemorrhage in the pregnant patient is governed almost entirely by neurosurgical factors and is more clearly defined than the management of AVMs. After an initial hemorrhage, the risk of subsequent bleeding from an aneurysm approaches 50% and is associated with high mortality. Dias and Sekhar demonstrated that after aneurysmal SAH, mortality can be significantly reduced by surgical intervention during pregnancy: the maternal mortality rate was 63% in the nonoperative group and 11% in the surgical group; fetal mortality improved from 27% in the nonoperative group to 5% in the surgical group.[68] After clipping of the aneurysm, the remainder of the pregnancy, including labor and delivery, can proceed normally without any specific modifications.[11] Women with SAH during active labor should be delivered by emergent cesarean section. This can be immediately followed by aneurysm surgery.[11]

The management of an incidentally discovered aneurysm during pregnancy is uncertain, and no guidelines yet exist. The size of the aneurysm appears to be the most important factor in the decision to operate. If the aneurysm is going to be clipped during pregnancy, many neurosurgeons choose to operate during the second trimester, when the risks of fetal malformation and premature labor are relatively low[78] and before the risk of aneurysmal rupture reaches its peak in the third trimester.

Although surgical repair of symptomatic aneurysms during pregnancy is recommended, some situations preclude this approach as an option. An aneurysm may be surgically inaccessible, or multiple aneurysms may be present. If no therapeutic possibilities exist, the patient must be counseled regarding the risks of hemorrhage during subsequent pregnancies. Women with inoperable aneurysms can give birth by either vaginal or cesarean deliveries. Some obstetricians prefer the latter,[11] although the route of delivery has no proven relationship to maternal and fetal mortality.[68]

Patients with catastrophic (Hunt and Hess grade IV and V) hemorrhages (described elsewhere) are usually treated conservatively with supportive intensive care. Ventricular catheterization and drainage may improve the patient's grade and level of consciousness. Salvage of a viable fetus by cesarean section should be considered early in the course of catastrophic SAH once the mother is hemodynamically stable.[77]

Vasospasm complicates the management of aneurysmal SAH in about one-third of patients, but it is rare after hemorrhage from AVM.[77] It can occur from 3 days to 3 weeks after the initial SAH and is associated with delayed neurologic deficits and possibly death associated with cerebral ischemia. Transcranial Doppler studies can measure mean and peak velocities in the major vessels and are useful in evaluating vasospasm. Nimodipine, a calcium-channel blocker, reduces the incidence and severity of deficits due to vasospasm after SAH in nonpregnant patients. However, nimodipine is teratogenic and embryotoxic in animals[79] and has not been rigorously tested in human beings. It may be considered for use in pregnancy if the benefits are deemed to outweigh the risks.[68, 77, 78] Nimodipine is generally administered after the initial hemorrhage and continued for 21 consecutive days.

Other measures used to treat vasospasm include volume expansion with colloid solutions and induced hypertension with dopamine or norepinephrine. When vasospasm persists despite maximal medical management, selective balloon angioplasty has been employed to dilate constricted vessels[78] (see also Chapter 11). However, this interventional technique has not been studied during pregnancy.

Metastatic Choriocarcinoma

Choriocarcinoma, a gestational trophoblastic neoplasm, is a malignancy that is virtually unique to pregnancy. It is rare in normal term pregnancies, occurring at a rate of 1 in 50,000, but complicates 1 in 30 molar pregnancies.[80] Conversely, about half of choriocarcinomas are associated with moles and the other half with normal gestations.[80] About 80% are metastatic to remote sites via the hematogenous route, especially to lungs and brain.[81] The metastatic lesions are highly prone to spontaneous hemorrhage and are an important diagnostic consideration in the pregnant or postpartum woman with SAH or parenchymal hemorrhage. The mechanism of hemorrhage appears to be related to the formation of cerebral aneurysms in response to tumor invasion of vascular walls, although this has been rarely demonstrated by angiography or pathology.[81, 82] Serum and urine levels of human chorionic gonadotropin are useful in establishing the diagnosis and can be followed to monitor response to therapy. Treatment consists of aggressive chemotherapy and whole-brain radiation therapy, although surgery may become required to manage an expanding hematoma.[80, 81] The mortality rate in patients with brain involvement is approximately 50%.[80]

Pituitary Apoplexy

The physiologic changes of pregnancy are associated with enlargement of the normal pituitary gland and a tenfold increase in serum prolactin concentration.[83] Prolactinoma is the most common pituitary tumor associated with pregnancy, and women who harbor this tumor have an increased risk of developing symptoms during pregnancy. Approximately 15%–35% of macroadenomas become symptomatic, although only about 5% of microadenomas become clinically evident.[84] If the adenoma grows slowly, the patient may complain only of headache, which may later be followed by visual deficits. Bromocriptine is safe in pregnancy and can effectively shrink the lesion.[83–85] Trans-sphenoidal tumor resection may be required in patients with symptomatic macroadenomas and can be performed during pregnancy without undue fetal risk.[83, 85]

Pituitary apoplexy is an infrequent complication of pituitary adenoma but appears to also have a predilection for the hypertrophic glands of pregnant women. Pituitary apoplexy is a neuroendocrine catastrophe that occurs in about 2% of patients with adenomas, although it may be encountered asymptomatically in a much higher percentage.[86] Acute hemorrhage and infarction into the enlarged anterior pituitary gland occurs spontaneously and clinically manifests as sudden onset of severe headache, nausea, vomiting, and neck rigidity. Often, acute visual field defects and ocular motor palsies become apparent (see also Chapter 18), followed by progression to stupor and coma. This clinical picture is consistent with that of SAH and should be evaluated by CT or MRI. The latter is far more sensitive to abnormalities of the pituitary region.[86] Lumbar puncture may reveal blood or xanthochromia and may reveal pleocytosis in response to necrotic debris in the CSF.[87] Serum should be obtained for measurement of cortisol, thyroid hormone, prolactin, growth hormone, and gonadotropins. Profound hypotension, tachycardia, hypoglycemia, hyponatremia, hyperkalemia, and acidosis may become evident as the hallmarks of an Addisonian crisis.

Initial emergent management is directed toward correction of the panhypopituitarism. Glucocorticoids and fluids are required to control the derangements of secondary adrenocortical insufficiency. Steroids have also been shown to decrease the size of the apoplectic pituitary gland[88] and may minimize the inflammatory response to necrotic material. Hydrocortisone is given at a dose of 100 mg every 8 hours for 24 hours (or an equivalent regimen of another glucocorticoid is administered), followed by a slow taper until hormonal homeostasis is restored.[84] Thyroid and other hormone replacement may become necessary later. Patients with severe or rapidly progressive neurologic deficits and impaired level of consciousness may require urgent surgical removal of the necrotic tumor.[86, 87] This can be performed via either a subfrontal or a trans-sphenoidal approach, depending on the extent of the tumor and hemorrhage, although the latter is associated with lower morbidity.[86] If pituitary apoplexy occurs late in the third trimester and the fetus is mature, delivery may be therapeutic, because the adenoma typically recedes after parturition. The choice of vaginal or cesarean delivery should be based on the clinical status of mother and fetus. Mortality due to pituitary apoplexy is not known, but it is generally believed to be high in patients who present with blindness or a declining level of consciousness.[86]

Pituitary necrosis may also occur in the postpartum period in association with maternal hypotension and obstetric hemorrhage during delivery. This is known as Sheehan's syndrome and usually does not become apparent until several months later, when the patient presents with agalactorrhea and amenorrhea.[84] A more acute form has been described, but this is clinically indistinguishable from pituitary apoplexy. For additional information on pituitary apoplexy, please refer to Chapters 7 and 18.

Surgical and Anesthetic Considerations

Surgery poses special risks to the fetus; therefore, intraoperative management must be modified accordingly. Manipulations of maternal blood pressure and volume status can interfere with fetal blood supply. Medications used perioperatively may also adversely affect the fetus. Continuous fetal monitoring during surgery is recommended, and the operating room should be prepared for emergent cesarean section if this becomes necessary. Intracranial surgery can be temporarily suspended for delivery of the fetus in distress.

The patient should be placed in the lateral decubitus position for craniotomy if possible, because the supine position is associated with compression of the inferior vena cava by the gravid uterus and may cause unexpected maternal hypotension.[89] Anesthetic induction with inhaled agents is faster during pregnancy because of the increase in maternal minute ventilation and may result in acute fetal toxicity.[89] Controlled hypotension with sodium nitroprusside has been used successfully during pregnancy to minimize bleeding and decrease the risk of aneurysmal rupture during surgery,[77, 89, 90] but this drug should be avoided if possible because of potential fetal ischemia. Sodium nitroprusside may also have a direct toxic effect on the fetus.[91] Hypothermia during surgery is used to decrease cerebral metabolism and edema. Although hypothermia causes a reduction in uterine blood flow, there is a concomitant decrement in fetal metabolism, such that hypothermia can be used safely during pregnancy.[11] Hyperventilation decreases maternal cerebral blood flow and intracranial pressure and does not injure the fetus. The acute use of corticosteroids is also safe during pregnancy for control of cerebral edema. Hyperosmolar diuresis with mannitol is relatively contraindicated in pregnancy because profound fetal dehydration may result.

SEIZURES AND STATUS EPILEPTICUS

Epilepsy affects approximately 0.5% of the entire population and is therefore one of the most common neurologic disorders that complicate pregnancy. The effect of pregnancy on epilepsy varies. About half of patients report no significant change in their seizure patterns, whereas one-quarter improve and another quarter worsen during pregnancy.[92, 93] No criteria exist to successfully predict how epileptic patients will respond to pregnancy. The physiologic changes associated with pregnancy appear to play an important role in the course of epilepsy. High levels of estrogen and progesterone, hyperventilation, and respiratory alkalosis may all increase susceptibility. Moreover, accelerated hepatic metabolism, reduced serum protein concentration, and impaired gastrointestinal absorption may result in subtherapeutic antiepileptic drug (AED) levels and poor seizure control.[94] Often, a 30%–50% increase in AED dosage is required to maintain stable levels. After parturition, the dosage should be reduced to prevent toxicity.

The initial onset of seizures during pregnancy suggests a structural abnormality and therefore warrants a thorough investigation for cerebral vascular malformation, venous thrombosis, tumor, and infection. Gestational epilepsy is a rare seizure disorder, distinct from eclampsia, that is unique to pregnancy and represents a diagnosis of exclusion.[94] The incidence of this disorder peaks in the late second and early third trimesters. Seizures may be partial or generalized, and the electroencephalogram (EEG) typically reveals a temporal or parietal focus. Recurrences in subsequent pregnancies are uncommon.[94] Chronic AED therapy is not indicated for gestational epilepsy.

Epilepsy and AEDs may adversely affect pregnancy. Phenytoin, phenobarbital, carbamazepine, valproic acid, and diazepam have all been associated with significant fetal anomalies. Valproate in particular is associated with neural tube defects and should be avoided during pregnancy. The others are more commonly associated with craniofacial abnormalities, dysmorphic limbs, impaired intrauterine growth, and mental retardation.[93, 95] In addition, congenital malformations are observed in the offspring of epileptic mothers even if they are not treated with AEDs during gestation.[95] The children of epileptic fathers also have an increased incidence of malformation.[95] A genetic etiology has been proposed to explain the connection between idiopathic epilepsy and congenital anomalies, but the mechanism is unknown. The highest rate of malformation occurs in children of women with refractory epilepsy who are taking multiple medications during pregnancy.[93, 95] Overall, congenital anomalies are twice as likely to occur in the offspring of epileptic women than in those of nonepileptic women. Nevertheless, about 90% of these pregnancies have normal outcomes.[92, 93] In patients who require AEDs to control their seizures, the benefits of therapy generally outweigh the risks. The management of chronic epilepsy during pregnancy and the choice of AED is too extensive a topic to discuss further here.

Maternal convulsions may cause fetal hypoxia and acidosis, although single brief seizures are seldom associated with any permanent sequelae.[94] A prolonged seizure during active labor may be an indication for urgent cesarean section, because the fetus is especially prone to hypoxia and distress at this time, and because the mother will no longer be able to cooperate with delivery.[93, 96] Persistent or recurrent seizures may evolve into status epilepticus, a neurologic emergency that results in mortality rates of about 30% (maternal) and 50% (fetal).[97] The causes of status epilepticus are protean, but during pregnancy the most common etiologies are noncompliance with medication in women who fear teratogenic side effects and subtherapeutic medication levels due to the altered metabolism of the AEDs,[78, 96] as described previously.

Status epilepticus is medically managed during pregnancy in the same fashion as in the general population. Benzodiazepines, phenytoin, phenobarbital, and barbiturate coma are indicated until seizures cease or a burst-suppression pattern is achieved on EEG. Supportive therapy with intubation, ventilation, fluids, and pressors is administered as needed. Status epilepticus does not necessarily mandate that the fetus be delivered unless the fetus is in distress or if the status is associated with eclampsia.[92, 97–99] Delivery can be performed by either the vaginal or the cesarean route.[98–101] However, delivery during status epilepticus has been associated with very high risk for both mother and fetus in some series.[97] For additional information on acute seizure disorders, please refer to Chapter 4.

ECLAMPSIA

The complex disorder of pregnancy characterized by hypertension, edema, and proteinuria is variably known as preeclampsia or toxemia gravidarum. The onset of seizures classically defines the entity of eclampsia, and progression of the disease may result in multiorgan dysfunction. Cerebral injury is by no means limited exclusively to convulsions. The word *eclampsia* is Greek for "a shining forth,"[102] which underscores the frequent flashing visual symptoms and potentially widespread neurologic manifestations of the disease. The pathophysiology of the disorder remains uncertain, and the optimal strategy for management is intensely debated.

Preeclampsia complicates about 5%–20% of otherwise normal pregnancies and 20% of pregnancies in women with chronic hypertension or renal disease.[103–105] Primigravid women are at highest risk for the disorder, particularly if they are malnourished or obese.[106] Multiparous women over the age of 35 are also at increased risk. Other predisposing factors include twin gestations, ectopic pregnancies, and hydatidiform moles. The incidence of eclampsia is between 1 in 100[107] and 1 in 3000 pregnancies.[108]

Diagnosis

Diagnostic criteria for pregnancy-induced hypertension have been established by the American College of Obstetrics and Gynecology.[109] Blood pressure must be 140/90 mm Hg or higher in a gravid woman who was previously normotensive. Alternatively, a 30 mm Hg increase in systolic pressure or a 15 mm Hg rise in diastolic pressure is acceptable. These measurements must be recorded on at least two occasions separated by a minimum of 6 hours. Preeclampsia is diagnosed when, in addition to pregnancy-induced hypertension, the patient demonstrates proteinuria greater than 300 mg in a 24-hour period or significant edema during the second half of pregnancy. Preeclampsia is further regarded as severe if blood pressure climbs to higher than 160/110 mm Hg, if proteinuria exceeds 5 g per day, or if any of the following develop: oliguria, headache, visual changes, altered consciousness, thrombocytopenia, pulmonary edema, cyanosis, and hepatic dysfunction or enlargement. In women with chronic hypertension, the appearance of these symptoms and signs after the twentieth week of pregnancy is often recognized as superimposed pregnancy-induced hypertension or pregnancy-aggravated hypertension.[110]

According to obstetric criteria, the disease is only identified as eclampsia when seizures appear in a woman who has no additional or pre-existing cause for seizures.[109] This distinction between preeclampsia and eclampsia carries significant prognostic value, because the latter is associated with a much higher risk of maternal morbidity and mortality.[106] However, the underlying neuropathology (described later) suggests that other neurologic manifestations should also be included in the category of eclampsia. Although the definition of eclampsia suggests that it follows in the natural history of preeclampsia, this is not universally true, because many cases of eclampsia occur without proteinuria or edema.

Eclamptic seizures are often generalized tonic-clonic events with focal or multifocal onset and may be associated with a focal postictal neurologic deficit. However, in the absence of other features of preeclampsia, no specific characteristics distinguish eclampsia from other causes of seizures in pregnant women. Eclamptic seizures may become apparent before, during, or after birth. Onset prior to the third trimester is rare.[111] Approximately 25% occur during the first 48 hours after parturition.[111] Although some authors demarcate an outside limit of 2 postpartum days for eclampsia,[112, 113] women have been reported to seize as late as 3 weeks afterward without evidence for an alternative etiology.[111, 114] The existence of this delayed postpartum eclampsia remains controversial among obstetricians, because many believe that the pathophysiologic abnormalities imposed by pregnancy should resolve rapidly after delivery.[113, 114]

Neuro-ophthalmologic symptoms and signs dominate the remainder of the eclamptic syndrome.[106, 115] Patients complain of blurred vision, headache, photophobia, photopsias, and scotomata. Ocular funduscopic abnormalities include angiospasm, retinal arteriolar narrowing, and central retinal artery occlusion. Retinal hemorrhages and retinal exudates may occur, and severe injury may culminate in serous retinal detachment. The finding of papilledema suggests brain swelling and mass effect rather than direct ocular involvement. Visual field defects and cortical blindness may occur because of bilateral occipital lobe damage (see also Chapter 7).

Long tract signs of hyperreflexia, clonus, quadriparesis, and extensor plantar responses may also be observed. These may be due to diffuse brain swelling, bilateral hemispheric involvement, or hydrocephalus. Impairment of the level of consciousness may occur, even resulting in coma, without any associated focal neurologic deficit or seizure. Severe cerebral involvement usually occurs in parallel with severe multiorgan dysfunction elsewhere.

The differential diagnosis of hypertension, headache, blurred vision, and seizures in a pregnant woman can be broad. Connective tissue disorders, disseminated intravascular coagulation, thrombotic thrombocytopenic purpura, and sepsis may mimic toxemia if they occur during the third trimester.[42] Postpartum cerebral venous thrombosis may resemble delayed eclampsia. Several patients with cocaine intoxication have presented with the clinical picture of preeclampsia/eclampsia, but their signs and symptoms improved as the drug effect waned.[116]

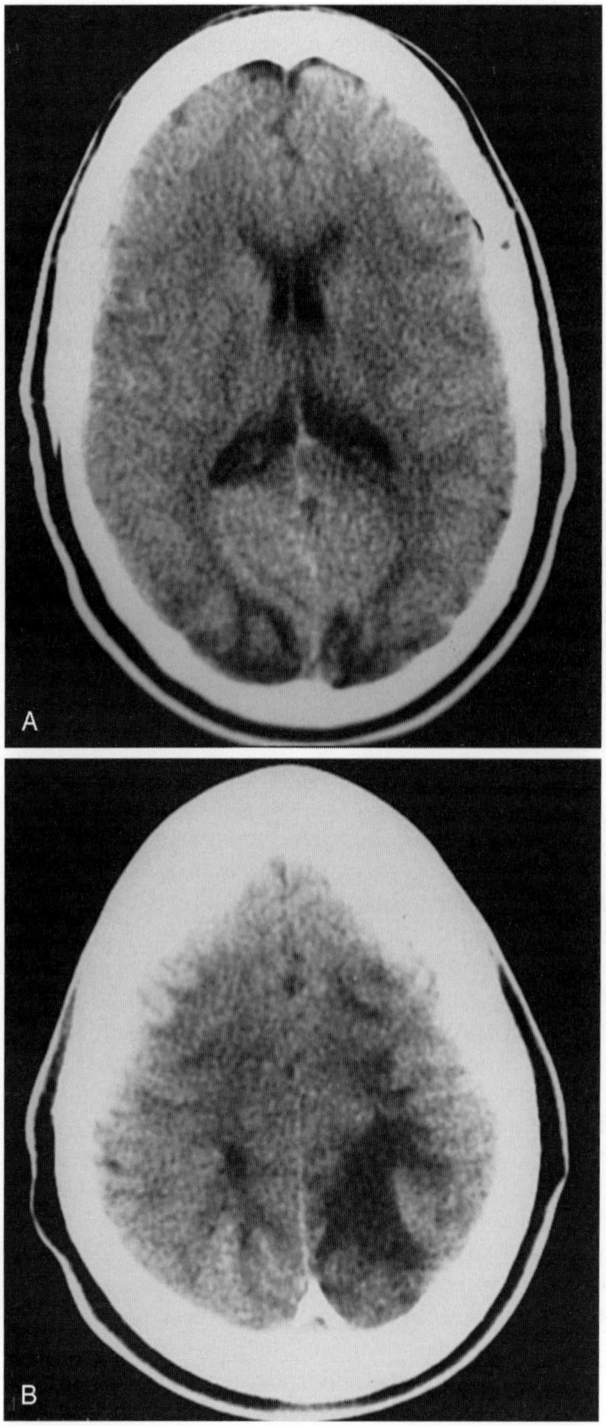

FIGURE 6-3 • *A, B,* Computed tomography (CT) in eclampsia. A 24-year-old woman presented near term with eclampsia manifesting as cortical blindness and headache. Noncontrast CT demonstrated areas of hypodensity in the parieto-occipital regions bilaterally.

Several neuroimaging techniques have been used in the evaluation of eclampsia. CT can be performed quickly for an acutely ill patient but may be of low yield, depending on the severity of the disease. Diffuse brain swelling with narrowed ventricles is a common finding on CT.[117–119] Symmetric hypodense bands in the posterior watershed areas may appear later as a result of local vasogenic edema[117, 118] (Fig. 6–3). Large parenchymal and subarachnoid hemorrhages also occur and are readily seen on CT. MRI of eclamptic patients has demonstrated both focal and diffuse brain edema as well, even early in the disease. These are evident as multiple regions of nonspecific hyperintense signal on T2-weighted images and are predominantly located in the cortex and deep white matter tracts.[120–122] The posterior watershed territories are most frequently involved.[120–124] The MRI occasionally additionally demonstrates multifocal areas of increased T2-weighted signal at the gray-white junction and in the basal ganglia that are hypointense on T1-weighted images, and are consistent with multifocal regions of cerebral ischemia and edema[122, 123] (Fig. 6–4). Some authors have proposed that this collection of findings is unique and therefore diagnostic of eclampsia.[122] Typically, these MRI abnormalities are completely reversible.[123, 124] Conventional cerebral arteriography may demonstrate vasospasm in medium and large vessels in a characteristic beading pattern[117, 125] (Fig. 6–5). Poor distal filling of terminal arteries may also be seen, with relatively poor perfusion of the parieto-occipital watershed territories. These findings have been called peripartum angiopathy or vasculopathy.[124, 126]

The CSF is usually normal in preeclampsia. In eclampsia, CSF protein is often moderately elevated to 60–100 mg/dL, and CSF pressure may be increased. The fluid may also be mildly blood-tinged in eclampsia, but the presence of grossly bloody fluid suggests that a major cerebral hemorrhage has occurred.[106] Although lumbar puncture is now rarely used in the diagnosis, it was once advocated as therapy for eclampsia but later abandoned.[106]

The baseline EEG in women who subsequently develop eclamptic seizures is typically normal, although up to one-half have diffuse slowing in association with significant preeclampsia alone.[127] The eclamptic EEG typically reveals intermittent spike-wave and polyspike-wave discharges with excessive diffuse background slowing.[127] Slowing in the posterior regions may persist for up to 6 months after delivery.

Pathophysiology

Many theories have been offered to explain the pathogenesis of preeclampsia, but none has been

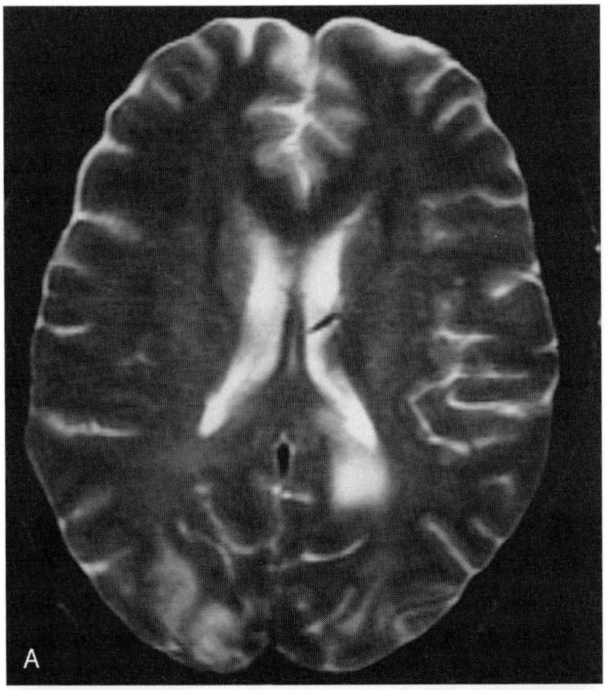

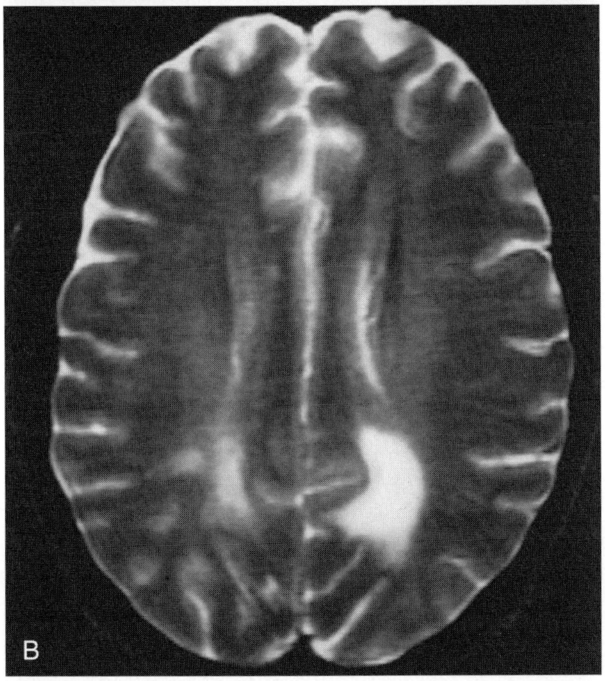

FIGURE 6–4 • *A, B,* Magnetic resonance imaging (MRI) in eclampsia. A 37-year-old woman presented 2 weeks after delivery with a left inferior quadrantanopsia and generalized seizures. T2-weighted MRI demonstrated hyperintense changes in the parieto-occipital white matter bilaterally. These changes were not visible on computed tomography. Follow-up MRI obtained 3 months later showed complete resolution of these abnormalities.

proven. Abnormalities of vasomotor tone, prostaglandin function, immunologic regulation, and placental trophoblastic formation are all currently implicated as primary etiologic factors in pregnancy-induced hypertension.[110] Progression to multiple organ injury is promoted by generalized arteriolar vasospasm, increased peripheral vascular resistance, reduced plasma volume, and increased serum viscosity. Systemic disease may also result from endothelial damage and disseminated intravascular coagulation. The HELLP syndrome (*h*emolysis, *e*levated *l*iver enzymes, and *l*ow *p*latelets) constitutes a severe form of preeclampsia with multiorgan dysfunction.[128]

The development of eclamptic seizures and other neurologic deficits has been traditionally attributed to transient cerebral vasospasm, resulting in cerebral ischemia. This view has been challenged as an insufficient explanation for the clinical and pathological features of the disorder, and a mechanism of eclampsia as a disorder of cerebral hemodynamic autoregulation has been proposed.[129, 130]

The neuropathological findings of eclampsia[115, 131] include petechial cortical and small subcortical parenchymal hemorrhages, microinfarctions, subarachnoid hemorrhage, and brain edema. Cortical petechiae and microinfarctions tend to occur in major arterial watershed areas, most frequently between the distributions of the middle and posterior cerebral arteries. Small hemorrhages are also found at the gray-white junction in a similar vascular distribution. Microscopically, precapillaries are occluded with fibrin and engorged with red cells. Arteriolar walls become edematous and necrotic. Ring hemorrhages are identified around thrombosed vessels because of diapedesis of red cells from intravascular into Virchow-Robin spaces. In some patients, massive cerebral parenchymal hemorrhage may occur in the basal ganglia, pons, or cerebral cortex in association with densely packed microhemorrhages in those regions. Rupture into the ventricles with subarachnoid hemorrhage may follow. Diffuse brain edema may be associated with gyral effacement and transtentorial or uncal herniation.

The formation of ring hemorrhages around thrombosed vessels is a consequence of dysregu-

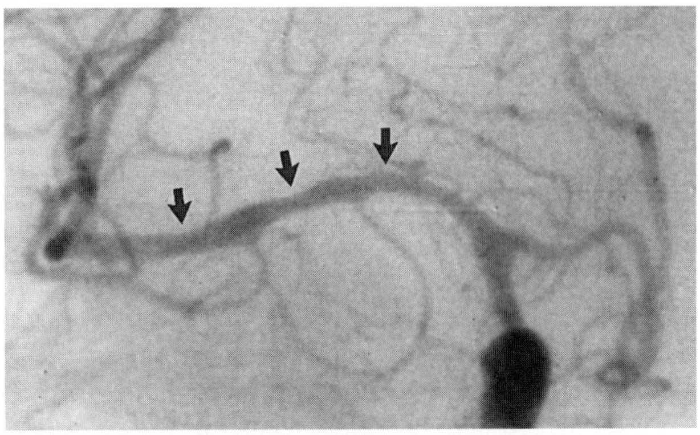

FIGURE 6–5 • Late postpartum angiopathy. Cerebral arteriography (performed on the patient from Fig. 6–4) demonstrated multifocal areas of segmental narrowing (arrows) and dilatation in the middle cerebral artery.

lated cerebral blood flow (CBF).[130] Normally, cerebral hemodynamic autoregulation maintains a constant CBF for a broad range of systemic blood pressures through a mechanism of arteriolar dilatation and constriction. In the normotensive patient, CBF is autoregulated for mean arterial pressures between 60 and 140 mm Hg, but in a young healthy woman whose usual blood pressure is relatively low, the upper limit may be only 120 mm Hg.[106] On the other hand, chronically hypertensive patients have substantially higher limits of this range. At the upper boundary of autoregulation, arterioles are maximally constricted to maintain stable CBF. In an individual patient, there is no well-defined method to predict this threshold, and an estimate can only be based on the patient's baseline pressure. Consequently, the blood-pressure criteria used in the definitions of pregnancy-induced hypertension and preeclampsia are arbitrary and unable to distinguish which patients are likely to develop cerebral and other systemic involvement.[103, 105, 111, 132, 133]

Brain insult occurs when the blood pressure exceeds the upper limit of autoregulation. This feature is associated with the time when a preeclamptic woman becomes physiologically eclamptic. She may develop seizures or other neurologic deficits, such as visual field defects and cortical blindness. Although the disease is only classified as eclampsia if seizures appear, the process that results in cortical visual symptoms is identical[106, 115] and should have the same clinical implications. An alternating pattern of arteriolar constriction and dilatation occurs both angiographically and pathologically and is described as the sausage-string phenomenon.[134] Small foci of cerebral infarction may occur in the territory of severely constricted vessels with subsequent formation of thrombus in the vessels. Once the profound vasoconstriction resolves, perfusion may resume to these areas, but they will be susceptible to perivascular extravasation and microhemorrhage around the thrombosed vessel.[130, 131, 134] Recurrent vascular injury occurs with each successive rise in mean arterial pressure. The pathological finding of ring hemorrhages is consistent with this mechanism of impaired cerebral hemodynamic autoregulation and is a typical feature of hypertensive encephalopathy.[131] More fulminant or persistent hypertension may lead to intracerebral or subarachnoid hemorrhage.

The microinfarctions and microhemorrhages of eclampsia are most common in the major arterial watershed zones and the occipital lobes. These areas are at particularly high risk for hypertensive encephalopathy. The anastomotic vessels undergo the greatest change in arteriolar size during normal cerebral hemodynamic autoregulation and are most likely to be damaged when blood pressure exceeds its limit.[131, 135]

Management

The treatment of eclampsia is directed toward the concomitant control of hypertension, prevention and treatment of seizures, delivery of the fetus, and supportive care. The presence of the fetus complicates management in two ways. First, the aggressive treatment of maternal hypertension and convulsions may result in fetal hypotension and distress. Second, the fetus and placenta must be removed in order to effectively treat the underlying cause of this pregnancy-induced disease. However, the mother must be stabilized before delivery can be attempted. The most appropriate therapy for eclampsia has long been debated. Obstetricians have favored the use of magnesium sulfate, citing extensive empiric data; neurologists have advocated treatment with anticonvulsant agents, arguing that eclampsia is fundamentally no different from other causes of epilepsy. Some authors have further argued that aggressive control of blood pressure is the key to preventing seizures, and that magnesium and anticonvulsants treat only the signs and symptoms and not the cause of the disease.[106, 136, 137]

Magnesium Sulfate

Eclampsia has been treated by obstetricians in the United States with magnesium sulfate for nearly a century. A standardized protocol established by Pritchard and colleagues in 1955[138] demonstrated efficacy with minimal maternal and fetal mortality. Magnesium sulfate was given as an intravenous 4 g loading dose followed by a 10 g intramuscular dose and arrested convulsions in the vast majority of cases. Additional intravenous doses (2 g) were administered if convulsions persisted. Maintenance doses of 5 g were then given every 4 hours thereafter. In their series of 245 patients,[112] there was only a single maternal death, compared with the nearly 30% mortality rate from eclamptic seizures prior to the widespread use of magnesium sulfate. Perinatal mortality was approximately 10% in this study. Alternative regimens of magnesium administration, including continuous intravenous infusion (1–3 g per hour), have been recommended with similar outcomes.[111, 139, 140]

The normal serum magnesium level is approximately 1.5–2.5 mEq/L. Maternal levels of serum magnesium after a loading dose typically approach 4–8 mEq/L. Although this has been purported to be the therapeutic range, not all patients remain seizure-free with these levels.[111, 112, 127] Magnesium toxicity may occur when the serum level is greater than 9 mEq/L.[141] The magnesium ion blocks neuromuscular transmission, and toxicity may therefore manifest as a myasthenic syndrome. Depression or loss of deep tendon reflexes is often the earliest sign, followed by weakness and respiratory paralysis. Obstetricians carefully follow the activity of tendon reflexes as a clinical indicator of the serum magnesium level. Complete heart block may also occur. Impairment of uterine contractility may prevent a vaginal delivery. Finally, magnesium crosses the placenta, and neonatal hypermagnesemia may occur after prolonged maternal exposure,[141] although this is rare.[139] Affected newborns may be hypotonic with a weak cry, poor sucking, and respiratory depression. Ventilatory support may be required for 1–2 days until the magnesium is adequately excreted. Severe hypermagnesemia may also be temporarily treated with intravenous calcium as an antidote,[113] although this maneuver usually does not obviate intubation.[141] Because magnesium exerts profound effects on the neuromuscular junction, some obstetricians have suggested that its mechanism of action in eclampsia may be peripherally mediated.[113] Donaldson and other staunch critics have suggested that magnesium does not control seizures at all but instead creates that illusion by causing a profound neuromuscular blockade and abolishing tonic-clonic movements.[142, 143]

Magnesium does not appear to cross the blood-brain barrier in sufficient quantity to affect the central nervous system. In control patients in whom acute severe hypermagnesemia was induced, their cognition, sensation, and EEG results remained normal despite complete neuromuscular paralysis.[144] The magnesium level in the CSF is regulated independently of the serum level, and acute dramatic increases in serum magnesium only cause a delayed and minimal increase in the CSF level.[138] However, when given as an intrathecal bolus dose, magnesium has actually caused seizures, spinal anesthesia, and stupor.[142] Several animal studies have yielded inconsistent results in attempts to demonstrate a significant anticonvulsant effect of magnesium, even at toxic levels.[145–147]

Many obstetricians continue to assert that magnesium is effective in arresting and preventing seizures, even in spite of evidence that it neither penetrates the blood-brain barrier in significant quantity nor exerts any definite antiepileptic effect, even when applied directly to neuronal tissue. The strength of the empiric data validating the use of magnesium sulfate appears to greatly influence their perspective. A case in point is the study by Sibai and colleagues,[127] in which the EEG was analyzed from 36 eclamptic patients treated with magnesium sulfate. The overwhelming majority of the abnormal EEG results of eclamptic patients were unchanged by the administration of magnesium. Furthermore, several of the patients continued to have clinical and electrographic seizures despite therapeutic and supratherapeutic serum magnesium levels. The authors surmised that the mechanism by which magnesium suppresses seizure activity does not alter the EEG results, and the EEG is therefore not reliable for patient evaluation.[127] An alternative conclusion: The EEG is sensitive enough, but the antiseizure effect of magnesium is negligible. Nevertheless, the excellent success rate attributed to magnesium sulfate in the management of eclampsia has established it as the standard of care among obstetricians in the United States. The empiric use of magnesium in this capacity will likely continue until controlled trials are performed to compare its efficacy with that of antiepileptic and antihypertensive medications (see Addendum).

Anticonvulsants

Outside the United States, eclamptic seizures are rarely treated with magnesium sulfate. Obstetricians in the United Kingdom and Australia usually use antiepileptic drugs, and this practice is favored by many neurologists worldwide.[106, 143] Until recently, chlormethiazole, barbiturates, and diazepam were the drugs of choice overseas.[148–150] These agents all are associated with significant maternal and fetal sedation and respiratory distress. Phenytoin was introduced into the treatment of eclampsia with the hope that it would be effective without significant central nervous system depression.[151] Phenytoin has been proven to control various seizure types caused by many etiologies, but its use in eclampsia remains controversial because large clinical trials are lacking. Phenytoin can be loaded in about 20 minutes (at a dose of 10–15 mg/kg with an infusion rate of up to 50 mg/min) with low risk to mother and fetus.[151–153] Higher loading doses may lead to toxicity, because a higher proportion of phenytoin is unbound in preeclamptic patients because of hypoalbuminemia.[152, 153] The serum level reaches a peak rapidly after the infusion is complete. The method of drug administration and the time to attain peak levels are similar to those of magnesium.

Several small studies have demonstrated safety and efficacy for phenytoin. Slater and colleagues[151] treated 26 patients with phenytoin. Only two were diagnosed with eclampsia; the remainder had preeclampsia. No seizures were reported during or after the infusion of phenytoin, nor were there any major maternal or fetal side effects. However, other studies found that 15%–25% of patients with eclampsia developed recurrent seizures after phenytoin administration.[154, 155] Other investigators then attempted to determine if an optimal dosing regimen[152, 156] or specific therapeutic level[153] existed for phenytoin but discovered that several patients continued to have seizures after treatment. Even when free phenytoin levels were monitored and controlled, a small number of patients proved refractory.[153] Friedman and colleagues[157] performed a prospective randomized trial comparing phenytoin (45 patients) and magnesium sulfate (60 patients). Among the preeclamptic patients, no seizures occurred in either group. However, two patients with eclampsia who received phenytoin had additional convulsions. Overall, fewer maternal side effects were demonstrated in the phenytoin-treated group, and labor was noted to be briefer with less blood loss. To date, no study has successfully demonstrated superiority of phenytoin over magnesium, and a large blinded randomized clinical trial seems warranted (see Addendum).

Diazepam is recommended as an acute treatment for recurrent eclamptic seizures and eclamptic status epilepticus. Because of the risks of fetal oversedation and neonatal respiratory depression, many physicians only use diazepam as a temporizing measure to halt ongoing seizures.[113, 140, 158] Given intravenously, it arrests convulsions rapidly, and its effects are short-lived. Single or divided doses up to a total of 10 mg may be used relatively safely until another agent can be administered.[129, 158] Other benzodiazepines, including lorazepam, have not been studied extensively in this setting but can presumably be used with similar profiles of potential risk and benefit (see also Chapter 4).

Antihypertensive Agents

Appropriate management of the hypertensive encephalopathy of eclampsia requires careful reduction in systemic blood pressure without causing fetal ischemia and hypoxia. The perfusion to the uteroplacental vascular bed is already compromised and may collapse in response to some antihypertensive agents. A precipitous decline in blood pressure may cause cerebral ischemia in the mother, because the cerebral arterioles are maximally constricted and cannot quickly dilate. Aggressive therapy requires continuous fetal monitoring and maternal hemodynamic monitoring.[159]

Diuretics are contraindicated in preeclampsia and eclampsia.[113, 140, 159] Patients may have profound intravascular volume depletion, and further reduction of volume may result in widespread tissue ischemia. Oliguria can only be worsened by diuresis. Instead, plasma volume should be expanded,[160] although overhydration may result in pulmonary edema. Colloid may be preferable to crystalloid, because the latter may worsen brain edema.[107]

Hydralazine is the most widely used antihypertensive agent for toxemia in the United States. It was included in Pritchard's original treatment protocol with magnesium sulfate[138] and has been deemed safe and effective in the vast majority of patients.[112] Hydralazine is a direct arterial vasodilator that theoretically dilates uteroplacental vessels in parallel with other vascular beds and thus avoids fetal ischemia.[112] It also has no direct cardiac effects, although reflex tachycardia and ventricular arrhythmias may occur.[161] Hydralazine can be administered in small bolus doses of 5–10 mg every 20 minutes until diastolic blood pressure is brought below 100 mm Hg.[112, 159] The risk of maternal hypotension and fetal distress in response to a dose of hydralazine is usually less than 10% but can be as high as 50% if the mother is not well hydrated.[162] No other significant fetal side effects have been associated with intrauterine exposure to hydralazine.[159]

Diazoxide is another direct arterial vasodilator without direct cardiac effects that has been effective in the management of eclampsia.[163] It can be given in doses of 30 mg every 1–2 minutes or 75 mg every 30 minutes, although the former regimen seems to pose a lower risk of maternal hypotension.[159, 163] Although the fetus is potentially at risk for hyperglycemia caused by diazoxide, this has not been clinically evident. When given close to term, diazoxide may also complicate labor and delivery because of its substantial tocolytic effects.[159] Pharmacologic induction is often necessary to resume active labor.

Labetalol is a combined alpha- and beta-adrenergic antagonist that has recently been demonstrated to be effective in eclampsia, particularly for controlling blood pressure during parturition.[159] A continuous intravenous infusion or intermittent small-bolus doses can be adjusted to maintain appropriate pressure control without significant acute side effects. Maternal hypotension is rare, and ventricular tachyarrhythmias are prevented by the beta$_1$-antagonist activity.[161] This pharmacologic mechanism also reduces the myocardial oxygen requirement and may reduce the risk of myocardial ischemia. Labetalol has been shown to control blood pressure as efficiently as hydralazine with fewer untoward effects.[161] However, the possibility of an association between labetalol and low birth weight has been suggested[164, 165] and requires further investigation.

Sodium nitroprusside is a rapidly acting and extremely potent dilator of arterial and venous smooth muscle. It is administered by continuous intravenous infusion and should be started at a low infusion rate of 0.25 μg/kg per minute. The dose can then be gradually titrated to the desired blood pressure. Intra-arterial pressure monitoring is required. The role of nitroprusside in pregnancy remains controversial because of its potential toxicity. Its metabolism produces cyanide, which is subsequently converted into thiocyanate. High infusion rates of nitroprusside may produce toxic quantities of thiocyanate that the fetus is unable to adequately excrete.[159] However, this complication has not been observed in human pregnancies.[166] Nitroprusside may also cause elevation of intracranial pressure, an unwanted effect in an eclamptic patient with brain swelling and pre-existing intracranial hypertension. Nevertheless, nitroprusside has been shown to improve blood pressure in preeclamptic and eclamptic patients whose hypertension was refractory to hydralazine and was associated with relatively minimal fetal risk.[166]

Several other antihypertensive medications have been suggested to have at least a hypothetical role in the treatment of preeclampsia and eclampsia. However, these agents present risks that may not be outweighed by their benefits. Calcium channel blockers have also been shown to be effective antihypertensive agents in preeclampsia,[136, 137, 167] but additional investigation is required to better assess safety. Nifedipine may interact with magnesium sulfate to cause profound hypotension and muscle weakness.[168] In addition, animal studies have found that these agents reduced the proportional blood flow to the uterus and placenta, resulting in fetal acidosis and hypercarbia.[159] Nitroglycerin has been rarely used in toxemia and may cause dose-related elevation of intracranial pressure. Angiotensin-converting enzyme inhibitors are associated with poor fetal outcome and are also contraindicated in pregnancy.[159] The cause of their toxicity is unknown.

Labor and Delivery

The definitive treatment of eclampsia is delivery of the fetus and placenta. Safe and successful delivery relies on expert obstetric, medical, and anesthetic management. Convulsions and severe hypertension must be stabilized before controlled delivery can take place. Metabolic derangements such as hypoxia, acidosis, and hypovolemia should be corrected. Anesthesia can be administered by either inhalation or epidural catheter infusion, each with their respective risk profiles. Many obstetricians currently prefer epidural anesthesia, but this issue remains controversial.[91, 110] Parenteral narcotics are commonly prescribed as well, although they cross the placenta and may cause neonatal sedation and respiratory depression. Throughout the delivery, fetal heart rate is continuously monitored for signs of distress. Invasive hemodynamic monitoring of the mother may be required in order to optimize blood pressure control. Delivery can proceed by the vaginal route in many cases, and cesarean section is performed in accord with standard obstetric indications.[110] Emergent operative delivery is mandated by acute fetal distress, maternal hemorrhage, and profound maternal hypotension, as well as other maternal or fetal emergencies. Emergent cesarean section requires general endotracheal anesthesia in all cases.

Preeclampsia and eclampsia usually resolve 24–48 hours after delivery. The mother should continue to be monitored and treated intensively until blood pressure, volume status, and urine output return toward normal. Coagulation study results and liver enzyme measurements should also normalize. Women who received magnesium therapy prior to delivery are often continued on this medication for 1 or more days. The role of long-term anticonvulsant therapy is controversial, and few obstetricians recommend this practice. Patients with persistent elevation of blood pressure can be treated with any effective antihypertensive agent once the pregnancy is completed. Hypertension lasting longer than 4–6 weeks warrants an evaluation for other causes of chronic hypertension. The majority of patients have an uncomplicated postpartum course and are discharged from the hospital within several days.[110]

Prognosis

Toxemia is the third most common cause of direct obstetric maternal mortality and causes about 10% of all maternal deaths.[70] Only severe obstetric hemorrhage and infection are more deadly. The long-term prognosis for both mother and child is good, however, if they survive the acute illness. Mothers rarely suffer permanent neurologic deficit or experience recurrent seizures except when intracerebral hemorrhage and stroke complicate the eclampsia.[111, 112] Abnormal neuroimaging study results usually return to normal within weeks.[121, 123, 124]

Women who develop eclampsia during their first pregnancy are unlikely to have recurrence with subsequent gestation, although they are at moderately increased risk for recurrent preeclampsia.[169] Older patients who become toxemic after multiple births have an increased incidence of chronic hypertension as well.[110] Women with toxemia superimposed on severe chronic hypertension, heart disease, or renal disease have such a markedly elevated risk of recurrent severe toxemia and death that they are frequently counseled against further pregnancy.[110]

NEUROMUSCULAR EMERGENCIES

The pathophysiology, diagnosis, and treatment of acute neuromuscular diseases is discussed at length in Chapter 13. However, the gravid patient requires special care that makes the management of these disorders even more challenging.

Myasthenia Gravis

Myasthenia gravis (MG) affects women of childbearing age. The peak incidence is in the third decade of life, and it affects twice as many females as males.[170] The clinical course of MG during pregnancy is unpredictable. About one-third of patients with MG worsen during pregnancy, one-third improve, and one-third remain unchanged.[171] Exacerbations appear to occur with equal frequency in all three trimesters. However, approximately 30% of patients with MG experience an exacerbation of their disease during the puerperium, often with sudden and severe manifestations.[171] The frequent occurrence of postpartum exacerbations of MG may be related to the levels of circulating alpha-fetoprotein. This factor appears to bind to acetylcholine receptor antibodies (AChR-Ab) and exert a protective effect during pregnancy that wanes as the levels fall after parturition.[171, 172] The exact mechanism of this effect remains unknown.[173]

Specific issues that arise in the treatment of the pregnant patient with MG include choice of medications, management of labor and delivery, and risks to the fetus and neonate. Anticholinesterase medications such as pyridostigmine (Mestinon) can be administered safely throughout pregnancy. However, alterations in intestinal absorption, metabolism, and renal excretion during pregnancy cause erratic changes in the level and duration of the drug effect. Many patients require frequent dosage adjustments throughout the pregnancy. Pyridostigmine should be given parenterally (at approximately one-thirtieth of the equivalent oral dose) during the critical period of labor and delivery in order to avoid inadequate levels.[171, 174, 175] Corticosteroids are the mainstay of chronic therapy during pregnancy. Although their prolonged use is associated with a small risk of cleft lip and palate, steroids have been proven to prevent exacerbations. Pregnant women should be maintained on the lowest effective dose or on an alternate-day dosing regimen.[171, 176] The antimetabolite immunosuppressive agents, such as azathioprine and cyclophosphamide, are potentially teratogenic and therefore contraindicated during pregnancy. Thymectomy can be performed during pregnancy if indicated but is more commonly performed before attempting pregnancy.[66] Intravenous immunoglobulin may be useful in the treatment of MG. Although not evaluated for its effect on MG during pregnancy, intravenous immunoglobulin has been used for the prevention of recurrent abortion (due to antiphospholipid antibodies syndrome) without success.[177] Intravenous immunoglobulin has also been associated with neonatal neutropenia[178] and cannot be recommended at this time.

Myasthenic crisis may occur in the setting of profound stress, and pregnancy is no exception. Moreover, the pregnant patient has an already reduced lung capacity, for which she compensates by breathing at an increased rate and tidal volume. A moderate degree of fatigability can be clinically silent until the patient suffers acute respiratory compromise. Declining vital capacity or inability to protect the airway from secretions is an indication for intubation and mechanical ventilation. Plasmapheresis has been used successfully to treat myasthenic crisis during pregnancy.[171, 176] The fluctuating volume status and coagulopathy are managed as in the nonpregnant myasthenic patient. Infection is a frequent precipitant of myasthenic crisis and must be treated aggressively. However, aminoglycosides as well as several other antibiotics must be avoided in MG.

Labor and delivery are usually normal, because smooth muscle is not affected by MG. The route of delivery depends entirely on obstetric considerations. The development of preeclampsia/eclampsia in a woman with MG is rare,[175, 179, 180] and the use of magnesium sulfate is contraindicated in MG because it further contributes to neuromuscular junction blockade and has been reported to precipitate severe myasthenic crisis.[180, 181] Beta-blockers such as labetalol are also contraindicated in MG.

The effects of maternal MG on the fetus vary. Most mothers report normal spontaneous fetal movements. However, several infants have been born with diffuse or focal joint contractures, or arthrogryposis.[171] Fetal movement is a challenge to quantitatively assess in utero by ultrasonography, and early detection is therefore difficult. Neonatal MG occurs in the offspring of 10%–20% of myasthenic mothers as a result of transplacental transport of AChR-Ab.[171, 174] Symptoms and signs, which may not become apparent for the first several days of life, include respiratory depression, bronchial obstruction, aspiration, impaired cry and suck, and diffuse hypotonia.[66, 171] The delayed onset of symptoms and signs has been attributed to the effects of alpha-fetoprotein, as described earlier.[172] The association between maternal titers of AChR-Ab and fetal or neonatal disease is uncertain, again making any attempts at risk stratification impossible. Regardless of the titers, infants should be closely observed for a minimum of 4 days.[66, 174] For myasthenic mothers with a history of poor fetal outcome, some authors have recommended serial plasmapheresis during pregnancy as prophylaxis against the fetal effects of the disease.[176]

Guillain-Barré Syndrome

Acute inflammatory demyelinating polyneuropathy, or the Guillain-Barré syndrome (GBS), is a rare and random event during pregnancy. About 40 patients have been reported. Pregnancy does not appear to alter the clinical manifestations or the course of the disease. Plasmapheresis may reduce the need for prolonged ventilation if started within 7 days of onset.[66, 182] Delivery is usually uncomplicated, because uterine contractions are not affected. However, severe autonomic neuropathy may prevent effective contractions and necessitate operative delivery. If the uterine smooth muscle is normal but the mother is unable to adequately participate with bearing down and pushing, an instrumented delivery can be performed. The fetus is not affected by maternal Guillain-Barré syndrome, and the fetal survival rate is 96%.[94, 183]

METABOLIC ENCEPHALOPATHY

Maternal nutritional status may be compromised by the needs of the fetus, and deficiencies in several vitamins and minerals are common during pregnancy. Nausea and vomiting is a common problem of early pregnancy that can only intensify the mother's nutritional depletion, and hyperemesis gravidarum further complicates the picture. Prolonged courses of hyperemesis gravidarum for 4–12 weeks have been associated with Wernicke's encephalopathy in the first half of pregnancy.[184, 185] This deficiency of thiamine may present with ophthalmoplegia, nystagmus, confusion, and ataxia. Mild polyneuropathy may also be apparent. Treatment of the malnourished patient with supplemental intravenous glucose may aggravate the biochemical deficit and precipitate acute onset of the syndrome. The diagnosis is generally based on the clinical response to thiamine, although the red-cell transketolase activity can also be assayed. Thiamine should be administered prior to any carbohydrate loading and then parenterally repleted at a dose of at least 100 mg daily for 1 week, followed by an oral regimen. The fetal mortality rate in Wernicke's encephalopathy is about 40%, and the cause of demise is unknown. The maternal mortality rate is estimated at 10%.[184]

Hyperemesis gravidarum may also result in severe electrolyte and acid-base disturbances and has further been associated with central pontine myelinolysis. The pathophysiology of this disorder is uncertain, but it is commonly regarded as a consequence of rapid correction of hyponatremia. Central pontine myelinolysis has occurred in a few pregnant patients with only mild hyponatremia but who also had Wernicke's encephalopathy.[185–187] It is believed that these disorders coexist more frequently than would be expected by chance. Some authors have suggested that thiamine deficiency predisposes pontine myelin to metabolic injury.[185] Hyponatremia, even if mild, should be corrected slowly, and thiamine supplementation is a reasonable adjunctive therapy that presents little risk and enormous potential benefit.

Liver disease can present during pregnancy as acute hepatic encephalopathy. Acute fatty liver of pregnancy is an uncommon phenomenon of the third trimester that can lead to hepatic failure, encephalopathy, and death. The cause is unknown. It occurs at a rate of one case per 10,000 to 20,000 pregnancies.[188] Primigravidas and women with multiple gestations may be at increased risk. Early symptoms include malaise, lethargy, nausea, vomiting, abdominal pain, and jaundice. The features of the encephalopathy are nonspecific, and the finding of asterixis is inconsistent. Many patients also have signs of hypertension, proteinuria, and edema, thereby mimicking or coinciding with preeclampsia or the HELLP syndrome, as described earlier.[188–190] The situation may be further complicated by severe coagulopathy, pulmonary edema, respiratory arrest, renal failure, or diabetes insipidus. The diagnosis is based on the clinical picture, elevation of transaminases, and abdominal CT or ultrasonography, but may require liver biopsy in atypical cases. Treatment is limited to supportive care measures, including administration of cathartics, blood products, mechanical ventilation, and dialysis. Many authors favor early delivery, which has been demonstrated to dramatically improve maternal and fetal survival.[188, 191] Liver transplantation has been used in several cases of fulminant hepatic failure with some success.[190] Recurrence of acute fatty liver of pregnancy during subsequent pregnancies is extraordinarily rare.[188, 191]

MATERNAL HEAD TRAUMA

Maternal injuries during pregnancy complicate approximately 7% of all pregnancies, and trauma is the leading nonobstetric cause of death in pregnancy.[70, 192] Motor vehicle accidents are the most frequent, followed by falls and assaults. Although abdominal trauma is a major cause of concern during pregnancy, traumatic brain injury considerably affects the patient's ability to perform as a mother.

Management of head trauma depends on the mechanism and severity of injury. Careful and frequent assessments of fetal well-being are required, but the primary focus of management is the mother. The examination, laboratory investigations, and radiologic evaluation of a gravid trauma patient are identical to those of a nongravid patient. Neurosurgical interventions are also similar but with the specific alterations described in regard to aneurysm and AVM surgery.[192] Treatment of elevated intracranial pressure with hyperventilation is appropriate, but the use of mannitol should be restricted. The risk of fetal death correlates with the severity of maternal trauma, unless injury is limited to the head only. If the mother dies, the fetus will also die unless delivered rapidly. Maternal death from head injury is associated with a better fetal outcome than is death from more extensive trauma or systemic illness.[192] If the fetus is viable, postmortem cesarean section may result in a good fetal outcome if performed within 5 minutes and in a poor outcome after 20 minutes.[193]

MATERNAL BRAIN DEATH

Severe brain insult as a consequence of infarction, hemorrhage, or trauma may result in deep coma, persistent vegetative state, or brain death. Prolonged life support can be maintained indefinitely in many instances unless the patient succumbs to medical complications of sepsis, hypotension, or adult respiratory distress syndrome. When the patient is pregnant, management of two lives must be considered. Predictors of outcome and the criteria for the diagnosis of brain death are presumably the same in pregnancy as in the general population. However, even if the mother's prognosis is dismal, in the absence of systemic maternal injury or disease the fetus may still be saved. If pregnancy has advanced beyond the 28th week, the viable fetus can be delivered by cesarean section with a good chance of being normal. This presents little ethical dilemma, because the fetal patient is mature and the procedure exposes the mother to relatively little risk.[194]

Management of the brain-dead gravida with an immature fetus is a difficult moral issue. Many brain-dead or comatose women have been maintained on life support for extended periods, up to several months, as incubators for their unborn offspring.[194] This practice clearly requires careful discussion and informed consent from the next-of-kin. However, informed consent can be based only on hope and speculation, because no data support or refute this type of management. Moreover, the next-of-kin must make the decision while coming to terms with the death of the mother and possibly the responsibility of raising her infant, if he or she survives. Although a discussion on the ethics of this issue is outside the scope of this chapter, it is certain that the neurologist plays a critical role in estimating the prognosis of the mother that will influence all subsequent decisions regarding her care and that of her fetus.

ADDENDUM

Since the submission of this chapter, a large clinical trial has compared magnesium sulfate with phenytoin in the prevention of eclampsia.[195] A total of 2138 pregnant women participated in the study. All had blood pressure of at least 140/90 mm Hg and had no prior history of seizures. Patients randomly received either magnesium sulfate (according to a protocol nearly identical to that described in this chapter) or phenytoin (1 g intravenously over 60 minutes followed by a maintenance dose) until 1 day post partum. If a patient developed seizures during the study period, she was treated with magnesium regardless of initial treatment regimen. Patients in each group were well matched in terms of risk factors for eclampsia. A significantly greater number of patients treated with phenytoin developed eclampsia compared with those treated with magnesium (0.9% vs. 0.0%; $P = .04$). The results of this trial have been criticized[196–198] because of several methodical flaws: (1) the study was not blinded and was performed in only one center; (2) there were significantly more surgical deliveries in the magnesium-treated patients; (3) the majority of phenytoin-treated patients had subtherapeutic levels at the time when seizures occurred (free levels were not measured); (4) electroencephalographic data were lacking; and (5) blood pressure management was not specified. Nevertheless, the importance of magnesium in the prevention and treatment of eclampsia has been upheld, and it maintains its long-standing position as the current standard of care in the United States.

References

1. Hume RF, Killam AP: Maternal physiology. In Scott JR, DiSaia PJ, Hammond CB, et al (eds): Danforth's Obstetrics and Gynecology, 6th ed, pp 93–100. Philadelphia, JB Lippincott, 1990.
2. Gibbs CE: Maternal death due to stroke. Am J Obstet Gynecol 1974;119:69–75.
3. Maternal and Neonatal Haemostasis Working Party of the Haemostasis and Thrombosis Task: Guidelines on the prevention, investigation and management of thrombosis associated with pregnancy. J Clin Pathol 1993;46:489–496.
4. Crowley J: Coagulopathy and bleeding in the parturient patient. R I Med J 1989;72:135–143.
5. Wilterdink JL, Easton JD: Cerebral ischemia. In Devinsky O, Feldmann E, Hainline B (eds): Neurological Complications of Pregnancy, pp 1–11. New York, Raven Press, 1994.
6. De Lia JE: Placental and fetal development. In Scott JR, DiSaia PJ, Hammond CB, et al (eds): Danforth's Obstetrics and Gynecology, 6th ed, pp 101–121. Philadelphia, JB Lippincott, 1990.
7. Wilkening RB, Meschia G: Fetal oxygen uptake, oxygenation, and acid-base balance as a function of uterine blood flow. Am J Physiol 1983;244:H749–H755.
8. Wiebers DO: Ischemic cerebrovascular complications of pregnancy. Arch Neurol 1985;42:1106–1113.
9. Cross J, Castro P, Jennett W: Cerebral strokes associated

with pregnancy and the puerperium. BMJ 1968;3:214–218.
10. Wiebers DO, Whisnant JP: The incidence of stroke among pregnant women in Rochester, Minn, 1955 through 1979. JAMA 1985;254:3055–3057.
11. Donaldson JO: Cerebrovascular disease. In Neurology of Pregnancy, 2nd ed, pp 137–184. London, WB Saunders, 1989.
12. Kittner SJ, Hebel R, Feeser B, et al: Stroke risk associated with pregnancy and the post-partum period. Stroke 1995;26:183.
13. Sharshar T, Lamy C, Mas JL: Incidence and causes of strokes associated with pregnancy and the puerperium. A study in public hospitals of Ile de France. Stroke 1995;26:930–936.
14. Schwartz RB: Neurodiagnostic imaging of the pregnant patient. In Devinsky O, Feldmann E, Hainline B (eds): Neurological Complications of Pregnancy, pp 243–248. New York, Raven Press, 1994.
15. Brent RL: The effect of embryonic and fetal exposure to x-ray, microwaves, and ultrasound: Counselling the pregnant and nonpregnant patient about these risks. Semin Oncol 1989;16:347–368.
16. Mattison CR, Angtuaco T: Magnetic resonance imaging in prenatal diagnosis. Clin Obstet Gynecol 1988;31:353–389.
17. Lechat P, Mas JL, Lascault G, et al: Prevalence of patent foramen ovale in patients with stroke. N Engl J Med 1988;318:1148–1152.
18. Jones HR, Caplan LR, Come PC, et al: Cerebral emboli of paradoxical origin. Ann Neurol 1983;13:314–319.
19. Lynch JJ, Schuchard GH, Gross CM, et al: Prevalence of right-to-left atrial shunting in a healthy population: Detection by Valsalva maneuver contrast echocardiography. Am J Cardiol 1984;53:1478–1480.
20. Webster MWI, Chancellor AM, Smith HJ, et al: Patent foramen ovale in young stroke patients. Lancet 1988;i:11–12.
21. Salazar E, Zajarias A, Gutierrez N, et al: The problem of cardiac valve prostheses, anticoagulants, and pregnancy. Circulation 1984;70(Suppl 1):169–177.
22. Procacci PM, Savran SV, Schreiter SL, et al: Prevalence of clinical mitral-valve prolapse in 1,169 young women. N Engl J Med 1976;294:1086–1088.
23. Degani S, Abinader EG, Scharf M: Mitral valve prolapse and pregnancy: A review. Obstet Gynecol Surv 1989;44:642–649.
24. Cruikshank DP: Cardiovascular, pulmonary, renal, and hematologic diseases in pregnancy. In Scott JR, DiSaia PJ, Hammond CB, et al (eds): Danforth's Obstetrics and Gynecology, 6th ed, pp 433–459. Philadelphia, JB Lippincott, 1990.
25. Hart RG, Foster JW, Luther MF: Stroke in infective endocarditis. Stroke 1990;21:695–700.
26. Kaplan E, Anthony B, Bisno A, et al: AHA committee report: Prevention of bacterial endocarditis. Circulation 1977;56:139–143.
27. Homans D: Peripartum cardiomyopathy. N Engl J Med 1985;312:1432–1437.
28. Hodgman M, Pessin M, Homans D: Cerebral embolism as the initial manifestation of peripartum cardiomyopathy. Neurology 1982;32:668–671.
29. Brady K, Duff P: Rheumatic heart disease in pregnancy. Clin Obstet Gynecol 1989;32:21–39.
30. Wiebers DO, Mokri B: Internal carotid artery dissection after childbirth. Stroke 1985;16:956–959.
31. Bruno A, Adams H, Biller J, et al: Cerebral infarction due to moyamoya disease in young adults. Stroke 1988;19:826–833.
32. Wong V, Wang R, Tse T: Pregnancy and Takayasu's arteritis. Am J Med 1983;75:597–601.
33. Brick JF: Vanishing cerebrovascular disease of pregnancy. Neurology 1988;38:804–806.
34. Call G, Fleming M, Sealfon S, et al: Reversible segmental vasoconstriction. Stroke 1988;19:1159–1170.
35. Geraghty JJ, Hoch DB, Robert ME, et al: Fatal puerperal cerebral vasospasm and stroke in a young woman. Neurology 1991;41:1145–1147.
36. Francis RB: Large-vessel occlusion in sickle cell disease: Pathogenesis, clinical consequences, and therapeutic implications. Medical Hypotheses 1991;35:88–95.
37. Birdsall MA, Pattison NS: Antiphospholipid antibodies in pregnancy: Clinical associations. Br J Hosp Med 1993;50:251–260.
38. Unander AM, Norberg R, Hahn L, et al: Anticardiolipin antibodies and complement in ninety-nine women with habitual abortion. Am J Obstet Gynecol 1991;156:114–119.
39. Birdsall M, Pattison N, Chamley L: Antiphospholipid antibodies in pregnancy. Aust N Z J Obstet Gynaecol 1992;32:328–330.
40. Branch DW: Antiphospholipid antibodies and pregnancy: Maternal implications. Semin Perinatol 1990;14:139–146.
41. Menashe Y, Ben-Baruch G, Greenspoon JS, et al: Successful pregnancy outcome with combination therapy in women with the antiphospholipid antibody syndrome. J Reprod Med 1993;38:625–629.
42. Martin JN, Stedman CM: Imitators of preeclampsia and HELLP syndrome. Obstet Gynecol Clin North Am 1991;18:181–198.
43. Pinette MG, Vintzileos AM, Ingardia CJ: Thrombotic thrombocytopenia purpura as a cause of thrombocytopenia in pregnancy: Literature review. Am J Perinatol 1989;6:55–57.
44. Upshaw J, Reidy T, Groshart K: Thrombotic thrombocytopenia purpura in pregnancy: Response to plasma manipulations. South Med J 1985;78:677–680.
45. Ginsberg JS, Hirsh J: Use of antithrombotic agents during pregnancy. Chest 1992;102(Suppl):385S–390S.
46. Greaves M: Anticoagulants in pregnancy. Pharmac Ther 1993;59:311–327.
47. Calhoun BC, Hesser JW: Heparin-associated antibody with pregnancy: Discussion of two cases. Am J Obstet Gynecol 1987;156:964–966.
48. Melissari E, Parker CJ, Wilson NV, et al: Use of low molecular weight heparin in pregnancy. Thromb Haemostas 1992;68:652–656.
49. Ramamurthy S, Talwar KK, Saxena A, et al: Prosthetic mitral valve thrombosis in pregnancy successfully treated with streptokinase. Am Heart J 1994;127:446–448.
50. Fagher B, Ahlgren M, Astedt B: Acute massive pulmonary embolism treated with streptokinase during labor and the puerperium. Acta Obstet Gynaecol Scand 1990;69:659–661.
51. Sturm JT, Toro C, Snyder BD: Emergency carotid artery thrombectomy for postpartum hemiplegia. Am J Emerg Med 1987;5:291–293.
52. Chambers CE, Clark SL: Cardiac surgery during pregnancy. Clin Obstet Gynecol 1994;37:316–323.
53. Cantu C, Barinagarrementeria F: Cerebral venous thrombosis associated with pregnancy and the puerperium: Review of 67 cases. Stroke 1993;24:1880–1884.
54. Turkewitz LJ, Jacobs AK, Bidwell JK: Atypical MRI findings of venous sinus thrombosis in pregnancy: Clinical significance relating to episodic vascular headache. Headache 1991;31:240–243.
55. Srinivasan K: Cerebral venous thrombosis and arterial thrombosis in pregnancy and puerperium: A study of 135 patients. Angiology 1983;34:731–746.
56. Bousser M, Chiras J, Bories J, et al: Cerebral venous thrombosis—A review of 38 cases. Stroke 1985;16:199–213.
57. Turkewitz LJ, Jacobs AK, Bidwell K: Atypical MRI findings of venous sinus thrombosis in pregnancy: Clinical significance relating to episodic vascular headache. Headache 1991;31:240–243.
58. Mattle HP, Wentz KU, Edelman RR, et al: Cerebral venography with MR. Radiology 1991;178:453–458.
59. Beal MF, Wechsler LR, Davis KR: Cerebral vein thrombosis and multiple intracranial hemorrhages by computed tomography. Arch Neurol 1982;39:437–438.
60. Halpern JP, Morris JGL, Driscoll GL: Anticoagulants and

cerebral venous thrombosis. Aust N Z J Med 1984;14:643–648.
61. Einhaupl KM, Villringer A, Meister W, et al: Heparin treatment in sinus venous thrombosis. Lancet 1991;338:597–600.
62. Castaigne P, Laplane D, Bousser MP: Superior sagittal sinus thrombosis. Arch Neurol 1977;34:788–789.
63. DiRocco C, Iannelli A, Leone G, et al: Heparin-urokinase treatment in aseptic dural sinus thrombosis. Arch Neurol 1981;38:431–435.
64. Scott JA, Pascuzzi RM, Hall PV, et al: Treatment of dural sinus thrombosis with local urokinase infusion. J Neurosurg 1988;68:284–287.
65. Horowitz M, Purdy P, Unwin H, et al: Treatment of dural sinus thrombosis using selective catheterization and urokinase. Ann Neurol 1995;38:58–67.
66. Donaldson JO: Neurologic emergencies in pregnancy. Obstet Gynecol Clin North Am 1991;18:199–211.
67. Wilterdink JL, Feldmann E: Cerebral hemorrhage. In Devinsky O, Feldmann E, Hainline B (eds): Neurological Complications of Pregnancy, pp 13–23. New York, Raven Press, 1994.
68. Dias MS, Sekhar LN: Intracranial hemorrhage from aneurysms and arteriovenous malformations during pregnancy and the puerperium. Neurosurgery 1990;27:855–866.
69. Barno A, Freeman DW: Maternal deaths due to spontaneous subarachnoid hemorrhage. Am J Obstet Gynecol 1976;125:384–392.
70. Varner MW: Maternal mortality in Iowa from 1952 to 1986. Surg Gynecol Obstet 1989;168:555–562.
71. Horton JC, Chambers WA, Lyons SL, et al: Pregnancy and the risk of hemorrhage from cerebral arteriovenous malformations. Neurosurgery 1990;27:867–872.
72. Verweij RD, Wijdicks EFM, van Gijn J: Warning headache in aneurysmal subarachnoid hemorrhage: A case-control study. Arch Neurol 1988;45:1019–1020.
73. Robinson JL, Hall CS, Sedzimer CB: Arteriovenous malformations, aneurysms, and pregnancy. J Neurosurg 1974;41:63–70.
74. Lanzino G, Jensen ME, Cappelletto B, et al: Arteriovenous malformations that rupture during pregnancy: A management dilemma. Acta Neurochir 1994;126:102–106.
75. Sadasivan B, Malik GM, Lee C, et al: Vascular malformations and pregnancy. Surg Neurol 1990;33:305–313.
76. Buckley TA, Yau GHM, Poon WS, et al: Cesarean section and ablation of a cerebral arterio-venous malformation. Anaesth Intensive Care 1990;18:248–251.
77. Dias MS: Neurovascular emergencies in pregnancy. Clin Obstet Gynecol 1994;37:337–354.
78. Raps EC, Galetta SL, Flamm ES: Neuro-intensive care of the pregnant woman. Neurol Clin 1994;12:601–611.
79. Physicians' Desk Reference, 49th ed. Montvale, NJ, Medical Economics, 1995.
80. Athanassiou A, Begent RHJ, Newlands ES, et al: Central nervous system metastases of choriocarcinoma: 23 years' experience at Charing Cross Hospital. Cancer 1983;52:1728–1735.
81. Fujiwara R, Mino S, Nagao S, et al: Metastatic choriocarcinoma with neoplastic aneurysms cured by aneurysm resection and chemotherapy. J Neurosurg 1992;76:148–151.
82. Watanabe AS, Smoker WRK: Computed tomography and angiographic findings in metastatic choriocarcinoma. J Comput Assist Tomogr 1989;13:319–322.
83. Nader S: Pituitary disorders and pregnancy. Semin Perinatol 1990;14:24–33.
84. Molitch ME: Endocrine emergencies in pregnancy. Bull Clin Endocrinol Metab 1992;6:167–191.
85. Sipes SL, Malee MP: Endocrine disorders in pregnancy. Obstet Gynecol Clin North Am 1992;19:655–677.
86. Onesti ST, Wisniewski T, Post KD: Clinical versus subclinical pituitary apoplexy: Presentation, surgical management, and outcome in 21 patients. Neurosurgery 1990;26:980–986.
87. Reid RL, Quigley ME, Yen SSC: Pituitary apoplexy. Arch Neurol 1985;42:712–719.
88. Armstrong MR, Douek M, Schellinger D, et al: Regression of pituitary macroadenoma after pituitary apoplexy: CT and MR studies. J Comput Assist Tomogr 1991;15:832–834.
89. Pedersen H, Finster M: Anesthetic risk in the pregnant surgical patient. Anesth 1979;51:439–451.
90. Minielly R, Yuzpe AA, Drake CG: Subarachnoid hemorrhage secondary to ruptured cerebral aneurysm in pregnancy. Obstet Gynecol 1979;53:64–70.
91. Ramanathan J: Anesthetic considerations in preeclampsia. Clin Perinatol 1991;18:875–889.
92. Patterson RM: Seizure disorders in pregnancy. Med Clin North Am 1989;73:661–665.
93. Delgado-Escueta AV, Janz D: Consensus guidelines: Preconception counseling, management, and care of the pregnant woman with epilepsy. Neurology 1992;42(Suppl 5):149–160.
94. Rolfs A, Bolik A: Guillain-Barré syndrome in pregnancy: Reflections on immunopathogenesis. Acta Neurol Scand 1994;89:400–402.
95. Janz D: On major malformations and minor anomalies in the offspring of parents with epilepsy: Review of the literature. In Janz D, Dam M, Richens A, et al (eds): Epilepsy, Pregnancy, and the Child, pp 211–222. New York, Raven Press, 1982.
96. Hiilesmaa VK: Pregnancy and birth in women with epilepsy. Neurology 1992;42(Suppl 5):8–11.
97. Teramo K, Hiilesmaa VK: Pregnancy and fetal complications in epileptic pregnancies: Review of the literature. In Janz D, Dam M, Richens A, et al (eds): Epilepsy, Pregnancy, and the Child, pp 53–59. New York, Raven Press, 1982.
98. Fougner AC, Wilson SJ, Seltzer VL: Status epilepticus in pregnancy: A case report. J Reprod Med 1985;30:948–950.
99. Mendez-Quijada J, Mores AF, Juviano N: Status epilepticus in pregnancy: A case report. J Reprod Med 1990;35:289–291.
100. Grunert GM, Field DR: Refractory status epilepticus in pregnancy: A case report. J Reprod Med 1985;30:69–73.
101. Goetting MG, Davidson BN: Status epilepticus during labor: A case report. J Reprod Med 1987;32:313–314.
102. Skinner HA: The Origin of Medical Terms, 2nd ed, p 149. New York, Hafner, 1970.
103. Redman CWG, Jefferies M: Revised definition of preeclampsia. Lancet 1988;i:809–812.
104. Gleicher N, Boler LR, Norusis M, et al: Hypertensive diseases of pregnancy and parity. Am J Obstet Gynecol 1986;154:1044–1049.
105. Villar MA, Sibai BM: Clinical significance of elevated mean arterial blood pressure in second trimester and threshold increase in systolic or diastolic blood pressure during third trimester. Am J Obstet Gynecol 1989;160:419–423.
106. Donaldson JO: Eclampsia. Neurology of Pregnancy, 2nd ed, pp 269–310. London, WB Saunders, 1989.
107. Richards AM, Moodley J, Graham DL, et al: Active management of the unconscious eclamptic patient. Br J Obstet Gynaecol 1986;93:554–562.
108. Moller B, Lindmark G: Eclampsia in Sweden, 1976–1980. Acta Obstet Gynecol Scand 1986;65:307–314.
109. American College of Obstetricians and Gynecologists: Management of preeclampsia. Tech Bull 1986;91.
110. Scott JR, Worley RJ: Hypertensive disorders of pregnancy. In Scott JR, DiSaia PJ, Hammond CB, et al (eds): Danforth's Obstetrics and Gynecology, 6th ed, pp 411–431. Philadelphia, JB Lippincott, 1990.
111. Sibai BM: Eclampsia VI. Maternal-perinatal outcome in 254 consecutive cases. Am J Obstet Gynecol 1990;163:1049–1055.
112. Pritchard JA, Cunningham FG, Pritchard SA: The Parkland Memorial Hospital protocol for treatment of eclampsia: Evaluation of 245 cases. Am J Obstet Gynecol 1984;148:951–963.
113. Pritchard JA: Management of preeclampsia and eclampsia. Kidney Int 1980;18:259–266.
114. Tso E, Reid RP, Barish RA, et al: Late postpartum eclampsia. Ann Emerg Med 1987;16:907–909.

115. Sheehan HL, Lynch JB: Pathology of Toxemia of Pregnancy. Baltimore, Williams & Wilkins, 1973.
116. Towers CV, Pircon RA, Nageote MP, et al: Cocaine intoxication presenting as preeclampsia and eclampsia. Obstet Gynecol 1993;81:545–547.
117. Lewis LK, Hinshaw AD Jr, Will AD, et al: CT and angiographic correlation of severe neurological disease in toxemia of pregnancy. Neuroradiology 1988;30:59–64.
118. Naheedy MH, Biller J, Schiffer M, et al: Toxemia of pregnancy: Cerebral CT findings. J Comput Assist Tomogr 1985;9:497–501.
119. Kirby JC, Jaindl JJ: Cerebral CT findings in toxemia of pregnancy. Radiology 1984;151:114
120. Crawford S, Varner MW, Digre KB, et al: Cranial magnetic resonance imaging in eclampsia. Obstet Gynecol 1987;70:474–477.
121. Schwaighofer BW, Hesselink JR, Healy ME: MR demonstration of reversible brain abnormalities in eclampsia. J Comput Assist Tomogr 1989;13:310–312.
122. Digre KB, Varner MW, Osborn AG, et al: Cranial magnetic resonance imaging in severe preeclampsia vs eclampsia. Arch Neurol 1993;50:399–406.
123. Sanders TG, Clayman DA, Sanchez-Ramos L, et al: Brain in eclampsia: MR imaging with clinical correlation. Radiology 1991;180:475–478.
124. Raps EC, Galetta SL, Broderick M, et al: Delayed peripartum vasculopathy: Cerebral eclampsia revisited. Ann Neurol 1993;33:222–225.
125. Trommer BL, Homer D, Mikhael MA: Cerebral vasospasm and eclampsia. Stroke 1988;19:326–329.
126. Bogousslavsky J, Despland PA, Regli R, et al: Postpartum cerebral angiopathy: Reversible vasoconstriction assessed by transcranial Doppler ultrasound. Eur Neurol 1989;29:102–105.
127. Sibai BM, Spinnato JA, Watson DL, et al: Effect of magnesium sulfate on electroencephalographic findings in preeclampsia-eclampsia. Obstet Gynecol 1984;64:261–266.
128. Barton JR, Sibai BM: Care of the pregnancy complicated by HELLP syndrome. Obstet Gynecol Clin North Am 1991;18:165–179.
129. Donaldson O: Eclampsia. In Devinsky O, Feldmann E, Hainline B (eds): Neurological Complications of Pregnancy, pp 25–33. New York, Raven Press, 1994.
130. Donaldson JO: Eclamptic hypertensive encephalopathy. Semin Neurol 1988;8:230–233.
131. Richards A, Graham D, Bullock R: Clinicopathological study of neurological complications due to hypertensive disorders of pregnancy. J Neurol Neurosurg Psychiatry 1988;51:416–421.
132. Chesley LC: Diagnosis of preeclampsia. Obstet Gynecol 1985;65:423–425.
133. Sibai BM: Pitfalls in diagnosis and management of preeclampsia. Am J Obstet Gynecol 1988;159:1–5.
134. Byrom FB: The pathogenesis of hypertensive encephalopathy and its relation to the malignant phase of hypertension. Lancet 1954;2:201–211.
135. Hatashita S, Hoff JT, Ishii S: Focal brain edema associated with acute arterial hypertension. J Neurosurg 1986;64:643–649.
136. Ramsay MM, Rimoy GH, Rubin PC: Are anticonvulsants necessary to prevent eclampsia? Lancet 1994;343:540–541.
137. Chua A, Redman CWG: Are prophylactic anticonvulsants required in severe pre-eclampsia? Lancet 1991;337:250–251.
138. Pritchard JA: The use of the magnesium ion in the management of eclamptogenic toxemias. Surg Gynecol Obstet 1955;100:131–140.
139. Sibai BM, Lipshitz J, Anderson GD, et al: Reassessment of intravenous $MgSO_4$ therapy in preeclampsia-eclampsia. Obstet Gynecol 1981;57:199–202.
140. Zuspan FP: Problems encountered in the treatment of pregnancy-induced hypertension. Am J Obstet Gynecol 1978;131:591–597.
141. Lipsitz PL: The clinical and biochemical effects of excess magnesium in the newborn. Pediatrics 1971;47:501–509.
142. Donaldson JO: Does magnesium sulfate treat eclamptic convulsions? Clin Neuropharmacol 1986;9:37–45.
143. Kaplan PW, Lesser RP, Fisher RS, et al: No, magnesium sulfate should not be used in treating eclamptic seizures. Arch Neurol 1988;45:1361–1364.
144. Somjen G, Hilmy M, Stephen CR: Failure to anesthetize human subjects by intravenous administration of magnesium sulfate. J Pharmac Exp Ther 1966;154:652–659.
145. Borges LF, Gucer G: Effect of magnesium on epileptic foci. Epilepsia 1978;19:81–91.
146. Koontz WL, Reid KH: Effect of parenteral magnesium sulfate on penicillin-induced seizure foci in anesthetized cats. Am J Obstet Gynecol 1985;153:96–99.
147. Koontz WL, Reid KH: The effect of pretreatment with magnesium sulfate on the initiation of seizure foci in anesthetized cats. Am J Obstet Gynecol 1989;160:508–509.
148. Hutton JD, James DK, Stirrat GM, et al: Management of severe pre-eclampsia and eclampsia by UK consultants. Br J Obstet Gynaecol 1992;99:554–556.
149. Trudinger BJ, Parik I: Attitudes to the management of hypertension in pregnancy: A survey of Australian fellows. Aust N Z J Obstet Gynaecol 1982;22:191–197.
150. Campbell DM: Clinical experiences and a review of chlormethiazole in the management of pre-eclampsia and eclampsia. Acta Psychiatr Scand Suppl 1986;73:175–181.
151. Slater RM, Wilcox FL, Smith WD, et al: Phenytoin infusion in severe pre-eclampsia. Lancet 1987;i:1417–1420.
152. Ryan G, Lange IR, Naugler MA: Clinical experience with phenytoin prophylaxis in severe preeclampsia. Am J Obstet Gynecol 1989;161:1297–1304.
153. Naidu S, Moodley J, Botha J, et al: The efficacy of phenytoin in relation to serum levels in severe pre-eclampsia and eclampsia. Br J Obstet Gynaecol 1992;99:881–886.
154. Tuffnell D, O'Donovan P, Lilford RJ, et al: Phenytoin in pre-eclampsia. Lancet 1989;ii:273–274.
155. Slater RM, Wilcox FL, Smith WD, et al: Phenytoin in pre-eclampsia. Lancet 1989;2:1224.
156. Lucas MJ, DePalma RT, Peters MT, et al: A simplified phenytoin regimen for preeclampsia. Am J Perinatol 1994;11:153–156.
157. Friedman SA, Lim KH, Baker CA, et al: Phenytoin versus magnesium sulfate in preeclampsia: A pilot study. Am J Perinatol 1993;10:233–238.
158. Crowther C: Magnesium sulphate versus diazepam in the management of eclampsia: A randomized controlled trial. Br J Obstet Gynaecol 1990;97:110–117.
159. Silver HM: Acute hypertensive crisis in pregnancy. Med Clin North Am 1989;73:623–638.
160. Rafferty TD, Berkowitz RL: Hemodynamics in patients with severe toxemia during labor and delivery. Am J Obstet Gynecol 1980;138:263–270.
161. Bhorat IE, Naidoo DP, Rout CC, et al: Malignant ventricular arrythmias in eclampsia: A comparison of labetalol with dihydralazine. Am J Obstet Gynecol 1993;168:1292–1296.
162. Vink GJ, Moodley J, Philpott RH: Effect of dihydralazine on the fetus in the treatment of maternal hypertension. Obstet Gynecol 1980;55:519–522.
163. Dudley DKL: Minibolus diazoxide in the management of severe hypertension in pregnancy. Am J Obstet Gynecol 1985;151:196–200.
164. Hjertberg R, Faxelius G, Lagercrantz H: Neonatal adaptation in hypertensive pregnancy—A study of labetalol vs hydralazine treatment. J Perinat Med 1993;21:69–75.
165. Sibai BM, Gonzalez AR, Mabie WC, et al: A comparison of labetalol plus hospitalization versus hospitalization alone in the management of preeclampsia remote from term. Obstet Gynecol 1987;70:323–327.
166. Stempel JE, O'Grady JP, Morton MJ, et al: Use of sodium nitroprusside in complications of gestational hypertension. Obstet Gynecol 1982;60:533–538.
167. Fenakel K, Fenakel G, Appelman Z, et al: Nifedipine in the treatment of severe preeclampsia. Obstet Gynecol 1991;77:331–337.
168. McCombs J: Treatment of preeclampsia and eclampsia. Clin Pharm 1992;11:236–245.

169. Sibai BM, El-Nazer A, Gonzalez-Ruiz A: Severe preeclampsia-eclampsia in young primigravid women: Subsequent pregnancy outcome and remote prognosis. Am J Obstet Gynecol 1986;155:1011–1016.
170. Kurtzke JF: Epidemiology of myasthenia gravis. Adv Neurol 1978;19:545–566.
171. Plauche WC: Myasthenia gravis in mothers and their newborns. Clin Obstet Gynecol 1991;34:82–99.
172. Hatada Y, Munemura M, Matsuo I, et al: Myasthenic crisis in the puerperium: The possible importance of alpha-fetoprotein. Case report. Br J Obstet Gynaecol 1987;94:480–482.
173. Heininger K, Edler C, Toyka KV: Alpha-fetoprotein and neonatal transient myasthenia gravis. Neurology 1984;34:403–404.
174. Mitchell PJ, Bebbington M: Myasthenia gravis in pregnancy. Obstet Gynecol 1992;80:178–181.
175. Piura B: The association of preeclampsia and myasthenia gravis: Double trouble. Isr J Med Sci 1994;30:243–244.
176. Carr SR, Gilchrist JM, Abuelo DN, et al: Treatment of antenatal myasthenia gravis. Obstet Gynecol 1991;78:485–489.
177. Heine O, Mueller-Eckhardt G: Intravenous immune globulin in recurrent abortion. Clin Exp Immunol 1994;97(Suppl 1):39–42.
178. Lassiter HA, Bibb KW, Bertolone SJ, et al: Neonatal immune neutropenia following the administration of intravenous immune globulin. Am J Pediatr Hematol-Oncol 1993;15:120–123.
179. Benshushan A, Rojansky N, Weinstein D: Myasthenia gravis and preeclampsia. Isr J Med Sci 1994;30:229–233.
180. Cohen BA, London RS, Goldstein PJ: Myasthenia gravis and preeclampsia. Obstet Gynecol 1976;48(Suppl 1):35S–37S.
181. Bashuk RG, Krendel DA: Myasthenia gravis presenting as weakness after magnesium administration. Muscle Nerve 1990;13:708–712.
182. Hurley TJ, Brunson AD, Archer RL, et al: Landry Guillain-Barré Strohl syndrome in pregnancy: Report of three cases treated with plasmapheresis. Obstet Gynecol 1991;78:482–485.
183. Nelson LH, McLean WT: Management of Landry-Guillain-Barré syndrome in pregnancy. Obstet Gynecol 1985;65:25S–29S.
184. Rotman P, Hassin D, Mouallem M, et al: Wernicke's encephalopathy in hyperemesis gravidarum: Association with abnormal liver function. Isr J Med Sci 1995;30:225–228.
185. Bergin PS, Harvey P: Wernicke's encephalopathy and central pontine myelinolysis associated with hyperemesis gravidarum. Br Med J 1992;305:517–518.
186. Fraser D: Central pontine myelinolysis as a result of treatment of hyperemesis gravidarum. Br J Obstet Gynaecol 1988;95:621–623.
187. Peeters A, Van de Wyngaert F, Van Lierde M, et al: Wernicke's encephalopathy and central pontine myelinolysis induced by hyperemesis gravidarum. Acta Neurol Belg 1993;93:276–282.
188. Usta IM, Barton JR, Amon EA, et al: Acute fatty liver of pregnancy: An experience in the diagnosis and management of fourteen cases. Am J Obstet Gynecol 1994;171:1342–1347.
189. Sjögren MH: Hepatic emergencies in pregnancy. Med Clin North Am 1993;77:1115–1127.
190. Amon E, Allen SR, Petrie RH, et al: Acute fatty liver of pregnancy associated with preeclampsia: management of hepatic failure with post partum liver transplantation. Am J Perinatol 1991;8:278–279.
191. Reyes H, Sandoval L, Wainstein A, et al: Acute fatty liver of pregnancy: A clinical study of 12 episodes in 11 patients. Gut 1994;35:101–106.
192. Jordan BD: Maternal head trauma during pregnancy. In Devinsky O, Feldmann E, Hainline B (eds): Neurological Complications of Pregnancy, pp 131–138. New York, Raven Press, 1994.
193. Buchsbaum HJ, Cruikshank DP: Postmortem cesarean section. In Buchsbaum HJ (ed): Trauma in Pregnancy, pp 236–249. Philadelphia, WB Saunders, 1979.
194. Loewy EH: The pregnant brain dead and the fetus: Must we always try to wrest life from death? Am J Obstet Gynecol 1987;157:1097–1101.
195. Lucas MJ, Leveno KJ, Cunningham FG: A comparison of magnesium sulfate with phenytoin for the prevention of eclampsia. New Engl J Med 1995;333:201–205.
196. Sankar R, Licht EA: Magnesium sulfate versus phenytoin for the prevention of eclampsia [Letter]. New Engl J Med 1995;333:1638.
197. Friedman MN: Magnesium sulfate versus phenytoin for the prevention of eclampsia [Letter]. New Engl J Med 1995;333:1638.
198. Duggan K, Macdonald G. Magnesium sulfate versus phenytoin for the prevention of eclampsia [Letter]. New Engl J Med 1995;333:1638–1639.

7

Neuro-Ophthalmologic Emergencies

Daniel T. Laskowitz, M.D. • Steven L. Galetta, M.D. • Eric C. Raps, M.D.

Neuro-ophthalmologic findings may serve as the cornerstone of neurologic and neurosurgical diagnosis, especially in the critically ill or obtunded patient in whom a detailed history and physical examination may not be possible. Subtle neuro-ophthalmologic findings may have exquisite localizing value and often provide the earliest clue of incipient neurologic catastrophe, such as acute hydrocephalus or impending transtentorial herniation. The initial portion of this chapter is devoted to the neuro-ophthalmologic signs and symptoms that are frequently encountered in the emergency setting; the latter part outlines specific entities in which neuro-ophthalmologic findings may play a prominent role in the diagnosis of neurologic emergencies.

A SYMPTOM-ORIENTED APPROACH TO NEURO-OPHTHALMOLOGIC EMERGENCIES

The Abnormal Optic Disc

Detection of an abnormal optic disc is a frequent cause of concern in the acute care setting. Although disc swelling due to increased intracranial pressure constitutes a neurologic emergency that should not be missed, there is a wide differential of less ominous causes of optic disc elevation that should be considered. The most common reasons for abnormal disc appearance include congenital anomalies, inflammatory processes, and ischemia (Table 7–1).

Although papilledema is a term that is often misapplied to any swelling of the optic disc, it should be limited to define optic disc swelling resulting from increased intracranial pressure. Several funduscopic features help to distinguish true papilledema from other causes of disc swelling. Disc elevation from papilledema often occurs first in the superior-inferior axis and is associated with disc hyperemia. Opacification of the nerve fiber layer may cause obscuration of retinal vessels as they leave the disc. Hemorrhages, cotton-wool spots, and exudates are common as papilledema progresses (Fig. 7–1*A* and *B*). Although an inconsistent finding, the presence of spontaneous retinal venous pulsations makes the presence of increased intracranial pressure less likely. Because spontaneous venous pulsations are a dynamic finding, partly reflecting the cerebrospinal fluid (CSF) pressure at the time of viewing, they may be occasionally observed in patients with increased intracranial pressure. Finally, the optic cup is preserved until papilledema is well developed. Papilledema is usually bilateral, although findings occasionally are asymmetric. Visual acuity and color perception are usually preserved until late papilledema, and the presence of an afferent pupillary defect (APD) is uncommon unless markedly asymmetric visual field loss has occurred. Unilateral disc swelling, loss of visual acuity or color perception, or the presence of an APD should suggest an alternative diagnosis, such as optic neuritis or optic nerve ischemia. The most common visual field abnormality of papilledema is enlargement of the blind spot, although inferior nasal defects and visual constriction may also appear early in the course. The presence of other clinical features compatible with increased intracranial pressure, such as transient visual obscurations, morning headache, nausea, ataxia, or abduction deficits, suggest that papilledema is responsible for the disc swelling.

Detection of papilledema constitutes a medical emergency, and immediate neuroimaging studies should be performed to rule out an intracranial mass lesion. In the absence of any structural etiol-

TABLE 7–1 **DIFFERENTIAL DIAGNOSIS OF THE ABNORMAL OPTIC DISC**

CAUSE	HISTORY	FUNDUSCOPIC APPEARANCE	VISUAL EXAMINATION	ANCILLARY DIAGNOSTIC TESTS
Increased ICP (papilledema)	Morning headache, ataxia, nausea, transient visual obscurations	Usually bilateral; disc hyperemia, cup preserved (early), absence of SVP, cotton-wool spots, exudates, blurring of vessels in peripapillary area	No APD, central acuity spared, no color loss, enlarged blind spot, visual field constriction and inferior nasal defect	MRI or CT of head; lumbar puncture (document OP, rule out infection)
Drusen (pseudo-papilledema)	Usually asymptomatic	Glistening hyaline bodies, +SVP, absence of disc hyperemia, hemorrhage or exudate; anomalous retinal vessels with central origination and trifurcations, irregular disc border, absent cup	Irregular peripheral contraction, enlarged blind spot; normal visual acuity	CT or orbital ultrasonography may visualize calcified hyaline bodies
Optic neuritis	History of MS; retro-orbital pain on eye movement, may worsen with heat (Uhtoff's phenomena)	Variable disc swelling (disc appears normal with retrobulbar involvement); Unilateral (adults)	APD; loss of central acuity and color discrimination; central or centrocecal scotoma	MRI for evidence of demyelination; CSF for pleocytosis and oligoclonal bands
Ischemia (anterior ischemic optic neuropathy)	Sudden painless loss of vision; >50 yrs of age; hypertension, diabetes mellitus, history of hypotensive episode	Usually unilateral; segmental disc edema; other eye may show absent cup	Variable field abnormality; often altitudinal; acuity variably affected; APD common	Work up for hypertension, diabetes mellitus, vasculitis (glucose, BP, ESR, RPR)

ICP, intracranial pressure; MS, multiple sclerosis; SVP, spontaneous venous pulsation; APD, afferent pupillary defect; MRI, magnetic resonance imaging; CT, computerized tomography; OP, opening pressure; CSF, cerebrospinal fluid; BP, blood pressure; ESR, erythrocyte sedimentation rate; RPR, rapid plasma reagin.

ogy, a lumbar puncture should be performed to document the opening pressure and to exclude infection. Pseudotumor cerebri, or idiopathic increased intracranial pressure, is strongly associated with obesity, and symptoms may remit with weight loss. Other conditions, including pregnancy, chronic obstructive pulmonary disease, Addison's disease, and treatment with glucocorticoids, tetracycline, or nalidixic acid, have also been reported in association with pseudotumor, although these relationships are less clear. After baseline visual fields are performed, treatment with diuretics, such as acetazolamide and furosemide, may improve headache and visual loss. In cases of progressive field loss, or when visual impairment is severe at onset (i.e., visual acuity less than 20/40), optic nerve fenestration may be indicated.

Congenital disc elevation, which may also be bilateral, is a frequent source of confusion and unnecessary alarm in the emergency room. There are several funduscopic features that may help to differentiate pseudopapilledema, or drusen, from swelling due to increased intracranial pressure. Congenital elevation of the optic disc is usually not associated with cotton-wool spots, peripapillary swelling, or hemorrhage, although the latter may rarely occur. Anomalous discs tend to be small and hyperemic, with an absent or reduced physiologic cup. The retinal vessels may appear to originate from a common point at the center of the disc and have prominent trifurcations and quadrifurcations. The disc margins may appear irregular, and glistening hyaline bodies may be directly visualized (see Fig. 7–1*C*). The presence of spontaneous venous pulsations provide further evidence against increased intracranial pressure. Calcified drusen may be seen on computerized tomography (CT) or ultrasound examination of the orbits. Although obviously not a medical emergency, the presence of drusen is not entirely benign either, and progressive symptomatic field loss and subretinal hemorrhage may occur as the patient ages.

Optic neuritis is another common cause of disc swelling. The patient typically presents with several days of unilateral visual deterioration associated with retro-orbital pain upon eye movement. Symptoms often progress for the first 5–7 days and then begin to improve spontaneously during the next several weeks. On confrontational testing, a central or centrocecal scotoma is the most common field defect. In the optic neuritis treatment trial, computer fields most commonly showed a generalized depression.[1] Central acuity and color discrimination are affected, and an APD is common in the involved eye. Funduscopic examination initially yields normal results in about 70% of patients, because the inflammatory process is primarily retrobulbar. The remainder of optic neuritis patients have some degree of disc swelling. In adults, optic neuritis is usually unilateral, and evidence of pallor in the contralateral eye suggests subclinical demyelinating disease. Approximately three-quarters of patients with multiple sclerosis have optic neuropathy at some point during their illness. Optic neuropathy may be the initial symptom of multiple sclerosis, and approximately one-third of men and two-thirds of women who initially present with optic neuritis have subsequent episodes of demyelination characteristic of multiple sclerosis.[2] The optimal treatment of optic neuritis remains somewhat controversial, with some studies suggesting that oral prednisone may actually be deleterious.[1] At our institution, if there is significant visual impairment or brain magnetic resonance imaging (MRI) shows demyelinating plaques, the patient is offered a short course of intravenous methylprednisolone.

Ischemic optic neuropathy is the most common cause of acute painless monocular visual loss in the elderly population. The most important predisposing factor may be a congenitally anomalous disc with a small cup-to-disc ratio.[3] Ischemic optic neuropathy is also commonly associated with diabetes and hypertension, although atherosclerosis, hypotension, or arteritis may predispose to this condition as well (see Fig. 7–1*D*). The presence of pain should strongly suggest the diagnosis of temporal arteritis. Acuity of the affected eye is variably affected, and an APD may be present. Altitudinal visual field defect with corresponding segmental edema is common. Simultaneous bilateral involvement is uncommon with nonarteritic ischemic neuropathy, and its presence should suggest underlying arteritis or an alternative explanation for the disc edema. At present, there is no clear indication that medical or surgical intervention improves visual recovery after an ischemic event. Certainly, because of the danger of fellow eye involvement, aggressive management of predisposing factors, such as diabetes mellitus, hypertension, and underlying collagen-vascular disease, should be initiated.

In addition to papilledema, congenital elevation, demyelination, and ischemia, there are a myriad of other conditions causing optic disc abnormalities that are beyond the scope of this discussion. In general, infectious etiologies—such as acquired immunodeficiency syndrome (AIDS), syphilis, or Lyme disease—and infiltrative lesions—such as sarcoid, lymphoma, or hematogenous malignancy—should

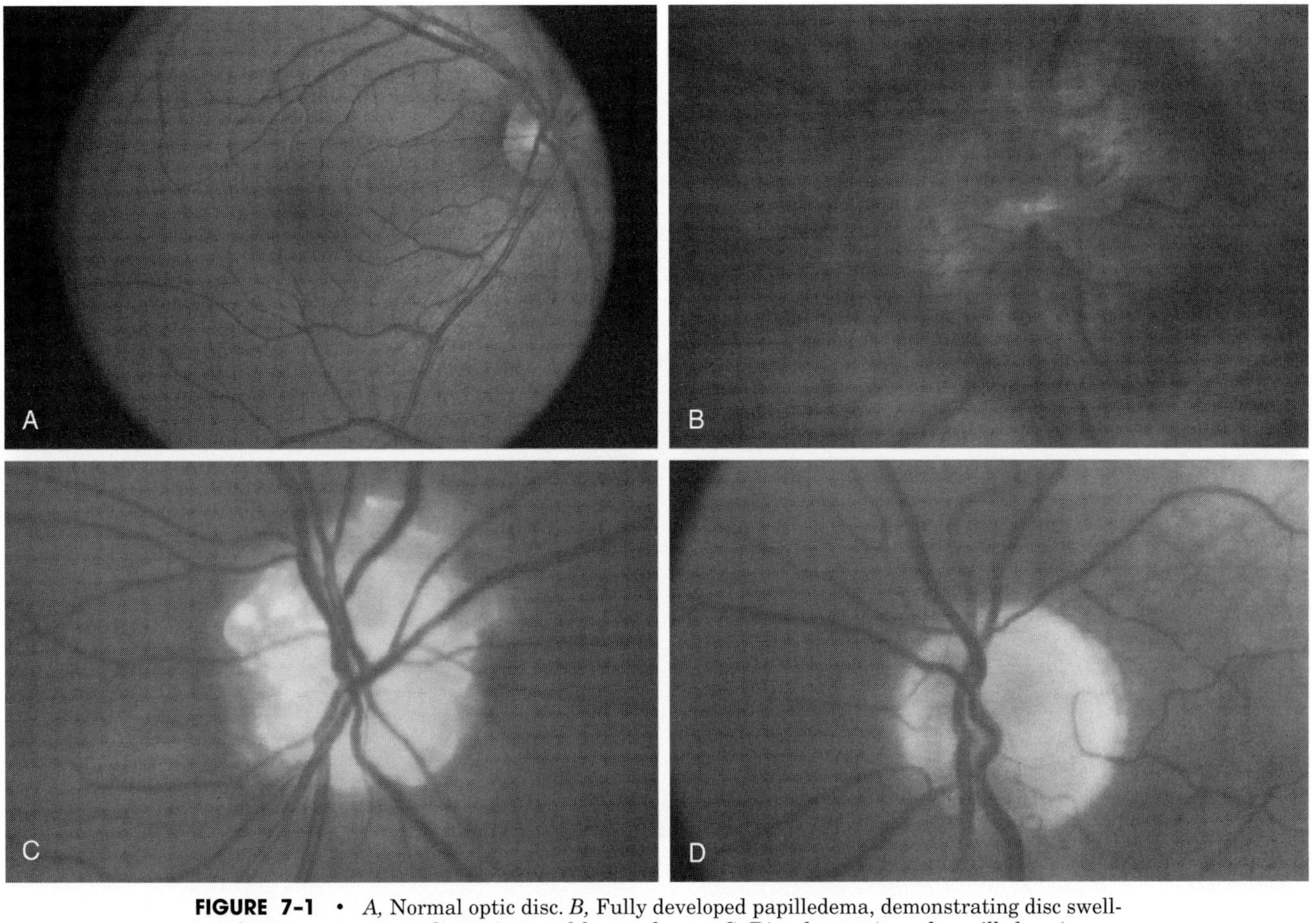

FIGURE 7–1 • *A,* Normal optic disc. *B,* Fully developed papilledema, demonstrating disc swelling, hyperemia, venous distention, and hemorrhages. *C,* Disc drusen (pseudopapilledema): note central origination of vessels and absence of peripapillary nerve fiber layer swelling. *D,* Segmental atrophy secondary to anterior ischemic optic neuropathy. (See color plate.)

be considered in patients with unexplained disc swelling. Certainly, neurologic or neuro-ophthalmologic consultation is appropriate in the patient with disc swelling of unclear etiology.

Visual Loss

The initial evaluation of unexplained visual loss should be directed toward establishing whether symptoms are due to neurologic or optic causes (Table 7–2). The most important test in this regard is the pinhole examination. If acuity improves when the patient looks through a pinhole, there is a high probability that the symptoms are optic and not neurologic. The most common ocular causes of reduced vision are uncorrected refractive error, lens or corneal opacity, and vitreous disease. If there remains a high index of suspicion that the problem is neuroretinal, clues to localization may be provided by careful funduscopic examination, the swinging flashlight test, and visual field testing.

Once it has been established that acuity does not improve with pinhole testing, the patient should be examined for a relative APD. The swinging flashlight test is performed by the brisk and alternate stimulation of the eyes with a strong light source. An APD is present if there is paradoxical pupillary dilation to direct stimulation, establishing that consensual response is greater than direct response. The presence of an APD strongly suggests optic nerve disease, although extensive retinal disease may cause this finding as well. The presence of optic nerve disease is also supported by the presence of decreased color perception and central acuity in the involved eye. Funduscopic examination may also be helpful in revealing retinal or optic nerve abnormalities. The most common causes of acquired disc abnormalities are inflammatory lesions and ischemia (see under The Abnormal Optic Disc). Disc swelling due to increased intracranial pressure usually does not cause an APD or decreased central acuity.

Visual field testing, either by confrontation or formal perimetry, may also provide valuable localizing information. Optic nerve disease most commonly causes central or centrocecal scotomas, although arcuate defects, generalized depression, and altitudinal defects may also occur. Chiasmal compression from parasellar masses classically present with bitemporal hemianopsia, although the visual fields may be asymmetric. Compressive lesions of the anterior chiasm may present in a similar fashion to optic nerve disease, with ipsilateral decreased acuity, central or centrocecal scotoma, and an APD. It cannot be overemphasized that the contralateral (asymptomatic) eye should be tested carefully. If the contralateral superior temporal quadrant defect is not detected, the diagnosis of a parasellar mass may be missed.

Homonymous hemianopsia suggests retrochiasmal disease. Interruption of the optic tract usually causes incongruous hemianopsia (congruity cannot be assessed if the hemianopsia is complete). An APD may be present in the eye with greater field loss. Furthermore, optic atrophy in association with a homonymous field defect suggests a lesion of the optic tract or lateral geniculate body. Lesions of the temporal geniculocalcarine radiations (Meyer's loop) most commonly cause a superior field defect, whereas interruption of parietal radiations causes an inferior field defect. Parietal lesions may also

TABLE 7–2 **CAUSES OF VISUAL LOSS**

LESION	CAUSE	FINDINGS
Optical	Refractive error, media opacities, vitreous abnormalities	No APD; usually unilateral; improvement with pinhole
Optic nerve	Inflammatory lesions (MS, sarcoid); ischemia (atherosclerotic, hypoperfusion, vasculitic); infiltrative/infectious (neoplastic, CMV, syphilis)	APD present; central, centrocecal, arcuate, or wedge field defect with apex at blind spot; disc swelling may be visualized if papillitis is due to inflammatory, ischemic, infiltrative lesion
Chiasm	Parasellar mass (pituitary adenoma, craniopharyngioma, mengioma, aneurysm); chiasmal neuritis	Bitemporal hemianopsia, may be asymmetric; junctional lesion may cause ipsilateral APD, central or centrocecal scotoma and contralateral superior temporal defect
Optic tract	Neoplastic, inflammatory, ischemic, infectious	APD variable; incongruous hemianopsia; "bow-tie" disc atrophy if long-standing
Lateral geniculate	Infarction, AVM, neoplastic	Incongruous hemianopsia, optic atrophy late; horizontal sectoranopsia or quadruple quadrantanopia suggestive of infarction
Optic radiations (parietal)	Neoplastic, inflammatory, ischemic, infectious	No APD; inferior contralateral quadrantanopia; ipsilateral smooth-pursuit abnormalities; spasticity of conjugate gaze
Optic radiations (temporal)	Neoplastic, inflammatory, ischemic infectious	No APD; superior contralateral quadrantanopia
Occipital	Ischemic, neoplastic, infectious, inflammatory	No APD; congruous contralateral hemianopsia; macular sparing and Riddoch's phenomenon may be present

MS, multiple sclerosis; CMV, cytomegalovirus infection; AVM, arteriovenous malformation; APD, afferent pupillary defect.

cause an ipsilateral smooth pursuit defect, which is best observed when the patient is asked to follow an optokinetic strip directed toward the side of the lesion. Another clue to parietal disease is spasticity of conjugate gaze. This refers to the observation that the eyes may deviate superiorly and away from the side of the lesion during eye closure, rather than the normal Bell's phenomenon (in which each eye is usually deviated superiolaterally). Occipital lesions usually cause hemianopsias that are extremely congruous. Macular sparing may be present because of the dual blood supply of the occipital poles, where the macula is represented. Another clue to the occipital lesion is the relative preservation of vision in the hemianopic field when kinetic stimuli are presented, as opposed to stationary targets (Riddoch's phenomenon).

Double Vision and Disorders of Gaze

Double vision is a common symptom of neuro-ophthalmologic disease and has many potential etiologies. The initial assessment should establish whether the diplopia is monocular or binocular. Monocular diplopia is rarely a sign of neurologic disease and is much more likely to be due to refractive error or lens opacity. Monocular diplopia caused by these conditions typically resolves when a pinhole is placed over the affected eye. Monocular diplopia not improved by a pinhole suggests a functional disorder (see later). Once it has been established that the double vision is binocular, the patient should be asked whether the double vision is horizontal or vertical, and in which direction of gaze the two images are most widely divergent. In general, symptoms worsen as the patient looks into the field of the paretic or restricted muscle. Ocular misalignment may be due to palsy of one or more cranial nerves innervating the extraocular musculature, restrictive processes such as thyroid eye disease or post-traumatic nerve entrapment, or brain stem disease causing internuclear ophthalmoplegia or skew deviation. The diagnosis of ocular motility defects may be confusing, and the importance of history cannot be overemphasized. For example, painless diplopia that fluctuates with fatigue should raise the clinical suspicion of myasthenia, especially if ptosis or signs of bulbar weakness are present. Finally, one should try to determine whether the motility disturbance is paretic or restrictive. Forced duction testing, performed by anesthetizing the eye and manually pushing the globe in the direction of limitation with a cotton-tip applicator, determines whether a restrictive process is present, as may be seen with thyroid eye disease or muscle entrapment syndromes.

The third nerve innervates the superior, medial, and inferior rectus, as well as the levator, the pupil, and inferior oblique muscles. A patient with complete third-nerve dysfunction manifests ptosis, a dilated pupil, and an eye that is deviated out and down (Fig. 7–2). The nerve may be damaged anywhere in its course as it leaves the third-nerve nucleus, travels ventrally through the midbrain, traverses the subarachnoid space, and travels through the cavernous sinus to enter the orbit via the superior orbital fissure. Although third-nerve dysfunction has many causes (Table 7–3), this syndrome is most commonly due to aneurysmal compression or ischemia from microvascular disease. Because the former may be life-threatening if missed, a considered approach to the management of third-nerve palsies is extremely important. In general, the most helpful features on initial examination are the presence or absence of other neurologic deficits, the status of the pupil, and the presence of aberrant regeneration.

All patients with new onset of third-nerve dysfunction should undergo a careful neurologic examination, because the presence or absence of other neurologic signs is the single most important factor in determining location and etiology. For example, if the nucleus of the third nerve is involved (because of infarct or an intrinsic brain stem lesion), there usually are bilateral ptosis and weakness of the contralateral superior rectus (the innervation to the superior rectus is crossed, and the levator complex is midline). If the third-nerve fascicle is involved in the midbrain as it passes adjacent to the red nucleus and corticospinal tracts, there may be a contralateral rubral tremor or hemiparesis. Involvement in the subarachnoid space may be associated with other cranial nerve deficits, meningismus, or constitutional symptoms. Compression against the free tentorial edge may occur with impending uncal

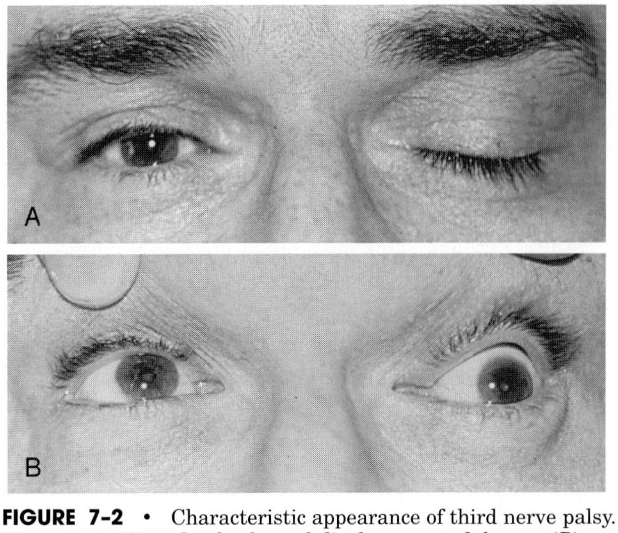

FIGURE 7-2 • Characteristic appearance of third nerve palsy. Note ptosis (*A*) and inferolateral displacement of the eye (*B*).

TABLE 7–3 **DIFFERENTIAL DIAGNOSIS OF THIRD-NERVE PALSY**

DIFFERENTIAL DIAGNOSIS	ASSOCIATED SYMPTOMS AND HISTORY	SIGNS	ANCILLARY DIAGNOSTIC TESTS
Aneurysmal compression	Retro-orbital pain, headache, stiff neck	Pupillary involvement common; aberrant regeneration may be present	Angiography, neuroimaging (if immediately available)
Uncal herniation	Trauma, hemorrhage, neoplasm	Altered mentation, pupillary involvement, ipsilateral hemiparesis	Neuroimaging (MRI, CT)
Vasculopathic	Over age 50 years; DM, hypertension, headache, retro-orbital pain may be indistinguishable from aneurysm	No aberrant regeneration, pupil usually spared	ESR, RPR, BP, blood glucose
Chronic meningitis	Immunocompromised constitutional symptoms, meningismus	Other cranial nerves may be involved	Lumbar puncture, MRI may show nerve, meningeal enhancement
Cavernous sinus neoplasm		Pupil may be spared; CSS	MRI
Cavernous-carotid fistula	Vasculopathy, trauma	Orbital bruit, CSS, chemosis, exophthalmus	MRI, angiography
Cavernous aneurysm	Vasculopathy, trauma	CSS, pupil may be spared	MRI, angiography
Cavernous sinus inflammation (Tolosa-Hunt)	Retro-orbital pain; may be associated with collagen-vascular disease	CSS, pupil may be spared	MRI may document cavernous sinus enhancement
Pituitary apoplexy	Severe headache, meningismus	CSS, ophthalmoparesis (may be bilateral), vision may be involved	MRI, lumbar puncture may document RBC, WBC
GBS (Miller-Fisher variant)	Preceding viral illness; painless	Areflexia, ataxia, extremity weakness	Lumbar puncture, electrodiagnostic studies
Ophthalmoplegic migraine	Adolescent or child; family history of migraine; headache		MRI to exclude other etiologies
Myasthenia gravis	Painless, fluctuates with fatigue; dysarthria	Pupil spared; jaw weakness, ptosis	Tensilon test, electrodiagnostic studies
Midbrain lesion (infarct, tumor, demyelination)	Hypertension, DM, cardiogenic emboli	Contralateral hemiparesis, rubral tremor	MRI
Wernicke's encephalopathy	History of alcohol abuse	Nystagmus, abduction deficit, ataxia, confusion	Improvement with thiamine

GBS, Guillain-Barré syndrome; DM, diabetes mellitus; CSS, cavernous sinus syndrome (may include involvement of cranial nerves IV, V, VI, and oculosympathetics); RBC, red blood cell count; WBC, white blood cell count; MRI, magnetic resonance imaging; CT, computed tomography; ESR, erythrocyte sedimentation rate; RPR, rapid plasma reagin; BP, blood pressure.

herniation. This is usually associated with a change in the level of consciousness, contralateral or ipsilateral hemiparesis, and a history of trauma or supratentorial mass lesion (see under Herniation Syndromes). Involvement of cranial nerves IV, V1, V2, or VI suggests cavernous sinus pathology (see under Cavernous Sinus Syndromes). Visual involvement suggests a lesion at the orbital apex or rapidly expanding parasellar lesion, such as may occur in pituitary apoplexy (see Chapter 18).

Careful examination of the pupil may help distinguish between aneurysmal compression and microvascular disease, the two most common causes of third-nerve palsy encountered in the emergency room. In general, compressive lesions in the subarachnoid space tend to damage the parasympathetic fibers traveling on the periphery of the oculomotor nerve, leading to early pupillary involvement. Vasculopathic lesions, on the other hand, tend to spare the pupil. Patients with clear risk factors for small-vessel disease such as hypertension or diabetes, who are over the age of 50, and who demonstrate pupillary sparing, may be managed expectantly; any pupillary involvement calls for urgent angiography. This rule of thumb has several caveats, however. Patients who initially present with pupillary sparing and a *partial* ocular motility defect may go on to have pupillary involvement; for this reason, they should be observed daily on an outpatient basis for 1 week.[4] Lesions of the cavernous sinus may not cause pupillary involvement. However, because the cavernous sinus does not communicate with the subarachnoid space, a delay in the diagnosis of cavernous carotid aneurysm is rarely life-threatening. The importance of pupillary findings in the setting of third-nerve palsy is discussed more fully under Aneurysms of the Posterior Circulation and Posterior Communicating Artery.

The presence of aberrant regeneration of the third nerve is a useful finding that is frequently overlooked. Aberrant regeneration suggests chronic denervation with reinnervation and misdirection of third-nerve fibers and suggests a slowly growing compressive lesion, such as aneurysm or meningioma. Aberrant regeneration does not occur after vasculopathic injury. Clinically, signs of aberrant regeneration may be elicited by having the patient adduct or depress the involved eye and by watching for lid retraction (Fig. 7–3). Alternatively, retraction of the globe may be seen upon attempted vertical gaze, or pupillary constriction may be seen with adduction.

The fourth cranial nerve innervates the superior oblique muscle, whose action is to intort and depress the adducted eye. Thus, a fourth-nerve palsy results in oblique diplopia that is worse in downgaze, especially when the affected eye is adducted. Patients with acute fourth-nerve palsy may find that diplopia resolves with contralateral head tilt and may unconsciously assume this position. Conversely, exacerbation of diplopia with ipsilateral head tilt suggests a fourth-nerve lesion. The most common cause of acquired fourth-nerve palsy is trauma (approximately 40%), although the nerve may also be affected by microvascular disease or inflammation in the subarachnoid space. Neoplasms rarely cause isolated fourth-nerve palsies. The diagnosis of fourth-nerve palsy requires a certain degree of neurologic sophistication, and undoubtedly the diagnosis is often missed in the acute setting. It is important to distinguish fourth-nerve palsy from skew deviation, another cause of vertical diplopia, because the latter is usually related to brain stem disease (see later).

The sixth cranial nerve innervates the lateral rectus muscle, and sixth-nerve dysfunction manifests as an esotropia, with exacerbation of horizontal diplopia with far and ipsilateral gaze. Sixth-nerve palsies are widely recognized as a nonlocalizing sign of increased intracranial pressure, but a variety of other conditions may produce an abduction deficit (Table 7–4). Trauma, microvascular disease, and neoplasm are the three most common causes of isolated sixth-nerve paresis. As with all motility deficits, associated neurologic signs and symptoms may give important clues as to the location and etiology of the problem. The presence of ipsilateral facial weakness and contralateral hemiparesis (Millard-Gubler's syndrome) localizes the disease to the ventral pons, whereas involvement of ipsilateral cranial nerves V and VII (Foville's syndrome) localizes to the pontine tegmentum. The abducens nerve is also vulnerable as it traverses the subarachnoid space and may be affected in basilar meningitis because of fungus, tuberculosis, or sarcoid. Tumors of the skull base, such as meningioma, chordoma, nasopharyngeal carcinomas, or chondromas, may cause direct compression of the sixth nerve against the clivus. The abducens nerve may be compressed by carotid aneurysms or cavernous sinus neoplasms. The presence of a Horner's syndrome with an isolated sixth-nerve palsy typically localizes the lesion to the cavernous sinus, where the oculosympathetic fibers travel with the sixth nerve for a short distance.

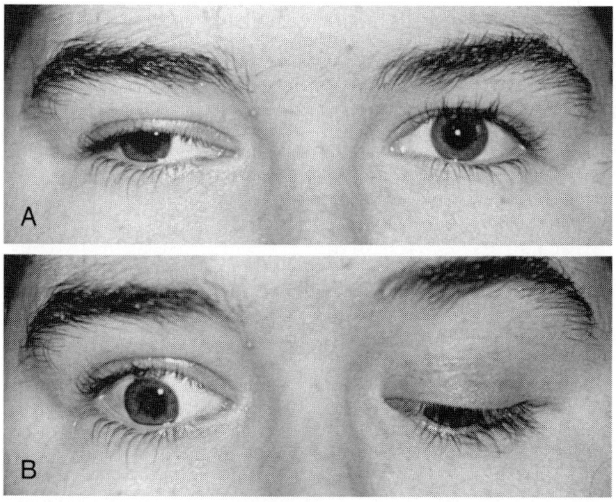

FIGURE 7–3 • *A,* Aberrant regeneration: patient with chronic third nerve dysfunction demonstrates right ptosis in primary position. *B,* There is paradoxical lid retraction when she attempts to look down.

The presence of bilateral sixth-nerve palsy is an ominous finding and should raise the suspicion of neoplasm or increased intracranial pressure. Several entities may masquerade as sixth-nerve palsies, including ocular myasthenia, the Miller-Fisher variant of the Guillain-Barré syndrome (GBS), and restrictive diseases such as thyroid eye disease or medial rectus entrapment. Convergence spasm refers to voluntary convergence, which may simulate bilateral abduction deficits. One clue to convergence spasm is the intermittent and fluctuating nature of the esotropia, because it requires a good deal of effort to maintain. Miosis is also present during periods of voluntary convergence. A benign cause of esotropia is decompensation of a latent esophoria. This most often occurs in the elderly patient after illness or trauma.

Management of isolated sixth-nerve palsies parallels that of isolated third-nerve palsies. If the patient is over age 50 and has risk factors for small-vessel disease (diabetes mellitus, hypertension) but no associated neurologic findings, close observation is appropriate. If the deficit does not improve in 2–3 months, MRI should be performed to rule out more malignant etiologies. There have been several recent reports of sixth-nerve palsies that spontaneously resolved and then recurred because of skull base tumors.[5] Early neuroimaging is prudent for any abduction deficit that follows a chronic or atypical course, as well as those that present bilaterally, or in association with any other neurologic deficit.

TABLE 7–4 **DIFFERENTIAL DIAGNOSIS OF ABDUCTION DEFICITS**

DIFFERENTIAL DIAGNOSIS	ASSOCIATED SYMPTOMS AND HISTORY	SIGNS	ANCILLARY DIAGNOSTIC TESTS
Brain stem disease (infarction, tumor, demyelination)	Vertigo, dysarthria, perioral numbness	Ipsilateral gaze paresis, internuclear ophthalmoplegia, involvement of ipsilateral CN VII, contralateral hemiparesis	MRI
Meningitis (carcinomatous, tuberculosis, fungal, sarcoid, Lyme, syphilis)	Systemic/constitutional symptoms; history of tuberculosis, syphilis, or malignancy; meningismus; headache	Other cranial nerves may be involved	Lumbar puncture; MRI may show enhancement of meninges or nerve
Increased intracranial pressure	Headache, nausea, ataxia	Papilledema, enlarged blind spots; often bilateral	CT, lumbar puncture (?)
Trauma	History of trauma	Battle's sign, cerebrospinal fluid otorrhea, hemotympanum, CN VII or VIII involvement with fracture of middle cranial fossa (petrous apex)	Head (with or without orbital) CT; rule out basilar skull fracture, orbital fracture with muscle entrapment; consider angiography to rule out carotid-cavernous fistula in the case of orbital chemosis, exophthalmus
Microvascular	Over age 50 yrs; diabetes mellitus, hypertension with or without headache	Unilateral, isolated	Rapid plasma reagin, erythrocyte sedimentation rate, blood pressure, blood glucose
Neoplasm	Hearing loss	Involvement of CN V or VII; ataxia, papilledema, serous otitis	MRI
Thyroid eye disease	May be worse in early morning; other signs of hyperthyroidism	Proptosis, restriction on forced duction; lid retraction and lag	Orbital CT to rule out entrapment or mass; thyroid function tests
Wernicke's disease	History of alcohol abuse	Often bilateral; confusional state, ataxia	Response to thiamine
Convergence spasm		Symptoms improve when patient is distracted, fluctuating esotropia, miosis	Oculocephalics
Myasthenia	Dysarthria; symptoms fluctuate with fatigue	May mimic any ocular motor palsy	Tensilon test, antiacetylcholine receptor antibodies, electrodiagnostics

CN, cranial nerve; MRI, magnetic resonance imaging; CT, computed tomography.

Bilateral ophthalmoplegia is a striking finding, which understandably creates a great deal of concern (Table 7–5). Fortunately, relatively few entities produce this motility disturbance. A history of excessive alcohol consumption should be sought, and the diagnosis of Wernicke's disease should be considered, particularly if the associated signs of gait ataxia and confusional state are present (see under Wernicke-Korsakoff). Pituitary apoplexy may cause ophthalmoplegia, because blood and necrotic tissue expands laterally to involve both cavernous sinuses (see under Pituitary Apoplexy). Consideration should also be given to neuromuscular diseases such as myasthenia gravis or botulism (see under Myasthenia Gravis; see also under Botulism). The Miller-Fisher variant of GBS is less common but should not be overlooked (see under Guillain-Barré syndrome and Chapter 13). Brain stem stroke is usually self-evident (see under Basilar Infarction and Chapter 8), but occasionally fulminant GBS with severe axonal involvement may be confused with the acute "locked-in" state.

Skew Deviation

Skew deviation is a vertical misalignment of the eyes that commonly occurs from acute brain stem dysfunction. Occasionally, skew deviation may also result from peripheral vestibular or cerebellar lesions. The presence of other neurologic signs often helps to distinguish skew deviation from other causes of vertical misalignment such as third- and fourth-nerve palsies. For instance, a vertical deviation of the eyes with other signs of pontomedullary dysfunction usually suggests a skew deviation.

The combination of skew deviation with ocular torsion and a head tilt is known as the ocular tilt reaction. This triad of signs is typically observed with lesions of the lateral pontomedullary junction or the paramedian thalamic-mesencephalic region and results from dysfunction of the utricular pathways that begin in the labyrinths and terminate in the rostral brain stem.[6] Although the exact neuroanatomic pathways that mediate the ocular tilt reaction or its component skew deviation remain uncer-

TABLE 7–5 **COMMON CAUSES OF BILATERAL OPHTHALMOPARESIS**

DIFFERENTIAL DIAGNOSIS	ASSOCIATED SYMPTOMS AND HISTORY	SIGNS	ANCILLARY DIAGNOSTIC TESTS
Pituitary apoplexy	Severe headache, menigismus	CN IV, V1, V2, or VI involvement (may be bilateral); visual loss may be present	MRI, lumbar puncture
Myasthenia gravis	Painless, fluctuates with fatigue, dysarthria	Pupil spared; signs of bulbar weakness, ptosis	Tensilon test, electrodiagnostic studies, antiacetylcholine receptor antibody
Botulism	May be associated with GI symptoms: anorexia, nausea, vomiting	Dilated, unreactive pupil, bradycardia, constipation	Electrodiagnostic studies; serum bioassay
Wernicke's encephalopathy	History of alcohol abuse	Nystagmus, ataxia, confusional state, physical stigmata of long-term ethanol abuse	Improvement with thiamine
Guillain-Barré syndrome (Miller-Fisher variant)	Preceding GI or upper respiratory illness	Areflexia, ataxia, extremity weakness	Lumbar puncture, electrodiagnostic studies
Brain stem stroke	History of cardiac arrhythmia, vascular disease	Bilateral long tract signs, skew deviation	MRI

GI, gastrointestinal; CN, cranial nerves; MRI, magnetic resonance imaging.

tain, the localizing value of skew deviation has evolved through clinical and experimental observation[7] (Table 7–6).

Both the utricular and semicircular pathways that regulate vertical gaze synapse in the vestibular nuclei cross the midline to ascend in the medial longitudinal fasciculus. The utricular pathway ultimately connects to the nuclei that activate the four vertically acting muscles—namely, the superior rectus, superior oblique, inferior rectus, and inferior oblique. It should be remembered that the superior rectus subnucleus and trochlear nucleus control the *contralateral* superior rectus and superior oblique muscles, respectively. Thus, a right utricular nerve lesion would result in a left hypertropia as a result of impaired action of the left inferior rectus muscle and the right superior rectus muscle. If the lesion occurs in the medial longitudinal fasciculus, the hypertropia is ipsilateral unless lateral pontomedullary structures are also affected. In this situation, the hypertropia may be contralateral to the internuclear ophthalmoplegia.

TABLE 7–6 **LOCALIZING VALUE OF SKEW DEVIATION**

LESION LOCATION	TYPE OF SKEW	ASSOCIATED SIGNS
Lateral pontomedullary	Contralateral hypertropia	Ipsilateral excyclotorsion; ipsilateral facial numbness; ipsilateral Horner's; lateropulsion
Midline cervico-medullary junction	Bilateral inferior rectus	Downbeat nystagmus
Medial longitudinal fasciculus	Ipsilateral hypertropia	Internuclear ophthalmoplegia
Rostral midbrain	Ipsilateral hypertropia	Vertical gaze palsy; conjugate cyclotorsion

Skew deviation may also develop after selective damage to the posterior or anterior semicircular canal pathways. For instance, injury to the right posterior semicircular canal projections would lead to left hypertropia and right-eye excyclotorsion from impaired innervation to the left inferior rectus and superior oblique muscles, respectively.[8] Damage to the crossing posterior semicircular projections in the dorsal medulla may lead to alternating hypertropia (i.e., right hypertropia in right gaze from impaired action of the right inferior rectus muscle, and left hypertropia in left gaze from disturbed function of the left inferior rectus muscle).[9] Although brain stem stroke and tumors are the most common causes of skew deviation, this motility disturbance may be rarely encountered as a false localizing sign from increased intracranial pressure.[10]

CERVICAL AND SUPRATENTORIAL LESIONS

Carotid Dissection

Carotid dissection accounts for at least 5% of cerebral ischemic episodes in young adults.[11] It is becoming increasingly recognized that dissection of the internal carotid artery may occur spontaneously or after trivial trauma such as vigorous nose blowing, coughing, or chiropractic manipulation.[12–14] Dissection may also occur as the result of hyperextension injuries, which stretch the internal carotid as it passes over the cervical vertebral bodies. When a clear precipitating event can be identified, neurologic signs and symptoms may not develop for hours or even days after the injury. Although carotid dissection usually occurs in the younger patient with no clear predisposing factors, it may be associated with vasculopathies such as Marfan's disease, cystic medial necrosis, syphilitic arteritis, Ehlers-Danlos syndrome, or fibromuscular dysplasia.[15] Of these conditions, fibromuscular dysplasia is the most common association, with carotid angiography suggestive of this disorder in 15% of patients with unilateral spontaneous dissection and perhaps as many as one-half of patients with bilateral dissections.[16]

The most common site of origin for dissection is several centimeters distal to the carotid bifurcation. Blood may dissect within the media or between the media and the adventitia, creating a pseudoaneurysm. In either case, the lumen may narrow sufficiently to cause progressive neurologic signs and symptoms. Dissections usually terminate proximal to the petrous bone, which physically restricts further extension.

The most common manifesting features of carotid dissection are head and neck pain, Horner's syndrome, and symptoms of cerebral ischemia (Fig. 7–4). In a review of 140 cases reported between 1975 and 1982, 79% of patients presented with nonthrobbing ipsilateral head and neck pain, which often preceded ischemic symptoms by 2 or 3 days. This pain was often associated with scalp tenderness. Classic carotodynia, or isolated lateral neck and ear pain, was described by one-quarter of the patients. Ischemic symptoms were also common, with just under one-half of patients reporting transient ischemic attacks in the carotid distribution and one-third progressing to cerebral infarction. One-half of the patient population presented with Horner's syndrome, due to interruption of the oculosympathetic fibers in the pericarotid plexus.[17] Although the triad of headache, Horner's syndrome, and anterior circulation ischemia is classic for dissection, this study also found other helpful signs and symptoms, such as pulsatile bruit (present in one-quarter of cases) and pulsatile tinnitus (present in one-third). Lingual paresis and dysgeusia occasionally occurs as well. Symptoms may also result from artery-to-artery embolization, and episodes of amaurosis fugax,[16] central retinal, ophthalmic artery occlusion,[16, 18] and ischemic optic neuropathy[18, 19] have been described in the literature. Occasionally, patients present with signs of orbital ischemia, including proptosis, motility restriction, injection, chemosis, and optic disc swelling.[20]

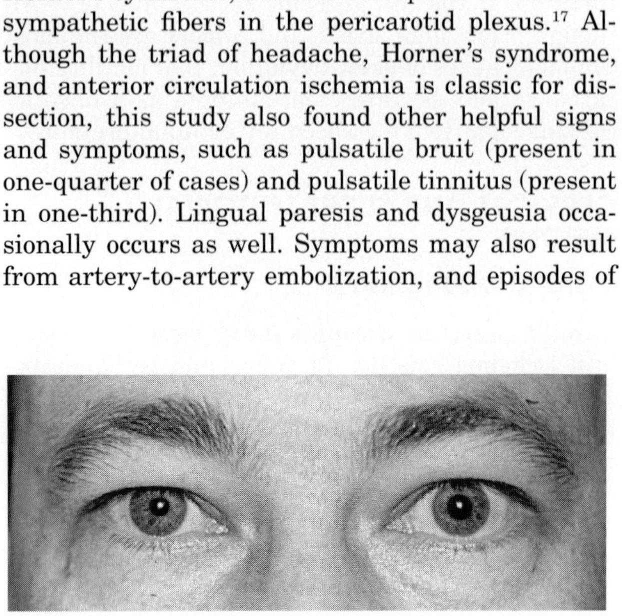

FIGURE 7–4 • Right Horner's syndrome secondary to carotid dissection.

Dissection of the intracranial carotid may also occur, although this is distinctly less common and more likely to be related to significant head trauma. Intracranial carotid dissection is usually associated with more precipitous symptoms of severe ipsilateral headache, signs of cerebral ischemia, and possible subarachnoid hemorrhage.

Management options for symptomatic carotid dissection include anticoagulation, antiplatelet agents, surgical exploration, proximal occlusion using interventional techniques, and observation. None of these therapies has been exposed to rigorous systematic investigation, and one study found complete recovery in 85% of patients regardless of treatment modality.[15] At our institution, symptomatic carotid dissections are initially treated with anticoagulation when not contraindicated. There may be a higher rate of hemorrhagic complications in the treatment of intracranial dissection, and anticoagulation is still controversial in this setting. Long-term therapy is individualized based on serial carotid noninvasive studies and patient course.

Cavernous Sinus Syndromes

Lesions of the cavernous sinus may cause a wide range of neuro-ophthalmologic findings, and knowledge of cavernous sinus anatomy is essential to understand the clinical manifestations of these lesions. The cavernous sinus is a triangular trabecular venous channel located on either side of the pituitary fossa and bounded anteriorly by the superior orbital fissure. The sinus is encapsulated in dura mater and does not communicate directly with the subarachnoid space. The carotid siphon, oculosympathetic complex, and cranial nerves III, IV, V1, V2, and VI pass through the sinus. All of these cranial nerves, with the exception of the abducens, are found in the lateral wall of the sinus, with the third nerve dividing into superior and inferior divisions anteriorly (Fig. 7–5). Under normal physiologic conditions, the cavernous sinus receives blood from the superior and inferior ophthalmic and middle meningeal veins. Venous blood exits posteriorly via the superior and inferior petrosal sinuses or inferiorly via the pterygoid sinus. The two cavernous sinuses are connected medially via the anterior and posterior coronary sinuses.

Distinctive neuro-ophthalmologic syndromes may evolve with cavernous sinus lesions because of the

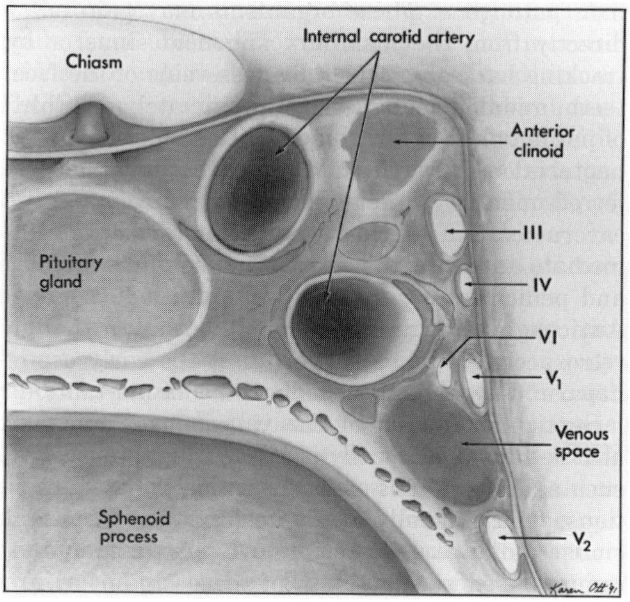

FIGURE 7–5 • Coronal section of cavernous sinus anatomy. (From Galetta SL: Cavernous sinus syndromes. In Margo CE, Hamed LM, Mames RN [eds]: Diagnostic Problems in Clinical Ophthalmology, pp 609–615. Philadelphia, WB Saunders, 1994.)

unique intracranial arrangement of a major artery passing within a venous structure and the close association of cranial nerves. Any combination of cranial nerves III, IV, V1, V2, or VI may be involved with cavernous sinus pathology. Involvement of the maxillary branch of the trigeminal nerve localizes the lesion to the posterior cavernous sinus. Horner's syndrome may also occur because of interruption of the oculosympathetic fibers within the sinus. It is worth noting that the pupil may be spared with slowly growing mass lesions of the cavernous sinus, as opposed to aneurysms of the posterior communicating artery, which usually cause pupillary dysfunction.

Meningiomas are the most common neoplasms originating from within the cavernous sinus, although epidermoids, dysgerminomas, craniopharyngiomas, and chordomas may occur as well.[21] More commonly, contiguous lesions such as nasopharyngeal carcinomas invade the sinus. Intracavernous neoplastic or aneurysmal masses may cause chronic denervation and misdirection of the oculomotor nerve. Signs of aberrant regeneration, such as eyelid retraction with adduction or globe retraction upon vertical gaze, suggest a slowly growing aneurysmal or neoplastic mass lesion. Rarely, a cavernous sinus syndrome is caused by an idiopathic granulomatous inflammatory reaction (Tolosa-Hunt syndrome). This frequently overdiagnosed condition is usually steroid-responsive.

Carotid-cavernous fistulas may present with a dramatic cavernous sinus syndrome. The male predominance of this disorder reflects the increased incidence of trauma in this population. Pseudoaneurysms and carotid-cavernous fistulas occasionally occur spontaneously or after trivial trauma, but this is usually assumed to be due to a pre-existing defect in the arterial wall of the intracavernous carotid or one of its branches. As many as 60% of spontaneous cavernous carotid fistulas are associated with a vasculopathy such as Ehlers-Danlos syndrome, pseudoxanthoma elasticum, fibromuscular dysplasia, or pre-existing aneurysms of the internal carotid artery.[22]

The presentation of carotid-cavernous fistulas may be divided into cranial nerve deficits and local orbital signs. If the fistula drains anteriorly into the ophthalmic vein, the classic presentation of a painful red eye with chemosis, exophthalmus, and arterialization of the episcleral vessels may result (Fig. 7–6). A bruit may be heard over the orbit. Occasionally, collateral flow via the coronary sinus results in contralateral orbital signs as well. The increased venous pressure and reduced ophthalmic artery pressure may also cause venous stasis retinopathy, characterized by engorged retinal veins, swelling of the optic disc, and retinal hemorrhage. Visual loss may occur on the basis of glaucoma, optic neuropathy, or retinopathy.[23] On the other hand, if the fistula drains posteriorly via the pterygoid or petrosal sinuses, or if the vascular abnormality has relatively low flow as may occur with a

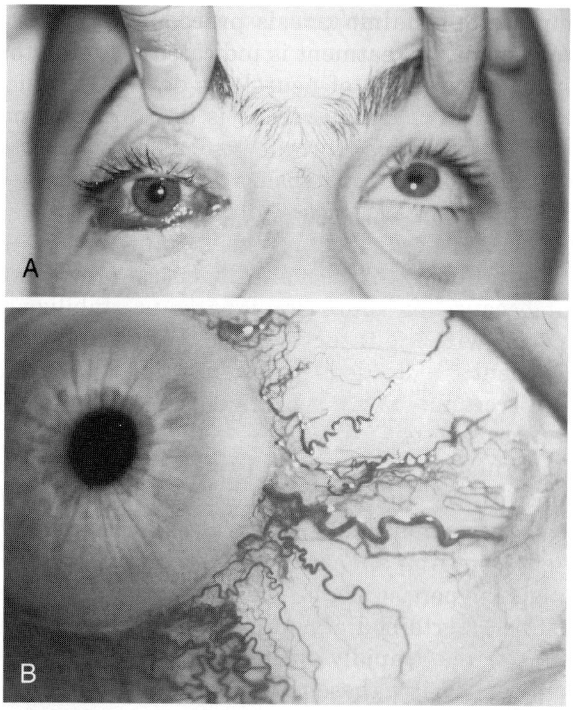

FIGURE 7–6 • *A,* Arterialized conjunctival and scleral vessels, exophthalmos, and chemosis due to orbital congestion from carotid-cavernous fistula. Impaired eye elevation may be from muscle and nerve dysfunction. *B,* Close up of arterialized conjunctival vessels. (See color plate.)

contralateral temporal quadrantanopsia or hemianopsia.[42] Less commonly, a posteriorly projecting aneurysm compressing the optic tract causes a homonymous defect. Afferent pupillary defects and signs of optic pallor are also common ipsilateral to the lesion.[41] The course of visual loss is highly variable. The majority of patients with giant unruptured aneurysms describe slowly progressive visual loss over a period of years, although visual deterioration may be rapid because of sudden aneurysm expansion, rupture, or Terson's syndrome (described later).

The definitive treatment for ophthalmic aneurysms is surgical clipping when a direct approach is possible. Four-vessel angiography is mandatory, because more than one-quarter of these patients have at least one other aneurysm, most commonly on the opposite carotid-ophthalmic junction.[40] Early surgery is indicated for patients with visual symptoms, because the natural history of these aneurysms is to cause progressive visual loss. Although aneurysms at the carotid-ophthalmic junction may have less of a tendency to rupture than those at other locations, surgery is usually recommended at most centers for aneurysms that are larger than 5 mm.[43] When the aneurysm is successfully collapsed, visual recovery may begin immediately, although the course of visual return is variable, and improvement may continue for several years. Overall visual function improves in about one-half of patients, although vision occasionally worsens.[41] In general, preoperative blindness is usually not reversible, and recovery is greatest in those patients whose visual symptoms have been of the shortest duration.[43]

Carotid Bifurcation Aneurysms

Aneurysms at the bifurcation of the internal carotid artery and middle cerebral artery may also manifest with visual signs and symptoms. Carotid bifurcation aneurysms account for 4% of all intracranial aneurysms and usually present in the fourth and fifth decade of life, without sex predominance.[44] In general, they present with the same visual signs and symptoms as carotid-ophthalmic aneurysms due to compression of the ipsilateral posterior optic nerve, chiasm, or tract. The most common visual deficit is an ipsilateral central scotoma, although contralateral temporal hemianopsia may also be present. Rarely, the aneurysms project posteriorly, causing optic tract defects. Definitive treatment is surgical clipping.

Aneurysms of the Anterior Communicating Complex

Anterior communicating aneurysms are relatively common and account for approximately one-third of all intracranial aneurysms. The typical presentation is subarachnoid hemorrhage, although visual symptoms may be present in more than one-quarter of patients.[26] Anterior communicating artery aneurysms usually cause visual loss by producing chiasmal compression.[45] Occasionally, a posteriorly projecting giant aneurysm causes tract compression.[46]

There are several patterns of visual loss in patients with anterior communicating artery aneurysms. Patients may have slowly progressive visual loss due to aneurysm enlargement. As is often the case with slowly growing lesions, the patient may not be aware of the extent of the visual deficit. Rupture of a posteriorly projecting aneurysm may cause precipitous and irreversible loss of vision due to hemorrhage into the chiasm and posterior optic nerve. Acute visual loss may also be due to Terson's syndrome, which constitutes vitreous, subhyaloid, or retinal bleeding in association with subarachnoid hemorrhage (Fig. 7–8). The exact mechanism by which this occurs is unclear, although it has been postulated that it may be due to subarachnoid blood tracking down the optic sheath, or outflow obstruction due to the sudden rise in intracranial pressure causing venous engorgement and hemorrhage. Although Terson's syndrome is most common in association with anterior communicating artery aneurysms, it may occur after subarachnoid hemorrhage from any etiology.

As with all intradural aneurysms, definitive treatment is by surgical clipping when possible. The perioperative morbidity rate is about 25% when subarachnoid hemorrhage has preceded surgery,

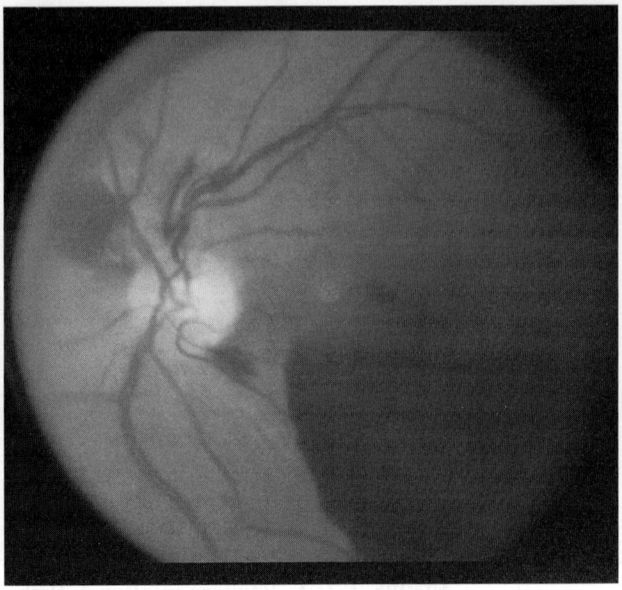

FIGURE 7–8 • Terson's syndrome: subhyaloid "boat-shaped" hemorrhage secondary to rupture of anterior communicating artery aneurysm. (See color plate.)

and only about one-half of patients return to employment.[47] Visual recovery is variable, and patients with long-standing lesions and severe optic atrophy may not demonstrate improvement. Visual loss due to Terson's syndrome, on the other hand, carries an excellent prognosis, and vision may return completely as blood is reabsorbed in the months following the hemorrhage.

Temporal Arteritis

Temporal arteritis is a systemic disease characterized by transmural granulomatous inflammation of intracranial arteries that may lead to sudden and irreversible blindness if not promptly recognized and treated. Temporal arteritis is mainly a disease of the elderly and is rare before 60 years of age. The hallmark of temporal arteritis is inflammation of extracranial carotid or vertebral vessels, and the diagnosis should be considered in any elderly patient complaining of new headaches and temporal tenderness. Jaw claudication and pain in the muscles of mastication may also be a presenting symptom. Diplopia is experienced by 10%–15% of patients and may be caused by cranial-nerve or extraocular-muscle ischemia.[48] Temporal arteritis is associated with polymyalgia rheumatica, a disorder characterized by anemia, elevated sedimentation rate, proximal joint pain, and nonspecific constitutional symptoms of fatigue, low-grade fever, and weight loss.

The first step in assessing temporal arteritis is to evaluate the sedimentation rate, which must be adjusted for hematocrit and age. A good rule of thumb is that the erythrocyte sedimentation rate should be less than one-half the age of a male patient, and less than half the sum of the age plus 10 for women. Although an excellent screening tool, the sedimentation rate occasionally is normal in patients with temporal arteritis, and the gold standard of diagnosis remains biopsy of the superficial temporal artery. The pathognomonic finding in temporal arteritis is transmural inflammation of the vessel. The media often has the most extensive involvement, with multinucleated giant cells, monocytes, neutrophils, and eosinophils. The elastin content of the vessel wall may account for the predilection of this disorder to affect some vessels, such as the ciliary arteries, while sparing contiguous ones. Interestingly, approximately one-third of patients with abnormal biopsies have no evidence of temporal artery tenderness upon physical examination.[49] Unfortunately, skip lesions may be present, and the false-negative rate of biopsy is 5%–15%.[50] For this reason, some authorities have suggested bilateral biopsy to improve yield. Although temporal artery biopsy is the standard, several noninvasive studies may have a role in diagnosis as well. Calculated ocular blood flows of less than 0.6 mL/min via ocular pneumoplethysmography strongly suggest the diagnosis.[51] Fluorescein angiography may also be useful, because patients with arteritis have a marked delay in choroidal filling.[52, 53]

When visual symptoms result from temporal arteritis, they are usually precipitous and permanent. Severe visual loss occurs in one-third to one-half of patients with temporal arteritis and systemic symptoms.[54] Visual loss may be heralded by several days of repeated amaurosis fugax in the involved eye, although in retrospect, symptoms suggestive of the diagnosis usually have been present for several months. The fellow eye is involved within 3 weeks in up to one-third of patients with visual loss.[55] Fixed visual loss is caused by ischemic optic neuropathy in 90% of patients and by central retinal artery occlusion in 3%–5% of the remainder.[48] When visual loss is present, we recommend intravenous methylprednisolone, 250 mg every 6 hours for 3 days, followed by prednisone, 1 mg/kg. Most patients require a daily maintenance dose of 10–15 mg for several years after diagnosis. In a retrospective review, Liu et al. showed that visual improvement is more likely in those treated initially with intravenous steroids over an oral regimen.[56] This latter trend did not reach statistical significance, in part because of the small number of patients included in the study.

Central Retinal Artery Occlusion

Occlusion of the central retinal artery, which is most common in the elderly population, may cause sudden and irreversible visual impairment. Although central retinal artery occlusion is usually caused by atherosclerotic thrombosis or embolization, alternative etiologies, such as arteritis or hypercoagulable state, should be considered as well. Approximately 20% of patients have significant carotid disease.[57] The clinical picture is usually one of sudden, painless monocular loss of vision. When pain is present, it should raise the possibility of carotid dissection or temporal arteritis. Funduscopic examination reveals a pale retina with attenuation of the vessels and a macular "cherry red spot" (Fig. 7–9). Emboli tend to lodge most frequently in the temporal retinal circulation.

Prognosis for visual recovery is poor, because irreversible ischemic damage to the retina occurs after the first several hours. Approximately 20% of patients are fortunate enough to have a patent cilioretinal artery, which may provide sufficient macular perfusion for the patient to retain central vision. Acute intervention is geared toward re-establishing retinal perfusion. Ocular massage, and attempts to

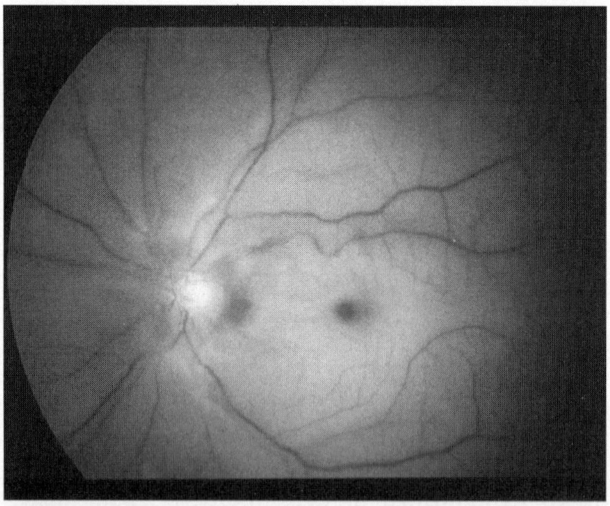

FIGURE 7-9 • Central retinal artery occlusion. Note pale retina, with attenuation of vessels. (See color plate.)

dilate the retinal vessels with carbon-dioxide inhalation, intravenous acetazolamide, and nitrates, have met with only limited success. Paracentesis of the anterior chamber is often recommended during the first 24 hours when more conservative measures fail. A recent study of 14 patients suggested that the selective intra-arterial infusion of urokinase may hold promise when treatment is initiated within the first 6 hours of the event. Four of these patients experienced marked improvement, and five experienced slight improvement as compared with a matched control group of 41 patients demonstrating essentially no improvement.[58, 59]

VASCULAR LESIONS OF THE POSTERIOR CIRCULATION AND POSTERIOR COMMUNICATING ARTERY

Basilar Infarction

Atherosclerotic disease most commonly affects the origin of the basilar artery, and correlates well with systemic atherosclerosis. Basilar occlusion may be heralded by bilateral signs of transient brain stem ischemia, including episodes of intermittent diplopia, dysarthria, bilateral weakness, and dizziness (most frequently described as presyncopal as opposed to true vertigo). Occipital headache may also be present for several days prior to occlusion.

Eye findings may help to establish the diagnosis of progressive pontine ischemia due to proximal basilar occlusion. Unilateral ischemia to the parapontine reticular formation or abducens nucleus causes ipsilateral gaze paresis. When there is bilateral involvement, a complete horizontal gaze palsy, with absent reflex oculocephalic and vestibulo-ocular responses, results. A lesion of the medial longitudinal fasciculus causes an ipsilateral adduction deficit (internuclear ophthalmoplegia). When both the parapontine reticular formation and adjacent medial longitudinal fasciculus are involved, a "one-and-a-half" syndrome is produced. This is clinically defined as a complete horizontal gaze palsy to the side of the lesion and an ipsilateral adduction deficit in contralateral gaze. Signs of oculosympathetic disruption and skew deviation may also be present if there is more rostral involvement of the mesencephalon.

The rostral tip of the basilar artery tends to have less atherosclerotic disease than the proximal and middle section, and occlusion here is more likely a result of embolization. The "top of the basilar syndrome" may result in prominent neuro-ophthalmologic signs due to bilateral ischemia of the midbrain, thalamus, and occipital lobes. The essential features of this syndrome include pupillary abnormalities, vertical gaze palsy, field defects, and changes in level of consciousness. Pupillary size may be variable. The pupils are usually large and poorly reactive to light with a brisk near response due to disruption of the afferent projection from the optic tract to the Edinger-Westphal nucleus. If the Edinger-Westphal nucleus is infarcted, the pupils will be fixed and dilated. Corectopia refers to the eccentric pupils that may be present after midbrain infarction. Occasionally, the pupils are in mid-position and poorly reactive as the result of concurrent sympathetic and parasympathetic pathway interruption.

Skew deviation is common after rostral basilar infarction. Although there has been debate over the localizing significance of skew deviation, it has been suggested that when the lesion extends to the midbrain, the ipsilateral eye will be hypertropic (Fig. 7–10). Upgaze paresis may occur when fibers projecting from the rostral interstitial nucleus of the medial longitudinal fasciculus are disrupted. The patient may also appear to have bilateral esotropia, or "pseudo-sixth-nerve palsy." This is believed due to the disruption of projections inhibiting convergence, although the anatomic substrate has not been clearly defined. Eyelid retraction, when present, is due to damage to the nucleus of the posterior commissure.

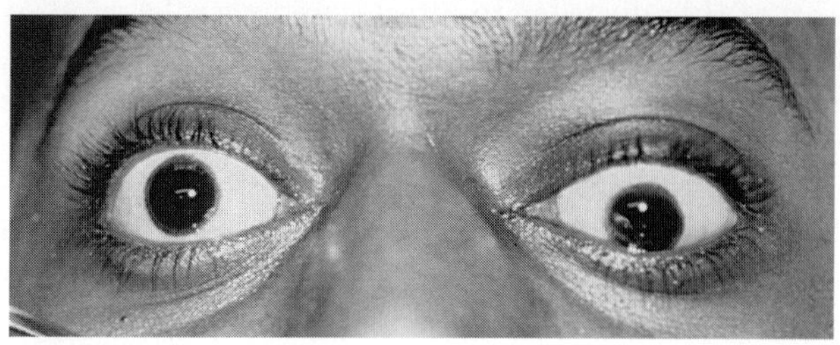

FIGURE 7-10 • Skew deviation after basilar infarction. Note pretectal eyelid retraction.

Hallucinations have also been described following top of the basilar infarction. These hallucinations, dubbed *peduncular hallucinosis,* are primarily visual and often composed of vividly colored, formed objects. These symptoms are almost always observed in patients who have disruptions of their sleep/wake cycle. If the embolus continues to travel distally, it may cause occlusion of one or both posterior cerebral arteries, resulting in unilateral or bilateral occipital infarction.

The sequelae of basilar occlusion can vary highly, depending on the nature of the collateral blood supply. Proximal basilar occlusion may be a catastrophic event, causing extensive infarction of the basis pontis. The resultant destruction of corticospinal and corticobulbar projections may lead to a locked-in state. Because of the potentially catastrophic consequences of completed brain stem infarction, progressive symptoms of brain stem ischemia constitute a medical emergency. Unfortunately, no therapy has been definitively shown to alter the course of evolving basilar thrombosis. Nonetheless, it has been our policy to anticoagulate these patients with the hope of preventing further propagation of clot. Symptoms of basilar ischemia are often perfusion-dependent, and tenuous blood supply to ischemic areas may be maximized by intravascular expansion with crystalloid or albumin solutions. At our institution, several patients have been treated acutely with selective intra-arterial urokinase, with promising results. Unfortunately, because of small patient numbers, it is premature to speculate whether this treatment will ultimately play a role in the management of acute posterior circulation stroke (see also Chapters 8 and 11).

Aneurysms of the Posterior Circulation and Posterior Communicating Artery

Aneurysms of the posterior circulation account for 10%–15% of all intracranial aneurysms; they occur commonly at the posterior communicating artery, vertebrobasilar junction, tip of the basilar artery, and posterior inferior and superior cerebellar arteries.[60] The most common neurologic sign accompanying posterior circulation aneurysms is oculomotor palsy. The third cranial nerve passes between the superior cerebellar and posterior cerebral arteries, and aneurysmal dilation at either of these two locations may cause third-nerve dysfunction (Fig. 7–11). The third nerve may also be compressed by a giant aneurysm of the basilar tip; this is often associated with compression of the cerebral peduncle as well, causing contralateral hemiparesis (Weber's syndrome). By far, however, the most common site of aneurysmal third-nerve compression is at the junction of the posterior communicating artery and the internal carotid artery.[61]

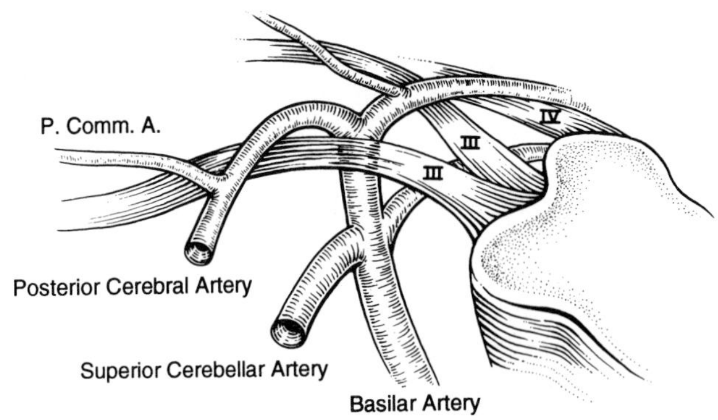

FIGURE 7-11 • Anatomic relationships between the third cranial nerve and the posterior circulation. P. Comm. A., posterior communicating artery; roman numerals, cranial nerves.

Given the potentially fatal implications of missing a cerebral aneurysm, appropriate evaluation and management of patients presenting with new third-nerve palsies is extremely important. In practice, it sometimes is difficult to definitively distinguish a vasculopathic from a compressive third-nerve palsy on clinical grounds alone. Retro-orbital pain of varying severity may be present in vasculopathic third-nerve palsies as well as those due to mass lesions, although the pain associated with vasculopathic lesions usually remits after several days, in contrast with the persistent pain of an aneurysm.

In general, pupillary involvement is an ominous finding and suggests a mass lesion compressing the parasympathetic fibers as they travel on the exterior of the third nerve. In contrast, the pupil is spared in 80% of all vasculopathic third-nerve palsies, probably because the center of the nerve is most vulnerable to ischemia from end vessels of the vasa vasorum. However, up to 14% of posterior communicating artery aneurysms present with a pupillary-sparing *partial* third-nerve palsy.[62] Furthermore, there has been at least one case described of a pupil-sparing complete third-nerve palsy resulting from a basilar aneurysm.[63] As recommended by Trobe, patients who are over the age of 50 years and who present with a pupil-sparing complete third-nerve palsy should be followed medically.[64] Risk factors for microvascular disease are assessed, including hypertension and diabetes mellitus. If spontaneous resolution is not noted within 90 days (as is typical for a vasculopathic lesion), an imaging study is performed. Patients under the age of 50 years receive an imaging study regardless of the status of their pupil, because other lesions are more common in this age group.

Patients who initially present with a pupil-sparing *partial* third-nerve palsy may go on to demonstrate signs of pupillary involvement over time, and close observation is mandatory. It is our policy to bring these patients back on a daily basis for 1 week. If any evidence of pupillary involvement evolves, we proceed to angiography. If the signs and symptoms do not resolve over a 3-month period, MRI of the head should be performed. Whenever a patient initially presents with a third-nerve lesion and any degree of pupillary dysfunction, an aneurysm is assumed until proven otherwise, and the subject should immediately undergo four-vessel angiography. Obviously, "the rule of the pupil" applies only to isolated third-nerve palsies, and a complete neurologic assessment must be performed to rule out any other localizing deficit. One exception to this rule is when patients present with an isolated superior division third-nerve palsy (e.g., ptosis and superior rectus dysfunction). This constellation of signs and symptoms carries a high probability of a structural lesion, usually in the anterior cavernous sinus, and neuroimaging should be performed without delay regardless of the pupillary status.[65]

There has been some debate over the role of magnetic resonance angiography in the management of these patients. In theory, a good-quality study may detect aneurysms as small as 3–4 mm, and most posterior communicating artery aneurysms that present with third-nerve dysfunction are in the range of 9–11 mm. At this point, however, conventional angiography remains the mainstay of diagnosis, and there have been several reports of patients presenting with third-nerve palsies due to posterior communicating artery aneurysms as large as 5–6 mm that were missed by magnetic resonance angiography.[66]

Third-nerve palsies are also relatively common after surgical clipping of posterior circulation aneurysms, due either to surgical manipulation of the nerve or to midbrain infarction. Several clinical features may help to differentiate transient from permanent postoperative third-nerve dysfunction. In a recent study, Solomon et al. found that bilateral ptosis and contralateral superior rectus dysfunction suggested nuclear involvement and correlated with poor neurologic recovery.[67]

Aneurysms of the posterior communicating artery may also cause visual compromise by compression of the intracranial optic nerve, chiasm, or optic tract. Sudden visual loss may also occur after aneurysmal rupture due to intraocular hemorrhage (Terson's syndrome), although this is less common than with rupture of an anterior communicating artery aneurysm.

INTRACEREBRAL HEMORRHAGE

Neuro-ophthalmologic findings may be extremely helpful in the localization and evaluation of intracerebral hemorrhages. Intracerebral hemorrhage accounts for 10% of all strokes, with a mortality rate of 25%–60%.[68] The main risk factor associated with parenchymal hemorrhage is hypertension. Other predisposing factors include vascular malformations, intracranial tumors, vasculitis, amyloid angiopathy, and use of sympathomimetic agents or systemic anticoagulation.

The most common site of intracerebral hemorrhage is the putamen, representing 35% of all cases.[69] Large putaminal hematomas may cause homonymous field defects. A contralateral gaze palsy is often present as well because of interruption of the projections from the frontal eye fields. Significant hemorrhages in this area usually cause dense hemiplegia and sensory loss. Ventricular extension, when present, carries a poor prognosis. Although most basal ganglia hemorrhages occur in the putamen, caudate hemorrhages may occur as well. These hemorrhages, which account for approximately 5% of all cases, may present similarly to rupture of an anterior communicating artery aneurysm. Signs of meningismus may be prominent because of early penetration of blood into the lateral ventricles. In general, involvement of the caudate has a more benign course than putaminal hemorrhage does. There are usually minimal neurologic or ophthalmologic signs after caudate hemorrhage, although mild hemiparesis and ipsilateral Horner's syndrome may be present with larger hematomas. The presence of normal oculocephalic responses may also provide valuable prognostic information. A recent study of post-traumatic basal ganglia hemorrhage showed that patients with normal oculocephalic responses had a 69% chance of good outcome, as opposed to 100% bad outcome in patients with absent responses.[70]

Lobar hemorrhages are the second most common site of intracerebral hemorrhage, accounting for about one-quarter of cases. These are the most likely to be due to predisposing factors other than hypertension, including vascular anomalies or amyloid angiopathy. Neuro-ophthalmologic manifestations depend on hemorrhage location. The most prominent sign of frontal hematoma is contralateral gaze palsy, which may be overcome with caloric stimulation. Acute frontal hemorrhage may also cause forced contralateral gaze. These cases of "wrong-way eyes" are due to the irritative effect of the hemorrhage. Pursuit abnormalities and contralateral inferior field cuts are common after parietal hemorrhage. Subtle pursuit abnormalities may be brought out by directing the optokinetic strip toward the lesion and noting impaired ipsilateral pursuit.

The thalamus is the third most common site of intracerebral hemorrhage, accounting for 10%–15%

of all cases.[69] These lesions may cause a variety of neuro-ophthalmologic findings. Bilateral esotropia (pseudo-sixth-nerve palsy) with downward gaze deviation is most common and is presumably due to loss of projections that inhibit convergence. Upward gaze palsy may also be present, due either to involvement of the nucleus or projections of the rostral interstitial medial longitudinal fasciculus. If the hemorrhage disrupts projections from the frontal eye fields prior to decussation, the eyes will be deviated conjugately toward the side of the hemorrhage, as is usually the case with a supratentorial lesion. If the hemorrhage is located more caudally, disruption of postdecussation fibers may result in "wrong-way eyes" or tonic deviation away from the side of the lesion. Signs of dorsal midbrain compression, including pupillary near-light disassociation, retraction nystagmus, upgaze paresis, and eyelid retraction, may be present after large hemorrhages. These symptoms usually remit after the edema and mass effect resolve. Damage to the lateral geniculate nucleus or proximal optic radiations may result in homonymous hemianopsia. Skew deviation and Horner's syndrome are common findings as well. Neurologic findings frequently include contralateral hemiparesis, hemisensory loss, and aphasia.

The cerebellum is the fourth most common site of intraparenchymal hemorrhage, accounting for 5%–10% of all cases.[71] Patients most often present with the triad of headache, ataxia, and vertigo. Vomiting is also a common symptom. Initially, neuro-ophthalmologic findings may be subtle, although ocular dysmetria and nystagmus may be present. The most common physical findings include ipsilateral appendicular ataxia with decreased tone. The most frequent life-threatening complication of cerebellar hemorrhage is compression of the adjacent brain stem by edematous tissue and blood. The late development of gaze palsy is ominous and may herald impending brain stem compression.

Brain stem hemorrhage is most common in the pons. Classic teaching is that "pontine pupils" are small and reactive. However, in a recent review, this was found to be the case only 21% of the time. Ocular bobbing was a slightly more common finding, occurring in one-quarter of patients.[72] Involvement of either the paramedian pontine reticular formation (PPRF) or the abducens nucleus causes ipsilateral gaze paresis. When the lesion is limited to the abducens nucleus, both ipsilateral voluntary gaze and oculocephalic reflexes are impaired. A slightly more rostral lesion, sparing the abducens nucleus and involving the PPRF, is associated with complete sparing of the ipsilateral oculocephalic reflex.[73] Interruption of the medial longitudinal fasciculus causes an ipsilateral adduction deficit (internuclear ophthalmoplegia). If the adjacent PPRF or abducens nucleus is involved as well, the one-and-a-half syndrome may result. This describes the combination of an ipsilateral gaze palsy and an ipsilateral adduction deficit (the only preserved motility is abduction of the contralateral eye).

Spontaneous mesencephalic or medullary hemorrhage is a rare event and should prompt a search for an underlying cause, such as a vascular malformation or tumor. Like thalamic hemorrhage, mesencephalic hemorrhage may present with features of a dorsal midbrain syndrome, including upgaze paresis, pupillary light-near disassociation, eyelid retraction, and retraction-convergence nystagmus. Bilateral ptosis may also be present because of involvement of the central caudal nucleus of the oculomotor complex. Medullary hemorrhage is also extremely rare and may present with features of a lateral medullary syndrome, including nystagmus and Horner's syndrome. Other features of the lateral medullary syndrome, including ipsilateral facial and contralateral body sensory loss, dysphagia, ataxia, and hiccups, may be present as well.

Initial management of intraparenchynal hemorrhage should be directed toward gentle blood pressure titration and identification and correction of increased intracranial pressure. Most patients are spontaneously hypertensive following significant parenchymal hemorrhage. Although the damaged area of brain may lose autoregulatory control and be directly dependent on pressure for adequate perfusion, it seems clear that significant hypertension may also increase the risk of rebleeding. For this reason, it has been recommended to keep systolic blood pressure below 160 mm Hg and mean arterial pressure below 110 mm Hg. Short-acting beta-blockers and angiotensin-converting enzyme inhibitors have become the preferred agents for controlling blood pressure, because nitrates and calcium channel blockers may cause cerebral vasodilation with a subsequent rise in the intracranial pressure. Patients with increased intracranial pressure should be managed with hyperventilation and osmotic therapy. There is no evidence that administration of glucocorticoids has any beneficial effect, and at least one study documented that administration of dexamethasone may be deleterious.[74] Phenytoin may be administered prophylactically to prevent seizures, especially if the hemorrhage is in a superficial location.

Hemorrhage location is an important factor in determining whether surgical intervention should be considered. Cerebellar hemorrhage may rapidly become life-threatening because of direct brain stem compression or acute hydrocephalus secondary to obstruction of the fourth ventricle. It is widely accepted that surgical evacuation of a posterior fossa hematoma is the treatment of choice for any patient experiencing neurologic deterioration. Some authors have advocated a somewhat more aggressive approach and recommend early neurosurgical intervention for all cerebellar hematomas larger than 3 cm, even in those patients who remain alert.[75] Surgery has less of a clearly defined role in the management of deep basal ganglia, thalamic, or pontine hemorrhages. Although evacuation of the hematoma may be considered in the rapidly deteriorating patient, there is scant evidence to suggest that these patients do better than those managed conservatively. The appropriate management of lobar hemorrhage also remains controversial, because these lesions are more superficial and may be more amenable to neurosurgical intervention. Initial medical management of lobar hemorrhage is usually directed toward preventing increases in intracranial pressure and maximizing perfusion via blood pressure control. Surgery should be considered for those patients who demonstrate evidence of neurologic deterioration despite maximal medical therapy. Clearly, however, waiting too long in the moribund patient offsets any potential advantages of surgical evacuation. Noncommunicating hydrocephalus due to obstruction of the fourth ventricle by clot or mass effect is another complication of parenchymal hemorrhage and may necessitate emergent ventriculostomy placement. Hydrocephalus is more common after basal ganglia, thalamic, or posterior fossa hemorrhage and may be heralded by early eye findings (see next section).

INCREASED INTRACRANIAL PRESSURE

Hydrocephalus

Neuro-ophthalmologic signs and symptoms may provide early clues to the diagnosis of impending hydrocephalus. Characteristic ocular motility, pupillary, and visual findings are often present before any radiologic evidence of ventriculomegaly. Knowledge of these eye findings may aid in the recognition of early hydrocephalus or impending shunt failure.

Features of the dorsal midbrain syndrome are the most sensitive and consistent neuro-ophthalmologic findings in early hydrocephalus. As mentioned previously, this syndrome consists of upgaze paresis, pupillary near-light dissociation, eyelid retraction, and convergence-retraction nystagmus. In the unshunted patient, other etiologies of midbrain compression must be considered, including neoplasms of the pineal (most commonly pinealoma) and aneurysms in the vein of Galen. The earliest feature of this syndrome is usually pupillary dysfunction, with loss of reaction to light and a spared near response. Upgaze paresis may then develop. In its most subtle form, the patient may be able to generate an initial upward saccade, only to have the eyes drift downward. This drift is followed by a corrective upward phase. Smooth pursuit is often affected last, and some patients who are unable to generate vertical saccades may still be able to track objects upward. Eventually, complete upgaze paresis may ensue.[76] Other features of the dorsal midbrain syndrome include pathologic eyelid retraction (Collier's sign) and convergence-retraction nystagmus. This latter feature describes the periodic retraction of the eyes into the orbits. This is best appreciated by viewing the patient on the side while having him or her track a downward-moving optokinetic strip. It is important to emphasize that the features of the dorsal midbrain syndrome are sensitive indicators of shunt failure and may precede any radiographic evidence of ventricular dilation.

Ocular motility deficits may also occur in the setting of early hydrocephalus. It is commonly recognized that unilateral or bilateral abduction deficits may be seen as a nonlocalizing sign of increased intracranial pressure due to downward displacement of the brain stem and stretching of the sixth cranial nerve. Mild bilateral abduction deficits may present as divergence insufficiency, with patients complaining of horizontal diplopia at distance. Fourth-nerve dysfunction, although much less common, has been reported in early shunt failure or hydrocephalus even before any changes are noted radiographically.[77] In a recent series of bilateral fourth-nerve palsies secondary to hydrocephalus, it was suggested that the mechanism was compression of the superior medullary velum by a dilated suprapineal recess.[78] Although there have been rare reports of third-nerve dysfunction in the setting of hydrocephalus, this is distinctly uncommon and should prompt a search for other etiologies.

Visual loss in the setting of increased intracranial pressure is relatively common and usually results from optic disc swelling. Papilledema characteristically causes enlarged blind spots, which may progress to inferior nasal arcuate defects and paracentral scotomas. Loss of central vision is a late finding. It appears as though the rate at which intracranial pressure rises may play a role in how well the optic disc swelling is tolerated. Perhaps for this reason, shunt failure may cause precipitous visual deterioration, with reports of complete blindness occurring even before any overt evidence of optic disc swelling.

Although papilledema is the most common cause of visual loss in hydrocephalus, unilateral and bilateral occipital infarction has also been reported after shunt failure. This is most likely due to compression of the proximal posterior cerebral arteries as they cross the tentorium.[79] Characteristic homonymous hemianopsias, often with sparing of macular vision, result from occipital infarction. Occasionally, bitemporal hemianopsia is due to compression of the chiasm superiorly by a dilated third ventricle.

Recovery of vision following decompression may vary highly. Although return of function is greatest in the weeks and months following decompression, there have been reports of visual recovery as late as 14 months after shunting. Ironically, shunting rarely is associated with further visual deterioration.[80] Although the mechanism by which this occurs is not understood, several reports have documented optic nerve dysfunction after a rapid decrease in intracranial pressure. Visual loss and motility deficits are uncommon in association with normal pressure hydrocephalus, and when they are present, another etiology should be sought.

Herniation Syndromes

The importance of monitoring the neuro-ophthalmologic examination in the critical care setting cannot be overemphasized, because the subtle progression of eye findings may herald a neurologic catastrophe such as compartmental herniation. Several patterns of cerebral herniation have been described. Subfalcian herniation refers to herniation of the cingulate gyrus under the falx. This is often accompanied by occlusion of the ipsilateral anterior cerebral artery, with ipsilateral gaze deviation and contralateral lower limb weakness. Eye findings may also be a sensitive predictor of impending central, uncal, or upward herniation.

Central transtentorial herniation is usually caused by a centrally placed mass lesion or diffuse swelling displacing the hemispheres downward. At its earliest stages, compression of diencephalic structures may cause the patient to become progressively lethargic, apathetic, and confused. Initially, the pupils are small and reactive, and oculocephalic reflexes are present. Roving conjugate or disconjugate eye movement may be present, indicating structural integrity of the midbrain. As hemispheric function and consciousness become progressively impaired, the oculocephalic reflex may become easier to elicit, although the rapid phase of nystagmus may be diminished or absent. The loss of reflexive upgaze is an ominous sign and suggests compression of the diencephalic pretectal area against the posterior tentorial incisura. Accompanying these eye findings, the patient may demonstrate extensor plantar responses, paratonia, ipsilateral decortication, and contralateral decerebration. It is important not to miss these early signs of central herniation, because they represent a reversible lesion; if missed, the patient is increasingly likely to suffer permanent neurologic deficit.

As rostral-caudal compression proceeds in the central syndrome, pupils dilate to midposition because of sympathetic and parasympathetic dysfunction. As the midbrain becomes progressively involved, the pupils may become irregular in shape. Reflex eye movements may become increasingly difficult to elicit, and transient internuclear ophthalmoplegia may occur. These eye findings are often accompanied by midbrain hyperventilation and decerebrate rigidity. As caudal brain stem compression evolves, autonomic dysregulation and death may occur. Pupils may dilate secondary to anoxia and circulating catecholamines but are at midposition at death.

The syndrome of uncal herniation is usually caused by a temporal lobe lesion that shifts the uncus medially and downward until it herniates over the tentorium, compressing the midbrain. The earliest sign of impending uncal herniation is a unilaterally dilated pupil secondary to compression of the parasympathetic fibers traveling on the periphery of the third nerve against the free tentorial edge. Initially, the patient may have no associated signs or symptoms except for moderate anisocoria with sluggish reaction to light. Because the diencephalon may be spared, the patient may initially be surprisingly alert. It is extremely important to recognize the early signs of uncal herniation, because permanent neurologic impairment and death may occur rapidly. As the syndrome progresses, the entire third nerve becomes dysfunctional. This is often associated with a rapid decrement in the level of consciousness and signs of contralateral or ipsilateral hemiplegia and extensor plantar response (due to ipsilateral or contralateral compression of the cerebral peduncle, respectively). The oculovestibular response may then disappear as the midbrain becomes ischemic. Eventually, bilateral pupillary dilation develops.

Both central transtentorial and uncal herniation may cause compression or kinking of the posterior cerebral artery against the free edge of the tentorium, resulting in unilateral or bilateral occipital infarction. When flow through the posterior cerebral artery is compromised because of herniation, superior visual field defects may be most prominent.[81] Unfortunately, it is often difficult to test visual fields in the acute setting because of the depressed level of consciousness. When reproducible testing to confrontation is possible, the Riddoch phenomenon may help to localize the field cut to the occipital lobe.[82] This refers to the finding that in occipital lesions, moving targets may be appreciated better than stationary targets when presented to the blind hemifield. Thus, by testing fields with wiggling fingers, one may miss an occipital lesion. In patients who have recovered sufficiently from transtentorial herniation to allow formal visual field testing, bilateral homonymous hemianopsia with macular sparing secondary to bioccipital infarction has been reported. The phenomenon of macular sparing is most probably caused by preservation of blood supply to the occipital pole by the middle cerebral artery. Hemorrhagic occipital infarcts are not uncommon and may result from secondary conversion of a bland infarct or obstruction of venous drainage from the calcarine cortex.[83]

Upward cerebellar herniation is a relatively uncommon syndrome that may result from tumor, infarct, or hemorrhage of the posterior fossa. This syndrome is usually associated with premonitory symptoms of headache, nausea, vomiting, and vertigo. As pontine compression occurs, abnormalities of ipsilateral gaze may develop, followed by an ipsilateral peripheral seventh-nerve palsy.

NEUROMUSCULAR EMERGENCIES

Guillain-Barré Syndrome

GBS is an acute inflammatory polyneuropathy that may rapidly progress to profound weakness and respiratory compromise. Although the cause is unknown, there is mounting evidence to support an autoimmune basis for this disease. Approximately two-thirds of afflicted patients give a history of trivial gastrointestinal or respiratory illness several weeks prior to symptom onset. GBS may also follow surgery, and the incidence is increased in patients with lymphoma, Hodgkin's disease, and systemic lupus.[84]

The most common clinical presentation of GBS is ascending weakness that progresses in a length-dependent fashion. Reflexes are lost early, and sensory symptoms may be variably present as well. Proximal back, limb girdle, and neck pain is not uncommon and most probably represents proximal nerve root inflammation. Symptoms peak at 10–14 days, and approximately one-third of patients need ventilatory assistance at some point in their course.

Although the motor, sensory, and autonomic dysfunction associated with GBS are well known, neuro-ophthalmologic signs and symptoms are often overlooked. In 1956, Fisher described a variant of GBS in which the primary features were ophthalmoplegia, areflexia, and ataxia.[85] Fisher's syndrome may occur in up to 5% of patients with GBS[86] and should always be considered when a patient presents with bilateral ophthalmoparesis, especially if the reflexes are absent. Typically, patients with Fisher's syndrome initially develop horizontal diplopia because of bilateral abduction deficits. Over the next several days, this may progress to complete ophthalmoparesis, and signs and symptoms of gait and limb ataxia may be noted.[86] Eye movement abnormalities may also accompany more typical cases of GBS; a prospective study demonstrated that over one-quarter of patients diagnosed at the Massachusetts General Hospital had some degree of ophthalmoparesis.[86] According to Ropper et al,[86] the most common limitation of eye movement is symmetric sixth-nerve palsy, with subjective diplopia at distance. Ptosis is usually present as well. Interestingly, Bell's phenomenon may be preserved even after upgaze is lost, suggesting a supernuclear mechanism.[87] Occasionally, patients present with isolated third- or sixth-nerve palsies without evidence of extremity weakness.[88] This may represent a variant of the Fisher's syndrome.

Pupillary abnormalities are relatively common as well and usually occur in the setting of ophthalmoparesis. The most common pupillary abnormality is a round dilated pupil with poor light reactivity.[86] Near-light dissociation may be present as well, especially during the recovery phase. Ptosis is common in the paretic eye and occasionally precedes weakness. Patients presenting with ptosis and mild motility disturbances as the initial signs occasionally are misdiagnosed as having myasthenia gravis. One clinical difference is that, even in the setting of facial diapiresis, the muscles of mastication are relatively spared in GBS and prominently involved in myasthenia. Lid lag occasionally occurs in GBS as well, although the cause of this is not entirely clear. Optic disc swelling has also been reported because of increased intracranial pressure. This complication, which should be considered in the patient complaining of headache and visual disturbance, usually occurs during the third week and is often associated with a high CSF protein.

The clinical diagnosis of GBS is confirmed by albuminocytologic disassociation in the CSF and electrodiagnostic studies. CSF protein is usually normal during the first few days of illness and slowly rises over the next several weeks to peak at 4–6 weeks. Occasionally, CSF protein remains normal throughout the illness.[89] The CSF is usually acellular, although this may not be the case when GBS occurs in the setting of AIDS. Electrodiagnostic studies demonstrate reduction in conduction velocity and block in motor nerves. Prolonged distal latencies, and the absence of F waves, reflecting proximal nerve root involvement, may be present as well.

The management of GBS is mostly supportive, and patients should be monitored closely early in the illness for signs of respiratory compromise. Plasmapheresis has been documented to reduce the length of hospitalization and necessity for mechanical ventilation when instituted within 2 weeks of symptom onset.[90] Intravenous gamma-globulin may also have a role in the treatment of GBS, especially in patients who are too unstable to undergo plasmapheresis. Although early studies have suggested that intravenous gamma-globulin may be as effective as plasmapheresis, other authors have raised concerns over the possibility of increased rates of relapse with this form of therapy.[91] In general, the prognosis is excellent, and approximately 85% of patients make a full recovery. Ten percent are left with significant residual deficit, and there is a 3% mortality rate. The most important prognostic factors in the acute setting are the patient's age, the degree of respiratory compromise, and the presence or absence of widespread denervation and severely reduced amplitudes of muscle action potentials.[84]

Myasthenia Gravis

Myasthenia gravis is an autoimmune disease characterized by fluctuating weakness due to impaired cholinergic transmission at the neuromuscular junction. This is believed to be due to binding of circulating antibodies to postsynaptic receptors. Myasthenia is associated with a bimodal pattern of onset, with a peak incidence in women between the ages of 20 and 30 years and men between the sixth and seventh decades of life.

The levator palpebrae and extraocular muscles are extremely vulnerable in myasthenia, and over 90% of patients have signs of extraocular motor palsies and ptosis at diagnosis. For this reason, myasthenia should always be considered in the differential diagnosis of diplopia, especially when there is a history of fluctuating symptoms that worsen with fatigue or show diurnal variation. When signs and symptoms are limited to the extraocular muscles for 1 year, there is a greater than 80% chance that progression to systemic involvement will not occur.[92] On the other hand, exacerbation of ocular weakness may herald potentially life-threatening progressive systemic involvement. Bulbar and facial weakness may also be prominent, and symptoms of dysphagia, dysarthria with nasal speech, and difficulty with mastication are common. Systemic involvement of myasthenia usually involves the shoulder and pelvic girdles, as well as neck flexors. When the diaphragm and accessory respiratory muscles become involved, the patient may experience respiratory failure necessitating emergent ventilatory support. Several studies have suggested that the danger of death is greatest in the year following diagnosis.[93]

The clinical presentation of fluctuating ocular, bulbar, and facial weakness should immediately raise the clinical suspicion of myasthenia gravis. Cogan's lid twitch sign may also be helpful in attributing ptosis to myasthenia. This sign is elicited by having the patient maintain downward gaze for 10 seconds and then quickly look up to a target at eye level. The sign is present if the previously ptotic lid overshoots, causing the momentary appearance of eyelid retraction before it settles down to the original ptotic position.[94] If there is a consistent deficit or easily fatigable muscle group, prompt and dramatic improvement with intravenous administration of edrophonium also strongly suggests the diagnosis. Antibodies directed against the acetylcholine receptor are present in 85%–90% of cases with generalized myasthenia and in 60% of patients whose signs and symptoms are associated with the ocular muscles.[95] Electrodiagnostic studies may also help to confirm the diagnosis. Characteristically, a decremental response in the amplitude of the compound muscle action potential occurs during stimulation at 3 Hz/sec. The finding of jitter, or variability of successive discharges from a single fiber, is sensitive for disease at the neuromuscular junction, but the process is time-consuming and should be performed by a skilled electromyographer.

Anticholinesterase agents remain the mainstay in the symptomatic treatment of myasthenia. Pyridostigmine is the most commonly used drug and is usually begun at a dose of 0.8–0.9 mg/kg twice daily. The dose may be titrated upward to 1.6–1.8 mg/kg every 3 hours. Symptoms of cramping and excessive salivation are not unusual, and judicious use of a peripheral anticholinergic agent such as glycopyrrolate may be beneficial. When the response to anticholinesterase agents is inadequate, a trial of corticosteroids is warranted. It should be kept in mind that prednisone may initially exacerbate the symptoms of myasthenia, and all unstable patients should be hospitalized for the initiation of therapy. Ideally, steroids should be given on alternating days and tapered once remission is induced. In patients with purely ocular myasthenia, one can often safely begin prednisone, 0.15 mg/kg every other day, with 0.15 mg/kg increments every 4–5 days on an outpatient basis. Once the ocular signs and symptoms have stabilized, the dose may be slowly tapered. However, most patients require a maintenance dose of 0.3 mg/kg every other day. In generalized patients with inadequate response to steroids and anticholinesterase agents, immunosuppression with azathioprine or cyclophosphamide may be attempted. Azathioprine is also commonly used as a steroid-sparing agent. Thymectomy may also be beneficial and is recommended in the 10% of patients with thymoma and in all postpubescent generalized myasthenic patients under the age of 60 years with inadequate response to medical therapy. Approximately one-third of patients experience remission after thymectomy, and another 45% show some clinical response.[96]

In acute myasthenic exacerbation, close monitoring of respiratory status is essential, because patients may undergo rapid deterioration and require ventilatory support. Plasmapheresis may induce temporary remission and is useful both in the setting of myasthenic crisis and in preoperative care. There is growing evidence that intravenous immunoglobulin (usually given in the dosage of 0.4 mg/kg for 5 days) may be beneficial in the acute setting as well.

Botulism

Botulism is a disorder of neuromuscular transmission caused by the exotoxin of *Clostridium botulinum.* The disease is food-borne and usually associated with home-preserved vegetables. Although outbreaks have been reported throughout the United States, it is much more common in the western portion of the country. Botulinum toxin is believed to interfere with the presynaptic release of acetylcholine, although the mechanism is not completely understood.

In the typical course of botulism, symptoms appear during the first several days after ingesting contaminated food. Prodromal gastrointestinal symptoms, including nausea, vomiting, and anorexia, may be present, but this is not always the case. Eye findings are usually the first sign of neurologic involvement and include intermittent extraocular muscle weakness, ptosis, and poorly reactive dilated pupils. Other signs of defective cholinergic transmission include dry mouth, urinary retention, orthostatic hypotension, and constipation. Neurologic deterioration usually occurs over the first 48–72 hours and may involve progressive bulbar and extremity weakness. The muscles of respiration may become involved as well; before supportive care was readily available, mortality rates of greater than 50% were usually due to respiratory compromise. In severe cases, weakness may progress to flaccid paralysis.

The initial findings of diplopia and ptosis, with signs of intermittent extraocular muscle and bulbar weakness, may cause the misdiagnosis of myasthenia gravis. One helpful distinction is that the pupils are poorly reactive in botulism. Occasionally, progressive weakness and loss of deep tendon reflexes may mimic GBS. In distinction to GBS, patients with botulism have normal CSF protein and no sensory involvement. The diagnosis of botulism may be confirmed by nerve conduction studies, which demonstrate an increase in amplitude with rapid repetitive stimulation (similar to the findings in Lambert-Eaton's myasthenic syndrome).

Treatment of patients with botulism is largely supportive. Respiratory involvement usually occurs during the first week of illness, and patients with progressive neurologic signs and symptoms should be placed under close observation. Trivalent antiserum should also be administered as soon as the diagnosis is clinically suspected. Full recovery may take weeks or months, with ocular motility usually showing the first signs of improvement.

Additional information on acute neuromuscular diseases may be found in Chapter 13.

METABOLIC DISTURBANCES

Wernicke-Korsakoff

Wernicke's disease is a medical emergency, and prompt diagnosis and treatment is necessary to prevent progressive, and often permanent, neurologic deterioration. Although it is often thought of as a complication of alcoholism, Wernicke's encephalopathy may occur in any chronically malnourished person and often occurs in the setting of chemotherapy, eating disorders, and elderly patients living alone and not maintaining their nutritional status. Wernicke's encephalopathy may also be precipitated in the chronically malnourished hospitalized patient in whom parenteral nutrition or dietary supplements are initiated. The onset of Wernicke's disease is most common in the fifth and sixth decades of life, and female alcoholics are disproportionately represented.

The characteristic clinical triad of confusion, eye findings, and ataxia was initially described by Carl Wernicke in 1881. Onset and progression of signs and symptoms may vary from patient to patient, and all three features may not be present. Eye findings are the most consistent feature of Wernicke's encephalopathy, and the diagnosis should be reconsidered in their absence. The most common neuro-ophthalmologic abnormality is horizontal nystagmus, which is worse in lateral gaze. Vertical nystagmus in upgaze is also relatively common. Sixth-nerve palsies are the next most common abnormality. Bilateral involvement is the rule, although both eyes are rarely involved symmetrically. Slightly less than one-half of patients have conjugate gaze palsies. In descending order of frequency, gaze palsies may involve horizontal gaze, upgaze, and downgaze. Internuclear ophthalmoplegia may also be present. Often, patients show a combination of these findings, and approximately one-quarter of patients have nystagmus, sixth-nerve palsy, and a paresis of conjugate gaze.[97] Isolated involvement of the third or fourth cranial nerve is distinctly unusual and, if present, should suggest an alternative etiology. Ptosis occasionally is encountered.

Although in his original observations of three patients, Carl Wernicke described optic disc swelling, this has rarely been reported subsequently. Optic atrophy and paracentral scotoma may occur from a chronic nutritional deficiency ("tobacco-alcohol amblyopia") but is not considered part of the acute disease process. Pupils are rarely involved until very late in the disease but may eventually become miotic and nonreactive.

In addition to ocular disturbances, mental status changes and ataxia complete the clinical triad of Wernicke's encephalopathy. Approximately 90% of patients present with some disturbance of mentation. This is usually manifested as a global confusional state, in which the patients may be disoriented, apathetic, and inattentive. Although patients are often lethargic and somnolent, they are rarely stuporous. Gait difficulties constitute the third prominent symptom and usually take the form of a moderately severe truncal ataxia. In its most severe form, patients may be unable even to stand without assistance. Occasionally, appendicular ataxia suggestive of cerebellar hemispheric disease may be present. To a large extent, this gait disturbance is probably due to bilateral vestibular hypofunction, and patients often demonstrate a defective oculocephalic response.[98] Symptoms of vertigo and deafness are uncommon, which suggests that the lesion is in the vestibular nuclei. Damage to the cerebellar vermis also contributes to the truncal ataxia, and patients may have persistent gait difficulties even after vestibular function has normalized.

On pathology, the mamillary bodies are almost universally involved with this disease process. Parenchymal lesions may be bilateral and widespread but usually involve the paraventricular regions of the hypothalamus and thalamus, floor of the fourth ventricle, and periaqueductal region of the midbrain. When the patient has evidence of Korsakoff's psychosis (anterograde amnesia, inability to consolidate new material, and confabulation), the dorsomedial nucleus of the thalamus is consistently involved. Pathologically, necrosis, microvascular hemorrhage, and reactive gliosis is found in the acute lesions. The capillaries in the involved region appear prominent because of endothelial hyperplasia, adventitial thickening, and luminal dilation. In the cerebellar cortex, loss of Purkinje cells is accompanied by a reactive increase in Bergmann's glia.[99]

The treatment of Wernicke's disease requires the immediate administration of thiamine. Although as little as 2 or 3 mg may be effective, in practice higher doses are given (most commonly 50–100 mg). Magnesium must also be supplemented when necessary. The prompt administration of thiamine reverses the biochemical lesion and prevents neurologic progression. Thiamine is also clearly effective in preventing progression to the Korsakoff's amnestic syndrome in patients who have little alteration of mentation. Ocular findings may respond dramatically to treatment. Abducens palsies are usually the first to recover, and dramatic improvement may be seen within hours to days. Conjugate gaze palsies have an excellent prognosis for full recovery as well. Nystagmus, ptosis, and vertical gaze palsies may take somewhat longer to recover, and improvement may continue for weeks or months after treatment. Ataxia and vestibular function also may take longer to recover, and improvement may continue for several months.

Toxic/Metabolic Encephalopathy

A careful neuro-ophthalmologic evaluation of the comatose patient may yield important diagnostic clues as to the etiology of the underlying disorder. In general, the pupillary light reflex is relatively resistant to metabolic insult and is usually preserved in metabolic coma. There are several common exceptions, however. Anticholinergic agents that are ingested in sufficient quantities to cause coma or delirium may cause dilated and poorly reactive pupils. This is especially important to keep in mind during the evaluation of post-arrest patients who may have received atropine as part of the resuscitation protocol. Severe anoxic injury may result in tonic upgaze and in fixed, dilated pupils due to parasympathetic denervation and high levels of circulating catecholamines.[100] The distinction between anticholinergic effect and anoxia may be made by the instillation of 1% pilocarpine. The miotic pupillary response is normal in the setting of anoxia but is diminished or absent if anticholinergic agents are present. Conversely, patients presenting with an alteration in their level of consciousness due to organophosphate toxicity demonstrate cholinergic effects, including miosis.

Other types of drug intoxication may cause relatively distinctive neuro-ophthalmologic findings as well. In general, overdose with sedative-hypnotic agents, such as benzodiazepines or barbiturates, causes small reactive pupils and impaired oculocephalic reflex. Decorticate or decerebrate posturing may be present. If the patient with barbiturate intoxication is conscious, prominent nystagmus may be noted. Barbiturate overdose is somewhat unusual in that reflex eye movements may be lost because of vestibular hypofunction even before the patient loses consciousness.[101] Severe barbiturate intoxication may cause a complete loss of pupillary reactivity. Phenytoin and tricyclic antidepressants are also potent vestibular suppressants and may diminish the oculovestibular response as well. Glutethimide, a sedative that is rarely used clinically, is atypical in that it may cause midposition or dilated unreactive pupils before respiration is impaired.[101] Opiate overdose characteristically produces pinpoint pupils; a strong light source and magnification may be necessary to document reactivity. Psychotomimetic drugs such as LSD, psilocybin, mescaline, and peyote cause pupillary dilation because of their sympathomimetic effect. Lithium toxicity may also cause mydriasis, as well as dry mouth and tachycardia, because of its anticholinergic properties. Patients presenting with mild ethanol intoxication usually have nystagmus. With severe intoxication, comatose patients may lose all reflex eye movements and demonstrate poorly reactive pupils.

Metabolic encephalopathies usually cause small reactive pupils, a nonspecific effect of sympathetic hypofunction. Patients with hepatic encephalopathy usually have brisk oculocephalic responses. Occasional patients with ocular bobbing, disconjugate eye movements, and tonic gaze deviation have been described in this setting.[102] Patients with hypercarbic encephalopathy due to chronic obstructive pulmonary disease or hypoventilation syndromes usually have full reflex eye movement as well. Ten percent of these patients have hypercarbic retinopathy, with evidence of disc swelling, engorged retinal veins, and hemorrhage on funduscopy.[103]

Disturbances of ocular motility rarely give any additional information as to the nature of the metabolic encephalopathy or intoxication. In general, asymmetric motility disturbances should be assumed to be due to a structural lesion until proven otherwise. Metabolic insult may cause surprisingly focal eye findings, however, and reversible internuclear ophthalmoplegia has been described in the setting of barbiturate intoxication and hepatic encephalopathy. In general, ice water caloric stimulation of the comatose patient causes a slow, sustained eye deviation toward the irrigated ear without the compensatory fast phase of nystagmus. When the fast phase of nystagmus is evident in an unresponsive patient, a psychogenic cause of the patient's coma should be considered. One exception to this rule is intoxication with phencyclidine or ketamine, in which the rapid phase of the nystagmus may be preserved.

THE NEURO-OPHTHALMOLOGY OF TRAUMA

Visual disturbances are a frequent consequence of trauma, and it has been estimated that 5% of patients describe visual symptoms following significant head or neck injury.[104] Although ocular motility deficits or pupillary dysfunction may occur, traumatic optic neuropathy often presents the most serious threat to vision. Although hemorrhage of the optic nerve sheath or traumatic avulsion of the optic nerve may occur, most cases of traumatic optic neuropathy are retrobulbar, and there is no initial or ophthalmoscopic evidence of injury. The intracanalicular portion of the optic nerve is most susceptible to indirect trauma, because it is tightly adherent to the dura lining the bony canal. It is believed that nerve injury results when a blow to the head causes bony deformity of the optic canal, damaging the small nutrient vessels and contusing the intracanalicular optic nerve.[105] There is a poor correlation between the severity of impact and the degree of visual loss, and relatively trivial trauma may cause symptoms. The inciting event is usually a blow to the ipsilateral forehead, and motorcycle and bicycle accidents are heavily represented in the literature. Visual deterioration may occur immediately or after a latency of several hours.[106] Traumatic optic neuropathy occasionally is associated with basilar or facial fractures, and high-resolution CT should be performed to rule out this posssibility.[107] Although optic neuropathy is almost always retrobulbar, there have been occasional reports of anterior ischemic optic neuropathy after trauma.[108] This also may occur as an indirect result of significant blood loss, usually in elderly and debilitated patients.

The management of traumatic optic neuropathy remains controversial. Extrapolating from studies on acute spinal injury, many authors advocate the use of high-dose steroids in the acute setting.[105] Although there is a good deal of anecdotal evidence that steroids may be of benefit in preserving vision, there is a paucity of controlled studies on this subject. Some studies have also demonstrated excellent results after decompressive surgery.[109] When a transethmoidal or trans-sphenoidal approach is used, optic nerve decompression can be performed without subjecting the patient to craniotomy. The role and timing of surgical intervention remains controversial, and most authorities would agree that decompression should be reserved for patients who fail to improve or show deterioration on steroid therapy.[105]

Although less common than optic neuropathy, chiasmal deficits may also occur after trauma. Chiasmal syndromes are more likely to accompany significant frontal head trauma, and one-third of patients have associated fractures of the frontal bone.[110] In this setting, the clinician should be alert for hypothalamic damage, including diabetes insipidus. MRI is the imaging modality of choice, and chiasmal tears, hemorrhage, or contusion may be seen. The most common visual field defect is bitemporal hemianopsia, although a junctional scotoma may be present in the patient with a postfixed chiasm. Subjective diplopia may be due to coexisting cranial-nerve palsies or the retinal slip phenomenon. The latter occurs when transection of the chiasm causes a complete bitemporal hemianopsia, preventing normal integration of the right and left visual fields. The delayed onset of chiasmal symptoms and evidence of hypothalamic dysfunction raises the possibility of chiasmal arachnoiditis, which may be a late complication of trauma, hemorrhage, or infection. Treatment of chiasmal injuries with high-dose steroids is often advocated, although there have been no well-controlled studies demonstrating their efficacy. Surgical intervention should be considered for chiasmal hemorrhage or fractures compressing the chiasm.

Cortical blindness is a less common consequence of head trauma. Instances of cortical blindness usually fall into two categories. In children and adolescents, cortical blindness may follow relatively trivial trauma including instances without loss of consciousness. Symptoms are transient, lasting minutes to hours, and prognosis for full recovery is excellent.[111] No structural lesions are usually demonstrated. In adults, cortical blindness is more likely to follow significant head injuries that are associated with other neurologic deficits. In this setting, prognosis for return of vision is guarded.

Ocular motility deficits following trauma may be caused by cranial-nerve palsies or mechanical restriction of the extraocular muscles. Orbital fractures of the inferior or medial wall may entrap the extraocular muscles and cause a limitation of abduction or upgaze. Forced duction testing, which involves anesthetizing the eye and applying pressure in the direction of muscle limitation with a cotton-tip applicator, helps to determine whether a restrictive process is present (Fig. 7–12). Orbital CT should be performed to rule out fracture or entrapment. Even in the absence of orbital fracture, intramuscular edema, hemorrhage, laceration, or avulsion may cause a mechanical restriction of gaze.

The most common ophthalmologic complaint after mild head trauma is difficulty focusing at near due to insufficiency of accommodation and convergence.[112] Although the exact anatomic lesion in convergence insufficiency has never been adequately described, these symptoms tend to be self-limited and show spontaneous resolution over weeks to months. Occasionally, complaints of blurred vision at near persist, requiring orthoptic exercises and, rarely, strabismus surgery. Fourth-nerve palsies are the most common cranial-nerve deficit following trauma.[113] The true incidence of post-traumatic fourth-nerve palsies may never be known, because the diagnosis requires a certain degree of neurologic sophistication and is almost certainly under-reported. Fourth-nerve palsies are most often unilateral, and when they are bilateral they are usually associated with a sustained loss of consciousness.[113] This is probably because of the fact that bilateral damage occurs as the fibers decussate in the superior medullary velum, and injury here may affect the adjacent reticular activating system. Post-traumatic third- and sixth-nerve palsies occur with roughly equal incidence.[114] The presence of a post-traumatic third-nerve or sixth-nerve palsy should prompt consideration of cavernous sinus aneurysm or carotid-cavernous fistula (described earlier). The exact mechanism of third- and sixth-nerve dysfunction is not clear, although it is probably related to stretching of the nerve by downward displacement of the brain stem. In the setting of blunt trauma, sixth-nerve palsies may also be seen after fracture of the middle cranial fossa involving the petrous tip. Signs and symptoms of seventh- or eighth-nerve dysfunction are common associated findings.[115] Approximately one-third to one-half of patients with traumatic cranial nerve palsies experience spontaneous improvement, although the number may be slightly higher for fourth-nerve palsies.[114]

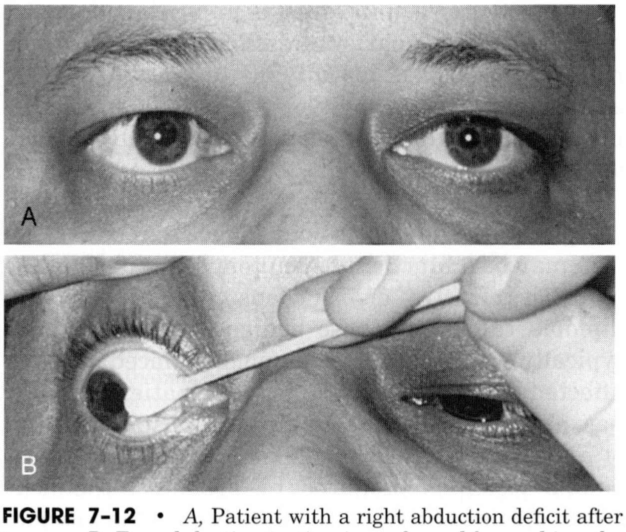

FIGURE 7–12 • *A,* Patient with a right abduction deficit after trauma. *B,* Forced duction testing is performed by pushing the globe in the direction of gaze limitation with a cotton-tip applicator after local anesthetic drops. In this case, the globe moves freely, demonstrating that there is no restrictive process.

Symptomatic relief of the diplopia accompanying traumatic nerve palsies may be obtained by eye patching. Alternate patching must be performed in children to prevent amblyopia but is not necessary in the adult. When the deficit remains fixed for at least 6 months, strabismus surgery may be considered. In general, the goals of surgery are to eliminate diplopia in the primary and reading positions. Surgical intervention is most beneficial for trochlear palsies, although there may be some improvement in third- and sixth-nerve palsies as well. Even when patients are not left with a useful range of fusion, surgery may have a beneficial cosmetic effect.

Pupillary abnormalities may be a frequent sequela of head trauma. After direct injury, the pupil may be either enlarged or small and poorly reactive because of ciliary dysfunction. This is frequently self-limited, and the pupil usually regains normal accommodation after several months. Disruption of oculosympathetic fibers may cause Horner's syn-

49. Lie JT, Gordon LP, Titus JL: Juvenile temporal arteritis: Biopsy study of four cases. JAMA 1975;234:496–499.
50. Allsop CJ, Gallagher PJ: Temporal artery biopsy in giant cell arteritis: A reappraisal. Am J Surg Pathol 1981;5:317–323.
51. Bosley TM, Savino PJ, Sergott RL, et al: Ocular pneumoplethysmography can help in the diagnosis of giant cell arteritis. Arch Ophthalmol 1989;107:379–381.
52. Mack E, O'Day J, Currie JN: Delayed choroidal perfusion in giant cell arteritis. J Clin Neuro-Ophthalmol 1991;11:221–227.
53. Siatkowski RM, Gass JD, Glaser JS, et al: Fluorescein angiography in the diagnosis of giant cell arteritis. Am J Ophthalmol 1993;115:57–63.
54. Grahm E, Holland A, Avery A, et al: Prognosis in giant cell arteritis. BMJ 1981;282:269–271.
55. Hollenhorst RW, Brown JR, Wagener HD: Neurologic aspects of temporal arteritis. Neurology 1960;10:490–498.
56. Liu GT, Glaser JS, Schatz NJ, et al: Visual morbidity in giant cell arteritis: Clinical characteristics and prognosis for vision. Ophthalmology 1994;101:1779–1785.
57. Sheng FC, Quinones-Baldrich W, Machleder HI, et al: Relationship of extracranial carotid occlusive disease and central retinal artery occlusion. Am J Surg 1986;152:175–178.
58. Schumaker M, Schmidt D, Wakhloo AK: Intra-arterial fibrinolytic therapy in central retinal artery occlusion. Neuroradiology 1993;35:600–605.
59. Schmidt D, Schumaker M, Wakhloo AK: Microcatheter urokinase infusion in central retinal artery occlusion. Am J Ophthalmol 1992;113:429–434.
60. Kistler JP, Ropper AA, Martin J: Cerebrovascular diseases. In Wilson J (ed): Harrison's Principles of Internal Medicine, 12th ed, pp 1977–2002. New York, McGraw-Hill, 1991.
61. Green WR: Neuro-ophthalmologic evaluation of ocular motor palsy. Arch Ophthalmol 1964;72:154–167.
62. Kissel JT, Burde RM, Klingele TG, et al: Pupil-sparing oculomotor palsies with internal carotid and posterior communicating artery aneurysms. Ann Neurol 1983;13:149–154.
63. Trobe JD: Isolated third nerve palsies. Semin Neurol 1986:135–141.
64. Trobe JD: Third nerve palsies and the pupil: Footnotes to the rule. Arch Ophthalmol 1988;106:601–602.
65. Guy JR, Day AL: Intracranial aneurysms with superior division paresis of the oculomotor nerve. Ophthalmology 1989;96:1071–1076.
66. Keane JR, Ahmadi J: Third nerve palsies and angiography. Arch Neurol 1991;48:470–472.
67. Solomon D, Schnee C, Raps E, et al: Benign and malignant ophthalmoparesis following basilar aneurysm surgery [abstract]. Neurology 1994;44(Suppl 2):227.
68. Kurtke JF.: Epidemiology of cerebrovascular disease. In Siekert RG (ed): Cerebrovascular Surgery Report, pp 135–176. Bethesda, National Institute of Neurological and Communicative Disorders and Stroke, 1980.
69. Kase CS, Mohr JP: General features of intracerebral hemorrhage. In Barnett H, Mohr JP (eds): Stroke: Pathophysiology, Diagnosis, and Management, pp 497–523. New York, Churchill Livingstone, 1986.
70. Lee JP, Wang AD: Post-traumatic basal ganglia hemorrhage: Analysis of 52 patients with emphasis on the final outcome. J Trauma 1991;31:376–380.
71. Heros R: Current concepts in cerebrovascular disease: Cerebellar hemorrhage and infarction. Stroke 1982;13:106–109.
72. Nakajima K: Clinicopathological study of pontine hemorrhage. Stroke 1983;14:485–493.
73. Pierrot-Deseilligny C: Brainstem control of horizontal gaze: Effects of lesions. In Kennard C, Rose F (eds): Physiological Aspects of Clinical Neuro-Ophthalmology, pp 209–235. Chicago, Year Book, 1988.
74. Poungvarin N, Bhoopat W, Viriyavejakul A, et al: Effects of dexamethasone in primary supratentorial intracerebral hemorrhage. N Engl J Med 1987;316:1229–1233.
75. Borges LF: Management of non-traumatic brain hemorrhage. In Ropper A (ed): Neurological and Neurosurgical Intensive Care, 3rd ed, pp 279–307. New York, Raven Press, 1993.
76. Corbett J: Neuro-ophthalmologic complications of hydrocephalus and shunting procedures. Semin Neurol 1986;6:111–123.
77. Cobbs WH, Schatz NJ, Savino PJ: Midbrain eye signs in hydrocephalus. Trans Am Neurol Assoc 1978;103:130–133.
78. Guy JR, Friedman WF, Mickle JP: Bilateral trochlear nerve paresis in hydrocephalus. J Clin Neuro-Ophthalmol 1989;105–111.
79. Arroyo HA, Jan JE, McCormick AQ, et al: Permanent visual loss after shunt malfunction. Neurology 1985;35:25–30.
80. Obenchain TG, Crandall PH, Hepler RS: Blindness following relief of increased intracranial pressure: A sequel to severe papilledema. Bull Los Angeles Neurol Soc 1970;35:147–152.
81. Digre K: Trauma to the brain with attention to the occipital lobe. North American Neuro-Ophthalmology Society Meeting, 1993.
82. Riddoch G: Dissociation of visual perceptions due to occipital injuries, with special reference to movement. Brain 1917;40:15–57.
83. Evans JP, Scheinker LM: Histologic study of the brain following head trauma: Post-traumatic infarction of cerebral arteries with consideration of the associated clinical picture. Arch Neurol Psychiatr 1943;50:258–268.
84. Asbury A, Bird S: Disorders of peripheral nerve. In Asbury A, McKhann G, McDonald W (eds): Diseases of the Nervous System: Clinical Neurobiology, 2nd ed, pp 252–269. Philadelphia, WB Saunders, 1992.
85. Fisher CM: An unusual variant of acute idiopathic polyneuritis (syndrome of ophthalmoplegia, ataxia, and areflexia). N Engl J Med 1956;255:57–59.
86. Ropper A, Wijdicks, Truax B: Ophthalmoplegia and other ocular signs. In Ropper A (ed): Guillain-Barré Syndrome, pp 90–94. Philadelphia, FA Davis, 1991.
87. Zasorin NL, Yee RD, Baloh RW: Eye movement abnormalities in ophthalmoplegia, ataxia, and areflexia (Fisher's syndrome). Arch Ophthalmol 1985;103:55–58.
88. Knox DL, Clark DB, Schuster FF: Benign VI nerve palsies in children. Pediatrics 1967;40:560–564.
89. Adams R, Victor M: Diseases of the peripheral nerve. In Adams R, Victor M (eds): Principles of Neurology, 5th ed, pp 1117–1169. New York, McGraw-Hill, 1993.
90. Guillain-Barré Study Group: Plasmapharesis and acute Guillain-Barré syndrome. Neurology 1985;35:1096–1104.
91. Kleyweg RP, Van der Meche FG, Meulstee J: Treatment of the Guillain-Barré syndrome with high dose gamma globulin. Neurology 1988;38:1639–1641.
92. Grob D, Brunner NG, Namba T: The natural course of myasthenia gravis and the effect of therapeutic measures. Ann N Y Acad Sci 1981;377:652–655.
93. Simpson JA: Myasthenia gravis and myasthenic syndromes. In Walton JN (ed): Diseases of Voluntary Muscle, 5th ed, pp 626–665. Edinburgh, Churchill Livingstone, 1988.
94. Cogan DG: Myasthenia gravis: A review of the disease and a description of lid twitch as a characteristic sign. Arch Ophthalmol 1965;74:217–219.
95. Newson-Davis J: Diseases of the neuromuscular junction. In Asbury AK, McKhann GM, McDonald WI (eds): Diseases of the Nervous System, 2nd ed, pp 197–212. Philadelphia, WB Saunders, 1992.
96. Adams RD, Victor M: Principles of Neurology, 5th ed, pp 1261–1262. New York, McGraw-Hill, 1993.
97. Victor M: Neurological disorders due to alcoholism and malnutrition. In Baker A, Baker L (eds): Clinical Neurology, 4th ed, pp 1–94. Philadelphia, JB Lippincott, 1992.
98. Ghez C: Vestibular paresis: A clinical feature of Wernicke's disease. J Neurol Neurosurg Psychiatry 1969;32:134–138.
99. Adams R, Sidman R: Metabolic, toxic, and nutritional disorders of the nervous system. In Adams R, Sidman R

(eds): Introduction to Neuropathology, p 256. New York, McGraw-Hill, 1968.
100. Keane JR: Sustained upgaze in coma. Ann Neurol 1983;9:409–412.
101. Plum F, Posner J: The pathologic physiology of signs and symptoms in coma. In Plum F, Posner J (eds): The Diagnosis of Stupor and Coma, 3rd ed, pp 1–86. Philadelphia, FA Davis, 1982.
102. Rai GS, Buxton-Thomas M, Scanlon M: Ocular bobbing in hepatic encephalopathy. Br J Clin Pract 1976;30:202–205.
103. Plum F, Posner J: Multifocal, diffuse, and metabolic brain diseases causing stupor or coma. In Plum F, Posner J (eds): The Diagnosis of Stupor and Coma, 3rd ed, pp 177–303. Philadelphia, FA Davis, 1982.
104. Gjerris F: Traumatic lesions of the visual pathways. In Vinken PJ, Bruyn CW (eds): Handbook of Clinical Neurology, pp 27–57. Amsterdam, North Holland, 1976.
105. Anderson RL, Panje WR, Gross CE: Optic nerve blindness following blunt forehead trauma. Ophthalmology 1982;89:445–455.
106. Lessel S: Indirect optic nerve trauma. Arch Ophthalmol 1989;107:382–386.
107. Federle MD, Brant-Zawadzki M: Computed Tomography in the Evaluation of Trauma. Baltimore, Williams and Wilkins, 1982.
108. Hedges TR, Gragoudas ES: Traumatic anterior ischemic neuropathy. Ann Ophthalmol 1981;13:625–628.
109. Joseph MP, Lessell S, Rizzo J, et al: Extracranial optic nerve decompression for traumatic optic neuropathy. Arch Ophthalmol 1990;108:1091–1093.
110. Tang RA: Chiasm trauma. North American Neuro-Ophthalmology Society Meeting, 1993.
111. Yamamoto LG, Bart RD: Transient blindness following mild head trauma. Clin Pediatr 1988;27:479–483.
112. Kowal L: Ophthalmologic manifestations of head injury. Austr N Z J Ophthalmol 1992;20:35–40.
113. Sydnor CF, Seaber JH, Buckley EG: Traumatic superior oblique palsies. Ophthalmology 1982;89:134–138.
114. Rush JA, Younge BR: Paralysis of cranial nerves III, IV, and VI: Cause and prognosis in 1000 cases. Arch Ophthalmol 1981;99:76–79.
115. Antoniades K, Karakasis D, Jaskos N: Abducens nerve palsy following transverse fracture of the middle cranial fossa. J Craniomaxillofac Surg 1993;21:172–175.
116. Thompson HS: Functional visual loss. Am J Ophthalmol 1985;100:209–213.
117. Slavin ML: The prism dissociation test in detecting unilateral functional visual loss. J Clin Neuro-Ophthalmol 1990;10:127–130.
118. Gittinger JW: Functional monocular temporal hemianopsia. Am J Ophthalmol 1986;101:226–231.
119. Keane JR: Neuro-ophthalmic signs and symptoms of hysteria. Neurology 1982;32:757–762.

propagates within the intracranial venous sinus system. This prevents normal venous drainage and causes edema and infarction. Central nervous system (CNS) venous infarctions usually involve the cortex and adjacent white matter in a bilateral fashion, and this occurs as a result of occlusion of the superior sagittal sinus and the lateral sinuses most frequently.[9] Hemorrhagic conversion of these infarcts is not uncommon.

Intracerebral hemorrhage can occur due to a variety of causes, with hypertension being the most common cause (50%–60%). Other causes (excluding trauma) include neoplastic disease (1%–2%),[10–12] arteriovenous malformations (AVM) and aneurysms (15%–25%),[13, 14] amyloid angiopathy (up to 10%),[15] drug abuse,[16, 17] vasculitis, primary and secondary coagulopathies (10%), and acute, severe alcohol intoxication.[18]

Lipohyalinosis and Charcot-Bouchard aneurysms are thought to underlie hypertensive intracerebral hemorrhage. In addition to these changes, there may be segmental fibrinoid degeneration of the vessel wall with plasmatic angionecrosis. A sudden rise in systemic blood pressure may cause the weakened cerebral blood vessel to rupture and cause an intraparenchymal hemorrhage.

CLINICAL PRESENTATION

The majority of patients admitted to the hospital with the diagnosis of acute stroke are initially evaluated by an emergency medicine physician in the emergency department (ED). The average time from onset of symptoms to arrival in the ED varies depending on the location of the hospital and the community knowledge of stroke signs and symptoms.[19] A thorough history and physical examination, followed by a diagnostic laboratory screening, should aid in ruling out other causes for acute neurologic deterioration such as trauma, seizures, metabolic disturbances, toxic ingestion, tumor, or syncope. Once the diagnosis of acute stroke is established and the patient is stabilized, a computed tomography (CT) scan of the head should be performed immediately. The purpose of this scan is to determine the presence or absence of hemorrhage, as well as edema and early signs of ischemic change.

Useful indicators of subarachnoid hemorrhage are complaints of a severe headache and a stiff neck. The presence or absence of headache, however, is not a sensitive indicator of the type or severity of the stroke in the context of primary intracerebral hemorrhage or cerebral infarction. This is due to the fact that (1) headache is not reported as an accompanying symptom in greater than 50% of these stroke patients; and (2) the percentage of patients who report headache is nearly equal in both hemorrhagic and ischemic strokes.[20, 21] Therefore, patients should not be categorized (as hemorrhagic or ischemic) based on this symptom.

Patients who present within minutes to hours after suffering a supratentorial stroke will generally present with acute onset of focal symptoms and signs that are typical for focal lesions within the area supplied by the involved vessel. The level of consciousness might be altered due to the primary insult if the stroke involves a significant portion of the thalamus or is accompanied by one or more of the following problems: midline location with associated midline shift or herniation, old or new parenchymal lesions in the opposite hemisphere, hydrocephalus secondary to intraventricular hemorrhage, or mass effect occluding the cerebral aqueduct. Alternatively, the level of consciousness might become depressed secondary to accompanying complex partial or generalized tonic-clonic seizures,[22] toxic-metabolic derangement, infection, or poor cerebral perfusion pressure due to systemic hypotension.

Most anterior circulation cortical infarctions are due to occlusions within the internal carotid artery or one of its main branches, such as the middle cerebral artery (MCA) and anterior cerebral artery (ACA). Infarctions within this territory generally present with a combination of neurologic deficits including aphasia, if the language cortex is involved; hemiparesis and/or hemisensory loss; apraxia; neglect; sensory extinction; and conjugate gaze deviation. A visual field deficit may be noted as a result of involvement of the optic radiations.

Infratentorial cerebral infarctions are due to posterior circulation vascular disease. The posterior circulation originates from both vertebral arteries, which come together to form the basilar artery. The basilar artery then bifurcates at the distal edge of the pons to form both posterior cerebral arteries. Vertebrobasilar artery disease may result in infarcts within the regions supplied by the posterior circulation, including the brain stem and cerebellum, occipital lobes, thalami, and medial temporal lobes. Infarctions in this territory more commonly present with one or more of the following: isolated homonymous hemianopsia due to occipital lobe infarction; an acute isolated gait disturbance; diplopia; dysarthria; dysmetria; dizziness or vertigo; sensory loss; and multiple cranial nerve deficits. Most patients present with a combination of brain stem deficits, and this should alert the physician that a vertebrobasilar distribution cerebral infarction has occurred. The level of consciousness might be altered in this setting due to acute basilar artery occlusion, or a lobar (cerebral or cerebellar) infarct with mass effect causing diencephalic shift or brain stem compression.

As discussed earlier, lacunar infarctions are due to small vessel occlusive disease and are generally located in the subcortical and brain stem regions. The four most common lacunar syndromes are pure motor stroke, pure sensory stroke, dysarthria–clumsy hand syndrome, and ataxic-hemiparesis syndrome. The changes may be very subtle with a lacunar infarct. Therefore, a careful and detailed history and neurologic examination are necessary to avoid a misdiagnosis.

Patients with intracerebral hemorrhage can present with a variety of neurologic disturbances, as well as alteration in level of consciousness. The focal neurologic abnormalities in this setting will vary depending on the vessel involved, as with cerebral infarctions (see above). The level of consciousness might be altered if the hemorrhage is large and associated with early edema or mass effect, if there is subarachnoid hemorrhage or intraventricular hemorrhage, or if there is increased intracranial pressure. Headache may be a frequent accompanying symptom, and its presence will depend on the anatomic location(s) that have been disrupted by the dissection of blood through the cerebral tissue.[22, 23]

In addition to the standard neurologic examination, a thorough general physical examination should be completed to search for signs of cardiovascular disease such as cardiac murmurs, pulmonary dysfunction, large vessel bruits, retinal changes, and hypertension. These findings may represent chronic complications of hypertension or may be acute findings associated with cardiac and pulmonary complications that are associated with stroke.

INITIAL MANAGEMENT AND PATIENT STABILIZATION

In the immediate period, it is important to establish an adequate airway, adequate ventilation, and adequate blood pressure, in all stroke patients. Certain stroke subtypes are associated with the risk of early deterioration due to inability to control the airway (e.g., brain stem strokes, large and/or deep intracerebral hemorrhages, and large infarcts with early edema). Inadequate ventilation can lead to hypoxemia and pneumonitis or pneumonia secondary to aspiration of oral contents. Maintaining stroke patients in an upright position (at about 30–45 degrees) and limiting oral intake help to avoid aspiration. Any patient who is somnolent or comatose (Glasgow Coma Scale score < 9), or is unable to protect the airway, should undergo endotracheal intubation immediately, despite the results of the arterial blood gases. Continuous ventilatory support should be reserved for those with persistent hypoxemia or carbon dioxide retention, due to lack of spontaneous breaths or inadequate tidal volumes.

Most acute stroke patients do not present with arterial hypotension unless there are underlying medical problems such as sepsis, myocardial infarction, or dehydration. When there is hypotension, the patients should undergo intravenous fluid resuscitation with 0.9% saline solution. Hypotonic fluids and fluids containing dextrose should be avoided because they may potentiate or exacerbate edema and cell death. If the blood pressure fails to respond to aggressive fluid resuscitation, pressor agents should be administered. The mean arterial pressure (MAP) should be increased to maintain a minimal cerebral perfusion pressure (CPP) of 70 mm Hg in a patient without a history of chronic hypertension. In patients with a history of chronic hypertension, there is a shift in their cerebral pressure autoregulation curve and they require a higher MAP to maintain an adequate CPP.[24, 25] In patients with chronic hypertension, the CPP should be about 90–110 mm Hg. The clinical examination may aid in determining the optimal MAP, as some patients will deteriorate if the MAP is insufficient and rapidly improve after the MAP is increased.

Calculation of the CPP requires quantification of the intracranial pressure (ICP). The ICP can be quantified through the use of a number of different monitoring devices, which are described later in this chapter. The CPP is calculated using the following equation: $CPP = MAP - ICP$.

Arterial hypertension is common with acute strokes. Approximately 80% of patients with acute stroke will present with hypertension.[26] This may be an acute phenomenon that represents a sympathetic reaction to acute stress. It may be a protective mechanism to prevent further cell death, as the shadow zone or penumbra (the marginally perfused area surrounding the core of infarction) is salvaged by the heightened perfusion pressure. The systemic blood pressure generally returns to a "baseline" level within the first week after the stroke.[27, 28] It is important to avoid sudden major drops ($>15\%$–25%) in blood pressure in the setting of intracerebral hemorrhage and cerebral infarction.[28, 29] Overly aggressive treatment of elevated blood pressure in the setting of acute stroke could have deleterious effects by affecting the ischemic penumbra and by causing additional areas of ischemia or infarction in hypertensive patients. Frequent neurologic checks should be correlated with the MAP to determine if there is evidence of worsening neurologic deficits as the MAP falls. In chronic hypertensive patients, MAPs of 120–130 mm Hg are often tolerated. No large-scale trials have been performed to determine the optimal management of hypertension in the setting of acute stroke.

When there is acute cerebral infarction and hypertension, the risk of intracerebral hemorrhage may be much greater with the infusion of heparin or a thrombolytic agent.[27] The following algorithm has been recommended[30] for acute treatment of hypertension in the setting of acute stroke:

1. If the diastolic blood pressure (BP) is greater than 140 mm Hg on two readings 5 minutes apart, start an infusion of sodium nitroprusside (0.5–10 μg/kg/minute).
2. If the systolic BP is greater than 230 mm Hg and/or diastolic BP is 121–140 mm Hg on two readings 20 minutes apart, give labetalol 20 mg intravenously over 1–2 minutes. The labetalol dose may be repeated or doubled every 10–20 minutes until a satisfactory BP reduction is achieved or until a cumulative dose of 300 mg has been administered by this minibolus technique. After the initial dosing schedule, labetalol doses may be administered every 6–8 hours as needed. Labetalol is preferably avoided in patients with asthma, cardiac failure, or severe cardiac conduction abnormalities, as this beta blocker may exacerbate these respective conditions.
3. If the systolic BP is 180–230 mm Hg and/or diastolic BP is 105–120 mm Hg, emergency therapy should be deferred in the absence of documented intracerebral hemorrhage or left ventricular failure. If the elevation persists, with two readings 60 minutes apart, use oral labetalol 200–300 mg two to three times daily as needed. Alternative treatments include oral nifedipine 10 mg every 6 hours or captopril 6.25–25 mg every 8 hours. If oral monotherapy is unsuccessful or if medication cannot be given orally, give labetalol as outlined above. Antihypertensive therapy is usually not indicated when the systolic BP is less than 180 mm Hg.
4. In acute stroke patients with a systolic BP of less than 180 mm Hg and/or a diastolic BP of less than 105 mm Hg, antihypertensive therapy is usually not indicated. Patients requiring heparin acutely should be anticoagulated after the BP has been cautiously lowered into an acceptable range of 150/85–95 mm Hg in patients without prior hypertension or 160–170/90–100 mm Hg in patients with a history of hypertension. Since the benefits of heparin are modest even when indicated, rapid lowering of the BP cannot be justified.

In treating hypertension, care should be taken to avoid the use of systemic vasodilators in patients with large strokes and edema. This will avoid exacerbation of increased intracranial pressure due to intracranial venous dilatation.[31] The resultant venous dilatation, with associated increased intracranial blood volume, may exacerbate intracranial hypertension.

Once adequate airway, ventilation, and circulation have been established, a bedside glucose screen should be performed. Both hyper- and hypoglycemia may cause or exacerbate focal neurologic deficits.[32–35] In the case of hypoglycemia, it should be immediately corrected with the use of 50% dextrose in water. In the case of hyperglycemia, insulin and normal saline solution should be administered to aim for a serum glucose concentration in the 100–200 mg/dL range.

In addition to continuous cardiac rhythm monitoring, all patients with acute stroke should have an electrocardiogram (ECG) to search for evidence of myocardial ischemia or infarction, arrhythmias, or conduction disturbances.[36] Patients with stroke will often have coexistent coronary and valvular heart disease. While only 2%–3% of those who present with an acute stroke will have an acute myocardial infarction, more than 50% of stroke survivors eventually die of heart disease. Acute stroke patients frequently will have cardiac conduction system disturbances and arrhythmias not attributable to coronary disease.[37, 38] The reason for these changes is not entirely clear but may reflect loss of hypothalamic regulation as a result of ischemia. This loss of regulation may result in a surge in catecholamine levels so high that detrimental cardiovascular effects may be observed. Any significant abnormality on the ECG, whether related to a conduction or rhythm disturbance, warrants a full evaluation to determine the cause and extent of the underlying problem. Treatment, in the form of nitrates, antihypertensives, and antiarrhythmic agents, is often necessary to halt deleterious cardiac rhythms or to prevent progression of myocardial damage. These drugs should be used cautiously in the setting of stroke due to the potential adverse CNS effects from the relative hypotension associated with their use.

The use of anticoagulant therapy is often necessary for treatment of a cardiac disease when it accompanies an acute stroke. Either of these drugs may contribute to extension of an intracerebral hemorrhage or hemorrhagic conversion of a large cerebral infarction. Patients with acute cerebral infarction who are treated with anticoagulation should be closely monitored for neurologic deterioration due to hemorrhagic conversion of the infarct. If significant neurologic deterioration occurs, the anticoagulant therapy should be stopped immediately. A head CT scan should be performed immediately to search for evidence of hemorrhagic conversion. In the case of intravenous heparin use for anticoagulation, if hemorrhagic conversion is present on the CT scan, protamine sulfate should be given to correct the partial thromboplastin time. In the case of oral warfarin use, fresh-frozen plasma and vitamin K should be given to correct the prothrombin time.

DIAGNOSTIC EVALUATION

Once the patient has been stabilized, it is important to obtain a head CT scan as soon as possible, to rule out hemorrhage and to determine if there is evidence of edema or mass effect. The head CT scan is the most reliable neuroimaging tool to detect intracranial hemorrhage within the first hours after stroke. Head magnetic resonance imaging (MRI) is more sensitive for the detection of early ischemia, brain stem infarcts, and lacunar infarcts. Routine MRI is nonspecific in its representation of early intracerebral hemorrhage, an equally critical problem in the acute period.

Hemorrhage appears bright on CT scan images (Fig. 8–1), and this is often described as "high-attenuation" change, or hyperdensity. Cerebral infarction appears dark on CT scan (Fig. 8–2) and is often described as "low-attenuation change," or hypodensity. In addition to detecting hemorrhage, the head CT scan obtained within the first 24 hours is often helpful in identifying early signs of cortical ischemia such as loss of the sulcal markings (see Fig. 8–2), unilateral loss of the gray-white matter differentiation, hypodensities, and mass effect. Detection of early ischemic changes is now more important than ever, as these changes were associated with a higher rate of hemorrhagic conversion in patients treated with recombinant tissue plasminogen activator (r-TPA) for acute ischemic stroke.[39]

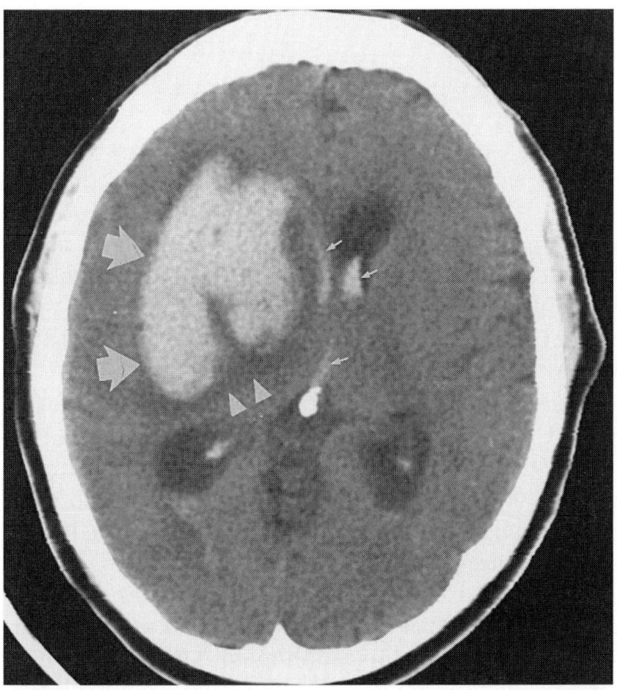

FIGURE 8–1 • Head computed tomography (CT) scan demonstrating a right basal gangliar hemorrhage (large white arrows) in a patient with known chronic hypertension. There is associated intraventricular blood (small white arrows), minimal surrounding edema (white arrowheads), and shift of the midline with effacement of the right lateral ventricle.

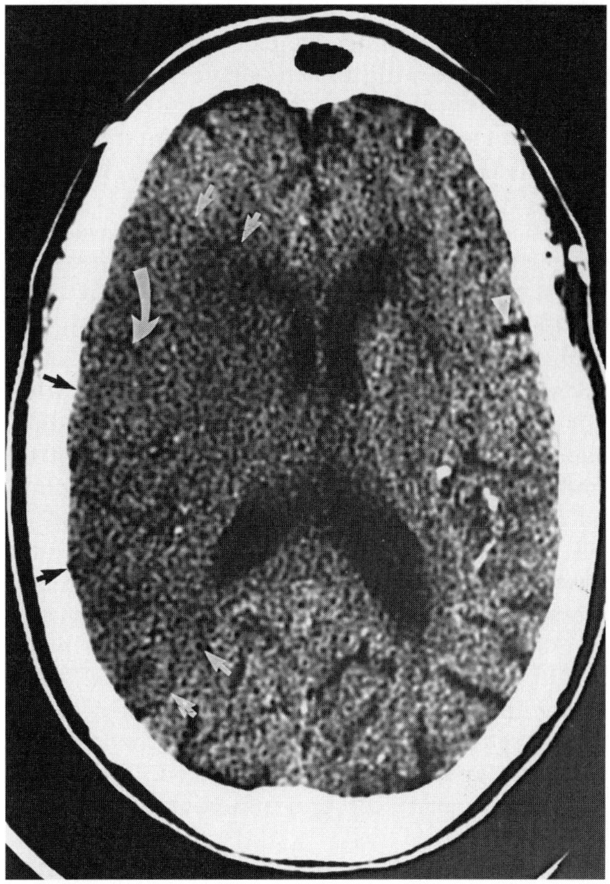

FIGURE 8–2 • Head CT scan of a patient with an acute right middle cerebral artery (MCA) distribution infarction. This image was obtained within 24 hours of the onset of stroke symptoms. There is demonstration of loss of sulcal markings (curved white arrow) and early low-attenuation change in the full MCA distribution (small white and black arrows). Note the normal sulcus on the left (white arrowhead).

Hypertensive intracerebral hemorrhages typically occur in four locations: putamen, thalamus, cerebellum, and pons. The demonstration of a hemorrhage in one of these typical locations (see Fig. 8–1), in a patient with a history of chronic hypertension, and an ECG and/or echocardiogram demonstrating hypertensive changes, is substantial evidence for the diagnosis of hypertensive intracerebral hemorrhage. This is further substantiated by the lack of history suggesting other etiologic possibilities.

After 24 to 72 hours, many supratentorial cerebral infarcts can be detected by head CT scan. These low-attenuation lesions may exhibit a variety of forms, from small, round, or ovoid lacunar infarctions to large, wedge-shaped cortical infarctions (see Fig. 8–2). Owing to bone artifact, many infratentorial cerebral infarcts are difficult to detect on CT scan imaging. If an infratentorial infarct is suspected, it can be imaged more optimally with the use of MRI.

A basic understanding of the imaging characteristics of MRI is necessary in order to realize its capabilities in the setting of acute stroke. For simplicity's sake, imaging characteristics for T2-weighted images will be described. Normal brain parenchyma appears gray on T2-weighted MRI, with gray matter appearing as a slightly lighter shade of gray compared with normal white matter. Cerebrospinal fluid (CSF) (Fig. 8–3) appears white and can be seen within the ventricular system as well as in the cortical sulci, basilar cisterns, and between the cerebellar folia. Blood flowing through a vessel does not project a magnetic resonance signal. As a result, patent blood vessels appear black on MRI (see Fig. 8–3). This characteristic of blood flowing through a vessel is described as a signal void, since the black image represents the lack of a projected signal from the flowing blood.

In general, acute cerebral infarctions, both small

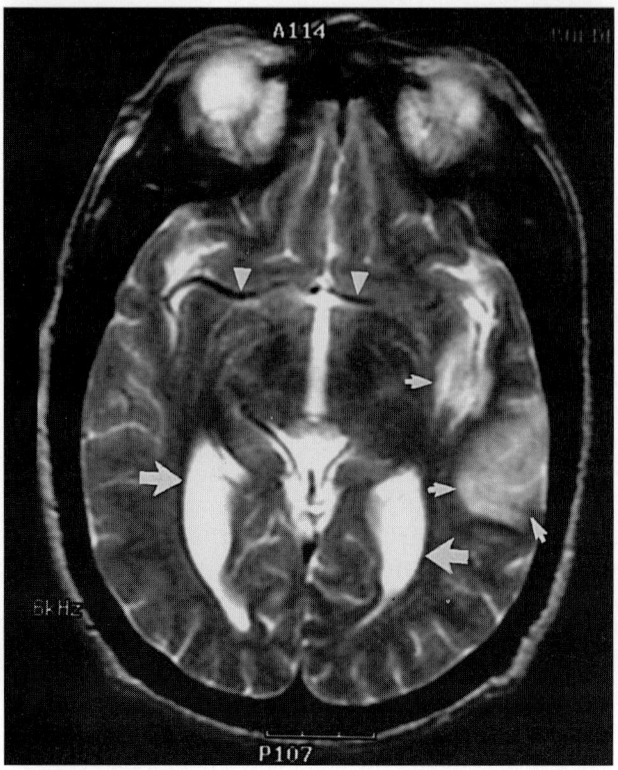

FIGURE 8–3 • Head magnetic resonance imaging (MRI) study that demonstrates a left MCA distribution cerebral infarction (small white arrows). This infarct involved portions of the perisylvian temporal and parietal lobes. Note the cerebrospinal fluid in the lateral ventricles (large white arrows) and normal signal void within the proximal MCAs (white arrowheads).

lacunar type and large cortical type infarctions, demonstrate an increased signal relative to brain and appear bright on T2-weighted MRI (see Fig. 8–3). The signal for cerebral infarction is slightly darker than for CSF. The infarct can be visualized on MRI as early as 4–6 hours after the onset of symptoms. In addition to the increased signal, moderate to large-sized infarctions may be accompanied by significant edema resulting in gyral enlargement or effacement of the ventricles or cisterns. Thrombosis of a large or medium-sized artery may be visualized in this setting. This usually appears as a bright signal within the vessel lumen on T2-weighted MRI, instead of the normal black signal void seen in patent vessels.

As stated above, in the setting of intracerebral hemorrhage the MRI signal abnormality is not specific enough to reliably confirm the diagnosis in the acute period. Therefore, a CT scan is recommended to confirm the diagnosis.

In addition to the simple documentation of a cerebral infarction or intracerebral hemorrhage, MRI has a number of other applications in the setting of stroke. Many patients who present with stroke signs and symptoms will have often had mild stroke symptoms well before their initial presentation. MRI can be used to determine the extent of cerebral damage due to small or silent infarcts that may have occurred much earlier than the presenting stroke. MRI has also demonstrated greater sensitivity than CT scan in identifying many vascular malformations and masses underlying intracerebral hemorrhages (Fig. 8–4).[40–42] Figure 8–5 illustrates a cerebral angiogram that was indicated because of the findings from Figure 8–4.

Identifying the cause of stroke is just as important as, if not more important than, documenting the location of the lesion through the use of brain imaging. Once the cause is identified, measures can be taken to prevent recurrent strokes, which are often more devastating. Therefore, all patients with stroke should undergo a diagnostic evaluation to determine the cause.

Patients with suspected embolic cerebral infarct should undergo an echocardiogram to look for evidence of an embolic source.[43] Many embolic sources can be identified through the use of a transthoracic echocardiogram (TTE), including mitral valve infectious or noninfectious endocarditis (Fig. 8–6), rheumatic valvular disease, and left ventricular thrombi (Fig. 8–7). Because of the anatomic location of the left atrium, the transesophageal echocardiogram (TEE) is usually required to identify thrombi within its chambers.[44, 45] A TTE color flow and bubble study is very useful in identifying a patent foramen ovale. This cardiac abnormality should be considered as a possible mechanism for cardioembolic stroke if no

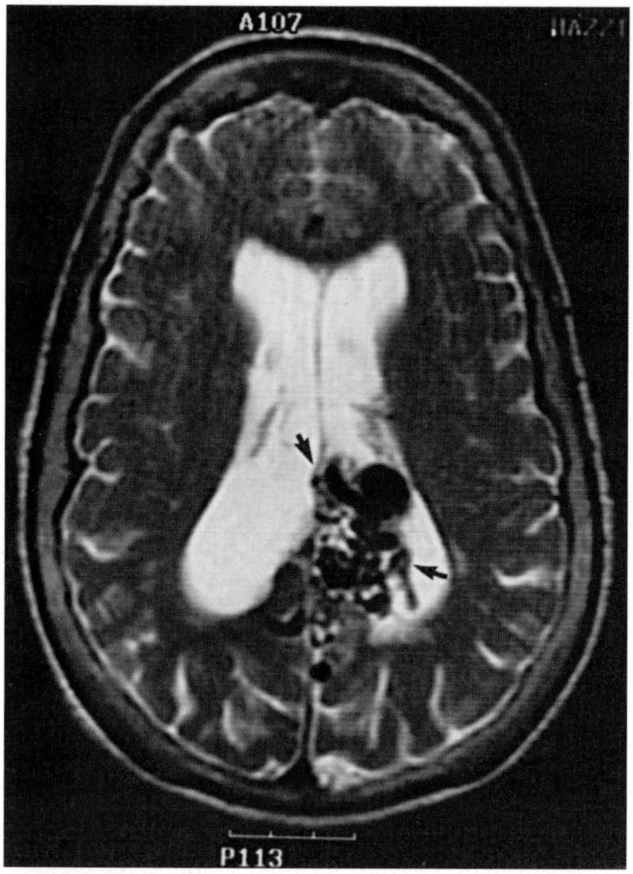

FIGURE 8–4 • Head MRI demonstrating an arteriovenous malformation (AVM) that extends into the left lateral ventricle (black arrows).

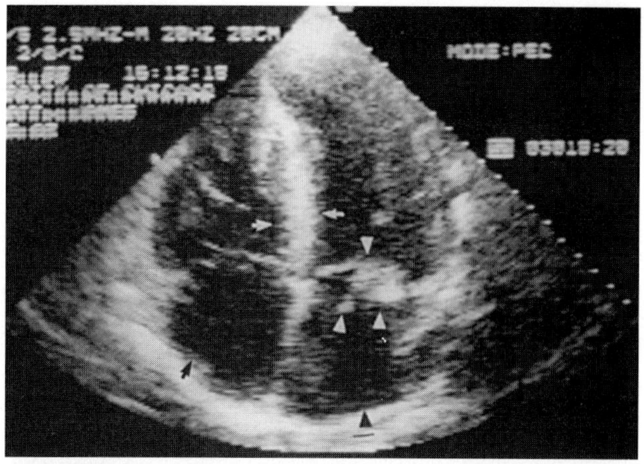

FIGURE 8–6 • Transthoracic echocardiogram demonstrating a mitral valve thrombus (white arrowheads). Note the left atrium (black arrowhead), right atrium (small black arrow), and ventricular septum (small white arrows).

other cause has been identified in a young person with stroke.[46]

In addition to echocardiography, patients with suspected embolic stroke or thrombotic stroke should undergo evaluation of the extracranial and intracranial large arteries to look for evidence of hemodynamically significant arterial stenosis. Patients are usually screened for extracranial stenosis through the use of carotid ultrasound. Carotid ultrasound technology uses blood flow velocities or frequencies and B-mode imaging (Fig. 8–8) to determine the degree of stenosis within a vessel.[47] Stenosis of 50% or greater is considered to be hemodynamically significant within the extracranial internal carotid artery (ICA) (Fig. 8–9). Carotid ultrasound is also useful in detecting other extracranial vascular abnormalities such as arterial dissection (Fig. 8–10), aneurysms, and fistulas. Since this

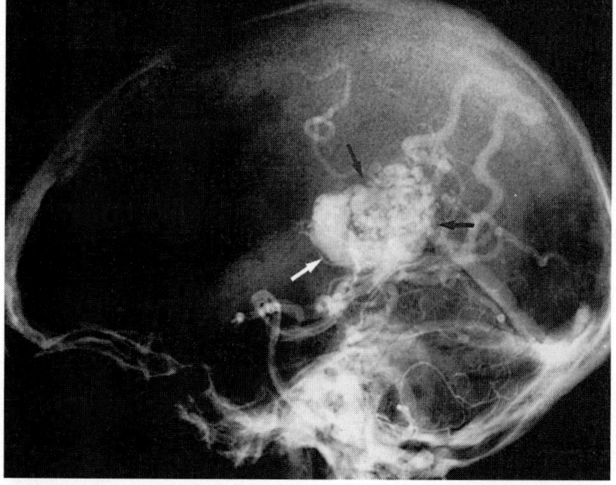

FIGURE 8–5 • Conventional cerebral angiogram of the left vertebral artery (same patient shown in Fig. 8–4). This study demonstrates the AVM supplied by the vertebrobasilar circulation (black arrows).

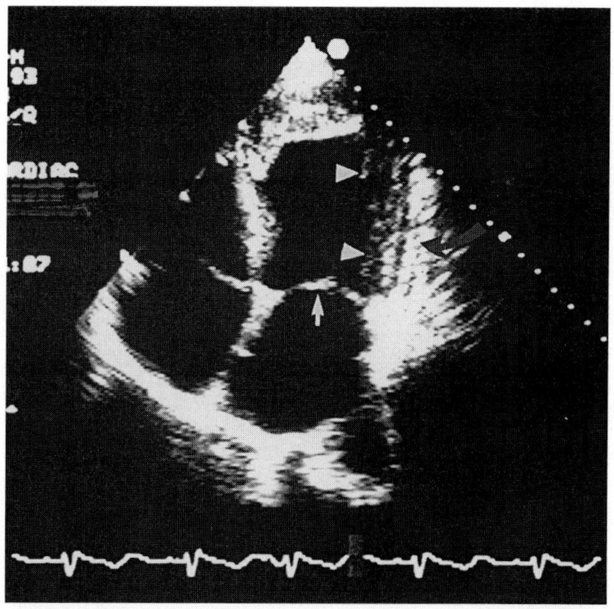

FIGURE 8–7 • Transthoracic echocardiogram demonstrating a left ventricular aneurysm (curved black arrow) and associated intraventricular thrombus (white arrowheads). Note the normal mitral valve (small white arrow).

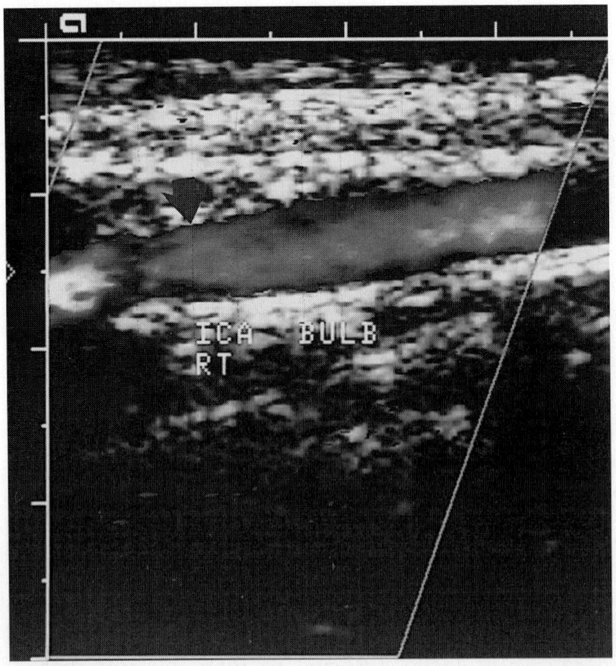

FIGURE 8–8 • Carotid ultrasound study demonstrating a normal internal carotid artery. Note the normal-vessel lumen (black arrow).

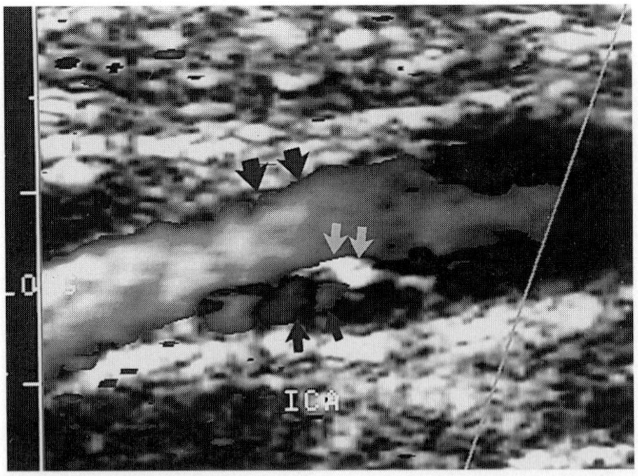

FIGURE 8–10 • Carotid ultrasound study demonstrating an internal carotid artery dissection. Note the true lumen (large black arrows), the dissected wall (white arrow), and the false lumen (small black arrows).

screening study is an indirect determination of stenosis and other vascular abnormalities, the results should be confirmed with cerebral angiography.

Transcranial Doppler (TCD) ultrasound technology is a modality that is becoming more widely used to identify intracranial arterial stenosis due to atherosclerotic vascular disease.[48] As with carotid ultrasound technology, stenosis within the intracranial large arteries is determined based on the TCD blood flow velocities (Figs. 8–11 and 8–12). B-mode imaging is not possible with the TCD machines currently in use. TCD is often used in combination with magnetic resonance angiography to screen for intracranial stenosis. If hemodynamically significant stenosis is suggested by TCD, confirmatory conventional cerebral angiography should be considered. In an effort to determine the clinical significance of a patent foramen ovale, some centers are now performing TCD with air contrast to obtain more direct evidence of paradoxic cerebral emboli in the setting of stroke (Fig. 8–13).[49]

Conventional cerebral angiography is generally reserved for a select population of patients with

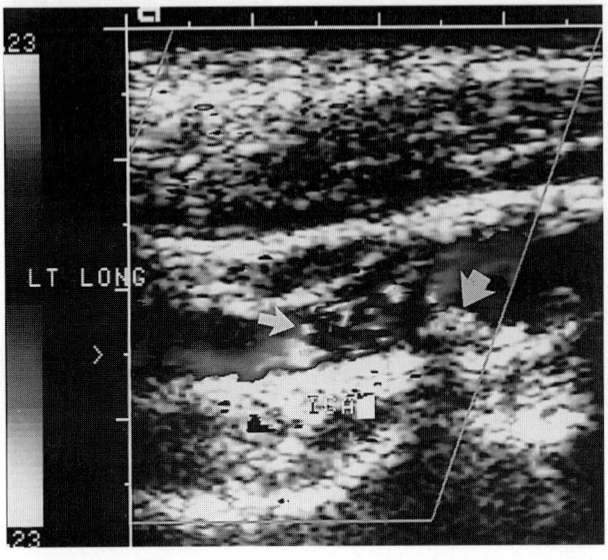

FIGURE 8–9 • Carotid ultrasound study demonstrating hemodynamically significant stenosis of the internal carotid artery. Note the atherosclerotic plaque (large white arrow) and the turbulent flow within the vessel lumen (small white arrow).

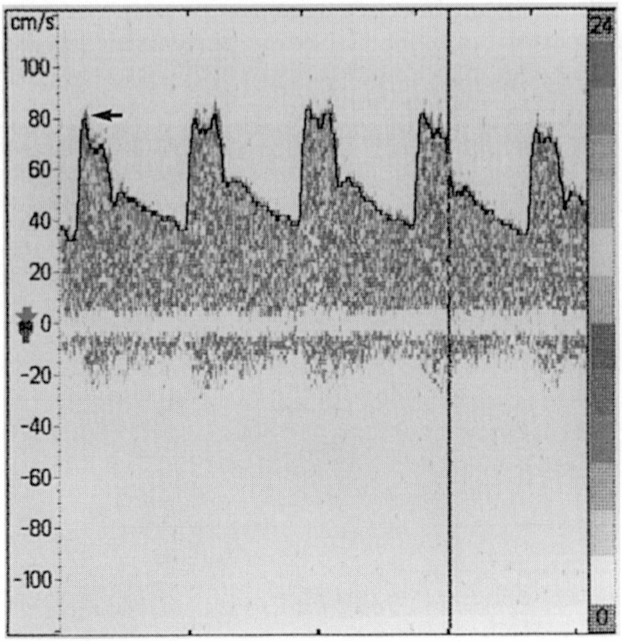

FIGURE 8–11 • Transcranial Doppler (TCD) ultrasound study demonstrating a normal signal and flow velocities within the middle cerebral artery.

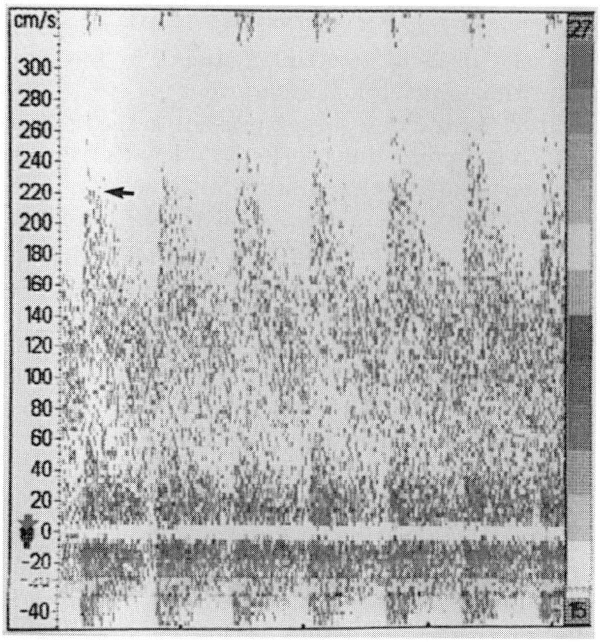

FIGURE 8–12 • TCD study of a patient with MCA stenosis. This study demonstrates elevated flow velocities within the MCA.

stroke. Individuals with intracerebral hemorrhage and a suspected aneurysm or arteriovenous malformation (see Fig. 8–5), progressive cerebral infarction believed to be due to medium to large vessel intracranial disease (Fig. 8–14) with a propagating clot, frequent transient ischemic attacks (TIAs), those with signs and symptoms suggestive of vasculitis or arterial dissection, or a young adult with a stroke of unknown etiology should be considered for cerebral angiography. Those individuals with evidence of significant ICA stenosis by carotid ultrasound should also be considered for conventional

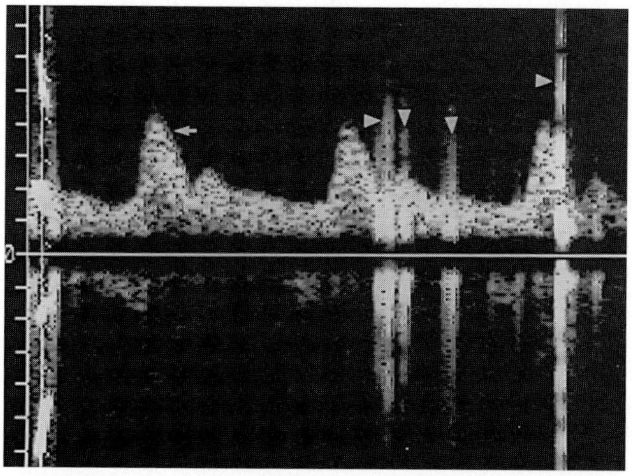

FIGURE 8–13 • TCD bubble study of the MCA. This study demonstrates high-intensity transient signals (HITS) (white arrowheads), a finding that is suggestive of a clinically significant patent foramen ovale. Note the normal signal and velocity of flow.

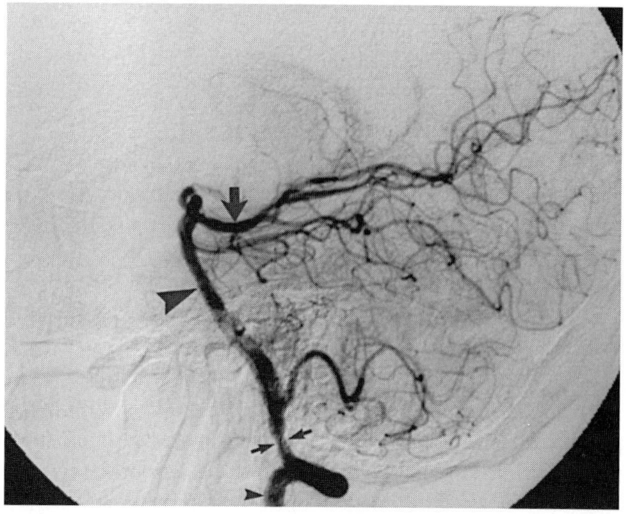

FIGURE 8–14 • Conventional cerebral angiography of the left vertebral artery (small arrowhead) demonstrating hemodynamically significant distal vertebral artery stenosis (small arrows). The basilar artery (large arrowhead) and posterior cerebral arteries (large arrow) are normal.

cerebral angiography. The purpose of angiography in the setting of suspected ICA stenosis is to confirm the ultrasound finding and to look for evidence of tandem stenosis distal to the ICA stenosis. When angiography is performed early, the presence of intra-arterial thrombus can also be identified in up to 80% of cases.

The risk of the conventional cerebral angiography procedure is relatively low, with the majority of complications being minor. Nevertheless, there is a risk of serious complications, predominantly stroke, of 0.5%–1% in patients with cerebrovascular disease.[50, 51] The risk of morbidity and mortality associated with conventional cerebral angiography may be much higher when the procedure is performed emergently by less experienced professionals. This fact should be kept in mind when deciding on the timing of angiography. Given the time required to perform the procedure, the associated costs, and the risks associated with this invasive procedure, its use should be reserved for those instances in which the management might be significantly altered by the result.

Magnetic resonance angiography (MRA) is a diagnostic tool that is currently being investigated for use in assessing patients with cerebrovascular disease. The technique involves converting the signal void from blood flowing within a vessel into a visual image. The signal from the brain parenchyma, CSF, and other soft tissue is erased. Both arterial and venous flow can be detected.

There is a tendency for the currently available MRA techniques to provide less detail and to overestimate the degree of arterial stenosis.[52–53] As a screening technique, MRA has been quite effective in detecting intracranial arterial stenosis and vascular malformations. It is the most reliable neuroimaging tool available for the detection of cavernous hemangiomas. MRA is useful in the setting of cerebral venous thrombosis because it fairly reliably detects lack of flow through the venous sinuses in this setting. Conventional cerebral angiography remains the gold standard for detection of cerebral venous thrombosis, intracranial arterial stenosis, and vascular malformations, other than cavernous hemangiomas.

The diagnostic studies recommended above will allow the clinician to document cardiovascular causes of acute stroke. While cardiovascular causes account for the majority of strokes, one must consider other causes as well, particularly with stroke in the younger population. Included in this category are coagulopathies,[54–59] systemic inflammatory diseases, hyperhomocysteinemia,[60] anemia and hyperviscosity syndromes, metabolic disturbances such as MELAS syndrome (mitochondrial encephalomyopathy with lactic acidosis and strokelike episodes),[61, 62] and illicit abuse of a variety of drugs, particularly cocaine.[16, 17] A diagnostic evaluation of each of these possibilities should be considered based on the clinical history and examination, and treatment should be directed at the underlying cause.

TREATMENT OPTIONS

A key factor in acute stroke treatment in the 1990s is the amount of time that has passed since the onset of the acute deficit. Individuals who present to the emergency department within 3 hours after the onset of their stroke signs and symptoms should be considered candidates for thrombolytic therapy.[63] Alteplase (r-TPA) has been approved by the United States Food and Drug Administration (FDA) for treatment of acute stroke. Selection of appropriate candidates is critical. Candidates for r-TPA should have an acute onset of a measurable, focal neurologic deficit that is not rapidly improving, and a head CT scan that demonstrates no evidence of hemorrhage or early ischemic change. In addition, there should be no evidence of a severe serum glucose abnormality, severe arterial hypertension, or hypertension that requires aggressive treatment to maintain the MAP within an acceptable range. Any factor(s) that might predispose the individual to intracranial bleeding or significant systemic bleeding serves as an exclusion criterion. This includes recent stroke; recent trauma or surgery; any history of intracranial hemorrhage; urinary tract or gastrointestinal hemorrhage; recent arterial puncture, lumbar puncture, or deep venous puncture; recent use of an anticoagulant; platelet count of $<100,000/\text{mm}^3$; seizure at the onset of the stroke; as well as other exclusions. Good clinical judgment should always be used in selecting patients to receive a drug with such a serious risk profile.

All r-TPA candidates must present to the hospital within a sufficient time period to allow assessment and determination of eligibility, a CT scan, and administration of the drug. All of these procedures must be accomplished within 3 hours of the onset of signs and symptoms. Rapid screening requires an integrated team of knowledgeable professionals who have expertise in hyperacute stroke care. This team must follow the eligibility guidelines approved by the FDA in an effort to avoid the very serious hemorrhagic risks associated with this drug.

Once full eligibility has been determined, the r-TPA can be given. The dose of r-TPA proven to be both safe and effective is 0.9 mg/kg, 10% of which is given as a bolus over 1 minute, followed by infusion of the remainder of the dose over 60 minutes. The dose should not exceed 90 mg. No antiplatelet or anticoagulant therapy should be given within the first 24 hours after infusion of the r-TPA. All patients should undergo frequent neurologic examinations in a neurointensive care unit when possible to detect early neurologic deterioration suggesting the possibility of intracranial bleeding.

If neurologic deterioration occurs after administration of the drug has begun, the infusion should be stopped. Hemodynamic and respiratory status should be assessed. An emergent head CT scan should be performed to rule out an intracranial hemorrhage. If an intracranial hemorrhage is identified, fresh-frozen plasma and cryoprecipitate should be given immediately. If the bleeding time is abnormal, platelets should be infused. A hematologic and neurosurgical consult should be obtained, and emergent evacuation of the blood should be considered when deemed appropriate. In addition to evaluation for hemorrhage by CT scan, other causes for clinical deterioration should be investigated, including extension of the infarction and the occurrence of seizures, hypoxemia, or a metabolic disturbance.

A number of other drugs are currently being investigated to provide improvement in outcome in those who present with signs and symptoms of an acute stroke. The presynaptic and postsynaptic excitatory amino acid inhibitors (e.g., lubeluzole and eliprodil) are among a number of neuroprotective agents that are currently being investigated for treatment of acute stroke.[64, 65] Low-molecular-weight heparin (ORG 10172) has been shown to have greater efficacy and a better safety profile for the treatment of deep venous thrombosis in the setting of acute cerebral infarction.[66, 67] It is currently being investigated for treatment of acute stroke. All physicians caring for acute stroke patients should be aware of the investigative drugs being tested within their respective regions and should consider recommending these trials to their patients.

Patients with frequent TIAs or progressive infarctions, suggesting recurrent emboli or a propagating thrombus, deserve emergent investigations to look for treatable vascular causes. Investigation with conventional cerebral angiography should be considered, particularly if the echocardiogram does not demonstrate an embolic source. Anticoagulant therapy (ACT) is indicated in the setting of stroke and a documented cardiac thrombus or cardioembolic source.[68, 69] The benefit of ACT for acute stroke or TIA outside of this setting has not been effectively proven.[70] Given the lack of strong supportive evidence for ACT in the setting of arterial stenosis, its use should be based on the best clinical judgment of the responsible physician. Patients with large cerebral infarcts are at a higher risk for clinically significant hemorrhagic conversion, regardless of the cause. This fact must be kept in mind when considering the use of ACT in this setting, as it might be associated with hemorrhagic conversion.[71] In the acute period, heparin is usually given intravenously as a continuous infusion at a rate of 10 units/kg/hour, without a bolus. This should be titrated to reach a partial thromboplastin time goal of 50–70 seconds. If the need for chronic anticoagulation is determined, treatment with oral warfarin should be considered. The goal International Normalized Ratio (INR) with warfarin therapy should be within the range of 2–3.

Treatment of cerebral infarction secondary to cerebral venous thrombosis is on the underlying cause. When the problem occurs in the setting of CNS infection, the patient should be treated with an antibiotic regimen that is based on culture results or empiric determination of the best antibiotic regimen. Institution of acute anticoagulation for this problem is controversial as a result of the risk of hemorrhagic conversion of the infarction. Clinical evidence to support the use of anticoagulation in this setting is increasing. On the other hand, surgical thrombectomy appears to provide no benefit for most patients with CVT and there is lack of evidence to support thrombolysis as its treatment.[9, 54, 72]

Carotid disease is said to account for 20%–75% of strokes.[73, 74] Patients with TIA or nondisabling cerebral infarction in the setting of tight carotid stenosis have a risk of 12%–13% and 5%–9% for an initial and recurrent stroke within the first year, respectively. Carotid endarterectomy (CEA) has been shown to provide greater risk reduction than medical therapy alone in this setting.[75–77] Therefore, if conventional cerebral angiography confirms hemodynamically significant internal carotid artery stenosis without associated tandem stenosis, these patients should be considered for CEA. Chronic anticoagulation might be of benefit in the setting of tight ICA stenosis if the patient cannot or will not undergo CEA.

Those patients with more disabling strokes and hemodynamically significant carotid stenosis should be re-evaluated for possible CEA several weeks later, given the risk of serious complications with surgery in this setting.

A significant number of stroke patients with ICA stenosis are considered to be poor operative candidates for CEA for a variety of reasons. This has resulted in the development of other approaches to address this problem. Currently, balloon angioplasty and intravascular stenting of the stenosed proximal internal carotid are being investigated as safe and reliable options to CEA.[78, 79]

As with anticoagulation, the benefit of antiplatelet therapy in the immediate setting of vascular causes for acute cerebral infarction or TIA is not clear, but its use in this setting is being investigated. Both aspirin and ticlopidine have been shown to be of benefit from a more chronic standpoint, in patients with TIA or mild ischemic stroke, decreasing the risk of recurrent stroke by 20%–30%.[54, 80–82]

Surgical management of intracerebral hemorrhage (ICH), in the form of clot evacuation, has been used in select cases. Cerebellar hematomas should be immediately evacuated, as this intervention can be life-saving.[83] The benefit of evacuation of clot from other areas of the brain has not been definitively proven, although both open and stereotactic evacuations of the clot have been performed.[84, 85] Owing to the uncertainty of this intervention, a multicenter trial is being considered to confirm its benefit.

In the instance of ICH due to an AVM that is approachable by surgery, surgical evacuation of the clot and resection of the AVM should be considered. These lesions are also being effectively treated with endovascular therapy.[86] ICH secondary to an aneurysm is rarely unaccompanied by subarachnoid hemorrhage. Early surgical clipping of the aneurysm is probably the best route of management for this problem.[87]

TREATMENT OF COMPLICATIONS

Acute stroke patients often experience a number of complications including massive brain swelling, seizures, deep venous thrombosis, pulmonary embolism, and aspiration pneumonia. Awareness of the potential complications is important because identification and early intervention may significantly improve the chances for a good outcome.

Cerebral Complications

Massive cerebral infarction secondary to anterior and middle cerebral artery occlusion is associated with a mortality rate of up to 80% or greater.[88] Nearly a third of these patients will die within the first 1–2 weeks due to herniation.[89–92] Clinical deterioration associated with brain swelling and increased ICP occurs in 10%–20% of patients with acute ischemic stroke. Maneuvers to prevent exacerbation of swelling and increased ICP should include keeping the patient in the upright position, as this will allow optimal jugular venous return. Venous return may also be compromised by maneuvers that cause an increase in intrathoracic pressure, such as coughing or the use of positive end-expiratory pressure, and measures should be taken to prevent or terminate these offenders.

The earliest sign of massive swelling and impending herniation, in the setting of cerebral infarction, is a depressed level of consciousness. Other signs include ipsilateral hemiparesis (or Kernohan's notch phenomenon), ipsilateral Babinski's reflex, and an ipsilateral fixed and dilated pupil. A CT scan should be obtained immediately to rule out massive swelling and impending herniation if this is suspected, based on the clinical examination.

Increased ICP may be a complication in 15%–20% of patients with acute massive cerebral infarction. If increased ICP is a concern, it should be monitored.[93] There are a variety of ICP monitoring devices available. The intraparenchymal fiberoptic monitoring device is reliable when CSF drainage is not necessary. If CSF drainage is necessary, an intraventricular catheter can be placed and will allow measurement of the ICP as well. Epidural catheters and subdural bolts and catheters have also been used to measure the ICP. There is a significant risk for bleeding and infection with each of these devices, especially the intraparenchymal and intraventricular ones. Therefore, serial assessment of the need for continued use of a device, and removal as early as possible, in a given patient is recommended.

Medical treatment of increased ICP may include the use of hyperventilation, hyperosmolar therapy, diuretic therapy, CSF drainage, and barbiturate therapy. Hyperventilation causes CSF alkalosis. The intracranial vessels constrict in association with the CSF alkalosis. Thus, hyperventilation decreases the ICP by decreasing the total intracranial blood volume through the mechanism of vasoconstriction. Its effect can be observed within minutes but may not be long lasting (duration of approximately 12–72 hours), most likely because brain swelling tends to exacerbate despite ongoing treatment. Therefore, hyperventilation represents a temporizing measure until more definitive treatment can be implemented. Rebound intracranial hypertension can be observed with rapid cessation of hyperventilation. Gradual tapering of the ventilatory rate, while observing the ICP values, is recommended to avoid rebound intracranial hypertension.

Hyperosmolar therapy for increased ICP is believed to work by creating an osmolar gradient between the intravascular space and the intraparenchymal space, which results in an overall loss of intracranial water content. Mannitol, urea, and glycerol have been used as hyperosmolar agents in this setting. Mannitol is the agent most commonly used in the United States. Mannitol also decreases blood viscosity, which may cause the intracranial vessels to constrict. This mechanism of vasoconstriction may also result in a decrease in ICP. The diuretic effect of mannitol causes an additional increase in the osmotic gradient. This effect can be augmented through the use of a loop diuretic such as furosemide.

Mannitol is usually infused intravenously as an initial bolus of 1 g/kg. This is usually followed by serial doses of 0.25–0.5 g/kg, given in dosing intervals of every 4 to 8 hours. The serum osmolality level should be checked every 8–12 hours, and the goal should be a plasma osmolality of 300–320 mOsm/L. The maintenance of osmolar levels beyond 320 mOsm/L should be avoided due to the risk of renal failure at higher levels. Mannitol may cause systemic hypotension as a result of excessive diuresis. To avoid hypotension, maintenance fluid in the form of 0.9% saline solution should be infused to maintain euvolemia.

CSF drainage can be an effective intervention for those cases complicated by acute hydrocephalus. In addition, ventricular catheterization provides a means of measuring the ICP. Its use is associated with a high rate of infection and intracranial hemorrhage. The catheter should be replaced or removed within 5 to 7 days to avoid infectious complications.

Barbiturate therapy is believed to decrease ICP by decreasing cerebral metabolism and intracranial blood volume. The high doses required to decrease the ICP are associated with significant risks. While it has been shown to be useful in the setting of acute stroke, owing to its potential risks barbiturate therapy is most commonly used only as a final treatment option in patients with refractory intracranial hypertension.[94, 95]

Hemicraniectomy, a therapeutic procedure that had fallen out of favor in this setting, is now being advocated as a life-saving intervention for treatment of brain swelling associated with massive strokes due to middle cerebral artery occlusion. In an animal study, this procedure was shown to significantly decrease mortality and improve functional outcome.[96] A prospective study in humans also showed a decrease in mortality and suggested improvement in functional outcome in patients who underwent hemicraniectomy versus conventional medical therapy.[97] The mechanism for improved outcome after this procedure is not entirely clear. It is thought to be due to prevention of death secondary to herniation, and a decrease in infarct size as a result of collateral flow augmentation.

Hemicraniectomy, in the setting of massive MCA infarction, involves removing a large portion of the skull overlying the infarcted brain tissue (Figs. 8–15 and 8–16).[98] A large incision is made in the dura mater, and the brain parenchyma is allowed to expand beyond the normal limits of the cranium. A dural graft is placed over the swollen brain to allow uniform expansion. The dura matter is then sutured over the graft. The scalp is then closed without the bone flap. Those patients who survive their stroke usually return to have the bone flap replaced after 8–12 weeks.

Hypotonic intravenous maintenance solutions may easily cross the vascular space (due to the osmotic gradient) and cause exacerbation of brain swelling. This same mechanism may be seen with the use of intravenous dextrose solutions. The latter may also exacerbate cell death through the formation of lactic acid within the anaerobic metabolic pathway.[34, 35] Therefore, intravenous hypotonic saline and dextrose solutions should be avoided in the setting of acute stroke, when possible.

Fevers can also exacerbate intracranial hypertension. Elevated body temperature causes an increase in cerebral metabolism that demands greater blood flow. Antipyretic and antibiotic therapy, when appropriate, should be instituted. Cooling blankets may cause an increase in ICP by inducing shivering, and this potential complication should be kept in mind when considering their use.

Seizures cause an increase in ICP by inhibiting venous return, through the Valsalva maneuver, and by increasing intracranial blood volume, through increasing cerebral metabolism. Less than 10% of stroke patients experience seizures. Most of these seizures occur within the first week and are short lived.[99, 100] Seizures have been observed more frequently in the setting of ICH when compared with cerebral infarction. Recurrent seizures can exacer-

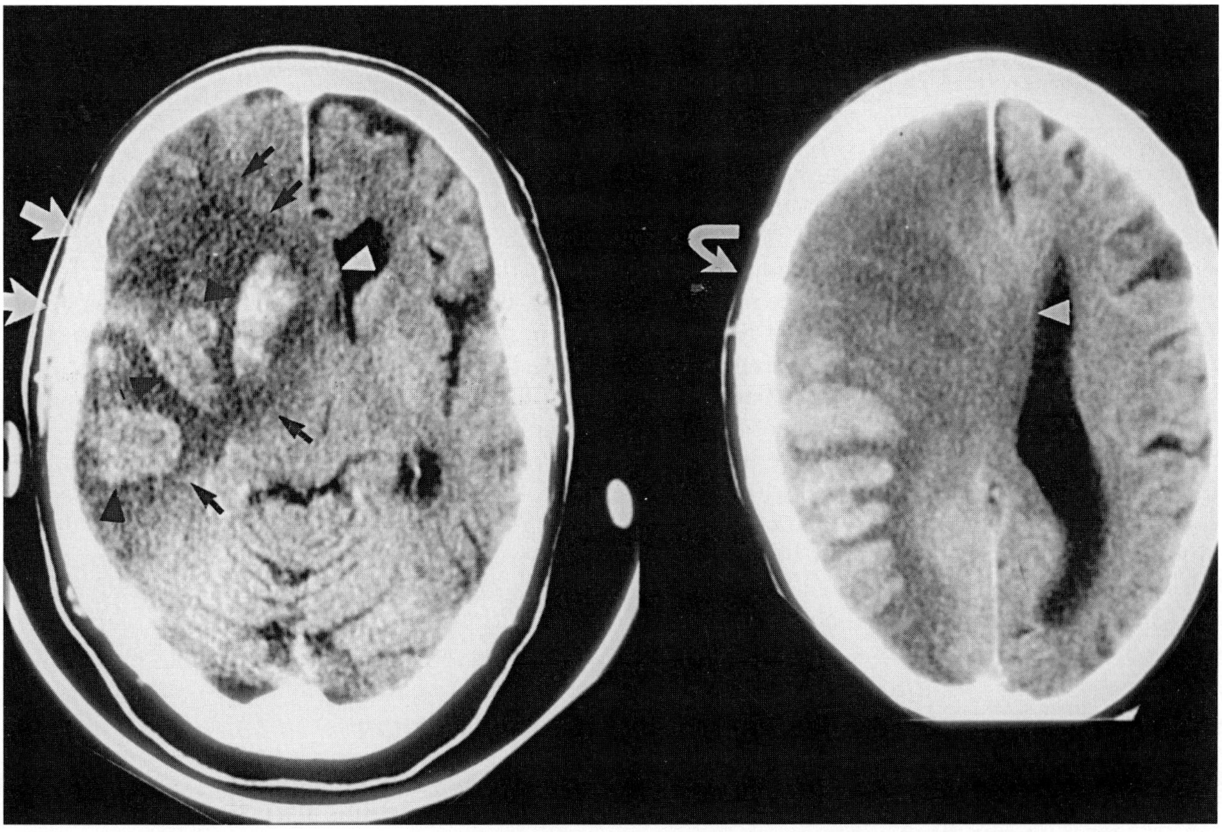

FIGURE 8–15 • Head CT scan demonstrating a right MCA distribution cerebral infarction (black arrows). This study was obtained 5 days after the onset of signs and symptoms and demonstrated hemorrhagic conversion of the infarction (black arrowheads), swelling with midline shift (white arrowhead), and obliteration of the right lateral ventricle. Note the intact skull (large white arrow). The figure to the right is an image of the same brain, taken at a higher level (curved arrow).

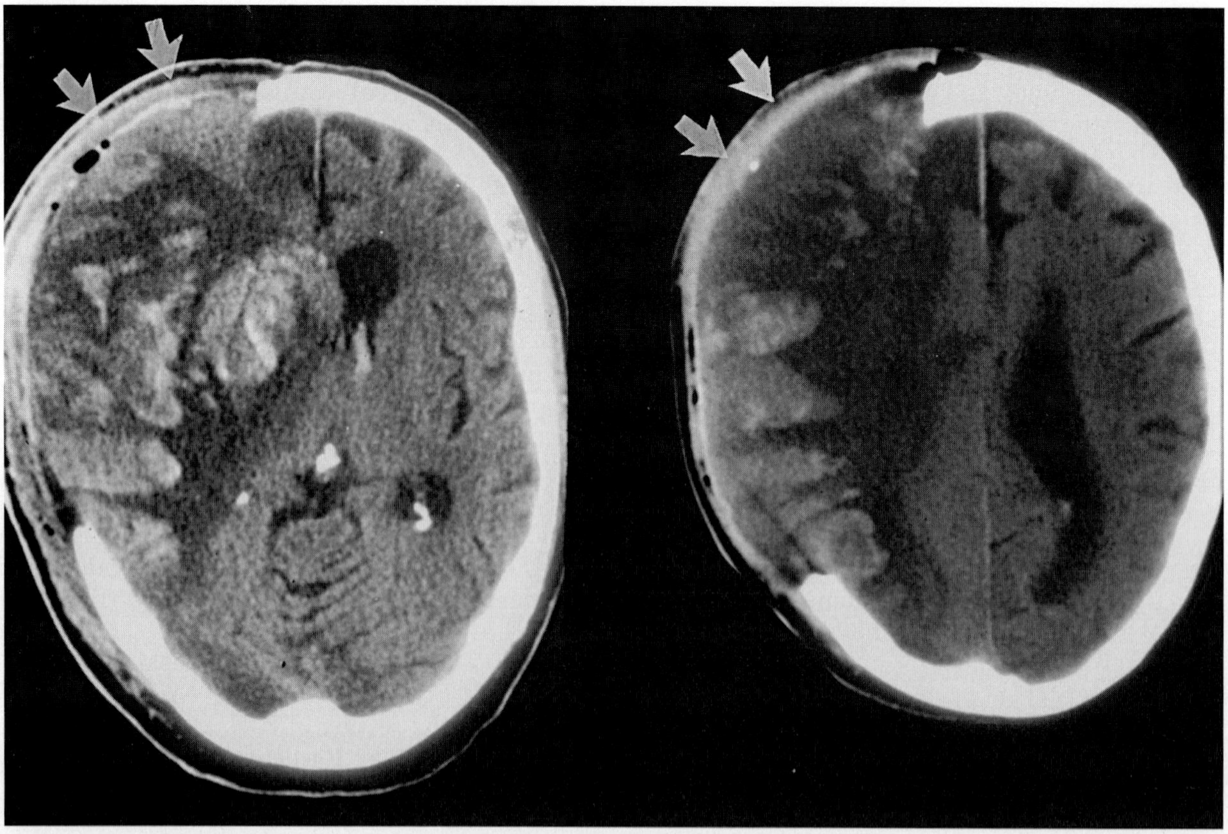

Figure 8-16 • Head CT scan of the same patient shown in Figure 8–15, after hemicraniectomy. That portion of the skull that covered the area of infarction has been removed (large white arrows), and the infarcted and swollen brain parenchyma has expanded well beyond the normal limits of the skull.

bate increased ICP in this setting. A protracted course of anticonvulsant therapy should be prescribed for those patients with significant risk. Intravenous phenytoin provides excellent anticonvulsant coverage for this problem. Phenytoin can be given with a loading dose of 20 mg/kg at a rate of 15–25 mg/minute in stable patients. Owing to the risk of cardiac arrhythmias and hypotension with rapid infusion of phenytoin, a faster rate of infusion (maximum 50 mg/minute) should be prescribed only for those patients in status epilepticus. Fosphenytoin may be a useful substitute in some patients.[101] Prophylactic anticonvulsant therapy is otherwise reserved for patients with cortical hemorrhages, or with ICH associated with an AVM, abscess, or neoplasm.

Other Complications

The peak period for deep venous thrombosis and pulmonary embolism is within the first week after the stroke.[102] Less than half of patients will demonstrate clinical findings. When the clinical suspicion is high, the demonstration of an abnormal noninvasive lower extremity venous flow study and an appropriately abnormal ventilation perfusion scan frequently establishes the diagnosis. Intravenous heparin with prolongation of the partial thromboplastin time is recommended, followed by oral warfarin therapy for 3–6 months.

All patients who are mechanically disabled from their stroke should receive prophylaxis for deep venous thrombosis in the form of subcutaneous heparin, low-molecular-weight heparin compounds, or pneumatic compression boots.

Pneumonia is a complication seen in approximately one third of stroke patients, with aspiration being the major cause. The precautions described earlier in this chapter should be taken to avoid aspiration. Identification of the offending agent and institution of the appropriate antibiotic therapy should be performed as soon as possible.

REHABILITATION

Evaluation for rehabilitation is optimally initiated as early as possible after the onset of stroke in stable patients.[103] This evaluation should include an assessment of motor, sensory/perceptual, language, and cognitive deficits. The plan of management and determination of post-stroke rehabilitation placement should be based on a combination of factors including cognitive ability, patient motivation, prior and present level of function, and medical stability.

CONCLUSION

With the advent of new diagnostic tools and therapies, the management of acute stroke is becoming increasingly complicated. A clear understanding of the pathophysiology of stroke, its complications, and the recommended approach to management, in combination with an experienced team of health care providers and a motivated patient, is the basic formula to the chance for a good outcome.

References

1. Gautier JC, Durr A, Koussa S, et al: Paradoxical cerebral embolism with a patent foramen ovale: A report of 29 patients. Cerebrovasc Dis 1991;1:193–196.
2. Van Camp G, Schulze D, Cosyns B, Vandenbossche JL: Relation between patent foramen ovale and unexplained stroke. Am J Cardiol 1993;71:596–598.
3. Hata JS, Ayres RW, Biller J, et al: Impact of transesophageal echocardiography on the anticoagulation management of patients with focal cerebral ischemia. Am J Cardiol 1993;72:707–710.
4. North American symptomatic carotid endarterectomy trial collaborators: Beneficial effect of carotid endarterectomy in symptomatic patients with high grade stenosis. N Engl J Med 1991;325:445–453.
5. Gasecki AP, Ferguson GG, Eliaszim, et al: Early endarterectomy for severe carotid artery stenosis after nondisabling stroke: Results from the North American Symptomatic Carotid Surgery Trial. J Vasc Surg 1994;20:288–265.
6. Fisher CM: The arterial lesions underlying lacunes. Acta Neuropathol 1968;12:1–15.
7. Fisher CM: Cerebral miliary aneurysms in hypertension. Am J Pathol 1972;66:313–330.
8. Fisher CM: Ataxic hemiparesis: A pathologic study. Arch Neurol 1978;35:126–128.
9. Bousser M, Barnett HJM: Cerebral venous thrombosis. In Barnett HJM, Mohr JP, Stein BM, et al (eds): Stroke: Pathophysiology, Diagnosis, and Management, 2nd ed, pp 523–537. New York, Churchill-Livingstone, 1992.
10. Wakai S, Yamakawa K, Manaka S, et al: Spontaneous intracranial hemorrhage caused by brain tumor: Its incidence and clinical significance. Neurosurgery 1982;10:437–444.
11. Niizuma H, Nakasato N, Yonemitsu T, et al: Intracerebral hemorrhage from a metastatic brain tumor. Importance of differential diagnosis preceding stereotaxic hematoma aspiration. Surg Neurol 1988;29:232–236.
12. Nutt SH, Patchell RA: Intracranial hemorrhage associated with primary and secondary tumors. Neurosurg Clin North Am 1992;3:591–599.
13. Rigamonti D, Spetzler RF: The association of venous and cavernous malformations. Report of four cases and discussion of the pathophysiological, diagnostic, and therapeutic implications. Acta Neurochir 1988;92:100–105.
14. Hyman RA, Black KS: Aneurysms and vascular malformations. Top Magn Reson Imag 1989;2:49–62.
15. Vinters HV, Gilbert JJ: Cerebral amyloid angiopathy: Incidence and complications in the aging brain. II. The distribution of amyloid vascular changes. Stroke 1983;14:924–928.
16. Levine SR, Brust JC, Futrell N, et al: Cerebrovascular complications of the use of the "crack" form of the alkaloid cocaine (comment). N Engl J Med 1990;323:699–704.
17. Levine SR, Brust JC, Futrell N, et al: A comparative study of the cerebrovascular complications of cocaine: Alkaloid versus hydrochloride—a review. Neurology 1991;41:1173–1177.
18. Juvela S, Hillbom M, Palomaki H: Risk factors for spontaneous intracerebral hemorrhage. Stroke 1995;26:1558–1564.
19. Alberts MJ, Perry A, Dawson DV, et al: Effects of public and professional education on reducing the delay in presentation and referral of stroke patients. Stroke 1992;23:352–356.
20. Mohr JP, Caplan LR, Melski JW, et al: The Harvard Cooperative Stroke Registry. Neurology 1978;28:754–762.
21. Edmeads J: The headache of ischemic cerebrovascular disease. Headache 1979;19:345–349.
22. Faught E, Peters D, Bartolucci A, et al: Seizures after primary intracerebral hemorrhage. Neurology 1989;8:141–147.
23. Ropper AH, Davis KR: Lobar cerebral hemorrhages: Acute clinical syndrome in 26 cases. Ann Neurol 1980;8:141–147.
24. Diringer MN: Intracerebral hemorrhage: Pathophysiology and management. Crit Care Med 1993;21:1591–1603.
25. Strandgaard S: Autoregulation of cerebral blood flow in hypertensive patients. Circulation 1976;53:720–727.
26. Broderick J, Brott T, Barsan W, et al: Blood pressure during the first minutes of focal cerebral ischemia. Ann Emerg Med 1993;22:1438–1443.
27. Wallace JD, Levy LL: Blood pressure after stroke. JAMA 1981;246:2177–2180.
28. Britton M, Carlsson A, Defaire U: Blood pressure course in patients with acute stroke and matched controls. Stroke 1986;17:861–864.
29. Phillips SJ: Pathophysiology and management of hypertension in acute ischemic stroke. Hypertension 1994;23:131–135.
30. Brott T, Reed RL: Intensive care for acute stroke in the community hospital setting: The first 24 hours. Curr Conc Cerebrovasc Dis Stroke 1989;24:1–5.
31. Rogers MC, Traystman RJ: Cerebral hemodynamic effects of nitroglycerin and nitroprusside. Acta Neurol Scand 1979;60(Suppl 72):600–602.
32. Montgomery BM, Pianer CA: Transient hypoglycemic hemiplegia. Arch Intern Med 1964;114:680–684.
33. Malouf R, Brust JCM: Hypoglycemia: Causes, neurological manifestations, and outcome. Ann Neurol 1985;17:421–430.
34. Dietrich WD, Alonso O, Busto R: Moderate hyperglycemia worsens acute blood brain barrier injury after forebrain ischemia in rats. Stroke 1993;24:111–116.
35. Wass CT, Lanier WL: Glucose modulation of ischemic brain injury: Review and clinical recommendations. Mayo Clin Proc 1996;71:801–812.
36. American Heart Association Stroke Council Special Writing Group: Guidelines for the management of patients with acute stroke. Stroke 1994;25:1901–1914.
37. Oppenheimer S, Hachinski V: Complications of acute stroke. Lancet 1992;339:721–724.
38. Hachinski VC: The clinical problem of brain and heart. Stroke 1993;24(12 Suppl): I1–2.
39. Fieschi C, Cavalletti C, Toni D, et al: Thrombolysis in acute ischemic stroke. Acta Neurochir Suppl 1996;66:76–80.
40. Chang KH, Han MC, Kim CW: Magnetic resonance imaging in neurologic diseases—comparison with computed tomography. J Korean Med Sci 1987;2:53–63.
41. Rigamonti D, Drayer BP, Johnson PC, et al: The MRI appearance of cavernous malformations. J Neurosurg 1987;67:518–524.
42. Rutka JT, Brant-Zawadzki M, Wilson CB, et al: Familial cavernous malformations. Diagnostic potential of magnetic resonance imaging. Surg Neurol 1988;29:467–474.
43. Sirna S, Biller J, Skorton DJ, et al: Cardiac evaluation of the patient with stroke. Stroke 1990;21:14–23.
44. Huain AM, Alter M: Transesophageal echocardiography in diagnosing cardioembolic stroke. Clin Cardiol 1995;18:705–708.
45. Rauh R, Fischereder M, Apengel FA: Transesophageal

echocardiography in patients with focal cerebral ischemia of unknown cause. Stroke 1996;27:1910–1911.
46. Lechat P, Mas JL, Lascault G, et al: Prevalence of patent foramen ovale in patients with stroke. N Engl J Med 1988;318:1148–1152.
47. Acker JD, Cole CA, Mauney KA, et al: Duplex carotid ultrasound. Neuroradiology 1986;28:608–617.
48. Dewitt LD, Wechsler LR: Transcranial Doppler. Stroke 1988;19:915–921.
49. Teague SM, Sharma MK: Detection of paradoxical cerebral echo contrast embolization by transcranial Doppler ultrasound. Stroke 1991;22:740–745.
50. Ernest F IV, Forbes G, Sandok BA, et al: Complications of cerebral angiography: Prospective assessment of risk. Am J Radiol 1984;142:247–254.
51. Dion JE, Gates PC, Fox JA, et al: Clinical events following neuroangiography: A prospective study. Stroke 1987;18:997–1003.
52. Ruggieri PM, Masaryk TJ, Ross JS: Magnetic resonance angiography: Cerebrovascular applications. Stroke 1992;23:774–780.
53. Riles TS, Eidelman EM, Litt AW, et al: Comparison of magnetic resonance angiography, conventional angiography and duplex scanning. Stroke 1992;23:341–346.
54. Landi G, D'Angelo A, Boccardi E, et al: Hypercoagulability in acute stroke: Prognostic significance. Neurology 1987;37:1667–1671.
55. Chancellor AM, Cull RE, Kilpatrick DC, et al: Neurologic diseases associated with anticardiolipin antibodies in patients without systemic lupus erythematosus: Clinical and immunologic features. J Neurol 1991;238:401–407.
56. Heistinger M, Rumpl E, Illiasch H, et al: Cerebral sinus thrombosis in a patient with hereditary protein S deficiency: Case report and review of the literature. Ann Hematol 1992;64:105–109.
57. Ginsburg KS, Liang MH, Newcomer L, et al: Anticardiolipin antibodies and the risk for ischemic stroke and venous thrombosis. Ann Intern Med 1993;118:986.
58. Barinagarrementeria F, Cantu-Brito C, De La Pena A, et al: Prothrombotic states in young people with idiopathic stroke. A prospective study. Stroke 1994;25:287–290.
59. Tatlisumak T, Fisher M: Hematologic disorders associated with ischemic stroke. J Neurol Sci 1996;140:1–11.
60. Verhoef P, Hennekens CH, Malinow MR, et al: A prospective study of plasma homocysteine and risk of ischemic stroke. Stroke 1994;25:1924–1930.
61. van Hellenberg Hubar JL, Gabreels FJ, Ruitenbeek W, et al: MELAS syndrome. Report of two patients, and comparison with data of 24 patients derived from the literature. Neuropediatrics 1991;22:10–14.
62. Zeviani M, Antozzi C: Defects of the mitochondrial DNA. Brain Pathol 1992;2:121–132.
63. The National Institute of Neurologic Disorders and Stroke r-TPA stroke study group: Tissue plasminogen activator for acute ischemic stroke. N Engl J Med 1995;333:1581–1586.
64. Muir KW, Lees KR: Clinical experience with excitatory amino acid antagonist drugs. Stroke 1995;26:503–513.
65. Diener HC, Hacke W, Hennerici M, et al: Lubeluzole in acute ischemic stroke. A double-blind, placebo-controlled phase II trial. Lubeluzole International Study Group. Stroke 1996;27:76–81.
66. Biller J, Massey EW, Marler JR, et al: A dose escalation study of ORG 10172 (low molecular weight heparinoid) in stroke. Neurology 1989;39:262–265.
67. Gordon DL, Linhardt R, Adams HP: Low-molecular-weight heparins and heparinoids and their use in acute or progressing ischemic stroke. Clin Neuropharm 1990;13:522–543.
68. Krayenbuhl HA: Cerebral venous and sinus thrombosis. Clin Neurosurg 1966;14:1–24.
69. Feinberg WM, Albers GW, Barnett JM, et al: Guidelines for the management of transient ischemic attacks: From the ad hoc committee on guidelines for the management of transient ischemic attacks of the stroke council of the American Heart Association. Circulation 1994;89:2950–2956.
70. Haley EC, Kassell NF, Torner JC: Failure of heparin to prevent progression in progressing ischemic infarction. Stroke 1988;19:10–14.
71. Furlan AJ, Cavalier SJ, Hobbs RE: Hemorrhage and anticoagulation in nonseptic embolic brain infarction. Neurology 1982;32:280–283.
72. Gettelfinger DM, Kokmen E: Superior sagittal sinus thrombosis. Arch Neurol 1977;34:2–6.
73. Anonymous: Endarterectomy for asymptomatic carotid artery stenosis. Executive Committee for the Asymptomatic Carotid Atherosclerosis Study. JAMA 1995;273:1421–1428.
74. Ferguson RD, Ferguson JG, Lee LI: Endovascular revascularization therapy in cerebral athero-occlusive disease. Angioplasty and stents, systemic and local thrombolysis. Neurosurg Clin North Am 1995;5:511–527.
75. Anonymous: Clinical Alert: benefit of carotid endarterectomy for patients with high grade stenosis of the internal carotid artery. National Institute of Neurologic Disorders and Stroke-Stroke and Trauma Division. North American Symptomatic Carotid Endarterectomy Trial (NASCET) investigators. Stroke 1991;22:816–817.
76. Anonymous: Beneficial effect of carotid endarterectomy in symptomatic patients with high-grade carotid stenosis. North American Symptomatic Carotid Endarterectomy Trial Collaborators. N Engl J Med 1991;325:445–453.
77. Treiman GS, Jenkins JM, Edwards WH, et al: The evolving surgical management of recurrent carotid stenosis. J Vasc Surg 1992;16:354–362.
78. Kachel R, Endert G, Basche S, et al: Percutaneous transluminal angioplasty (dilatation) of carotid, vertebral, and innominant artery stenoses. Cardiovasc Intervent Radiol 1987;10:142–146.
79. Diethrich EB, Ndiaye M, Reid DB: Stenting in the carotid artery: Initial experience in 110 patients. J Endovasc Surg 1996;3:42–62.
80. Horner J, Massey EW, Riski JE, et al: Aspirin following stroke: Clinical correlates and outcome. Neurology 1988;38:1359–1362.
81. Gent M, Blakely JA, Easton JD, et al: The Canadian American ticlopidine study (CATS) in thromboembolic stroke. Lancet 1989;1:1215–1220.
82. Hass WK, Easton JD, Adams HP, et al: A randomized trial comparing ticlopidine hydrochloride with aspirin for the prevention of stroke in high risk patients. N Engl J Med 1989;321:501–507.
83. Brennan RW, Bergland RM: Acute cerebellar hemorrhage. Analysis of clinical findings and outcome in 12 cases. Neurology 1977;27:527–532.
84. Kandel EI, Peresedov VV: Stereotactic evacuation of spontaneous intracerebral hematomas. J Neurosurg 1985;62:206–213.
85. Kaufman HH: Treatment of spontaneous intracerebral hematomas: A review. Stroke (Suppl I) 1993;24:I101–I106.
86. Dion JE, Mathis JM: Cranial arteriovenous malformations. The role of embolization and stereotactic surgery. Neurosurg Clin North Am 1994;5:459–474.
87. Haley EC, Kassell NF, Torner JC: The International Cooperative Study on the Timing of Aneurysm Surgery. The North American Experience. Stroke 1992;23:205–214.
88. Hacke W, Schwab S, Horn M, et al: "Malignant" middle cerebral artery territory infarction: Clinical course and prognostic signs. Arch Neurol 1996;53:309–315.
89. Shaw CM, Alvord EC, Berry GR: Swelling of the brain following ischemic infarction with arterial occlusion. Arch Neurol 1959;1:161–177.
90. Ropper AH, Shafran B: Brain edema after stroke. Arch Neurol 1984;41:26–30.
91. Silver FL, Norris JW, Lewis AJ, et al: Early mortality following stroke: A prospective review. Stroke 1984;15:492–496.
92. Frank JI: Large hemispheric infarction, deterioration, and intracranial pressure. Neurology 1995;45:1286–1290.
93. Ford GF, Bleck TP: Increased intracranial pressure. In

Parillo J (ed): Current Therapy in Critical Care Medicine, 3rd ed, pp 318–323. Toronto, BC Decker, 1997.

94. Woodcock J, Ropper AH, Kennedy SK: High-dose barbiturates in nontraumatic brain swelling: ICP reduction and effect on outcome. Stroke 1982;13:785–787.
95. Piatt JH, Schiff SJ: High-dose barbiturate therapy in neurosurgery and intensive care. Neurosurgery 1984;15:427–444.
96. Forsting M, Reith W, Schabitz WR, et al: Decompressive craniectomy for cerebral infarction. An experimental study in rats. Stroke 1995;26:259–264.
97. Reike K, Schwab S, Krieger D, et al: Decompressive surgery in space-occupying hemispheric infarction: Results of an open, prospective trial. Crit Care Med 1995;23:1576–1587.
98. Delashaw JB, Broaddus WC, Kassell NF, et al: Treatment of right hemispheric infarction by hemicraniectomy. Stroke 1990;21:874–881.
99. Kilpatrick CJ, Davis SM, Tress BM, et al: Epileptic seizures in acute stroke. Arch Neurol 1990; 47:157–160.
100. Drury I, Beydoun A: Seizure disorders of aging: Differential diagnosis and patient management. Geriatrics 1993;48:52–58.
101. Ramsay RE, DeToledo J: Intravenous administration of fosphenytoin: Options for the management of seizures. Neurology 1996;46:S17–9.
102. Roth EJ, Noll SF: Stroke rehabilitation. 2. Comorbidities and complications. Arch Phys Med Rehabil 1994;75:S42–S46.
103. Lorish TR, Sandin KJ, Roth EJ, et al: Stroke rehabilitation. 3. Rehabilitation and management. Arch Phys Med Rehabil 1994;75:S47–S51.

9

Parasurgical Management of Aneurysmal Subarachnoid Hemorrhage

David J. Langer, M.D. • Eric L. Zager, M.D. • Eugene S. Flamm, M.D.

Cerebral arterial aneurysms are relatively uncommon lesions with an estimated frequency of 1%–8% in the general population based on autopsy and angiographic series.[1–4] These aneurysms represent dilatations of the cerebral arteries and occur in several different forms within the central nervous system (Table 9–1). Their existence was first recognized in the mid-1800s; it was Hermann Lebert, in Breslau in 1866, who stated that "in a number of cases a diagnosis of cerebral aneurysm is possible" with the conclusion that "the prognosis in general is very gloomy."[5]

Since then a number of innovations have led to dramatic improvements in the diagnosis and treatment of cerebral aneurysms. With the introduction of cerebral angiography by Moniz in 1927,[6] diagnosis of aneurysms was greatly improved. Innovations in anesthetic and surgical techniques followed with anecdotal reports of successful surgical treatment, especially after the development of removable vascular clips in the 1950s.[5] However, it was not until the advent of microneurosurgery that acceptable rates of morbidity and mortality became possible. Despite these tremendous advances in the treatment of cerebral aneurysms, subarachnoid hemorrhage (SAH) remains a disease with extremely high morbidity and mortality; indeed, mortality alone in the first month after SAH in all patients, treated and untreated, approaches 50%. Our intention in this chapter is to describe the current thinking regarding the patient who has sustained an SAH and to describe our methods of managing these critically ill patients.

TABLE 9–1 **ANEURYSM TYPES**

Aneurysm types
Saccular
Fusiform (atherosclerotic)
Traumatic
Dissecting
Mycotic
Miliary

EPIDEMIOLOGY OF INTRACRANIAL ANEURYSMS

Saccular or berry aneurysms are the most commonly encountered form of cerebral arterial aneurysms. These are thought to be acquired lesions related to hemodynamic stress placed on the arterial wall arising at arterial bends or bifurcations.[7–9] Interestingly, saccular aneurysms occur solely in the intracranial circulation, and certain unique characteristics of these vessels may make them susceptible to their formation. Intracranial arteries have a very thin adventitia, lack an external elastic lamina, and lie in the subarachnoid space, unsupported by adjacent tissue. Histologic sections through aneurysms and their associated bifurcations show that the muscle coat and internal elastic lamina stop abruptly at the aneurysmal neck.[10] Most arise from the terminal portion of the internal carotid artery and from the major branches of the anterior portion of the circle of Willis[10] (Table 9–2). It is generally accepted that aneurysms are acquired. They are most commonly encountered clinically or at autopsy in persons between the ages of 40 and 70 years with a mean age of hemorrhage of 50 years.[9] Childhood aneurysms do occur, however, accounting for 0.5%–4.6% of cerebral aneurysms in epidemiologic aneurysm series.[11, 12] Although hypertension, smoking, alcohol, and oral contraceptives have been linked to the development of aneurysmal subarachnoid hemorrhage, certainly intrinsic vascular factors play a part in aneurysm formation as evidenced by their occurrence in children. Additionally, a number of disease states that either alter the arterial wall or result in abnormal blood flow or pressure through the affected artery are associated with an increased incidence of saccular aneurysms[10, 13] (Table 9–3). These disease states likely result in weakness of the vascular wall, resulting in an increased susceptibility to aneurysm formation.

The rupture of an intracranial aneurysm is a devastating occurrence. Weir concluded in a review of large autopsy and epidemiologic studies that 2% of the general population will have an intracranial aneurysm, 1% will have a rupture during their lifetime, and 0.5% will die because of SAH.[13] Although the morbidity and mortality from the surgical treatment of aneurysms has improved greatly over time, the overall outcome in patients with SAH has not: Less than 60% of patients who are alive upon admission have a favorable outcome.[14]

ACUTE ANEURYSMAL SUBARACHNOID HEMORRHAGE—INITIAL MANAGEMENT

The rupture of an intracranial aneurysm is a medical emergency, and rapid identification and stabilization of these patients is of paramount importance in their management. Unfortunately, the early mortality rate of the initial bleed alone approaches 30%, rendering medical intervention fruitless.[13, 15] However, expeditious management of the SAH patient clearly is important in order to limit the risk of subsequent morbidity and mortality.

Upon presentation to the emergency room or clinic, awake patients most commonly complain of the "worst headache of their life," the sine qua non of SAH. Patients commonly present in a moribund or comatose state; these patients in particular must be managed with great urgency to rule out immediate life-threatening, potentially reversible pathology.

A number of factors are thought to predispose the person harboring an aneurysm to SAH[16] (Table 9–4). Smoking, hypertension, and alcohol are associated with an increased risk of aneurysmal rupture.[17–20] It is likely that peaks of arterial hypertension and rapid oscillations in venous and cerebrospinal fluid (CSF) pressure increase the likelihood of aneurysmal rupture.[13] Interestingly,

TABLE 9–2 **ANEURYSM LOCATION**

LOCATION	PERCENTAGE
Anterior cerebral	35–40
Internal carotid	30
Middle cerebral	20–25
Posterior circulation	10

TABLE 9–3 **DISEASE STATES ASSOCIATED WITH FORMATION OF SACCULAR ANEURYSMS**

1. Increased blood pressure
   - Fibromuscular dysplasia
   - Polycystic kidney disease
   - Aortic coarctation
2. Increased blood flow
   - Cerebral arteriovenous malformation
   - Aplastic, hypoplastic, ligated contralateral vessel
   - Persistent carotid-basilar anastomosis
3. Blood vessel disorders
   - Granulomatous angiitis
   - Systemic lupus erythematosus
   - Moyamoya disease
4. Genetic
   - Ehlers-Danlos syndrome
   - Marfan's syndrome
   - Osler-Weber-Rendu syndrome
   - Pseudoxanthoma elasticum
   - Klippel-Trenaunay-Weber syndrome
5. Congenital
   - Persistent fetal circulation
   - Absent/hypoplastic arterial circulation
6. Metastatic tumors to cerebral arteries
   - Atrial myxoma
   - Choriocarcinoma
   - Undifferentiated carcinoma
7. Infectious
   - Bacterial
   - Fungal

TABLE 9–4 **RISK FACTORS FOR SUBARACHNOID HEMORRHAGE**

1. Hypertension
2. Cigarette smoking
3. Oral contraceptives
4. Alcohol consumption
5. Diurnal variations in blood pressure
6. Pregnancy and parturition
7. Slight increase during lumbar puncture, cerebral angiography, or both

TABLE 9–5 CLINICAL PRESENTATION FOLLOWING ANEURYSMAL RUPTURE

1. Meningismus (64%)
2. Coma (52%)
3. Nausea/vomiting (45%)
4. No localizing signs (39%)
5. Global headache (32%)
6. Occipital headache (21%)
7. Reflex changes (19%)
8. Motor deficit (17%)
9. Dysphasia (13%)
10. Confusion (12%)
11. Intraocular hemorrhage (12%)
12. Anisocoria (12%)
13. Papilledema (11%)
14. Homonymous hemianopsia (9%)
15. Lateralized headache (8%)
16. Third-nerve palsy (7%)
17. Sensory disturbance (5%)

though, 30% of aneurysmal SAHs occur during sleep. Various activities of daily living that raise intracranial pressure (ICP), such as defecation or coitus, are commonly thought to increase the risk of SAH, but this risk is difficult to quantify.

In the cooperative aneurysm study of 2621 cases of Sahs et al., it was found that 10%–15% of patients with ruptured aneurysms had symptoms related to their aneurysm prior to rupture.[21] Headache occurred in 48%, dizziness in 10%, orbital pain in 7%, diplopia in 4%, and visual loss in 4%. Signs that were present prior to SAH included sensory or motor disturbances in 6%, seizures in 4%, ptosis in 3%, bruits in 3%, and dysphasia in 2%. Other studies have suggested a slightly higher incidence of warning signs of up to 40%–50%, occurring an average of 10–20 days prior to aneurysmal rupture.[22, 23]

Upon presentation, a patient with possible SAH should be carefully examined and graded prior to undergoing computed tomography (CT) of the head. Patients most commonly present with meningismus, headache, or coma[24] (Table 9–5). Patients who present with a clinical history even remotely suggesting SAH ought to undergo head CT. Grading of the clinical condition of these patients is important when deciding on the appropriateness of surgical intervention while allowing the neurosurgical team to follow the patient's condition in a systematic and objective fashion. We use the Hunt-Hess classification of SAH (Table 9–6).[25] A second frequently used scale is the World Federation of Neurosurgical Societies (WFNS) grading of SAH. This scale was developed after analysis of data from the International Cooperative Aneurysm Study revealed that no difference in outcome was noted between Hunt-Hess grades 1 and 2. In addition, hemiparesis and aphasia had no effect on mortality. The WFNS scale relies on the Glasgow Coma Scale, incorporating the patient's level of consciousness along with the presence or absence of a major focal cortical deficit into a clinical grade (Table 9–7).[26] The modified Botterell grading scale is the third clinical scale commonly used and is similar in organization to the Hunt-Hess scale (Table 9–8).[27] The choice of scale is not as important as that the scale chosen must be used and understood by all caregivers, including emergency room personnel, neurosurgeons, neurologists, anesthesiologists, intensivists, and intensive care and perioperative nursing personnel.

The acute care management of the patient with a possible SAH must be tailored to the needs of each individual. Clearly, a patient becoming progressively obtunded should be handled differently from the awake, alert patient complaining of a headache; however, several points deserve special attention when evaluating a patient for the first time.

Most importantly, the patient must be stable in

TABLE 9–6 HUNT-HESS CLASSIFICATION OF SUBARACHNOID HEMORRHAGE

GRADE	DESCRIPTION
0	Unruptured
1	Asymptomatic/mild headache, nuchal rigidity
2	Cranial nerve palsy, moderate to severe headache, nuchal rigidity
3	Mild focal deficit, lethargy, confusion
4	Stupor, hemiparesis
5	Coma, extensor rigidity

TABLE 9–7 WORLD FEDERATION OF NEUROSURGICAL SOCIETIES GRADING SCALE FOR SUBARACHNOID HEMORRHAGE

GRADE	GCS	MAJOR FOCAL DEFICIT	COMMENTS
0	—	—	Unruptured
1	15	Absent	
2	13–14	Absent	
3	13–14	Present	
4	7–12	Present or absent	
5	3–6	Present or absent	

GCS, Glasgow Coma Scale.

TABLE 9–8 MODIFIED BOTTERELL GRADING SCALE FOR SUBARACHNOID HEMORRHAGE

GRADE	DESCRIPTION
0	Unruptured/no subarachnoid hemorrhage in past 30 days
1	Alert, oriented, with or without headache; no motor or sensory deficits
2	Severe headache, major meningeal signs, mild alteration of sensorium or focal deficits
3	Major alteration of sensorium or major focal deficit
4	Semi-comatose or comatose, with or without major lateralizing findings

regard to the Advanced Cardiac Life Support (ACLS) "ABCs"—airway, breathing, and cardiovascular systems. Patients should be intubated if their respiratory status is compromised or if their level of consciousness is such that their airway might be affected. Intubation commonly results in subsequent periodic sedation, rendering the neurologic examination difficult to interpret. If the ABCs are "A-OK," a directed neurologic examination should immediately ensue (Table 9–9). In order to grade the patient adequately, one should pay careful attention to the patient's level of consciousness, and in the awake patient, to the chief complaint. Nuchal rigidity is an important sign that is generally readily recognized and usually occurs within 6–24 hours post SAH.[16] Kernig's sign (pain in the hamstrings with hip flexion and knee extension) and Brudzinski's sign (involuntary hip flexion with neck flexion) can be easily evaluated as well, although we find these signs less useful than nuchal rigidity. Lateralization of headache should be noted, because the side of pain is often associated with the side of aneurysmal location and, in patients with multiple aneurysms, may aid in determining the location of the bleed.

The patient should be carefully checked for cranial nerve deficits (particularly cranial nerves II, III, and VII) and for evidence of cortical deficits (i.e., dysphasia or lateralizing motor weakness, sensory disturbance, or reflex changes). Cranial nerve II is often affected with aneurysms of the supraclinoid carotid artery, particularly with ophthalmic artery aneurysms.[28] Optic pallor is a common sign, as is an afferent pupillary defect on the side of these aneurysms.[29] Posterior communicating artery aneurysms often present with third cranial nerve dysfunction, with the vast majority of these involving pupillary function.[30] Facial asymmetry from "central" seventh-nerve palsy can be a subtle sign of cortical dysfunction; however, the cranial nerve itself is rarely affected by aneurysmal rupture or expansion. We find that testing for pronator drift is a particularly sensitive method for assessing subtle motor weakness and can be performed easily throughout the patient's therapeutic course with

TABLE 9–9 **DIRECTED NEUROLOGIC EXAMINATION OF THE POSSIBLE SUBARACHNOID HEMORRHAGE PATIENT**

1. Level of consciousness
2. Chief complaint
3. Presence of headache and its location
4. Presence of nuchal rigidity
5. Cranial nerve examination
6. Evaluation for motor weakness/pronator drift
7. Evaluation for sensory disturbance
8. Evaluation for reflex changes

good reproducibility. Even subtle changes in mentation or motor function may be early signs of arterial vasospasm, and a good baseline examination is invaluable in assessing clinical deterioration. If time permits, a stable and cooperative patient should be evaluated for subhyaloid hemorrhages, which occur in 10% of SAH patients.[31] Infrequently, blood extends into the vitreous humor (Terson's syndrome), which can lead to blindness. Prompt treatment with vitrectomy, photocoagulation, or both is indicated when vision is compromised.[32]

Prior to departing for head CT, the patient should be stabilized with regard to several other systems. SAH patients often present with hypertension, and gentle blood pressure control should be considered with systolic pressures above 180 mm Hg or diastolic pressure above 100 mm Hg. Careful attention should be paid to the medical history, because a previously hypertensive patient ought to be treated less aggressively than the normotensive patient. An electrocardiogram (ECG) ought to be obtained, because patients can present with cardiac ischemia thought to be related to massive sympathetic activation initiated by SAH and increased ICP. Abnormalities of T and U waves, as well as prolongation of the Q-T interval, are frequently identified.[33, 34] Szabo et al. studied 19 patients with thallium scans with confirmed SAH and abnormal ECG results and found that abnormal myocardial perfusion and possibly ischemia occur frequently following SAH, but no specific ECG characteristics identified these perfusion abnormalities.[35] In addition, arrhythmias occasionally occur with SAH patients and should be managed appropriately if they occur. Seizures have been historically reported to occur in the setting of SAH in approximately 24% of cases[36] and ought to be treated with anticonvulsants quickly to limit the attendant rise in blood and ICP in the acute phase. Patients with middle cerebral artery and anterior communicating artery aneurysms, parenchymal hematomas, hypertension, and significant cerebral infarcts are thought to have an increased risk of seizures after SAH.[37–39] No increase in morbidity or mortality was found in patients who have acute seizures with SAH.[36]

A battery of electrolyte tests should be performed because SAH patients can present with the syndrome of inappropriate anti-diuretic hormone (SIADH) (particularly ruptured anterior communicating artery aneurysms) and cerebral salt wasting. A PT/PTT profile should be performed to ensure adequate coagulation in the post-SAH patient. Derangements in coagulation can lead to a higher frequency of rebleeding, and any gross clotting abnormality ought to be treated when possible. At the first sign of an abnormal value, liver function tests ought to be performed and a hematologic consultation obtained so as to better understand and treat this potential complication. Lastly, pain control is often necessary in the awake, alert patient with a headache. We usually use acetaminophen alone if possible. Narcotics can affect the level of consciousness of the patient and are therefore used only for stable persons under close surveillance. Corticosteroids alone may relieve the headache in the SAH patient, and we continue to use steroids routinely in the perioperative period.

Radiologic Evaluation—Indications for Intervention

Hydrocephalus/Intracranial Blood

Once the question of subarachnoid hemorrhage is entertained based on history and examination, CT should be performed as rapidly as possible. CT is nearly 100% sensitive in detecting blood if performed on the day of the ictus, with the probability falling to 50% after 1 week, 30% after 2 weeks, and almost 0% after 3 weeks.[40] Particular attention should be paid to the location of the blood, the presence of hydrocephalus (20%),[41, 42] the presence of intraventricular blood (13%–28%),[43] intraparenchymal blood (20%–40%),[16] or subdural blood (1.3%–2.8%).[43] The goals of CT (Table 9–10) should be to diagnose the presence or absence and location of SAH, to identify any space-occupying clot that could be causing neurologic deterioration, and to evaluate the ventricles for the presence of hydrocephalus. It is imperative that space-occupying clot and hydrocephalus are ruled out in the acute phase, particularly for poor-grade cases, because rapid treatment of both is indicated and should supersede further evaluation in the comatose or rapidly deteriorating patient. The CT signs of acute hydrocephalus are distinctive and consist of ballooning of the frontal horns, rostral-caudal enlargement of the ventricles, and periventricular edema.[41] Enlargement of the temporal horns is commonly associated with hydrocephalus and may be the best indicator of significant hydrocephalus. Emergent craniotomy without angiogram is indicated in the poor-grade case with a space-occupying clot thought responsible for the patient's poor neurologic condition. In addition, rapid ventriculostomy is indicated for the poor-grade case with hydrocephalus, whereas semi-emergent ventriculostomy ought to be performed in the lethargic, awake patient with significant ventriculomegaly. We have seen many patients improve one or two Hunt-Hess grades with ventriculostomy alone.

TABLE 9–10 **GOALS OF EVALUATION WITH HEAD CT**

Determine whether the following are present:
1. Intracranial blood
2. Mass-occupying clot
3. Hydrocephalus

Mass Effect

CT often gives information concerning the aneurysm itself. Occasionally, aneurysms present with symptoms of mass effect, occurring in approximately 10% of patients. These aneurysms are most commonly large or giant; however, even small aneurysms can exert pressure against adjacent neural structures.[31] CT often reveals the presence of these aneurysms, and careful scrutiny ought to be given to anatomically distinct areas that the examination suggests as being affected. Space-occupying clot and the presence of midline shift can also be easily appreciated on CT. A large parenchymal clot thought to be responsible for a patient's neurologic deficits should be evacuated promptly.

Negative CT Results

Occasionally, patients present with a clinical history or examination consistent with SAH but have negative CT results. If the diagnosis of SAH is entertained and clinical suspicion is moderate or better, a lumbar puncture (LP) ought to be undertaken to rule out a possible bleed. Xanthochromia can appear in CSF within 3 hours following SAH, and its presence even in the absence of blood on CT is an indication for arteriography. Vermeulen et al. reported that CSF remained xanthochromic in 32 of 32 patients 2 weeks after SAH and in over 70% of their group after 3 weeks.[44] In addition, the concentrations of bilirubin and oxyhemoglobin in CSF continue to increase for 1 week after SAH, whereas the xanthochromic index can continue to rise for up to 3 weeks after the ictus.[44, 45] Whether the lack of xanthochromia with negative CT results truly rules out SAH is controversial. MacDonald and Mendelow argued that the absence of xanthochromia does not rule out SAH based on the fact that 7 of 20 patients with SAH and negative CT results had bloody CSF without xanthochromia.[46] This argument was countered by Vermeulen et al., who found that all 111 patients studied with proven SAH had xanthochromia.[44] In addition, only six patients over a period of 6 years had sudden headache, negative CT results, and bloody CSF without xanthochromia. Angiograms were carried out in three of these patients and yielded negative results as well. None of these patients was readmitted with headache over a 4-year period. Given their results, the authors concluded that normal CT results in the absence of xanthochromia does exclude SAH,[44] an opinion with which we agree. Significant mass effect from an infarct, tumor, blood clot, or hydrocephalus should be ruled out by CT prior to performing an LP. An LP may be safe in a patient with hydrocephalus provided it is of the communicating type.

Perimesencephalic Hemorrhage

A type of SAH known as perimesencephalic hemorrhage (PMH) has been defined that has an excellent long-term prognosis and uncommonly results in the discovery of an aneurysm by arteriography (2.7%).[47] CT of this entity characteristically shows cisternal blood with the center of bleeding located immediately anterior to the brain stem (Fig. 9–1). Extension to the ambient cistern or to the basal parts of the sylvian fissure is common. Intraventricular rupture does not occur.[48] Although delayed cerebral ischemia does not seem to be associated with PMH, acute hydrocephalus can occur, albeit at a lower frequency than is seen in aneurysmal SAH (5% vs. 10%–30%). The hydrocephalus in PMH is thought to be related to CSF blockage at the tentorial hiatus due to the presence of blood in the perimesencephalic cistern.[49, 50] We perform arteriography in all patients with PMH; however, we do not recommend follow-up angiograms for patients with negative study results. It must be stressed that PMH remains a diagnosis of exclusion. A high-quality four-vessel angiogram is mandatory prior to the entertainment of this diagnosis.

Dynamic Contrast Three-Dimensional CT

A new and relatively promising technology for the evaluation of intracranial aneurysms is three-dimensional (3D) contrast CT angiography (3D-CTA). This modality uses images obtained on standard contrast CT to generate three-dimensional images of the cerebrovascular system more rapidly and more cheaply than by magnetic resonance imaging (MRI) or contrast angiography. The relationship of vascular lesions to normal cerebral vessels and the cranial base are readily seen with 3D-CTA. The images generated can be rotated in all directions and thus aid the surgeon in surgical planning.[51, 52] This technique has been shown to be of particular help when evaluating the relationship of ophthalmic aneurysms with the anterior clinoid process.[52] Dorsch et al.[53] have identified five indications for CTA: (1) suspicion of an aneurysm on conventional CT; (2) follow-up of previously diagnosed aneurysm

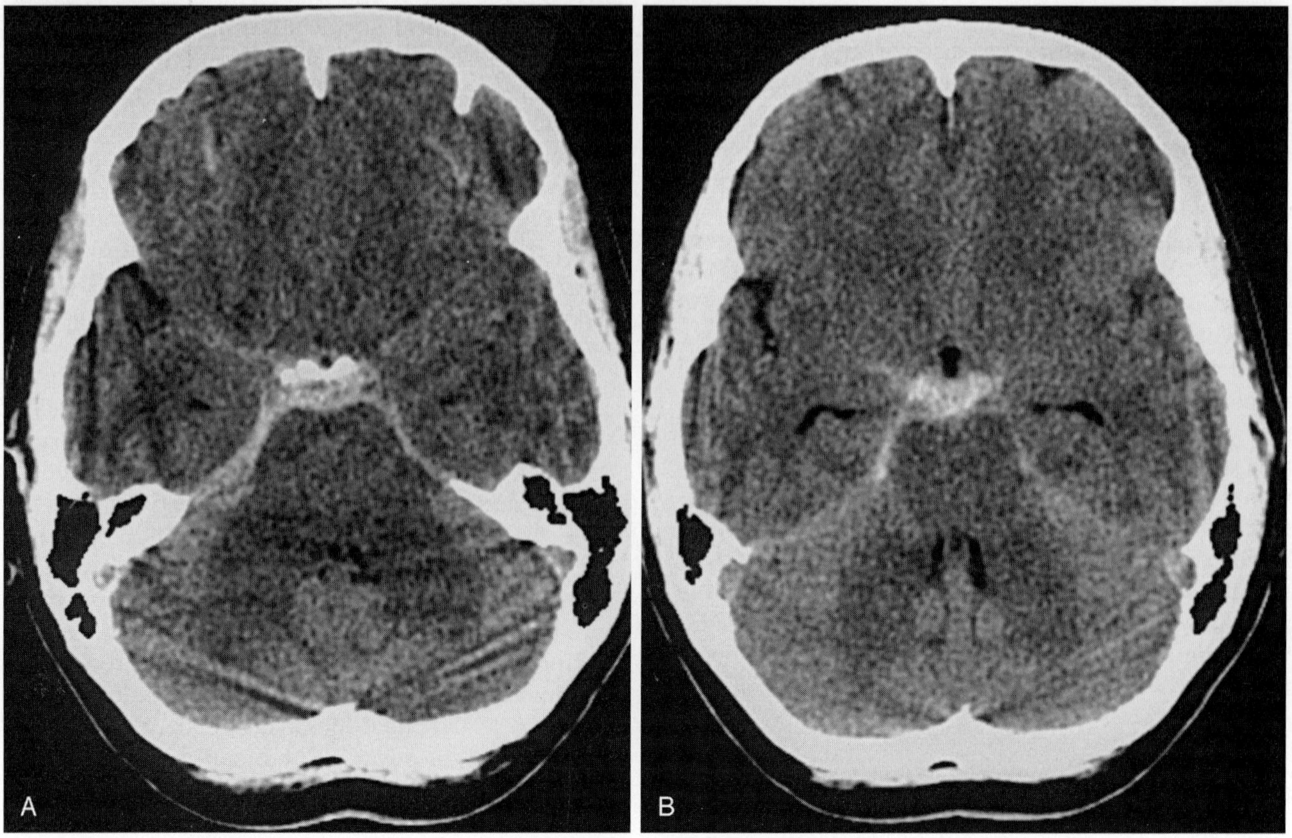

FIGURE 9–1 • Noncontrast axial head CT scan with subarachnoid hemorrhage in the prepontine *(A)* and perimesencephalic cisterns *(B)*. Subarachnoid blood in this location is consistent with a "perimesencephalic" type subarachnoid hemorrhage, infrequently associated with the presence of an aneurysm. Note the slight dilatation of the temporal horns consistent with early hydrocephalus.

not planned for surgery; (3) follow-up of aneurysm anatomy after surgical clipping; (4) detection of ruptured aneurysms; and (5) screening. These authors also point out some of the advantages of 3D-CTA over magnetic resonance angiography (MRA), including the ability to obtain fast scans and to scan patients who have contraindications to MRI. In addition, patients with aneurysm clips can undergo CT with impunity, regardless of the clip type.

Compared with angiography, 3D-CTA is faster, avoids arterial cannulation and, using computer reconstruction, improves the ability to visualize the aneurysm from any angle or vantage point. Disadvantages of this technique include the need for relatively large amounts of contrast and the technical expertise required in order to obtain quality images.[53] Although arteriography remains the standard in the evaluation of intracranial aneurysms, 3D-CTA holds promise in that it can be performed immediately following the noncontrast scan, can be accomplished with far less radiation exposure to both technician and patient than angiography and, as stated earlier, is cheaper than both MRA and conventional contrast angiography.

Angiography of Cerebral Aneurysms

A four-vessel angiogram remains the standard for the diagnosis of intracranial aneurysms. High-quality digitally subtracted images of all four vessels with anteroposterior, lateral, and oblique views must be obtained to adequately rule out the presence of an aneurysm. We routinely infuse both internal carotid arteries individually to assess the anterior circulation. The posterior circulation can often be cleared by injecting one vertebral artery as long as the reflux down the opposite vertebral allows precise visualization of the contralateral posterior inferior cerebellar artery (Fig. 9–2). The value of quality angiograms in surgical decision-making

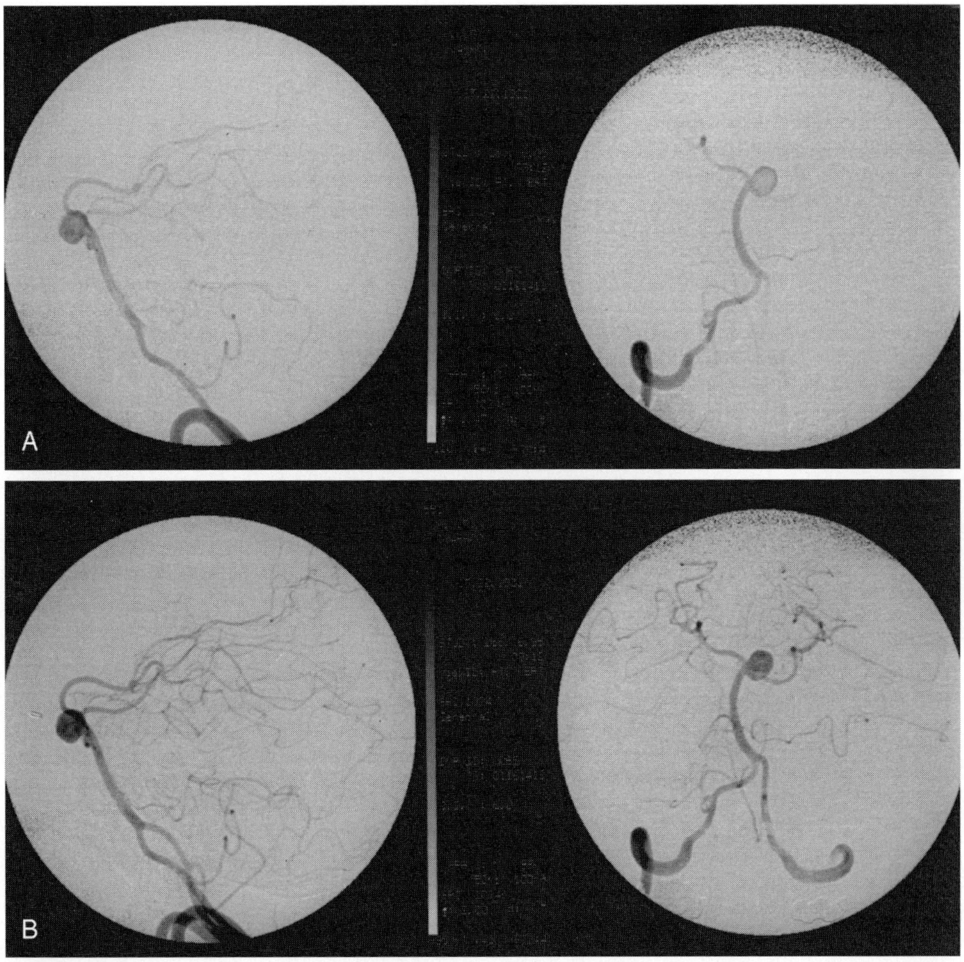

FIGURE 9-2 • Anteroposterior (right) and lateral (left) views of digitally subtracted right vertebral arteriogram in a patient status post–subarachnoid hemorrhage with the presence of a basilar tip aneurysm. *A*, Filling of the right vertebral artery early in the arterial phase without adequate filling of the contralateral vertebral artery. *B*, A later arterial phase image with reflux of contrast into the contralateral vertebral artery and left posterior inferior cerebellar artery, adequately ruling out the presence of a second aneurysm in the posterior circulation.

cannot be overemphasized. In the neurologically stable patient admitted at night, we often wait until morning for the angiogram so as to obtain the best possible study with only minimal delay in getting the patient to the operating room the next day. A quality angiogram can usually be completed in 90 minutes or less, and rushing a stable patient through a midnight angiogram for an operation the following morning is clearly not desirable. The main purpose of the angiogram is clearly to determine whether or not an aneurysm is present. Once an aneurysm is found, appropriate views should be obtained so as to highlight the aneurysm's anatomy, with particular attention paid to defining the neck of the lesion. Using the location of blood on the CT scan as a guide, the neuroradiologist injects contrast first into the vessel thought most likely to harbor the aneurysm, so that if the patient should become unstable over the course of the study, we have as much pertinent information as possible.

It is thought that angiography slightly increases the risk of a second bleed within the first 6 hours,[54] but the importance of obliterating the aneurysm early in the good-grade case so as to prevent a devastating rebleed far outweighs this possible, slightly increased risk. The angiogram should be used to evaluate the cerebrovasculature for the presence of vasospasm. Acute arterial vasospasm within the first day after SAH occurs occasionally and likely represents spasm secondary to an earlier undiagnosed bleed. It is vitally important that the neuroradiologist responsible for interpreting the angiogram have experience in diagnosing aneurysms and potential vasospasm following SAH. Vascular loops and bends can easily disguise themselves as aneurysmal lesions, and the correct oblique views must be obtained in order to adequately determine the true nature of what is thought to be an aneurysm. The diagnosis of vasospasm must be made at angiography as well, and although it is often clearly evident, confusion can occur because of vascular streaming artifact (Fig. 9–3), which can mimic arterial vasospasm.

Complications of Cerebral Angiography

Non-ionic contrast agents are generally used for evaluation of the cerebral vasculature by digital subtraction angiography (DSA). Fatalities associated with contrast agents occur in 1 in 20,000–40,000 doses.[55] The incidence of severe reactions to non-ionic contrast agents is 126 per 100,000.[55] Iodinated contrast agents are potentially nephrotoxic, with the likelihood for severe renal damage greatest in patients with pre-existing renal disease.[55] Pretreatment of these patients with intravenous hydration and mannitol appears to provide some protection from this nephrotoxicity.

Transient ischemic attacks and cerebral infarctions in "high-risk" patients occur in cerebral arteri-

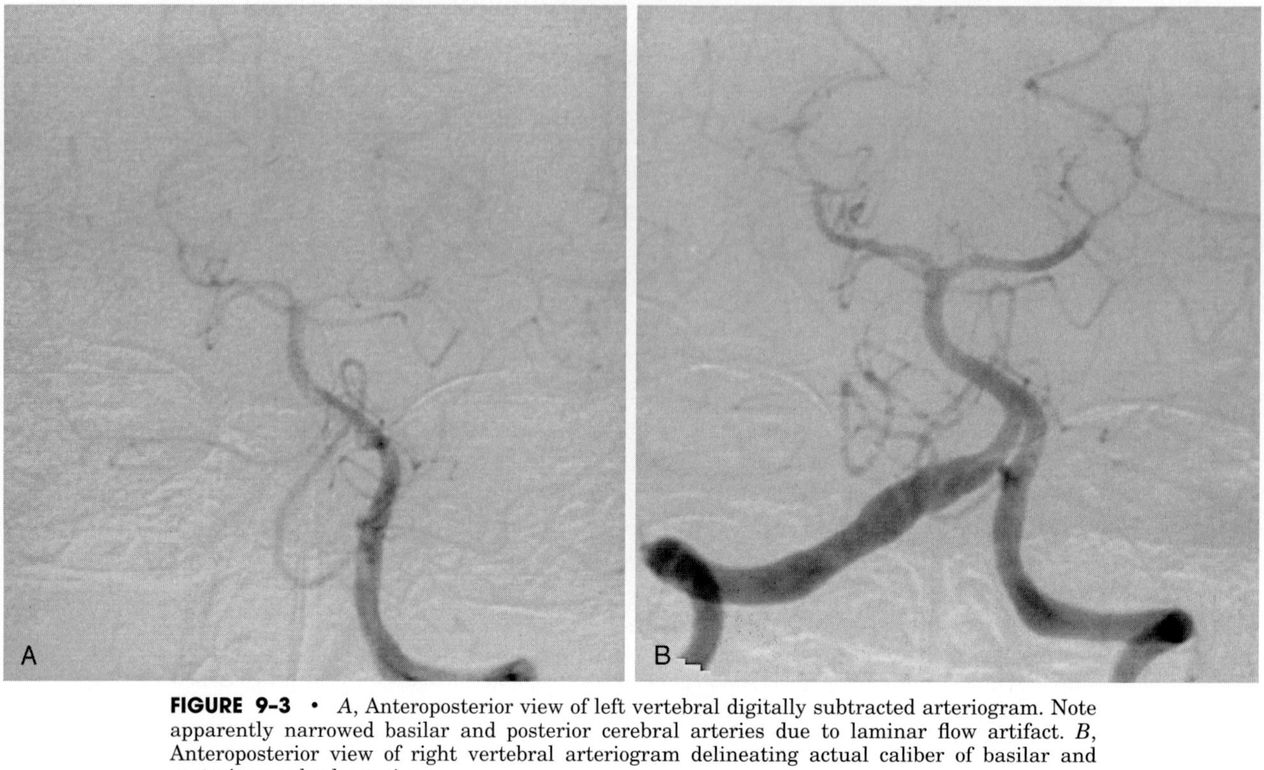

FIGURE 9–3 • *A*, Anteroposterior view of left vertebral digitally subtracted arteriogram. Note apparently narrowed basilar and posterior cerebral arteries due to laminar flow artifact. *B*, Anteroposterior view of right vertebral arteriogram delineating actual caliber of basilar and posterior cerebral arteries.

ography in 1.6% of patients using Omnipaque contrast, according to the package insert.[55] In addition, transient global amnesia (TGA), a syndrome in which a person becomes suddenly bewildered and disoriented with poor short-term memory,[56] has been reported during cerebral arteriography.[57, 58] The prognosis following these episodes is generally excellent, and the patient's symptoms usually resolve completely within a few hours.[55] The etiology of TGA is not clear, but cerebral blood flow studies suggest that it is related to temporal lobe, hippocampal, and possibly thalamic ischemia.[59–62]

Aneurysms and Angiograms

Grossman and Yousem have summarized the crucial information that should be conveyed to the neurosurgeon by the radiologist after evaluating a cerebral arteriogram (Table 9–11).[55] We rely heavily on the meticulousness of the neuroradiologists to help us answer these questions, and patients should not be taken to the operating room before these issues have been fully addressed unless a true emergency exists. Optimally, the neurosurgeon should review the angiogram with the neuroradiologist *as the study is being performed.* In that way, the neurosurgeon can be satisfied that the aneurysm neck has been adequately visualized and that all surgically relevant anatomic nuances have been defined.

Each aneurysm is unique in its anatomy and its relationship to other vessels. However, certain themes concerning aneurysms and their specific locations do exist and ought to be considered when evaluating an aneurysm. **Anterior communicating artery (AComA) aneurysms** are one of the most common types, accounting for 30% of aneurysmal SAHs in the 1966 Cooperative Study.[63] These aneurysms usually arise at the point where the AComA joins the dominant anterior cerebral artery most commonly projecting (in increasing order of frequency) inferiorly, anteriorly, and superiorly.[63]

TABLE 9–11 **CEREBRAL ANGIOGRAPHY—QUESTIONS TO BE ANSWERED**

1. Is there an aneurysm?
2. What is the exact location of the aneurysm?
3. Is there multiplicity?
4. If multiple, which aneurysm bled?
5. What is the size of the aneurysm?
6. From which vessel does the aneurysm arise?
7. Where is the aneurysm neck, and what is its size and its relationship to the aneurysm and the parent artery?
8. Is the aneurysm the source of the patient's subarachnoid hemorrhage?
9. Is there collateral flow to the area served by the aneurysm's parent artery?
10. Is any other lesion associated with the aneurysm?
11. Is there vasospasm?

TABLE 9–12 **ANATOMIC VARIANTS ASSOCIATED WITH ANTERIOR COMMUNICATING ARTERY ANEURYSM**

1. Dominant A1: fills both A2s
2. Unilateral hypoplasia of one A1
3. Exclusive filling of anterior communicating artery by one A1

AComA aneurysms are often associated with a relatively common anatomic variant (i.e., absence or hypoplasia of one anterior cerebral artery A1 segment with the aneurysm dome pointing away from the dominant contralateral A1 segment) (Fig. 9–4). This variant occurs in approximately 25% of patients with AComA aneurysms.[64] Charbel et al. found three variants associated with AComA aneurysms (Table 9–12).[65] In addition, Ogawa et al. reported that 21.4% of AComA aneurysms had vascular anomalies identified at surgery, including presence of a median artery of the corpus callosum, duplication of the AComAs, and duplication of an A1 segment.[66] Because of both the anatomic complexity and the high frequency of vascular variation, a quality angiographic examination of this region is extremely important. Often, multiple oblique views, cross-compression of the contralateral carotid artery, and submental vertex views are necessary to define the aneurysm's orientation and vascular relationships, so as to give the surgeon a fully three-dimensional understanding of this complex anatomic region.

Anterior cerebral artery (ACA) aneurysms distal to the AComA are uncommon, accounting for 4% of aneurysms in one series.[67] These aneurysms are often associated with vascular anomalies including multiple aneurysms, arteriovenous malformations (AVMs), and an azygous ACA. A larger percentage of distal ACA aneurysms occur as a result of infection and trauma than aneurysms in any other location.[68] The junction of the pericallosal with the callosomarginal artery is the most common site for distal ACA aneurysms.[69]

Aneurysms of the internal carotid artery are common, together accounting for nearly 30%–40% of aneurysms in most series.[13, 31, 70] These aneurysms include the ophthalmic artery aneurysm (OAA), superior hypophyseal artery aneurysm (SHAA), posterior communicating artery aneurysm (PComAA), anterior choroidal artery aneurysm (AChAA), and the carotid bifurcation aneurysm (CBA). OAA and SHAA occur proximally on the supraclinoid carotid artery, with OAAs projecting superiorly or superomedially and SHAAs projecting inferiorly or inferomedially.[71] OAAs and SHAAs are frequently large and can present with symptoms related to optic nerve and chiasmal compression, respectively.[28] In addition, they show a marked predominance in

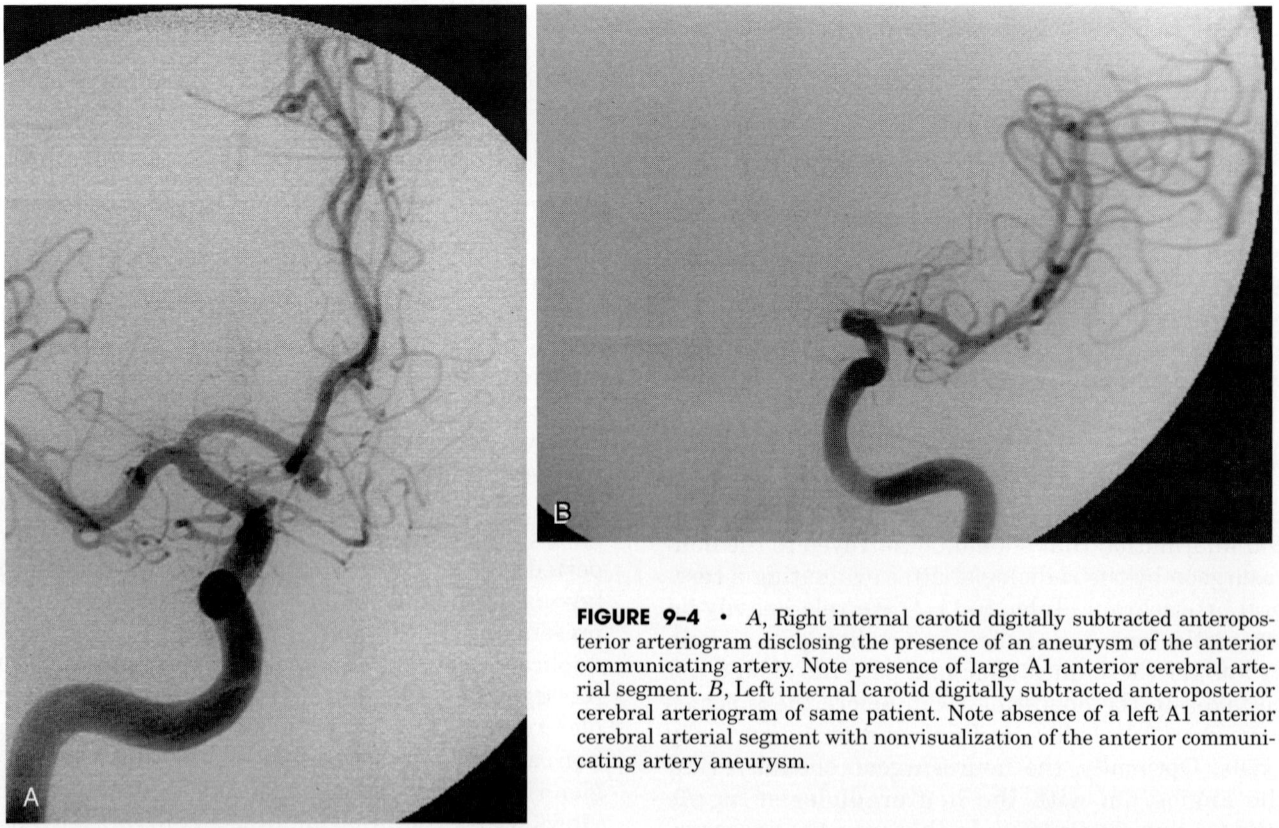

FIGURE 9–4 • *A*, Right internal carotid digitally subtracted anteroposterior arteriogram disclosing the presence of an aneurysm of the anterior communicating artery. Note presence of large A1 anterior cerebral arterial segment. *B*, Left internal carotid digitally subtracted anteroposterior cerebral arteriogram of same patient. Note absence of a left A1 anterior cerebral arterial segment with nonvisualization of the anterior communicating artery aneurysm.

women and are among the most frequent aneurysms associated with multiplicity.[28, 63] Angiographically, these aneurysms can be difficult to differentiate, and multiple oblique views may be needed to ascertain the location of the aneurysmal neck, if it can be determined at all. Occasionally the aneurysm neck of an OAA originates within the cavernous sinus, with varying portions of the aneurysm dome being intracavernous as well. It is important to attempt to delineate these features preoperatively to properly prepare for approaching these aneurysms surgically.

PComAAs and AChAAs are among the most common aneurysms, accounting for up to 35% of all anterior circulation lesions.[71] PComAA aneurysms classically present with third-nerve palsy in association with SAH symptoms consistent with third-nerve compression by the ruptured aneurysm. Occasionally, patients present with third-nerve palsy alone as their symptomatic complaint, which should alert the examining physician to possible impending aneurysmal rupture with third-nerve compression due to acute aneurysmal expansion. Minor head trauma can precipitate oculomotor palsies in patients with occult PComAA, and therefore these patients should not be excluded from further work-up.[72] Patients with third-nerve palsy that involves the pupil should undergo angiography to rule out an aneurysm. Although alternatives to angiography, including MRA and high-resolution contrast CT, have been investigated,[73–75] intra-arterial digital subtraction angiography continues to be the favored technique to rule out aneurysms at our institution.

Controversy surrounds the work-up of patients with pupil-sparing third-nerve palsy. Reports of aneurysms causing pupil-sparing third-nerve palsies do exist.[76–78] Capo et al. studied 41 patients with isolated third-nerve palsies with normal pupils.[79] They found that the 28 patients with a microvascular etiology, whether idiopathic or secondary to diabetes mellitus, all showed improvement in their symptoms by 12 weeks. They suggested that in patients with pupil-sparing third-nerve palsy, expectant management is indicated, and angiography should only be pursued in those patients who fail to improve after 4–8 weeks. We agree that patients with pupil-sparing third-nerve palsies should be managed expectantly, especially the elderly, hypertensive, or diabetic patient, and that angiography be reserved for those with persistent symptoms or without risk factors. It is of paramount importance, however, to study those patients with pupil-involving third-nerve palsies as expeditiously as possible, because if an aneurysm is present, the potential for rupture is high. In addition, studies have shown that the recovery of third-nerve function is related to the interval from time of onset of palsy to surgery.[80]

PComAAs often present without third-nerve

involvement.[21, 30] Angiograms in these patients should be carefully examined for evidence of an aneurysm projecting laterally into the medial temporal lobe rather than in the more common downward direction. Identification of this feature is of great importance because it would preclude retraction of the temporal lobe prior to identification of the aneurysm at surgery. In addition to identifying the aneurysm anatomy, it is also important to identify the posterior communicating and anterior choroidal arteries and their relationship to the aneurysm. Assessment of collateral circulation is important to evaluate, because potential temporary occlusion of the posterior communicating artery, internal carotid artery, or both at surgery cannot be tolerated as well by patients with absent or atretic A1 segments. In 20% of cases, the posterior communicating artery is the major origin of the posterior cerebral artery, making its sacrifice at surgery contraindicated.[30, 81]

It is equally important to assess the anatomy of the anterior choroidal artery on the angiogram. This vessel must be identified and preserved at surgery, and it is vitally important for the operating surgeon to have a good three-dimensional understanding of the anatomic relationship between the anterior choroidal artery and the posterior communicating artery prior to the surgical procedure. Anatomic variation has been reported in this area,[82] and special care to identify these two vessels on the angiogram is extremely important. AChAAs are much less common than PComAAs and do not present with third-nerve stigmata as frequently. Great emphasis should be placed on identification of the anterior choroidal artery and early branches, which are often intimately related.

CBAs are the most uncommon of the internal carotid aneurysms, accounting for approximately 5% of intracranial aneurysms.[30] They appear to have a predilection for children, adolescents, and young adults.[83] In addition, these aneurysms occasionally present with a parenchymal hematoma located slightly anterior and inferior to the classic putaminal and thalamic hemorrhages associated with hypertension.[83] Once again, local arterial anatomy should be well evaluated by angiography with multiple views in order to establish the anatomic relationships between the anterior and middle cerebral arteries, the anterior choroidal artery, and the internal carotid artery. Special attention should be paid to perforating arteries at or near the carotid bifurcation as well as the course of the anterior choroidal artery in relationship to the aneurysm.

Middle cerebral artery aneurysms (MCAAs) are found in the second most common aneurysm location and are the third most likely to bleed, accounting for 20%–25% of aneurysms in most series.[30, 81] These aneurysms often become large without compression of vital structures, rendering them clinically silent prior to rupture. Although rarely associated with aneurysms in general, temporal lobe epilepsy and transient ischemic attacks (TIAs) are commonly due to MCAAs when they do occur.[84] Subdural hematoma is a rare mode of presentation of a ruptured aneurysm, but when it occurs it is frequently due to an MCAA.[85] Additionally, ruptured MCAAs more often present with loss of consciousness, lateralizing headache, and severe neurologic deficits than do aneurysms in other locations.[84] Intracerebral hematomas secondary to ruptured aneurysms are most commonly due to MCAAs,[86] and it may be that this propensity to bleed into the brain itself is one of the reasons that these aneurysms present so commonly with focal neurologic deficits. A patient who presents with a hematoma extending into both the frontal and temporal opercula, bridging the sphenoid ridge on CT, should undergo angiography at once, because a hematoma in this location is virtually pathognomonic for MCAA.

The majority of MCAAs occur at the middle cerebral artery bifurcation/trifurcation and have a high rate of multiplicity. Aneurysms arising from the M1 segment are less common, accounting for 12.9% of MCAAs in one series.[87] Mirror MCAAs are not uncommon, making it important to use CT and clinical examination along with the angiogram in deciding which similarly sized aneurysm bled. Middle cerebral cortical branch aneurysms are the most common aneurysms associated with traumatic injury, and their presence should alert the surgeon to the possibility of previous trauma. In order to best delineate the vascular architecture of the bifurcation, oblique and submental views are often helpful.

Basilar artery apex aneurysms are the most common posterior circulation aneurysms, accounting for approximately 5% of all aneurysms.[88] Basilar apex aneurysms most commonly present with SAH. Occasionally these aneurysms cause third-nerve or chiasmal disruption due to aneurysmal compression[80] and may even present with Weber's syndrome when large enough to compress both the third cranial nerve and the ipsilateral cerebral peduncle,[89] or with oculomotor disturbances if large enough to cause pontine compression (Fig. 9–5). At angiography it is important to identify the aneurysm's relationship to a number of vascular and skull base structures. The location of thalamoperforators and thalamogeniculate arteries in relation to the aneurysm is important to assess. Additionally, the anatomy of the posterior communicating arteries should be evaluated with regard to collateral circulation in the event that temporary occlusion of the basilar or P1 segments is necessary during surgery. P1 anatomy is often difficult to resolve, especially when the

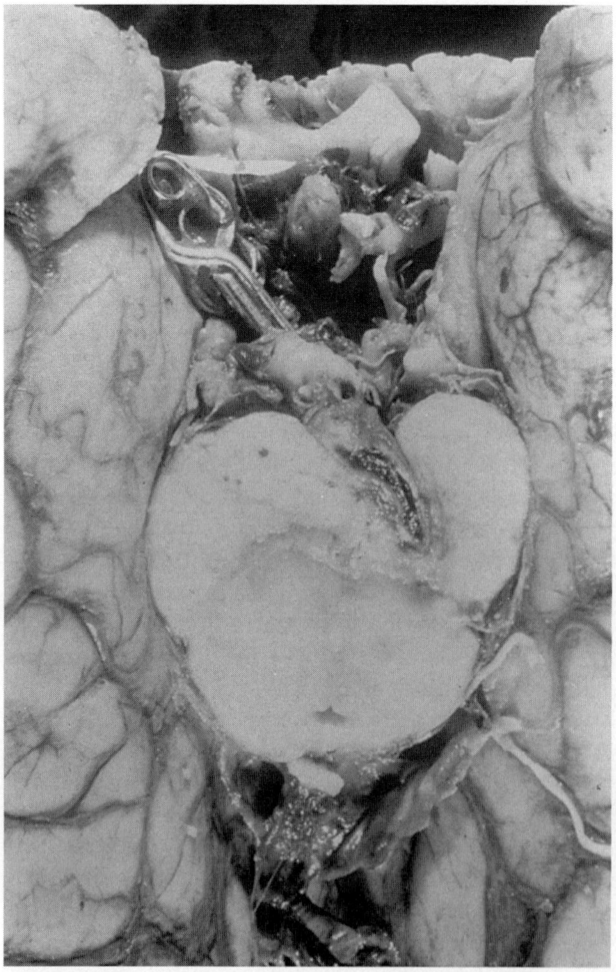

FIGURE 9–5 • Postmortem specimen of axial section through the midbrain of a patient with a basilar aneurysm that had been clipped prior to the patient's death. Note the significant amount of compression and displacement of the cerebral peduncle by the aneurysm. Note presence of optic chiasm anterior to the clip.

basilar tip aneurysm assumes larger sizes. At times the aneurysm neck cannot be well seen, and at surgery one finds that the large, broad-necked aneurysm actually originates from the P1 itself.

We also closely examine the relationship of the basilar apex to the posterior clinoid process, because its location dictates the likelihood of success of aneurysm clipping through a pterional versus a modified subtemporal approach (see Chapter 10). It is also important to examine carefully both anteroposterior and lateral views, because the superimposition of the P1 vessels on the basilar apex on lateral projection can be confused with an aneurysm. In addition, the basilar apex infrequently develops focal vasospasm and can be normal in size when the more proximal basilar artery is in spasm, resulting in a bulbous appearance of the basilar apex that can resemble an aneurysm.

Basilar tip aneurysms often present as giant aneurysms (>2.5 cm), and angiography frequently underestimates their true size because of the presence of intramural thrombus. MRI can often prove to be a useful diagnostic aid preoperatively for undergoing elective surgery, because the true size and complexity of the aneurysmal sac can be better appreciated. SAH secondary to posterior circulation aneurysms in general is less often associated with intracerebral hemorrhage than in anterior circulation aneurysms but results in vasospasm and hydrocephalus with the same frequency as in SAH from the supratentorial distribution.[90]

Other posterior circulation aneurysms in decreasing order of frequency include superior cerebellar artery (SCA) aneurysms and posterior inferior cerebellar artery (PICA) aneurysms. Aneurysms arising from the posterior cerebral artery, at the vertebrobasilar junction, midbasilar and in the region of the anterior inferior cerebellar artery, are even less common. As mentioned earlier, the only way to adequately clear the vertebrobasilar circulation is to insist on a four-vessel angiogram. Great care must be taken to adequately reflux contrast into the contralateral vertebral artery when only one vertebral artery is injected. If the contralateral vertebral or the posterior inferior cerebellar artery on that side is not well seen, the vertebral artery should be injected separately.

Multiple aneurysms have been detected in 14%–50% of patients with cerebral aneurysms.[13, 91–93] They are more common in women and in hypertensive persons[92, 94] as well as those with aneurysm-producing disease states (see Table 9–3). Because of this high rate of multiplicity, a four-vessel angiographic study is absolutely required in every patient presenting with SAH. When angiography reveals the presence of multiple aneurysms, it is important for the neurosurgeon and neuroradiologist to closely review the patient's examination, head CT, and angiogram so as to surmise accurately which aneurysm bled. Although simultaneous rupture of two intracranial aneurysms has been reported,[95] this is decidedly rare, and every effort should be made to determine with confidence which aneurysm bled. Patient history and examination can suggest which aneurysm bled because the headache often lateralizes to the side of rupture, particularly with middle cerebral artery aneurysms. Cranial nerve involvement and lateralizing weakness can direct the examiner to the symptomatic aneurysm as discussed earlier.

Angiographic size and appearance are two important aneurysm characteristics that help determine site of bleed. Larger aneurysms are more likely to bleed, whereas individual aneurysm anatomy may reveal a daughter lobe, a bleb, or a dome irregularity that implicates the aneurysm as the culprit. Certainly, location of blood on the CT scan is an important piece of information regarding the location of the aneurysm that bled, particularly when there is asymmetry in blood location or if the major clot burden is in a single location. Often, however, this is not the case; with symmetric SAH and multiple equivalently sized and shaped aneurysms, MRI can help to pinpoint the location of the symptomatic aneurysm. A number of case reports have shown MRI to be valuable in determining site of aneurysm rupture;[96, 97] however, MRI should be reserved only for neurologically stable, good-grade patients who can tolerate MRI without sedation.

Giant aneurysms (i.e., aneurysms >2.5 cm in diameter) are uncommon, accounting for less than 2% of all aneurysms.[13] These aneurysms can present with SAH; however, they also commonly present with signs and symptoms of mass effect.[98, 99] Giant aneurysms have been misdiagnosed as meningioma, pituitary adenoma, craniopharyngioma, and glioblastoma,[99] but with modern imaging techniques, particularly with the advent of high-resolution MRI, this has become less common. Characteristic features of these aneurysms on MRI are: round, extra-axial masses with a hypointense rim; signal void, paradoxical enhancement, or even echo rephasing due to blood flow; and laminated, eccentric thrombus with increased signal intensity when fresh, peri-aneurysmal hemorrhage occurs in the acute or subacute stage after aneurysmal rupture[100] (Fig. 9–6).

TABLE 9–13 **DIFFERENTIAL DIAGNOSIS OF DISTAL CEREBRAL ARTERIAL ANEURYSMS**

1. Infectious aneurysm
2. Traumatic aneurysm
3. Focal dissection

Angiography often underestimates the true size of these lesions, because intramural thrombus often occupies a significant amount of space within the aneurysmal sac (see Fig. 9–6). MRI can help to delineate the true anatomy of these lesions as well as help to define the blood flow through them.[100]

Mycotic or infectious aneurysms (Table 9–13) occur most commonly in association with bacterial endocarditis, accounting for 0.49%–4.3% of all intracranial aneurysms, with a 2%–10% incidence reported in patients with infective endocarditis.[101, 102] Other etiologies include meningitis and septic thrombophlebitis.[103] The proposed mechanism for their formation includes: (1) embolic occlusion of the vasa vasorum of affected arteries; (2) direct invasion of the arterial wall by blood borne bacteria; and (3) injury to the arterial wall by antigen-antibody complexes.[102] These aneurysms occur most commonly at distal branch points of the cerebral arteries, often in the distribution of the middle cerebral artery. However, they can occur on proximal

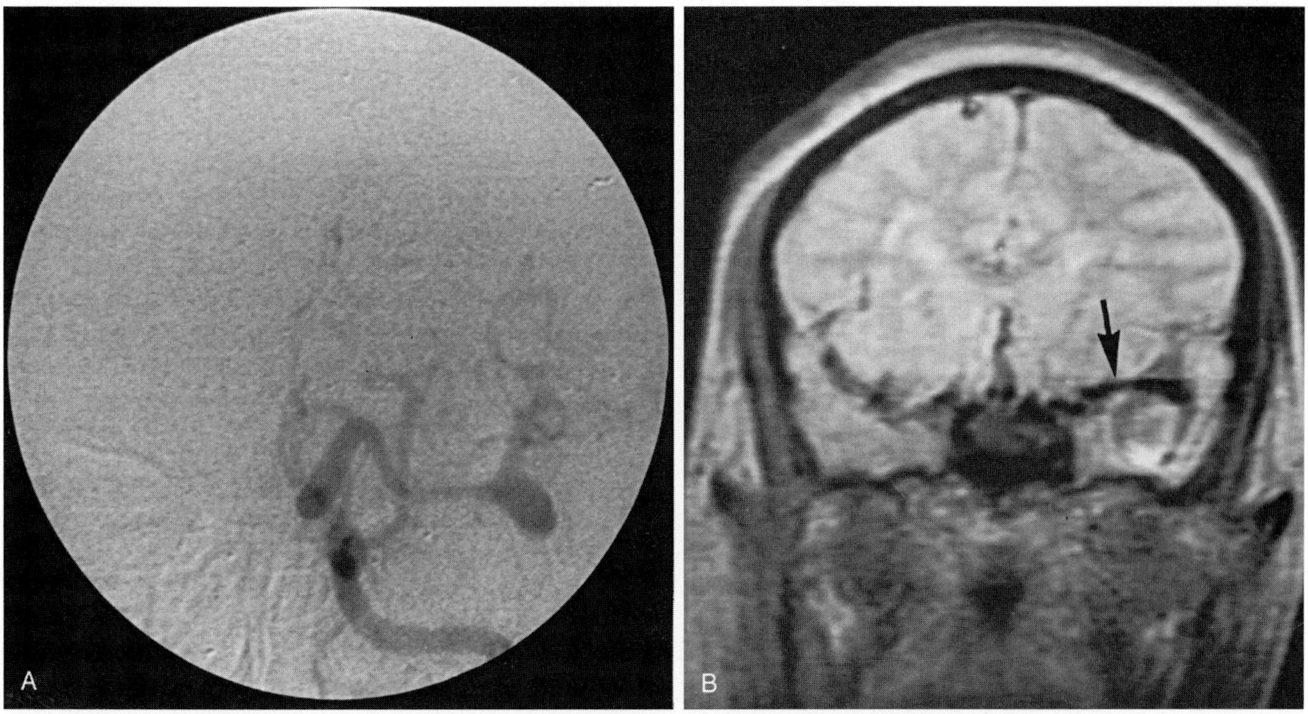

FIGURE 9–6 • *A*, Left internal carotid digitally subtracted anteroposterior cerebral arteriogram disclosing the presence of a large aneurysm at the middle cerebral artery bifurcation. *B*, Coronal proton gradient magnetic resonance image elucidating true size of this giant aneurysm (arrow). Note the presence of a hypointense rim with heterogeneous signal intensity within the aneurysmal lumen.

arterial segments including the intracavernous and extracavernous segments of the internal carotid artery as well.[103, 104] The most common pathogens associated with these aneurysms are *Streptococcus viridans* and *Staphylococcus aureus*, with infectious aneurysms usually appearing late in the course of disease.[102] Rare bacterial types associated with infectious aneurysms include *Neisseria, Enterococcus*, and *Pseudomonas*.

Fungal aneurysms are rare but will no doubt be seen with greater frequency because of more widespread use of immunosuppressive agents and the advent of AIDS. The most common pathogen is *Aspergillus,* although a case of *Coccidioides*-related mycotic aneurysms has been reported.[105] Virally induced aneurysms are rare, but aneurysms secondary to herpes zoster have been reported.[106] Infectious aneurysms are usually discovered following intracranial hemorrhage and carry a 39%–90% mortality rate.[101, 107] Frazee has suggested that most patients harboring infectious aneurysms present with signs and symptoms suggestive of the formation of a septic aneurysm prior to rupture, and that in a patient with endocarditis, even subtle neurologic symptoms ought to be investigated with angiography.[103] Following their discovery by angiography, there is some controversy as to their management. A prolonged course of antibiotic treatment with serial angiography has been the standard of care in the past because of the high morbidity and mortality of surgery, and because these aneurysms usually resolve with appropriate antibiotic therapy. However, Kojima et al. reviewed 149 cases of infectious intracranial aneurysms and found higher mortality rates among patients treated with antibiotics alone versus those treated with surgery.[101]

We believe that asymptomatic and certainly ruptured infectious aneurysms ought to be surgically managed whenever possible. Our decision-making regarding these lesions is similar to the management of non-infectious aneurysms, and conservative therapy ought to be reserved for surgically difficult or poor-grade cases. Unlike non-infectious saccular aneurysms, these lesions are usually not amenable to clip repair by obliteration of a neck. These lesions are pseudo-aneurysms that are friable and often require simple excision of the diseased vessel segment. The advent of stereotaxy and neurointerventional techniques has allowed safe treatment of otherwise surgically difficult or inaccessible lesions.[108–110] The use of these special techniques should be entertained when the potential morbidity of standard neurosurgical techniques is felt to be too high.

Traumatic intracranial aneurysms (see Table 9–13) are rare, occurring in approximately 3% of patients following *penetrating* head trauma and accounting for less than 0.5% of all intracranial aneurysms.[111, 112] Sixty percent to 70% of traumatic aneurysms are due to blunt head trauma, whereas 15%–25% are due to penetrating traumatic injury.[112] The mechanism of formation of these lesions is controversial. Blunt trauma can produce a vascular injury as a result of differential velocity between brain and skull with resultant shearing forces.[111, 113] Direct injuries to vessels can occur as they come into contact with bony or ligamentous protuberances within the intracranial compartment.[113] Traumatic tears due to traction injuries are also thought to be the cause of some of these aneurysms.[113] Trapping of the cortical vessel within a fracture has also been shown to be responsible for the genesis of some of these lesions.[113] Histologically, these aneurysms can either be "true" aneurysms with dilation secondary to partial disruption of the arterial wall, or "false" aneurysms in which the artery has a full-thickness tear, and scar from brain tissue or organized hematoma acts as an aneurysmal wall.[114] One study found seven of seven traumatic aneurysms secondary to penetrating trauma to be of the false type.[115]

Traumatic intracranial aneurysms can become angiographically apparent as early as 2 hours post injury and are thought to develop within the first hours to days following head trauma. There are a few case reports of delays in diagnosis of 14 months to 10 years.[114, 116] These lesions are 2–15 mm in diameter and occur most frequently on distal middle cerebral arterial branches and less commonly on the internal carotid and pericallosal arteries. Fewer than 10% occur in the posterior circulation, and they are multiple in 20% of patients.[112, 115, 117] Skull base traumatic aneurysms most commonly involve the petrous, cavernous, or supraclinoid carotid artery.[118] Traumatic cerebral aneurysms are accompanied by intracerebral hemorrhage in 80% of cases and by subdural hematoma in 26%. Haddad et al. recommend trapping or excision in all cases, given the propensity of these aneurysms to rebleed.[115] The morbidity and mortality of traumatic aneurysms is higher than that of nontraumatic aneurysms. The mortality rate is approximately 16% for operative management and ranges from 10% to 41% for nonoperative management.[112] The reasons for this higher morbidity and mortality are likely due to (1) characteristics of the aneurysm itself which, when subjected to surgery, has a high rate of intraoperative rupture due to the presence of dense arachnoid adhesions,[112] and (2) the attendant premorbid condition of the head-injured patient. The most common form of presentation of these patients is that of delayed SAH after head trauma with associated alteration of the patient's level of consciousness.[112] Other manifestations that should alert the physician to a possible traumatic aneurysm include delayed extracerebral hemorrhage after head trauma, unexplained arterial bleeding during surgical evacuation of "traumatically" induced hematoma, or delayed onset of cranial nerve palsy.[112]

The diagnosis of traumatic aneurysms in patients following head injury remains problematic. As noted by a number of authors, the replacement of angiography by CT as the diagnostic procedure of choice for head-injured patients since the late 1970s has resulted in a definite decline in the number of diagnosed traumatic aneurysms despite an overall increase in head injuries.[111–113] Traumatic aneurysms are therefore more likely to be missed given the relative insensitivity of CT in the diagnosis of these lesions. As Levy et al. point out, fewer than 30% of patients with traumatic aneurysms seeking treatment over a 20-year period in their institution were diagnosed after implementation of CT in 1976.[112]

It is clearly important to perform angiography on head-injured patients thought to be at high risk for the development of traumatic cerebral aneurysms. The incidence of SAH after closed head injury is approximately 40%[119] and, by itself, is not an indication for angiography. Du Trevou and van Dellen found a 12% incidence of traumatic aneurysms in a group of 181 patients suffering from stab wounds to the brain.[120] Patients who sustain head trauma with foreign-body penetration through the dura should be considered for angiography if they survive their initial injury. Other clinical criteria that should lead to immediate angiography in the head-injured patient include delayed SAH; detection of a delayed intracerebral hemorrhage on serial CT in a setting of mild head trauma, especially when associated with a delayed neurologic deficit, SAH, or both; delayed-onset cranial nerve palsy; moderate to severe epistaxis; or brisk intraoperative arterial bleeding.[112]

Rarely, an SAH is caused by cerebral arterial dissection (Tables 9–13 and 9–14), most frequently involving the middle cerebral or basilar arteries.[121] Intracranial arterial dissection is caused by blood extravasation from the true arterial lumen through the intima into the vessel wall, spreading between the intima and the media causing luminal narrowing and decreased flow.[121] Pathologically these lesions have been shown to have subadventitial hemorrhage, multiple noncontiguous intramural hemorrhages, and neovascular changes in and around the vessel wall.[122] Dissection may occur spontaneously or secondary to traumatic injury. Spontaneous dissection is associated with a number of vascular etiologies (see Table 9–14), as well as oral contraceptive use and migraine.[121, 123] Although most commonly associated with pain and embolic events, dissection can present with SAH, often in the posterior circulation.[121, 124] Angiographically, one most often finds focal narrowing of the vessel lumen (string sign) with a proximal dilatation of the same vessel (pearl sign), as well as fusiform dilatation and double lumen.[121, 125] Care must be taken in order to distinguish arterial dissection from a saccular aneurysm with attendant vasospasm.[121, 126] MRI has been shown to be valuable in assisting in diagnosis because it can show the dissecting hematoma within the vessel wall,[127] although it can fail to reveal hematoma in the acute phase.[126]

TABLE 9–14 **VASCULAR DISEASES ASSOCIATED WITH CEREBRAL ARTERIAL DISSECTION**

1. Fibromuscular dysplasia
2. Syphilitic arteritis
3. Polyarteritis nodosa
4. Mucoid degeneration of the media
5. Marfan's disease/cystic medial necrosis
6. Atherosclerosis
7. Takayasu's disease
8. Allergic arteritis

Angiogram-Negative Subarachnoid Hemorrhage

One of the most difficult diagnostic dilemmas in neurosurgery occurs when angiogram results following an SAH are negative. The incidence of normal cerebral angiograms in patients with CT-proven SAH is approximately 15%–20%.[128–130] In the case of perimesencephalic SAH, this result is somewhat expected.[47, 130] However, with evidence of classic SAH with diffuse subarachnoid blood or well-localized blood in areas other than the basal cisterns, a negative angiogram result can be somewhat worrisome for both physician and patient. The management of these patients is controversial, and decision-making relies heavily on the quality of the angiogram itself. Although overall long-term outcomes for this group of patients has been shown to be better than that of patients harboring aneurysms on their initial angiograms,[131–133] a number of studies have shown that the risk of subsequent hemorrhage in patients with angiogram-negative perimesencephalic hemorrhage differs from that of classic SAH involving blood localizing to areas other than the perimesencephalic region.[128–130, 134]

Rinkel et al. have suggested that patients with negative results on angiogram be divided into two groups managed differently according to the CT blood pattern: (1) those with perimesencephalic hemorrhage who are managed conservatively; and (2) those with more classic aneurysmal "like" SAH who should undergo at least one additional angiogram.[128, 130] Patients with classic SAH with negative angiogram results usually harbor an occult aneurysm; however, arterial dissection, trauma, dural arteriovenous malformation, mycotic aneurysm, bleeding disorder, substance abuse, and cervical origin of SAH should be considered.[130] Tatter et al. described a series of 40 patients with angiogram-negative SAH, of which 9 underwent exploratory surgery after review of their studies disclosed subtle angiographic abnormalities consistent with possible rupture sites.[133] In seven of these nine patients, an arterial abnormality was discovered at surgery and was thought to be the source of hemorrhage. Three of these abnormalities were small aneurysms, whereas four were microaneurysms too small for clipping. Although one could argue that these angiograms were not truly "negative," this study demonstrates that aneurysmal lesions, some treatable, are likely responsible for many of the angiogram-"negative" classic SAHs.

We feel that it is important to carefully correlate the CT findings with the angiographic result. Certainly, a patient with basal frontal interhemispheric blood should arouse more clinical suspicion than a patient with perimesencephalic-type hemorrhage. Patients with good-grade cases who can tolerate MRI can undergo MRA, which has been reported to demonstrate aneurysms in angiogram-negative SAH patients,[135, 136] although our experience with MRA to date would suggest that this is a very low-yield study in this situation.

Our current management of these patients is as follows: Patients with perimesencephalic-type SAH undergo conventional cerebral arteriography and, if results are negative, can be discharged when stable. These patients are not thought to be at risk for rebleed or vasospasm, and their risk of hydrocephalus is also low.[47, 128] Although the vast majority of these patients have negative angiogram results, the presence of aneurysms resulting in these types of hemorrhage is well documented,[47, 134, 137] and they must undergo at least one high-quality, four-vessel angiogram. Patients with "classic" aneurysmal SAH should be considered a separate entity when angiographic work-up is negative. Patients with focal clots on CT should undergo careful angiographic evaluations, including multiple oblique views of suspicious areas, before an angiogram result is interpreted as negative. In patients with diffuse subarachnoid blood, careful scrutiny should certainly be given to all vessels, especially in areas with high incidence of aneurysm formation (e.g., anterior communicating complex, middle cerebral bifurcation). If these patients are truly thought to have negative angiogram results, they should be kept in the intensive care unit for at least 2–5 days with close monitoring of their neurologic examination. Transcranial Doppler testing (see later) should be performed every other day to evaluate for possible vasospasm, because these patients have the same risk of developing delayed arterial vasospasm as do patients with documented aneurysmal SAHs.[128] If the initial angiogram is truly high-quality without vasospasm, mass effect from clot, or patient motion artifact, these patients should undergo one further angiogram electively in 4–6 weeks. The second study, if done too early, may be marred by vasospasm and could necessitate a third study after the spasm clears. The morbidity of an angiogram is low enough to warrant this sort of an aggressive approach to rule out the presence of an aneurysm.

Indications for Early Neuroradiologic Intervention

Once the diagnosis of intracranial aneurysm is made by angiography, the surgeon is next confronted with the decision concerning whether or not to prepare the patient for surgery. For a specific subset of aneurysms, this decision now includes the consideration of whether to treat the vascular lesion with a neurointerventional procedure (see Chapter 11). Technical improvements and advances in microcatheter technology and in design and delivery of thrombogenic coils have resulted in a new role for the neurointerventionalist in the treatment of cerebral aneurysms. Close cooperation between neurosurgeon and neurointerventionalist is necessary when planning these procedures. Although long-term study of the effects of a number of the techniques used has yet to be completed, interventional approaches may improve patient outcome and ought to be considered in certain situations that have yet to be fully defined (Table 9–15). The decision to initiate therapy by a neurointerventionalist depends on a number of factors that vary from institution to institution. The experience of the surgeon and neurointerventionalist, the aneurysm's anatomic features, and the grade of the case all play a role in this decision. At our institution, we consider a neurointerventional approach to cases of poor clinical grade or of severe systemic disease.

Endovascular detachable coil obliteration of aneurysms has been shown to be effective in the treatment of all sizes of aneurysms if there is a definitive

TABLE 9–15 **INDICATIONS FOR EARLY NEURORADIOLOGIC INTERVENTION FOLLOWING ANEURYSMAL SUBARACHNOID HEMORRHAGE**

1. Giant/inoperable aneurysm
2. Poor-grade condition
3. Severe vasospasm

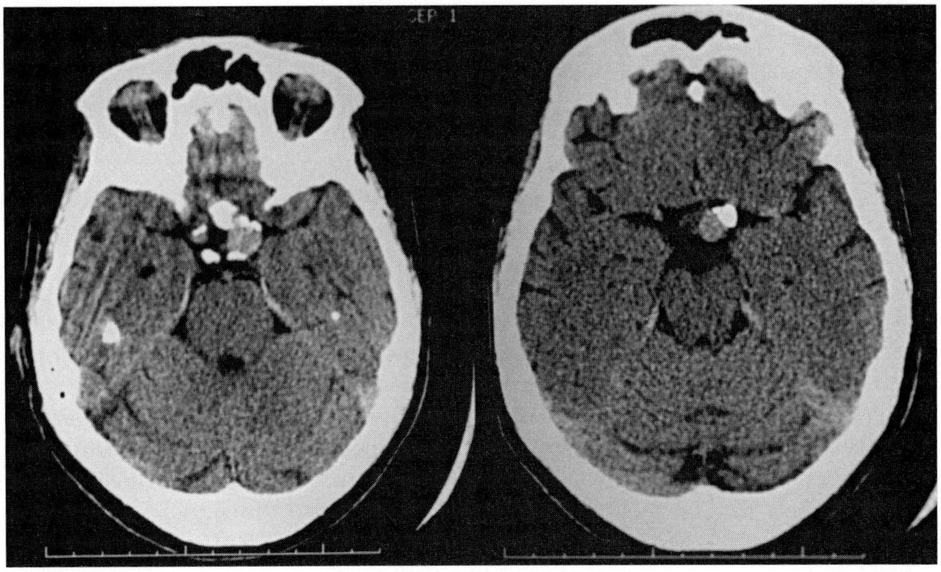

FIGURE 9–7 • Axial noncontrast head CT scan of a patient with a known left carotid–ophthalmic artery aneurysm. CT discloses the presence of a significant amount of high-density signal consistent with calcification associated with the aneurysm.

neck.[138] These aneurysms are often giant, are in the posterior circulation, and may possess significant amounts of atherosclerosis and calcium appreciated on CT, making their repair by direct clipping nearly impossible (Fig. 9–7). A similar group of indications has been described by others.[139–144] A poor-grade patient not considered a candidate for early surgery ought to be evaluated for possible neurointerventional therapy. These patients carry a high risk of early rebleeding with its attendant morbidity, and therefore even partial obliteration of the ruptured aneurysm may decrease this risk, although protection is not guaranteed.[140] We have treated a number of poor-grade cases with basilar tip aneurysms in this way without a single episode of early rebleeding to date (Fig. 9–8). These patients all require follow-up angiography to determine whether the aneurysm is growing, and some patients require further coil placement or craniotomy for direct clipping. Unfortunately, the aneurysms that are often most difficult to repair by direct clipping (i.e., aneurysms with broad necks) are also the most challenging for coil embolization. The coils tend to reflux out through the broad neck and thus increase the risk of parent vessel occlusion.

The last group of patients we consider for early neuroradiologic intervention are patients with significant deficits thought potentially secondary to se-

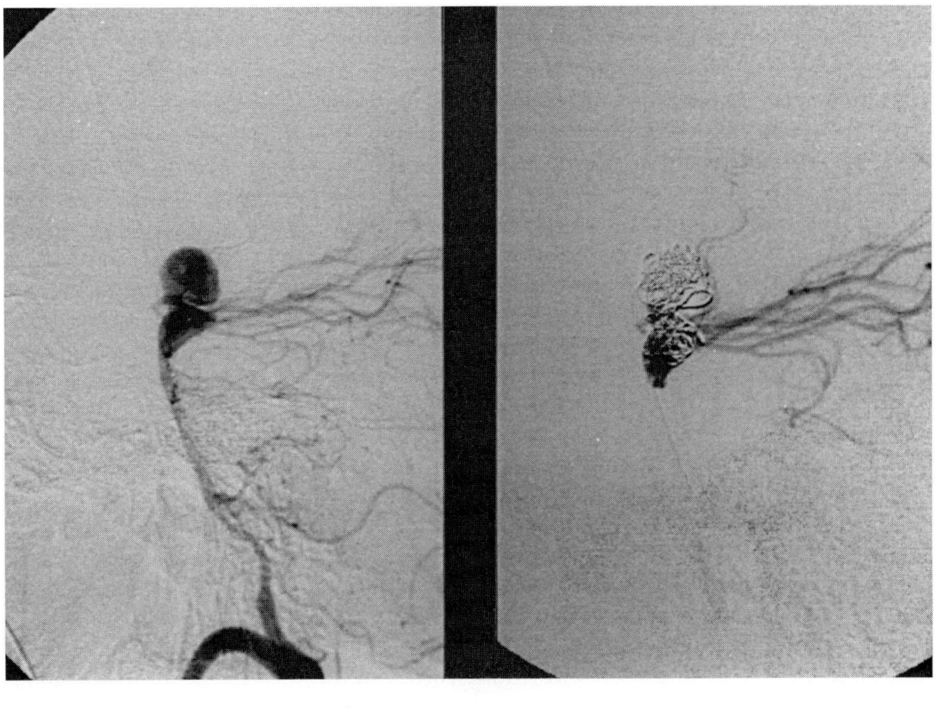

FIGURE 9–8 • Right vertebral artery digitally subtracted lateral cerebral arteriogram in patient with a basilar tip aneurysm. Image on left shows aneurysm prior to coil embolization. Image on right shows the same aneurysm following partial obliteration with detachable thrombogenic coils. Note preservation of posterior cerebral arterial flow.

vere vasospasm who, despite their poor condition, undergo surgery to allow balloon angioplasty of the aneurysm's feeding vessel (see Chapter 11). Proximal vessel balloon angioplasty has become a new tool in our armamentarium in treating vasospasm; however, angioplasty of vessels feeding unclipped ruptured aneurysms is relatively contraindicated. Angioplasty produces long-lasting dilatation of narrowed vasospastic vessels with few reports of recurrent vasospasm following treatment,[145] although its mechanism of action is not entirely clear. Newell et al. proposed that angioplasty is effective because it disrupts the increased collagenous and fibrous deposition observed in vasospasm.[146] Its permanent effects may be due to irreversible endothelial and smooth muscle damage[145, 147] with simple disruption of the degenerative muscle and proliferative nonmuscle and connective tissue components of the media[148] preventing transmission of contractile forces to the vessel wall.[149]

On a number of occasions we have gone ahead with surgery with poor-grade cases to allow institution of aggressive neuroradiologic intervention in the setting of severe vasospasm, hoping that reversal of vasospasm with balloon angioplasty and intra-arterial papaverine infusion will improve the neurologic outcome in these severely disabled patients. Le Roux et al. have described a similar approach in treating patients with severe symptomatic vasospasm and unsecured aneurysms with good outcome in four of five such patients.[150] Balloon angioplasty should be performed with the utmost caution by an experienced neurointerventionalist, because it can cause vessel rupture or embolic stroke.[151] This technique should be reserved for symptomatic patients with dense deficits that correlate with the distribution of the radiographic vasospasm (see later).

Occlusion of feeding vessels as a therapy for ruptured aneurysms is usually a treatment of last resort. Treatment of infectious aneurysms through endovascular means with proximal vessel occlusion can be effective. A number of case reports attest to its efficacy, particularly in cases of anatomically difficult aneurysms or in aneurysms in unstable patients.[108, 109, 152] In treating inoperable internal carotid aneurysms, carotid occlusion has been used for some time. In 1805, Sir Astley Cooper used this technique in a patient with an extracranial internal carotid artery aneurysm.[153] The goal of carotid occlusion is to decrease internal carotid flow enough so that the aneurysms thrombose, excluding themselves from the intracranial circulation. As surgical techniques have improved and historically inoperable aneurysms have become operable, indications for carotid occlusion have become fewer. However, a small subset of patients with internal carotid aneurysms remain candidates for this form of therapy if preoperative testing predicts tolerance of such a procedure. Aneurysms requiring emergent treatment are those that have caused SAH. Extradural aneurysms do not cause SAH and can be managed conservatively, depending on the severity of their signs and symptoms (e.g., cranial nerve compression, pain).[154] Care must be taken, however, when evaluating these lesions radiographically, because extradural intracavernous aneurysms can extend into the subarachnoid space along the distal dural ring of the cavernous sinus, thus placing them at risk for subarachnoid bleed.[155]

Carotid occlusion has now largely fallen under the domain of the neurointerventionalist, because technological improvements in catheter and coil design and delivery now allow routine entry and obliteration of aneurysms of the internal carotid artery, as well as the internal carotid itself. The risk of this procedure depends largely on collateral circulation rather than size of the aneurysm. A direct open surgical approach using bypass techniques combined with direct clipping or trapping of the aneurysm has been recommended for patients with poor collateral flow who are thought to be unlikely to tolerate internal carotid occlusion.[156] The morbidity of surgical ligation of the common or internal carotid artery has been estimated to be between 7.5% and 20%.[157] Miller et al. determined that inadequate collateral reserve, a "low-flow" state, would occur in approximately 20% of patients after acute carotid occlusion.[158] Swearingen and Heros, however, suggested that most ischemic complications after carotid ligation seemed to be thromboembolic rather than due to low-flow states, arguing that common carotid occlusion was preferable to internal carotid occlusion.[159] Following common carotid occlusion, the internal carotid artery frequently remains patent, with a decrease in incidence of stump emboli hypothesized.[159]

Although common carotid occlusion did not gain wide acceptance, the problem of stump emboli has remained with us and is certainly a major source of morbidity with endovascular occlusion of the internal carotid artery. When being evaluated for potential carotid occlusion, patients undergo balloon test occlusion with systemic heparinization along with angiographic evaluation of collateral circulation and frequent neurologic examinations. Other centers use a variety of parameters when evaluating these patients, including cerebral blood flow measurements, single photon emission computed tomography (SPECT), electroencephalographic monitoring, and induced hypotension.[156, 160–165] The literature suggests that in unselected normotensive patients, abrupt occlusion of the internal carotid artery will result in infarctions in approximately 26% of patients.[165] The rate of infarction in patients undergoing internal carotid occlusion who tolerated balloon test occlusion clinically without blood flow testing is approximately 13%, halving the expected rate of stroke in these patients.[165] Linskey et al. showed no further improvement in morbidity rates in patients undergoing internal carotid occlusion who tolerated test occlusion both clinically and by cerebral blood flow testing.[165]

During balloon test occlusion, cerebral cortical deficits are the most common deficits observed, although monocular blindness, ocular ischemic syndrome, and crossed cerebellar diaschisis have been reported, reaffirming the importance of close and compulsive neurologic monitoring of the patient.[166–168] Certainly clinical examination can help to predict low-flow phenomena resulting from internal carotid occlusion; however, thromboembolic events remain the most common cause of postocclusive stroke, and the risk of embolic stroke cannot be predicted. We treat our patients with low-dose intravenous heparin (500 U/hour) after carotid occlusion for approximately 48 hours and continue the patient on enteric-coated aspirin each day unless contraindicated for other medical reasons. Carotid occlusion is also associated with potential long-term risk to the patient. Occlusion of the internal carotid artery results in concomitant increased cerebral blood flow through the contralateral carotid and vertebral arteries. This increased flow may cause enlargement and rupture of occult aneurysms as well as lead to the de novo generation of cerebral aneurysms.[169, 170] In addition, hypertension has been reported to have an increased incidence in patients with carotid occlusion.[171] Overall, these risks are much lower than the risk of living with an untreated, ruptured aneurysm. These risks are also acceptably low when considering the morbidity of a symptomatic and often painful cavernous carotid aneurysm or carotid-cavernous fistula.

Currently the delivery of thrombogenic coils to the internal carotid lumen is the method of choice for endovascular internal carotid occlusion. This method is somewhat time-consuming compared with balloon occlusion, because multiple coils must be delivered individually in order to adequately occlude the vascular lumen. Balloon occlusion is currently not being used as frequently because the Food and Drug Administration has not approved it for use in this setting.

ACUTE INTENSIVE CARE UNIT MANAGEMENT OF THE SUBARACHNOID HEMORRHAGE PATIENT: PREOPERATIVE MANAGEMENT

Once an intracranial aneurysm has been diagnosed following SAH, a specific protocol is followed for every patient that is tailored to the needs of each individual. All therapeutic measures have been developed with the three most important sources of morbidity in mind—rebleeding, vasospasm, and hydrocephalus. By keeping these three cardinal factors in mind, the physician can manage these patients as efficiently and safely as possible.

Rebleeding

Rebleeding is the most dreaded complication that can occur in the post-SAH patient, carrying a mortality rate of 51%–80%.[172–174] Its incidence is generally accepted to be greatest in the first 24–48 hours following initial rupture (approximately 6%), with a rate of 1.5% per day for the rest of the initial 2 weeks.[173, 175, 176] Inagawa et al. reported this risk to be highest in the first 6 hours,[54] but some controversy does surround this issue. Hijdra et al., in a prospective study of 176 patients, found the peak incidence of rebleeding to be at the end of the second and third weeks after SAH; risk of rebleeding was significantly increased in survivors of a first rebleed.[172] Rosenorn et al. followed 1076 patients with ruptured intracranial aneurysms prospectively and found the risk of rebleed to be greatest at days 4–9. Two of these studies found the highest risk of rebleeding to be in poorer-grade cases,[54, 174] a finding disputed by others.[173]

Regardless of the actual peak incidence, one can safely say that the risk is greatest in the first 2 weeks with a cumulative 2-week risk of approximately 20%–30%. A penchant for delayed surgery combined with the desire to lower the rebleeding risk during the waiting period led to the liberal use of antifibrinolytic agents (epsilon-aminocaproic acid and tranexamic acid) by the early 1980s. These agents slow the access of the fibrinolytic protein plasmin to the fibrin clot.[177] Interestingly, antifibrinolytic drugs likely have little effect on preventing rebleeding in the first 48 hours, the period with the highest risk of rebleed.[177] These early bleeds are not thought to be due to lysis of fibrin clot but rather are "blow out" hemorrhages due to the unstable nature of the aneurysmal thrombus.[177] The recent International Cooperative Study on the Timing of Aneurysm Surgery suggested that early surgery was no more dangerous to patients than late surgery, and gradual acceptance of early operation led to a decline in the use of antifibrinolytics.[31, 178–181] In addition, these drugs were shown to increase the morbidity of delayed ischemia and were associated with a higher incidence of hydrocephalus.[182–185] Although the use of antifibrinolytics has waned, a number of other medical interventions are thought to be important in helping to prevent rebleeding.

The clinical factors that can increase the likelihood of rebleeding are hypertension, anxiety, agitation, and seizure with their attendant rise in blood pressure. All acute patients are kept in the intensive care unit under "SAH precautions." This designation results in the patient being kept flat in a quiet, dark room with a strict limitation of visitors. In order to limit these factors' contribution to the risk of recurrent hemorrhage, we aggressively treat hypertension, but careful management and observation is necessary because the chance of rebleeding and the risk of iatrogenic hypoperfusion must be carefully balanced. Blood pressure should be closely monitored in the intensive care unit. Often, sedation and mild pain control can lower blood pressure to tolerable levels. Previously hypertensive patients should be continued on their antihypertensive medications with intravenous forms of oral drugs given, if possible. For patients refractory to drugs given at regular intervals, intravenous esmolol or sodium nitroprusside can be given as an infusion, with doses titrated to specific blood-pressure parameters. We also find that sublingual nifedipine is useful in the preoperative patient and can be given as needed for specific blood-pressure values. In some instances, particularly in poor-grade cases, a ventricular catheter with lowering of ICP can reduce blood pressure.[15]

Seizures are not uncommon following SAH, occurring in 13%–24% of patients, most commonly within the first 24 hours after bleeding.[15, 36] We load all post-SAH patients with 1 g (15 mg/kg) of phenytoin, usually intravenously, at a rate of not more than 50 mg/minute. We maintain patients on an anticonvulsant for 4–12 weeks after their ictus, depending on the perceived risk of a seizure. In patients who have no further seizures during this period, drugs are tapered off. A recent report by Baker et al. suggests that anticonvulsant therapy can be safely limited to the immediate postoperative period in those patients without parenchymal clot, ischemic infarct, or postoperative hematoma.[37] Older series of surgically treated aneurysms after SAH have reported the incidence of seizure to be 10%–27%.[37] However, recent data show a much lower incidence of postoperative epilepsy, calling into question long-term prophylactic treatment with anticonvulsants.[37, 186–188]

Volume expansion is initiated early in the course of treatment, with insertion of a central venous catheter preoperatively if time permits. We routinely maintain central venous pressure (CVP) of 8–12 mm Hg with isotonic saline solution running continuously and albumin given as needed for CVP of less than 8 mm Hg. Some have argued for placement of Swan-Ganz catheters with pulmonary capillary wedge pressure monitoring in all patients.[189] We have reserved pulmonary arterial monitoring for patients with pre-existing conditions such as congestive heart failure or pulmonary hypertension, and for especially debilitated patients in whom more intensive left-sided cardiac monitoring is desirable. Volume expansion with blood-pressure control has been shown to improve survival after aneurysmal subarachnoid hemorrhage,[15] despite a theoretical increase in rebleeding one might fear from volume expansion. Hasan et al. prospectively evaluated the effects of volume expansion on outcome and found that increased fluid intake along with antihypertensive therapy only in those with pre-existent high blood pressure helped to prevent cerebral ischemia.[190] Prior to aneurysm clipping, we manage the blood pressure aggressively, but after surgery, particularly in the early surgery patient, we are more conservative with antihypertensive therapy, allowing systolic pressures of up to 160–180 mm Hg without intervention.

Rebleeding remains the most significant source of morbidity and mortality for the SAH patient in the early period following the initial ictus. Obliteration of the aneurysm, either through surgical clipping or endovascular occlusion, remains the only factor truly associated with significant improvements in lowering the risk of this dreaded complication.

Hydrocephalus

Hydrocephalus secondary to SAH occurs in two distinct forms. We will address the treatment of the first, acute form here and will discuss management of the delayed form in the postsurgical section. The acute form, occurring immediately or up to 7 days following subarachnoid bleed, is caused by compromise of CSF circulation pathways, resulting in increased ICP and ventricular dilatation. Patients with acute hydrocephalus following SAH are more often of a lower preoperative grade and have a poorer prognosis than do SAH patients without hydrocephalus.[42] Symptomatic hydrocephalus most often results in a decreased level of consciousness, which is thought to be secondary to decreased basal blood flow.[41, 191–193] This condition may improve spontaneously without intervention.[193] The patient's level of consciousness remains the best clinical measure of intracranial pressure.[15] This condition can be diagnosed by careful clinical observation and CT. Patients with intraventricular blood are at higher risk for developing hydrocephalus,[42, 194] although cisternal blood alone may increase the risk slightly[194] and patients with perimesencephalic hemorrhage have been shown to develop hydrocephalus.[49, 50] In the International Study on the Timing of Aneurysm Surgery, it was concluded that the risk of development of acute hydrocephalus was related to a number of clinical and radiographic factors (Table 9–16).[185] Cisternal blood, although predisposing the patient to hydrocephalus, similarly increases the risk of cerebral arterial vasospasm, and these two sequelae of SAH often occur together.[195] Recent experimentation in cats with intrathecal fibrinolytic agents has suggested that they may be beneficial in helping to prevent the development of hydrocephalus, but no clear benefit has yet been demonstrated in humans.[196]

The treatment of acute hydrocephalus largely depends on its severity, both clinically and radiographically. Certainly, an obtunded patient with dilated ventricles deserves immediate ventriculostomy; however, often we are confronted with patients with minimally dilated cerebral ventricles and subtle compromise of level of consciousness. Given that there may be some increased risk of rebleeding associated with ventriculostomy placement along with the known infectious risks,[193, 197–199] we may opt to treat these patients conservatively but will intercede promptly should their clinical condition decline. Some have used serial lumbar punctures,[192] which we reserve for the postoperative patient to attempt to avoid the necessity of inserting an indwelling shunt. Despite these risks, urgent ventriculostomy should be performed in all SAH patients with altered level of consciousness and CT evidence of acute hydrocephalus.[197] Ventriculostomy, when performed correctly, is a relatively low-morbidity procedure that can result in prompt and often dramatic clinical improvement in approximately two-thirds of patients.[41] This clinical improvement often leads to changes in management strategy in poor-grade cases, because if clinical grade improves enough, patients may become candidates for early surgery. One must be careful in grading patients clinically, in that reversible deficits related to hydrocephalus may be contributing to a patient's poor condition. Bailes et al. inserted ventriculostomies in 47 poor-grade aneurysm patients without CT evidence of irreversible brain destruction.[200] Thirty-five of these patients underwent aggressive surgical and postoperative therapy with a good outcome in 19, suggesting that early control of ICP and aggressive management may be desirable in a subset of poor-grade cases. These authors also point out that a number of these patients had high ICP without ventriculomegaly on CT.

TABLE 9–16 **FACTORS RELATED TO THE DEVELOPMENT OF CLINICAL HYDROCEPHALUS FOLLOWING SUBARACHNOID HEMORRHAGE**

1. Increasing age
2. Pre-existing hypertension
3. Admission blood pressure
4. Postoperative hypertension
5. Intraventricular hemorrhage
6. Diffuse subarachnoid blood
7. Thick focal collection of subarachnoid blood
8. Posterior circulation site of aneurysm
9. Focal ischemic deficits
10. Preoperative use of antifibrinolytic drugs
11. Hyponatremia
12. Decreased level of consciousness on admission
13. Low score on the Glasgow Outcome Scale

Vasospasm

Cerebral arterial vasospasm occurs 3–14 days following SAH. It appears angiographically in 30%–70% of patients, becoming symptomatic in 20%–30% with permanent morbidity or death occurring in 10%–20%.[201] Vasospasm is thought to be induced by thick subarachnoid clots coating the adventitial surfaces of cerebral arteries. The vascular distribution and severity of vasospasm correlate closely with the location and size of the subarachnoid clot.[202] Its true etiology and pathophysiology remain poorly understood despite many years of intense investigation.

Cerebral vasospasm is characterized by significant pathomorphologic changes in the cerebral arterial blood vessels. Animal models suggest that most vasospasm occurs in large arteries and arterioles.[203–207] Seifert et al. point out that the endothelium of cerebral vessels undergoes significant changes following SAH, potentially leading to an alteration in the balance between vasoconstrictive and vasoreactive substances.[205] These pathomorphologic changes include infolding and corrugation of the endothelium, disorientation and desquamation of endothelial cells, and vacuolation and ingrowth of fibrous tissue between the endothelial and muscular layers.[205] Mayberg et al. suggest that these morphologic and structural changes may act in concert with contractile mechanisms to alter normal physiologic responses and maintain a narrowed lumen.[206]

The question of what substance induces these profound effects is yet unanswered, but certainly a large body of evidence points to oxyhemoglobin as the most likely candidate.[202] Hemoglobin has been shown to penetrate the basilar arterial wall in a rabbit model of SAH, penetrating the smooth muscle and endothelial cell layers, with the degree of vasospasm correlating with the total amount of hemoglobin present.[208] Iron chelating agents have been shown to inhibit arterial vasospasm, suggesting perhaps that it is the ferric moiety of the hemoglobin molecule that is the inducing agent.[209] The precise mechanism whereby oxyhemoglobin unleashes a cascade of molecular biologic, biochemical, and physiologic changes is unclear. A number of

a number of factors. One must first consider the condition of the patient preoperatively. Certainly, a patient intubated preoperatively should not be extubated in the immediate postoperative period, whereas a grade I alert patient can be extubated if the operation has gone smoothly. Once a patient is awake in the operating room and he or she can follow commands bilaterally without obvious deficit, we commonly extubate the patient before going to the intensive care unit.

We delay extubation if the patient has undergone a posterior fossa operation with manipulation of the lower cranial nerves, because airway protection may be compromised. We ask our otolaryngologists to evaluate the movement of the vocal cords immediately upon extubation to ensure adequate airway protection. The other group of patients that often require delayed extubation are those who have been intentionally cooled intraoperatively, often with prolonged temporary arterial occlusion. These patients should be transported quickly to the intensive care unit, where they can be rapidly warmed and extubated when stable. Patients with any apparent compromise of ventilation or oxygenation also ought to be brought to the intensive care unit intubated. It is of paramount importance to prevent pulmonary complications, particularly in patients with vasospasm or high ICP. Significant hypoxemia, hypercarbia, or acidosis can significantly worsen cerebral ischemia and cerebral edema.

Upon arrival in the intensive care unit, patients should be stabilized with reinstitution of all relevant noninvasive monitoring. Patients are maintained with the head of the bed elevated 30–45 degrees. Arterial blood pressure, central venous pressure, respiratory parameters with pulse oximetry, core body temperature and, if applicable, ICP should be immediately assessed. Great care must be taken to ensure that all lines are cared for and secured adequately. A full set of electrolytes, coagulation profile, complete blood count, anticonvulsant level, and arterial blood gas should be tested.

As alluded to earlier, we liberalize our tight control of blood pressure in the postoperative period. However, during the first 24–48 hours postoperatively, elevations of systolic pressure above 180 mm Hg ought to be treated to prevent intracranial hemorrhage. Patients are continued on high-dose steroid therapy, anticonvulsant of choice (usually phenytoin), H_2 blocker, and nimodipine. An antibiotic, usually a first-generation cephalosporin such as cefazolin, is continued for the first 24 hours after surgery. Liberal volume expansion after surgery is the rule with central venous pressure (or pulmonary capillary wedge pressure, if indicated) serving as the measure of intravascular volume status. Replacement of all measured and insensible losses (important to consider in a mechanically ventilated patient) plus an additional 1000–1500 mL/day is recommended.[189] We use isotonic saline solution running continuously at 100–150 mL/hour (depending on the size of the patient) and supplement this infusion with albumin boluses every 4 hours as needed for central venous pressure values of less than 8 mm Hg. This schedule can be increased or decreased in frequency; depending on the individual patient and clinical circumstance. Patients should undergo an initial postoperative anteroposterior portable chest radiograph to assess lung fields and position of the endotracheal tube, if applicable.

Once the patient has been stabilized, a careful neurologic evaluation should ensue with particular importance paid to level of consciousness, relevant cranial nerves, and focal cortical deficits such as aphasia and motor weakness. Preoperative neurologic deficits are often somewhat more pronounced in the immediate postoperative period, and careful, frequent evaluation is important, because deficits should slowly improve with time as the patient warms and the effects of anesthesia wane. If deficits do not improve or if new deficits appear, we have a low threshold to perform immediate postoperative head CT.

All of our patients undergo head CT within the first 24 hours postoperatively. However, early CT within the first few hours after surgery is occasionally necessary and is important to obtain in patients with new or worsening deficits. The decision to reoperate on an intracranial clot should be based on the patient's condition as well as the size and degree of mass effect of the clot. Immediate assessment of the patient's platelet count and coagulation parameters ought to be made and any abnormality corrected as quickly as possible. In patients with significant mass effect either from clot or cerebral swelling, volume expansion therapy should be curtailed somewhat so as not to increase the degree of mass effect. Patients who deteriorate should be reintubated if necessary and treated with mannitol therapy prior to being taken to the operating room for decompressive craniotomy. Patients with severe progressing deficits with negative CT results ought to undergo angiography as soon as possible. Vasospasm, embolic arterial occlusion, and obliteration of arteries by the aneurysm clip are all possible causes of early deterioration, and each entity is managed differently.

Vasospasm

We routinely obtain TCD evaluations of cerebral blood flow velocity either daily or every other day to follow flow velocities noninvasively in post-SAH patients. TCD provides a noninvasive method for recording blood flow velocity in the basal cerebral arteries and allows prediction of vasospasm in patients at risk.[250] TCD examination technique is easily learned but should be performed by experienced persons to achieve consistent and useful results. Normal velocity for the anterior cerebral artery is 49–60 cm/sec, slightly less than that of the middle cerebral artery. A velocity of 120 cm/sec is generally used as the value above which vasospasm is diagnosed.[251, 252] Hutchison and Weir found that the best single parameter for judging a patient's susceptibility to clinically significant vasospasm is middle cerebral artery velocity.[253] They also found that patients whose velocities stayed below 100 cm/sec are highly unlikely to suffer from significant vasospasm, whereas patients with velocities over 200 cm/sec were at high risk for the development of clinically significant vasospasm.[253]

Interestingly, in one study 90% of all patients undergoing surgery in the acute period showed some degree of localized acceleration of blood flow velocity as measured by TCD; however, only 38% of patients developed delayed deficits.[254] TCD velocities have been shown to accelerate during the third to twelfth days after SAH, whereas Harders and Gilsbach found peak velocity occurring during days 11–20 after bleed.[254–256] It is important to keep these numbers in mind when managing postoperative patients. Clinically stable patients who are discharged to home should be advised about the importance of returning for evaluation should new-onset headache or lethargy occur, because patients can develop vasospasm after the usual postoperative hospital stay. We have seen patients develop ischemic deficits as late as 18–21 days post SAH. We also have the clinical impression that smokers and abusers of cocaine may be susceptible to more severe and prolonged vasospasm. It is also crucial not to discharge patients to home or to rehabilitation who maintain high TCD velocities until their velocities have been shown to peak and return toward normal. Patients who maintain high velocity but who are clinically stable can undergo some rehabilitation therapy while in the hospital, as long as it is done under the supervision of experienced therapists who are familiar with the signs and symptoms of cerebral ischemia.

It is of utmost importance to maintain consistency of TCD examination and to perform the studies often, so as to follow not only mean velocity but to observe the relative change in velocities from one day to the next. Grosset et al. studied TCD measurements in 121 SAH patients and found that rapid increases of greater than 50 cm/sec per day indicated significant vasospasm. Mizuno et al. confirmed that rapid rise was important but also pointed out that when vasospasm was in vessels distal to the segments evaluated by TCD, no rapid increases in flow velocities were observed.[257] Variability in vascular anatomy, proximal vasospasm, distal vasospasm, defective autoregulation, and infarction with distal hyperperfusion can all confound TCD results, making interpretation of velocities difficult.[250] Sloan et al. studied 34 patients with SAH undergoing angiography during the period of risk of vasospasm.[252] TCD was performed within 24 hours of these patients' angiograms and correctly diagnosed vasospasm in 17 of the 34 without false-positives.[252] There were, however, 12 false-negatives, frequently due to vasospasm in vessels not well evaluated by TCD.[252] These data suggest that TCD is highly specific (100%) but relatively insensitive (58.6%) in detecting vasospasm.[252] Information such as this reinforces the importance of the physical examination in evaluating patients for possible vasospasm. A low threshold for angiography should be the rule in high-risk patients with delayed neurologic deficits regardless of the TCD results.

Hypervolemic, hypertensive, hemodilutional (so-called triple H) therapy is an effective method of elevating and sustaining cerebral blood flow.[258] Elevation of cerebral blood flow using triple H therapy is thought to be effective both as a preventative measure and as a form of treatment of cerebral ischemia from vasospasm following aneurysmal SAH.[231, 259] Levy and Giannotta favor the use of dobutamine therapy with Swan-Ganz pulmonary arterial catheterization for the treatment of medically refractory symptomatic vasospasm with enhancement of fluid volume status until pulmonary arterial wedge pressure of approximately 14 mm Hg is maintained.[189] This degree of volume expansion maximizes cardiac performance, whereas wedge pressures above 14 mm Hg resulted in no improvement in cardiac indices.[189] Constant monitoring of cardiac performance is used in each patient in order to reduce complications such as cerebral edema, congestive heart failure, and pulmonary edema.[189] Enhanced cardiac output, perhaps independent of cerebral perfusion pressure changes, apparently improves blood flow to ischemic brain tissue,[260] lending credence to the hypothesis of Levy and Giannotta that cardiac output and pulsatility are important determinants of flow to dysautoregulated brain.[189]

In most patients, we currently use an isotonic saline solution and albumin protocol, as mentioned earlier, with less invasive central venous pressure (CVP) monitoring, to maintain a CVP of 8–12 mm Hg. Hypertensive therapy is initiated when patients are refractory to volume alone. Our first-line agents for increasing blood pressure are phenylephrine and dopamine, two alpha-receptor agonists. We have seen a number of patients develop significant hypotension using dobutamine and therefore reserve its use for patients unresponsive to the alpha agonists. Patients refractory to aggressive triple H therapy constitute a group with a poor prognosis, and few effective medical therapeutic options exist. Phlebotomy has been attempted rarely to decrease hematocrit; however, the evidence for an independent beneficial effect of hemodilution is not persuasive.[189, 231] Other options include ventricular catheterization with reduction of ICP and maximization of cerebral perfusion pressure using mannitol and removal of CSF.

Questions do arise regarding the use of triple H therapy in postoperative patients who harbor other unclipped, unruptured aneurysms. Swift and Solomon, in a study of 31 patients with one or more unprotected aneurysms, showed that not one rupture occurred during therapy, and they concluded that the benefit of triple H therapy warrants its use even in patients with unprotected aneurysms.[261] Although reports of complications such as aneurysm recurrence exist,[262] hypervolemic, hypertensive therapy is thought to be safe when patients are carefully managed by experienced neurointensivists. Although there have been no randomized controlled trials of hypervolemia and hypertensive therapy, most neurosurgeons employ this therapy based on their own clinical experience, as well as on the strong support that these methods have received in the literature.[231]

Once a presumptive diagnosis of vasospasm is made on the basis of deteriorating neurologic function along with significant elevation of TCD cerebral blood flow velocities, we approach the treatment of the patient in a stepwise fashion. If maximal medical therapy has been initiated, and if neurologic function does not improve or continues to decline, immediate angiography is considered. Mechanical dilation of the cerebral arteries via balloon angioplasty is an invasive and potentially dangerous procedure. Prior to considering angioplasty, other causes of clinical deterioration must be ruled out. Patients should undergo emergent head CT to check for the presence of an intracranial clot, stroke, or hydrocephalus as the cause of the neurologic decline. Simultaneously, the patient's electrolytes, blood count, and blood gases ought to be evaluated to ensure that electrolyte imbalance, sepsis, or hypoventilation is not responsible. Once these other potential sources of neurologic deterioration have been excluded, an angiogram should be obtained. Patients should be kept flat in bed once high ICP has been ruled out. If severe vascular spasm is diagnosed in a distribution that correlates with the patient's neurologic deficit, angioplasty ought to be considered.

Successful treatment of patients with cerebral vasospasm following SAH is predicated on prophylactic volume expansion, the initiation of hypertensive therapy as symptoms arise, and early intervention with angioplasty when indicated. Despite the effectiveness of triple H therapy and calcium channel blockade, 40% of patients with ischemic deficits due to vasospasm do not respond to this therapy, either remaining stable with their deficits or continuing to decline.[202] Definitive benefit has been shown in treating refractory vasospasm with angioplasty (see Chapter 11), particularly when therapy is initiated early in its course.[263–266] Approximately 60%–70% of patients undergoing balloon dilatation for vasospasm demonstrate clinical improvement, with most patients sustaining their improvements and continuing to do well.[267] Once signs and symptoms appear, the therapeutic window for successful angioplasty appears to be between 12 and 18 hours.[267] There is also a suggestion that spastic vessels are more easily dilated early in the course of vasospasm.[263, 267] Delayed angioplasty has been reported to be beneficial in selected cases,[268] but vessel dilatation after more than 48 hours has been found to be associated with a poor outcome. Balloon angioplasty should generally be limited to cases in which it can be performed shortly after the onset of neurologic deterioration.[263–266]

Intra-arterial papaverine therapy has been shown to be beneficial as an adjunct to cerebral angioplasty.[269–271] This intra-arterial vasodilator has been advocated for several situations: (1) when a balloon catheter cannot be passed through a spastic arterial segment; (2) when certain arterial branches cannot be reached with a balloon microcatheter (e.g., commonly the A1 or A2 segments of the anterior cerebral arteries); and (3) when dilatation of distal or perforating vessels is desired.[271] Clouston et al., in a series of 14 patients with vasospasm treated with intra-arterial papaverine, showed angiographic improvement in 95% of treatments, with 50% showing marked clinical improvement. Clinical results, however, did not directly correlate with the degree of angiographic response.[271] Our clinical experience with papaverine has not been as gratifying. Vasospasm can and does recur following papaverine therapy. We have on a number of occasions retreated patients who showed initial clinical improvement following papaverine therapy only to decline secondary to recurrent vasospasm. We commonly now combine balloon angioplasty for proximal spasm (e.g., internal carotid artery, M1 segment of the middle cerebral artery) with intra-arterial papaverine infusion for distal spasm. There are some suggestions that intra-arterial papaverine may elevate ICP in certain patients, occasionally into a dangerous range.

Neurointerventional therapy for vasospasm is a new method in ameliorating cerebral arterial vasospasm due to SAH. It is imperative, however, when using these therapies, to maintain standard hypertensive, hypervolemic therapy to ensure the best possible outcome.

Hydrocephalus

Hydrocephalus occurs in both the immediate and the early phases, as well as in a later delayed phase after SAH. This delayed, communicating form of hydrocephalus occurs days or weeks after a subarachnoid bleed, often with an indolent presentation, with symptoms and signs mimicking the syndrome of normal pressure hydrocephalus (NPH), including dementia, lethargy, gait ataxia, and urinary incontinence.[272] The development of delayed hydrocephalus is related to the same factors as those associated with the acute form (see Table 9–16)[185] and is thought to occur in approximately 10%–15% of patients following SAH.[31]

Unlike the acute form, which is due to obstruction of CSF drainage pathways, the chronic form is a communicating hydrocephalus with its etiology likely due to scarring of the arachnoid granulations by blood breakdown products. Fibrin deposition has been implicated as a possible contributor to the development of delayed hydrocephalus by reducing CSF circulation and absorption.[272] In a study by Gjerris et al., late hydrocephalus (more than 1 month after SAH) was associated with normal pressure but a high resistance to CSF outflow.[273] In addition, they found that patients who had a long interval from SAH to onset of hydrocephalus can often have normal CSF flow dynamics without the characteristic increased frequency of B pressure waves seen in patients with NPH and high outflow resistance. Although patients with abnormal CSF flow dynamics ought to be shunted, these authors argue that patients without these derangements can be managed non-operatively. Recently, high levels of transforming growth factor–beta 1, released by platelets into the CSF following SAH, have been found in patients with ventricular dilatation following bleeding.[274] Tada et al. had previously shown that intracisternal injection of this multifunctional polypeptide can induce communicating hydrocephalus in mice, suggesting that it may play a major role in its development after SAH.[275]

The treatment of hydrocephalus in large part is determined by its clinical severity. Acute hydrocephalus occurring with SAH must often be treated with emergent ventriculostomy. Some patients remain asymptomatic from their hydrocephalus and are managed without intervention. Patients who develop delayed hydrocephalus either in the early post-hemorrhagic period or later are treated symptomatically as well. Although data suggest that drainage of CSF in patients with communicating hydrocephalus after SAH improves cerebral blood flow, other research has determined that aggressive drainage can also increase the risk of cerebral infarction secondary to vasospasm, as well as result in an increased incidence of shunt dependence.[272]

Patients with acute hydrocephalus who are treated with early ventriculostomy are maintained on drainage for approximately 3–7 days. Patients are treated with prophylactic intrathecal gentamicin with CSF samples sent daily for cell count, glucose, and culture. Other centers favor different management regimens. Ventriculostomy drainage heights are maintained between 10 and 15 cm above the tragus to give us some idea as to the likelihood of the patients being shunt-dependent. Patients who drain only small amounts of CSF at these levels undergo ventriculostomy clamping with ICP monitoring and serial head CT to check for changes in ventricular size. In patients who tolerate this clamping regimen with normal ICP without neurologic decline or change in ventricular size, the ventricular catheters are removed. Patients who become symptomatic with clamping or who develop significant change in their ventricular size are shunted as early as possible to decrease the risk of infection with prolonged external drainage. Obtunded patients who have external drains are most commonly shunted so as to treat presumed high ICP and give these debilitated patients every chance for a meaningful recovery. With large amounts of intraventricular clot, external drains often malfunction, and sluggish drainage may be due to catheter blockage rather than low CSF pressure. To check for this, one can lower the drainage apparatus to evaluate catheter patency so as to ensure that low flow is truly due to low pressure. In addition, placement of an internal shunt in patients with highly proteinaceous CSF is somewhat problematic because they have a higher incidence of shunt obstruction. We often keep patients with proteins over 500 mg% on external drainage, with ventriculostomy change if necessary, to wait for clearance of the blood protein load.

When evaluating the ventricular dilatation of delayed hydrocephalus, one must determine whether surgical intervention is necessary. Some patients present with the classic signs and symptoms of NPH, whereas others are relatively asymptomatic. Improvement of the patient's symptoms following a high-volume lumbar puncture is good evidence that the patient will benefit from an internal shunt. However, occasionally patients have no objective symptomatic relief after CSF drainage and are followed with serial head CT. Patients who have continued enlargement of their ventricular system ought to be shunted despite lack of benefit after lumbar puncture, whereas those whose ventricular size remains stable can be followed as outpatients. We rarely use radionuclide scans as part of our decision-making process, but others have reported their usefulness.[276–278]

Postoperatively, patients often complain of headaches; the persistence of this symptom after the first few days ought to prompt investigation. Head CT can rule out hydrocephalus as the cause, whereas TCD can provide help in determining whether cerebral vasospasm is the etiology. Once these two possible causes have been ruled out, the patient can be followed clinically. Headache alone is no real cause for concern. Should the patient develop other symptoms, such as neck stiffness or fever, lumbar puncture is indicated to rule out meningitis. CSF should be sent for cell count with differential, glucose, protein, and culture with immediate institution of intravenous antibiotics including a third-generation cephalosporin in patients with significant CSF pleocytosis. If cultures return negative, the antibiotic can be discontinued; however, persistent symptoms with negative cultures may be due to aseptic meningitis, particularly following posterior fossa surgery. The clinical presentation of aseptic meningitis is similar to bacterial meningitis and is characterized by spiking fever and meningismus.[279] Its differentiation from bacterial meningitis may be difficult. Ross et al. point out that no laboratory or clinical criterion or combination of criteria were sensitive and specific enough to reliably differentiate bacterial from aseptic meningitis in the majority of patients.[280] Blomstedt, however, showed in a prospective study of 24 patients with postoperative meningitis and sterile cultures that termination of antibiotics following return of cultures resulted in no difference in outcome between treated and untreated groups.[281] Given that aseptic meningitis probably represents a sterile inflammatory process, we have treated these patients with both intravenous and oral nonsteroidal anti-inflammatory therapy as well as with intravenous and oral steroid therapy in refractory cases.

Unfortunately, poor outcomes after SAH, both with and without surgery, remain all too common. Patients are often left with severe disability affecting their activities of daily living, resulting in significant effects on their families and care givers. It is vitally important to limit morbidity related to their neurologic injury by initiating occupational and physical therapy as early as safely possible and to compulsively attend to skin care (to prevent pressure ulcers) and bowel regimen. Patients with significant compromise of their airway protection ought to undergo early tracheostomy and feeding tube placement where indicated. In order to limit risk of aspiration, our nutritional support service often recommends the insertion of a jejunostomy tube rather than a gastric tube; however, the indications for each in an individual patient ought to be discussed with the general surgeon and the patient's family, as well as the patient, if possible.

FAMILIAL INTRACRANIAL ANEURYSMS

Familial aneurysm is defined by the presence of intracranial aneurysms in two or more first- to third-degree relatives. Familial aneurysms present with rupture at an earlier age than do nonfamilial aneurysms (42.3 years versus 50–54 years), occur at the same site or mirror site in sibling pairs, and occur in identical twins, suggesting a genetic basis for their occurrence.[282] A Finnish study of 215 familial intracranial aneurysms (FIAs) showed that, in addition to earlier rupture, FIAs tend to be on average smaller in size than nonfamilial aneurysms at the time of rupture.[283] The authors also found that males presented with their aneurysms at a younger age than did females with FIAs (44 versus 50 years) and that the location of FIAs was more commonly on the middle cerebral artery than was observed in non-FIAs (49% versus 30%).[283] A retrospective analysis among patients with ruptured intracranial aneurysms estimated a familial frequency of 6.7%.[282]

The development of sensitive screening of patients felt to be at risk for harboring a cerebral aneurysm could significantly affect outcome from this devastating illness. MRA screening for the presence of intracranial aneurysms has been examined. In an evaluation of patients with polycystic kidney disease, aneurysms were successfully found in 11.7% of the study group and in 25.8% of patients who had a family member with an aneurysm.[284] Although MRA screening has been studied with reasonable success, conventional digitally subtracted contrast angiography remains the gold standard for diagnosis, but its use as a screening tool should likely be reserved for those felt to be at highest risk. A study of 12 affected families found that the highest rate of familial occurrence was in the siblings of those with aneurysms with angiographic detection of lesions in 29% of 51 asymptomatic relatives.[285] Interestingly, it was found that siblings of affected males were at higher risk to have an aneurysm than siblings of affected females (22% versus 9%).[285] MRA or high-resolution contrast CT should likely be the screening tool of choice solely for patients with polycystic kidney disease, because angiography in this group is thought possibly to result in an unacceptably high complication rate.[286]

Currently, we use MRA to screen family members with at least two first-degree relatives with cerebral aneurysms. The patient is advised as to the limitations of MRA as well as the morbidity of angiography, resulting in answers that are not 100% certain. We use both time-of-flight and phase contrast MRA when screening for an aneurysm. Time-of-flight MRA is useful for diagnosing small aneurysms but often misses large aneurysms with turbulent flow, because the flow signal from these aneurysms is lost using this technique. Phase contrast MRA, however, is excellent for larger aneurysms (> 15 mm) with turbulent flow but can often miss smaller, less well-demarcated aneurysms. Phase contrast imaging is also less susceptible to T1-related artifacts such as blood as well as hemosiderin and vascular clips.[287] A number of studies have been designed to estimate the sensitivity of MRA in delineating cerebral aneurysms. Korogi et al. showed time-of-flight MRA to be useful for identifying aneurysms larger than 5 mm (77%–94% sensitive) while being clinically inadequate for aneurysms of less than 5 mm (50%–60% sensitive).[288] Horikoshi et al. showed a similar sensitivity of time-of-flight MRA of 79% with a specificity rate of 92%. False-positive results all involved the internal carotid artery.[289]

One other potential use of MRA is in the prediction of an aneurysm's likelihood of rupturing. Meyer et al. used ciné phase contrast MRA to show that ruptured aneurysms demonstrate a much larger increase in volume between cardiac diastole and systole than do unruptured aneurysms (51% increase versus 17%).[290] Information such as this could be useful in predicting the identity of a ruptured aneurysm in a patient with subarachnoid blood and multiple aneurysms, as well as the potential for rupture in a patient with an unruptured aneurysm.

THE UNRUPTURED ANEURYSM

The management of patients harboring unruptured aneurysms found incidentally has received increased attention recently, because these lesions have been discovered with greater regularity. Prior to the advent of MRI and CT screening, these aneurysms were only discovered incidentally in patients with ruptured aneurysms studied by angiography. Identification of people who harbor unruptured aneurysms might have great impact, because the incidence of SAH could be reduced significantly by repairing these asymptomatic lesions. The sensitivity of MRI and MRA in particular has led to an increased frequency of incidental discovery of intracranial aneurysms. Controversy has surrounded the management of these patients, because the risks of surgery are weighed against the attendant morbidity and mortality of potential SAH.

Aneurysm size has often been closely evaluated when weighing surgical options, because size was felt to be the most accurate indicator of risk of rupture. Unruptured aneurysms are often small, with one study of 44 asymptomatic aneurysms showing a mean diameter of 4.8 mm, with 80% smaller than 6 mm.[291] Wiebers et al. found 10 mm to be the critical cutoff for risk of bleeding,[292] whereas others have recommended surgery for lesions larger than 3–5 mm.[293, 294] Although size remains an important characteristic when evaluating these lesions, any aneurysm regardless of size ought to be considered for surgery, because aneurysms can enlarge over time, and almost all aneurysms are at risk for subsequent rupture.[295, 296]

The natural history of these lesions was evaluated in Finland with 142 patients followed with 181 unruptured aneurysms until death or SAH intervened, or for at least 10 years after diagnosis.[296] An annual rupture rate of 1.4% was found with 14 episodes of fatal SAH. The cumulative bleeding rate was found to be 10% at 10 years, 26% at 20 years, and 32% at 30 years. Additionally, the authors concluded that an unruptured aneurysm should be subjected to surgery irrespective of size if technically possible, as long as no patient factors are contraindications to surgery. Given the risks of SAH over time, a number of groups have attempted to quantify surgical risk so as to better estimate which subgroup of patients benefit most from surgery while identifying those patients who should be managed nonoperatively. In a study of 202 consecutive operations for attempted clipping of unruptured aneurysms, Solomon et al. showed excellent or good outcome in 100% of aneurysms less than 10 mm, 95% with aneurysms 11–25 mm, and 79% with aneurysms greater than 25 mm.[297] King et al. performed a meta-analysis of the literature on morbidity and mortality from elective surgery for asymptomatic unruptured intracranial aneurysms between 1966 and 1992.[298] The estimated morbidity and mortality rates were found to be 4.1% and 1.0%, respectively.[298] Given the relatively significant cumulative bleeding risk with a reported low surgical morbidity/mortality as stated, surgery would appear to be indicated in most otherwise healthy patients harboring an unruptured intracranial aneurysm.

In managing these patients, we most often use age and, in particular, "physiologic age" as the most specific criterion for recommending surgery. Clearly, a blanket statement regarding a specific age as a cutoff for surgery would be inappropriate. The physician must evaluate each patient as an individual. The aneurysm and its size, location, and appearance must be weighed against the patient's medical condition and likelihood of living for at least 10 more years. As the cumulative risk of bleeding surpasses the inherent risk of surgery, the recommendation for surgery becomes more appropriate. Patients over 60 years of age with larger aneurysms, greater than 1.5 cm in diameter, and in less accessible locations (particularly posterior circulation aneurysms) may not benefit from surgery because surgical morbidity for these lesions is higher and, with advancing age, the lifetime risk of rupture decreases.[299] This decision, however, must be carefully discussed with the patient and the patient's family with an in-depth explanation of the risks of both options. One cannot discount the patient's own fears of living with an unclipped cerebral aneurysm and how that could potentially affect his or her own quality of life. King et al. attempted to quantify these various factors using mathematical modeling techniques to determine the relative cost-effectiveness of surgery on asymptomatic, unruptured, intracranial aneurysms.[300] Their findings support surgery on these lesions provided that surgical morbidity and mortality remain at approximately 5%, the patient has a life expectancy of at least 13 years, and the patient experiences a decreased subjective quality of life as a result of harboring this aneurysm.

Today, the management of an unruptured aneurysm without surgery does not necessarily mean no treatment. With the advent of interventional neuroradiologic techniques, aneurysmal obliteration potentially can be accomplished without the risks of surgery. Certainly, other risks exist with neurointerventional therapy and long-term outcomes of coiled aneurysms have yet to be analyzed. However, in a high-risk surgical patient or in a patient who refuses surgery, neurointerventional techniques may be an excellent alternative and may provide long-term protection from SAH.

Summary • The treatment of patients with aneurysmal SAH remains a challenge to the entire neurosurgical team. In this chapter we have tried to emphasize the importance of a number of factors when caring for these critically ill patients.

Patients must be evaluated quickly and with great urgency. Once the diagnosis of SAH is made, treatment options should be well thought out and discussed with the patient and his or her family. Significant steps should be taken as early as possible to limit the risk of possible complications, including rebleeding, hydrocephalus, seizure, and vasospasm. Patients should be meticulously examined and stabilized, with each patient optimally treated so as to ensure smooth transition into and out of surgery. Postoperatively, aggressive prophylaxis against vasospasm and seizures should continue. Constant vigilance is necessary on the part of the entire treatment team, because patient outcome can only benefit from rapid diagnosis and institution of appropriate therapy.

The future challenge for the neurosurgeon will be to incorporate new modalities of diagnostic imaging and neurointerventional therapies intelligently into mainstream strategies of clinical decision-making. Although outcomes after aneurysm surgery have improved greatly since the 1970s, interventional approaches in the treatment of aneurysms and cerebral vasospasm have become an important consideration. Lastly, in order to have the greatest impact on the morbidity and mortality of aneurysmal SAH, we must continue to search for ways to better identify aneurysms prior to rupture. Advances in imaging techniques, as well as possible identification of high-risk patients with genetic screening, may someday allow us to identify early even more of these potentially life-threatening lesions.

References

1. Atkinson JL, Sundt TM Jr, Houser OW, et al: Angiographic frequency of anterior circulation intracranial aneurysms. J Neurosurg 1989;70:551.
2. McCormick WF, Nofzinger JD: Saccular intracranial aneurysms: An autopsy study. J Neurosurg 1965;22:155.
3. Pakarinen S: Incidence, aetiology, and prognosis of primary subarachnoid haemorrhage: A study based on 589 cases diagnosed in a defined urban population during a defined period. Acta Scand (Suppl) 1967;29:1.
4. Sekhar LN, Heros RC: Origin, growth and rupture of saccular aneurysms: A review. Neurosurgery 1981;8:248.
5. Ljundgren B, Sharma S, Buchfelder M: History of aneurysm surgery. In Ratcheson RA, Wirth FP (eds): Ruptured Cerebral Aneurysms: Perioperative Management, vol 6: Concepts in Neurosurgery, p 1. Baltimore, Williams and Wilkins, 1994.
6. Moniz E: Léncephalographie arterielle: Son importance dans la localisation des tumeurs cerebrales. Rev Neurol (Paris) 1927;2:72.
7. Rhoton AL Jr: Anatomy of saccular aneurysms. Surg Neurol 1990;14:59.
8. de la Monte SM, Moore GW, Monk MA, et al: Risk factors for the development and rupture of intracranial berry aneurysms. JAMA 1985;78:957.
9. Stehbens WE: Etiology of intracranial berry aneurysms. J Neurosurg 1989;70:823.
10. Adams JH, Duchen LW (eds): Greenfield's Neuropathology, 5th ed, pp 282–301. New York, Oxford University Press, 1992.
11. Ostergaard JR: Aetiology of intracranial saccular aneurysms in childhood. Br J Neurosurg 1995;5:575.
12. Meyer FB, Sundt TM, Fode NC, et al: Cerebral aneurysms in childhood and adolescence. J Neurosurg 1989;70:420.
13. Weir B: Intracranial aneurysms and subarachnoid hemorrhage: An overview. In Wilkins RH, Rengachary SS (eds): Neurosurgery, p 1308. New York, McGraw-Hill, 1985.
14. Saveland H, Hillman J, Brandt L, et al: Overall outcome in aneurysmal subarachnoid hemorrhage. A prospective study from neurosurgical units in Sweden during a 1-year period. J Neurosurg 1992;76:729.
15. Crowell RM, Gress DR, Ogilvy CS, et al: Principles of management of subarachnoid hemorrhage: General

management. In Ratcheson RA, Wirth FP (eds): Ruptured Cerebral Aneurysms: Perioperative Management, vol 6: Concepts in Neurosurgery, p 59. Baltimore, Williams and Wilkins, 1994.
16. Greenberg MS: Handbook of Neurosurgery, 2nd ed, pp 603–604. Lakeland, Greenberg Graphics, 1991.
17. Morris KM, Shaw MD, Foy PM: Smoking and subarachnoid haemorrhage: A case control study. Br J Neurosurg 1992;6:429.
18. Bonita R: Cigarette smoking, hypertension and the risk of subarachnoid hemorrhage: A population-based case-control study. Stroke 1986;17:831.
19. Longstreth WT Jr, Nelson LM, Koepsell TD, et al: Cigarette smoking, alcohol use, and subarachnoid hemorrhage. Stroke 1992;23:1242.
20. Juvela S, Hillbom M, Numminen H, et al: Cigarette smoking and alcohol consumption as risk factors for aneurysmal subarachnoid hemorrhage. Stroke 1993;24:639.
21. Sahs AL, Perret GE, Locksley HB, et al (eds): Intracranial Aneurysms and Subarachnoid Hemorrhage: A Cooperative Study. Philadelphia, JB Lippincott, 1969.
22. Leblanc R: The minor leak preceding subarachnoid hemorrhage. J Neurosurg 1987;66:35.
23. Okawara SH: Warning signs prior to rupture of an intracranial aneurysm. J Neurosurg 1973;38:575.
24. Sarner M, Rose FC: Clinical presentation of ruptured intracranial aneurysm. J Neurol Neurosurg Psychiatry 1967;30:67.
25. Hunt WE, Hess RM: Surgical risk as related to time of intervention in the repair of intracranial aneurysms. J Neurosurg 1968;28:14.
26. Drake CG: Report of World Federation of Neurological Surgeons Committee on a universal subarachnoid hemorrhage grading scale. J Neurosurg 1988;68:985.
27. Botterell EH, Lougheed WM, Scott JW, et al: Hypothermia, and interruption of carotid, or carotid and vertebral circulation, in the surgical management of intracranial aneurysms. J Neurosurg 1956;13:1.
28. Day AL: Aneurysms of the ophthalmic segment. A clinical and anatomical analysis. J Neurosurg 1990;72:677.
29. Ferguson GG: Carotid-ophthalmic artery aneurysms. In Wilkins RH, Rengachary SS (eds): Neurosurgery, p 1385. New York, McGraw-Hill, 1985.
30. Flamm ES: Aneurysms of internal carotid and anterior communicating arteries. In Wilkins RH, Rengachary SS (eds): Neurosurgery, p 1394. New York, McGraw-Hill, 1985.
31. Meyer FB, Morita A, Puumala MR, et al: Medical and surgical management of intracranial aneurysms. Mayo Clin Proc 1995;70:153.
32. Roux FX, Panthier JN, Tanghe YM, et al: Terson's syndrome and intraocular complications in meningeal hemorrhages (26 cases). Neurochirurgie 1991;37:106.
33. Rudehill A, Olsson GL, Sundqvist K, et al: ECG abnormalities in patients with subarachnoid haemorrhage and intracranial tumours. J Neurol Neurosurg Psychiatry 1987;50:1375.
34. Salvati M, Cosentino F, Artico M, et al: Electrocardiographic changes in subarachnoid hemorrhage secondary to cerebral aneurysm. Report of 70 cases. Ital J Neurol Sci 1992;13:409.
35. Szabo MD, Crosby G, Hurford WE, et al: Myocardial perfusion following acute subarachnoid hemorrhage in patients with an abnormal electrocardiogram. Anesth Analg 1993;76:253.
36. Sundaram MB, Chow F: Seizures associated with spontaneous subarachnoid hemorrhage. Can J Neurol Sci 1986;13:229.
37. Baker CJ, Prestigiacomo CJ, Solomon RA: Short-term perioperative anticonvulsant prophylaxis for the surgical treatment of low-risk patients with intracranial aneurysms. Neurosurgery 1996;37:863.
38. Ohman J: Hypertension as a risk factor for epilepsy after aneurysmal subarachnoid hemorrhage and surgery. Neurosurgery 1990;27:578.
39. Keranen T, Tapaninaho A, Hernesniemi J, et al: Late epilepsy after aneurysm operations. Neurosurgery 1985;17:897.
40. van Gijn J, van Dongen KJ: Time course of aneurysmal haemorrhage on computed tomograms. Neuroradiology 1982;23:153.
41. Milhorat TH: Acute hydrocephalus after aneurysmal subarachnoid hemorrhage. Neurosurgery 1987;20:15.
42. van Gijn J, Hijdra A, Wijdicks EF, et al: Acute hydrocephalus after aneurysmal subarachnoid hemorrhage. J Neurosurg 1985;63:355.
43. Tresser SJ, Selman WR, Ratcheson RA: Pathophysiological alterations following aneurysm rupture. In Ratcheson RA, Wirth FP (eds): Ruptured Cerebral Aneurysms: Perioperative Management, vol 6: Concepts in Neurosurgery, p 23. Baltimore, Williams and Wilkins, 1994.
44. Vermeulen M, Hasan D, Blijenberg BG, et al: Xanthochromia after subarachnoid haemorrhage needs no revisitation. J Neurol Neurosurg Psychiatry 1989;52:826.
45. Vermeulen M, van Gijn J, Blijenberg BG: Spectrophotometric analysis of CSF after subarachnoid hemorrhage: Limitations in the diagnosis of rebleeding. Neurology 1983;33:112.
46. MacDonald A, Mendelow AD: Xanthochromia revisited: A re-evaluation of lumbar puncture and CT scanning in the diagnosis of subarachnoid haemorrhage. J Neurol Neurosurg Psychiatry 1988;51:342.
47. Pinto AN, Ferro JM, Canhao P, et al: How often is a perimesencephalic subarachnoid haemorrhage CT pattern caused by ruptured aneurysms? Acta Neurochir (Wien) 1993;124:79.
48. Rinkel GJ, Wijdicks EF, Vermeulen M, et al: Nonaneurysmal perimesencephalic subarachnoid hemorrhage: CT and MR patterns that differ from aneurysmal rupture. AJNR 1991;12:829.
49. Rinkel GJ, Wijdicks EF, Vermeulen M, et al: Acute hydrocephalus in nonaneurysmal perimesencephalic hemorrhage: Evidence of CSF block at the tentorial hiatus. Neurology 1992;42:1805.
50. Rinkel GJ, Wijdicks EF, Vermeulen M, et al: The clinical course of perimesencephalic nonaneurysmal subarachnoid hemorrhage. Ann Neurol 1991;29:463.
51. Harbaugh RE, Schlusselberg DS, Jeffery R, et al: Three-dimensional computed tomographic angiography in the preoperative evaluation of cerebrovascular lesions. Neurosurgery 1995;36:320.
52. Tampieri D, Leblanc R, Oleszek J, et al: Three-dimensional computed tomographic angiography of cerebral aneurysms. Neurosurgery 1995;36:749.
53. Dorsch NWC, Young N, Kingston RJ, et al: Early experience with spiral CT in the diagnosis of intracranial aneurysms. Neurosurgery 1995;36:230.
54. Inagawa T, Kamiya K, Ogasawara H, et al: Rebleeding of ruptured intracranial aneurysms in the acute stage. Surg Neurol 1987;28:93.
55. Grossman RI, Yousem DM: Neuroradiology: The Requisites, pp 16–17. St. Louis, Mosby, 1994.
56. Victor M, Adams RD: Confusion, delirium, amnesia and dementia. In Braunwald E, Isselbacher KJ, Petersdorf RG, et al (eds): Harrison's Principles of Internal Medicine, 11th ed, p 134. New York, McGraw-Hill, 1987.
57. Juni J, Morera J, Lainez JM, et al: Transient global amnesia after cerebral angiography with iohexol. Neuroradiology 1992;34:141.
58. Giang DW, Kido DK: Transient global amnesia associated with cerebral angiography performed with use of iopamidol. Radiology 1989;172:195.
59. Stillhard G, Landis T, Schiess R, et al: Bitemporal hypoperfusion in transient global amnesia: 99m-Tc-HM-PAO SPECT and neuropsychological findings during and after an attack. J Neurol Neurosurg Psychiatry 1990;53:339.
60. Tanabe H, Hashikawa K, Nakagawa Y, et al: Memory loss due to transient hypoperfusion in the medial temporal

lobes including hippocampus. Acta Neurol Scand 1991;84:22.

61. Goldenberg G, Podreka I, Pfaffelmeyer N, et al: Thalamic ischemia in transient global amnesia: A SPECT study. Neurology 1991;41:1748.
62. Laloux P, Brichant C, Cauwe F, et al: Technetium-99m HM-PAO single photon emission computed tomography imaging in transient global amnesia. Arch Neurol 1992;49:543.
63. Samson DS, Batjer HH: Intracranial Aneurysm Surgery: Techniques, pp 97–120. Mount Kisco, NY, Futura, 1990.
64. Osborne AG: Introduction to Cerebral Angiography, pp 143–165. Philadelphia, Harper and Row, 1980.
65. Charbel FT, Seyfried D, Mehta B, et al: Dominant A1: Angiographic and clinical correlations with anterior communicating artery aneurysms. Neurol Res 1991;13:253.
66. Ogawa A, Suzuki M, Sakurai Y, et al: Vascular anomalies associated with aneurysms of the anterior communicating artery: Microsurgical observations. J Neurosurg 1990;72:706.
67. Wisoff JH, Flamm ES: Aneurysms of the distal anterior cerebral artery and associated vascular anomalies. Neurosurgery 1987;20:735.
68. Fleischer AS, Barrow DL: Distal anterior cerebral artery aneurysms. In Wilkins RH, Rengachary SS (eds): Neurosurgery, pp 1383–1384. New York, McGraw-Hill, 1985.
69. Rhoton AL Jr: Microsurgical anatomy of saccular aneurysms. In Wilkins RH, Rengachary SS (eds): Neurosurgery, p 1330. New York, McGraw-Hill, 1985.
70. Flamm ES: Anterior circulation aneurysms. In Long DM (ed): Current Therapy in Neurological Surgery, 2nd ed, p 151. Toronto, BC Decker, 1989.
71. Batjer HH, Kopitnik TA, Giller CA, et al: Surgery for paraclinoidal carotid artery aneurysms. J Neurosurg 1994;80:650.
72. Walter KA, Newman NJ, Lessell S: Oculomotor palsy from minor head trauma: Initial sign of intracranial aneurysm. Neurology 1994;44:148.
73. Tomsak RL, Masaryk TJ, Bates JH: Magnetic resonance angiography (MRA) of isolated aneurysmal third nerve palsy. J Clin Neuroophthalmol 1991;11:16.
74. Gouliamos A, Gotsis E, Vlahos L, et al: Magnetic resonance angiography compared to intra-arterial digital subtraction angiography in patients with subarachnoid haemorrhage. Neuroradiology 1992;35:46.
75. Teasdale E, Statham P, Straiton J, et al: Non-invasive radiological investigation for oculomotor palsy. J Neurol Neurosurg Psychiatry 1990;53:549.
76. Good EF: Ptosis as the sole manifestation of compression of the oculomotor nerve by an aneurysm of the posterior communicating artery. J Clin Neuroophthalmol 1990;10:59.
77. Kwan ES, Laucella M, Hedges TR, et al: A cliniconeuroradiologic approach to third cranial nerve palsies. AJNR 1987;8:459.
78. Ranganadham P, Dinakar I, Mohandas S, et al: A rare presentation of posterior communicating artery aneurysm. Clin Neurol Neurosurg 1992;94:225.
79. Capo H, Warren F, Kupersmith MJ: Evolution of oculomotor nerve palsies. J Clin Neuroophthalmol 1992;12:21.
80. Fujiwara S, Fujii K, Nishio S, et al: Oculomotor nerve palsy in patients with cerebral aneurysms. Neurosurg Rev 1989;12:123.
81. Samson DS, Batjer HH: Aneurysms of the posterior internal carotid artery wall. In Samson DS, Batjer HH (eds): Intracranial Aneurysm Surgery: Techniques, p 55. Mt. Kisco, NY, Futura, 1990.
82. Moyer DJ, Flamm ES: Anomalous arrangement of the origins of the anterior choroidal and posterior communicating arteries. Case report. J Neurosurg 1992;76:1017.
83. Samson DS, Batjer HH: Aneurysms of the internal carotid artery bifurcation. In Samson DS, Batjer HH (eds): Intracranial Aneurysm Surgery: Techniques, p 69. Mt. Kisco, NY, Futura, 1990.
84. Heros RC: Middle cerebral artery aneurysms. In Wilkins RH, Rengachary SS (eds): Neurosurgery, p 1376. New York, McGraw-Hill, 1985.
85. Page RD, Richardson PL: Emergency surgery for haematoma-forming aneurysmal haemorrhage. Br J Neurosurg 1990;4:199.
86. Pasqualin A, Bazzan A, Cavazzani P, et al: Intracranial hematomas following aneurysmal rupture: Experience with 309 cases. Surg Neurol 1986;25:6.
87. Hosoda K, Fujita S, Kawagushi T, et al: Saccular aneurysms of the proximal (M1) segment of the middle cerebral artery. Neurosurgery 1995;36:441.
88. Weir B: Aneurysms Affecting the Nervous System, p 188. Baltimore, Williams and Wilkins, 1987.
89. Peerless SJ, Drake CG: Posterior circulation aneurysms. In Wilkins RH, Rengachary SS (eds): Neurosurgery, p 1422. New York, McGraw-Hill, 1985.
90. Weir B: Posterior circulation aneurysms. In Long DM (ed): Current Therapy in Neurological Surgery, 2nd ed, p 157. Toronto, BC Decker, 1989.
91. Rinne J, Hernesniemi J, Puranen M, et al: Multiple intracranial aneurysms in a defined population: Prospective angiographic and clinical study. Neurosurgery 1994;35:803.
92. Wilson FM, Jaspan T, Holland IM: Multiple cerebral aneurysms—A reappraisal. Neuroradiology 1989;31:232.
93. Inagawa T, Hirano A: Ruptured intracranial aneurysms: An autopsy study of 133 patients. Surg Neurol 1990;33:117.
94. Ostergaard JR, Hog E: Incidence of multiple intracranial aneurysms. Influence of arterial hypertension and gender. J Neurosurg 1985;63:49.
95. Joslyn JN, Williams JP, White JL, et al: Simultaneous rupture of two intracranial aneurysms: CT diagnosis. Stroke 1985;16:518.
96. Stone JL, Crowell RM, Gandhi YN, et al: Multiple intracranial aneurysms: Magnetic resonance imaging for determination of the site of rupture. Report of a case. Neurosurgery 1988;23:97.
97. Hackney DB, Lesnick JE, Zimmerman RA, et al: MR identification of bleeding site in subarachnoid hemorrhage with multiple intracranial aneurysms. J Comput Assist Tomogr 1986;10:878.
98. Hamburger C, Schonberger J, Lange M: Management and prognosis of intracranial giant aneurysms. A report on 58 cases. Neurosurg Rev 1992;15:97.
99. Vorkapic P, Czech T, Pendl G, et al: Clinico-radiological spectrum of giant intracranial aneurysms. Neurosurg Rev 1991;14:271.
100. Matsumura K, Saito A, Nakasu Y, et al: Magnetic resonance imaging of large and giant intracranial aneurysms. Neurol Med Chir (Tokyo) 1990;30:382.
101. Kojima Y, Saito A, Kim I: The role of serial angiography in the management of bacterial and fungal intracranial aneurysms—Report of two cases and review of the literature. Neurol Med Chir (Tokyo) 1989;29:202.
102. Stumacher RJ: Clinical Infectious Diseases, p 150. Philadelphia, WB Saunders, 1987.
103. Frazee JG: Inflammatory intracranial aneurysms. In Wilkins RH, Rengachary SS (eds): Neurosurgery, p 1440. New York, McGraw-Hill, 1985.
104. Hurst RW, Choi IS, Persky M, et al: Mycotic aneurysms of the intracavernous carotid artery: A case report and review of the literature. Surg Neurol 1992;37:142.
105. Hadley MN, Martin NA, Spetzler RF, et al: Multiple intracranial aneurysms due to Coccidioides immitis infection. Case report. J Neurosurg 1987;66:453.
106. O'Donohue JM, Enzmann DR: Mycotic aneurysm in angiitis associated with herpes zoster ophthalmicus. AJNR 1987;8:615.
107. Clare CE, Barrow DL: Infectious intracranial aneurysms. Neurosurg Clin North Am 1992;3:551.
108. Frizzel RT, Vitek JJ, Hill DL, et al: Treatment of a

287. Huston J, Rufenacht DA, Ehman RL, et al: Intracranial aneurysms and vascular malformations: Comparison of time-of-flight and phase-contrast MR angiography. Radiology 1991;181:721.
288. Korogi Y, Takahashi M, Mabuchi N, et al: Intracranial aneurysms: Diagnostic accuracy of three-dimensional, Fourier transform, time-of-flight MR angiography. Radiology 1994;193:181.
289. Horikoshi T, Fukamachi A, Nishi H, et al: Detection of intracranial aneurysms by three-dimensional time-of-flight magnetic resonance angiography. Neuroradiology 1994;36:203.
290. Meyer FB, Huston J, Riederer SS: Pulsatile increases in aneurysm size determined by cine phase-contrast MR angiography. J Neurosurg 1993;78:879.
291. Ujiie H, Sato K, Onda H, et al: Clinical analysis of incidentally discovered unruptured aneurysms. Stroke 1993;24:1850.
292. Wiebers DO, Whisnant JP, O'Fallon WM: The natural history of unruptured intracranial aneurysms. N Engl J Med 1981;304:696.
293. Kassel NF, Torner JC: Size of intracranial aneurysms. Neurosurgery 1983;12:291.
294. Asari S, Ohmoto T: Natural history and risk factors of unruptured cerebral aneurysms. Clin Neurol Neurosurg 1993;95:205.
295. Lindley JG, Wirth FP: Epidemiology of cerebral aneurysms. In Ratcheson RA, Wirth FP (eds): Ruptured Cerebral Aneurysms: Perioperative Management, vol 6: Concepts in Neurosurgery, p 15. Baltimore, Williams and Wilkins, 1994.
296. Juvela S, Porras M, Heiskanen O: Natural history of unruptured intracranial aneurysms: A long-term follow-up study. J Neurosurg 1993;79:174.
297. Solomon RA, Fink ME, Pile-Spellman J: Surgical management of unruptured intracranial aneurysms. J Neurosurg 1994;80:440.
298. King JT, Berlin JA, Flamm ES: Morbidity and mortality from elective surgery for asymptomatic, unruptured, intracranial aneurysms: A meta-analysis. J Neurosurg 1994;81:837.
299. Wirth FP: Surgical treatment of incidental intracranial aneurysms. Clin Neurosurg 1986;33:125.
300. King JT Jr, Glick HA, Mason TJ, et al: Elective surgery for asymptomatic, unruptured, intracranial aneurysms: A cost-effectiveness analysis. J Neurosurg 1995;83:403.

10

Surgical Management of Spontaneous Intracranial Hemorrhage

Eric L. Zager, M.D. • Eugene S. Flamm, M.D.

Spontaneous intracranial hemorrhage (ICH) comprises a diverse set of clinical syndromes and pathological entities. Virtually any intracranial compartment can be subject to spontaneous hemorrhage, and there is a wide array of possible etiologies that vary in incidence, most notably according to the patient's age. Other factors that may play an important role in the pathological type and anatomic site of hemorrhage include the patient's sex, racial background, and cerebrovascular risk factors. In this chapter we specifically exclude all hemorrhages related to cerebral trauma or surgery, topics that are discussed in other chapters. Included in this discussion are specific vascular lesions, in particular cerebral aneurysms and arteriovenous malformations (AVMs). Spontaneous ICH is responsible for a large proportion of the major morbidity and mortality related to stroke in general. The major goal of this chapter is to discuss the role for surgical intervention in appropriate cases of spontaneous ICH.

Epidemiology

Spontaneous ICH is the third leading cause of stroke, following thrombosis and embolism. Spontaneous ICH accounts for 15%–20% of all strokes, but patients in this group are devastated. The mortality rate may be as high as 35%–50%, and these hemorrhages account for a disproportionate amount of the major morbidity from stroke.[1] Advanced age is clearly the most important risk factor for ICH overall, but this statement oversimplifies a complex relationship. Hypertensive (often called *primary*) intracerebral hemorrhage is rare in patients younger than 45, and the incidence rises substantially with increasing age. In the elderly (over 80 years), the incidence of hypertensive hemorrhage is approximately 350 per 100,000 per year, which is nearly 25 times the incidence for the general population.[2, 3] Vascular malformations and aneurysms cause a higher percentage of hemorrhages in younger adult patients, whereas hemorrhages due to brain tumors and vasculopathies are more common in the elderly. There are reports that identify a higher incidence of primary intracerebral hemorrhage in Japanese, Chinese, and African-American populations.[4–7] Gender differences have been reported, but the results of these studies have been conflicting.[4, 5, 8] Aneurysmal subarachnoid hemorrhage (SAH) shows a slight female preponderance of approximately 1.6:1.[9] The overall incidence of spontaneous ICH has declined since the 1950s; the reasons for this trend are not well understood. It is hopeful to conclude, as many have, that this declining incidence is due to more aggressive management of hypertension, but it is not clear that this explanation is entirely satisfactory.

General Clinical Features

The general clinical features of patients with spontaneous ICH vary widely and are well known to most clinicians. The classic presentation includes the sudden onset of a severe neurologic deficit, often associated with headache and alteration in the level of consciousness. However, the majority of cases do not fit this classic presentation. Patients may range in clinical condition from asymptomatic to deeply comatose, with virtually unlimited degrees of deficit in between these two extremes. The nature and severity of the deficit depend entirely on such factors as the size and location of the hematoma, the eloquence of adjacent structures, the age and general health of the patient, and the underlying pathophysiology of the lesion. Some patients may rapidly deteriorate following the initial ictus, whereas others may have a transient deficit that clears, similar to a transient ischemic attack. Either focal or generalized seizures may occur, as in occlusive cerebrovascular disease, and ultimately nothing in the presentation is specific enough to definitively diagnose a spontaneous ICH prior to imaging studies.

As in all patients, the history often is the most telling aspect of the initial evaluation, particularly with regard to a history of such factors as hypertension, compliance with antihypertensive medication, treatment with anticoagulant medication, use of illicit drugs or excessive amounts of alcohol, the presence of a malignant tumor elsewhere in the body or a primary brain lesion such as a vascular malformation or tumor, a known vasculopathy or coagulopathy, and the presence of a prosthetic heart valve. The physical examination must be goal directed and tailored in its degree of urgency to the clinical condition of the patient. Not uncommonly, patients who have suffered a significant ICH present with seriously impaired mental status such that the initial management involves control of the airway and extremes of blood pressure. A presentation with coma and clinical signs of herniation warrants rapid stabilization of vital signs and treatment for presumed intracranial hypertension while simultaneously arranging for emergency head computed tomography (CT).

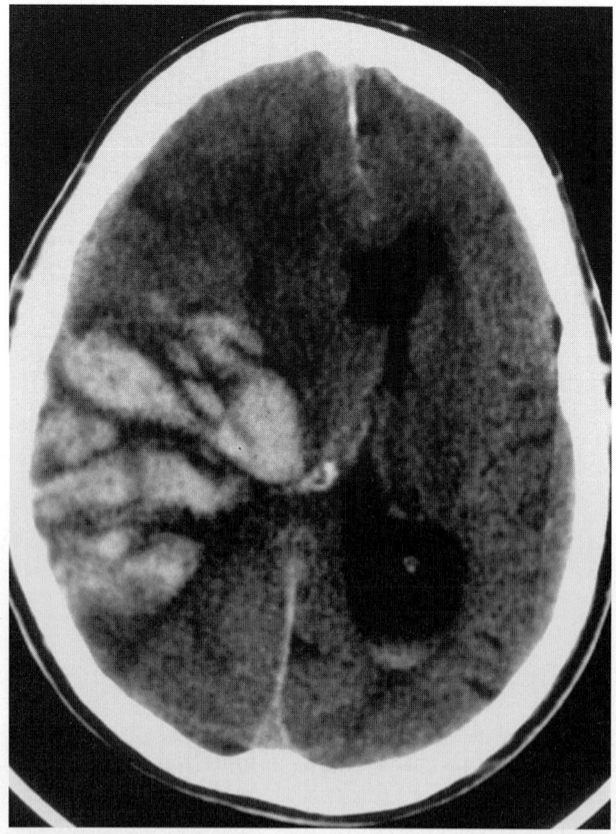

FIGURE 10-2 • Head computed tomography showing massive hemorrhagic transformation of a large right middle cerebral artery territory infarction in a patient treated with heparin.

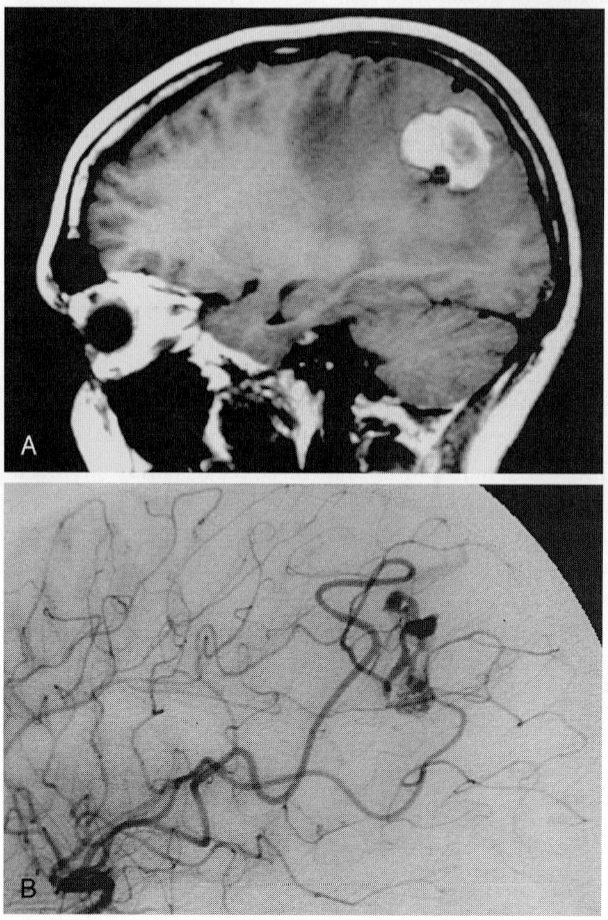

FIGURE 10-1 • *A,* Sagittal T1-weighted magnetic resonance image showing an acute right parietal hematoma in a young patient. *B,* Cerebral arteriogram (internal carotid artery injection, lateral view) from the same patient showing an underlying arteriovenous malformation.

Classification

Perhaps the simplest starting point for classification of spontaneous ICH is to categorize according to the anatomic location of the hematoma. The intracranial space may be divided into epidural, subdural, subarachnoid, intraparenchymal, and intraventricular spaces. Hemorrhages may occur in any one of these anatomic spaces or in combination, depending largely on the underlying pathology. The intracranial space may also be divided usefully into supratentorial and infratentorial compartments. When a spontaneous ICH is described by these anatomic features, it is possible to derive a meaningful differential diagnosis and plan for further evaluation. Among intraparenchymal hematomas, certain specific types present in characteristic clinical scenarios. For example, *lobar* (subcortical) *hemorrhages* account for 20%–50% of all intracerebral hemorrhages. These hematomas typically present with acute onset of headache, which may localize the involved lobe, as well as neurologic deficits that reflect the functional anatomy of adjacent parenchyma.[10, 11] For example, a dominant temporal lobe hematoma is likely to affect speech function, whereas a frontoparietal hematoma may impair contralateral motor function. In the elderly patient, recurrent lobar hemorrhages, particularly in the parietal and occipital lobes, strongly suggest the pathological diagnosis of amyloid angiopathy. In a younger patient, a single lobar bleed should raise the suspicion of a vascular malformation, a tumor, or a drug-induced hemorrhage (Fig. 10–1). Hemorrhagic transformation of an ischemic infarction, either with or without iatrogenic anticoagulation, closely follows a discrete vascular territory (Fig. 10–2).

A *putaminal* or *thalamic hemorrhage* usually presents with some degree of contralateral hemiparesis due to involvement of the internal capsule. Depending on the precise location, there may be hemianesthesia, speech dysfunction, gaze paresis, or hemianopia.[12] Larger hematomas may impair the level of consciousness because of a shift of midline structures or associated hydrocephalus (Fig. 10–3). Thalamic hemorrhages commonly extend into the upper brain stem and are then accompanied by vertical gaze palsy, retraction nystagmus, skew deviation, ptosis and miosis, unreactive pupils, and loss of convergence.[13, 14] Putaminal hemorrhages account for approximately 40%–50% of all intracerebral hemorrhages, whereas thalamic bleeds account for only 5%–20% of these lesions. These are most commonly hypertensive in etiology and have been well studied.[13] There may be no clear history of hypertension, but careful monitoring often reveals labile hypertension that has never been diagnosed.

Cerebellar hemorrhages account for 5%–10% of

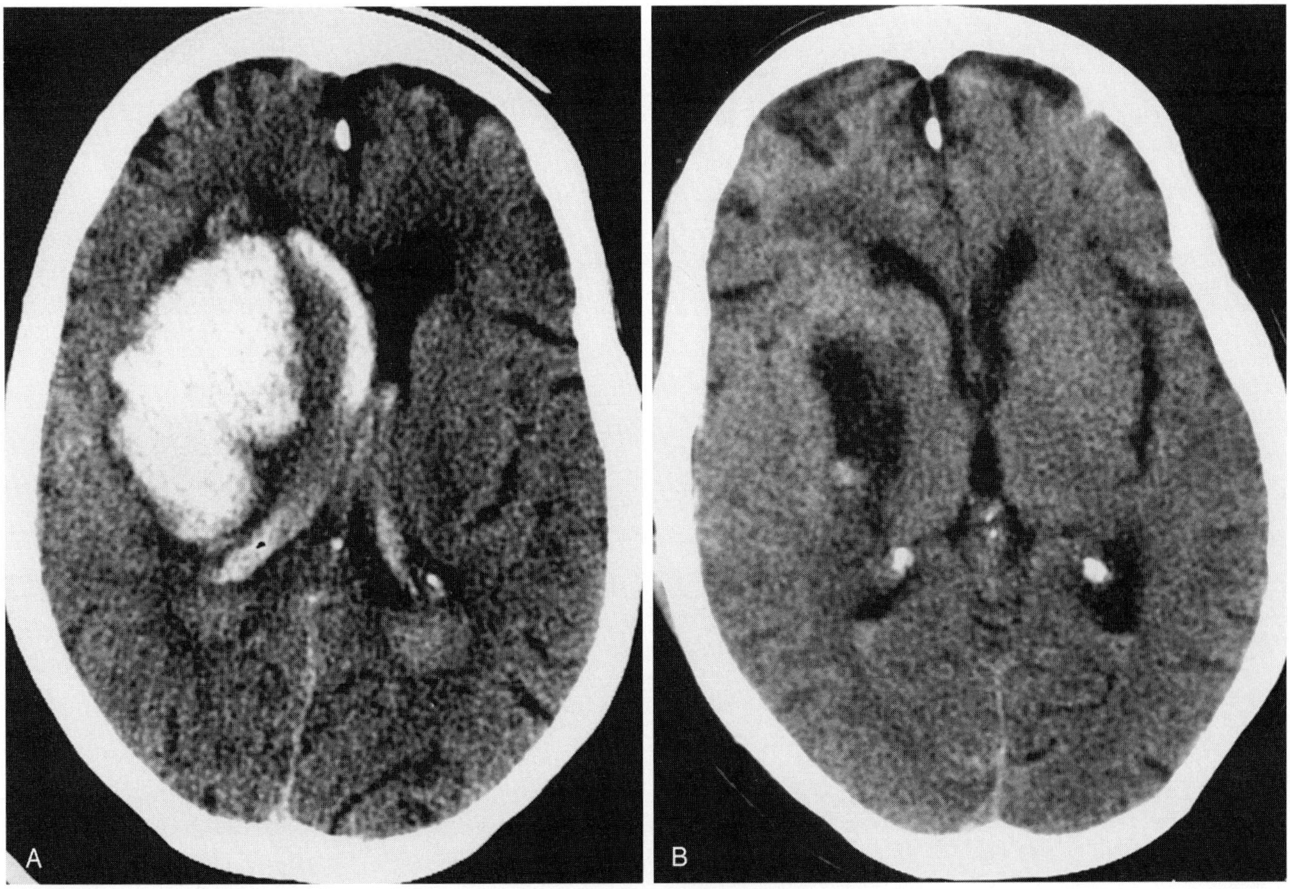

FIGURE 10–3 • *A,* Head computed tomography of a hypertensive patient with a large acute right putaminal hemorrhage. The patient was hemiplegic and became progressively obtunded with a dilating ipsilateral pupil. *B,* Postoperative scan 12 days after emergent evacuation of the clot. The patient recovered consciousness and had antigravity function on the left side.

all intracerebral bleeds, and because of the confined space of the posterior fossa, these are among the most dangerous. Cerebellar bleeds typically present with acute headache, nausea, dizziness, and balance difficulties. Findings on examination may include truncal and appendicular ataxia, nystagmus, ipsilateral gaze palsy, intention tremor, and scanning speech. With larger hematomas there may be signs of obstructive hydrocephalus, direct brain stem compression, or both.[15] There is often a history of hypertension in patients with deep nuclear cerebellar bleeds, but other etiologies are possible (Fig. 10–4).

Brain stem hemorrhages are distinctly uncommon, accounting for only 1%–5% of all intracerebral hemorrhages. Because of the compact and eloquent anatomy of the brain stem, even small bleeds may produce devastating neurologic deficits. The specific impairments depend entirely on the precise location of the hematoma and can vary from mild impairment of eye movements to irregular respiration, coma, or sudden death. The "locked-in" state (the patient is conscious but completely paralyzed, with the exception of eye movements) is one of the most feared outcomes of brain stem hemorrhage. Pontine hemorrhages classically occur in hypertensive patients (Fig. 10–5), but once again other etiologies are possible (see Fig. 10–9).

Intraventricular hemorrhages usually do not occur in isolation but rather in association with an

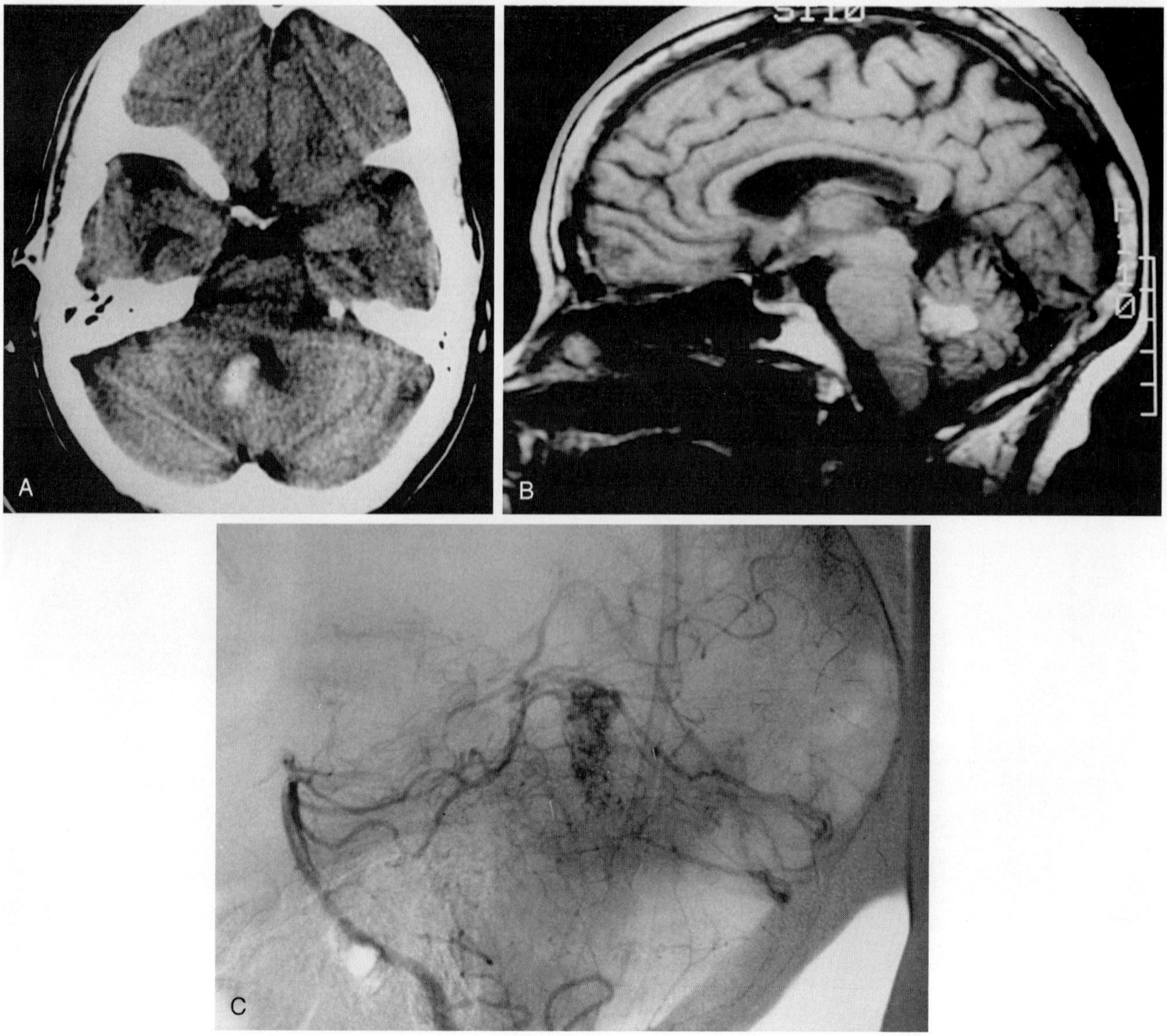

FIGURE 10–4 • *A,* Head computed tomography of an elderly nonhypertensive patient showing a deep cerebellar hematoma adjacent to the fourth ventricle. *B,* Sagittal T1-weighted magnetic resonance image of the same patient. *C,* Cerebral arteriogram (vertebral artery injection, lateral view) shows a cerebellar arteriovenous malformation.

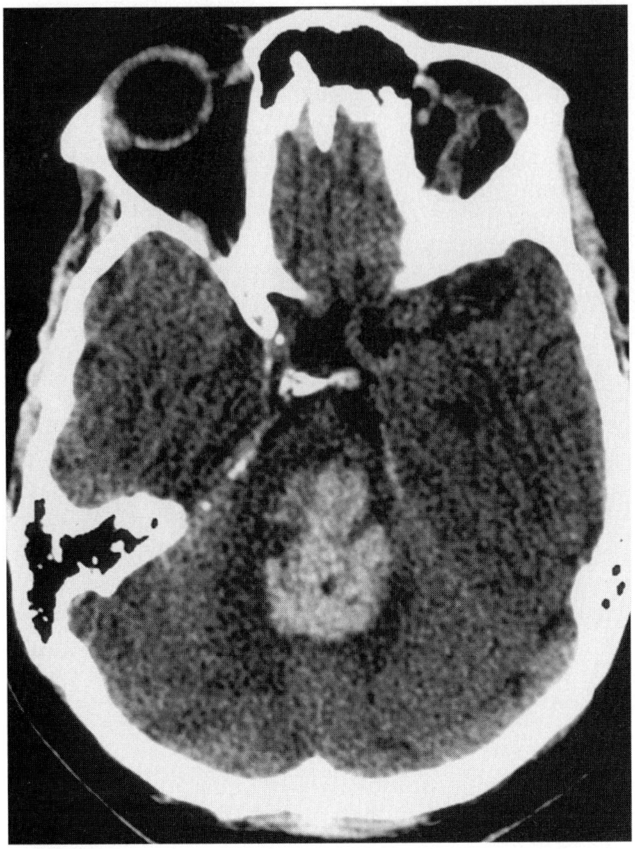

FIGURE 10–5 • Head computed tomography of an elderly hypertensive woman who presented in deep coma following this massive pontine and deep cerebellar hemorrhage.

adjacent intraparenchymal bleed. The most common such bleeds include hypertensive putaminal or thalamic hematomas. Purely intraventricular hemorrhages occur with certain AVMs, aneurysms, or intraventricular tumors (Fig. 10–6). Patients may present with a nonlocalizing headache or with acute hydrocephalus with dense impairment of level of consciousness.[16]

Spontaneous ICH may also be classified according to etiology. Table 10–1 lists one classification scheme according to the underlying etiology of the bleed. It is beyond the scope of this chapter to describe each of these entities in detail, and they have been reviewed elsewhere.[3, 17–19] The surgical management of aneurysmal SAH is discussed in some detail (see later).

Diagnostic Evaluation

The patient's clinical condition dictates the urgency of the diagnostic evaluation. As part of the patient's initial evaluation, routine preoperative laboratory studies are sent in an urgent fashion. These investigations should include a complete blood count, platelets, coagulation parameters, electrolytes, blood glucose, blood urea nitrogen (BUN) and creatinine, an electrocardiogram, chest radiograph, and urinalysis. In certain settings, blood, urine, or both should be screened for illicit drugs, particularly in search of cocaine or amphetamines. The index of suspicion should be highest for relatively young patients with no history of hypertension who present with apparently classic hypertensive-type bleeds. Cerebral aneurysms may also be provoked to rupture by these sympathomimetic agents.[20]

Head CT remains the initial imaging procedure of choice to evaluate ICH. This is the most reliable study to demonstrate acute hematoma, is widely available, and is faster than magnetic resonance imaging (MRI). In addition, no special arrangements need be made for performing CT on a patient who is intubated and on a ventilator, unlike the case with MRI. CT has more difficulty demonstrating a hematoma in the subacute or chronic phases because the fluid collection becomes isodense with brain. In the case of subarachnoid blood, the brain may merely look swollen in the subacute phase. With subacute subdural hematomas, the only telltale sign may be the mass effect of the isodense collection. Small parenchymal clots may be invisible to CT in the subacute stage. The chronic subdural hematoma is hypodense in relation to brain, and CT once again shows the collection well. In the subacute and chronic cases, MRI is much more sensitive than CT is. In addition, if an underlying lesion (e.g., tumor or AVM) is suspected, MRI with and without contrast material is the imaging modality of choice. There is a complex relationship between the age of the hematoma and its appearance on T1- and T2-weighted MR, based on the intracellular or extracellular location of the breakdown

TABLE 10–1 **ETIOLOGIES OF SPONTANEOUS INTRACRANIAL HEMORRHAGE**

Hypertension
Vascular lesions
- Cerebral aneurysm
- Arteriovenous malformation
- Cavernous malformation
- Venous angioma
- Capillary telangiectasia

Hemorrhagic transformation of ischemic infarction
Amyloid (congophilic) angiopathy
Neoplasia
- Primary tumor
- Metastasis
- Leukemia

Hemorrhagic disorders
- Constitutional (e.g., aplastic anemia, thrombocytopenic purpura, liver disease, hemophilia, hypofibrinogenemia)
- Medication

Drug abuse
Septic embolism, mycotic aneurysm
Other arteriopathies: Moya moya disease, dural venous sinus thrombosis, arterial dissection, inflammatory disease of cerebral arteries or veins

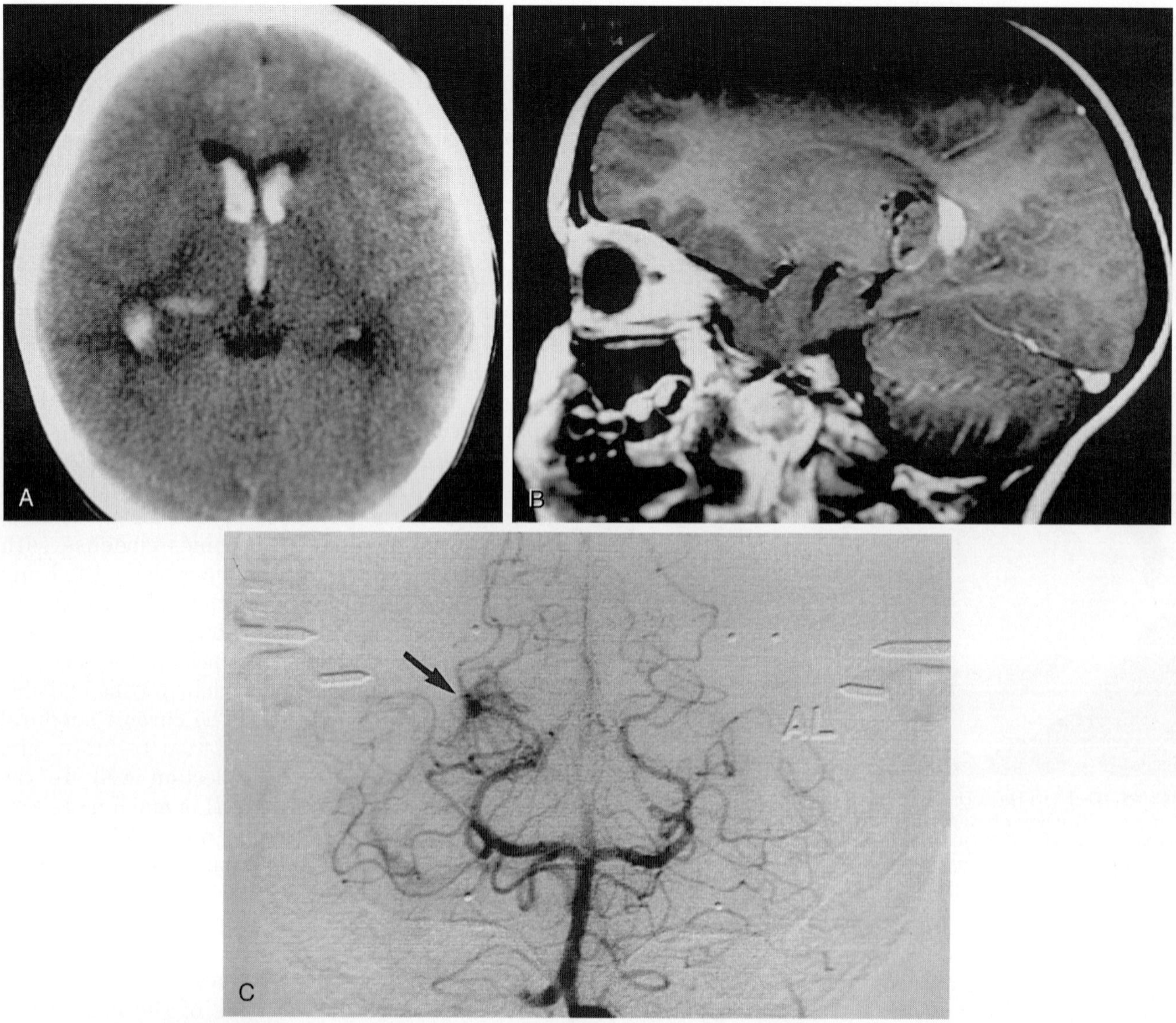

FIGURE 10–6 • *A,* Head computed tomography of a young boy showing an intraventricular hemorrhage (IVH). *B,* Sagittal T1-weighted magnetic resonance image showing the acute IVH along with associated flow-voids. *C,* Cerebral arteriogram (vertebral artery injection, anteroposterior view) demonstrates the small arteriovenous malformation (AVM) (arrow). The patient is in a stereotactic frame for radiosurgical treatment of the AVM nidus.

products of hemoglobin (deoxyhemoglobin, methemoglobin, hemosiderin).[21]

Magnetic resonance angiography (MRA) has developed substantially in recent years; in many centers it serves as a routine cerebrovascular screening examination. The flow-voids of an AVM are usually well demonstrated by MRI, but MRA may provide additional information regarding the size of the nidus, the feeding arteries, and the draining veins (Fig. 10–7). If time-of-flight methods are used, the presence of a hematoma may obscure the anatomic details of MRA. Cerebral aneurysms can also be demonstrated on high-resolution MRA, even small aneurysms in the 3 to 4 mm range (Fig. 10–8). However, for surgical planning in all cases of AVM and aneurysm, we still rely on the gold standard: high-resolution digital subtraction contrast angiography. An angiogram need not be obtained for an elderly hypertensive patient with a typical putaminal, thalamic, or cerebellar hemorrhage. However, younger patients with lobar hemorrhages, SAH, or parenchymal bleeds adjacent to the Sylvian fissure should undergo contrast angiography. In recent years, high-resolution infusion CT has been advocated for selected cases of presumed aneurysmal SAH in which the patient is in poor condition because of a large parenchymal clot.[22] This rapid study may provide enough anatomic information regarding the aneurysm to obviate the need for contrast angiography, and thus there is no significant delay in evacuating the hematoma and repairing the aneurysm.

of a ventriculostomy for treatment of acute hydrocephalus can often dramatically improve a patient's neurologic condition.

Once the diagnosis of aneurysmal SAH is established, the issue of timing of definitive surgical intervention becomes paramount. Despite the impressive recent advances in the technology of interventional neuroradiology, the only proven definitive treatment for a ruptured cerebral aneurysm at the present time remains a craniotomy for microsurgical clipping of the aneurysm neck. Balloon angioplasty for refractory, symptomatic vasospasm has rapidly become a crucial adjunctive intervention during the 2 to 3 week period following SAH. It is likely that interventional neuroradiologic techniques will play an increasingly important role in the overall management of these patients in the years ahead.

Chapter 9 discusses the perioperative management of patients with aneurysmal SAH. In this chapter we discuss the technical aspects of surgical intervention in these cases, including issues of timing of surgery, neuroanesthetic considerations, general neurosurgical guidelines and microinstrumentation, the role of various electrophysiologic monitoring techniques, specific operative approaches for each aneurysm location, and special problems posed by giant aneurysms.

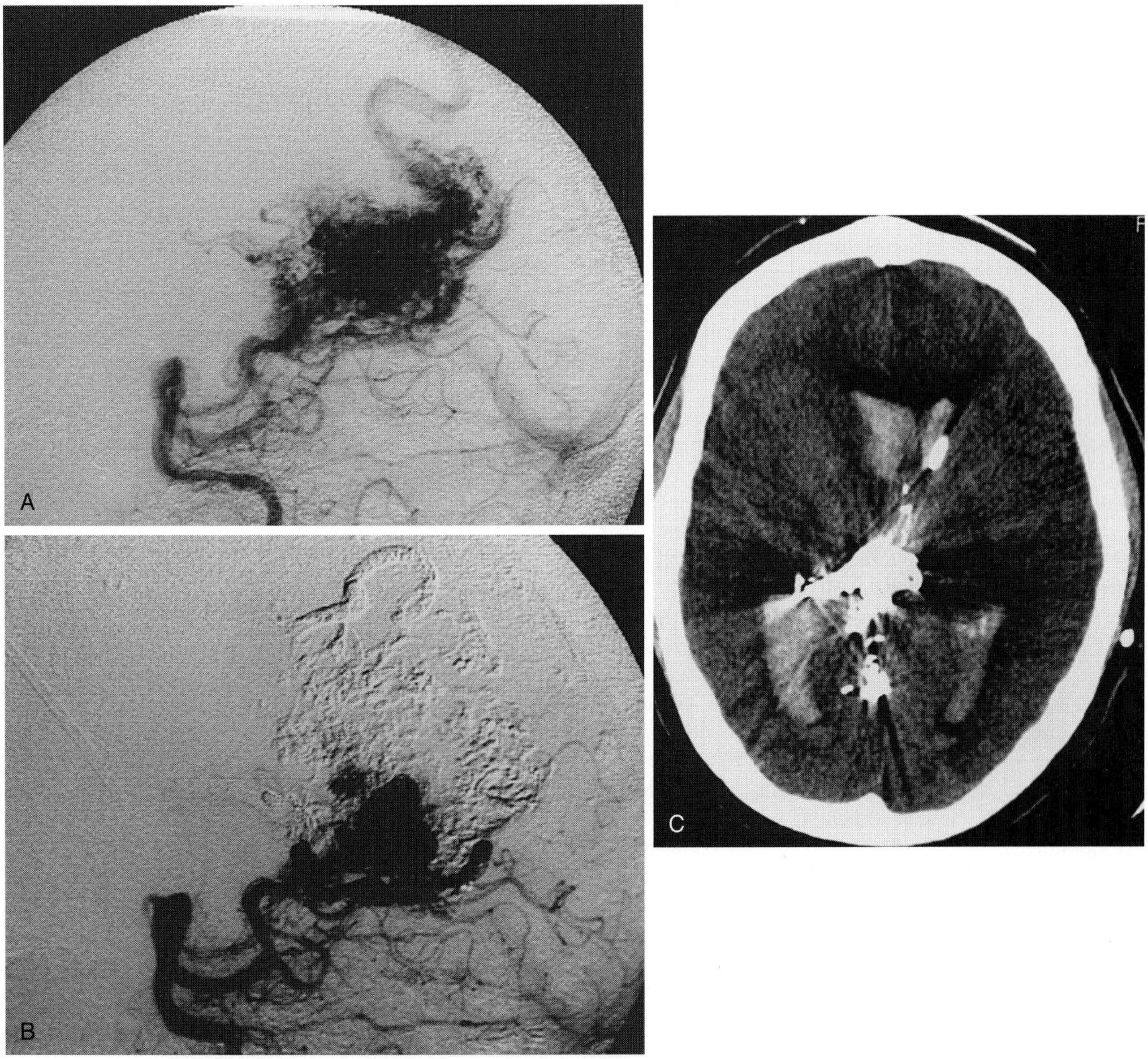

FIGURE 10–10 • *A,* Cerebral arteriogram (vertebral artery injection, lateral view) showing a large arteriovenous malformation (AVM) supplied by posterior and middle cerebral artery feeders. *B,* The same view following partial embolization of the AVM nidus, with loss of some superficial venous drainage. *C,* Postembolization head computed tomography showing a large acute hemorrhage from the residual nidus.

Timing of Aneurysm Surgery

The proper timing of surgical intervention for a ruptured cerebral aneurysm remains controversial. Until relatively recently, delayed surgery was the rule, usually 10–14 days following SAH, and sometimes later, depending on the patient's condition. Early surgery was thought to be associated with technical difficulties due to a swollen, recently injured brain. Retraction and dissection were more difficult, and thus adequate visualization of the aneurysm neck and surrounding vessels was compromised. Moreover, there was a serious concern that early surgery would exacerbate the delayed ischemic deficits due to vasospasm.[56] However, rebleeding is the most feared and often devastating complication of aneurysmal SAH and is common within the first 24–48 hours after the initial bleed.[57] Therefore, early surgery was not abandoned entirely. In addition, substantial improvements in neuroanesthesia and microsurgical technique have reduced the morbidity of early aneurysm surgery.

The International Cooperative Study on the Timing of Aneurysm Surgery examined these issues in detail in a series of 3521 patients treated at 68 neurosurgical centers.[9, 58] This study demonstrated that there was no significant difference in the surgical results between early (days 0–3) and late surgery (days 11–14). Good recovery rates were lowest and mortality was highest if surgery was performed in the 7 to 10 day period following SAH. The causes of morbidity and mortality were different in the early and late surgery groups: rebleeding was reduced in the early group, but surgical results were better in the patients who underwent surgery after day 10. Patients who were alert fared best if they underwent surgery early.

The results of this study changed the management strategy in many neurosurgical centers. Currently, most centers recommend early surgery for good-grade patients (usually Hunt-Hess grades 1 and 2, and sometimes grade 3). Despite the technical challenges of a "tight" brain and subarachnoid cisterns filled with clot, the surgical complication rate is acceptably low in experienced hands. In fact, the Cooperative Study showed that the intraoperative premature leak or rupture rate was not increased in the early surgery group. The major advantage of early surgery is the prompt elimination of the risk of recurrent hemorrhage. An additional benefit is the boost provided in the aggressive treatment of vasospasm. Once the aneurysm has been obliterated, the hypertensive portion of standard "triple H" therapy (hypervolemia, hypertension, hemodilution) can be pursued without concern regarding the risks of aneurysmal hemorrhage.

Moreover, by eliminating the recently ruptured aneurysm, the newer interventional neuroradiologic techniques of balloon angioplasty and intra-arterial papaverine infusion may be applied. Balloon angioplasty has been demonstrated to be a generally safe, effective, and durable technique for treatment of symptomatic vasospasm that has not responded to hypervolemic, hypertensive therapy.[59–64] In cases of distal spasm or in tortuous arteries that cannot be expanded by balloon, infusion of intra-arterial papaverine may be beneficial.[65–67] Our experience has been favorable with balloon angioplasty, less so with papaverine. Balloon angioplasty carries several important caveats: It should not be used in an arterial segment proximal to an unsecured aneurysm, in the immediate vicinity of an aneurysm clip, or in the arterial distribution of a recent major infarction (see also Chapters 9 and 11).

One additional theoretical advantage of early aneurysm repair is the possibility of prevention or amelioration of delayed vasospasm by early removal of clot from the subarachnoid cisterns.[68] Using conventional irrigation and suction alone, we generally do not remove a substantial clot burden. However, recent animal and clinical trials have demonstrated fairly impressive clearing of subarachnoid clot by the infusion of rt-PA,[69–75] with an accompanying reduction or elimination of subsequent vasospasm. The recent, relatively small randomized multicenter trial of intraoperative, intracisternal rt-PA for the prevention of vasospasm showed the treatment to be safe in terms of the risks of hemorrhagic complications, but there was no significant reduction in the severity of clinical vasospasm.[76] Subgroup analysis showed some encouraging trends, and therefore a larger randomized trial is planned.

The timing of surgery in poor-grade patients remains controversial.[77–79] Most centers do not intervene aggressively in grade 5 patients unless there is significant improvement, particularly with ventricular drainage. The rationale in some centers for aggressive, early surgical management in the grade 3 and 4 patients is based on the availability of the newer interventional neuroradiologic techniques (balloon angioplasty and intra-arterial papaverine infusion) discussed earlier.

In recent years, we have used an additional interventional neuroradiologic technique that may have an important effect on the management of poor-grade aneurysm patients. The development of flexible, thrombogenic coils of various sizes and configurations allows the early thrombosis of the aneurysm dome via the neuroradiologist's microcatheter. It has not yet been established whether these coils provide long-term protection against rebleeding, but our early experience and that of others[80] suggest that even partial obliteration of the thinnest portion of the aneurysm dome (including daughter lobes) provides some degree of protection. Subsequently, if the patient makes a reasonable neurologic recovery, either definitive clipping or further coil embolization may be considered. Some aneurysms may be curable through this technique, but the results to date leave room for improvement, even with the platinum electrothermocoagulation coils (Guglielmo detachable coils).[81] Interestingly, the broad-necked aneurysms that pose the greatest technical difficulty for the aneurysm surgeon also present a serious challenge for the interventionalist using coil embolization.

One group of critically ill patients deserves special comment with regard to timing of surgery. Certain aneurysms may rupture into the brain parenchyma directly and produce a sizable hematoma. Depending on the clot's location and size, the patient may present in extremis due to impending herniation. Perhaps the most common scenario for this urgent situation is the case of a middle cerebral artery (MCA) or posterior communicating artery (PComA) aneurysm that ruptures into the temporal lobe, with early uncal herniation and midbrain compression (Fig. 10–11). Depending on the rapidity of deterioration, three options can be considered: (1) In the most urgent case, the patient is taken directly from the CT scanner to the operating room, simultaneously receiving osmotic diuresis (mannitol) and perhaps barbiturates as well. The temporal lobe clot is urgently evacuated, either with or without immediate exploration of the internal carotid artery (ICA) and MCA for aneurysm repair.[82] (2) If the neurosurgeon determines by the clinical course that more time is available, a single-vessel carotid arteriogram may be obtained in order to delineate the anatomy of the lesion preoperatively. (3) Le Roux et al.[22] have recommended an intermediate approach with infusion CT that can be performed much more quickly than contrast angiography, adds little time to noncontrast CT, and often localizes the aneurysm accurately. Newer techniques of three-dimensional dynamic contrast CT angiography produce higher-resolution images of the aneurysm complex.[83–86]

Neuroanesthetic Considerations

The hallmarks of a good neuroanesthetic technique for intracranial aneurysm surgery are precise control of blood pressure and intravascular volume, adequate brain relaxation, deep anesthesia with neuromuscular blockade during intracranial microdissection, and rapid, smooth emergence to allow prompt postoperative neurologic evaluation. Preoperative mild sedation may be useful in alert patients to avoid the hypertension associated with

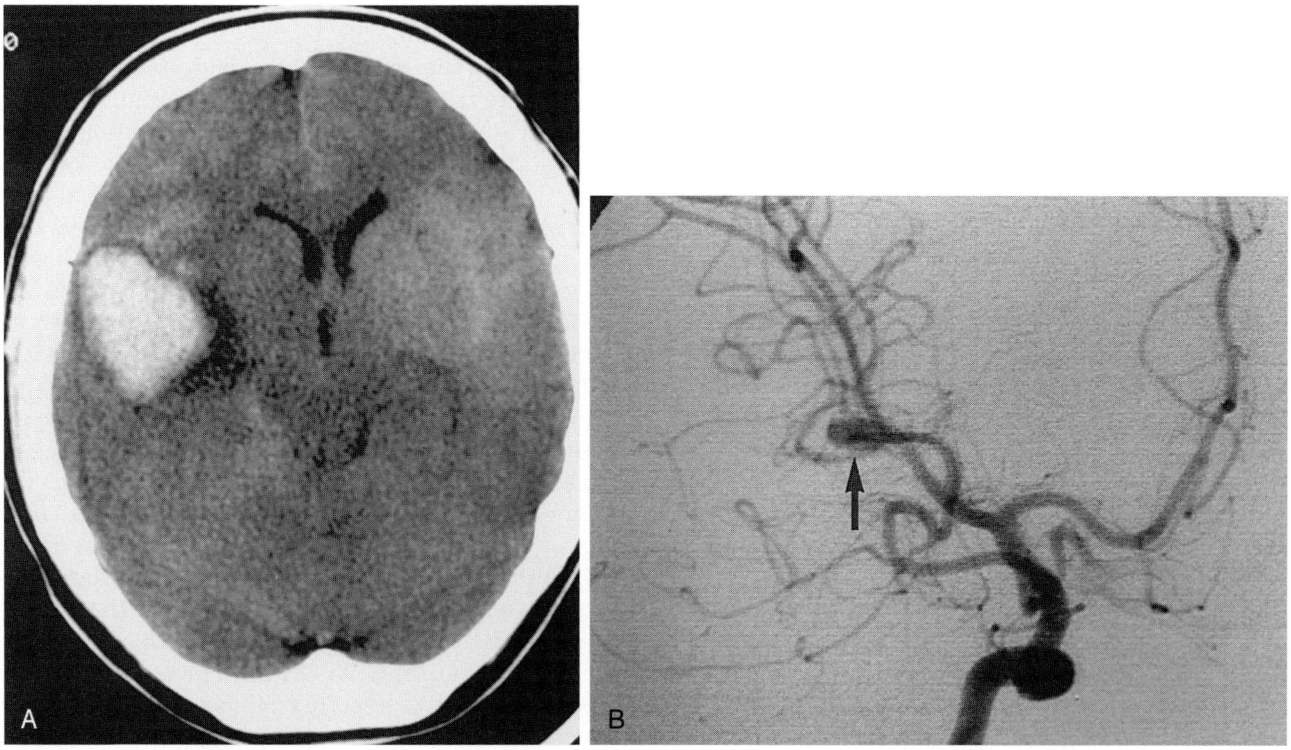

FIGURE 10–11 • *A,* Head computed tomography of a patient who presented with acute headache, left hemiparesis, and progressive obtundation. *B,* Cerebral arteriogram (internal carotid artery injection, anteroposterior view) shows a middle cerebral artery aneurysm (arrow) with displacement of vessels by the hematoma. The patient was stable enough for a single carotid injection and then was taken for immediate clot evacuation and aneurysm repair.

excessive anxiety. Heavy preoperative sedation is avoided so that constant neurologic evaluation is possible. Standard intraoperative monitoring includes electrocardiogram, esophageal stethoscope, temperature probe, pulse oximeter, noninvasive blood pressure cuff, and capnograph or mass spectrograph. A radial arterial catheter and large-bore intravenous lines are placed, usually including a central venous catheter. Patients with significant cardiac disease are often monitored with Swan-Ganz pulmonary artery catheters. Urinary bladder catheterization is required in all patients. Patients are usually already on an anticonvulsant such as phenytoin (Dilantin), and high therapeutic serum levels should be maintained during the perioperative period. Acute intravenous loading with phenytoin should be administered slowly (maximum of 50 mg/min) to avoid cardiac dysrhythmias, and interactions with nondepolarizing agents must be borne in mind. Many neurosurgeons (including us) use standard doses of glucocorticoids (e.g., 10 mg of dexamethasone or 250 mg of methylprednisolone every 6 hours) for these patients, although compelling clinical data supporting their usefulness in the management of SAH are not available.[87] The calcium channel antagonist nimodipine is now standard for all patients who have suffered an aneurysmal SAH,[88] and mild decreases in mean arterial pressure should be anticipated.

Prior to induction the patient is given an intravenous fluid bolus (5–10 mL/kg), which usually includes 5% albumin. Following preoxygenation, an induction dose of thiopental (4–7 mg/kg) is administered, followed by a nondepolarizing neuromuscular blocker (usually vecuronium, 0.1–0.2 mg/kg). Fentanyl (5–12 μg/kg) is added slowly during mask ventilation. Direct laryngoscopy is performed initially to check on depth of anesthesia and to apply topical lidocaine to the airway (1–1.5 mg/kg). Additional agents (e.g., induction agent, beta-blocker, narcotic) are administered if necessary, depending on the response to laryngoscopy. Once intubation is achieved and the endotracheal tube has been secured, anesthesia is maintained with nitrous oxide, low-dose isoflurane (0.2%–0.8%), and possibly a low-dose narcotic infusion (e.g., fentanyl, 2–3 μg/kg per hour). Arterial blood gases are monitored, with a goal $Paco_2$ of 28–30 torr (3.7–4 kPa). Mannitol (0.5–1 g/kg) and sometimes furosemide (10–20 mg) are administered during exposure for adequate brain relaxation.

The neurosurgeon may request a lumbar subarachnoid catheter for CSF drainage if a ventriculostomy tube is not in place, particularly for early aneurysm surgery when the brain is "full." In addition, for aneurysms that typically require significant amounts of brain retraction (e.g., basilar bifurcation, anterior communicating, and carotid bifurcation aneurysms), a lumbar CSF drain is often helpful even for the delayed or unruptured case. Some surgeons request drains for every aneurysm case. Following induction of anesthesia and intubation, the catheter is placed through a Tuohy needle, secured, and usually closed until dural opening. The patient is positioned so that there are no pressure points, particularly overlying the ulnar and common peroneal nerves, and with appropriate regard for brachial plexus traction in variants of prone and lateral positions. Excessive head turning, neck flexion, or neck extension is avoided in order to prevent compromise of venous drainage and cervical cord or root compression, particularly in the elderly patient with presumed cervical spondylosis. The eyes must always be carefully protected from compression or abrasion, usually with lubricant ointment and occlusive dressings. Sequential compression stockings are applied to the lower extremities for deep vein thrombosis prophylaxis. Local anesthetic is used in the scalp prior to placement of the head frame, along with additional general anesthetic as needed. Any hypertensive response to pin placement is promptly treated.

In recent years we have routinely used temporary occlusion of parent arteries for final aneurysm neck dissection and definitive clipping,[89] a technique introduced in 1960 by Pool and Housepian.[90] We use several putative cerebral protective measures that may help provide safe periods of temporary occlusion. First, the patient's core body temperature is lowered to the mild to moderate hypothermia range (32°–34° C), which requires passive cooling during exposure, followed by gradual, active rewarming after aneurysm repair. No randomized clinical trials support this approach in SAH patients, but we have been convinced by the wealth of animal studies[23–26] as well as extrapolation from nonrandomized and other related clinical studies[91, 92] that this intervention is protective. During emergence from anesthesia, the physiologic effects of hypothermia (peripheral vasoconstriction, shivering, increased oxygen consumption and CO_2 production, and increased risk of cardiac ischemia) must be anticipated. Our neuroanesthesiologists have become facile at managing this additional intervention, and few if any complications are encountered. The patients are usually warm enough for extubation at the completion of the procedure, generally with a goal core body temperature of 35°–37° C. The management of deeper degrees of hypothermia is considerably more complicated, and this approach is reserved for complex, giant aneurysms that require cardiac standstill (see later). We have not used intracerebral temperature monitoring as some have done in investigational settings,[93] but this may prove to be an important adjunct to optimize hypothermic management.

The ideal technique for safe, temporary arterial occlusion has not been determined. If technically feasible, we prefer to use several brief periods of temporary occlusion (up to approximately 15 minutes) with at least several minutes of intervening recirculation rather than one more prolonged occlusion period. Several animal studies[94, 95] support this approach, although it is certainly controversial.[96, 97] Intermittent reperfusion is not possible in certain situations (e.g., in giant, partially thrombosed aneurysms that require trapping, thrombectomy, and aneurysmorrhaphy). If the temporary occlusion period is anticipated to be prolonged (longer than 20–30 minutes), additional protective measures should be considered, including barbiturate boluses or infusion to achieve a burst-suppression electroencephalogram (EEG) pattern or even deep hypothermia with circulatory arrest. Deep hypothermic circulatory arrest for cerebral protection in cases in which prolonged temporary occlusion is anticipated (particularly giant vertebrobasilar aneurysms) has recently been revived in some centers,[98–100] but the safety of this technique has been questioned (for further discussion, see the section on giant aneurysms).

For temporary occlusion, we routinely ask the anesthesiologist to elevate the patient's blood pressure in order to enhance collateral circulation. We may also use a mannitol bolus for its putative rheologic properties[101, 102] and either a pentothal or a propofol bolus or infusion in order to reduce cerebral metabolic demand. We have preliminary data[103] that indicate that propofol infusion may significantly prolong the safe period of temporary occlusion as monitored by somatosensory evoked potentials (SSEPs). Other authors have advocated the use of etomidate for cerebral protection.[104–106]

Arterial blood pressure must be carefully controlled throughout the procedure. Painful stimuli such as laryngoscopy and intubation, head frame placement, and scalp incision must be anticipated. During the initial exposure, the mean arterial pressure is maintained within the patient's normal range. When the aneurysm is being dissected, mild hypotension in the range 90–110 mm Hg systolic is preferred, unless a temporary clip is to be placed. Intraoperative monitoring in the form of electroencephalography, SSEPs, and brain stem auditory evoked potentials may play an important role in determining the safe limits of temporary occlusion.[107, 108] Deep hypotension is now reserved for the rare cases in which proximal control is not possible (e.g., very low-lying basilar bifurcation aneurysms), or when uncontrollable bleeding from aneurysmal rupture is encountered.

Surgical Technique—General Considerations

The goals of surgical intervention for cerebral aneurysms include optimal exposure of the aneurysm and surrounding vital structures along with minimal trauma to the brain, cranial nerves, and vessels. Our general approach to most aneurysms has not changed dramatically in recent years. Interestingly, there are two recent trends in neurosurgical technique that are diametrically opposed: the concept of "minimally invasive" surgery, on the one hand, and so-called skull-base approaches. The least invasive technique for aneurysm surgery is the one that avoids craniotomy altogether—the endovascular techniques that currently are using flexible, thrombogenic microcoils for aneurysm obliteration.[81, 109, 110] The endoscopic techniques that are being popularized for intraventricular, pituitary, and spine surgery[111] have not yet found a routine application in aneurysm surgery, although flexible endoscopes may be useful as adjunctive tools for visualizing the "dark side" of complex aneurysms in the near future. The "key-hole" craniotomy has been advocated by various authors for certain aneurysms,[112, 113] but we have not yet been convinced that the temporary cosmetic advantages of a very small craniotomy hole outweigh the compromised operative exposure and working room. The various skull-base approaches, however, do enhance our ability to tackle more difficult aneurysms, particularly mid-basilar lesions, more safely by reducing the need for brain retraction while increasing vital working space.[114]

Patient positioning depends on the particular site of the aneurysm to be treated. Most patients are positioned horizontally with the head secured in a skeletal fixation headholder. We prefer the Sugita system with self-retaining retractors, but other acceptable systems are available. The head is generally elevated to some degree above the heart to enhance venous drainage, and the neck should not be rotated, flexed, or extended excessively. If possible, the head is positioned so that gravity assists in the exposure by allowing the brain to "fall away" from the skull base. In the pterional approach, for example, this translates into gentle neck extension, placing the zygoma uppermost to allow the ipsilateral frontal lobe to ease away from the anterior cranial base.

The importance of a meticulous pterional approach for most anterior circulation and many posterior circulation aneurysms cannot be overemphasized. The scalp incision begins at the level of the zygoma just anterior to the tragus and extends up over the superior temporal line behind the hairline toward the midline anteriorly. The incision is carried down to the temporalis fascia, and Raney or other hemostatic skin clips are placed. The temporalis fascia and muscle are incised in line with the incision and are elevated with the scalp flap using monopolar cautery in a subperiosteal fashion. The frontozygomatic junction must be well visualized for placement of the "key" burr hole. Additional burr holes may be placed in the low anterior temporal region and posteriorly just below the superior temporal line if necessary for dural separation from the inner table. The craniotomy must extend low anteromedially in order to provide an unobstructed view of the anterior cranial base, and the lateral sphenoid ridge should be removed aggressively with a rongeur and high-speed drill (we prefer the Midas Rex with an AM-8 or a B-1 cutting bur). A broad exposure along the frontotemporal base allows the operating microscope to be mobilized for a variety of views of the aneurysm complex. Once dural tenting sutures are placed and complete hemostasis is ensured, the dura is opened and firmly retracted anteriorly in order to allow full visualization along the anterior base. Generally, the lower the bony exposure anteriorly, the less brain retraction that is required. Indeed, some surgeons advocate the routine addition of orbitozygomatic osteotomy in order to reduce further the need for brain retraction. We have used this approach in selected cases rather than routinely.

The intradural exposure is started with gentle elevation of the frontal lobe using a handheld malleable retractor. Initially with headlight illumination and loupe magnification, the ipsilateral olfactory tract and optic nerve are visualized at the anterior clinoid process. Protective cottonoid patties are placed, and CSF is patiently aspirated from the basal cisterns in order to reduce brain tension and minimize retraction pressure. If a lumbar drain is in place, it is opened at the time of dural opening, and CSF is progressively withdrawn until the brain is slack enough to allow retraction without undue pressure on the brain. Temporal tip draining veins that are on tension are coagulated with the bipolar and divided. Self-retaining retractors are placed in a subfrontal and anterior medial temporal position, and the remainder of the dissection is performed under the operating microscope. If an aneurysm is suspected to be adherent to the temporal lobe (e.g., many posterior communicating and occasional anterior choroidal artery aneurysms), the temporal lobe retractor is not positioned until the ICA has been exposed for proximal control. This cautious approach avoids premature rupture of the aneurysm dome at a time when the important anatomy has not yet been visualized. The specific location of the aneurysm dictates the sequence of the microsurgical procedure from this point onward; this strategy will be detailed in each subsequent section.

Following aneurysm clipping, the clip blades are carefully inspected in order to confirm that the entire neck has been obliterated. Microendoscopes may be useful at this point to look at the deep side of the aneurysm complex, particularly for perforators or residual unclipped aneurysm neck. We then use a micro-Doppler probe to confirm patency of the parent vessel and any surrounding branches and to try to confirm lack of flow within the aneurysm sac. If we are confident that we can safely reposition the clip or add an additional clip, the dome is punctured. We have occasionally been misled by the micro-Doppler and may find persistent bleeding or refilling of the sac that requires clip adjustment or addition of another clip. If the dome is not punctured, the patient is committed to postoperative angiography. Intraoperative angiography is another option; the resolution of newer units has improved but still does not equal that obtained in the angiography suite.

Prior to closure, the vessels that have been manipulated are covered with a few small pledgets of Gelfoam soaked in papaverine. This relieves the mechanical spasm in the vessel walls. As hemostasis is being checked, we ask the anesthesiologist to rehydrate the patient with albumin and saline and to re-elevate the blood pressure into the high-normal range. The dense subarachnoid clot in the vicinity of the aneurysm is gently irrigated and aspirated away in cases of early aneurysm surgery in an attempt to reduce the severity of delayed vasospasm. We have already mentioned the recent reports of instillation of rt-PA into the subarachnoid cisterns following early aneurysm clipping in order to clear the cisterns of clot more effectively. At the time of this writing, the efficacy of this technique has not been clearly established, and therefore we do not yet use this adjunctive measure, pending further studies. As the self-retaining retractors are removed, the retracted surfaces of cortex are lined with either Surgicel or Oxycel cotton, and the subdural space is filled with antibiotic-containing saline. A water-tight dural closure is routinely obtained, and the remainder of the closure is standard.

Operative Approaches by Aneurysm Location

Anterior Circulation

INTERNAL CAROTID ARTERY

ICA aneurysms account for approximately one-third of all intracranial aneurysms, and they have been divided into anatomic segments in various ways. We have adopted one standard nomenclature that includes the following (from proximal to distal): petrous, cavernous, ophthalmic, paraclinoid, posterior communicating, anterior choroidal, and carotid bifurcation aneurysms. Other authors have further subdivided these categories (e.g., Kobayashi et al.[115]), and a new classification has recently been proposed.[116]

For *petrous* and *cavernous carotid aneurysms,* we do not generally recommend direct operative approaches, because there is virtually no risk of a life-threatening SAH. Cavernous ICA aneurysms have a benign natural history when compared with true subarachnoid aneurysms.[117, 118] When cavernous ICA aneurysms become symptomatic, usually in the form of a cavernous sinus syndrome with oculomotor palsies, with or without a carotid-cavernous fistula, then interventional neuroradiologic techniques are our first line of treatment. This intervention usually involves a 30-minute balloon test occlusion (BTO) of the ICA with close neurologic examination, followed immediately by permanent detachable balloon or, more recently, coil occlusion of the ICA. Various adjunctive measures have been proposed to augment the safety and predictive value of the BTO, including such procedures as controlled hypotension, EEG, single photon emission computed tomography or positron emission tomography, transcranial Doppler, ^{133}Xe cerebral blood flow studies, and stable xenon-enhanced CT cerebral blood flow studies.[119–123] If a patient cannot tolerate BTO of the ICA, an extracranial-intracranial bypass procedure is planned, followed by repeat BTO and then permanent ICA occlusion.[124] It is still debated whether the occasional delayed ischemic complication of acute carotid occlusion is primarily related to insufficient collateral flow (i.e., inadequate cerebrovascular reserve) or to embolic phenomena. We suspect that emboli are more often to blame, and therefore our patients are managed with 24–48 hours of low-dose intravenous heparin (500 units/hour) followed by aspirin. Other surgeons prefer to trap the involved segment of the ICA, reasoning that a surgical clip distally is more likely to prevent stump emboli. This controversy has not yet been resolved. Some cavernous and occasional petrous ICA aneurysms extend into the subarachnoid space, usually large and giant lesions. These aneurysms require an operative approach similar to that for ophthalmic-ICA aneurysms that may extend into the cavernous sinus. Thrombogenic coil occlusion of these aneurysms via the endovascular route is currently a leading therapeutic option. Common carotid artery occlusion is still a viable option for unclippable ICA aneurysms.[125]

Ophthalmic-ICA aneurysms (Fig. 10–12) arise from the medial or anteromedial wall of the ICA just distal to the origin of the ophthalmic artery (OA). These aneurysms are much more common in women (7:1), are frequently associated with other intracranial aneurysms (up to 50%), may be bilateral, and are often large or giant ($\geq$ 2.5 cm).[126, 127] They often present with SAH but may also cause visual compromise[128] and retro-orbital headache via local mass effect. Even in the largest aneurysms, exploration is virtually always worthwhile because the neck is usually much smaller than the dome, and direct clipping may then be possible. During the preoperative angiogram, multiple oblique views are often needed in order to visualize the aneurysm neck and its relationship to the OA. Either cross-

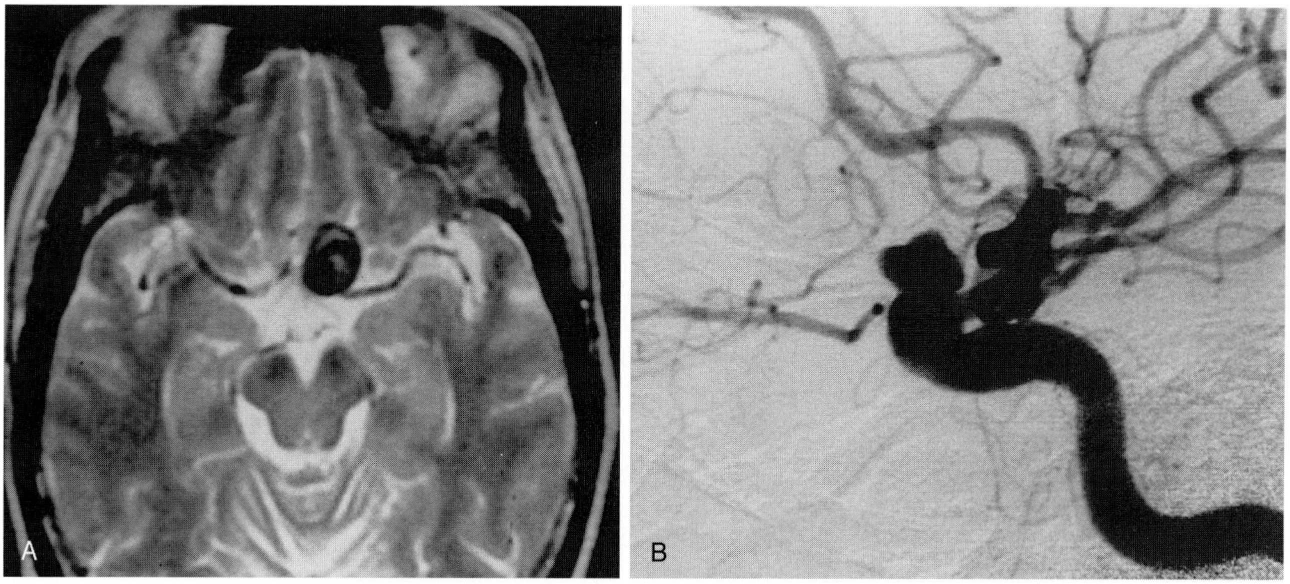

FIGURE 10–12 • Axial T2-weighted magnetic resonance image (*A*) and lateral internal carotid arteriogram (*B*) showing a large, partially thrombosed carotid-ophthalmic aneurysm.

compression or BTO should be considered in order to assess collateral circulation; temporary or occasionally permanent carotid occlusion may be necessary during the operation.

We generally begin the surgical procedure by exposing the cervical carotid artery in order to maintain proximal control. However, for small aneurysms we may only sterilely prepare and drape the patient's neck, anticipating that clipping of the aneurysm will be possible without the need for proximal control in the neck. The aneurysm is exposed through a standard pterional approach[129] with plans to drill the anterior clinoid process and adjacent skull base structures in order to visualize the proximal neck and OA. Many surgeons now prefer to drill the clinoid extradurally in the manner popularized by Dolenc.[130–132] We prefer to open the dura first so that we may inspect the ICA and the aneurysm directly while we drill. Occasionally, an ophthalmic-ICA aneurysm can be clipped directly without drilling the anterior clinoid process if the OA origin is quite distal on the ICA. The dura overlying the anterior clinoid and the optic nerve should be carefully palpated prior to coagulating it on low current. Often the optic nerve has no bony covering for several millimeters, and this area of dura should not be coagulated. The dura is incised in a semicircular fashion from the medial edge of the optic nerve laterally toward the entry of the third nerve into the cavernous sinus. This dural flap is reflected posteriorly to provide a protective covering over the ICA and the optic nerve during drilling. We prefer to drill the clinoid with a diamond burr under continuous saline irrigation to dissipate heat. It is important to thoroughly drill away the clinoid over the ICA as well as the optic canal roof and lateral wall; the remnants of the anterior clinoid process may be removed with a microcurette, a 1 mm Kerrison, or another fine rongeur. Often the cavernous sinus is entered during the drilling process, and venous bleeding is usually easily controlled with a few tiny wisps of Surgicel, Oxycel cotton, or Gelfoam and small pieces of bone wax. Rarely, excessive packing of the sinus results in injury of the oculomotor nerve within the cavernous sinus. Korosue and Heros[133] have pointed out that occasionally the anterior clinoid process is eroded by a "subclinoid" carotid aneurysm, and this variant, or a fully pneumatized clinoid (Fig. 10–13), should be recognized by inspection of the bone windows on preoperative head CT.

The carotid dural ring is then opened and the dural flap is resected in order to permit safe retraction of both the ICA and optic nerve. The OA origin and proximal ICA should be visualized in virtually all cases, and the proximal neck should be separated from the artery. In large aneurysms the optic nerve is often draped and distorted over the dome, which usually projects superiorly and medially. With the dura of the optic canal released, the nerve may be gently mobilized as needed to develop the aneurysm neck. For final neck dissection and clipping, we usually temporarily occlude the carotid artery in the neck except in cases of small aneurysms. If the dome is large and requires mobilization for optimal visualization of the neck, we do not hesitate to trap the aneurysm with temporary clips on the supraclinoid ICA and occasionally on the PComA if it is large. Either direct[134] or retrograde[135] suction decompression may be helpful in the largest aneurysms, and occasionally aneurysmorrhaphy is necessary (see discussion of giant aneurysms). We routinely use EEG and SSEPs for these cases in order to monitor the safety of ICA occlusion, aneurysm trapping, or both. The dome is usually punctured and decompressed following clip placement. The aneurysm clip may gently rest against the optic nerve without incurring a visual deficit.

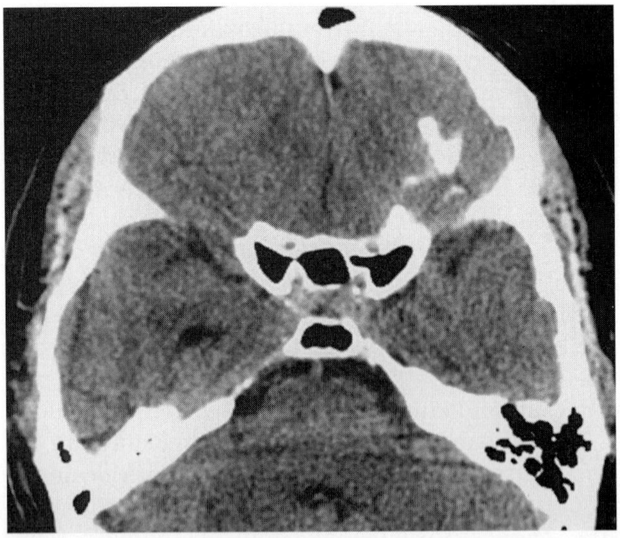

FIGURE 10–13 • Head computed tomography of a patient with a carotid-ophthalmic aneurysm. There is unusual pneumatization of the skull base, including the anterior clinoid process.

Paraclinoid-ICA aneurysms arise just distal to the ophthalmic-ICA aneurysms and proximal to the origin of the PComA (some authors include ophthalmic aneurysms in the paraclinoid group[127, 136]). These lesions often are related to the superior hypophyseal artery and project inferomedially,[137] and some are named for this small branch of the supraclinoid ICA.[126] Others project posteriorly and are associated with no obvious arterial branch site. These aneurysms have a much more variable projection from the ICA than ophthalmic aneurysms do and therefore warrant separate discussion. For many of these aneurysms, the surgeon must be prepared to drill the anterior clinoid process in order to visualize the proximal neck. It may still not be possible to gain proximal control of the ICA, and therefore consideration should be given to exposure of the carotid artery in the neck before beginning the intracranial exposure, as in ophthalmic cases. Particularly for large lesions with a broad neck, it is often safest to temporarily occlude the ICA or to trap the lesion for a few minutes at the time of final neck preparation and clipping. If trapping is elected, care should be exercised in distal clip placement to avoid injury to the anterior choroidal artery (AChA) and its branches and, if possible, to maintain collateral flow through the AChA. The permanent clip blades should be placed as close to parallel to the ICA as possible in order to avoid compromise of the lumen, particularly if there is atherosclerotic involvement of the ICA. For ventrally projecting aneurysms, an angled fenestrated aperture clip is usually best (Fig. 10–14). Prior to placement of the clip, the operating microscope should be moved both medially and laterally in order to identify and spare any perforating vessels arising from the ventral ICA and the PComA.

PComA aneurysms arise just distal to the origin of the PComA and project laterally, posteriorly, and inferiorly. These aneurysms constitute 25%–30% of all intracranial aneurysms and have a female/male ratio of 2:1.[138] Because of their proximity to the oculomotor (third cranial) nerve just prior to its entry into the cavernous sinus, these are the most common aneurysms to present with a cranial nerve palsy. A case of progressive third-nerve paresis involving pupillary dilatation with or without a retro-orbital headache generally should be evaluated as an emergency. This presentation signifies progressive expansion of a PComA aneurysm, often with a warning leak. Following head CT and angiography, we usually proceed directly to the operating room with these patients. Subarachnoid hemorrhage remains the most common presentation of these aneurysms, but occasionally an intraparenchymal clot in the temporal lobe is caused by a PComA aneurysm rupture. In rare cases the hemorrhage extends into the subdural space (Fig. 10–15).

For aneurysms that are not associated with third-nerve paresis, it must be assumed that the dome may be adherent to the medial surface of the temporal lobe. With that relationship in mind, we proceed cautiously during the pterional approach and initial exposure. We generally wait to position the temporal lobe retractor until the operating microscope has been brought in, and we do not search for deep temporal tip draining veins until the frontal retractor allows a view of the proximal ICA. The sylvian fissure is then opened, and dissection proceeds along the dorsomedial surface of the ICA to the level of the anterior choroidal artery. The distal aneurysm neck must be clearly seen distinct from the AChA origin, because compromise of this important small artery may result in devastating hemiparesis. Not infrequently, the AChA is duplicated or may have an early branch that must be separated from the distal neck of the aneurysm along the lateral aspect of the ICA.

We always search for the PComA origin and try to spare it as well, although because of its posterior cerebral artery (PCA) collateral supply, this is not

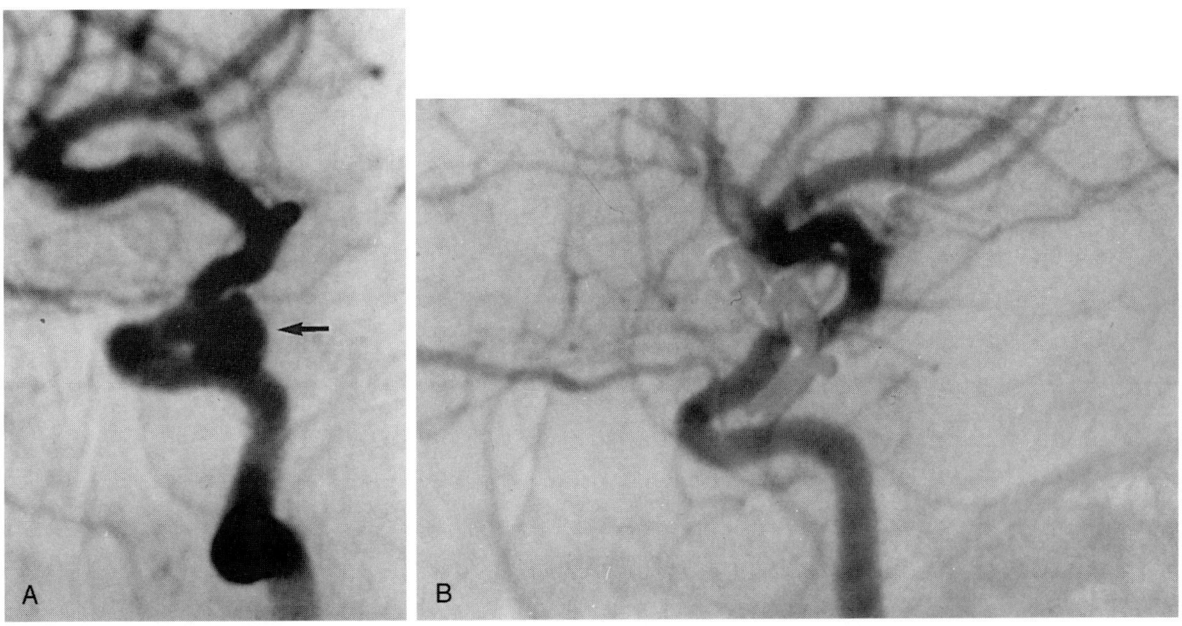

FIGURE 10–14 • *A,* Preoperative cerebral arteriogram (internal carotid artery injection, lateral view) showing a ventral paraclinoid carotid aneurysm (arrow). *B,* Postoperative arteriogram showing obliteration of the aneurysm with an angled fenestrated clip.

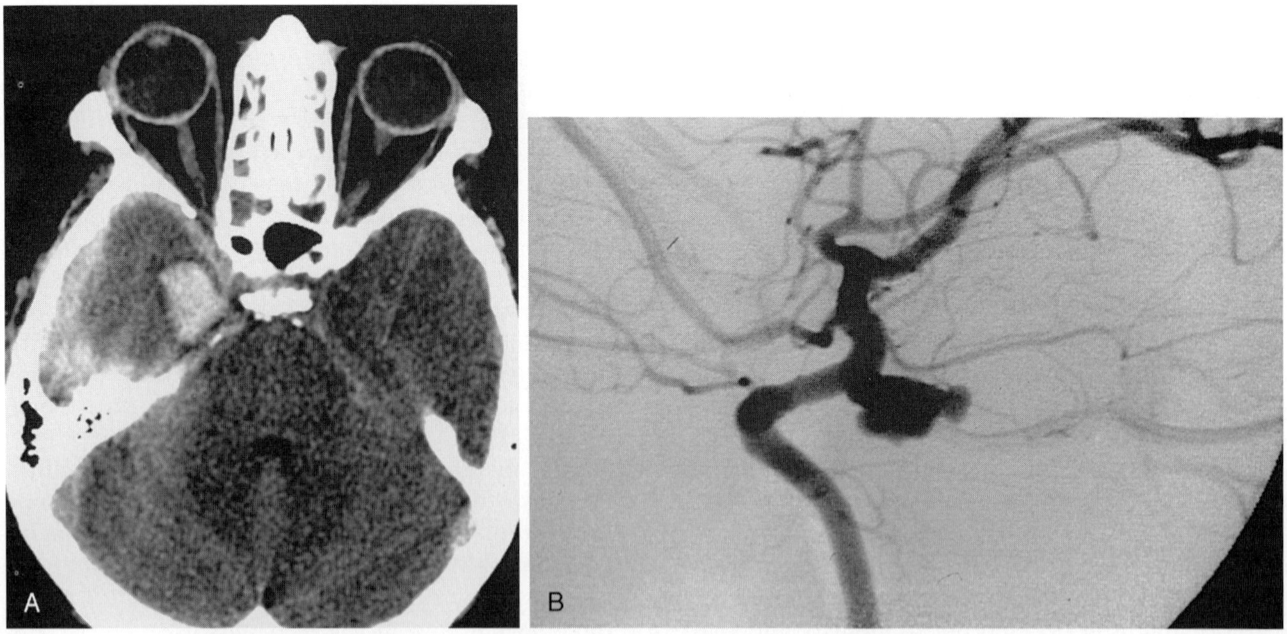

FIGURE 10–15 • Head computed tomography (*A*) and carotid arteriogram (*B*) of a patient with a ruptured posterior communicating artery aneurysm. There is intraparenchymal and subdural blood in addition to the subarachnoid hemorrhage.

as crucial as the AChA. The PComA may be difficult to visualize along the lateral aspect of the ICA, but often it can be seen by swinging the microscope medially and viewing between the optic nerve and the medial surface of the ICA. A myriad of perforating vessels usually arise proximally from the PComA, and these should not be disturbed if at all possible. It is not difficult to put these tiny vessels into spasm, which may produce deep ischemia in the thalamus or hypothalamus if there is inadequate collateral supply. Occasionally a PComA aneurysm originates very proximally from the ICA and may not be visible under the anterior clinoid process or the petroclinoid ligament. In these cases the anterior clinoid process is drilled as in cases of ophthalmic or paraclinoid aneurysms. Most PComA aneurysms are clipped from the lateral side of the ICA using either a straight or slightly curved clip with or without a bayoneted shaft. However, for very broad-necked aneurysms, thought should be given to the principle of placing the clip blades parallel to the ICA long axis by using a side-opening clip or even occasionally a fenestrated clip. In patients who present with third-nerve paresis, we always puncture the aneurysm dome after clip placement and evacuate the thrombus in order to decompress the third nerve. The vast majority of patients with third-nerve palsies recover within 6 months (some within a few days), although an occasional patient is left with mild persistent paresis.

Anterior choroidal artery aneurysms are much less common than PComA aneurysms (they constitute 1%–4% of all intracranial aneurysms),[138, 139] and they may be mistaken on angiography for their more proximal cousins (Fig. 10–16). Subarachnoid hemorrhage is the most common presentation; rarely, third-nerve paresis occurs. These aneurysms arise more superiorly than PComA aneurysms do and usually project posteriorly.[140] These may be treacherous lesions even when small because of their intimate relationship with, and often adherence to, the anterior choroidal artery (AChA) and its branches. AChA aneurysms are approached with the same considerations as for PComA aneurysms, including the caveat regarding possible adherence of the dome to the medial temporal cortex. The sylvian fissure requires more extensive opening for AChA aneurysms, because these lie surprisingly close to the carotid bifurcation. Excessively long clips should be avoided because of the risk of inadvertently occluding deep hidden perforators. Loss of the anterior choroidal artery often produces devastating flaccid hemiplegia.

ICA bifurcation aneurysms constitute approximately 5% of all intracranial aneurysms.[138] These aneurysms typically present with SAH, with no characteristic features that allow a specific diagnosis prior to angiography. Occasionally intraparenchymal hemorrhage occurs and can mimic basal ganglia hypertensive hemorrhages. Lying just inferior to the anterior perforated substance, most ICA bifurcation aneurysms are a direct continuation of the ICA, projecting upward and posteriorly (Fig. 10–17). These aneurysms require extensive opening of the sylvian fissure and deep retraction. The proximal anterior (A1) and middle (M1) cerebral artery segments must be identified, along with their crucial lenticulostriate vessels. These important perforating arteries arise at a variable distance from the actual carotid bifurcation and may bifurcate themselves early.[141] A distal bend in the ICA may project the aneurysm dome toward either the A1 or the M1 segment, and these aneurysms may appear on angiography to arise from the closer major branch. Careful inspection at surgery demonstrates the more common arrangement with the neck at

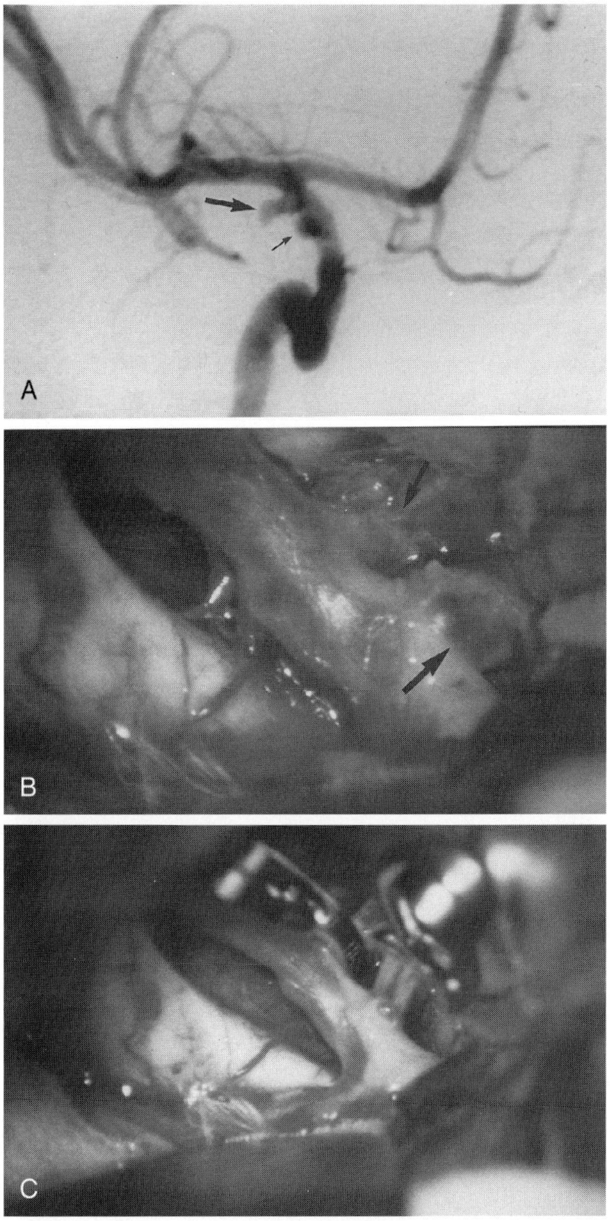

FIGURE 10–16 • *A,* Preoperative cerebral arteriogram (internal carotid artery injection, anteroposterior view) showing aneurysms of the posterior communicating artery (PComA) (small arrow) and anterior choroidal artery (AChA) (large arrow). *B,* Intraoperative photomicrograph showing both aneurysms (PComA aneurysm—small arrow; AChA aneurysm—large arrow). (See color plate.) *C,* Following clip obliteration of both aneurysms. (See color plate.)

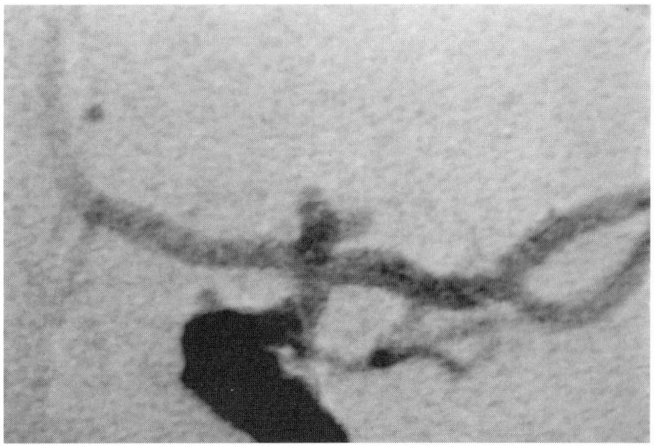

FIGURE 10–17 • Cerebral arteriogram (internal carotid artery injection, anteroposterior view) showing a bilobed internal carotid artery bifurcation aneurysm.

the ICA bifurcation itself.[142] If a large bifurcation aneurysm requires trapping before definitive clipping, the lenticulostriate arteries must not be injured by the temporary clips. If there is a broad neck, the clip may need to be placed slightly distal on the neck in order to avoid compromise of the A1 and M1 segments. If an excessively long clip is used, it may compromise the anterior choroidal artery or its branches that pass deep to the ICA bifurcation.

Anterior cerebral artery aneurysms may be divided into proximal (A1 segment) aneurysms, anterior communicating artery (AComA) aneurysms, and distal anterior cerebral artery or pericallosal artery aneurysms.

By far the most common in this group are the *AComA aneurysms,* which account for approximately 30%–35% of all cerebral aneurysms in most series. These aneurysms typically present with SAH, which has a characteristic appearance on CT with blood in the anterior interhemispheric fissure (Fig. 10–18). Blood is often in the ventricular system because of the intimate relationship with the lamina terminalis of the third ventricle. Patients who have bled are commonly confused with a characteristic amnestic and confabulatory syndrome, most likely due to direct injury to the septal nuclei of the hypothalamus or their connections.[143] The neuroradiologist performing angiography on these patients must be skillful and persistent in order to demonstrate the aneurysm neck and the highly variable anatomy in this region. Indeed, more anatomic variants are noted in the region of the AComA than in any other locus in the circle of Willis.[144] At times a submental vertex (base) view is helpful (Fig. 10–19) in addition to various oblique views. One important variant we have seen is that of the third, or accessory A2, segment arising from the AComA complex.[145] This vessel may be difficult to identify on angiography (except in retrospect), and inadver-

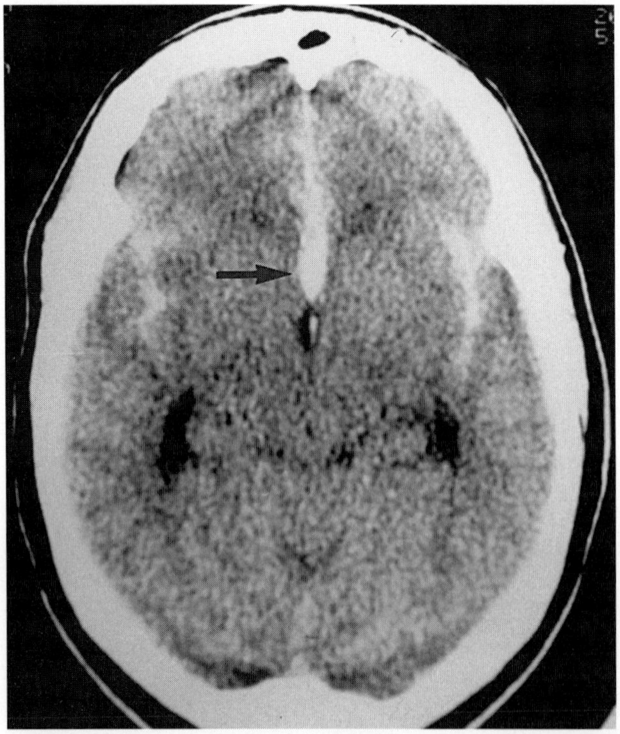

FIGURE 10–18 • Head computed tomography showing the typical pattern of subarachnoid hemorrhage following rupture of an anterior communicating artery aneurysm, with blood concentrated in the anterior interhemispheric fissure (arrow).

tent occlusion by the aneurysm clip can produce serious morbidity.

The majority of AComA aneurysms are associated with asymmetric A1 segments of the anterior cerebral artery, and not infrequently there is one atretic A1 (Fig. 10–20). Most surgeons choose to approach these aneurysms from the side of the dominant A1 segment for two reasons: (1) to establish early proximal control of the major feeder and (2) to approach the aneurysm from the side of the neck rather than toward the dome. Most domes project away from the dominant A1 segment and arise from the junction of the AComA and the A2 segment. In contrast, some surgeons choose to approach these aneurysms always from the right side in order to avoid retraction of the dominant frontal lobe and because a right-handed surgeon has more working room with the right hand from the right side. We tend to favor the first approach; if the A1 segments are balanced, we approach from the right side. If there is a sizable intraparenchymal frontal hematoma, it may be best to approach from that side in order to evacuate the hematoma on the way in and to avoid bifrontal injury. For smaller hematomas, we are guided by the dominant A1 segment and find that the hematoma can be evacuated from the contralateral side after clipping the aneurysm. Invariably the dome projects into the contralateral medial frontal lobe where the hematoma is found.

For early surgery on AComA aneurysms, most patients require either a ventricular catheter (if the ventricles are enlarged) or a lumbar subarachnoid drain to facilitate retraction. The standard pterional approach remains the most commonly used procedure for AComA aneurysms. The sylvian fissure is opened widely, and the interhemispheric fissure is also opened to allow more unrestricted elevation of the ipsilateral frontal lobe. The ipsilateral A1 segment is identified as it crosses the optic nerve, and it is prepared for temporary clipping if necessary. The recurrent artery of Heubner runs parallel to the A1 segment and originates from the distal A1, from the proximal A2, or from their junction with the AComA.[144] The other lenticulostriate arteries should not be disturbed. Many surgeons routinely resect a portion of the ipsilateral gyrus rectus during the approach to the AComA complex,[146, 147] but we do this only when necessary to avoid excessive retraction.

Ideally, the contralateral A1 segment is identified and prepared for temporary clipping so that there is true proximal control at that point. The neck is dissected next and is carefully separated from each A2 segment. Occasionally this requires sharp dissection because of tenacious adhesions. It is most important to work out the complex arterial anatomy in this region prior to clip placement. For final neck dissection, it is often helpful to occlude the two A1 segments temporarily so that the dome may be safely deflected to either side. If there is a premature rupture, there can be a surprising amount of bleeding despite temporary occlusion of both A1 segments alone. In this case, temporary clips may be needed on both A1 and A2 segments to completely trap the aneurysm for definitive repair. Ideal clip placement preserves the AComA and its important perforators.

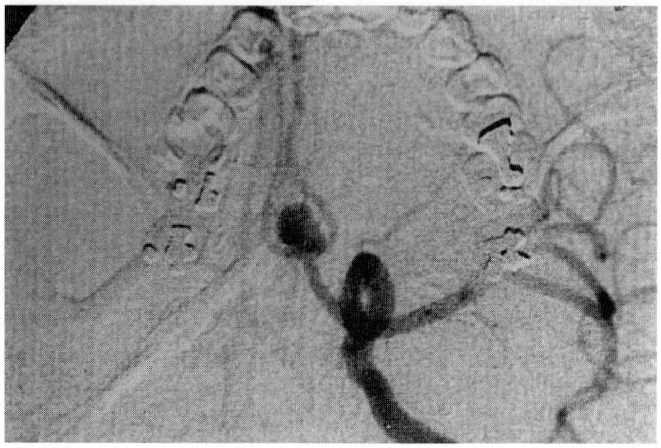

FIGURE 10–19 • Cerebral arteriogram (internal carotid artery injection, submental vertex view) showing an anterior communicating artery (AComA) aneurysm along with its relationship to the AComA artery and the A2 segments.

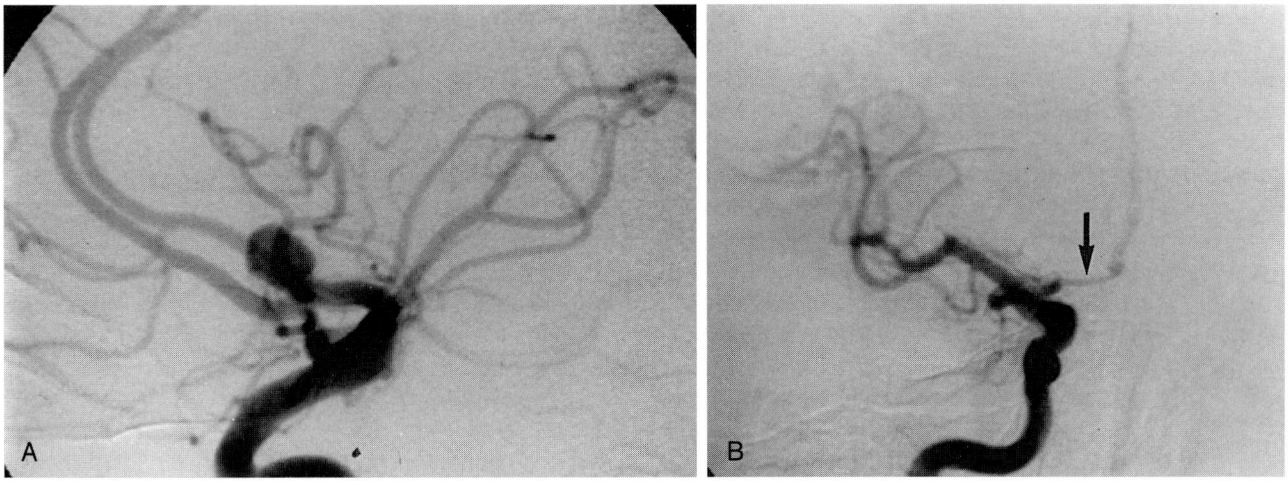

FIGURE 10-20 • *A,* Cerebral arteriogram (left internal carotid artery injection, lateral view) showing an anterior communicating artery (AComA) aneurysm and both A2 segments filling through a dominant left A1 segment. *B,* Right carotid injection showing an atretic right A1 segment (arrow), a typical asymmetric pattern associated with AComA aneurysms.

Occasionally the AComA must be sacrificed, but this may be tolerated if there are patent A1 segments bilaterally and if the perforators have been preserved. In aneurysms that project superiorly, the contralateral A2 segment usually is the most difficult to identify, particularly when large domes obstruct this view. The domes that project posteriorly endanger the perforators during dissection and clip placement. An inferiorly projecting dome may be adherent to the optic chiasm or even to the dura of the planum sphenoidale. In these cases the frontal lobe must be retracted with caution, because a premature rupture is a distinct possibility. In addition to clearing clot from the subarachnoid space following aneurysm repair, we often open the lamina terminalis in an attempt to enhance CSF circulation.

Several alternative approaches to AComA aneurysms have been advocated. The addition of orbital osteotomy to a standard pterional approach has been recently popularized.[114] We have used orbitozygomatic osteotomy on occasion, and we find that the angle of approach is modified to permit adequate exposure with somewhat less frontal lobe retraction. Some authors have demonstrated good results using a bifrontal anterior interhemispheric approach to AComA aneurysms.[148, 149] These surgeons argue that this approach minimizes brain retraction, and the olfactory tracts can be preserved. A modification of the pterional approach through the temporal fossa reduces the frontal lobe retraction needed, allows early proximal control, and protects the recurrent artery and perforators.[150] For most surgeons, the pterional approach is the most familiar, and a generous exposure along the anterior cranial base is important to allow adequate visualization of the relevant anatomy as well as sufficient working room.

Proximal anterior cerebral artery aneurysms of the A1 segment are decidedly uncommon and may pose challenging technical problems. The approach is the same as for AComA aneurysms, but the midline is not reached. These aneurysms may be challenging because of their intimate relationship with the medial lenticulostriate arteries that arise along the proximal A1 segment. Often there is a bend in the A1 segment or a particularly large perforating artery that arises adjacent to the aneurysm neck. The dissection of the neck often requires meticulous separation of these delicate perforators from the neck, dome, or both, and this may put these tiny vessels into spasm. Clip placement must be precise enough to spare all of these important end arteries in order to avoid a significant cognitive deficit postoperatively. The dome of these aneurysms may be adherent to the frontal cortex, and retraction must therefore be judicious with attention to proximal control.

Distal anterior cerebral artery or pericallosal aneurysms are also uncommon (2%–4.5% of all intracranial aneurysms),[127] and they pose unique technical challenges. These aneurysms present with SAH that characteristically includes a dense clot high in the anterior interhemispheric fissure. There may also be intraparenchymal hematoma which can produce a hemiparesis, lower extremity monoparesis, or even urinary incontinence and cognitive deficits if the clot is bifrontal. The aneurysm most often arises at the junction of the pericallosal and callosomarginal arteries (Fig. 10–21), not uncommonly in association with anatomic anomalies such as an azygous distal anterior cerebral artery.[144, 151]

The operative approach is interhemispheric through a relatively small parasagittal craniotomy centered just anterior to the coronal suture, usually

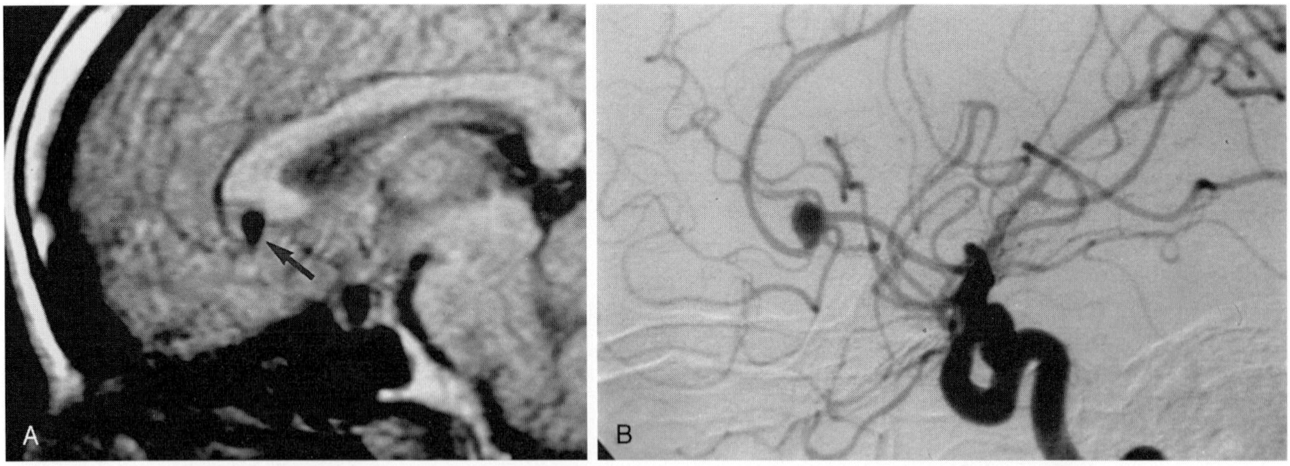

FIGURE 10–21 • *A,* Magnetic resonance image (sagittal plane) showing a distal anterior cerebral artery aneurysm (arrow) just inferior to the genu of the corpus callosum. *B,* Cerebral arteriogram (internal carotid artery injection, lateral view) showing the distal anterior cerebral artery aneurysm at a typical arterial bifurcation.

on the nondominant side with the medial limb on the midline.[152–154] If there is a sizable hematoma in the dominant frontal lobe, it may be prudent to approach from that side in order to avoid bifrontal injury. For the rare proximal pericallosal aneurysms that lie inferior to the genu of the corpus callosum, an approach through the basal interhemispheric fissure working superiorly may be best, and this allows early proximal control. Alternatively, a portion of the genu may be aspirated using an approach from above.[155, 156] The standard interhemispheric approach may require ventricular drainage through a catheter placed either preoperatively or at the time of surgery.

The venous anatomy should be examined on the preoperative angiogram, and it is generally possible to work between major veins draining into the superior sagittal sinus. It is usually considered safe to sacrifice one or two of these veins anterior to the coronal suture if necessary. The adhesions between the two frontal lobes are meticulously lysed, and gentle retraction is applied to the ipsilateral cingulate gyrus and, if needed, along the falx. A callosomarginal branch is usually found first and is traced proximally until the pericallosal arteries are identified overlying the corpus callosum. With close reference to the arteriogram, the pericallosal arteries are followed proximally until the aneurysm is identified. Proximal control has not yet been established, and therefore retractors must be placed with great care. The aneurysm dome is commonly imbedded in the frontal cortex and occasionally is adherent to the inferior edge of the falx. In order to gain proximal control and to dissect the proximal neck, it may be necessary to mobilize the aneurysm dome. The safest way to do this is by gentle aspiration of a small rim of surrounding cortex, leaving clot and scarred pia-arachnoid undisturbed on the dome. We have even cut the edge of the falx if necessary to avoid premature rupture when mobilizing the dome. The clip blades must be carefully inspected to be sure that there is no compromise of the pericallosal artery or its branches. We usually leave the ventricular drain in place postoperatively with external drainage as needed.

MCA aneurysms are among the most common intracranial aneurysms, constituting approximately 20% of all aneurysms[138, 157] (higher in some series[158]). Most (80%) occur at the MCA bifurcation, with smaller numbers along the M1 segment at a sharp bend in the artery, at the origin of the anterior temporal branch, or at the origin of a large lenticulostriate perforator (Fig. 10–22). Rarely, an aneurysm is found further distally in the MCA tree; often these aneurysms are mycotic. Patients with multiple intracranial aneurysms are highly likely to harbor at least one MCA aneurysm (Fig. 10–23).[158] MCA aneurysms most commonly present with SAH that characteristically produces a clot focally in the Sylvian fissure. Hemorrhage from MCA aneurysms is apparently less likely than from anterior communicating or ICA aneurysms.[159]

Ipsilateral headache and temporal lobe epilepsy are more often associated with MCA aneurysms than with other aneurysms. Focal ischemic symptoms are uncommon with any aneurysm, but MCA aneurysms are the most likely to result in these. These aneurysms also commonly produce an intraparenchymal hematoma in the temporal lobe, frontal lobe, or both (in up to 50% of ruptured cases); this often is associated with a focal cortical deficit (see Fig. 10–11).[158, 160] Occasionally a temporal lobe hematoma is large enough to produce acute uncal herniation with brain stem compression. These pa-

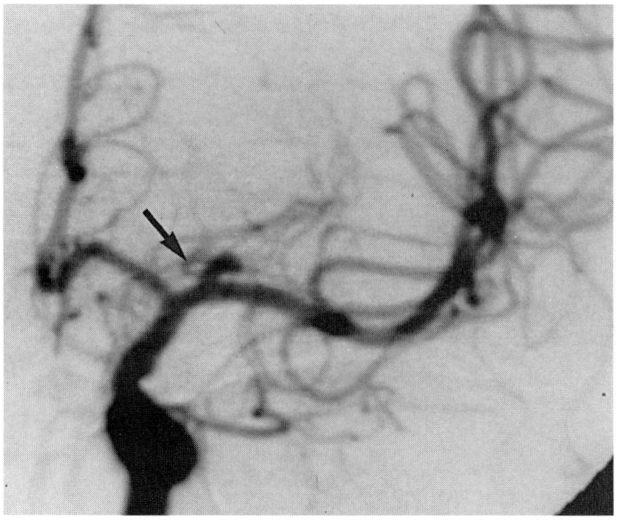

FIGURE 10-22 • Cerebral arteriogram (internal carotid artery injection, anteroposterior view) showing a small proximal M1 segment aneurysm arising at the origin of a large lenticulostriate branch (arrow).

tients may present in extremis and must be decompressed emergently in order to survive. The patient is given mannitol during emergency head CT. Infusion CT may show the aneurysm quickly and directs the exploration without the need for a time-consuming angiogram.[22] More recently, some authors have advocated the use of a three-dimensional computed tomographic angiography using dynamic scanning with spiral CT in order to obtain a "poor-man's angiogram" as the operating room is being prepared.[83–86] Emergent clot evacuation is followed immediately by microsurgical exploration of the MCA bifurcation for definitive repair of the aneurysm. Delaying aneurysm repair leads to a higher incidence of poor outcome, probably due to rebleeding.[161] Four-vessel angiography is performed postoperatively to confirm complete obliteration of the aneurysm and to search for other aneurysms.

In the more "elective" presentation, angiography is performed preoperatively with multiple oblique views in order to work out the complex and variable arterial anatomy of the MCA bifurcation region (trifurcation is not uncommon).[162] The operative approach is via frontotemporal craniotomy, which extends slightly more posteriorly in the temporal region than a standard pterional approach does. The patient's head is not rotated as much (approximately 30–45 degrees) in order to allow a balanced view through the sylvian fissure. We usually begin the microdissection by opening the fissure distally and identifying major distal MCA branches.[159] If the M1 segment is short, or if the aneurysm arises from the M1 segment itself, proximal control may be obtained by visualizing the ICA at the anterior clinoid process and opening the fissure medially. As the frontal and temporal retractors are adjusted, the aneurysm dome is usually seen bulging into the fissure, adherent to one bank of cortex. Proximal control is obtained at this point, usually the M1 segment deep to the aneurysm. Separation of the frontal and temporal lobes may require coagulation and division of bridging veins, but all arterial branches must be preserved. Dissection along the M1 segment is safest on its anterior inferior surface to avoid manipulation of the delicate lenticulostriate vessels. A site should be prepared for temporary clip placement on the M1 segment, preferably distal to the lenticulostriate arteries. Often three self-retaining retractors are useful at this point, particularly the tapered variety. The aneurysm must be circumferentially dissected in order to identify and

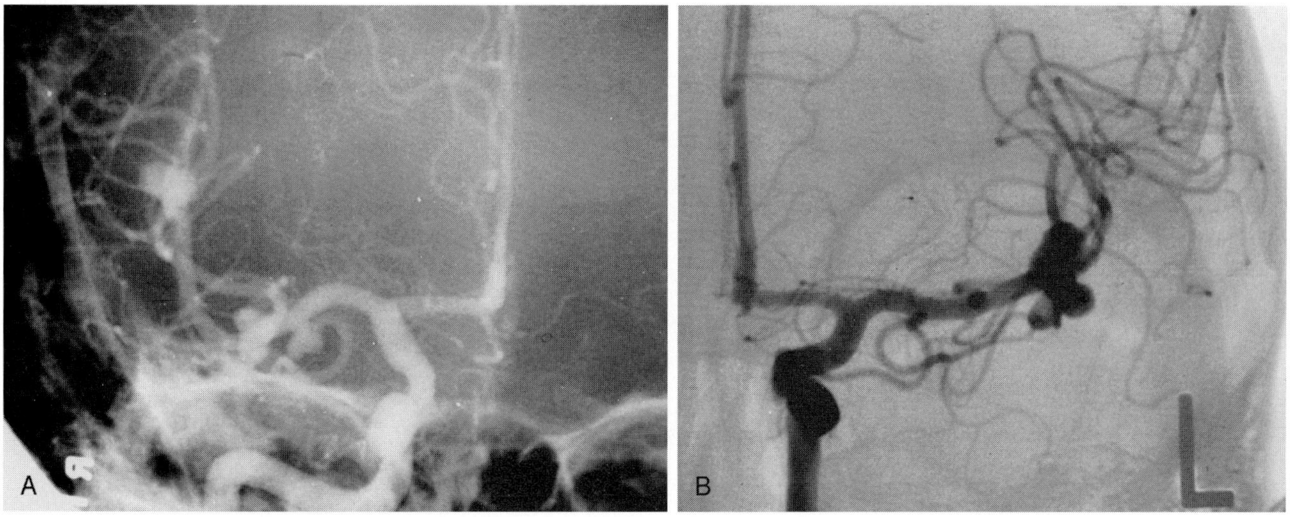

FIGURE 10-23 • Right (*A*) and left (*B*) internal carotid artery injections (anteroposterior views) showing multiple middle cerebral artery aneurysms on each side. A total of seven aneurysms were clipped in two sessions.

separate all MCA branches from the dome. These branches may be strongly adherent, and sharp dissection is frequently necessary. Temporary clipping of the M1, and occasionally both M2 segments, may be helpful in completing the dissection prior to permanent clip placement.

For broad-necked aneurysms, particularly those associated with atherosclerotic changes in the major branches, clip selection and placement must avoid compromise or kinking of the major arterial branches. This usually requires that the clip blades be placed as close to parallel to the M1 segment as possible. Multiple clips may be needed, often including the fenestrated design, to preserve the branches and to occlude the neck optimally. EEG and SSEP monitoring may be useful during the temporary occlusions and in evaluating flow following permanent clipping of the neck. If necessary, we do not hesitate to resect a small amount of cortex in order to provide full exposure of the aneurysm neck and all of the arterial branches. However, we do not favor the superior temporal gyrus approach[163] unless there is a temporal lobe hematoma.

The overall management outcome of patients with MCA aneurysms appears to be unfavorable when compared with the outcomes of other anterior circulation aneurysms. Epilepsy, severe hemiparesis, and visual field deficits are the most common neurologic disabilities seen in survivors of these aneurysms.[158]

Posterior Circulation

Aneurysms of the posterior circulation (i.e., the vertebrobasilar system) constitute 5%–15% of most series but usually account for a higher percentage of aneurysms seen in a cerebrovascular referral center (up to 35% of our practice). We divide these aneurysms anatomically by level of the vertebrobasilar system in a fairly traditional classification scheme: basilar apex (also called the basilar tip, caput, or bifurcation), PCA, superior cerebellar artery (SCA), midbasilar or basilar trunk (including the anterior inferior cerebellar artery—AICA), vertebrobasilar junction (VBJ), and vertebral artery–posterior inferior cerebellar artery (PICA) aneurysms. Because the surgical approaches are virtually the same, we will consider the basilar tip, PCA, and SCA aneurysms together.

Basilar bifurcation, posterior cerebral, and SCA aneurysms together constitute the most common group of posterior circulation aneurysms. Of these, the basilar bifurcation aneurysms are by far the most common, accounting for about one-third to one-half of all posterior circulation aneurysms and 5%–8% of all intracranial aneurysms.[164] These aneurysms usually present with SAH, with blood concentrated in the interpeduncular cistern (Fig. 10–24). Basilar tip aneurysms may rupture directly upward through the floor of the third ventricle, and thus the majority of blood may be intraventricular

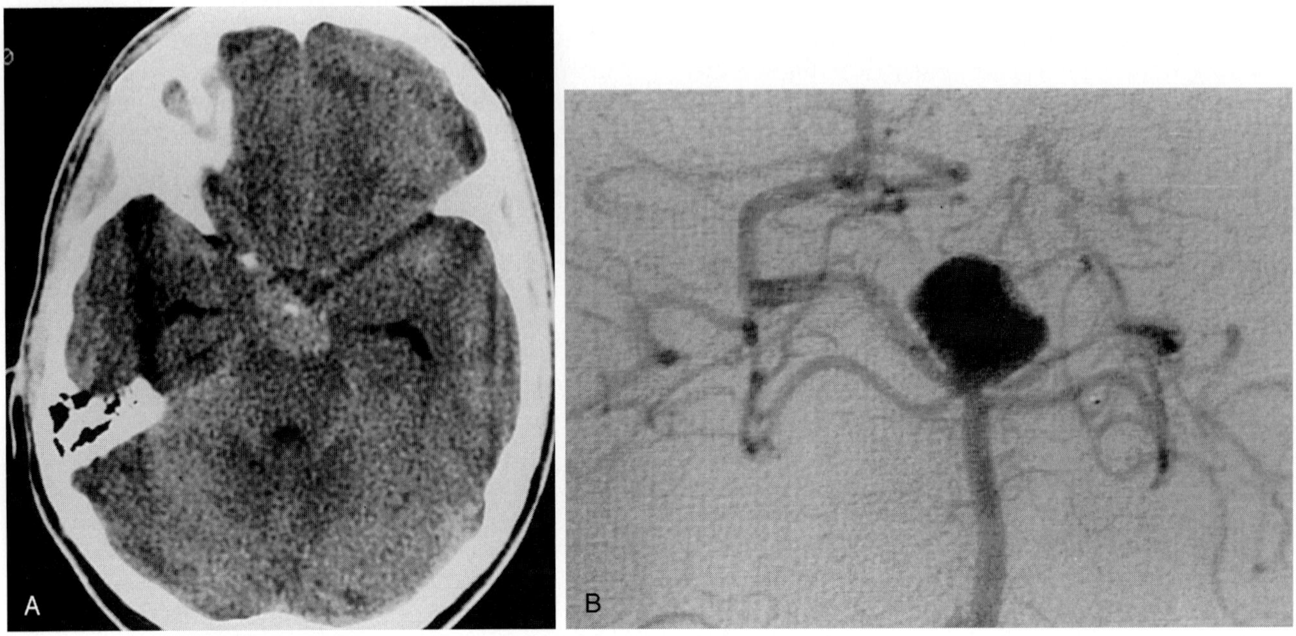

FIGURE 10–24 • *A,* Head computed tomography of a patient following an acute subarachnoid hemorrhage showing blood concentrated in the interpeduncular cistern, a pattern typical of a ruptured basilar tip aneurysm. *B,* Cerebral arteriogram (vertebral artery injection, anteroposterior view) showing the large basilar tip aneurysm.

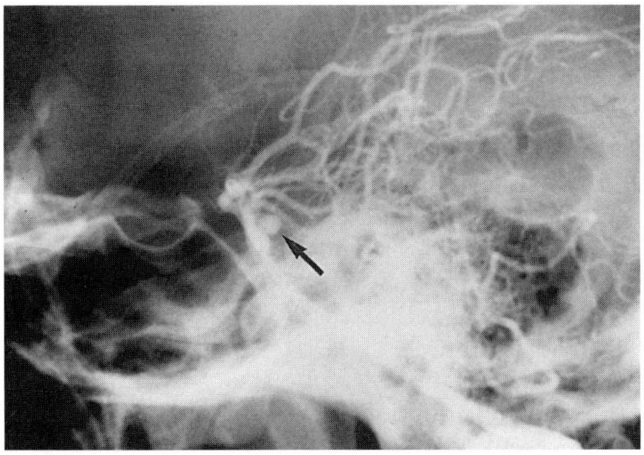

FIGURE 10–25 • Cerebral arteriogram (vertebral artery injection, lateral view) showing a small basilar apex aneurysm (arrow) that originates low relative to the posterior clinoid processes and projects posteriorly. This aneurysm may be approached either subtemporally or, as in this case, through a pterional/trans-sylvian approach with drilling of the ipsilateral posterior clinoid process.

but almost invariably with some subarachnoid component. Early obstructive hydrocephalus is common, and the timely placement of a ventriculostomy may be life-saving. Patients are commonly confused if awake following SAH from a basilar tip aneurysm, and oculomotor and pupillary disturbances are common.[165–168] Occasionally, large or giant basilar tip aneurysms present with oculomotor palsy, contralateral hemiparesis, or both (Weber's syndrome) due to local mass effect.[169, 170] The larger aneurysms are often seen on CT, and MRI may be helpful in identifying thrombus within an aneurysm dome, which appears much smaller on angiography. A complete four-vessel study is mandatory, with attention to oblique views that define the aneurysm neck. The larger aneurysms may have a broad base that extends downward so that the PCAs originate from an aneurysmally dilated top of the basilar artery. Large perforating arteries can often be visualized on high-resolution angiography, but their usual sites of origin from the distal basilar artery and proximal P1 segments may not be identified. On the lateral unsubtracted view it is important to carefully examine the relationship between the aneurysm and the dorsum sellae. For aneurysms that originate below the level of the posterior clinoid processes, either a subtemporal approach should be used or the surgeon should plan to drill the ipsilateral posterior clinoid during the pterional/trans-sylvian approach for exposure of the neck and distal basilar artery (Fig. 10–25). The carotid artery injections should be inspected carefully for the presence of additional aneurysms, which may influence the choice of approach. The posterior communicating arteries should be examined as well, in that a fetal type PCA may require preservation of the communicating segment.

Ruptured basilar tip aneurysms should be treated aggressively: Their natural history is devastating. In Peerless and Drake's series of 26 patients with posterior circulation aneurysms followed nonoperatively, all of these patients died because of recurrent hemorrhage within 3 years.[171] Decisions regarding the timing of surgery are similar to cases of anterior circulation aneurysms (i.e., if the patient is awake, generally a "good" grade 3 or better, early surgery is planned). A lumbar drain is used in all cases, unless ventriculostomy has already been performed. Intraoperative electrophysiologic monitoring has been useful in most cases. We generally plan a *pterional/trans-sylvian approach*[172] from the right side, but we extend the bone flap inferiorly and posteriorly to the temporal fossa floor to reserve the option of switching to a *subtemporal approach* if necessary.[170] The Sylvian fissure is opened widely, and the ICA is exposed to the level of its bifurcation. The arachnoid surrounding the optic nerve is also opened widely so that the space between the nerve and the ICA may be used for some of the dissection. Some surgeons advocate routinely drilling the *anterior* clinoid process and opening the optic canal so that the optic nerve may be safely mobilized, thus enhancing the working space between the nerve and ICA. A second potential working space is between the A1 and M1 segments just below the optic tract. We usually find the best working space between the ICA and the oculomotor nerve. This route may be enlarged by retracting the temporal lobe laterally and occasionally dividing the tentorium between the third and fourth nerves.[170, 172] In addition, we often place a self-retaining tapered retractor gently on the lateral wall of the ICA to retract it medially. SSEP changes are occasionally noted with the placement of this retractor, thus notifying the surgeon that ICA territory perfusion has been impaired and that the retractor must be adjusted. The arachnoid surrounding the oculomotor nerve is widely dissected, which allows the nerve to be manipulated, often with no postoperative third-nerve palsy.

In low-lying basilar aneurysms, proximal control of the basilar artery may be obtained by working between the third nerve and the tentorial edge; the tentorium is either retracted with a suture or divided. The membrane of Liliequist, which is often thick and adherent to clot, is opened widely to enter the interpeduncular cistern. The PComA is followed back to its junction with the PCA. Some authors[157] routinely sacrifice a small PComA distal to its perforators if it interferes with access to the basilar tip, but we usually preserve it unless it poses a major impediment. The PCA is then followed proximally to the top of the basilar artery (BA), initially avoiding the region of the aneurysm neck. The top of the BA should be followed proximally until the SCA is visualized; this exposure may require drilling of the posterior clinoid process in order to gain proximal control. Additional working space may be found lateral and inferior to the third nerve, similar to the subtemporal approach. Some authors call this view the "half-and-half" modified pterional (anterior temporal) or temporopolar approach.[157, 170, 173–175] Partial sectioning or suturing of the tentorial edge may enhance this more lateral window. The contralateral SCA can be found by looking across the anterior aspect of the BA. A site on the BA just proximal or distal to the SCA origins should be prepared for later temporary clip placement, avoiding any perforators that may arise from this segment. The dissection across the top of the BA should then allow visualization of the contralateral P1 segment. Usually the reach across the midline is performed anterior to the aneurysm neck, except in the unusual case of an anteriorly projecting basilar tip aneurysm, which may be adherent to the clivus.

Once these landmarks have been identified, the aneurysm neck itself may be dissected. Often there are arachnoid adhesions between the neck and the P1 segments, and the perforating arteries must be preserved during this dissection. The most difficult step is usually the dissection behind the aneurysm neck where the plane with the ventral aspect of the brain stem must be established. Perforators must be gently mobilized away from the neck during this step, and the contralateral P1 segment is usually seen to confirm that the entire neck has been visualized. The final steps in neck dissection often require mobilization of the aneurysm itself, which is safest if a temporary clip is placed on the BA. We attach a fine suture (4-0 braided nylon) to the handle of this temporary clip, which serves as a "leash" for retrieval with the clip remover when the clip occasionally disappears behind the clivus. Selection of a permanent clip and clip applier depends on the specific anatomic relationships in each case. Often it is helpful to use a long clip and a side-opening clip applier so that the handle of the clip and the clip applier do not obstruct the surgeon's view during the final placement of the clip.

The trans-sylvian approach may be expanded in order to enhance exposure of the upper BA in the *transcavernous trans-sellar approach.*[132] Following a standard pterional bone flap, the sphenoid wing is removed extradurally, and the anterior clinoid process and orbital roof are removed either extradurally or intradurally. The distal dural ring is incised, and the optic nerve and proximal ICA may be mobilized. The dura over the third and fourth nerves is opened, and a broad exposure over the anterior cranial base is afforded. Once the sylvian fissure and membrane of Liliequist have been opened, the posterior clinoid process is drilled away, and the upper basilar complex is then well visualized.

The *subtemporal approach* to basilar tip aneurysms may be performed with the patient either supine with a shoulder roll or in the lateral decubitus position. In either case the head is positioned so that the temporal squama is parallel to the floor. If the trans-sylvian exposure is not to be used, the scalp incision may be linear from the level of the zygoma to just above the superior temporal line. A small temporal bone flap is turned with a broad base along the zygoma, which extends to the temporal floor.[176] We have at times removed the zygoma in order to mobilize the temporalis further inferiorly. This step adds a small amount of time to both the exposure and the closure, but it reduces the amount of temporal lobe retraction that is required. It is particularly useful for high-riding basilar bifurcations. The temporal lobe is elevated from the temporal floor, and the free edge of the tentorium is identified. Small bridging veins may be sacrificed, and the vein of Labbé is usually far enough posterior so that it is not at risk. The tentorial edge anterior to the insertion site of the fourth nerve is sutured to the dura of the temporal floor. Alternatively, the tentorial edge may be divided just posterior to the insertion site of the fourth nerve.[177] The third nerve is identified through the arachnoid and is allowed to elevate with the temporal lobe. As the arachnoid that forms the lateral border of the interpeduncular cistern is opened under the microscope, the SCA is identified. The SCA is followed proximally to the BA, preserving all perforating arteries in the process. The ipsilateral P1 segment is identified just distally arising from the top of the BA. Dissection anterior to the aneurysm neck allows identification of the contralateral P1 segment (for the unusual anteriorly projecting domes, this step is performed last). Final neck preparation is similar to the trans-sylvian procedure and may be safer with a temporary clip on the BA either proximal or distal to the SCAs.

Because the subtemporal approach is more lateral, the ipsilateral PCA is more often in the line of permanent clip placement. Therefore, the most useful clip design for this approach is a fenestrated (or aperture) clip with the PCA in the fenestration. Although the subtemporal approach may allow somewhat easier identification of perforators, visualization of the contralateral P1 segment is usually more difficult than in the trans-sylvian approach. The exposure is somewhat shallower with the subtemporal approach, but it requires more temporal lobe retraction and does not allow the surgeon to address any anterior circulation aneurysms, unlike the pterional approach. With time, the two approaches have evolved so that they are actually similar, and they are actually fused in the half-and-half approach.[157, 170, 173–175, 178] In general, the choice of approach depends on the height of the basilar bifurcation (the lower bifurcation is best addressed by a subtemporal approach, the higher bifurcation by the pterional approach) and, importantly, the surgeon's training and experience.

PCA aneurysms may arise from the P1 segment, from the junction of the PComA and the P1 segment, or further distally (Fig. 10–26). These uncommon lesions may be approached either pterionally or subtemporally. The more distal lesions are only suitable for the subtemporal approach and may at times present difficulties in localization. If the aneurysm is fusiform, this may require trapping of the lesion with sacrifice of the distal PCA. If this is performed distal to the junction with the PComA, the P1 perforators are spared and collateral circulation usually permits a good neurologic outcome.[176]

SCA aneurysms (more accurately, BA-SCA aneurysms) present just distal to the SCA origin from the BA and usually project laterally and somewhat posteriorly. They are often imbedded into the cerebral peduncle and occasionally are intimately associated with the third nerve. Large SCA aneurysms may present with either partial third-nerve paresis or Weber's syndrome. If the subtemporal approach is used, it must be from the side of the aneurysm. The pterional approach from the right side may readily address SCA aneurysms on either side. A low-lying SCA aneurysm may be difficult to reach via the pterional approach, and therefore the surgeon must be prepared either to drill the posterior clinoid process or to switch to the subtemporal approach. In contrast with basilar tip or P1 aneurysms, SCA aneurysms usually are free of crucial perforating arteries that arise from the proximal P1 segment (Fig. 10–27).[176]

Midbasilar or basilar trunk aneurysms are fortunately uncommon (fewer than 5% of all intracranial aneurysms), because they are among the most technically difficult and potentially dangerous lesions in cerebrovascular surgery (Fig. 10–28). These aneurysms present either with SAH or with symptoms and signs related to direct brain stem compression. Operative access to these lesions presents the surgeon with a formidable challenge, and once access

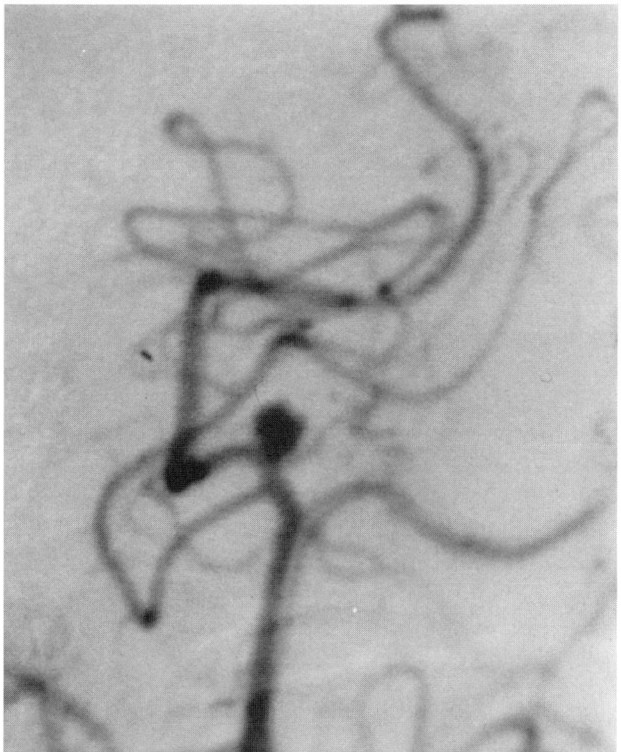

FIGURE 10–26 • Cerebral arteriogram (vertebral artery injection, anteroposterior view) showing a posterior cerebral artery aneurysm. This aneurysm was repaired via a pterional/trans-sylvian approach.

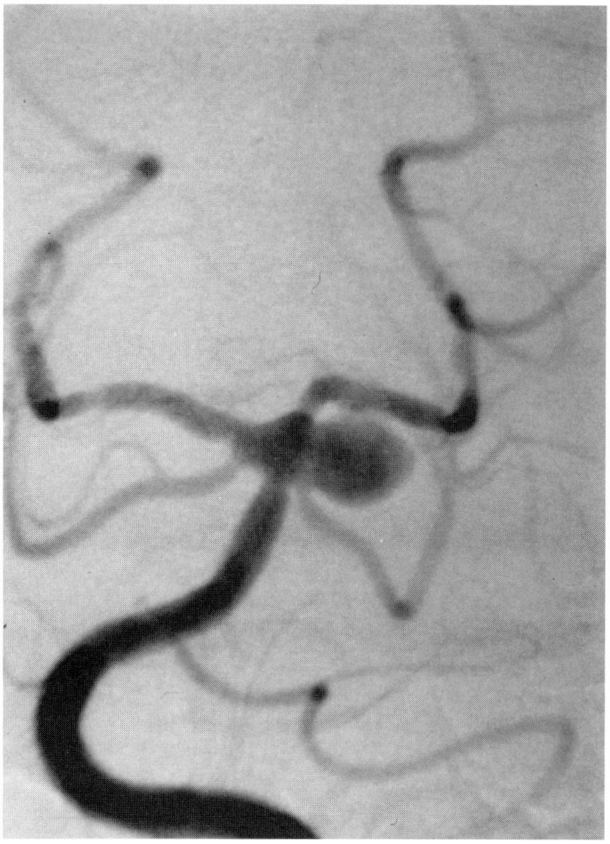

FIGURE 10–27 • Cerebral arteriogram (vertebral artery injection, anteroposterior view) showing a left superior cerebellar artery aneurysm. This can be repaired pterionally from either side or subtemporally from the left side. In this case, the patient also had a left internal carotid artery bifurcation aneurysm, and therefore a left pterional approach was selected.

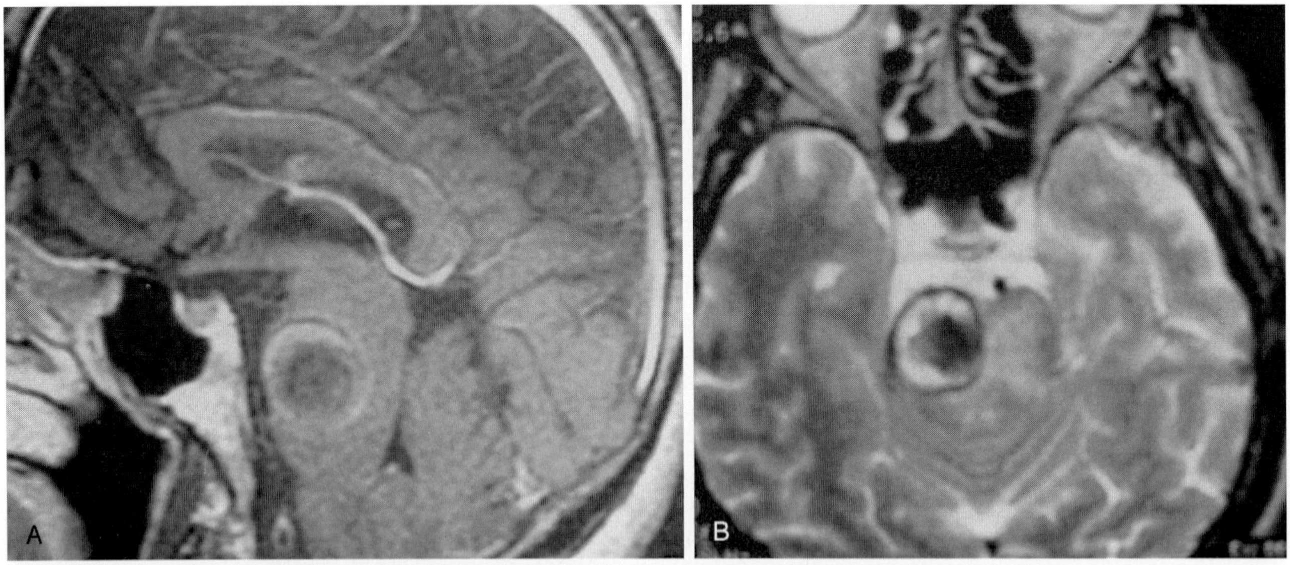

FIGURE 10–28 • Magnetic resonance image in the (*A*) sagittal and (*B*) axial planes showing a giant midbasilar artery aneurysm with brain stem compression. This aneurysm was repaired through a transpetrosal approach.

is achieved, the working space is extremely limited. The adjacent brain stem and cranial nerves, along with crucial perforating arteries, make technical errors extremely costly in terms of neurologic morbidity.

Several options are available for the surgical approach to aneurysms of the basilar trunk, and the selection of approach depends on the anatomic level of the aneurysm and its relationship to the cranial base. Indeed, the recent proliferation of creative skull base approaches for challenging tumors has carried over to the management of these difficult vascular lesions.[114] For upper to middle third basilar trunk lesions that involve the BA at or above the origin of AICA (we considered the BA-SCA aneurysms together with basilar tip and PCA aneurysms earlier), the traditional *subtemporal transtentorial approach* was popularized by Peerless and Drake.[176, 179] The patient is positioned laterally, and spinal drainage is employed. We use somatosensory and brain stem auditory evoked potential monitoring for virtually all posterior circulation aneurysms. A generous temporal craniotomy is made, which extends to the temporal floor with two-thirds of the bone flap positioned posterior to the external auditory canal. The midtemporal lobe is elevated with care taken to preserve the vein of Labbe. The tentorium is sectioned just behind the insertion of the fourth nerve and 1–2 cm posterior to the petrous ridge. The anterior leaflet of the tentorium is sutured to the dura of the floor of the middle fossa, and the fourth and fifth cranial nerves are identified and protected. The petrosal vein is coagulated and divided, and the retractor is gently positioned so that the anterior aspect of the cerebellum is retracted away from the clivus. This retraction rotates the brain stem so that the basilar trunk is visualized. The midbasilar aneurysm is generally approached through the relatively narrow space between the fifth nerve and the seventh/eighth nerve complex. For BA-AICA aneurysms, the sixth nerve is often intimately associated with the dome and must be gently mobilized to expose the neck.[176] Because of the narrow operative window, either a narrow clip applier or an extra long clip may be needed.

The *transpetrosal approach,* a modification of the subtemporal transtentorial approach,[180] involves an extradural resection of a portion of the petrous ridge followed by ligation of the superior petrosal sinus. This modification serves to protect the venous drainage of the temporal lobe and reduces temporal lobe retraction. The anatomy of the petrous apex must be carefully studied in order to avoid serious complications with this approach, including injury to the trigeminal nerve and ganglion, the petrous ICA, the cochlea, and the seventh/eighth nerve complex.

An expansion of the subtemporal approach for basilar trunk aneurysms has been called the *extended middle fossa* or *rhomboid approach.*[181] In this approach, an extradural dissection of the temporal floor identifies a rhomboid-shaped area of bone bordered by the greater superficial petrosal nerve, cochlea, foramen ovale, dura of the internal auditory canal, and superior petrosal sinus. The greater superficial petrosal nerve is followed to the geniculate ganglion in order to unroof the internal auditory canal. The intradural portion includes ligation and division of the superior petrosal sinus. These maneuvers greatly enhance the exposure of the basilar trunk in order to provide proximal control of the BA in most midbasilar aneurysms.

For low-lying basilar trunk aneurysms, the *combined supratentorial and infratentorial exposure* is usually best.[127, 182] The patient is placed in the park-bench position, and the incision extends into the temporal region from the linear retromastoid suboccipital incision. A suboccipital craniectomy is then combined with a temporal craniotomy. The transverse sinus is skeletonized and divided, provided there is adequate venous drainage on the contralateral side. The cerebellum is retracted so that the pons is gently rotated, providing a view of a lengthy segment of the BA. Various modifications of this approach have been described.[183, 184] With further drilling of the mastoid, the dura anterior to the sigmoid sinus is exposed, and the superior petrosal sinus may be ligated at its junction with the sigmoid. This approach allows the transverse sinus to be preserved, and less rotation of the brain stem is needed. More radical temporal bone resection, including the labyrinth and cochlea, can further enhance exposure of the basilar trunk for complex lesions in which proximal and distal control is critical.

Aneurysms of the lower basilar trunk, VBJ, and vertebral-PICA junction usually present with SAH that is concentrated in the posterior fossa cisterns. The patient is more likely to complain of neck pain and occipital headache than are patients with anterior circulation aneurysms. The ruptured vertebral-PICA aneurysms often have a signature CT appearance, with blood ballooning the fourth ventricle (Fig. 10–29). The angiographic evaluation in these cases should include injection of both vertebral arteries, if possible; we have seen PICA aneurysms missed on single vertebral injections even with reflux of contrast into the opposite vertebral artery. Because there is often little blood around the vessels of the circle of Willis, vasospasm is usually less severe in these cases, and early surgery is the rule in most patients.

A *retromastoid suboccipital craniectomy* approach is standard for most aneurysms of the vertebral-PICA junction (generally called PICA aneurysms). The patient is positioned either three-quarters prone or laterally, and the craniectomy is familiar to most neurosurgeons.[127, 185, 186] The cerebellar hemisphere is retracted upward, and the PICA is followed to its junction with the vertebral artery. At this point, dissection of the aneurysm involves some manipulation of the lower cranial nerves and variable retraction of the medulla. Distal control is often limited, but the working space is generally adequate for most aneurysms. Following these procedures, the patient's airway must be carefully evaluated prior to extubation because of the risk of vocal cord paresis and aspiration.

The *extreme lateral inferior transcondylar exposure* is a modification of this standard approach, which allows exposure of the midline with less brain stem retraction.[187, 188] A park-bench position is used, and the incision extends from the retromastoid region to approximately C3. The vertebral artery is identified extradurally, and the craniectomy includes the inferior mastoid and the rim of the foramen magnum. The lateral aspect of the posterior arch of C1 is removed, and the occipital condyle is drilled until the hypoglossal canal and jugular tubercle are exposed. The dura is opened, and the

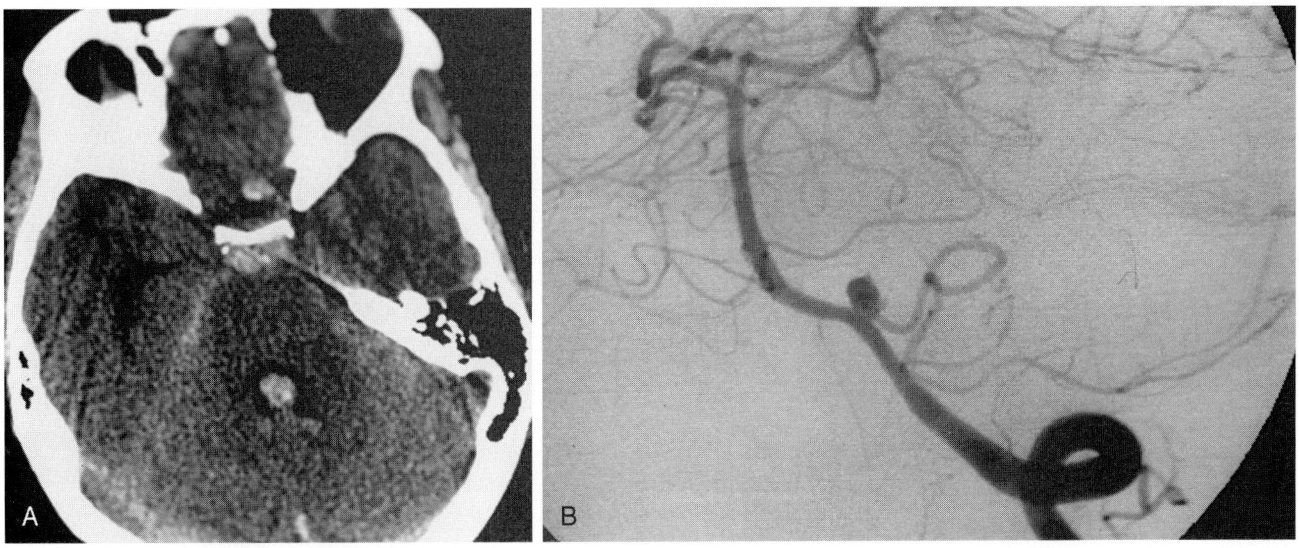

FIGURE 10–29 • *A,* Head computed tomography following rupture of a posterior inferior cerebellar artery (PICA) aneurysm with blood within the fourth ventricle and early hydrocephalus. *B,* Cerebral arteriogram (vertebral artery injection, anteroposterior view) showing the aneurysm arising from the vertebral artery at the origin of the PICA.

vertebral artery can be followed distally to the VBJ, requiring minimal cerebellar and brain stem retraction. A watertight dural closure is often difficult, and the distance to the VBJ is lengthy, but this approach avoids sacrifice of the sigmoid sinus when the venous anatomy does not safely allow it.[181]

A *retrolabyrinthine trans-sigmoid approach* is selected for difficult basilar trunk and VBJ aneurysms in which competent contralateral venous drainage is present. This approach preserves hearing and minimizes retraction on the cerebellum and brain stem. The patient is positioned supine with a roll under the ipsilateral shoulder and the head turned far toward the opposite side. Partial mastoidectomy is performed, which preserves the labyrinth and exposes the posterior fossa dura both anterior and posterior to the sigmoid sinus. The sinus is ligated and divided, and the dural opening provides exposure of the AICA and BA. Usually a self-retaining retractor is not needed, and the aneurysm may be dissected by working on either side of the seventh/eighth nerve complex.[181, 189]

For sake of completeness, we mention the *transoral-transclival approach* for midbasilar aneurysms. This approach has the advantage of avoiding brain stem retraction entirely, but several disadvantages make it less than desirable. The exposure requires extensive drilling of the clivus and special instrumentation because of the long reach.[190] The problem of dural closure and the contaminated exposure through the oropharynx make postoperative meningitis an ongoing threat.

Giant Aneurysms

Cerebral aneurysms larger than 25 mm in diameter are somewhat arbitrarily defined as giant.[191] Giant aneurysms account for approximately 5% of all intracranial aneurysms (20% of our referral practice) and they tend to present clinically in the same age range or perhaps slightly later than other aneurysms, with a peak in the fourth through sixth decades of life.[192, 193] In certain locations, particularly the more confined posterior fossa, large aneurysms in the 15 to 25 mm range pose similar technical problems. Although there is a slight female preponderance for aneurysms in general, the sex incidence for giant aneurysms appears to be roughly equal except for carotid-ophthalmic and paraclinoid aneurysms, which are far more common in females.[128, 194] Most giant aneurysms are saccular and therefore are often amenable to direct repair. Giant fusiform and serpentine aneurysms pose severe technical problems for attempts at direct repair,[195, 196] and these types have generally been managed either nonoperatively or by proximal ligation,[197] by

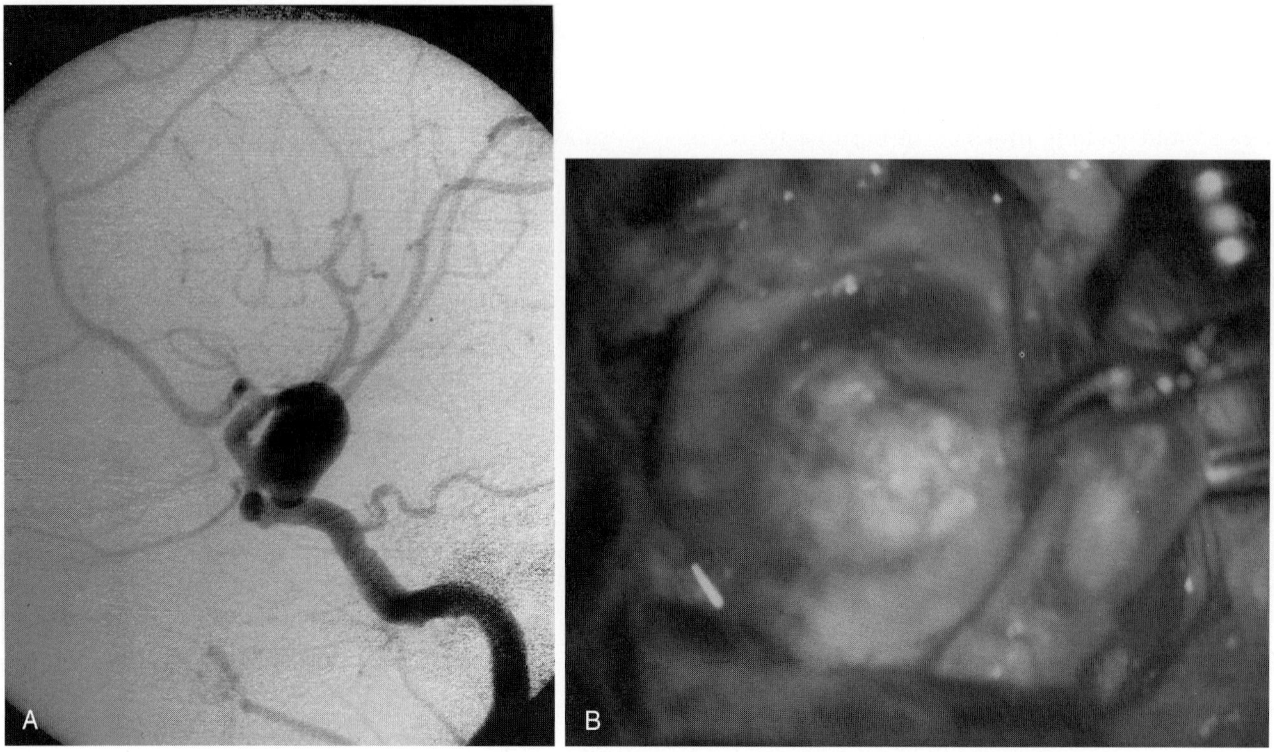

FIGURE 10-30 • *A,* Cerebral arteriogram (internal carotid artery injection, oblique view) showing a giant paraclinoid carotid aneurysm in an elderly patient. *B,* Intraoperative photomicrograph showing the heavily calcified, atherosclerotic aneurysm dome, which was repaired with an angled fenestrated clip. (See color plate.)

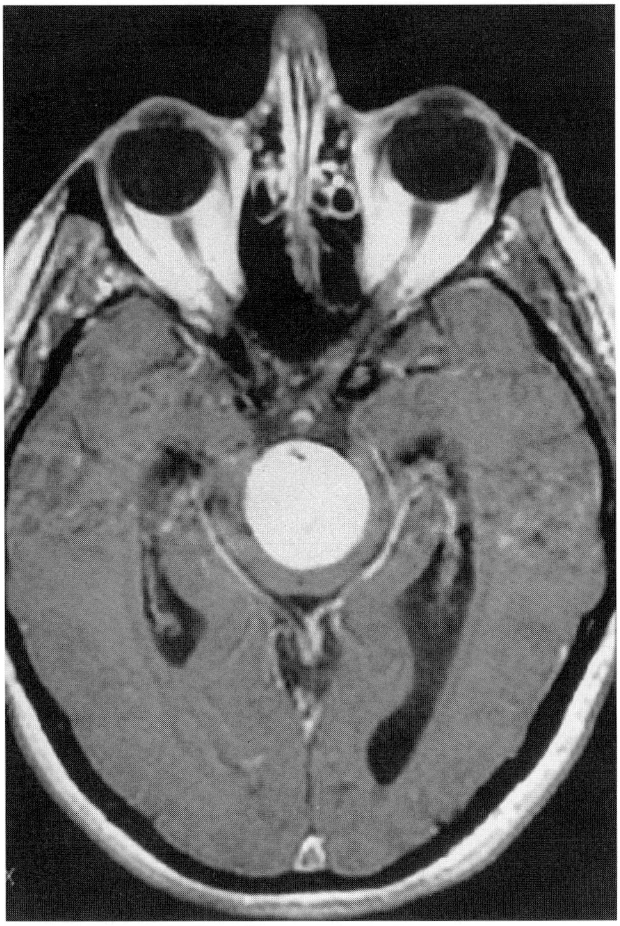

FIGURE 10–31 • Magnetic resonance image of a young woman who presented with headaches and mild gait instability. The giant basilar artery aneurysm causes massive brain stem compression. While obtaining second opinions regarding management, the patient suddenly became deeply comatose and never regained consciousness.

trapping,[198] by wrapping,[199] or via interventional neuroradiologic techniques.[200] Some form of revascularization procedure is often performed in conjunction with these indirect repairs.[198, 201, 202]

Atherosclerosis and calcification of the neck and fundus of giant aneurysms are common, as is partial thrombosis (Fig. 10–30). These factors serve to protect a portion of the aneurysmal wall from hemorrhage, but there are invariably very thin portions that are just as prone to hemorrhage as are nongiant aneurysms.[201] Up to 35% of giant aneurysms present with SAH. Other forms of presentation include headaches, seizures (particularly with MCA aneurysms), focal neurologic deficits from mass effect, and rarely ischemic episodes that may be due to embolic phenomena from the intra-aneurysmal thrombus. In fact, the most common form of presentation is due to mass effect, which occurs in 65%–85% of patients. Anterior circulation giant aneurysms commonly present with visual deficits due to compression of the optic pathways. Occasionally a giant aneurysm (usually off the MCA) presents with massive surrounding edema similar to that seen with a primary or metastatic tumor. There is virtually universal agreement that these lesions, once symptomatic, have a treacherous natural history and should be treated somehow if at all possible (Fig. 10–31).

As in nongiant aneurysms, the optimal treatment entails definitive clipping and exclusion of the fundus from the circulation, if possible. An additional goal in the treatment of giant aneurysms is to decompress the brain and cranial nerves. Preoperative imaging studies should include MRI in addition to high-resolution four-vessel contrast angiography, because the true size and anatomic relationships of the giant dome are often not appreciated by angiography alone because of the intra-aneurysmal thrombus (Figs. 10–32 and 10–33). It is particularly important to study the earliest angiographic images in order to determine the true location and breadth of the aneurysmal neck. In some cases a discrete neck cannot be visualized despite multiple oblique views. Nevertheless, most of these cases should be explored; a clippable neck may well be identifiable at surgery. In giant carotid aneurysms, BTO of the ICA should be considered, because the sufficiency of collateral circulation may determine the surgical options if direct repair of the aneurysm is not possible. Many surgeons do not recommend early surgery for giant aneurysms, even in patients who are "good grades" following a SAH. The sheer size of a giant fundus may necessitate extensive retraction and dissection, as well as temporary vessel occlusion, trapping of the lesion, or both; therefore, a "slack" brain is absolutely essential in these cases.

For the safe exposure and dissection of giant aneurysms, temporary proximal vessel occlusion or trapping should be considered a routine maneuver.[193] Trapping is preferable in aneurysms with intraluminal thrombus in order to minimize the risk of distal embolization and to allow opening of the dome for thrombectomy prior to definitive clip placement.[203] Thrombectomy may be facilitated at times by the Cavitron ultrasonic aspirator.[204] When the aneurysm neck is calcified or heavily atherosclerotic, endarterectomy at the neck and proximal dome may be necessary prior to clip placement.[205] If the period of temporary occlusion is anticipated to be prolonged (i.e., more than 20–30 minutes), some authors advocate a prior bypass procedure to provide collateral flow, even if the parent vessel is spared.[206] Others more recently have reported good success with circulatory arrest and deep hypothermia,[98, 99] but this undertaking certainly poses a variety of serious risks. Samson and colleagues have tried to establish parameters for safe periods of temporary occlusion,[96] but this is a complex analysis

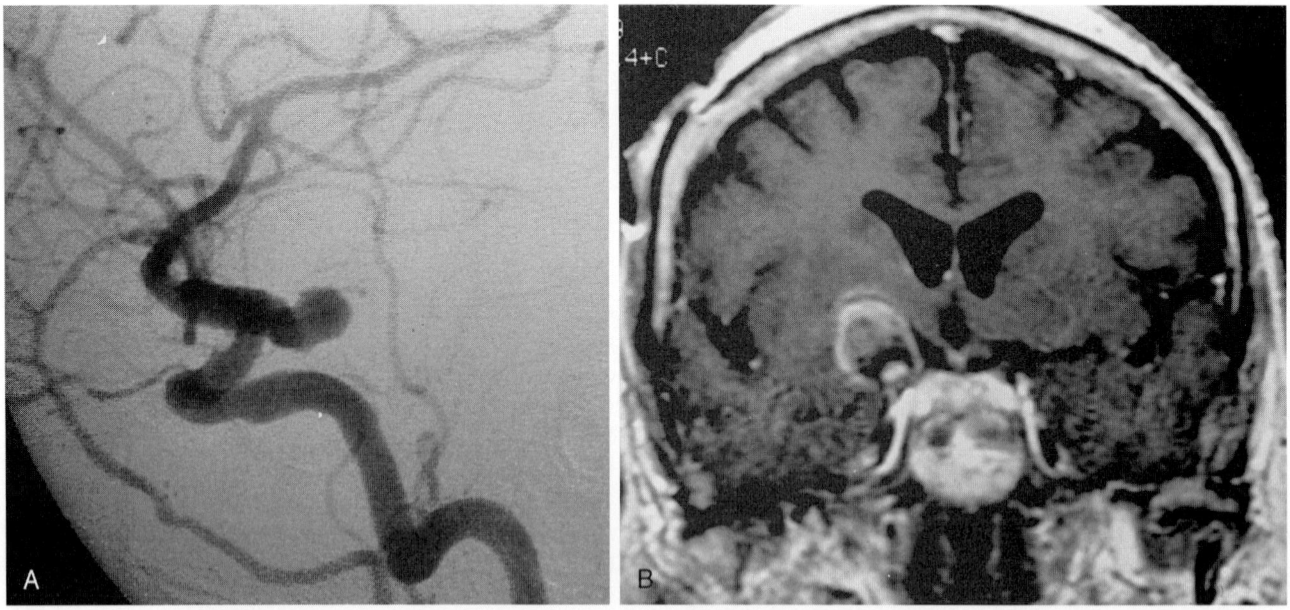

FIGURE 10-32 • Cerebral arteriogram (*A*) and coronal magnetic resonance image (*B*) demonstrating a giant carotid aneurysm. Only a small portion of the giant dome fills on the arteriogram. The magnetic resonance image is important for operative planning.

with so many variables that rigid guidelines are virtually impossible. Further research, both laboratory and clinical, is desperately needed in this important area, particularly in search of a reliable cerebral protective regimen.

For giant carotid-ophthalmic and paraclinoid carotid aneurysms, the ICA should be exposed in the neck to provide proximal control, and suction may be applied through a catheter to decompress the aneurysm.[135] Alternatively, direct suction decompression through a 21-gauge butterfly needle inserted into the dome may be more effective.[134] For most basilar apex aneurysms, proximal temporary occlusion may be established directly by either the pterional or the subtemporal approach, but occasionally this is not possible, and a brief period of moderate hypotension may be helpful.

When direct repair of a giant aneurysm is not

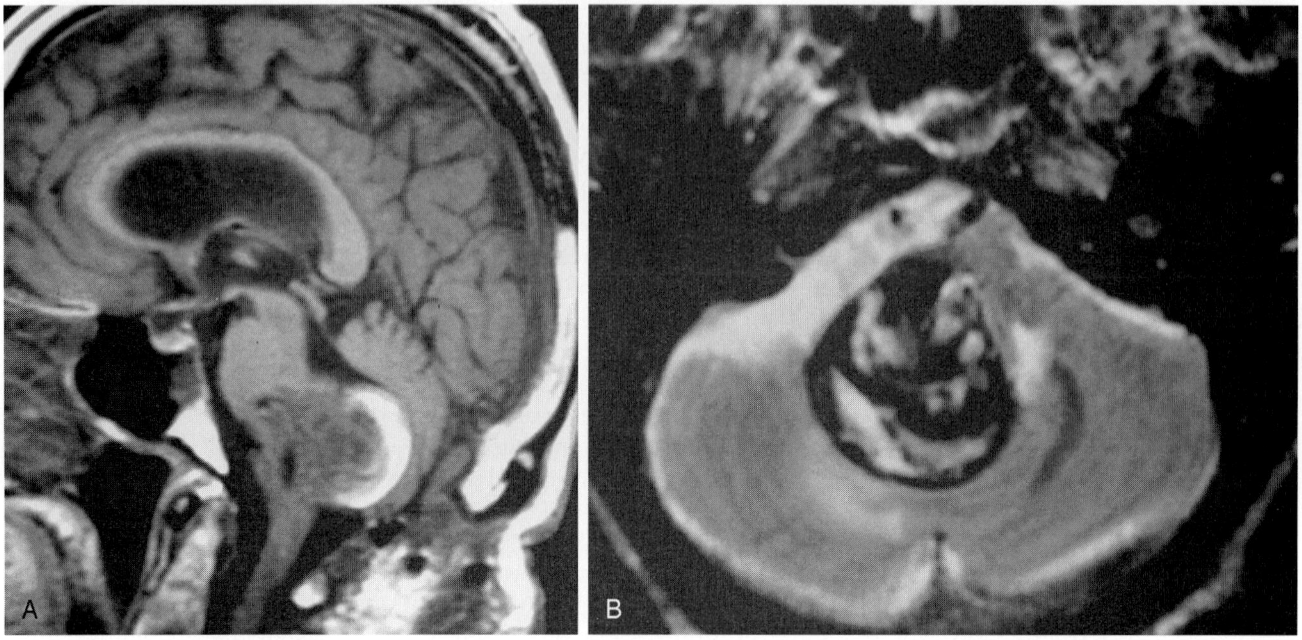

FIGURE 10-33 • Magnetic resonance image in the (*A*) sagittal and (*B*) axial planes demonstrating a giant basilar artery aneurysm with severe brain stem compression and obstructive hydrocephalus. Note the thrombus of varying ages within the giant dome.

possible, a variety of indirect techniques should be considered.[193] Wrapping and coating procedures may provide some early protection against rebleeding, but long-term studies have demonstrated the inadequacy of these techniques.[199] Acrylic in particular should be avoided, because it seriously impedes future attempts to expose and repair the dome, which commonly enlarges with time. Direct intramural thrombosis[207] has largely been replaced by modern interventional techniques using thrombogenic coils.[80, 81] Common carotid ligation, either open or via interventional neuroradiologic techniques, is a viable option for unclippable carotid aneurysms.[125, 208, 209] ICA occlusion or trapping, with or without bypass, is an effective alternative.[157, 198, 201, 206] Proximal vessel occlusion has been used in the vertebrobasilar system as well.[201, 210]

References

1. Brott T, Thalinger K, Hertzberg V: Hypertension as a risk factor for spontaneous intracerebral hemorrhage. Stroke 1986;17:1078.
2. Mohr JP, Caplan LR, Melski JW, et al: The Harvard Cooperative Stroke Registry: A prospective registry of patients hospitalized with stroke. Neurology 1978;28:754–762.
3. Hamilton MG, Zabramski JM: Intracerebral hematomas. In Carter LP, Spetzler RF, Hamilton MG (eds): Neurovascular Surgery, pp 477–496. New York, McGraw-Hill, 1995.
4. Kojima S, Omura T, Wakamatsu W, et al: Prognosis and disability of stroke patients after 5 years in Akita, Japan. Stroke 1990;21:72.
5. Ueda K, Hasuo Y, Kiyohara Y, et al: Intracerebral hemorrhage in a Japanese community, Hisayama: Incidence, changing pattern during long-term follow-up, and related factors. Stroke 1988;19:48.
6. Shi F, Hart RG, Sherman DG, Tegeler CH: Stroke in the People's Republic of China. Stroke 1989;20:1581.
7. Broderick JP, Brott T, Tomsick T, et al: Intracerebral hemorrhage more than twice as common as subarachnoid hemorrhage. J Neurosurg 1993;78:188–191.
8. Sacco RL, Wolf PA, Bharucha NE, et al: Subarachnoid and intracerebral hemorrhage: Natural history, prognosis, and precursive factors in the Framingham study. Neurology 1984;34:847.
9. Kassell NF, Torner JC, Haley EC, et al: The International Cooperative Study on the Timing of Aneurysm Surgery. Part 1: Overall management results. J Neurosurg 1990;73:18–36.
10. Kase CS, Williams JP, Wyatt DA, Mohr JP: Lobar intracerebral hematomas. Clinical and CT analysis of 22 cases. Neurology 1982;32:1146–1150.
11. Tanaka Y, Furuse M, Iwasa H, et al: Lobar intracerebral hemorrhage: Etiology and a long-term follow-up study of 32 patients. Stroke 1986;17:51–57.
12. Ojemann RG, Mohr JP: Hypertensive brain hemorrhage. Clin Neurosurg 1975;23:220–244.
13. Fisher CM: The pathologic and clinical aspects of thalamic hemorrhage. Trans Am Neurol Assoc 1959;84:56–59.
14. Walshe TM, Davis KD, Fisher CM: Thalamic hemorrhage: A computed tomographic–clinical correlation. Neurology 1977;27:217–222.
15. Ott KH, Kase CS, Ojemann RG, Mohr JP: Cerebellar hemorrhage: Diagnosis and treatment. A review of 56 cases. Arch Neurol 1974;31:160–167.
16. Little JR, Blomquist GA Jr, Ethier R: Intraventricular hemorrhage in adults. Surg Neurol 1977;8:143–149.
17. Minematsu K, Yamaguchi T: Management of intracerebral hemorrhage. In Fisher M (ed): Stroke Therapy, pp 351–372. Boston, Butterworth-Heinemann, 1995.
18. Caplan L: Intracerebral hemorrhage revisited. Neurology 1988;38:624–627.
19. Adams RD, Victor M: Cerebrovascular diseases. In Adams RD, Victor M (eds): Principles of Neurology, 4th ed, pp 663–682. New York, McGraw-Hill, 1989.
20. Wojak JC, Flamm ES: Intracranial hemorrhage and cocaine use. Stroke 1987;18:712–715.
21. Thulborn KR, Atlas SW: Intracranial hemorrhage. In Atlas SW (ed): Magnetic Resonance Imaging of the Brain and Spine, pp 175–222. New York, Raven Press, 1991.
22. Le Roux PD, Dailey AT, Newell DW, et al: Emergent aneurysm clipping without angiography in the moribund patient with intracerebral hemorrhage: The use of infusion computed tomography scans. Neurosurgery 1993;33:189–197.
23. Busto R, Dietrich WD, Globus MYT, et al: Small differences in intraischemic brain temperature critically determine the extent of ischemic neuronal injury. J Cereb Blood Flow Metabol 1987;7:729–738.
24. Chopp M, Chen H, Dereski MO, Garcia JH: Mild hypothermic intervention after graded ischemic stress in rats. Stroke 1991;22:37–43.
25. Minamisawa H, Nordstrom CH, Smith ML, Siesjo BK: The influence of mild body and brain hypothermia on ischemic brain damage. J Cereb Blood Flow Metab 1990;10:365–374.
26. Moyer DJ, Zager EL, Welsh FA: Spontaneous cerebral hypothermia diminishes focal infarction in rat brain. Stroke 1992;23:1812–1816.
27. Batjer HH: Timing of operation for ruptured aneurysms: Early surgery. In Ratcheson RA, Wirth FP (eds): Ruptured Cerebral Aneurysms: Perioperative Management, pp 46–53. Baltimore, Williams and Wilkins, 1994.
28. Onesti ST, Baker CJ, Sun PP, Solomon RA: Transient hypothermia reduces focal ischemic brain injury in the rat. Neurosurgery 1991;29:369–373.
29. Poungvarin N, Bhoopat W, Viriyavejakul A, et al: Effects of dexamethasone in primary supratentorial intracerebral hemorrhage. N Engl J Med 1987;316:1229–1233.
30. Weir BKA: Results of burr hole and open or closed suction drainage for chronic subdural hematomas in adults. Can J Neurol Sci 1983;22–26.
31. Camel M, Grubb RL Jr: Treatment of chronic subdural hematoma by twist-drill craniostomy with continuous catheter drainage. J Neurosurg 1986;65:183–187.
32. Markwalder TM: Chronic subdural hematoma: A review. J Neurosurg 1981;54:637–645.
33. Hamilton MG, Frizzell JB, Tranmer BI: Chronic subdural hematoma: The role for craniotomy reevaluated. Neurosurgery 1993;33:67–72.
34. Svien HJ, Gelety JE: On the surgical management of encapsulated subdural hematoma. A comparison of the results of membranectomy and simple evacuation. J Neurosurg 1964;21:172–177.
35. O'Lavoire SA, Crockard HA, Thomas DGT, Gordon DS: Brain stem hematoma. A report of six surgically treated cases. J Neurosurg 1982;56:222–227.
36. Fahlbusch R, Strauss C, Huk W: Pontine-mesencephalic cavernomas: Indications for surgery and operative results. Acta Neurochir Suppl (Wien) 1991;53:37–41.
37. Scott RM, Barnes P, Kupsky W, Adelman LS: Cavernous angiomas of the central nervous system in children. J Neurosurg 1992;76:38–46.
38. Wascher TM, Spetzler RF: Cavernous malformations of the brain stem. In Carter LP, Spetzler RF, Hamilton MG (eds): Neurovascular Surgery, pp 541–556. New York, McGraw-Hill, 1995.
39. Zimmerman RS, Spetzler RF, Lee KS, et al: Cavernous malformations of the brain stem. J Neurosurg 1991;75:32–39.
40. Heros RC: Cerebellar hemorrhage and infarction. Stroke 1982;13:106–109.
41. Kobayashi S, Sato A, Kageyama Y, et al: Treatment of hy-

pertensive cerebellar hemorrhage—Surgical or conservative management? Neurosurgery 1994;34:246–251.
42. Andrews BT, Chiles BW, Olsen WL, Pitts LH: The effect of intracerebral hematoma location on the risk of brainstem compression and on clinical outcome. J Neurosurg 1988;69:518–522.
43. Batjer HH, Reisch JS, Allen BC, et al: Failure of surgery to improve outcome in hypertensive putaminal hemorrhage. A prospective randomized trial. Arch Neurol 1990;47:1103.
44. Waga S, Yamamoto Y: Hypertensive putaminal hemorrhage: Treatment and results. Is surgical treatment superior to conservative one? Stroke 1985;14:480–485.
45. Kanno T, Sano H, Shinomya Y, et al: Role of surgery in hypertensive intracerebral hematoma. A comparative study of 305 nonsurgical and 154 surgical cases. J Neurosurg 1984;61:1091–1099.
46. Auer LM, Deinsberger W, Niederkorn K, et al: Endoscopic surgery versus medical treatment for spontaneous intracerebral hematoma: A randomized study. J Neurosurg 1989;70:530–535.
47. Juvela S, Heiskanen O, Poranen A, et al: The treatment of spontaneous intracerebral hemorrhage. A prospective randomized trial of surgical and conservative treatment. J Neurosurg 1989;70:755–758.
48. Nehls DG, Mendelow AD, Graham DI, Teasdale GM: Experimental intracerebral hemorrhage: Early removal of a spontaneous mass lesion improves late outcome. Neurosurgery 1990;27:674–682.
49. Niizuma H, Shimizu Y, Yonemitsu T, et al: Results of stereotactic aspiration in 175 cases of putaminal hemorrhage. Neurosurgery 1989;24:814.
50. Nguyen JP, Decq P, Brugieres P, et al: A technique for stereotactic aspiration of deep intracerebral hematomas under computed tomographic control using a new device. Neurosurgery 1992;31:330–335.
51. Matsumoto K, Hondo H: CT-guided stereotaxic evacuation of hypertensive intracerebral hematomas. J Neurosurg 1984;61:440–448.
52. Spetzler RF, Martin NA, Carter P, et al: Surgical management of large AVM's by staged embolization and operative excision. J Neurosurg 1987;67:17–28.
53. Cunha e Sa MJ, Stein BM, Solomon RA, et al: The treatment of associated intracranial aneurysms and arteriovenous malformations. J Neurosurg 1992;77:853–859.
54. Brown RD Jr, Wiebers DO, Forbes GS: Unruptured intracranial aneurysms and arteriovenous malformations: Frequency of intracranial hemorrhage and relationship of lesions. J Neurosurg 1990;73:859–863.
55. Sahs AL, Nibbelink DW, Torner JC (eds): Aneurysmal Subarachnoid Hemorrhage: Report of the Cooperative Study. Baltimore, Urban and Schwarzenberg, 1981.
56. Auer L: Unfavorable outcome following early surgical repair of ruptured cerebral aneurysms: A critical review of 238 patients. Surg Neurol 1991;35:152–158.
57. Kassell NF, Torner JC: Aneurysmal rebleeding: A preliminary report from the cooperative aneurysm study. Neurosurgery 1983;13:479.
58. Kassell NF, Torner JC, Jane JA, et al: The International Cooperative Study on the Timing of Aneurysm Surgery. Part 2: Surgical results. J Neurosurg 1990;73:37–47.
59. Konishi Y, Maemura E, Sato E, et al: A therapy against vasospasm after subarachnoidal haemorrhage: Clinical experience of balloon angioplasty. Neurol Res 1990;12:103.
60. Higashida RT, Halbach VV, Dowd CF, et al: Intravascular balloon dilatation therapy for intracranial arterial vasospasm: Patient selection, technique, and clinical results. Neurosurg Rev 1992;15:89.
61. Newell DW, Eskridge J, Mayberg M, et al: Endovascular treatment of intracranial aneurysms and cerebral vasospasm. Clin Neurosurg 1992;39:348.
62. Le Roux PD, Mayberg MR: Management of vasospasm: Angioplasty. In Ratcheson RA, Wirth FP (eds): Ruptured Cerebral Aneurysms: Perioperative Management, pp 155–167. Baltimore, Williams and Wilkins, 1994.
63. Le Roux PD, Newell DW, Eskridge J, et al: Severe symptomatic vasospasm: The role of immediate postoperative angioplasty. J Neurosurg 1994;80:224.
64. Barnwell SL, Higashida RT, Halbach VV, et al: Transluminal angioplasty of intracerebral vessels for cerebral arterial spasm: Reversal of neurological deficits after delayed treatment. Neurosurgery 1989;25:424.
65. Kaku Y, Yonekawa Y, Tsukahara T, et al: Superselective intra-arterial infusion of papaverine for the treatment of cerebral vasospasm after subarachnoid hemorrhage. J Neurosurg 1992;77:842.
66. Kassell NF, Helm G, Simmons N, et al: Treatment of cerebral vasospasm with intra-arterial papaverine. J Neurosurg 1992;77:848.
67. Clouston JE, Numaguchi Y, Zoarski GH, et al: Intraarterial papaverine infusion for cerebral vasospasm after subarachnoid hemorrhage. Am J Neuroradiol 1995;16:27.
68. Mizukami M, Kawase T, Usami T, Tazawa T: Prevention of vasospasm by early operation with removal of subarachnoid blood. Neurosurgery 1982;10:301–307.
69. Findlay JM, Weir BKA, Steinke D, et al: Effect of intrathecal thrombolytic therapy on subarachnoid clot and chronic vasospasm in a primate model of SAH. J Neurosurg 1988;69:723–735.
70. Findlay JM, Weir BKA, Kanamaru K, et al: Intrathecal fibrinolytic therapy after subarachnoid hemorrhage: Dosage study in a primate model and review of the literature. Can J Neurol Sci 1989;16:28–40.
71. Findlay JM, Weir BKA, Kanamaru K, et al: The effect of timing of intrathecal fibrinolytic therapy on cerebral vasospasm in a primate model of subarachnoid hemorrhage. Neurosurgery 1990;26:201–206.
72. Findlay JM, Weir BKA, Kassell NF, et al: Intracisternal recombinant tissue plasminogen activator after aneurysmal subarachnoid hemorrhage. J Neurosurg 1991;75:181–188.
73. Ohman J, Servo A, Heiskanen O: Effect of intrathecal fibrinolytic therapy on clot lysis and vasospasm in patients with aneurysmal subarachnoid hemorrhage. J Neurosurg 1991;75:197–201.
74. Stolke D, Seifert V: Single intracisternal bolus of recombinant tissue plasminogen activator in patients with aneurysmal subarachnoid hemorrhage: Preliminary assessment of efficacy and safety in an open clinical study. Neurosurgery 1992;30:877–881.
75. Macdonald RL, Weir BK: Management of vasospasm: Tissue plasminogen activator. In Ratcheson RA, Wirth FP (eds): Ruptured Cerebral Aneurysms: Perioperative Management, pp 168–181. Baltimore, Williams and Wilkins, 1994.
76. Findlay JM, Kassell NF, Weir BKA, et al: A randomized trial of intraoperative, intracisternal tissue plasminogen activator for the prevention of vasospasm. Neurosurgery 1995;37:168–178.
77. Bailes JE, Spetzler RF, Hadley MN, et al: Management of morbidity and mortality of poor-grade aneurysm patients. J Neurosurg 1990;72:559–566.
78. Shucart W, Wu J: Timing of operation for ruptured aneurysms: Delayed surgery. In Ratcheson RA, Wirth FP (eds): Ruptured Cerebral Aneurysms: Perioperative Management, pp 54–58. Baltimore, Williams and Wilkins, 1994.
79. Winn HR, Newell DW, Mayberg MR, et al: Early surgical management of poor grade patients with intracranial aneurysms. Clin Neurosurg 1990;36:289–298.
80. Graves VB, Strother CM, Duff TA, et al: Early treatment of ruptured aneurysms with Guglielmi detachable coils: Effect on subsequent bleeding. Neurosurgery 1995;37:640–648.
81. Guglielmi G, Vinuela E, Dion J, et al: Electrothrombosis of saccular aneurysms via endovascular approach. 2. Preliminary clinical experience. J Neurosurg 1991;75:8–14.
82. Batjer HH, Samson DS: Emergent aneurysm surgery without cerebral angiography for the comatose patient. Neurosurgery 1991;28:283–287.
83. Dorsch NWC, Young N, Kingston RJ, et al: Early experience with spiral CT in the diagnosis of intracranial aneurysms. Neurosurgery 1995;36:230.

84. Harbaugh RE, Schlusselberg DS, Jeffery R, et al: Three-dimensional computed tomographic angiography in the preoperative evaluation of cerebrovascular lesions. Neurosurgery 1995;36:320.
85. Hsiang JNK, Liang EY, Lam JMK, et al: The role of computed tomographic angiography in the diagnosis of intracranial aneurysms and emergent aneurysm clipping. Neurosurgery 1996;38:481–487.
86. Tampieri D, Leblanc R, Oleszek J, et al: Three-dimensional computed tomographic angiography of cerebral aneurysms. Neurosurgery 1995;36:749.
87. Lee SH, Heros RC: Principles of management of subarachnoid hemorrhage: Steroids. In Ratcheson RA, Wirth FP (eds): Ruptured Cerebral Aneurysms: Perioperative Management, pp 77–85. Baltimore, Williams and Wilkins, 1994.
88. Kemper CM, Allen GS: Management of vasospasm: Calcium channel-blocking agents. In Ratcheson RA, Wirth FP (eds): Ruptured Cerebral Aneurysms: Perioperative Management, pp 146–154. Baltimore, Williams and Wilkins, 1994.
89. Charbel FT, Ausman JI, Diaz FG, et al: Temporary clipping in aneurysm surgery: Technique and results. Surg Neurol 1991;36:83–90.
90. Pool JL, Housepian E: Temporary clip occlusion of major cerebral arteries during intracranial aneurysm surgery. Surg Forum 1960;10:791–794.
91. Mellergard P, Nordstrom CH, Christensson M: A method for monitoring intracerebral temperature in neurosurgical patients. Neurosurgery 1990;27:654–657.
92. Suzuki J, Kwak R, Okudaira Y: The safety time limit of temporary clamping of cerebral arteries in the direct surgical treatment of the intracranial aneurysm under moderate hypothermia. Brain Nerve 1973;25:407–416.
93. Mellergard P, Nordstrom CH: Intracerebral temperature in neurosurgical patients. Neurosurgery 1991;28:709–713.
94. Goldman MS, Anderson RE, Meyer FB: Effects of intermittent reperfusion during temporal focal ischemia. J Neurosurg 1992;77:911–916.
95. Steinberg GK, Panahian N, Sun GH, et al: Cerebral damage caused by interrupted, repeated arterial occlusion versus uninterrupted occlusion in a focal ischemic model. J Neurosurg 1994;81:554–559.
96. Samson D, Batjer HH, Bowman G, et al: A clinical study of the parameters and effects of temporary arterial occlusion in the management of intracranial aneurysms. Neurosurgery 1994;34:22–29.
97. Tomida S, Nowak TS Jr, Vass K, et al: Experimental model for repetitive ischemic attacks in the gerbil: The cumulative effect of repeated ischemic insults. J Cereb Blood Flow Metab 1987;7:773–782.
98. Spetzler RF, Hadley MH, Rigamonti D, et al: Aneurysms of the basilar artery treated with circulatory arrest, hypothermia, and barbiturate cerebral protection. J Neurosurg 1988;68;868–879.
99. Solomon RA, Smith CR, Raps EC, et al: Deep hypothermic circulatory arrest for the management of complex anterior and posterior circulation aneurysms. Neurosurgery 1991;29;732–738.
100. Ausman JI, Malik GM, Tomecek FJ, et al: Hypothermic circulatory arrest and the management of giant and large cerebral aneurysms. Surg Neurol 1993;40:289–298.
101. Jafar JJ, Johns LM, Mullan SF: The effect of mannitol on cerebral blood flow. J Neurosurg 1984;64:754–759.
102. Suzuki J, Yoshimoto T: The effect of mannitol in prolongation of permissible occlusion time of cerebral arteries: Clinical data of aneurysm surgery. In Suzuki J (ed): Cerebral Aneurysms: Experiences with 1000 Directly Operated Cases, pp 330–337.Tokyo, Neuron, 1979.
103. Zager EL, Stecker M, Weil R, et al: Congress of Neurological Surgeons annual meeting, Oct. 1995, San Francisco (abstract).
104. Batjer HH, Frankfurt AI, Purdy PD, et al: Use of etomidate, temporary arterial occlusion, and intraoperative angiography in surgical treatment of large and giant cerebral aneurysms. J Neurosurg 1988;68:234–240.
105. Batjer HH: Cerebral protective effects of etomidate: Experimental and clinical aspects. Cerebrovasc Brain Metab Rev 1993;5:17–32.
106. Wauquier A: Brain protective properties of etomidate and flunarizine. J Cereb Blood Flow Metab 1982;2(Suppl 1):S53–S56.
107. Little JR, Lesser RP, Luders H: Electrophysiological monitoring during basilar aneurysm operation. Neurosurgery 1987;20:421–427.
108. Schramm J, Koht A, Schmidt G, et al: Surgical and electrophysiological observations during clipping of 134 aneurysms with evoked potential monitoring. Neurosurgery 1990;26:61–70.
109. Choi IS, Morris PP: Endovascular treatment of intracranial aneurysms. In Cohen AR, Haines SJ (eds): Minimally Invasive Techniques in Neurosurgery, pp 154–165. Baltimore, Williams and Wilkins, 1995.
110. Livingston K, Guterman LR, Gibbons KJ, et al: Endovascular therapy of cerebral aneurysms. In Carter LP, Spetzler RF, Hamilton MG (eds): Neurovascular Surgery, pp 789–806. New York, McGraw-Hill, 1995.
111. Manwaring KH, Hamilton AJ: Neurosurgical endoscopy. In Tindall GT, Cooper PR, Barrow DL (eds): The Practice of Neurosurgery, pp 233–242. Baltimore, Williams and Wilkins, 1996.
112. Van Lindert E, Perneczky A: The supraorbital keyhole. A surgical window to supratentorial aneurysms. 4th International Workshop on Cerebrovascular Surgery. Chicago, Forefront Publications, 1995.
113. Sato S, Toya S, Suga S: Key hole surgery for patients with a ruptured aneurysm in the acute stage. 4th International Workshop on Cerebrovascular Surgery. Chicago, Forefront Publications, 1995.
114. Sekhar LN, Kalia KK, Yonas H, et al: Cranial base approaches to intracranial aneurysms in the subarachnoid space. Neurosurgery 1994;35:472–483.
115. Kobayashi S, Kyoshima K, Gibo H, et al: Carotid cave aneurysms of the internal carotid artery. J Neurosurg 1989;70:216–221.
116. Bouthillier A, van Loveren HR, Keller JT: Segments of the internal carotid artery: A new classification. Neurosurgery 1996;38:425–433.
117. Kupersmith MJ, Hurst R, Berenstein A, et al: The benign course of cavernous carotid artery aneurysms. J Neurosurg 1992;77:690–693.
118. Linskey ME, Jungreis CA, Yonas H, et al: Stroke risk after abrupt internal carotid artery sacrifice: Accuracy of preoperative assessment with balloon test occlusion and stable xenon-enhanced CT. AJNR 1994;15:829–843.
119. Eckard DA, Purdy PD, Bonte FJ: Temporary balloon occlusion of the carotid artery combined with brain blood flow imaging as a test to predict tolerance prior to permanent carotid sacrifice. AJNR 1992;13:1565–1569.
120. Erba SM, Horton JA, Latchaw RE, et al: Balloon test occlusion of the internal carotid artery with xenon/CT cerebral blood flow imaging. AJNR 1988;9:533–538.
121. Latchaw RE, Madison MT: Imaging, vascular assessment, and embolization of skull base tumors. In Tindall GT, Cooper PR, Barrow DL (eds): The Practice of Neurosurgery, pp 901–927. Baltimore, Williams and Wilkins, 1996.
122. Linskey ME, Sekhar LN, Hirsch WL Jr, et al: Aneurysms of the intracavernous carotid artery: Natural history and indications for treatment. Neurosurgery 1990;26:933–938.
123. Origitano TC, Al-Mefty O, Leonetti JP, et al: Vascular considerations and complications in cranial base surgery. Neurosurgery 1994;35:351–363.
124. Gelber BR, Sundt TM Jr: Treatment of intracavernous and giant carotid aneurysms by combined internal carotid ligation and extra- to intracranial bypass. J Neurosurg 1980;52:1–10.
125. Swearingen B, Heros RC: Common carotid occlusion for unclippable carotid aneurysms: An old but still effective operation. Neurosurgery 1987;21:288.
126. Day AL: Aneurysms of the ophthalmic segment. A clinical and anatomical analysis. J Neurosurg 1990;72:677–691.
127. Ojemann RG, Heros RC, Crowell RM: Surgical Manage-

ment of Cerebrovascular Disease. Baltimore, Williams and Wilkins, 1988.
128. Ferguson GG, Drake CG: Carotid-ophthalmic aneurysms: The surgical management of those cases presenting with compression of the optic nerves and chiasm alone. Clin Neurosurg 1980;27:263–308.
129. Yasargil MG, Gasser JC, Hodosh RM, et al: Carotid-ophthalmic aneurysms: Direct microsurgical approach. Surg Neurol 1977;8:155–165.
130. Dolenc V: Direct microsurgical repair of intracavernous vascular lesions. J Neurosurg 1983;58:824–831.
131. Dolenc VV: A combined epi- and subdural direct approach to carotid-ophthalmic artery aneurysms. J Neurosurg 1985;62:667–672.
132. Dolenc VV: Anatomy and Surgery of the Cavernous Sinus. Wien/New York, Springer-Verlag, 1989.
133. Korosue K, Heros RC: "Subclinoid" carotid aneurysm with erosion of the anterior clinoid process and fatal intraoperative rupture. Neurosurgery 1992;31:356–360.
134. Flamm ES: Suction decompression of aneurysms. Technical note. J Neurosurg 1981;54:275–276.
135. Batjer HH, Samson DS: Retrograde suction decompression of giant paraclinoid aneurysms. J Neurosurg 1990;73:305.
136. Batjer HH, Kopitnik TA, Giller CA, et al: Surgery for paraclinoidal carotid artery aneurysms. J Neurosurg 1994;80:650–658.
137. Krisht AF, Barrow DL, Barnett DW, et al: The microsurgical anatomy of the superior hypophyseal artery. Neurosurgery 1994;899–903.
138. Sahs AL, Perret GE, Locksley HB, et al (eds): Intracranial Aneurysms and Subarachnoid Hemorrhage. A Cooperative Study. Philadelphia, JB Lippincott, 1969.
139. Najjar JA, Carter LP: Saccular aneurysms of the internal carotid artery. In Carter LP, Spetzler RF, Hamilton MG (eds): Neurovascular Surgery, pp 649–658. New York, McGraw-Hill, 1995.
140. Yasargil MG, Yonas H, Gasser JC: Anterior choroidal artery aneurysms: Their anatomy and surgical significance. Surg Neurol 1978;9:129–138.
141. Gibo H, Lenkey C, Rhoton AL Jr: Microsurgical anatomy of the supraclinoid portion of the internal carotid artery. J Neurosurg 1981;55:560.
142. DaPian R, Pasqualin A, Scienza R: Direct microsurgical approach to aneurysms of the internal carotid bifurcation. Surg Neurol 1980;13:27.
143. DeLuca J, Diamond BJ: Aneurysm of the anterior communicating artery: A review of neuroanatomical and neuropsychological sequelae. J Clin Exp Neuropsych 1995;17:100–121.
144. Perlmutter D, Rhoton AL Jr: Microsurgical anatomy of the anterior cerebral–anterior communicating–recurrent artery complex. J Neurosurg 1976;45:259–272.
145. Gibbons K, Hopkins L, Heros RC: Occlusion of an "accessory" distal anterior cerebral artery during treatment of anterior communicating artery aneurysms. Report of two cases. J Neurosurg 1991;74:133.
146. VanderArk GD, Kempe LG, Smith DR: Anterior communicating aneurysms: The gyrus rectus approach. Clin Neurosurg 1974;21:210–233.
147. Crowell RM, Ogilvy CS: Anterior communicating artery aneurysms and distal anterior cerebral artery aneurysms. In Tindall GT, Cooper PR, Barrow DL (eds): The Practice of Neurosurgery, pp 2061–2074. Baltimore, Williams and Wilkins, 1996.
148. Suzuki J, Mizoi K, Yoshimoto T: Bifrontal interhemispheric approach to aneurysms of the anterior communicating artery. J Neurosurg 1986;64:183.
149. Yeh H, Tew J: Anterior interhemispheric approach to aneurysms of the anterior communicating artery. Surg Neurol 1985;23:98.
150. Poletti C: A temporal approach to anterior communicating artery aneurysms. Technical note. J Neurosurg 1989;71:144.
151. Fujimoto K, Waga S, Kojima T, et al: Aneurysm of distal anterior cerebral artery associated with azygos anterior cerebral artery. Acta Neurochir (Wien) 1981;59:65–69.
152. Wisoff JH, Flamm ES: Aneurysms of the distal anterior cerebral artery and associated vascular anomalies. Neurosurgery 1987;20:735–741.
153. Hernisniemi J, Tapaninaho A, Vapalahti M, et al: Saccular aneurysms of the distal anterior cerebral artery and its branches. Neurosurgery 1992;31:994–999.
154. Yasargil MG, Carter LP: Saccular aneurysms of the distal anterior cerebral artery. J Neurosurg 1974;40:218–221.
155. Traynelis VC, Dunker RO: Interhemispheric approach with callosal resection for distal anterior cerebral artery aneurysms. Technical note. J Neurosurg 1992;77:481–483.
156. Dickey PS, Bloomgarden GM, Arkins TJ, et al: Partial callosal resection for pericallosal aneurysms. Neurosurgery 1992;30:136–137.
157. Sundt TM Jr: Surgical Techniques for Saccular and Giant Intracranial Aneurysms. Baltimore, Williams and Wilkins, 1990.
158. Rinne J, Hernesniemi J, Niskanen M, et al: Analysis of 561 patients with 690 middle cerebral artery aneurysms: Anatomic and clinical features as correlated to management outcome. Neurosurgery 1996;38:2–11.
159. Solomon RA: Middle cerebral artery aneurysm surgery. In Carter LP, Spetzler RF, Hamilton MG (eds): Neurovascular Surgery, pp 687–700. New York, McGraw-Hill, 1995.
160. Lougheed WM, Marshall BM: Management of aneurysms of the anterior circulation by intracranial procedures. In Youmans JR (ed): Neurological Surgery, vol 2, pp 742–750. Philadelphia, WB Saunders, 1973.
161. Wheelock B, Weir B, Watts R, et al: Timing of surgery for intracerebral hematomas due to aneurysm rupture. J Neurosurg 1983;58:476–481.
162. Gibo H, Carver CC, Rhoton AL Jr, et al: Microsurgical anatomy of the middle cerebral artery. J Neurosurg 1981;54:151.
163. Heros RC, Ojemann RG, Crowell RM: Superior temporal gyrus approach to middle cerebral aneurysms: Techniques and results. Neurosurgery 1982;10:308–313.
164. Fisher CM: Clinical syndromes in cerebral thrombosis, hypertensive hemorrhage, and ruptured saccular aneurysms. Clin Neurosurg 1975;22:117.
165. Pia HW: Classification of vertebro-basilar aneurysms. Acta Neurochir 1979;47:3.
166. Koga H, Mori K, Kawano T, et al: Parinaud's syndrome in hydrocephalus due to a basilar artery aneurysm. Surg Neurol 1983;19:548.
167. Batjer HH, Purdy PD: Enlarging thrombosed aneurysm of the distal basilar artery. Neurosurgery 1990;26:695.
168. Stark RJ: Supranuclear ophthalmoplegia with basilar artery aneurysms. Surg Neurol 1979;12:447.
169. McKinna AJ: Eye findings in 611 cases of posterior fossa aneurysms: Their diagnostic and prognostic value. Can J Ophthalmol 1983;18:3.
170. Wascher TM, Spetzler RF: Saccular aneurysms of the basilar bifurcation. In Carter LP, Spetzler RF, Hamilton MG (eds): Neurovascular Surgery, pp 729–752. New York, McGraw-Hill, 1995.
171. Peerless SJ, Drake CG: Management of aneurysms of the posterior circulation. In Youmans JR (ed): Neurological Surgery. A Comprehensive Reference Guide to the Diagnosis and Management of Neurosurgical Problems, 3rd ed, pp 1764–1806. Philadelphia, WB Saunders, 1990.
172. Yasargil MG, Antic J, Laciga R, et al: Microsurgical pterional approach to aneurysms of the basilar bifurcation. Surg Neurol 1976;6:83.
173. Solomon RA, Stein BM: Surgical approaches to aneurysms of the vertebral and basilar arteries. Neurosurgery 1988;23:203.
174. Sano K: Temporopolar approach to aneurysms of the basilar artery at and around the distal bifurcation: Technical note. Neurol Res 1980;2:361–367.
175. Heros RC, Lee SH: The combined pterional/anterior temporal approach for aneurysms of the upper basilar complex: Technical report. Neurosurgery 1993;33:244–251.
176. Peerless SJ, Drake CG: Posterior circulation aneurysms. In Wilkins RH, Rengachary SS (eds): Neurosurgery, pp 1422–1437. New York, McGraw-Hill, 1985.

177. Drake CG: The surgical treatment of aneurysms of the basilar artery. J Neurosurgery 1968;29:436.
178. Drake CG: Microsurgical evaluation of the pterional approach to aneurysms of the distal basilar circulation. Neurosurgery 1978;3:140–141.
179. Drake CG: The treatment of aneurysms of the posterior circulation. Clin Neurosurg 1979;26:96.
180. Kawase T, Toya S, Shiobara R, et al: Transpetrosal approach for aneurysms of the lower basilar artery. J Neurosurg 1985;63:857.
181. Schneider JH, Giannotta SL: Basilar trunk and vertebrobasilar junction aneurysms. In Carter LP, Spetzler RF, Hamilton MG (eds): Neurovascular Surgery, pp 753–762. New York, McGraw-Hill, 1995.
182. Kasdon DL, Stein BM: Combined supratentorial and infratentorial exposure for low-lying basilar aneurysms. Neurosurgery 1979;4:422.
183. Spetzler RF, Daspit CP, Pappas CTE: The combined supra- and infratentorial approach for lesions of the petrous and clival regions: Experience with 46 cases. J Neurosurg 1992;76:588.
184. Samii M, Ammirati M, Mahran A, et al: Surgery of petroclival meningiomas: Report of 24 cases. Neurosurgery 1989;24:12.
185. Chou SN, Ortiz-Suarez HJ: Surgical treatment of arterial aneurysms of the vertebrobasilar circulation. J Neurosurg 1974;41:671.
186. Hammon WM, Kempe LG: The posterior fossa approach to aneurysms of the vertebral and basilar arteries. J Neurosurg 1972;37:339.
187. Heros RC: Lateral approach for vertebral and vertebrobasilar artery lesions. J Neurosurg 1986;64:559.
188. Sen CN, Sekhar LN: An extreme lateral approach to intradural lesions of the cervical spine and foramen magnum. Neurosurgery 1990;27:197.
189. Giannotta SL, Maceri DR: Retrolabyrinthine transsigmoid approach to basilar trunk and vertebrobasilar junction aneurysms. J Neurosurg 1988;69:461.
190. Crockard H, Koksel T, Watkin N: Transoral transclival clipping of an anterior inferior cerebellar aneurysm using new rotating appliers. Technical note. J Neurosurg 1991;75:483.
191. Locksley HB: Report of the cooperative study of intracranial aneurysms and subarachnoid hemorrhage. Section V, part II. Natural history of subarachnoid hemorrhage, intracranial aneurysms and arteriovenous malformations based on 6368 cases in the cooperative study. J Neurosurg 1966;23:321.
192. Heros RC: Giant intracranial aneurysms. In Long DM (ed): Current Therapy in Neurological Surgery, pp 80–84. Philadelphia, BC Decker, 1985.
193. Atkinson JLD, Piepgras DG: Giant aneurysms: Supratentorial. In Carter LP, Spetzler RF, Hamilton MG (eds): Neurovascular Surgery, pp 815–828. McGraw-Hill, New York, 1995.
194. Heros RC, Nelson PB, Ojemann RG, et al: Large and giant paraclinoid aneurysms: Surgical techniques, results and complications. Neurosurgery 1983;13:153–163.
195. Dolenc VV: Treatment of fusiform aneurysms of the peripheral cerebral arteries. Report of two cases. J Neurosurg 1978;49:272–277.
196. Samii M, Turel KE: Possibility of the excision of aneurysms in the vertebrobasilar system followed by end-to-end anastomosis for the maintenance of circulation. Neurol Res 1985;7:39–45.
197. Drake CG, Peerless SJ, Ferguson GG: Hunterian proximal arterial occlusion for giant aneurysms of the carotid circulation. J Neurosurg 1994;81:656–665.
198. Lawton MT, Hamilton MG, Morcos JJ, et al: Revascularization and aneurysm surgery: Current techniques, indications, and outcome. Neurosurgery 1996;38:83–94.
199. Todd NV, Tocher JL, Jones PA, et al: Outcome following aneurysm wrapping: A 10-year follow-up review of clipped and wrapped aneurysms. J Neurosurg 1989;70:841–846.
200. Gobin YP, Vinuela F, Gurian JH, et al: Treatment of large and giant fusiform intracranial aneurysms with Guglielmi detachable coils. J Neurosurg 1996;84:55–62.
201. Drake CG: Giant intracranial aneurysms: Experience with surgical treatment in 174 patients. Clin Neurosurg 1979;26:12–95.
202. Ausman JI, Diaz FG, Sadasivan B, et al: Giant intracranial aneurysm surgery: The role of microvascular reconstruction. Surg Neurol 1990;34:8–15.
203. Sinson G, Philips MF, Flamm ES: Intraoperative endovascular surgery for cerebral aneurysms. J Neurosurg 1996;84:63–70.
204. Flamm ES, Ransohoff J, Wuchinich D, et al: Preliminary experience with ultrasonic aspiration in neurosurgery. Neurosurgery 1978;2:240–245.
205. Hylton PD, Reichman OH: Endaneurysmal microendarterectomy in the treatment of giant cerebral aneurysms: Technical note. Neurosurgery 1988;23:674–679.
206. Sundt TM Jr, Piepgras DG: Surgical approach to giant intracranial aneurysms. Operative experience with 80 cases. J Neurosurg 1979;51:731–742.
207. Hosobuchi Y: Direct surgical treatment of giant intracranial aneurysms. J Neurosurg 1979;51:743.
208. Giannotta SL, McGillicuddy JE, Kindt GW: Gradual carotid artery occlusion in the treatment of inaccessible internal carotid artery aneurysms. Neurosurgery 1979;5:417.
209. Fox AJ, Vinuela F, Pelz DM, et al: Use of detachable balloons for proximal artery occlusion in the treatment of unclippable cerebral aneurysms. J Neurosurg 1987;66:40.
210. Steinberg GK, Drake CG, Peerless SJ: Deliberate basilar or vertebral artery occlusion in the treatment of intracranial aneurysms. Immediate results and long-term outcome in 201 patients. J Neurosurg 1993;79:161–173.

11

Cervicocerebral Interventional Neuroradiology

Robert W. Hurst, M.D.

Techniques of interventional neuroradiology have found increasing use in the treatment of disorders affecting the blood vessels of the head, neck, and central nervous system (CNS). A number of clinical conditions involving vascular damage or disease may require urgent endovascular management and treatment. Control of hemorrhage, treatment of acute cerebral ischemia, and closure of arteriovenous fistulas are a few instances in which interventional techniques may play a significant role in management of both traumatic and nontraumatic cervicocephalic vascular disease. This chapter is designed to give an overview of situations in which acute application of techniques of interventional neuroradiology should be considered. It also mentions diagnostic considerations in emergent conditions for which interventional techniques are potentially useful.

NEURORADIOLOGIC EVALUATION AND TREATMENT IN NECK AND SKULL BASE INJURIES

Vascular injuries resulting from trauma to the neck and skull base are significant causes of morbidity and mortality. This is especially true in cases of penetrating cervical trauma, wherein the most common serious injuries are vascular injuries.[1, 2]

Because the specific location of penetrating neck injury has major implications for the evaluation and treatment of underlying vascular injuries, the neck has been divided into three anatomic zones to facilitate management. Zone I includes the area between the sternal notch and the cricoid cartilage. Vascular structures within this region include the subclavian, common carotid, and vertebral arteries as well as the jugular veins. Zone II, the most common region for injury, lies between the cricoid cartilage and the angle of the mandible. Carotid, vertebral, and jugular injuries may result from penetrating trauma to zone II. Zone III, between the angle of the mandible and the skull base, is an area in which the common, internal, and external carotid arteries as well as the vertebral arteries and jugular veins are exposed to injury.

Surgical exposures for exploration of injuries involving zone I or zone III are extensive and carry significant risks. Management of zone I injuries, for example, frequently requires thoracotomy for proximal control of vessels. Surgical exploration of injuries in zones I or III is not recommended in the absence of preoperative angiography. Emergent angiographic evaluation is therefore routine in patients with penetrating injuries of zone I or zone III to determine the presence and extent of vascular damage prior to surgical exploration.

In contrast with zone I or III injuries, controversy surrounds the role of preoperative angiographic evaluation in the patient with penetrating injury involving zone II. The rate of significant arterial injury with penetrating trauma to zone II is approximately 12%. As expected by the anatomy, the common carotid artery (CCA) is the vessel most often affected, although injuries to other major vessels, including the internal carotid artery (ICA), external carotid artery (ECA), vertebral artery, and subclavian artery, occur in approximately 1%–2% of this patient population.[3] Two approaches have been developed for the acute management of penetrating injuries in this region: One approach recommends routine exploration of all penetrating injuries associated with violation of the platysma; the second advocates selective exploration based on preoperative evidence of injury to vascular, respiratory, or gastrointestinal structures. Factors cited to support routine exploration include the ease of relatively complete evaluation of injuries at the time of surgical exploration, the difficulty of delineating significant injuries prior to exploration, and the low morbidity of a surgical approach to this region.

A number of authors, however, recommend a more selective approach to zone II injuries, with a decision to operate based on clinical indications or radiographic findings suggesting vascular injury. Studies comparing the two methods of management have failed to show significant differences in outcome or cost of one method over the other. The varying opinions have led to the suggestion that arteriography be reserved for hemodynamically stable patients with clinical or radiographic features raising suspicion of carotid or vertebral injury.[3]

Therefore, in penetrating neck trauma, emergent angiographic evaluation is undertaken routinely for injuries above the angle of the mandible or below the cricoid cartilage (zones I or III). For penetrations between these levels (within zone II), the management, including the need for emergent angiography, must be individualized.

Vascular damage may also result from blunt head and neck trauma, particularly when associated with hyperextension of the neck or basal skull fracture. Although extracranial vessels are more often affected, intracranial vascular damage may occur as well.[4] Vascular injuries from blunt trauma are similar to those resulting from penetrating injury and include dissection, intimal disruption, vessel laceration, or pseudoaneurysm. Injury to the vessel wall may permit thrombus formation with occlusion of the vessel or the development of emboli to the CNS. Vascular injuries may remain asymptomatic or result in acute or delayed sequelae (including the formation of fistula or pseudoaneurysm) or the development of ischemic neurologic deficits. Most often the ICA is injured in its upper cervical portion or the region of the skull base, although other vessels, including external carotid branches and the vertebral artery, may also be damaged.

Dissection of the extracranial ICA occurring spontaneously and in association with head and neck trauma has been recognized with increasing frequency in recent years. The pathogenesis of "spontaneous" ICA dissection remains unclear and may represent a combination of factors, including both underlying vessel abnormality and mechanical factors including unrecognized trauma. A number of conditions affecting the vessel wall have been associated with spontaneous ICA dissection, including fibromuscular dysplasia, redundancy of the cervical ICA, hypertension, syphilis, familial occurrence of intracranial aneurysms with cervicocephalic dissection, and connective tissue disorders, including the Ehlers-Danlos and Marfan syndromes.[5–7] Such underlying abnormalities may increase the likelihood of vessel damage in association with minimal and otherwise subclinical trauma. In contrast with patients with spontaneous ICA dissection, evidence of underlying arterial disease is uncommon in patients with traumatic dissection.

ICA dissection in the setting of blunt trauma most often results from motor vehicle accidents. The upper cervical ICA at the level of C1–C2 is most commonly affected. Dissection should be suspected and angiographic evaluation performed if focal neurologic deficits, either acute or delayed, are not explained by traumatic lesions on computed tomography (CT) of the head. Additional clinical evidence for ICA dissection includes Horner's syndrome, amaurosis, or the presence of a bruit in a young patient.

Damage to the vertebral artery may also occur with blunt trauma of the neck, particularly in association with cervical spine injuries. Recent clinical and autopsy series have suggested that vertebral artery injury may accompany up to 46% of cases with fractures involving the foramen transversarium or subluxation with locked facets. The vertebral artery injury often remains asymptomatic and unrecognized. The most common angiographic finding has been complete occlusion, either at the origin of the vertebral artery or at the level of injury.[8] Adequate vertebrobasilar blood flow through the opposite vertebral artery accounts for the rarity of neurologic symptoms. Nevertheless, symptomatic brain stem ischemic symptoms have been reported to occur either acutely or with delay following injury, probably as a result of emboli formation in a patent but injured vessel.[9]

Angiographic evaluation in patients with trauma of the skull base and neck is tailored to the region of suspected injury. Imaging studies often considerably help to ensure complete angiographic evaluation of potential injuries. Evaluation may include the aortic arch to visualize the origins of the great vessels but often requires more selective catheterization for best imaging of head and neck vessels. Caution is necessary prior to placing a catheter into a potentially damaged vessel. More proximal injections should be performed initially if injury to a vessel origin is suspected.

Angiographic irregularity or stenosis of the lumen is the most common finding in arterial dissection. The angiographic finding may represent a spectrum of underlying vessel wall injury, ranging from arterial spasm to severe injury with dissection or laceration. Other cases may involve complete vessel occlusion, often with a tapered distal configuration in the acute phase. Other findings include abrupt widening of a more proximally narrowed vessel, pseudoaneurysm, or occasional visualization of an intimal flap. Arteriovenous shunting indicates fistula formation (see later). The intracranial circulation should be closely scrutinized for evidence of compromise, including slowing of intracranial flow or branch occlusion.[10] Traumatic vessel injury is often a dynamic process in which initial injury with narrowing or even angiographic occlusion may be followed by reopening and later development of chronic wall abnormalities including pseudoaneurysm.[11] Neurologic deficits may develop from perfusion compromise in luminal stenosis or from thromboembolic phenomena, often delayed, if persistent flow is present (Fig. 11–1).

Cervicocephalic arterial dissection infrequently requires emergent endovascular therapy. Nevertheless, appreciation of the condition and diagnostic findings is important should delayed neurologic deficits develop either as a result of flow compromise or embolization from the injured segment of the vessel. Often medical treatment of dissection with anticoagulants must be avoided or delayed in the face of other traumatic injuries. Such patients may be candidates for endovascular occlusion of the damaged vessel to prevent further neurologic damage.

Traumatic vascular injuries resulting in hemorrhage may require emergent neuroangiographic treatment. Facial injuries with damage to the ECA branches often present problems in localization of the site of bleeding. Angiographic identification of the exact site of hemorrhage using selective injections may be necessary, with endovascular treatment accomplished at the same time. Evidence

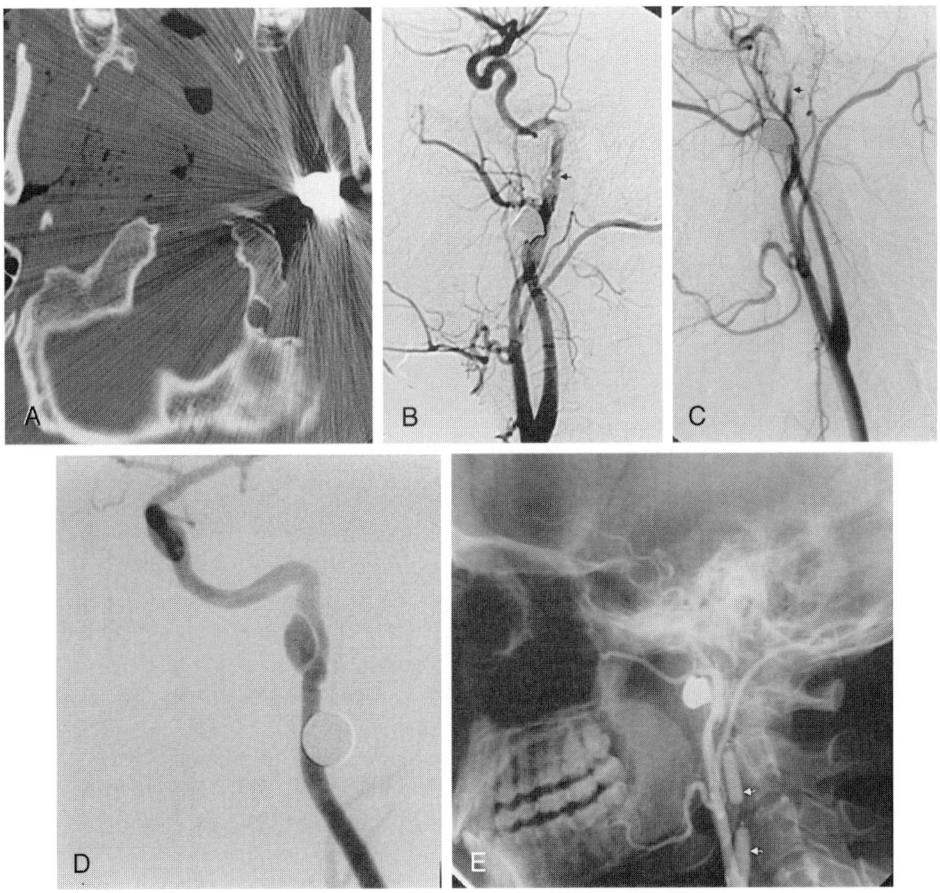

FIGURE 11-1 • A 23-year-old male admitted with a gunshot wound of the left side of the neck. *A,* Axial computed tomography (bone windows) shows location of bullet adjacent to the course of the left internal carotid artery (ICA). *B,* Left common carotid artery injection demonstrates mild irregularity just distal to the bullet location (arrow). *C,* Repeat angiogram 1 month later—increased narrowing of the upper cervical and petrous ICA (arrow) with delay in flow through the vessel. The patient was treated with anticoagulants. *D,* Left ICA injection 3 months later—development of pseudoaneurysm at the location of the previously noted irregularity of the vessel. The patient had experienced several transient episodes of right-sided weakness. *E,* Following 30-minute test occlusion of the ICA, permanent balloon occlusion was performed (arrow, balloon).

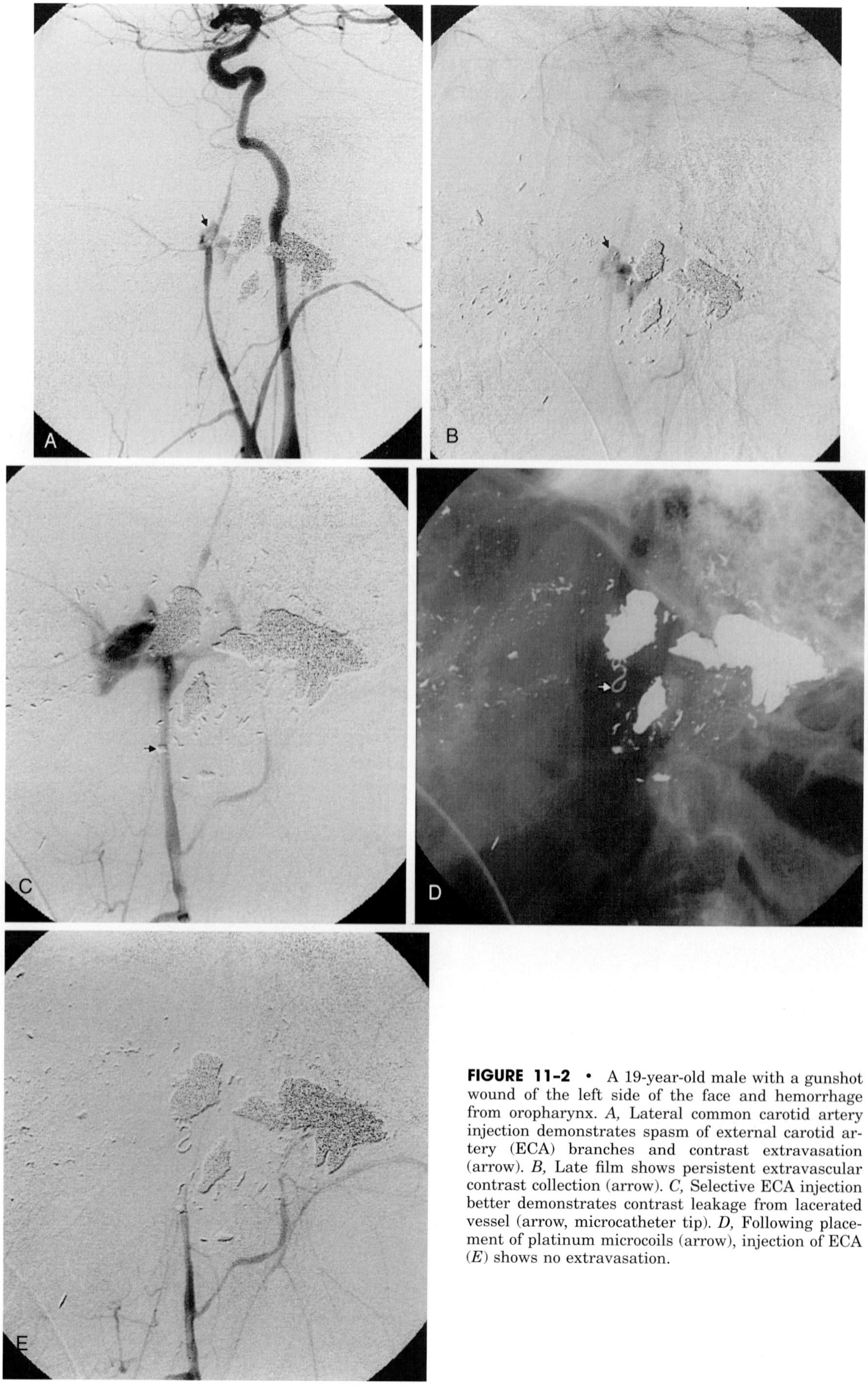

FIGURE 11–2 • A 19-year-old male with a gunshot wound of the left side of the face and hemorrhage from oropharynx. *A,* Lateral common carotid artery injection demonstrates spasm of external carotid artery (ECA) branches and contrast extravasation (arrow). *B,* Late film shows persistent extravascular contrast collection (arrow). *C,* Selective ECA injection better demonstrates contrast leakage from lacerated vessel (arrow, microcatheter tip). *D,* Following placement of platinum microcoils (arrow), injection of ECA (*E*) shows no extravasation.

of vascular injury, including vessel irregularity or pseudoaneurysm, is usually present; late-phase films should be evaluated to identify contrast extravasation. Hemorrhage originating from branches of the ECA often is best controlled by endovascular occlusion of the involved vessel. A microcatheter is selectively placed into the affected vessel, and the site of hemorrhage is confirmed with injection of contrast. Platinum microcoils or Gelfoam plugs are useful for acute hemorrhage control and may be precisely placed within the damaged branch, thereby sparing undamaged vessels in the vicinity (Figs. 11–2 and 11–3).

Traumatic ECA injury may also result in delayed hemorrhage following formation of pseudoaneurysm. Diagnosis requires angiographic evaluation. Occlusion of the involved ECA branch may be performed at the time of angiography (Fig. 11–4).

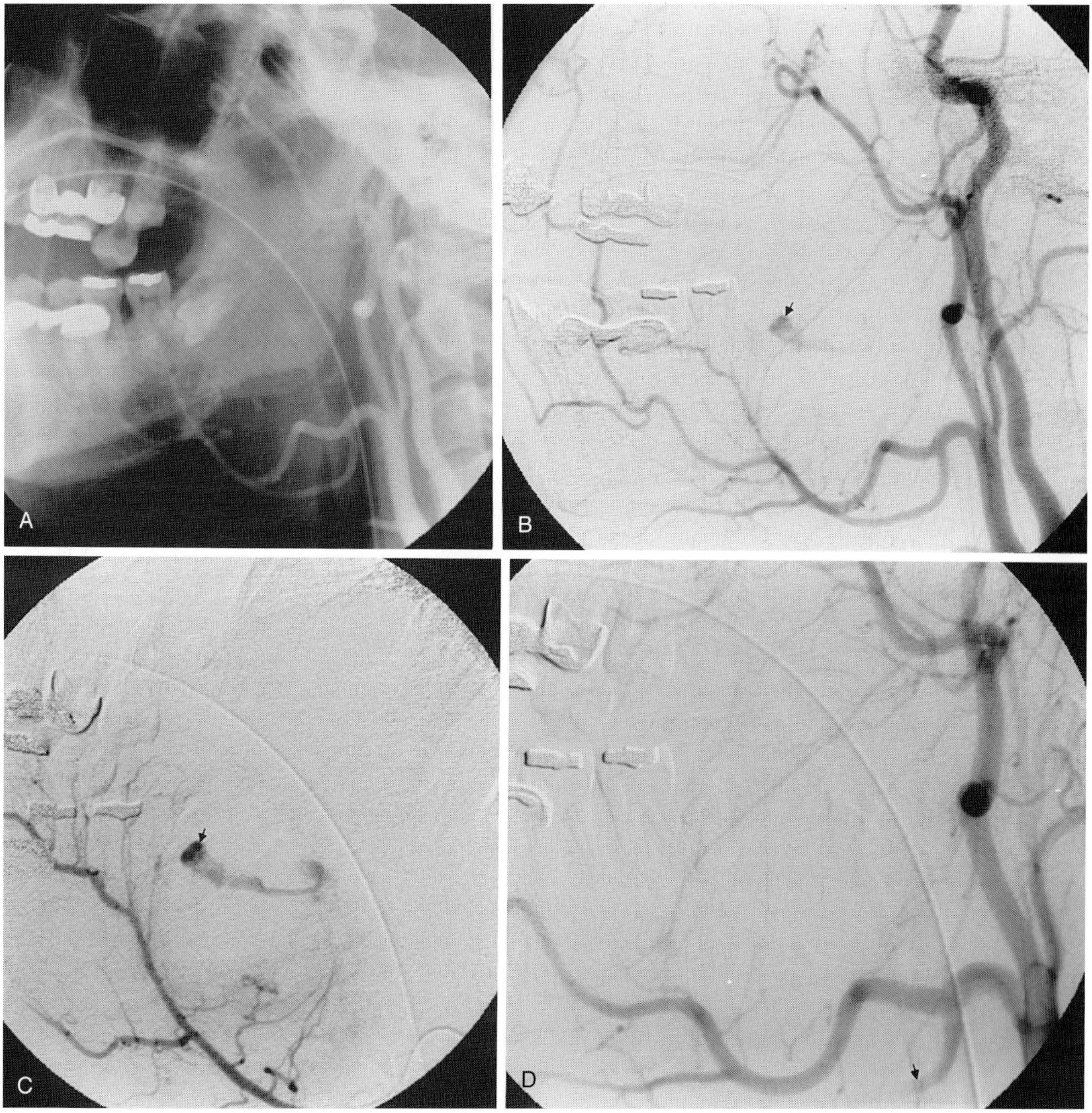

FIGURE 11–3 • A 21-year-old male post trauma with a mandibular fracture and severe hemorrhage from the mouth. Lateral unsubtracted (*A*) and subtracted (*B*) angiographic view of common carotid artery injection demonstrate extravasation of contrast into oral cavity (arrow) from external carotid artery branches. *C*, Subtracted lateral view of selective lingual artery injection identifies the site of extravasation (arrow). Selective embolization of lingual artery with Gelfoam was accomplished. D, Postembolization film shows stump of lingual artery (arrow) and no further extravasation.

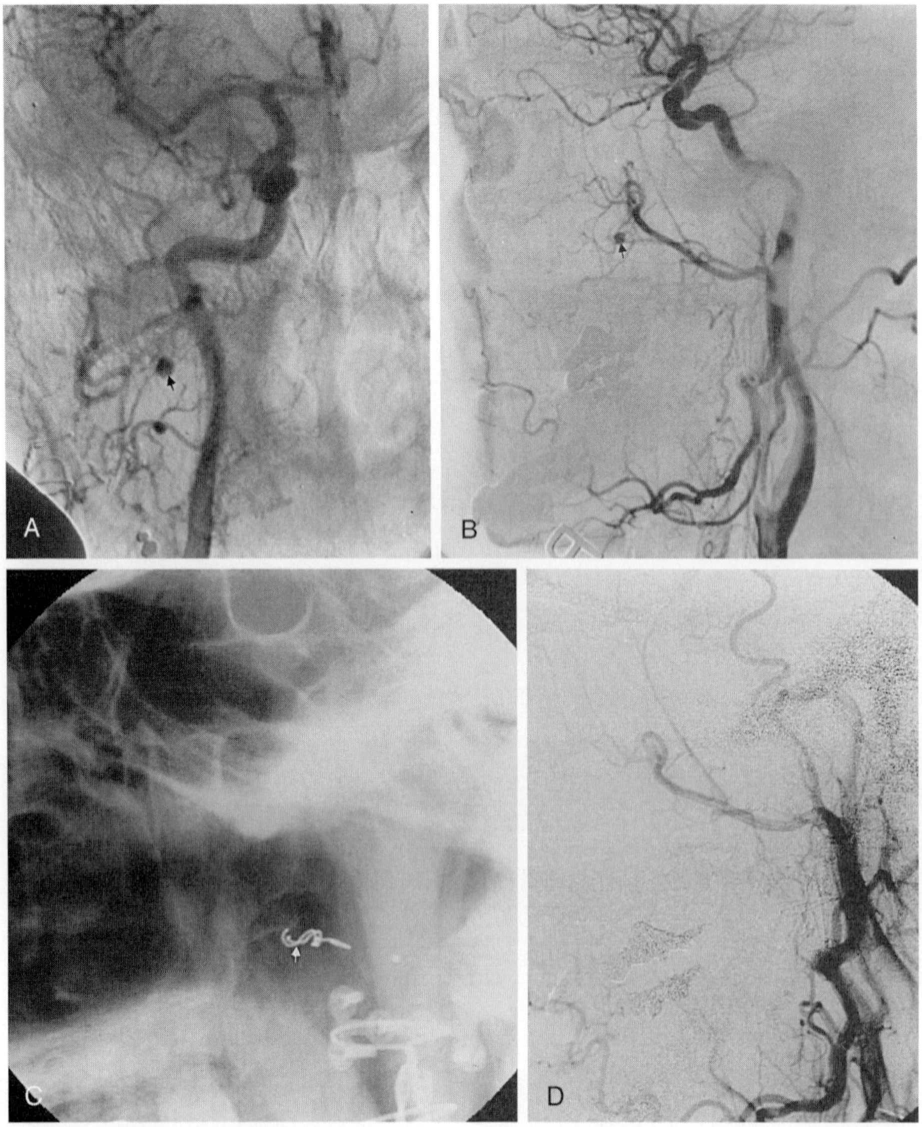

FIGURE 11–4 • A 43-year-old male with multiple facial trauma status following multiple reconstructive surgeries. New-onset severe epistaxis is present. Anteroposterior (*A*) and lateral (*B*) right common carotid artery injection shows aneurysm of the superior alveolar branch of the external carotid artery (arrow). *C,* Plain film following selective catheterization and placement of platinum microcoils (arrow) to occlude the vessel. *D,* Postembolization angiogram—no filling of the aneurysm.

Although extradural dissection of the internal carotid or vertebral arteries is infrequently associated with hemorrhage, laceration of these large vessels may result in life-threatening bleeding. In the petrous portion of the ICA or foraminal (second) portion of the vertebral artery, surrounding bony structures may prevent control of hemorrhage by direct compression, even in the operating room. Lacerations of the petrous or cavernous ICA can hemorrhage into the sphenoid sinus with resultant epistaxis. Petrous or cavernous ICA injury may result from surgical trauma or rarely from rupture of preexisting aneurysms (Fig. 11–5). The vertebral artery may also sustain damage from surgical or other penetrating trauma with life-threatening hemorrhage that requires emergent occlusion.

Endovascular occlusion of ICA or vertebral artery laceration is best performed by "trapping" or occluding the vessel both distally and proximally to the site of hemorrhage. Distal occlusion prevents retrograde flow from the intracranial circulation, which may allow continued hemorrhage if only proximal occlusion is performed.

CAROTID-CAVERNOUS FISTULA

A carotid-cavernous fistula (CCF) is an abnormal communication between the carotid arterial system and the cavernous sinus. A number of classifications for CCFs have been based on various features of the fistula, including: etiology of the fistula (traumatic versus spontaneous); speed of arteriovenous shunting (high versus low flow); and anatomy of the arterial supply (direct versus dural; internal carotid versus external carotid).

The type of CCF most commonly encountered as a result of trauma is the direct type of CCF. In contrast, dural arteriovenous fistulas involving the cavernous sinus are spontaneously developing lesions characterized by slower flow and are fed by dural

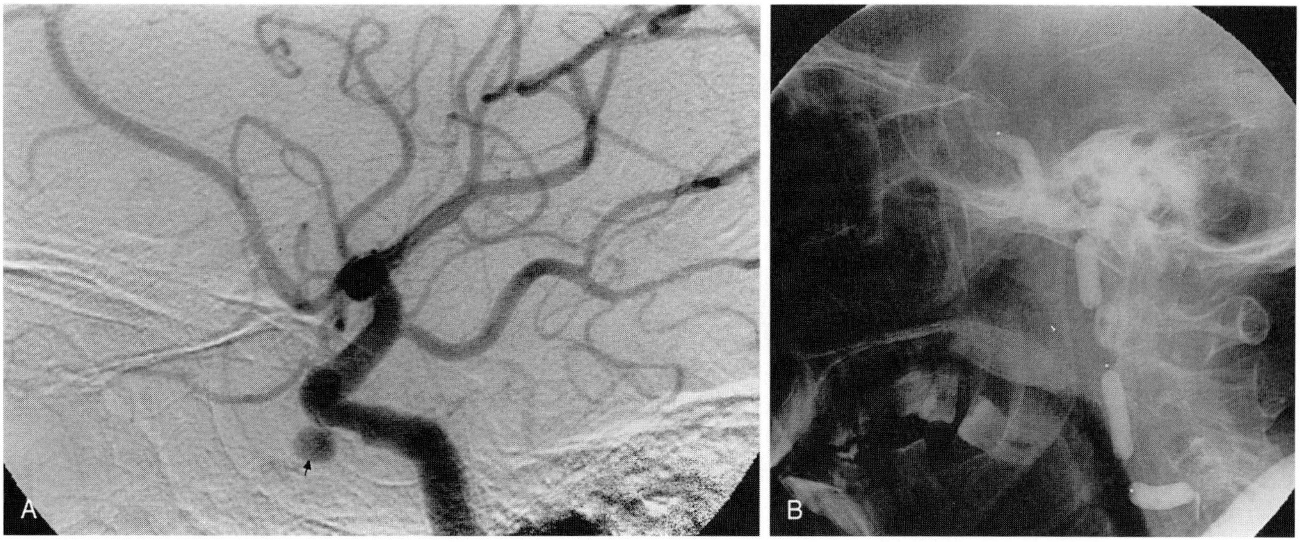

FIGURE 11-5 • While undergoing trans-sphenoidal hypophysectomy, this patient experienced uncontrollable hemorrhage within the sphenoid sinus. *A,* Angiogram shows pseudoaneurysm (arrow) of cavernous internal carotid artery (ICA). *B,* Immediate balloon occlusion of the ICA was performed with resolution of hemorrhage.

branches of the ICA or ECA. Dural arteriovenous fistulas are not further discussed in this chapter.

Direct CCFs most commonly arise following head trauma with laceration of the cavernous portion of the ICA. Because the cavernous ICA is surrounded by the venous channels of the cavernous sinus, arteriovenous shunting into the cavernous sinus is the result. The increased flow and pressure within the cavernous sinus results in retrograde filling of its venous tributaries as well as distention and dilation of the cavernous sinus itself.

Traumatic direct CCFs usually result from blunt trauma and are frequently associated with more obvious injuries, such as basal skull fracture, epidural hematoma, or cervical spine injury. Penetrating injuries to the orbit are a less common setting in which CCF may develop. As expected from the traumatic etiology, males are more frequently affected by traumatic CCF. Less frequently, iatrogenic injuries, including sinus surgery, percutaneous treatment of trigeminal neuralgia, and thromboendarterectomy of the ICA, have been associated with the development of CCF.

A direct CCF may uncommonly occur in the absence of trauma, usually from rupture of a preexisting aneurysm involving the cavernous ICA. Because of the higher female predominance of cavernous ICA aneurysm, spontaneous direct CCF affects females more frequently than males. Spontaneous development of a direct CCF has also been associated with congenital vascular anomalies, including persistent trigeminal artery and connective tissue disorders, such as fibromuscular dysplasia or Ehlers-Danlos syndrome.

Signs and symptoms of direct CCF may develop immediately following injury, but are commonly delayed in onset for days to weeks. Although signs and symptoms are most often ipsilateral to the CCF, drainage into the contralateral cavernous sinus may occur via the intercavernous sinuses. The drainage pattern can result in contralateral or even bilateral signs and symptoms. The increased flow through the fistula usually results in a bruit over the ipsilateral orbit. The pulse-synchronous bruit may appear prior to any other manifestations of the CCF.

Ocular manifestations are the most significant clinical features of CCF and result from retrograde flow into the superior and inferior ophthalmic veins. Engorgement of the orbital veins as well as congestion and edema of intraorbital soft tissue structures results. Manifestations include red eye, proptosis, diplopia, and visual loss. Proptosis affects virtually all patients with orbital drainage from a CCF and is most often associated with palpable ocular pulsation. Chemosis of the conjunctiva is usually present. Diplopia affects over 80% of patients with CCF and may result from mechanical impairment of ocular movement secondary to intraorbital congestion or from dysfunction of cranial nerves III, IV, and VI. Diplopia usually improves somewhat following endovascular treatment of the CCF. Complete resolution of diplopia occurs in only one-third of cases following treatment, however.

Visual loss associated with traumatic CCF is relatively common and has been noted in up to 21% of cases. Mechanisms of visual loss include traumatic optic neuropathy, reversible optic neuropathy due to arterial steal, venous stasis retinopathy, central retinal artery occlusion secondary to increased intraocular pressure, and glaucoma.[12]

Imaging findings in CCF include enlargement of the cavernous sinus and superior ophthalmic vein. Associated traumatic injuries may be identified, including fractures, cerebral contusion, or extracerebral hematoma.

Although best treated electively, CCF has several indications for emergent treatment. Progressive decline in vision is a major indication for emergent embolization of a CCF. Arterial steal from the CCF may cause symptomatic ischemia of the ipsilateral cerebral hemisphere. Although uncommon, this latter condition may also require emergent treatment to restore hemispheral perfusion. Retrograde venous drainage from the CCF into the pial veins of the brain is an additional indication for urgent treatment, to decrease the risk of intracranial hemorrhage.

Treatment of a CCF is directed toward closure of the abnormal arteriovenous shunt with preservation of the involved ICA. Currently available endovascular techniques make both goals feasible in approximately 80% of direct CCFs. Pre-embolization angiographic examination must evaluate a number of features of the cerebrovascular anatomy, including: the location and size of the fistula; the routes of venous drainage; collateral arterial routes to the involved cerebral hemisphere; and associated vascular injuries or anomalies.

Initial angiographic injections are directed at locating the site of the fistula. Locating the site of shunting enables more precise direction of embolization material into the arteriovenous shunt. The high flow through the CCF with rapid venous filling is frequently an impairment to exact localization of the fistula site. A number of techniques can assist in localization, including high-speed filming (15 frames per second), which sometimes permits localization of the arteriovenous shunt. In addition, ICA injection during manual compression of the ipsilateral CCA often slows filling of the fistula sufficiently to allow visualization of the site of arterial damage. Injection of the dominant vertebral artery during compression of the CCA ipsilateral to the fistula sometimes permits visualization of both the ICA distal to the fistula and the site of fistulization itself. Dissection, aneurysm, or other abnormality of the involved ICA must also be identified.

Injection of the opposite ICA is performed to permit evaluation of cross-filling via the anterior communicating artery. Damage to the opposite ICA, including aneurysm, atherosclerotic disease, or other arteriovenous fistulas, must be identified.

CCF treatment with detachable balloons results in successful fistula occlusion with preservation of the ICA in approximately 80% of cases. The balloon is placed across the fistula into the cavernous sinus and inflated, sealing the hole in the ICA while preserving flow through the vessel. The balloon is then detached within the cavernous sinus (Fig. 11–6). When balloon placement across the fistula is not possible, selective catheterization of the cavernous sinus with a microcatheter and placement of microcoils into the cavernous sinus may seal the fistula with preservation of the ICA. Recent reports suggest that a venous approach may be useful in some cases of CCF that cannot be closed via the arterial route. This technique may be more technically difficult and less frequently successful than the arterial approach.

Preservation of the involved ICA is not always feasible. In such cases, trapping of the fistula is necessary by closing the ICA both distal *and* proximal to the fistula. In no case should proximal occlusion of the ICA be performed in an attempt to treat a CCF. If only proximal occlusion is performed, arteriovenous shunting through the open fistula will continue from the intracranial circulation, possibly exacerbating symptoms of hemispheral ischemia. When trapping of the fistula is to be performed, the involved artery should undergo test occlusion under full systemic heparinization for a minimum of 30 minutes. The patient is closely monitored for development of neurologic deficits during the period of temporary carotid occlusion. After it has been demonstrated that the patient will tolerate ICA occlusion and if no abnormality of the contralateral carotid artery is present, trapping of the fistula is performed using detachable balloons placed both above and below the site of the fistula.

VERTEBROVENOUS FISTULA

Analogous to CCF, vertebral artery trauma may result in fistula formation to the vertebral venous plexus, most often in the upper cervical region. In contrast with CCF, however, penetrating trauma, including stab and bullet wounds, is most often the cause of a vertebrovenous fistula (VVF). Spontaneous VVF has also been associated with connective tissue disorders, as is the case with CCF.[7]

VVFs often present in a delayed fashion after trauma with a cervical bruit and neck pain. Neurologic deficits may result from arterial steal from the vertebrobasilar system or from compression of the cervical spinal cord or nerve roots by distended arterialized veins.

Angiographic evaluation of suspected VVF includes injection of both vertebral arteries. It is necessary to both evaluate the size of the contralateral vertebral artery and to determine the presence of retrograde filling of the fistula from the opposite vertebral artery. Evaluation of adjacent vessels, including ascending and deep cervical arteries as well as external carotid arteries, may be necessary to

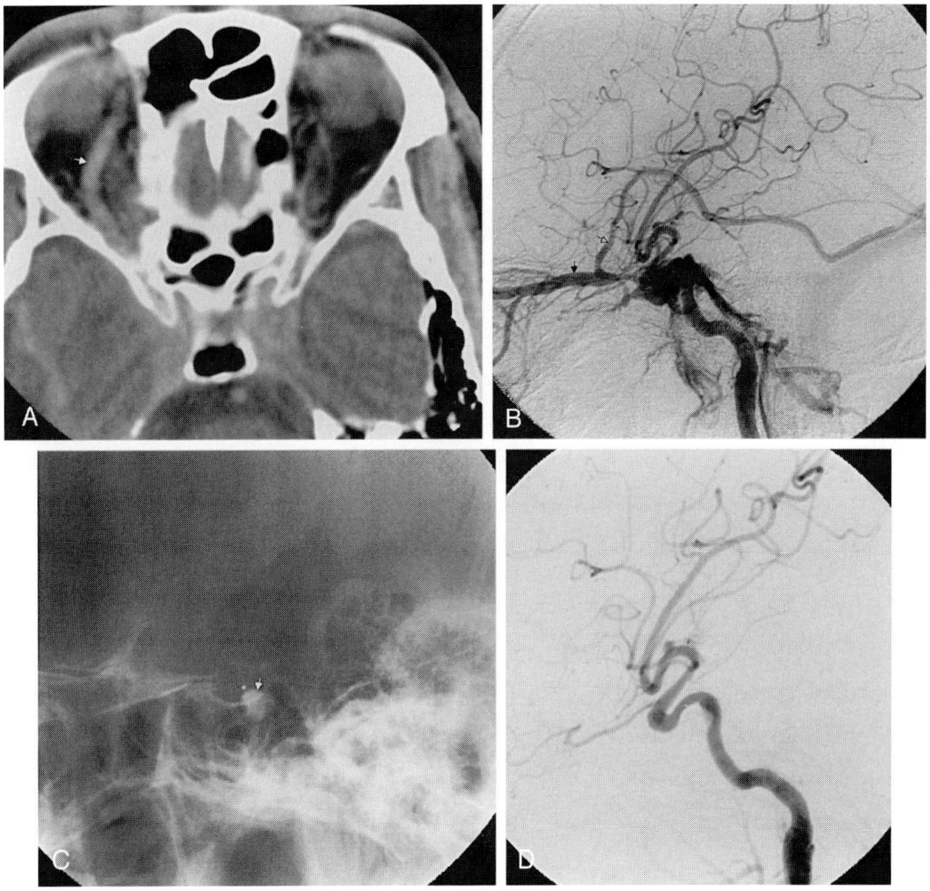

FIGURE 11–6 • A 57-year-old male developed right proptosis and orbital bruit following head trauma. *A,* Computed tomography demonstrates enlargement of the right superior ophthalmic vein (arrow). *B,* Lateral view of right internal carotid artery injection shows immediate filling of right cavernous sinus with retrograde filling of superior ophthalmic vein (arrow), superficial middle cerebral vein (open arrow), inferior petrosal sinus, and pterygoid venous plexus. *C,* Plain film shows contrast-filled balloon (arrow) placed across fistula into cavernous sinus. *D,* Post embolization film shows no further arteriovenous shunting.

exclude multiple sources of supply to the fistula. In the most common case of a single-hole VVF, detachable balloons or coils are placed across the fistula with preservation of the involved vertebral artery.[13] In cases with associated vertebral artery pseudoaneurysm or dissection wherein preservation of the involved vertebral artery is not possible, trapping of the fistula is performed. Occlusion of the vertebral artery above the fistula is followed by subsequent placement of balloons or coils across and proximal to the fistula (Fig. 11–7). Simple proximal occlusion of the vertebral artery without closure of the fistula must be avoided because it results in continued filling of the fistula from above with no route of vascular access.

REVASCULARIZATION PROCEDURES

Cerebral revascularization procedures refer to interventional neuroradiologic techniques for reperfusion of regions of the CNS that have been deprived of adequate blood flow. In all cases of cerebral ischemia, revascularization should be performed at the earliest possible time following the onset of ischemia to maximize the potential for recovery and minimize potential complications. Acute revascularization procedures include (1) intra-arterial thrombolysis for acute cerebral occlusion and pharmacologic dilation and (2) balloon angioplasty of intracranial vasospasm associated with subarachnoid hemorrhage (SAH).

Intra-Arterial Thrombolysis for Acute Cerebral Ischemia

The term *stroke* refers to a sudden-onset, nonconvulsive neurologic deficit of cerebrovascular origin. Strokes result from various mechanisms, including both ischemia and hemorrhage. Nearly 80% of strokes are ischemic, with the vast majority of ischemic strokes resulting from atherothrombotic or thromboembolic occlusion of large vessels supplying the CNS.[14] Emboli responsible for ischemic strokes usually originate from the extracranial carotid arteries or the heart. When patients with ischemic stroke are studied angiographically within 6 hours of onset, an occlusive vascular lesion correlating with the clinical deficit may be found in over 75%.[15, 16]

“Transient ischemic attacks” (TIAs) are ischemic neurologic deficits that, by definition, resolve completely within 24 hours. Determining whether an ischemic neurologic deficit is likely to resolve spontaneously is difficult but important in candidates

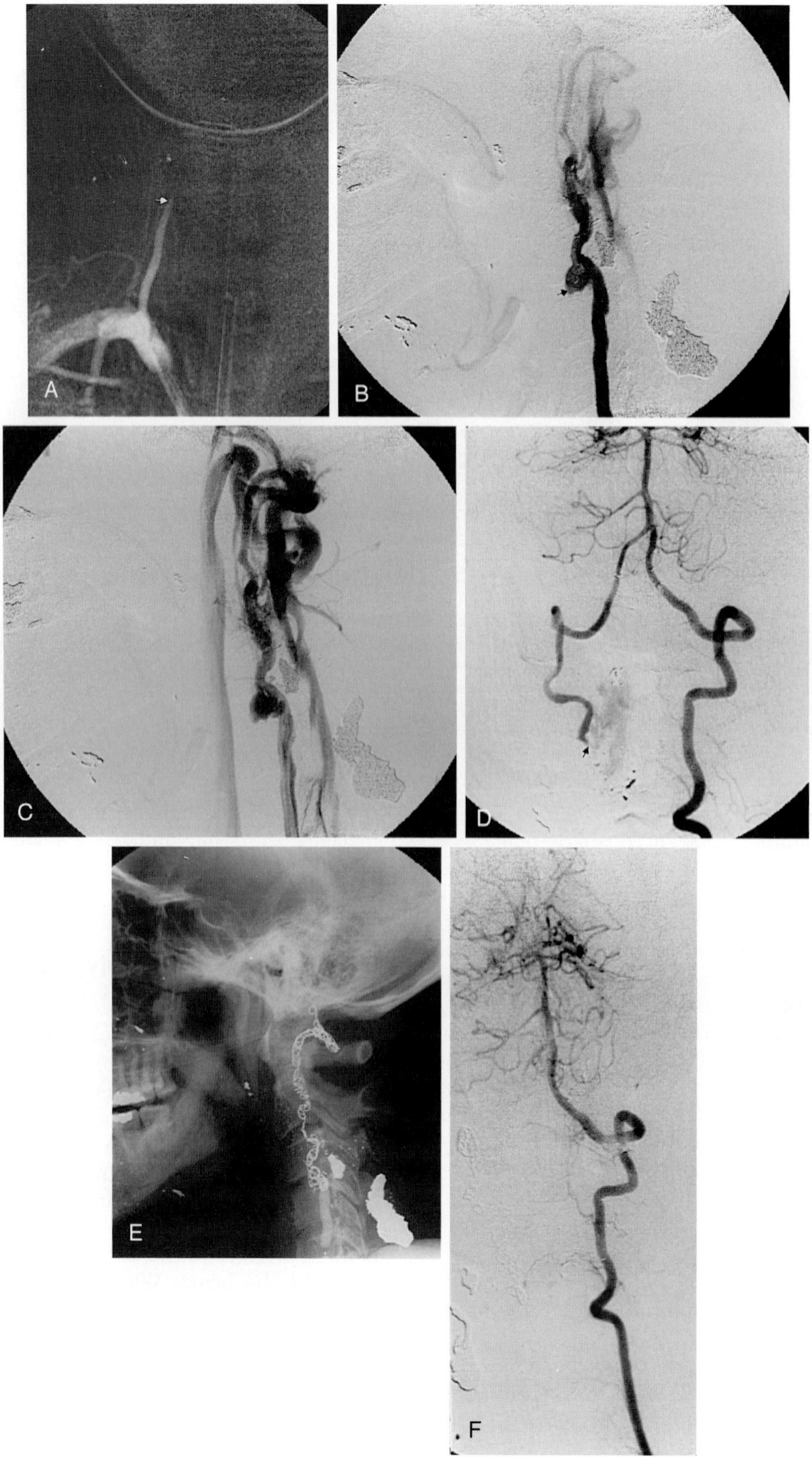

FIGURE 11-7 • *See legend on opposite page*

sponsible for nearly 80% of nontraumatic SAH. The mortality rate of aneurysmal SAH is estimated to be as high as 50%–65%, with the prognosis for survivors also grim. In addition, nearly two-thirds of patients discharged from the hospital never regain the quality of life experienced prior to rupture.[42] The risk of recurrent rupture following aneurysmal SAH is high, up to 2% per day for the first 2 weeks, with up to 50% in the first 6 months. A significant mortality rate, estimated to be as high as 60%, is also associated with each episode of rebleeding. Early surgical clipping of ruptured aneurysms minimizes rebleeding as a cause of significant morbidity. Currently, the leading contributor to both morbidity and mortality in patients surviving aneurysmal SAH is delayed ischemic deficit from intracranial vasospasm.

Following an episode of SAH, spasm is initiated by the presence of blood in the subarachnoid space. The pathophysiology of intracranial vasospasm is incompletely understood, although evidence has implicated a number of substances, including oxyhemoglobin, as potential etiologic agents.[43] Narrowing of the vessel lumen decreases blood flow to the cerebral parenchyma with consequent ischemia and infarction.

Angiographic vasospasm is common and may occur in as many as 75% of patients following aneurysmal SAH. Clinically symptomatic ischemic deficits are less common but occur in up to 30% of cases, usually between the fourth and twelfth day following SAH.

CT at the onset of SAH often suggests the risk of later development of vasospasm, with localized clot or a layer of subarachnoid blood greater than 1 mm thick indicating a particularly high risk. The hemorrhage location on CT correlates with both the distribution and the severity of the vasospasm.[44, 45]

Transcranial Doppler (TCD) permits noninvasive evaluation of flow velocities within the major intracranial arteries. Narrowing of the vessel lumen from vasospasm results in a proportional increase in flow velocity as long as constant flow is maintained. As vasospasm develops, increasing flow velocities are seen on serial TCD studies. Elevated flow velocities precede clinical ischemic deficits; patients who develop velocities indicative of severe spasm on or before the fifth day post hemorrhage appear to be at particularly high risk of subsequent infarction.[46] TCD monitoring permits close observation of high-risk patients for rapid institution of therapy if clinical vasospasm develops.

Medical management of vasospasm includes presurgical prophylactic treatment with calcium channel blockers. If clinical spasm develops after surgical clipping, volume expansion and induced hypertension have been found effective, with reversal of neurologic symptoms in over 80% of patients. Should delayed ischemic deficits fail to resolve with maximal medical treatment, interventional neuroradiologic therapy, including angioplasty and intra-arterial pharmacologic dilation, should be promptly considered.

Dilation or angioplasty of intracranial vessels with a balloon catheter was first reported in 1984 by Zubkov. Since then, multiple series have confirmed the clinical usefulness of intracranial angioplasty in the treatment of selected patients with symptomatic vasospasm.[47–49]

Intracranial angioplasty should be considered when ischemic neurologic deficits resulting from vasospasm persist despite medical therapy. Prior to angiography, CT is performed to exclude the most common differential causes for new-onset neurologic deficits, including rehemorrhage, hydrocephalus, and infarction. As with any treatment for cerebral ischemia, angioplasty should be performed as soon as possible after the onset of signs and symptoms.

Angiography is performed using a transfemoral approach with local anesthesia. The symptomatic vessel distribution is studied to confirm the presence of vasospasm. The smoothly contoured narrowing of the intracranial vessel lumen representing spasm is usually most severe in the distribution harboring the aneurysm. Angiographic spasm may result in either focal or diffuse narrowing of the contrast column. Irregular discontinuous areas of spasm may occur along a single vessel, often with a "beaded" appearance. With severe spasm, present in most symptomatic patients, slowing or delay of flow through the involved vessel distribution may occur[50, 51] (Figs. 11–10 and 11–11). Because intracranial vessel dilation should be performed only in vessel distributions not harboring an unclipped,

FIGURE 11–9 • A 57-year-old female with acute-onset right hemiplegia and aphasia. The patient had known atrial fibrillation. *A,* Anteroposterior view of left internal carotid artery injection demonstrates abrupt cutoff of superior trunk of the left middle cerebral artery (arrow) just distal to the origin from embolus. *B,* Microcatheter tip (arrow) at the origin of the occluded vessel and reflux of contrast into lenticulostriate arteries and into intact inferior trunk branches (open arrow). Abrupt cutoff of the superior trunk by the embolus is shown. *C,* Selective placement of catheter into the occluded trunk shows embolic occlusion (open arrow). *D,* After urokinase infusion was started, the occluded segment partially opened with some distal filling (open arrow). *E,* Following thrombolysis, good filling of previously occluded trunk is seen (arrow). The patient made excellent neurologic recovery.

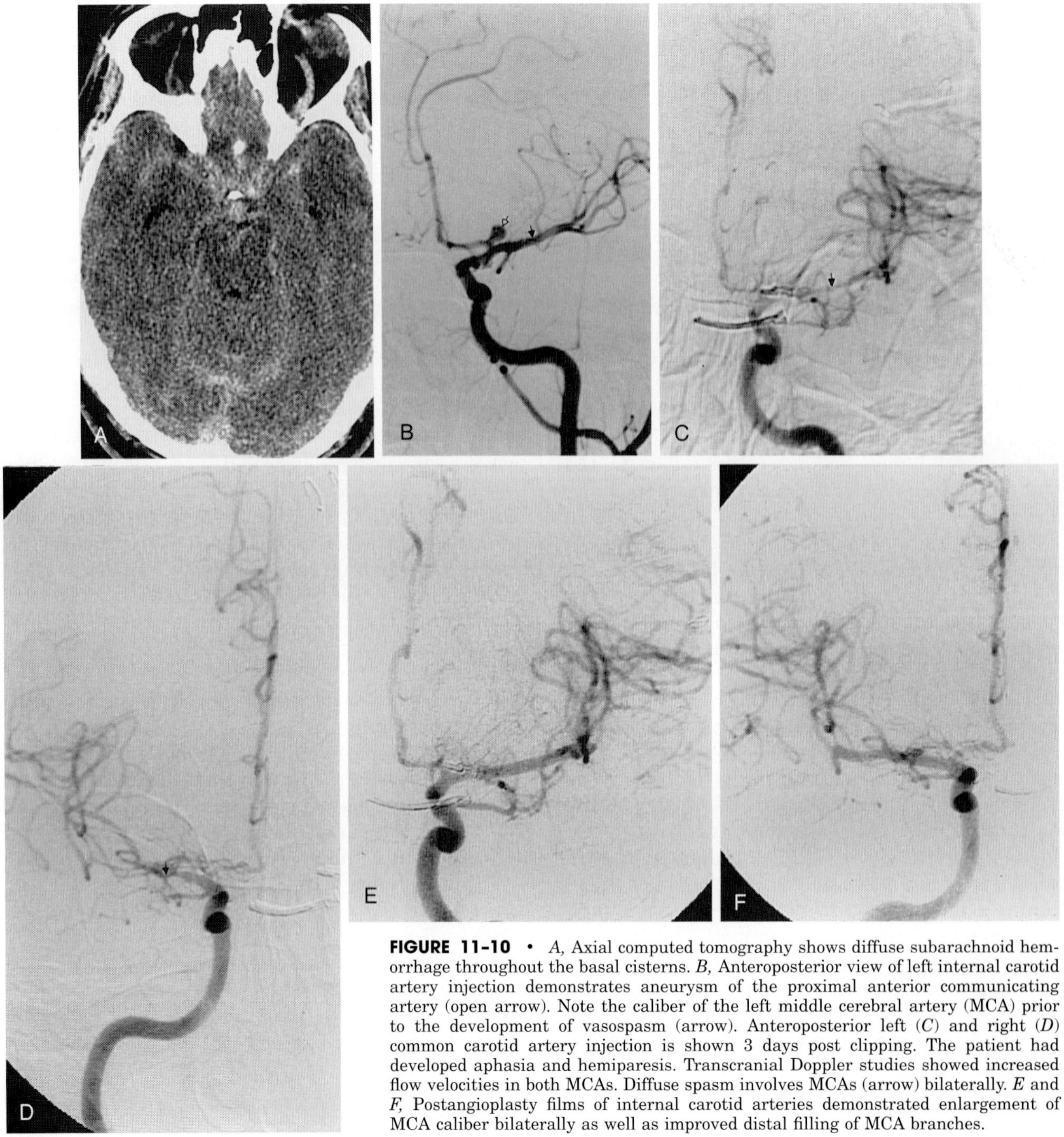

FIGURE 11-10 • *A,* Axial computed tomography shows diffuse subarachnoid hemorrhage throughout the basal cisterns. *B,* Anteroposterior view of left internal carotid artery injection demonstrates aneurysm of the proximal anterior communicating artery (open arrow). Note the caliber of the left middle cerebral artery (MCA) prior to the development of vasospasm (arrow). Anteroposterior left (*C*) and right (*D*) common carotid artery injection is shown 3 days post clipping. The patient had developed aphasia and hemiparesis. Transcranial Doppler studies showed increased flow velocities in both MCAs. Diffuse spasm involves MCAs (arrow) bilaterally. *E* and *F,* Postangioplasty films of internal carotid arteries demonstrated enlargement of MCA caliber bilaterally as well as improved distal filling of MCA branches.

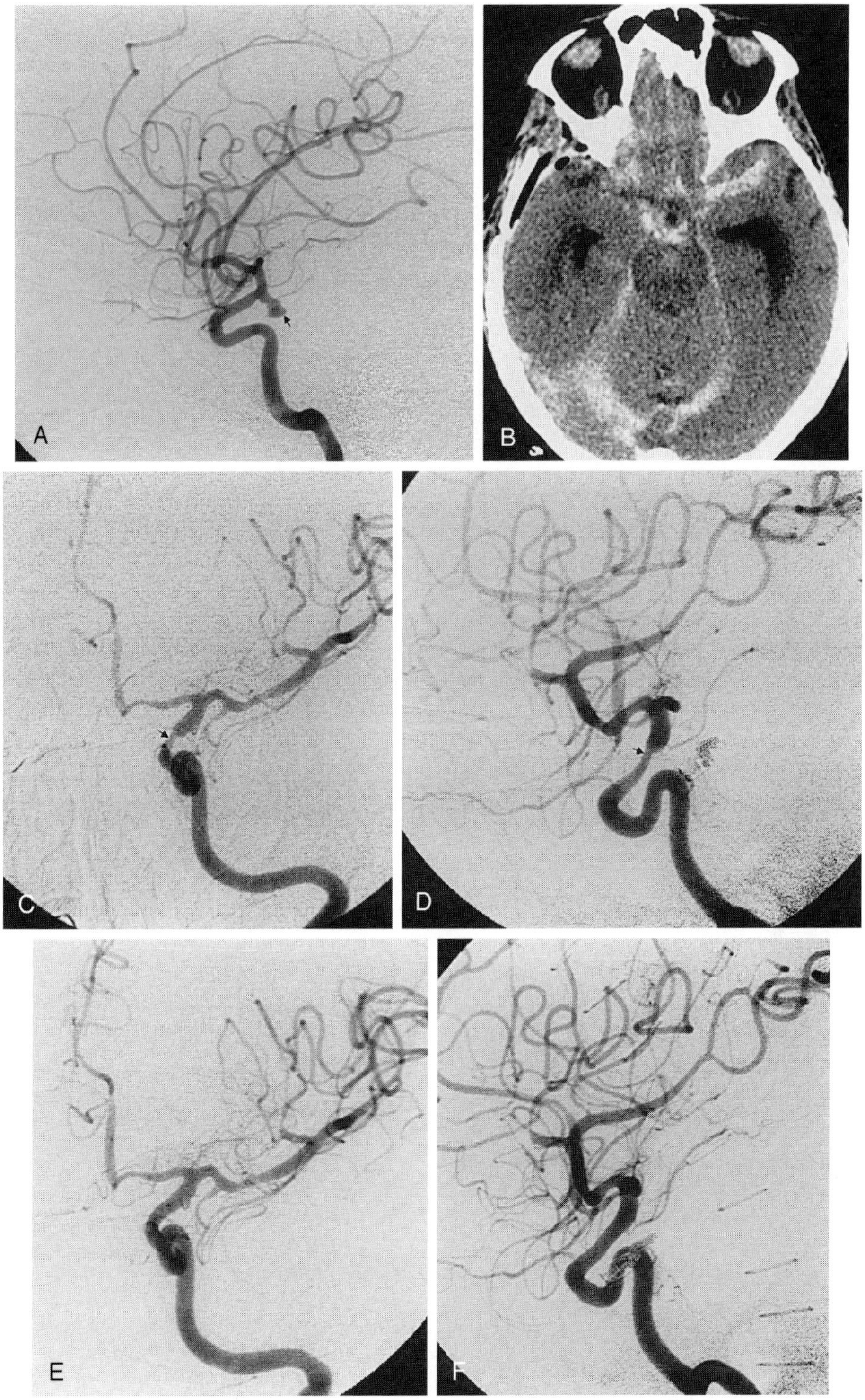

FIGURE 11-11 • A 47-year-old female experienced severe headache and nuchal rigidity. An angiogram (*A*) demonstrated an aneurysm of the posterior communicating artery (arrow). *B,* Computed tomography post clipping with considerable residual subarachnoid hemorrhage throughout basal cisterns. Left internal carotid artery (ICA) injection, in anteroposterior (*C*) and lateral (*D*) views, demonstrates a focal area of vasospasm (arrow) involving the supraclinoid ICA. Anteroposterior (*E*) and lateral (*F*) views post angioplasty show dilation of focal spasm. Transcranial Doppler velocities returned to normal, with resolution of aphasia.

previously ruptured aneurysm, exclusion of residual aneurysm is important before performing angioplasty.

Prior angiograms are helpful to exclude other uncommon etiologies of intracranial vessel narrowing, including intracranial atherosclerotic disease and vessel hypoplasia. A1 segment hypoplasia is associated with aneurysms of the anterior communicating artery complex and must be recognized, if present (Fig. 11–12).

Nondetachable microballoons for intracranial angioplasty include both silicone and latex types.

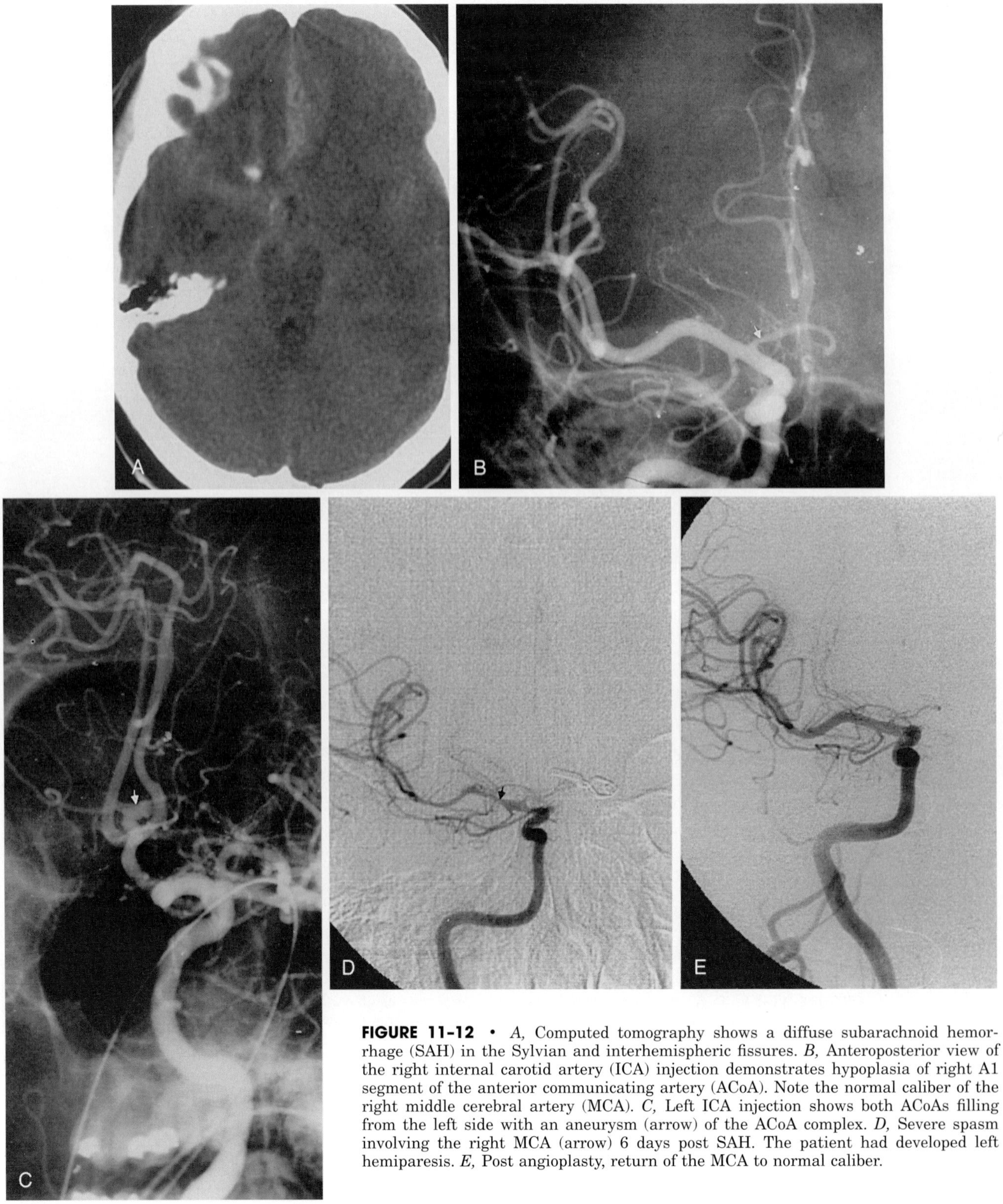

FIGURE 11-12 • *A,* Computed tomography shows a diffuse subarachnoid hemorrhage (SAH) in the Sylvian and interhemispheric fissures. *B,* Anteroposterior view of the right internal carotid artery (ICA) injection demonstrates hypoplasia of right A1 segment of the anterior communicating artery (ACoA). Note the normal caliber of the right middle cerebral artery (MCA). *C,* Left ICA injection shows both ACoAs filling from the left side with an aneurysm (arrow) of the ACoA complex. *D,* Severe spasm involving the right MCA (arrow) 6 days post SAH. The patient had developed left hemiparesis. *E,* Post angioplasty, return of the MCA to normal caliber.

Roadmapping is used to positively identify both the caliber of the vessel involved by the spasm and the length of the segment involved in spasm. After the involved vessel segment is roadmapped, the angioplasty catheter is advanced into the vessel either with or without the aid of a guidewire. Vessel dilation for vasospasm is performed with multiple transient gentle inflations of the balloon. Care is taken not to overinflate the balloon to a size larger than the normal caliber of the involved portion of the vessel. As dilation progresses, the balloon is advanced more distally to gain access to undilated segments of the artery. Following angioplasty for vasospasm, no angiographic evidence of dissection or anatomic disruption of the vessel wall should be present. Restoration of normal luminal caliber occurs throughout the treated portion of the vessel. Recurrence of vasospasm has not been observed in vessel segments treated by angioplasty.[52]

The size of available balloons limits intracranial angioplasty to the larger vessels, including the supraclinoid ICA, intracranial vertebral arteries, basilar artery, and proximal segments of anterior, middle, and posterior cerebral arteries. Attempts to subject more distal segments to angioplasty incur a high risk of vessel rupture with currently available balloon catheters. Angioplasty in the immediate vicinity of an aneurysm clip is also to be avoided because of the potential for clip dislodgment. Angiographically invisible vessel-wall defects have also been documented adjacent to intracranial aneurysms, which have resulted in vessel rupture when angioplasty is performed in the immediate vicinity.[53]

Following dilation, postangioplasty contrast injection is performed to ensure that all treatable segments of the involved vessel have been dilated. Following angioplasty of proximal vessels, filling of the more distal portions of the vascular distribution usually is improved.

Clinical improvement is reported in over 60% of patients treated with intracranial angioplasty. Infrequent instances of complications, including rare vessel rupture, have been reported, particularly if more distal segments are treated.[47–49] Postangioplasty, hypertensive hypervolemic therapy in the intensive care unit is continued. TCD studies following successful angioplasty show decreases in flow velocity in the treated vessel distributions. Persistently increased velocity on follow-up TCD studies suggests the development of new areas of spasm in previously uninvolved portions of the vessel.[54]

When vasospasm involves arterial branches that cannot be selectively catheterized or more distal branches where angioplasty is unsafe, intra-arterial infusion of vasodilating medication may be performed. A number of studies have documented the usefulness of intra-arterial papaverine infusion for the treatment of post-SAH vasospasm.[55, 56] Papaverine (300 mg) in 100 mL of normal saline solution is infused over 20 minutes to 1 hour. Infusion is directly into the involved vessel through a microcatheter. Results indicate a 65%–90% success rate in dilating arterial distributions involved by vasospasm.

Several reports of significant alterations in blood pressure, respiratory rate, and intracranial pressure during papaverine infusion indicate the necessity for close monitoring during the procedure. Unlike angioplasty, the effects of papaverine infusion are not necessarily permanent, and recurrent symptomatic vasospasm may develop in treated vessel distributions, requiring retreatment.

Interventional neuroradiologic treatment offers significant benefit to patients with intracranial vasospasm in whom medical treatment fails. These patients would otherwise be expected to sustain severe neurologic deficits resulting in permanent disability. Early identification of patients likely to develop vasospasm and aggressive application of interventional techniques in appropriate patients is important for the optimal management of post-SAH vasospasm.

SUMMARY

Recent developments in interventional neuroradiology have permitted new or improved treatments in a number of urgent situations involving cerebrovascular damage or disease. All physicians involved in the evaluation and treatment of patients with cerebrovascular and neurologic disorders should be aware of the potential benefits offered by these techniques, as well as the clinical situations in which their use should be considered.

References

1. Pinson C: The neck. In Trunkey D, Lewis F (eds): Current Therapy of Trauma. Baltimore, BC Decker, 1991.
2. Salander J, Coffey J: Cervical vascular injury. In Trunkey D, Lewis F (eds): Current Therapy of Trauma. Baltimore, BC Decker, 1991.
3. Asensio J, Valenziano C, Falcone R, Grosh J: Management of penetrating neck injuries. Surg Clin North Am 1991;71:267–396.
4. Morgen M, Besser M, Johnson I: Intracranial carotid injury in closed head trauma. J Neurosurg 1987;66:192–195.
5. Hart R, Easton J: Dissections of cervical and cerebral arteries. Neurol Clin 1983;1:155–182.
6. Barbour P, Castaldo J, Rae-Grant A, et al: Internal carotid artery redundancy is significantly associated with dissection. Stroke 1994;25:1202–1206.
7. Schievink W, Michels V, Piepgras D: Neurovascular manifestations of heritable connective tissue disorders. Stroke 1994;25:889–903.
8. Willis B, Greiner F: The incidence of vertebral artery injury after midcervical spine fracture or subluxation. Neurosurgery 1994;34:435–442.

9. Tulyapronchote R, Selhorst J, Malkoff M, Gomez C: Delayed sequelae of vertebral artery dissection and occult cervical fractures. Neurology 1994;44:1397–1399.
10. Fisher C, Ojemann RG, Roberson G: Spontaneous dissection of the cervicocerebral arteries. Can J Neurol Sci 1978;5:9–19.
11. Steinke W, Rautenberg W, Schwartz A, Hennerici M: Noninvasive monitoring of internal carotid artery dissection. Stroke 1994;25:998–1005.
12. Kupersmith M: Neurovascular Neuro-Ophthalmology, pp 69–108. Berlin, Springer-Verlag, 1993.
13. Halbach V, Higashida R, Hieshima G: Treatment of vertebral arteriovenous fistulas. AJNR 1988;9:741–749.
14. Mohr J, Caplan L, Melski J, et al: The Harvard cooperative stroke registry: A prospective registry. Neurology 1978;28:28–35.
15. Fieschi C, Argentino C, Lenzi G, et al: Clinical and instrumental evaluation of patients with ischemic stroke within the first six hours. J Neurol Sci 1989;91:311–321.
16. Sloan M: Thrombolysis and stroke. Arch Neurol 1987;44:748–768.
17. Levy D: How transient are transient ischemic attacks? Neurology 1988;38:674–677.
18. Koudstaal P, van Gijn J, Frenken C, et al: TIA, RIND, minor stroke: A continuum, or different subgroups. JNNP 1992;55:55–69.
19. Astrup J, Siesjo B, Symon L: Thresholds in cerebral ischemia—The ischemic penumbra. Stroke 1981;12:723–725.
20. Skyhoj-Olson T, Larsen B, Herring M, et al: Blood flow and vascular reactivity in collateral perfused brain tissue: Evidence of an ischemic penumbra in patients with acute stroke. Stroke 1983;14:332–341.
21. Teal P, Pessin M: Hemorrhagic transformation. Neurosurg Clin North Am 1992;3:601–610.
22. Liebeskind A, Chinichian A, Schechter M: The moving embolus seen during serial cerebral angiography. Stroke 1971;2:440–443.
23. Dalal P, Shah P, Sheth S, Deshpande C: Cerebral embolism angiographic observations in spontaneous clot lysis. Lancet 1965;i:61–64.
24. Lodder J: CT-detected hemorrhagic infarction: Relation with the size of the infarct and the presence of midline shift. Acta Neurol Scand 1984;70:329–335.
25. Okada Y, Yamaguchi T, Minematsu K: Hemorrhagic transformation in cerebral embolus. Stroke 1989;20:598–602.
26. Pessin M, Del Zoppo G, CJ E: Thrombolytic agents in the treatment of stroke. Clin Neuropharmacol 1990;13:271–289.
27. Hornig C, Dorndorf W, Agnoli A: Hemorrhagic cerebral infarction: A prospective study. Stroke 1986;17:174–185.
28. Weisberg L: Nonseptic cardiogenic cerebral embolic stroke: Clinical-CT correlations. Neurology 1985;35:896–900.
29. Levine S, Brott T: Thrombolytic therapy in cerebrovascular disorders. Prog Cardiovasc Dis 1992;34:235–262.
30. Mori E, Masayasu T, Yoshida T, Yamadori A: Intracarotid urokinase with thromboembolic occlusion of the middle cerebral artery. Stroke 1988;19:802–812.
31. Barnwell S, Clark W, Nguyem T, et al: Safety and efficacy of delayed intraarterial urokinase therapy with mechanical clot disruption for thromboembolic stroke. AJNR 1994;15:1817–1822.
32. Hacke W, Zeumer H, Ferbert A, et al: Intra-arterial thrombolytic therapy improves outcome in patients with acute vertebrobasilar occlusive disease. Stroke 1988;19:1216–1222.
33. Jungreis C, Wechsler L, Horton J: Intracranial thrombolysis via a catheter embedded in the clot. Stroke 1989;20:1578–1580.
34. Zeumer H, Freitag H, Gryska U, Neunzig H: Local intraarterial thrombolysis in acute vertebrobasilar occlusion. Neuroradiology 1989;31:336–340.
35. del Zoppo G, Ferbert A, Otis S, et al: Local intra-arterial fibrinolytic therapy in acute carotid territory stroke. Stroke 1988;19:307–313.
36. Wardlaw J, Warlow C: Thrombolysis in acute ischemic stroke: Does it work? Stroke 1992;23:1826–1839.
37. Matsumoto K, Satoh K: Topical intraarterial urokinase infusion for acute stroke. In Hacke W, del Zoppo G, Hirschberg M (eds): Thrombolytic Therapy in Acute Ischemic Stroke, pp 207–212. Berlin, Springer-Verlag, 1990.
38. Theron J, Courtheoux P, Casasco A: Local intraarterial fibrinolysis in carotid territory. AJNR 1989;10:753–756.
39. Mobius E, Berg-Dammer H, Kuhne D, Ahser H: Local thrombolytic therapy in acute basilar artery occlusion: Experience in 18 patients. In Hacke W, del Zoppo G, Hirschberg M (eds): Thrombolytic Therapy in Acute Ischemic Stroke, pp 213–215. Berlin, Springer-Verlag, 1991.
40. Sasaki O, Shifekazu T, Koike T, et al: Fibrinolytic therapy for acute embolic stroke: Intravenous, intracarotid, and intra-arterial local approaches. Neurosurgery 1995;36:246–253.
41. Saito I, Segawa H, Shiokawa Y: Middle cerebral artery occlusion: Correlation of computed tomography and angiography and clinical outcome. Stroke 1987;18:863–868.
42. Mohr J, Kistler J, Zabramski J, et al: Intracranial aneurysms. In Stroke Pathophysiology, Diagnosis and Management, Vol 2, pp 643–677. New York, Edinburgh, London, Melbourne, Churchill Livingstone, 1986.
43. Findlay J, MacDonald RL, Weir B: Current concepts of pathophysiology and management of cerebral vasospasm following aneurysmal subarachnoid hemorrhage. Cerebrovasc Brain Metab Rev 1992;3:336–361.
44. Kistler J, Crowell R, Davis R, et al: The relation of cerebral vasospasm to the extent and location of subarachnoid blood visualized by CT scan: A prospective study. Neurology 1983;33:424–436.
45. Adams H, Kassell N, Torner J, Haley E: Predicting cerebral ischemia after aneurysmal subarachnoid hemorrhage: Influences of clinical condition, CT results, and antifibrinolytic therapy. Neurology 1987;37:1586–1591.
46. Seiler R, Grolimund P, Aslid R, et al: Cerebral vasospasm evaluated by transcranial ultrasound correlated with clinical grade and CT visualized subarachnoid hemorrhage. J Neurosurg 1986;64:594–600.
47. Newell D, Eskridge J, Mayberg M, et al: Angioplasty for the treatment of symptomatic vasospasm following subarachnoid hemorrhage. Neurosurgery 1989;71:654–660.
48. Higashida R, Halbach V, Dowd C, et al: Intravascular balloon dilation therapy for intracranial arterial vasospasm: Patient selection, technique, and clinical results. Neurosurg Rev 1992;15:89–95.
49. Higashida R, Halbach V, Cahan L, et al: Transluminal angioplasty for treatment of intracranial arterial vasospasm. J Neurosurg 1989;71:648–653.
50. Kwak R, Niizuma H, Ohi T, Suzuki J: Angiographic study of cerebral vasospasm following rupture of intracranial aneurysms: Part 1. Time of appearance. Surg Neurol 1979;11:257–261.
51. Kwak R, Niizuma H, Ohi T, Suzuki J: Angiographic study of cerebral vasospasm following rupture of intracranial aneurysms: Part 2. Relation between the site of aneurysm and the occurrence of vasospasm. Surg Neurol 1979;11:263–267.
52. Yamamoto Y, Smith R, Bernanke D: Mechanism of action of balloon angioplasty in cerebral vasospasm. Neurosurgery 1992;30:1–6.
53. Linskey M, Horton J, Rao G, Yonas H: Fatal rupture of the intracranial carotid artery during transluminal angioplasty for vasospasm induced by subarachnoid hemorrhage. J Neurosurg 1991;74:985–990.
54. Hurst R, Schnee C, Raps E, et al: Role of transcranial Doppler in neuroradiological treatment of vasospasm. Stroke 1993;24:299–303.
55. Kaku Y, Yonekawa Y, Tsukahara T, Kazekawa K: Superselective intra-arterial infusion of papaverine for the treatment of cerebral vasospasm after subarachnoid hemorrhage. J Neurosurg 1992;77:842–847.
56. Kassell N, Helm G, Simmons N, et al: Treatment of cerebral vasospasm with intra-arterial papaverine. J Neurosurg 1992;77:848–852.

12

Pediatric Neuroemergencies With Intracranial Hypertension

Derek A. Bruce, M.B., Ch.B.

Many neurosurgical emergencies have—as at least a part of their pathophysiology—raised intracranial pressure (ICP) as a direct result of the central nervous system (CNS) lesion. The poor airway reflexes and reduced ventilation that often accompany unconsciousness cause a further elevation of the ICP. Thus, a clear understanding of the normal homeostasis inside the cranium is important for anyone caring for the child with an acute CNS emergency. Although raised ICP is only one of many physiologic and chemical disturbances that occur with CNS emergencies, it is one that lends itself to prevention and treatment and that is often the cause of death. It is simple to measure the ICP, making it a parameter that is easy to follow both in the emergency room and in the intensive care unit. Thus, although the importance of elevated ICP may be overstressed, it remains one of the causes of secondary brain injury that can be prevented.

Normal Intracranial Homeostasis

The intradural space (intracranial and intraspinal) contains three main components: cerebral tissue and spinal cord, cerebrospinal fluid (CSF), and cerebral blood volume (CBV).[1] The neural tissue accounts for 80% of the volume, CSF for 10%, and blood volume for 10%. Young infants and children have a relatively greater volume of CSF than do older children and adults.[2] There are normal variations in the ICP with each heart beat and with respiration. During cardiac systole, CBV increases; this is balanced somewhat by displacement of CSF from the cranium into the spinal subarachnoid space. During diastole, CSF returns from the spinal dural sack to the cranial cavity, thus limiting the alterations in pressure that occur. The primary factor that allows for any increase in the intradural volume is the compressibility of the epidural veins in the spinal canal. Under normal equilibrium conditions, the spinal epidural veins are distended and the spinal dura is not completely expanded. Thus, when volume increases in the cranium, CSF is displaced into the spinal dural sack until it is fully expanded. Up to this point, there is a small but real increase in the intradural volume accompanied by a small increase in ICP (Fig. 12–1).[3–7] The presence of an open fontanelle in the infant does permit small increases in intracranial volume as the fontanelle is distended, but this is inadequate to prevent acute intracranial hypertension. *The presence of an open fontanelle is no protection against raised ICP.*

The CSF is free to move from the lateral ventricles through the foramens of Monro into the third ventricle; through the aqueduct into the fourth ventricle; through the foramens of Luschka and Magendie into the subarachnoid spaces of the spine and cranium; and thence over the surface of the cerebrum to be absorbed predominately at the arachnoid villi in close relationship to the sagittal sinus.[8] The patency of these communicating spaces is important for the normal control of ICP. If the free communication of CSF through the ventricular system, into the spinal and cerebral subarachnoid spaces, through the tentorial hiatus, and across the arachnoid villi is impeded, the ability of the CSF to act as a major buffer for alteration in the volume of the other intracranial components is impeded, and the ICP will rise. Many of the acute pathologies associated with neuroemergencies result in interfer-

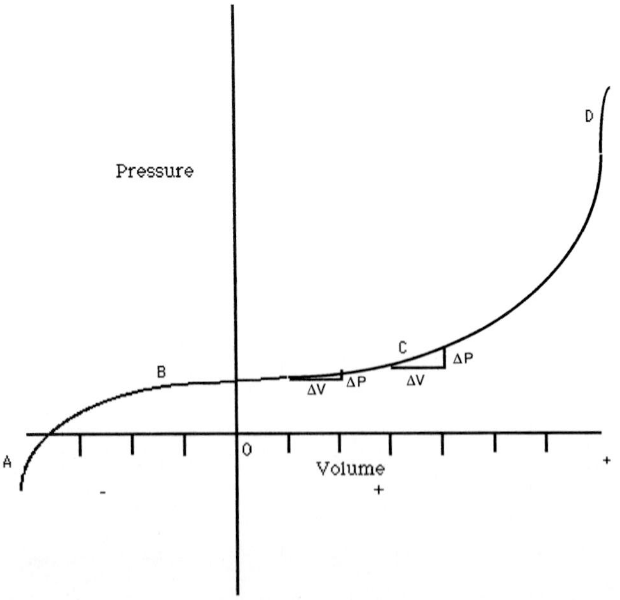

FIGURE 12-1 • A–B depict a period of decreasing spinal venous volume with increasing intradural volume and a small increase in intracranial pressure (ICP). B–C depict a period of compensation in which increase in volume of one component is offset by decreasing volume of the others, resulting in no change in ICP. C–D depict a period of lost compensation wherein further increases in intracranial volume cannot be compensated for by decreases in other components, resulting in a rapid increase in ICP. This portion of the curve is governed by the compressibility of the intracranial components.

ence with the circulation and absorption of CSF. When the CSF pathways are patent, displacement and absorption of CSF account for 80% of the buffering ability of the intradural space; thus, when the pathways are occluded, elevated ICP is common.

The CBV is the second factor in buffering within the intradural space.[9, 10] The majority of the intracranial blood is in the arachnoid veins, and much of this can be displaced into the venous sinuses with little increase in resistance to blood flow. Compression of the venous sinuses to compensate for increased ICP happens only late in the course of elevated ICP and only at very high ICPs.

The third factor in compensation is the cerebral tissue itself.[11] Although for many years the teaching has been that the brain is minimally compressible, this concept has to be revised. In the face of an expanding mass lesion, the brain is in fact quite compressible, even acutely, as is often the case when an acute epidural hematoma is scanned (Fig. 12–2). The brain can be compressed by several centimeters within a matter of minutes or hours. The compressibility of the brain depends on the elastic modulus of the cerebral tissue, and that is affected by the water content (e.g., edema), the presence of tumor or hematoma in the tissue, and the systemic arterial pressure. The higher the pressure and the poorer the vessel autoregulation, the stiffer the brain (i.e., the less easily it is compressed).

As a result of the ability of the three intracranial components to alter their volumes reciprocally, a certain volume can be added to the intracranial space without the ICP rising. The additional volume (e.g., a growing tumor) can be compensated for by decreased CSF, decreased venous blood volume, and cerebral distortion or compression up to some finite value. The actual tolerated volume depends on the rate of expansion, the location of the expanding lesion, and its effect on the spinal fluid pathway patency (see Fig. 12–1). The pressure-volume index is a measure of the amount of volume that is required to raise the ICP by a factor of 10.[12] This volume varies with the location of the patient's value on the pressure-volume curve and brain stiffness; therefore, any given increase in volume may be differently tolerated at different times in the patient's course. It is important to remember that the pathology varies over time and that treatment may need to be modified as time passes after the acute event has taken place.

The normal ICP in infants with open fontanelle is 5 mm Hg. The normal ICP once the fontanelle is closed is 10–15 mm Hg. The deleterious effects of elevated ICP appear to be predominantly related to the effect on local and general blood flow to the brain. The cerebral blood vessels exhibit pressure autoregulation such that under normal and many

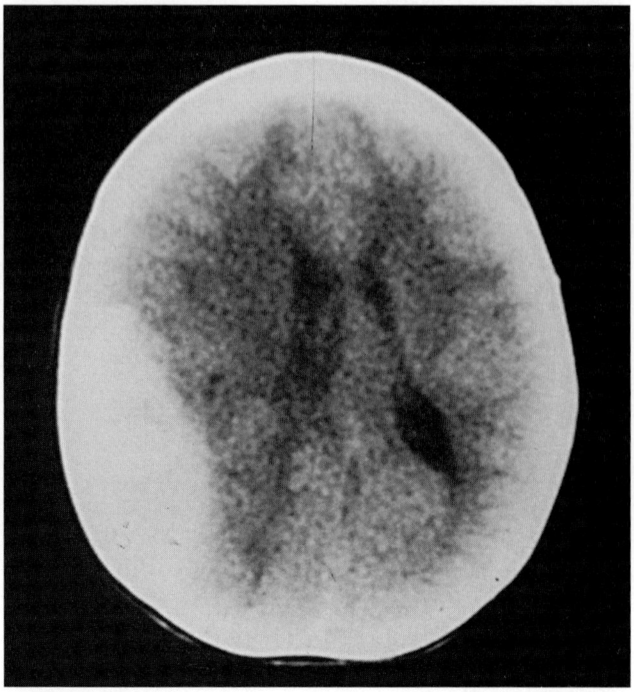

FIGURE 12-2 • Computed tomography of the head disclosing a large right temporoparietal acute epidural hematoma producing marked parenchymal and ventricular compression, as well as a midline shift.

ataxia, poor school performance, or occasionally mild dementia. They may also present in coma with no focal signs. In each of these situations, it is vital to consider the diagnosis of raised ICP and to perform the appropriate radiologic study. The sooner the child is treated, the better the chance of visual recovery. The appropriate therapy is a shunt, usually ventriculoperitoneal. Using mannitol, steroids, and hyperventilation is of no value unless the child is comatose and these measures are used to gain time to perform a scan to obtain the diagnosis. Currently, children who have acute hydrocephalus as a result of aqueductal stenosis may be treated by third-ventriculostomy and a temporary ventricular drain. If this works, it avoids the need for a permanent shunt.

If the hydrocephalus is secondary to another pathology (e.g., tumor or hemorrhage), the treatment of the acute hydrocephalus depends on the clinical state of the child. If the child has disturbed consciousness, a ventricular drain, a shunt, or a third-ventriculostomy is required to relieve the pressure. If the level of consciousness is normal, the child may be treated with steroids for several days prior to definitive neurosurgical removal of the primary tumor.

Most of these children do not require intubation and ventilation but require acute relief of the hydrocephalus. Intravenous steroids and acetazolamide (Diamox) may help control the ICP for a day or two to allow for a full neuroradiologic evaluation and selection of the best surgical therapy.

Chronic subdural collections do occur in infants and often result in an acute presentation with vomiting, irritability or somnolence, failure to thrive, anemia, and a bulging fontanelle. The diagnosis is made by CT. If acute therapy to lower the ICP is required, this is best done with a fontanelle tap. Although the condition of a few of these children may be the result of abuse, this is rare; we currently do not know the etiology of these lesions that usually present in the first few months of life. They may well be the result of tearing of a bridging vein at birth and repeated hemorrhage with crying and straining. The definitive therapy is usually a subdural-peritoneal shunt.

The most frequent presentation of acute hydrocephalus is a child with a blocked or malfunctioning shunt. Because these children are used to having relatively low pressures and have an inadequate ability to absorb their CSF, they can rapidly go from being awake with only complaints of waves of pressure to respiratory arrest; an accurate diagnosis is vital as early in the course of the shunt block as possible. A pumping device is incorporated into most shunt systems, and because there are many types of shunts on the market the ER physician has to be aware of the kind of device used by the local neurosurgeons. If there is any doubt, a plain radiograph will show the shunting device. The clue to the correct diagnosis is always the history. The parents must be listened to; even if the story sounds strange, they must be given attention. If a child has had a previous shunt block and the parent says "this is just like the last time" or "this is always how he presents when the shunt blocks," listen to the parent and check the shunt. The clinical examination may help by showing listlessness or coma. Papilledema may be present or CSF collected around the shunt. Usually, however, the history and the parent's observations are the best clues. If the shunt has a pump, this can be depressed and should empty and refill easily. However, interpretation of the pumping device can be difficult, and CT and shunt survey are required. Interpretation of the CT scan can be difficult if no previous scan is available for comparison. Some children never develop significant ventriculomegaly, whereas others normally have enlarged ventricles even if the shunt is working. If the shunt is blocked, the next step is neurosurgical consultation. Often the shunt is tapped to establish whether the pressure can be acutely relieved and which end of the shunt, proximal or distal, is likely to be the problem. If the proximal end or valve is the problem, the shunt is usually revised acutely that day or night. If the distal end is the problem, CSF can be drained, the pressure lowered, and often surgical revision postponed until a cell count and Gram's stain are performed. Abdominal ultrasonography may be indicated to seek the reason for the distal block, which is often due to infection. If the child's symptoms recur while waiting, the shunt must be re-tapped and more CSF removed. The child should not be treated with narcotics for the headache. Headache is a sign of raised ICP, and the correct therapy is to lower the ICP. If the headache recurs frequently, it is safer to go ahead and revise the shunt. All children with shunt obstruction are at risk for pressure waves and sudden respiratory arrest.

There is a group of children who have been referred to as having "slit ventricle" syndrome.[33, 34] This defines a group of children in whom, even when the shunt is not working, ventricular dilatation does not occur. These children can be difficult to diagnose and manage. The major difficulty in an emergency is to try to decide whether the child's symptoms are due to low or high ICP, because the finding of small ventricles can be the result of overdrainage of the shunt as well as a manifestation of slit ventricle syndrome, in which the symptoms are due to high pressure. These children require pediatric neurosurgical consultation.

Pseudotumor Cerebri

In this condition, the presentation is usually severe headaches, progressive visual loss (central scotomas and color vision first), and third- or sixth-nerve palsy. The examination must include evaluation of the optic fundi, because papilledema or optic pallor may be the only definitive sign. There are children in whom headache is only a minor or minimal problem, yet vision is severely compromised. Often these children have been seen by a physician and, because no funduscopic examination was performed, the diagnosis was missed. The setting is often of an overweight child, preteen, or teenager, but pseudotumor can occur in toddlers. CT or MRI shows no focal abnormality with normal or small ventricles. The diagnosis is then confirmed by a spinal tap that shows markedly elevated CSF pressure. Acute therapy is with steroids and acetazolamide or furosemide (Lasix). If the visual examination shows central scotomas, loss of acuity, or chronic papilledema with optic atrophy, acute decompression is necessary; this is usually accomplished by lumboperitoneal shunt. If only one nerve is severely involved, decompression of the optic nerve sheath may be successful. The underlying pathology appears to be an increase in outflow resistance to CSF with normal brain elastance, such that ventriculomegaly does not occur.[35–37] This can occur after withdrawal of steroids, after use of antibiotics, and with excess vitamin A, but in most cases the etiology is not known. The challenge is to make the diagnosis before there is irreversible visual loss.

Neoplasia

Most brain tumors have a chronic presentation, but some present as an acute neurologic emergency. These are most frequently the result of decompensation of chronically increased ICP. The mechanisms are: acute hydrocephalus; cerebral herniation from mass effect; hemorrhage into the tumor; cortical tumor or metastases producing seizures; and acute stroke due to vessel occlusion by the tumor.

The most common acute presentation is that of decompensation of hydrocephalus. This is similar to the signs and symptoms of any acute hydrocephalus. It is most frequent with midline tumors—intraventricular, peri-aqueductal, or in the posterior fossa. There may be long history of morning headaches, vomiting, or both, and there may be local neurologic findings related to the location of the tumor. The investigation involves either CT or MRI with and without contrast. The treatment is as described earlier for children with acute hydrocephalus and may include steroids, ventricular drainage, third-ventriculostomy, or shunt or tumor resection, depending on the state of the child, the size of the ventricles, and the size and location of the tumor. If no intracranial tumor is seen on scan it must be remembered that spinal cord tumors occasionally present with hydrocephalus. Thus, a complete neurologic examination is mandatory.

Children who present with headache and an acute decrease of level of consciousness with or without signs of cerebral herniation (pupil dilatation, extraocular palsies, or vital sign changes) are likely to have a large supratentorial mass, often with surrounding edema. There is usually a past history of headaches. The major thrust is to establish an airway and ventilation if the child is in coma followed by CT or MRI, preferably MRI. If the child is not severely obtunded and the airway is preserved, a scan is obtained without prior endotracheal intubation. Once again, the therapy depends on the rate of change of consciousness, current responsiveness and location of tumor, and degree of midline shift on the scan. Emergency tumor resection often is warranted in this setting. As with all other acute ICP problems associated with mass lesions, it is ideal to calm down the ICP prior to definitive surgery, but this is not always possible.

Hemorrhage into a pre-existing tumor occurs in 5%–10% of pediatric tumors. Usually the tumor is rapidly growing (e.g., primitive neuroectodermal tumors—medulloblastoma). The presentation is usually of headache and an acutely deteriorating level of consciousness. The symptoms and signs are just like any other intracerebral bleed but often there is a pre-existing history of headache or focal neurologic deficit. Management is standard—the ABCs. The scan can easily be misinterpreted as a bleed due to a ruptured AVM unless the possibility of a tumor is considered and contrast given. Treatment depends on the condition of the child and may be surgical or medical with or without ICP monitoring.

Seizures as a presentation of brain tumor are uncommon but certainly occur with cortical tumors or when there are tumor metastases over the cortex. They are more common with tumor recurrence; thus, it is important to seek a history of any previous CNS involvement. The cortical metastases may be hard to see on standard scans, and initially only an inferential diagnosis may be made. If there is no intracranial mass effect, a lumbar puncture or shunt tap to look for cells in the CSF is performed. Treatment of the seizures is as for any other seizure problem. Treatment of the metastases is usually elective, and most of these children do not have elevated ICP unless there is a recurrent tumor mass or acute hydrocephalus as a result of CSF pathway obstruction from the metastases.

Stroke is an uncommon presentation in children

with brain tumors but can occur in two settings. The first is usually in an infant or toddler with a chiasmatic hypothalamic glioma that produces elongation and then occlusion of the carotid artery or one of its major branches. The stroke is usually hemispheral and therefore can be associated with brain swelling, herniation, and raised ICP. Many of these children have a large tumor already taking up room in the cranium and may also have hydrocephalus such that the additional volume of the swollen hemisphere can produce decompensation and high ICP. The second setting is in a child who has been irradiated in the suprasellar area years previously for tumor, usually chiasmatic hypothalamic glioma or craniopharyngioma. These children can develop Moya-Moya disease with occlusion of the major vessels and hemispheral stroke, hemorrhage, or both.

Infections

Although meningitis is often accompanied by mild elevations in ICP because of blocked arachnoid villi and poor flow of CSF through the inflamed subarachnoid spaces,[38] it is rarely a major problem, and ICP monitoring and therapy for elevated ICP are usually not necessary. In tuberculous meningitis, acute hydrocephalus is common, and ventricular drainage or a ventriculoperitoneal shunt may be required. Acute hydrocephalus can occur in other forms of meningitis; in the child who is not doing well, CT may show acute hydrocephalus that requires drainage.

If severe cerebritis is leading to seizures that require ventilation and paralysis for control, an ICP monitor may be helpful because the level of consciousness can no longer be used as a measure. Chronic fungal meningitis can present with hydrocephalus.

In most cases of encephalitis, the ICP is not elevated. However, in the hemorrhagic encephalitides (e.g., herpes simplex, Rocky Mountain spotted fever), the ICP may be very high and ICP monitoring helpful in the overall care of the child.

Brain abscesses are not common but account for a small percentage of mass lesions in the United States in children. In Mexico, cysticercosis is one the most frequent causes of an intracranial mass lesion. Thus, the incidence of intracranial mass lesion due to an infectious etiology varies widely from country to country. In the United States, sinus infections are the most common association with brain abscesses in children, especially from the frontal sinus. Spread is probably through septic thrombophlebitis with a resultant frontal lobe abscess. Other associations are with congenital heart disease and endocarditis. Presentation is usually severe headache with or without fever. The presence of localizing neurologic findings depends on the location of the abscess. The white cell count and sedimentation rate are usually elevated, but not always. Diagnosis is made by history and scan with contrast. Once again, depending on the location, size, and number of the abscesses, therapy varies.[39, 40] If the patient is showing an altered level of consciousness with a large mass lesion with edema, acute needle aspiration of the lesion is necessary to relieve the herniation and ICP. Repeated aspiration may be needed and with appropriate antibiotics usually is all that is required. It is uncommon to have to perform craniotomy and excision of the abscess. Another reason for acute aspiration of the abscess is to obtain pus for culture and to select the appropriate antibiotic. Acute onset of coma can occur with rupture of the abscess into the ventricle. This is usually manifested by high fever and a severely "toxic" child.

Subdural or subarachnoid high-protein CSF collections are common in infants treated for meningitis. These collections are probably not subdural but in fact subarachnoid. They are usually identified after several days of therapy in a child who is continuing to have fever despite assumed adequate antibiotic therapy. These rarely ever produce raised ICP and are rarely the site of residual organisms. Contrast CT can help in that if the membranes enhance, the risk of an infected collection is higher and surgical drainage and culture may be warranted. Most of the time these collections resolve spontaneously and do not need therapy.

Epidural empyema is rare but presents usually after cranial surgery, sinus infection, or trauma. Symptoms and signs are of severe headache, possible obtundation, and rarely focal abnormalities unless there is underlying septic venous thrombosis or subdural empyema. Treatment in the past has always been emergency craniotomy. This is not always necessary and depends on the patient's condition, the presence of other positive cultures (e.g., blood), and the size and location of the lesion.[41] If the lesion is small, burr holes and irrigation may be adequate; if it is larger, craniotomy is required.

Subdural empyema usually results from meningitis or sinusitis with cerebral venous thrombophlebitis. The lesion, especially in small children, is often diffuse in the interhemispheric fissure as well as over both hemispheres.[41, 42] The cause of the elevated ICP is usually underlying cerebritis and brain swelling rather than just the mass of the empyema. This plays a role in the decision to perform surgery or not, because the brain can be swollen and inflamed, and surgery can result in further cortical injury. Seizures that are difficult to control often accompany subdural empyema. Although classic teaching has been that acute craniotomy is required, this is no longer true. If the infection can be treated with antibiotics and usually steroids and if the clinical condition improves, it is possible to avoid surgery altogether in some children. In others, surgery is needed but can be performed once the acute cerebritis and raised ICP are controlled.

Miscellaneous Conditions

Craniofacial syndromes rarely present as acute emergencies, but children with Crouzon's, Apert's, or Pfeiffer's syndromes are at risk for intracranial hypertension as a result of hydrocephalus, inadequate intracranial space because of the sutural synostosis, and Chiari I malformation that can result in compression at the foramen magnum and acute exacerbation of the pre-existing ventriculomegaly. In these children a major part of the problem is believed to be cerebral venous hypertension as a result of venous outlet obstruction at the skull base foramens. This can produce cerebellar swelling and ventriculomegaly to add to the already increased venous volume. The symptoms may be headache and vomiting or apnea, swallowing difficulties, sleep apnea, lower cranial nerve palsies and signs of spinal cord compression, spasticity, and gait problems. The fundi may show papilledema, there may be a cracked-pot sound to the head, the head may be small or large, and there may be local signs of brain stem and medullary compression. These presentations are usually in the middle to late years of childhood and are unusual in newborns except those with kleiblatschadel. The synostosis needs surgical reconstruction and expansion of the cranium, the hydrocephalus needs a shunt, and the Chiari malformation requires a posterior fossa decompression and possible tonsillar resection.

Other congenital intracranial mass lesions can present as emergencies. Occasionally a child with an arachnoid cyst presents with headache and papilledema, as well as acute intracranial hypertension. This is often precipitated by an injury to the head days to weeks before, which results in expansion of a middle fossa arachnoid cyst over the hemisphere with intracranial decompensation due to the focal mass effect. Arachnoid cysts in other locations rarely present acutely. If the ICP is diffusely elevated, the lesion may need urgent surgical therapy: shunt or excision.

Venous sinus thrombosis, which is often accompanied by dehydration or a hypercoagulable state, produces acute intracranial hypertension as a result of increased venous volume, increased sinus pressure resulting in increased outflow pressure for the CSF, and venous cortical infarctions. If intracranial hypertension is severe, anticoagulation may be required. Care must be taken not to convert the venous infarctions into hemorrhagic infarctions. Direct intrasinus delivery via femoral catheterization with thrombolytic agents is helpful. For this to work, the diagnosis must be made early in the course of the disease.

Systemic diseases that can result in intracranial hypertension are superior vena cava obstruction, congestive heart failure, and acute liver failure. After treatment for diabetic ketoacidosis, ICP elevation can occur; if the patient's level of consciousness deteriorates after therapy or fails to improve as the glucose falls to near normal levels, brain swelling must be ruled out.

Summary • Many of the acute signs and symptoms of neuroemergencies in children are the result of intracranial hypertension. Intracranial hypertension can cause secondary brain damage and death if not controlled, and local or general brain ischemia can be prevented by timely therapy. Whenever intracranial hypertension is suspected, the cause needs to be defined as soon as possible. This is usually done by neuroimaging (CT or MRI). In unconscious children the primary therapy to prevent or treat intracranial hypertension is immediate establishment of an adequate airway and ventilation. Further treatment depends on the cause of intracranial hypertension and varies from immediate surgery to medical management. The pathophysiology that results in intracranial hypertension varies over time in any given child, and therefore the selection of best therapy also varies. Appropriate therapy and indeed the need for any therapy must be frequently evaluated during the course of the child's illness. A number of monitoring techniques can help define the intracranial dynamics and help select best therapy. The selection of monitoring depends on the availability of the equipment and the physician's experience. Although control or prevention of high ICP does not guarantee a good outcome, it is one of the main contributing factors to good recovery in many children. The height of the elevated ICP is not as important as the length of time during which it is elevated and the state of cerebrovascular autoregulation. Control of the ICP remains one of the most important aspects of care in children with neuroemergencies.

References

1. Avezaat CJJ, Van Eijhdhoven JHM: Cerebrospinal Fluid Pulse Pressure and Craniospinal Dynamics. A Theoretical and Experimental Study. Hague, A Gonabloed en zoon, 1984.

2. Bruce DA: Pathophysiology of intracranial pressure. In Asbury AK, McKhann GM, McDonald WI (eds), Diseases of the Nervous System, Clinical Neurobiology, vol II, pp 1044–1062. Philadelphia, WB Saunders, 1986.
3. Razumovsky AY, Hanley DF: Intracranial pressure measurement/cranial vault mechanics: Clinical and experimental observations. Curr Opin Neurol Neurosurg 1992;5:818–825.
4. Miller JD: Volume and pressure in the craniospinal axis. Clin Neurosurg 1975;22:76–105.
5. Shapiro K, Morris WJ, Teo C: Intracranial hypertension: Mechanisms and management. In Cheek WR (ed): Pediatric Neurosurgery, 3rd ed, pp 307–319. Philadelphia, WB Saunders, 1994.
6. Marmarou A, Shulman K, LaMorgese J: Compartmental analysis of compliance and outflow resistance of the cerebrospinal fluid system. J Neurosurg 1975;43:523–534.
7. Marmarou A, Shulman K, Rosende R: A non-linear analysis of the cerebrospinal fluid system and intracranial pressure dynamics. J Neurosurg 1978;48:332–334.
8. Greitz D: Cerebrospinal fluid circulation and associated intracranial dynamics. A radiologic investigation using MR imaging and radionuclide cisternography. Acta Radiol Suppl 1993;386:1–23.
9. Barie PS, Ghajar JB, Firlik AD, et al: Contribution of increased cerebral blood volume to posttraumatic intracranial hypertension. J Trauma 1993;35:88–95.
10. Czosnyka M, Pickard J, Whitehouse H, Piechnik S: The hyperaemic response to a transient reduction in cerebral perfusion pressure. A modelling study. Acta Neurochir 1993;115:90–97.
11. Doczi T: Volume regulation of the brain tissue—A survey. Acta Neurochir 1993;121:1–8.
12. Shapiro K, Marmarou A, Shulman K: Characterisation of clinical CSF dynamics and neural axis compliance using the pressure-volume index. 1. The normal volume-pressure index. Ann Neurol 1980;7:508–511.
13. Paulson OB, Strandgaard S, Edivinsson L: Cerebral autoregulation. Cerebrovasc Brain Metab Rev 1990;2:161–192.
14. Hauerberg J, Juhler M: Cerebral blood flow autoregulation in acute intracranial hypertension. J Cereb Blood Flow Metab 1994;14:519–525.
15. Chan KH, Miller JD, Dearden NW, et al: The effect of changes in cerebral perfusion pressure upon middle cerebral artery blood flow velocity and jugular bulb venous oxygen saturation after severe brain trauma. J Neurosurg 1992;77;55–61.
16. Niwa K, Lindauer U, Villringer A, Dirnagl U: Blockade of nitric oxide synthesis in rats strongly attenuates the CBF response to extracellular acidosis. J Cereb Blood Flow Metab 1993;13:535–539.
17. Tanaka K, Gotoh F, Gomi S, et al: Inhibition of nitric oxide synthesis induces a significant reduction in local cerebral blood flow in the rat. Neurosci Lett 1991;27:129–132.
18. Bouma GJ, Muizelaar JP, Stringer WA, et al: Ultra-early evaluation of regional cerebral blood flow in severely head injured patients using xenon-enhanced computerized tomography. J Neurosurg 1992;77:360–368.
19. Bruce DA, Alavi A, Bilaniuk L, et al: Diffuse brain swelling following head injury in children: The syndrome of "malignant brain edema." J Neurosurg 1981;54:170–178.
20. Muizelaar JP, Marmarou A, DeSalles AA, et al: Cerebral blood flow and metabolism in severely head injured children, Part I: Relationship with GCS, outcome, ICP and PVI. Part II: Autoregulation. J Neurosurg 1989;71:63–71.
21. Lundberg N: Continuous recording and control of ventricular fluid pressure in neurosurgical practice. Acta Psychol Neurol Scand 1960;36(Suppl):149.
22. Portnoy HD, Chopp M: Intracranial fluid dynamics. Interrelationships of CSF and vascular phenomena. In Concepts in Pediatric Neurosurgery 3, pp 133–144. Basel, S Karger, 1983.
23. Bruce DA, Raphaely RC, Goldberg AI, et al: Pathophysiology, treatment and outcome following severe head injury in children. Childs Brain 1979;5:174–191.
24. Bruce DA: Head injuries in the pediatric population. Curr Prob Pediatr 1990;20:61–107.
25. Alberico AM, Ward JD, Choi SC, et al: Outcome after severe head injury, relationship to mass lesions, diffuse injury and ICP course in pediatric and adult patients. J Neurosurg 1987;67:648–856.
26. Humphreys RP: Special article—Hemorrhagic stroke in childhood. Rev Neurosci Pediatr 1986;2:1.
27. Schoenberg BS, Meelinger JF, Schoenberg DG: Cerebrovascular disease in infants and children: A study of incidence, clinical features and survival. Neurology 1978;28:763–768.
28. Meyer FB, Sundt TM, Fode NC, et al: Cerebral aneurysms in childhood and adolescence. J Neurosurg 1989;70:420–425.
29. Kassell NF, Torner JC, Haley C Jr, et al: The international cooperative study of the timing of aneurysm surgery. Part 1: Overall management results. J Neurosurg 1990;73:18–36.
30. Kassell NF, Torner JC, Jane JA, et al: The international cooperative study of the timing of aneurysm surgery. Part 2: Surgical results. J Neurosurg 1990;73:37–47.
31. Kassell NF, Peerless SJ, Durward QJ, et al: Treatment of ischemic deficits from vasospasm with intravascular volume expansion and induced arterial hypertension. Neurosurgery 1982;11:337–343.
32. Petruk KC, West M, Mohr G, et al: Nimodipine treatment in poor grade aneurysm patients; results of a multicenter double-blind placebo controlled trial. J Neurosurg 1988;68:505–517.
33. Coker SB: Cyclic vomiting and the slit ventricle syndrome. Pediatr Neurol 1987;3:297–299.
34. Serlo W, Heikkinen E, Saukkonen AL, von-Wendt L: Classification and management of the slit ventricle syndrome. Childs Nerv Syst 1985;1:194–199.
35. Sklar FH, Beyer CY, Ramanathau M, et al: Cerebrospinal fluid dynamics in patients with pseudotumor cerebri. Neurosurgery 1979;5:208–216.
36. Frank JI: Management of intracranial hypertension. Med Clin North Am 1993;77:61–76.
37. Janny P, Chazal J, Colnet G, et al: Benign intracranial hypertension and disorders of CSF circulation. Surg Neurol 1981;15:168–174.
38. Tunkel AR, Scheld WM: Pathogenesis and pathophysiology of bacterial meningitis. Clin Microb Rev 1993;6:118–136.
39. Hirsch JF, Roux FX, Sainte-Rose C, et al: Brain abscess in childhood. A study of 34 cases treated by puncture and antibiotics. Childs Brain 1983;10:251–255.
40. Neilsen H: Cerebral abscess in children. Neuropediatrics 1983;14:76–81.
41. Smith HP, Hendrick EB: Subdural empyema and epidural abscess in children. J Neurosurg 1983;58:392–395.
42. Hockley AD, Williams B: Surgical management of subdural empyema. Childs Brain 1983;10:294–297.

13

Acute Neuromuscular Diseases

Alberto A. Gabbai, M.D. • Acary S. B. Oliveira, M.D. • Ayrton R. Massaro, M.D. • Suzana M. F. Malheiros, M.D.

The neuromuscular system that comprises the motor neuron, its axon, the neuromuscular junction (NMJ), and the skeletal muscle is the site of many acute injuries or insults that may lead to a variety of morbid states. The most important and threatening of these is the paralysis of the respiratory muscles. We have divided the acute involvement of the neuromuscular system into four groups:

1. Diseases that have a genetic background
   - The periodic paralyses
   - Malignant hyperthermia
   - The porphyrias
2. Autoimmune diseases
   - Acquired myasthenia gravis
   - Guillain-Barré syndrome
3. Infectious diseases
   - Diphtheritic polyneuritis
   - Tick paralysis
   - Lyme disease
   - Poliomyelitis
   - Tetanus
   - Botulism
   - Acute viral myositis
4. Involvement due to drugs, metals, and toxins
   - Involvement of peripheral nerves
   - Involvement of the NMJ
   - Involvement of muscle

DISEASES THAT HAVE A GENETIC BACKGROUND

Periodic Paralyses

Definition

Periodic paralyses (PP) is the name given to a variety of diseases of different etiologies characterized by recurrent episodes of flaccid weakness. Respiratory and cranial muscles tend to be spared. The attacks are usually self-limited and recede spontaneously, although the condition rarely evolves to immobility of the respiratory muscles.[1]

Classification

PP may be divided into primary and secondary diseases. The primary forms are genetically transmitted, usually in an autosomal dominant form. The secondary forms are due to a variety of conditions that alter the normal potassium metabolism.

Another classification is based on the potassium level during the paralytic attack, as hypokalemic, normokalemic, or hyperkalemic.[2]

Primary Periodic Paralyses

Primary Hypokalemic

Primary hypokalemic PP is the most common of the PPs. Its prevalence has been estimated as 1.25 per 100,000 population.[3] The disease is transmitted as an autosomal dominant trait and was linked to chromosome 1. The defective gene has been identified as the dihydropyridine-sensitive receptor calcium channel.[4] The disease presents as late as the third decade of life. The majority of cases start before age 16, but severe cases start during early childhood.[5] An attack generally occurs in the early morning hours or at night. It is usually generalized and, if severe, leads to a reduction in vital capacity with possible death from ventilatory failure.[6]

The trigger for an attack is often a carbohydrate-rich meal or intense physical activity. Slight physical activity, on the other hand, can prevent mild attacks. During attacks, the serum potassium decreases, but not necessarily below the normal range. When serum potassium is low, bradycardia and electrocardiographic signs of hypokalemia can be detected.[7, 8]

The diagnosis of primary hypokalemic PP is suspected in a patient with a positive family history who presents with a major attack associated with a decrease in the serum potassium level. The serum phosphorus may decrease in parallel to a decrease in serum potassium. The serum creatine kinase is usually not elevated during the attacks.[1]

Pathogenesis

The hypokalemia present is caused by an uptake of potassium from the extracellular space into the sarcoplasm. It has been established that the uptake is insulin-dependent.[9] The muscle fiber inexcitability in hypokalemic PP is due to a membrane depolarization. The lower extracellular potassium levels in patients with PP (which in normal persons would produce hyperpolarization) produces an abnormal depolarization of the muscle fibers and initiates the attacks.[10]

Most physiologic studies of primary hypokalemic PP to date have been based on the assumption that the primary defect would be in the potassium channel. With the recent discovery of the basic defect located in a calcium channel, a substantial aspect of the pathogenesis will have to be reviewed.

Treatment

ATTACK

Mild paralytic attacks are self-limited. Muscle strength returns to normal in a matter of hours. If the potassium level is so low as to alter the electrocardiogram with bradycardia, the appearance of U waves, flattening of T waves, and depression of ST segment, intravenous potassium should be given with caution to avoid the overshooting of life-threatening hyperkalemia.[11] In the case of generalized paralysis, potassium chloride should be given by mouth in an unsweetened 25% aqueous solution. Potassium chloride (0.2–0.4 mMol/kg) causes muscle strength to be regained in about 1 hour. The dose may be repeated after 3 hours, if there are no signs of recovery.[12]

PREVENTIVE MEASURES

After the attacks, preventive measures include the avoidance of carbohydrate-rich meals and the avoidance of strenuous exercises.

Drugs that may be used with some success are acetazolamide, dichlorphenamide, diazoxide, verapamil, or lithium.[1]

Primary Hyperkalemic

Primary hyperkalemic PP clinically resembles hypokalemic PP, but during an attack the serum potassium levels are increased.

The disease may present without myotonia or with clinical or electromyographic myotonia. Both forms have the same genetic defect.[1]

Primary hyperkalemic PP is an autosomal dominant disease, linked to the long arm of chromosome 17, with complete penetrance in both sexes; it is due to a defect in the SCN4A gene, which encodes the alfa-subunit of the tetrodotoxin-sensitive sodium channel of the skeletal muscle.[13]

Clinical Features

The disease usually begins in the first decade of life. The attacks are usually mild and short (15 minutes to 1 hour) and tend to involve segments of the body instead of being generalized. They may be worse in pregnancy, with the use of glucocorticoids, and especially in cold environments.[14] Rest after strenuous exercises may precipitate the weakness that is often accompanied by an increase in serum potassium levels. Cardiotoxic levels of serum potassium are rare, but may be high enough to cause cardiac dysrhythmia.[15]

The diagnosis is made in a patient with episodes of weakness or paralysis who has a positive family history and who may or not have myotonia or paramyotonia. Serum creatinine kinase (CK) elevation is not rare during the attacks.[1] Provocative tests may be used: Either potassium chloride may be administered, or the patient may be subjected to intense exercise followed by complete rest in bed.[16]

Normokalemic

Patients with clinical features of familial hyperkalemic PP rarely present with normokalemic crises. It is questionable whether the hyperkalemia was missed, because some patients with normokalemic PP develop weakness when challenged with oral potassium salts.[17] Furthermore, at least in one family with normokalemic PP, the same genetic mutation that occurs in hyperkalemic PP was demonstrated.[1]

Pathogenesis

Hyperkalemic PP is today classified as one of the muscle sodium channelopathies.[18] A sustained muscle membrane depolarization seems to be the under-

a decrease in the number of AChRs to as low as one-third of healthy controls,[64] and in general the degree of reduction of AChR is proportional to the severity of the disease.[65] Patients with MG also depict morphologic changes in their NMJs, namely simplification of the pattern of postsynaptic membrane folding and an increased gap between the nerve terminal and the postsynaptic muscle membrane. The clinical and electrophysiologic features of MG are fully explained by these changes at the NMJ.[66]

Diagnosis

A detailed history along with the physical findings are the most important clues to the diagnosis. In patients who relate a typical history, a positive anticholinesterase drug test result[67] and a decremental electromyographic response[68] are the simplest tests used to confirm the diagnosis. In patients with no involvement of the external ocular muscles, with symptoms that do not fluctuate, or with unusual associated clinical or neurologic findings in whom the earlier-mentioned tests produce negative results, further studies are needed to confirm or exclude the diagnosis. In these patients, it is important to determine the anti-AChR antibody titer.[69] If positive, there is no need to proceed with single-fiber electromyographic testing[70] or ultrastructural analysis of the NMJ.[54]

In the differential diagnosis, the conditions that may acutely cause weakness of the cranial and somatic musculature include intracranial mass lesions, congenital myasthenic syndromes,[54] drug-induced myasthenia,[71, 72] hyperthyroidism, botulism,[66] and organophosphate intoxication.[73]

Treatment

The methods of treatment currently in use are anticholinesterase agents, prednisone, immunosuppressants other than prednisone, surgical thymectomy, plasmapheresis, and intravenous immunoglobulin.

Anticholinesterase agents are still the first drugs of choice in the treatment of MG. Pyridostigmine bromide, in 60 mg tablets, is the most widely used, but neostigmine bromide, 15 mg tablets, may be used as well in an equivalent basis per tablet. The effective dose may vary from one-half of a tablet every 6 hours to three tablets every 3 hours. Both drugs are also available for parenteral administration when medications cannot be given orally. The parenteral dosage should be approximately one-thirtieth of the oral dose.[54] Neostigmine methylsulfate may also be effectively used intranasally.[74]

Prednisone, immunosuppressants, and thymectomy are indicated in patients who do not respond favorably to moderate doses of anticholinesterase drugs. Months are usually the minimum time before these therapeutic approaches produce clear and sustained improvement. The reader is referred to excellent reviews on the long-term management of MG.[54, 66]

A cholinergic crisis is defined when an excessive amount of ACh is present at the NMJ, desensitizing the AChR, leading to increasing weakness.[54]

A myasthenic or cholinergic crisis is usually heralded by a progressive muscle weakness in spite of increasing amounts of anticholinesterase drug administered. Although a cholinergic crisis can be distinguished when the patient also exhibits marked muscarinic side effects, cholinergic and myasthenic impairment at the NMJ may coexist in different muscles or in different fibers of the same muscle. Hence, it is best to withdraw all anticholinesterase drugs when the condition evolves to a crisis in a short period. These patients must be treated with ventilatory support and parenteral feeding. After a few days, transmission at the NMJ usually improves again to the action of anticholinesterase drugs.[54]

Plasmapheresis[75] or intravenous immunoglobulin[76] is the therapeutic modality of choice for quickly stabilizing the patient in acute, severe, and generalized crisis. Neither is intended for long-term use.

Plasmapheresis is not an easy procedure. Complications include infection of the indwelling catheter, pulmonary embolism, and severe hypotension. Its beneficial effects are rapid, occurring within days, but are temporary, lasting only weeks. The number of exchanges, the interval between the exchanges, and the amount of plasma exchanged per session vary.[77] Usually, daily exchanges of 28–30 mL/kg each are performed. Others prefer to exchange a volume of plasma equal to 5% of the body volume at each treatment, repeating at 2- to 15-day intervals, depending on the patient's clinical status.[78] Improvement is associated with a decrease in the anti-acetylcholine-receptor antibody titers, but even patients with antibody-negative MG have improved after the procedure.[79]

Intravenous immunoglobulin is also used for stabilizing an acute myasthenic crisis. Usually, 400 mg/kg/day are infused for 5 consecutive days, or 1 g/kg/day for 2 consecutive days. Improvement begins after about 5 days and lasts for weeks, rarely months.[80] Complications that occur in about 10% of patients include headache, fluid overload, renal failure, aseptic meningitis,[81] and cerebral infarction.[82] Immunoglobulin's mechanism of action is unknown but may involve anti-idiotypic antibodies that bind to pathogenic anti-AChR antibodies.[54]

Both plasmapheresis and intravenous immunoglobulin are costly procedures. The cost and the sizable risks should be weighed against the possible rapid improvement paralleled with the fact that usually neither modality confers long-term protection.

Guillain-Barré Syndrome

In 1859, Landry[83] reported the presenting symptoms, course, and outcome of GBS. Guillain, Barré, and Strohl, in 1916, added further elucidation by reporting acute flaccid paralysis with areflexia and elevated spinal fluid protein.[84]

Epidemiology

The annual incidence of GBS is about one or two cases per 100,000 population,[85–87] slightly more common in males than females.[88]

At least two-thirds of GBS cases have been preceded by infections or other antecedent events during the 1–3 weeks before. An extensive retrospective survey of 1100 cases of GBS from 1949 to 1966 listed more than 700 possible associations.[89]

There are several reports of GBS being associated with viral infections, such as cytomegalovirus,[90] or Epstein-Barr virus infection[91]; segmental herpes zoster[92]; herpes simplex[93]; hepatitis A,[94] B,[95] and C[96]; and influenza.[97]

Bacterial infections are also described preceding GBS, and of these, the most reliable concern *Campylobacter.*[98] Some of the serologic evidence of *Campylobacter* infection in GBS nevertheless may be nonspecific, especially in older patients.[99] The incidence of *Campylobacter* preceding GBS is approximately 14%.[100]

Numerous cases of GBS have been reported after swine influenza vaccine[101] and oral polio vaccine.[102]

Several cases of GBS have also been reported at pregnancy or the puerperium.[103] Surgery has been emphasized as a trigger for GBS.[104] Type of operation, duration of surgery, mode of anesthesia, postoperative wound infection, or blood transfusion have not consistently been associated with GBS.

GBS cases following drug administration are usually acute axonal neuropathies. Isolated case reports of GBS occurring during treatment with commonly used drugs have to be dismissed as probably coincidental. There are some reports of GBS following captopril,[105] streptokinase,[106] and other drugs.

Diagnostic Criteria

Since the demonstration of inflammation in autopsy[107] and the recognition that most cases demonstrate both physiologic and pathological criteria for demyelination,[108, 109] GBS has often been considered synonymous with acute inflammatory demyelinating polyneuropathy. This view was made explicit in the criteria for diagnosis of GBS.[109] In these criteria, the presence of demyelination, as inferred from electrodiagnosis, is included for diagnosis of GBS.

Similar clinical and spinal-fluid patterns occur in persons with different electrophysiologic and pathological findings—findings underlying a different pathophysiology. This is illustrated in the axonal GBS cases[110] and the acute motor axonal neuropathy described in northern China.[111, 112] Otherwise, different clinical pictures can be seen in patients who appear to have similar pathophysiologic features.[113]

Cases fulfilling the clinical criteria[108, 109] should be called *GBS clinically defined.* Cases with electrophysiologic or pathological criteria of demyelination are called *demyelinating GBS.* If the clinical picture differs from that described by Guillain, Barré, and Strohl, as in Fisher syndrome, a preferable term is *acute demyelinating neuropathy.* In most cases of GBS clinically defined but with nondemyelinating features, terms such as *GBS of axonal type* and *acute motor axonal neuropathy* can be used.

Pathophysiology

GBS is an inflammatory peripheral neuropathy, involving the early appearance of lymphocytes and macrophages surrounding endoneural vessels, with predilection for nerve roots, causing adjacent demyelination.[107]

Both immune mechanisms, T-cell and B-cell, participate in the macrophage-induced demyelination. The primary lymphocytic T-cell mechanism probably is an aberrant response to a precipitating stimulus. Activated T cells expressing several surface receptors circulate during the acute illness, and serum levels of interleukin-2 and its soluble receptor are greatly increased.[114] According to one hypothesis, an early antibody attack on myelin occurs in some cases and a mainly inflammatory process occurs in others, both leading to a macrophage response that causes myelin destruction.[115] Circulating antineural antibodies have been demonstrated in GBS, occasionally against P-2 or cerebroside.[116] IgM antibodies against ganglioside GM1 have been found in GBS after *Campylobacter* infection.[117]

Clinical Features

GBS or acute inflammatory polyneuropathy frequently occurs after a preceding infection and begins with a combination of pain, sensory symptoms, and weakness.

Weakness is first noted in the legs. All limbs become symmetrically weak as the illness progresses, but weakness may be markedly asymmetric at the onset. The hips and shoulders tend to be involved earlier and more intensively than do the feet and hands.[118] Facial weakness (Fig. 13–2) becomes evident after a few days. Oropharyngeal weakness usually appears after all limbs have been affected. The weakness of shoulder elevation and neck flexion correlates with diaphragmatic weakness and respiratory failure. Diplopia occurs in 10%–20% of cases. Some patients may simulate a "locked-in" syndrome.[119]

Sensory symptoms often precede weakness by 1 or 2 days, and more than weakness, paresthesias truly ascend, but generally remain distal to the wrists and ankles.

Areflexia, an essential feature of GBS, sometimes is delayed until weakness and paresthesias are well developed.

Pain may be symmetric in the large muscles of the hips, upper legs, and back with intense paresthesias or burning, or it may present as severe dorsal midline pain.[120]

Most patients worsen over 1 or 2 weeks, some for up to 4 weeks, and a few are quadriplegic within a day or two. Some patients show a temporary halt in progression, followed by rapid worsening over several days. Patients who continue to worsen after 4 weeks usually experience a chronic progressive or relapsing course.[121]

Dysautonomia is more frequent in patients with severe motor deficits and respiratory failure. Numerous cases of sudden death in GBS have been attributed to dysautonomia, although secondary causes, including hypoxia, pulmonary embolism, gastrointestinal bleeding or fluid electrolyte disturbances, must be excluded.

Paroxysmal hypertension often occurs in combination with orthostatic hypotension. The frequency of orthostatic hypotension varies from 5% to 10%.[122] Urinary retention[118] and ileus have also been reported.[123]

Some unusual features have been described, such as facial palsy with myokymia[124]; meningismus and headache without a cerebrospinal fluid (CSF) cellular reaction[125]; ophthalmoplegia,[126] sometimes with pupillary abnormalities; and retrobulbar optic neuritis.[127] Papilledema with pseudotumor cerebri has been reported in GBS,[128, 129] more often in patients with lupus erythematosus, and in chronic inflammatory demyelinating polyneuropathy.

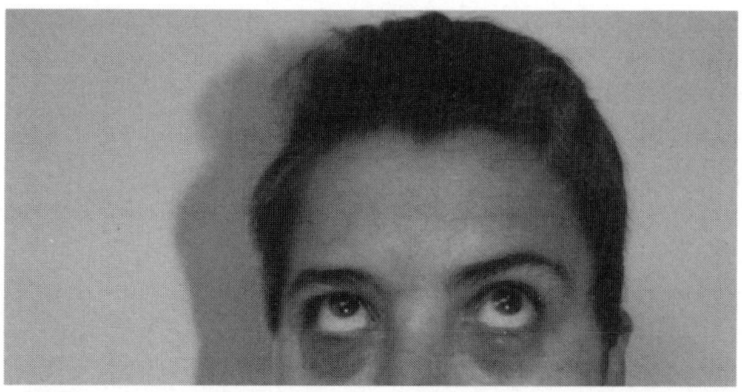

FIGURE 13–2 • Bilateral facial paralysis in Guillain-Barré syndrome. The patient is attempting to close both eyes. Note the impossibility of upper-lid closure with bilateral Bell's sign. Bilateral facial drooping was also noted, most evident on the right. (See color plate.)

Variant Syndromes

PURE MOTOR

Preferential inflammation of ventral roots probably accounts for pure motor GBS,[130] with no sensory signs or symptoms.

SENSORY GBS

Fewer cases retain the initial predominantly sensory quality, with areflexia but with little or no weakness. One autopsy case showed infiltrates and demyelination of posterior roots, contrasted with entirely normal anterior roots.[131]

PANDYSAUTONOMIA

In typical cases, gastrointestinal dysfunction or orthostatic dizziness is the initial symptom.[132] Additional features include an atonic bladder, diminished sweating, salivation and lacrimation, and pupillary abnormalities.

MILLER-FISHER SYNDROME

In 1956, Fisher[133] described three patients with total external ophthalmoplegia, severe ataxia, and loss of the tendon reflexes. Ropper and Shahani proposed that the ataxia was due to a mismatch of information from muscle spindles and other proprioceptors to the cerebellum.[134]

Although some of the physical signs of this syndrome can be mimicked by a brain stem lesion, the typical cases have never been documented as involving a central nervous system (CNS) lesion.[134–136] CSF protein concentration is elevated in most cases in the late course of the illness.[137] All conventional electrophysiologic studies of Miller-Fisher syndrome have shown a peripheral neuropathy.[138]

AXONAL

The issue of axonal GBS remains controversial. Supportive evidence comes from pathological examination of peripheral nerve (PN) in four cases that showed severe axonal degeneration without inflammatory demyelination.[110, 139] These patients often become severely and rapidly paralyzed and ventilator-dependent, and eventually they experience profound atrophy and a prolonged recovery.

Support for the concept of axonal GBS comes also from the recent studies of the seasonal acute motor axonal neuropathy seen in northern China.[112] Physiologic studies have demonstrated prominent motor axonal loss with only modest features of demyelination.

Laboratory Investigation

In 1916, Guillain, Barré, and Strohl[84] did not mention many typical features of GBS, but they introduced albuminocytologic dissociation as a laboratory marker. The absence of cells in the CSF supports the diagnosis of GBS, and the increased level of protein is often detectable only after 5–10 days of illness.

Within 24–48 hours of the onset of GBS, electrophysiologic studies are often characteristic enough to indicate the presence of demyelinating polyneuropathy.[140, 141] The presence of conduction block, either proximally or distally,[142] and the characteristic finding of motor unit potentials that fire rapidly and in decreased numbers in weak muscles, strongly suggest demyelination, even though standard motor and sensory nerve conduction study results may be relatively normal. Absent or delayed F wave latencies are also an early sign.[143] Phrenic nerve conduction studies and needle electromyography of the diaphragm are particularly valuable in establishing the type and severity of the involvement of phrenic nerve and diaphragm.[144] Serial studies to follow the course of the treatment, such as plasmapheresis, hyperimmunoglobulin, or steroids, are valuable. However, in our experience, symptomatic improvement may precede electrophysiologic improvement.

Magnetic resonance imaging has become increasingly useful in the study of PN disease, including GBS.[145, 146] The abnormal enhancement of nerve roots is nonetheless nonspecific.

Differential Diagnosis

Botulism, tick paralysis, AIP, acute toxic neuropathies, and myelopathic causes of acute flaccid paralysis are the major differential possibilities.

Fever at onset and CSF pleocytosis may suggest poliomyelitis syndrome. The presence of pleocytosis should raise the possibility of associated HIV infection.[147]

A meningoradiculitis syndrome with facial palsy, pain, sensory loss, weakness, areflexia, and mononuclear CSF pleocytosis, called Bannwarth's syndrome in Europe, may simulate acute GBS.[148] The peripheral neuropathy in Lyme disease is generally not ascending and is typically asymmetric or monoparetic. The CSF has markedly elevated cell counts (many of the CSF cells in Lyme disease are immunoblasts or plasmacytes). The significance of isolated reports of GBS following this infection is difficult to evaluate.[149]

Peripheral nerve disorders that resemble acute GBS are common in patients with malignancies and paraneoplastic or paraproteinemic neuropathy. The clinical features in Hodgkin's-related GBS have been identical to those of the idiopathic variety and inconsistent with other neuropathies, such as vincristine neuropathy.

Approximately 10% of patients with systemic lupus erythematosus have a peripheral neuropathy, often mononeuritis multiplex or relapsing demyelinating polyneuropathy. When acute progressive ascending weakness does occur, however, the pathological findings resemble those in GBS.

Several reports describe a GBS-like illness and sarcoidosis with paresthesias, pain, and rapid limb weakness, with some patients experiencing a meningeal reaction.

An axonal polyneuropathy of yet unknown etiology may complicate critical illness, most often in patients who are intubated or present with multiple organ dysfunction. The electrophysiologic and CSF features distinguish the neuropathy from GBS.[150]

Prognosis

Winer and coworkers reported 100 patients with GBS and defined poor outcome as either prolonged disability confining the patient to bed 3 months after onset or inability to perform manual work 12 months after onset.[118] No relationship was found between poor outcome and sensory deficit, facial weakness, sex, incontinence, or CSF results. Features significantly associated with poor outcome as defined were age over 40 years, disease severity (reaching a bed-bound state in < 4 days after onset), requiring mechanical ventilation, and a small muscle evoked potential.

The results of the North American Guillain-Barré Syndrome Trial[151] defined poor outcome as an inability to walk after 6 months. Several factors were found to have predictive value: distal muscle evoked potential ($> 20\%$ or $< 20\%$ of the lower limit of normal); type of treatment; prior length of illness (> 7 or < 7 days); and age. Plasmapheresis had an effect on prognosis even in the face of all other predictive factors suggesting a poor prognosis. A worse prognosis is associated with need for ventilatory support, especially if required for more than 1 month, and age over 70 years.

Preliminary reports of the Dutch Guillain-Barré Syndrome Study Group[152] on prognosis in GBS found that age, serologic evidence of recent *Campy-*

lobacter jejuni infection, and anti-GM1 antibodies were related to prognosis.

Treatment

GENERAL MEDICAL MANAGEMENT

The management of GBS requires special expertise in medical and intensive care. Unfortunately, there are no simple methods of predicting early worsening.

The dramatic reduction in mortality of GBS reflects the improvements in respiratory and critical care. The keys to management are hospitalization of even mildly affected patients and close observation for respiratory failure, bulbar weakness, and difficulties with swallowing and handling secretions.

Autonomic disturbance is one of the main contributors to mortality and additional morbidity in GBS. It includes sudden cardiac arrest during intubation or extubation, severe arrhythmias, hypertension, and ileus. Since the first reports of cardiac arrest in GBS, the question has been raised about the routine use of transthoracic cardiac pacemakers in GBS patients with autonomic problems. The treatment of severe autonomic dysfunction with unstable blood pressures or bowel dysfunction often requires the insertion of central venous catheters.

GBS patients in an intensive care unit are also at high risk of acquiring nosocomial infections.

Stress ulcers and acute erosive gastritis are potential complications in the immobilized GBS patient. Sucralfate has been shown to be an alternative to antacids and H_2 blockers.

Pulmonary embolism has occurred in up to 5% of bed-bound patients with GBS. Prophylaxis with subcutaneous heparin and intermittent calf pneumatic compression have been effective in preventing pulmonary embolism.

Intravenous suxamethonium should be avoided during tracheostomy and other procedures because, in patients with severe weakness, it may lead to the release of large amounts of potassium, causing serious ventricular arrhythmia.[153]

Hyponatremia is usually attributable to the syndrome of inappropriate antidiuretic hormone secretion and is more common in patients on a ventilator. Seldom severe, it responds to fluid restriction. In some patients with natriuresis, NaCl infusion is appropriate.

Pain is often alleviated when the knees and hips are slightly flexed. Some patients have benefited from cold or warm packs. Acetaminophen and aspirin may provide temporary and incomplete relief. A narcotic (meperidine) has been the most effective treatment, although it may contribute to ileus.

Enteric tube feeding should be started after several days in patients with normally functioning gastrointestinal tracts who have difficulty swallowing. Antral placement is usually safe. Full nutritional supplementation through a central venous catheter is indicated when ileus, sepsis, or bowel perforation is evident.

Daily attention to the eyes is necessary in order to prevent corneal ulcerations.

Care of the GBS patient involves psychologic support. During the progressive phase, severe anxiety, fear, and even panic can be reinforced by the patient's lack of knowledge about the disease.

RESPIRATORY SUPPORT

Acute respiratory failure due to ventilatory muscle dysfunction is the major life-threatening complication in patients with GBS. Expiratory effort, maintenance of airway patency, and inspiratory muscle strength may all be compromised in GBS. Weakness of laryngeal and glottic muscle causes difficulty in swallowing and coughing, and it increases the risk of aspiration.[154] Respiratory function may be compromised before clinical signs of ventilatory insufficiency are obvious. Serial assessment of ventilatory status is essential to determine the need for intubation and mechanical ventilation. Monitoring maximum inspiratory force, forced vital capacity, and arterial blood gases or oxygen saturation is useful in assessing ventilatory function. If vital capacity falls bellow 15 mL/kg, the risk for ventilatory failure increases.[155] Practice should tend toward earlier intubation and mechanical ventilation to minimize pulmonary complications.[154–156]

Early tracheostomy may be indicated in patients with severe GBS who show clinical and electromyographic evidence of axonal involvement, ventilatory failure, and dysautonomia, but it is better to wait till the end of the second week of mechanical ventilation in patients with evolving illness, when plasmapheresis is completed and the disease course can be predicted more accurately.

SPECIFIC TREATMENT

Since the recognition that demyelination in GBS has an autoimmune substrate, the emphasis on specific treatment has been to modulate the host immune response.

Plasma exchange (PE) was the first therapy demonstrated to benefit GBS and remains a mainstay of therapy.[157–159] Both the American and the French studies found that patients who had undergone PE required shorter periods of ventilation and began to walk unaided earlier than did those who had not been treated.[158,159] In the French study, the treated group was further randomized to either plasma or albumin as the replacement fluid, and these were equally efficacious, suggesting that PE works by removing a substance (probably antibodies) rather than by delivering a compound that modulates immune function. Patients treated within a week of onset and those requiring ventilation derived a greater benefit from PE. PE is expensive, requires skilled personnel and special equipment not available in many hospitals, and is associated with a small amount of morbidity (hypotension, arrhythmias, and line complications), which makes it unsuitable for those patients with severe autonomic defects or septicemia.

Intravenous human immunoglobulin (HIG) has been demonstrated to be efficacious.[160] The results showed that HIG therapy, an easier procedure, was as good as, or possible better than, PE.

Multicenter trials of corticosteroids have demonstrated no efficacy, despite initial enthusiasm for steroids in the 1960s. Corticosteroid as the primary therapy should be regarded as contraindicated in GBS.[161, 162]

The decision of which therapy to use is aided by some considerations. First, the effectiveness of PE has been confirmed in multiple studies,[158, 159] whereas the data available to suggest that HIG is effective in GBS are more limited. The HIG study[160] has been criticized because the PE group seemed to do particularly worse than that group from the North American trial. In addition, there were imbalances between the HIG and the PE group at admission that could have biased the conclusion. There are also some uncontrolled data suggesting that the incidence of relapses may be higher in the HIG-treated group,[163] as well as others showing the lack of HIG efficacy.[164]

PE should be used as the first-choice therapy if there are no contraindications. The recommended protocol is five exchanges of 50 mL/kg carried out over 5–10 days. If this is not available, or if it is contraindicated, intravenous HIG at a dose of 0.4 g/kg over 5 consecutive days should be used. Also, in patients with whom obtaining or maintaining the PE will be a problem, HIG may be used. Ongoing trials are assessing the combination of HIG with PE.

Once we have a better understanding of the pathogenesis of this disease, therapy will be more precisely targeted at the specific cellular or humoral agents, with better efficacy.

INFECTIOUS DISEASES

Diphtheritic Polyneuritis

Diphtheritic polyneuritis is a rare toxin-mediated sensorimotor neuropathy caused by *Corynebacterium diphtheriae,* a pleomorphic gram-positive, not invasive bacillus that remains superficial in the respiratory mucosa and skin, causing mild inflammatory local reaction.[165]

The disease occurs predominantly in winter. Airborne respiratory droplets or contact with respiratory secretions and skin lesions' exudates is the primary mode of transmission. Asymptomatic respiratory carriage, as well as skin carriage, may be important in perpetuating endemic and epidemic diphtheria.[165]

C. diphtheriae produces an extremely potent exotoxin that inhibits protein synthesis in mammalian cells, depending on the presence of a lysogenic B-phage, which carries the gene encoding for the toxin. It integrates into the host bacteria's genetic material as a prophage.[166]

The most common distant sites affected secondary to absorption and dissemination of the toxin are the heart, kidneys, and PNs, particularly the ganglia. Demyelination is the leading feature.[167]

After an incubation period of 2–4 days, diphtheria usually begins with abrupt fever, headache, sore throat, and cervical lymphadenopathy (also called "bull neck appearance"). A membranous exudate on the nares, tonsils, pharynx, or even tracheobronchial tree may become the adherent grayish (gray-brown) or black membrane typical of diphtheria, the extent of which correlates with the severity of the disease.[165] Most deaths have been related to myocarditis, polyneuritis, and other complications such as pulmonary embolism or bronchopneumonia,[168] although local air obstruction by edema, membrane involvement of the trachea, or even membrane aspiration can also be fatal.

Although variable, the incidence of neuropathy is about 20%[167] and seems to be proportional to severity and localization of diphtheritic primary infection.[168] Patients usually have difficulty swallowing related to the membranous exudate, although palatal and pharyngeal paralysis producing nasal speech and regurgitation is almost always the initial sign of neuritis within the first few days.[168, 169] The palatal paralysis, often asymmetric, is due to local action of the diphtheric toxin. Between 2 and 5 weeks, oculomotor and ciliary paralysis appear, causing blurred vision in half of patients. Patients usually notice difficulty in reading as a result of impaired accommodation to near objects.[167] This finding may also be the initial symptom in some cases of wound or cutaneous diphtheria. Pupillary responses to light and convergence are often normal, with impaired reaction to accommodation.[167] Limb weakness is usually symmetric and predominantly proximal and occurs between 5 and 7 weeks of disease,[168] although it may be a presenting feature. Respiratory failure is uncommon but may appear in severe cases when paresis affects intercostal and auxiliary respiratory muscles. Although rare,[170] muscle atrophy may occur. Diminished or absent deep tendon reflexes may precede severe weakness. All modalities of sensation may be affected: Mild paresthesia is the most common complaint, and sensory ataxia (pseudotabes) has been reported. Sphincteric dysfunction is uncommon and reported only in severe cases, but sinus tachycardia is frequent.[167–169]

Myocarditis may appear in the second week or occur simultaneously with the neuropathy, presenting with congestive heart failure, arrhythmia, T-wave changes, and atrioventricular or branch blocks.[171]

CSF albuminocytologic dissociation, with protein levels between 75 and 300 mg/dL, usually occurs in diphtheritic neuropathy. Mild CSF lymphocytosis may also occur.[167–169]

Electrophysiologic studies usually show increased distal motor latencies and decreased nerve conduction velocities (NCVs), characteristic of a demyelinating mixed sensory/motor polyneuropathy. Late responses and sensory action potentials may be affected. A remarkable dissociation between the time course of clinical and neurophysiologic abnormalities is described.[172, 173]

Diagnosis is based on clinical features and identification of *C. diphtheriae* in cultures.

Clinical, CSF, and electrophysiologic features are similar to those of GBS. Slower evolution, asymmetric palatal paralysis, accommodation paralysis, myocarditis, and epidemiologic aspects are important clues to the diagnosis.

No definite treatment is available for the neuropathy, except the specific treatment with diphtheric antitoxin (hyperimmune antiserum produced in horses) as soon as a presumptive diagnosis is suspected clinically, in order to avoid the development of the neuropathy and other complications. The antibody does not neutralize the toxin after its entry into cells. Antibiotic therapy is suggested to stop toxin production and to reduce the spread of the agent; penicillin and erythromycin are usually the most recommended. Close monitoring is necessary for early detection and management of respiratory and cardiac complications, the main cause of death. The prognosis of neuropathy is usually good with total recovery that may take months.[165, 167, 168]

The major clinical manifestations should be ideally prevented by immunization with formalin-inactivated toxin. Contacts should receive complete immunization, in addition to prophylactic antibiotics, if their immunization status is incomplete. Convalescent patients should also receive immunization, because infection may not produce adequate antibody levels.[165]

Tick Paralysis

Tick paralysis is a rare, usually acute form of progressive ascending flaccid paralysis caused by a neurotoxin presented in the saliva of the gravid female of certain species of tick.

Children between 2 and 5 years of age are mostly affected, with a seasonal incidence from April to June, when nymphs and mature ticks are more prevalent. The northwestern United States and western Canada, but also the southeastern United States, Australia, South Africa, Crete, France, and other European countries, have reported cases. Forty-three species of ticks have been reported, but wood and dog ticks were the most often implicated in the United States and Canada.[174, 175]

Clinical manifestations occur 2–7 days after tick attachment. Ataxia and areflexia may precede weakness, leading to a gait disorder. Acute ascending, symmetric, and flaccid paralysis begins in the lower limbs, affecting the trunk and upper limbs within a few hours, and may involve bulbar, extraocular, facial, and respiratory muscles. Although paresthesias may be common and affect the face and perioral region, objective sensory loss is rare. Autonomic dysfunction with sphincteric disturbances or tachycardia is unusual. Death may occur when respiratory muscles are affected.[176, 177]

CSF occasionally presents with mild pleocytosis or protein elevation. Electrophysiologic studies show a prominent reduction in the amplitude of muscle action potentials and mild to moderate slowing of motor conduction velocities, without impairment of neuromuscular transmission.[177–179]

A high index of suspicion and meticulous physical examination are crucial for diagnosis. Cure by removing the tick is nearly miraculous.[176, 177] Tick paralysis caused by *Ixodes holocyclus,* most prevalent in Australia, may be particularly severe even after tick removal and should be treated with hyperimmune serum.[175]

Protective clothing, insect repellents, and care with domestic animals are important prophylactic measures.

Lyme Disease

Lyme disease is the most common tick-borne disease in the United States. It is caused by the spirochete *Borrelia burgdorferi* and affects primarily the skin, nervous system, heart, and joints. Ixodes are the primary vectors, and the disease has a seasonal occurrence during the summer.[175,176]

Several different pathogenic mechanisms seem to be involved in the neurologic manifestations of Lyme disease: immune factors, indirect inflammatory factors, and toxic-metabolic factors are possible explanations.

Up to half of the infections are asymptomatic, depending on the host's immune system response. Clinical disease may occur during early or late infection.

The multisystemic disease begins with the classic erythema chronicum migrans, which may be accompanied by malaise, fatigue, and fever to further involve the heart, joints, and nervous system. A large number of neurologic manifestations have been associated with Lyme disease, particularly meningitis, meningoencephalomyelitis, encephalitis, peripheral neuritis, and radiculopathies. Cranial neuropathy may include optic neuritis, diplopia, facial numbness or pain, hearing loss, and mostly facial palsy, sometimes bilateral.[180, 181]

Encephalomyelitis is rare and may occur in an acute, relapsing-remitting, or chronic progressive course. Bannwarth's syndrome, the European Lyme disease, is characterized by painful lymphocytic meningoradiculitis.

CSF may show pleocytosis, with intrathecal antibody production,[182] elevated IgG, and oligoclonal bands, but may be normal in pure peripheral nervous system involvement or encephalopathy. Electromyographic results are consistent with a demyelinating or axonal neuropathy.[182]

The diagnosis is based on clinical criteria. Erythema migrans is the only pathognomonic marker. Antecedent of tick bite *(Ixodes),* with prolonged attachment, and systemic symptoms like joint and muscle pain, fatigue, and cardiac involvement are suggestive. The most important neurologic features are meningitis; cranial neuritis, particularly with facial nerve involvement; and radicular neuritis.[183]

Laboratory tests are based on the detection of serum or CSF antibodies, but there is no definitive and readily available test for active infection. Recently, CSF detection of *Borrelia burgdorferi* nucleic acids using polymerase chain reaction has been described.[183a]

The diagnosis should be accurate, because it has recently been shown that antibiotics should be avoided in the treatment of unsubstantiated Lyme disease.[184]

Poliomyelitis

Poliomyelitis is a systemic infection that mainly affects the CNS. Poliomyelitis may result from live-attenuated oral polio vaccine virus[185] in vaccine recipients or their contacts, especially if they are immunodeficient, as well as in an inadequately or non-immunized population[186]; it may also result from wild polio virus in inadequate or non-immunized populations. The three serotypes of the polioviruses, members of the genus *Enterovirus,* family Picornaviridae, are distinguished by neutralization tests.[187] Infection confers type-specific, lifelong immunity.[187] Though experimental disease and infection can be produced in primates, humans are the only natural host and reservoir of the virus.[187] Natural occurring strains vary largely in neurovirulence, whereas vaccine strains have lower neurovirulence and are distinguished by temperature sensitivity and subtle antigenic differences. The median incubation period may be shorter in vaccine recipients. Pregnancy, strenuous exercise, intramuscular injections, trauma, tonsillectomy, and genetic factors seem to be risk factors for the development of paralysis in infected subjects.[187]

After the implantation and replication in the gut, adjacent lymphoid tissue, and deep lymph nodes, the virus may elicit the formation of type-specific antibodies in asymptomatic infection, or it may replicate and cause viremia in a few subjects. The routes of CNS infection are still controversial; experimental studies suggest that the virus may spread from muscle to CNS through PNs.[188] Motor neurons of the anterior horn of the spinal cord, brain stem motor nuclei, and autonomic neurons are particularly damaged, accompanied by inflammatory infiltrates of polymorphonuclear leukocytes, lymphocytes, and macrophages. The dorsal root ganglia may be affected, although without sensory deficits. The anterior roots and PNs undergo axonal degeneration leading to denervation atrophy in skeletal muscles.[188]

At least 95% of infections are asymptomatic and recognized only by virus isolation from feces or oropharynx, or by raised serum antibodies.[187] Fever, headache, nausea, coryza, and sore throat are the first symptoms, often accompanied by diarrhea. Constipation or rash occurs in abortive poliomyelitis. A bimodal course with remission of prodromal symptoms and recurrence is frequent in children.[189, 190] Anxiety, photophobia, sonophobia, muscle pain, fever, headache, vomiting, and nuchal rigidity, with CSF pleocytosis, characterize the meningitic phase that usually precedes the paralytic phase, often accompanied by muscle pain. After 3–4 days, or seldom as the first symptom, flaccid paralysis, typically asymmetric, predominantly involving lower limbs and proximal muscles, occurs. Deep tendon reflexes may be briefly hyperactive and rapidly become absent in the paretic limb. Paralysis may involve abdominal, respiratory, paraspinal, and neck muscles, as well as facial, masticatory, extraocular, palatal, pharyngeal, and laryngeal muscles. Pure bulbar involvement is rare, causing dysphagia, nasal speech, and dyspnea. Respiratory and vasomotor centers may be affected, leading to an ominous prognosis.[191] Respiratory failure may result from paralysis affecting respiratory muscles and involvement of cranial nerve nuclei or brain stem respiratory centers.[191] Autonomic dysfunctions include hypertension, arrhythmia, thermoinstability, and urinary retention. Muscle atrophy may appear after the first week. Sensory symptoms without objective sensory loss may occur. Adults tend to have more widespread and severe paralysis with bulbar involvement than do children.[192]

Polioencephalitis is infrequent and may present with seizures, spastic paralysis, and impairment of consciousness. Myocarditis is rare.

CSF findings are those of an aseptic meningitis with mild to moderate pleocytosis and an increase in proteins. Nerve conduction studies may show no muscle response in a severely affected limb. When a response can be elicited, motor NCV is usually normal.[193] Electromyography shows a reduced interference pattern and reduced number of recruited motor units, but abnormal spontaneous activity is absent in early illness. Fibrillations generally begin after 1–4 weeks. Later motor unit action potentials become polyphasic and increased in duration and amplitude, characteristic of anterior horn cell disease. Decremental response of the compound muscle action potential (CMAP) amplitude to repetitive stimulation may occur.

The diagnosis is confirmed by isolation of the virus from the throat in the first weeks, from stool samples for several weeks, and rarely from the CSF. Identification of the virus isolate (wild or vaccine type) is important, mainly in areas of low incidence of the disease.[187] A fourfold or greater rise between acute and convalescent serum antibody titers supports the diagnosis. When the virus is not found in the gastrointestinal tract, and serum antibodies have reached a plateau, demonstration of IgM antibodies sometimes helps in indicating a recent infection.[194]

The scenario is different from that of GBS: Patients present typically with fever, signs of meningeal irritation, asymmetric paralysis without sensory loss, and CSF and electrophysiologic findings. Other diagnoses, like diphtheria, botulism, tick paralysis, acute transverse myelitis, and paralytic non-polio enterovirus disease, must be excluded.

Treatment is only symptomatic and supportive, because there are no specific antiviral agents against poliovirus. Pain relief and bed rest are important in the acute phase of the disease. Physiotherapy must wait until progression has stopped. Respiratory failure and bulbar paralysis usually require tracheal intubation and positive pressure ventilators. The mortality rate was higher, mainly in patients with bulbar and respiratory muscle involvement, before the critical care era.[195] Complete recovery seems to be rare in severe paralysis, whereas total recovery from bulbar paralysis may occur.[187]

Immunization is the best way to prevent the disease, despite occasional reports of paralytic poliomyelitis in trivalent oral vaccine recipients or contacts.[185, 196] Adoption of a sequential vaccination schedule with inactivated poliovirus vaccine preceding oral polio vaccine has been suggested in order to decrease the risk of vaccine associated paralytic poliomyelitis while retaining the benefits of oral vaccine.[186]

Recently, after the decline in the incidence of poliovirus, other enteroviruses, such as coxsackievirus, echovirus, and enterovirus-71, have emerged as relatively important causes of paralytic poliomyelitis.[197]

Tetanus

Clostridium tetani is an obligate anaerobic bacillus, gram-positive in fresh cultures.[198] Any wound, but particularly wounds contaminated with dirt, puncture wounds, burns, avulsions, and crush injuries, may be inoculated with tetanus spores.[198] *C. tetani* produces two toxins: tetanospasmin, also called tetanus toxin, and tetanolysin, which is of uncertain importance in the pathogenesis of the disease. Tetanospasmin is cleaved extracellularly into a light chain (fragment A) and a heavy chain, which can further be cleaved into fragments B and C. The heavy chain mediates binding to the cell surface receptors conferring target specificity and facilitates entry of the light chain, which produces clinical tetanus by causing a presynaptic inhibition of neurotransmitter release.[199] The toxin enters the nervous system by the presynaptic terminals of lower motor neurons (alpha motor neurons). It is carried to the cell bodies of the neurons in the brain stem and spinal cord by retrograde axonal transport.[198] In the CNS, the toxin spreads to inhibitory synapses like local glycinergic interneurons in the spinal cord and descending GABAergic neurons from the brain stem, impairing neurotransmitter release and causing muscular rigidity and spasms. Failure to inhibit adrenal release of catecholamines may also occur, producing a hypersympathetic state. Recovery depends on sprouting of the terminal neurons at the NMJ and probably other synapses.[200]

The four clinical types—generalized, localized, cephalic, and neonatal—probably reflect different host factors and sites of inoculation. They seem to have prognostic importance. Poorer prognoses are related to shorter incubation periods, as well as certain sites of inoculation, regardless of the clinical form. Generalized tetanus often begins with masseter rigidity (trismus) and rigidity of the abdominal and limb muscles. The generalized painful spasms are often triggered by sensory stimulus and cause opisthotonus. Respiratory dysfunction may result from upper airway obstruction and diaphragm spasm. Autonomic dysfunction includes hypertension, tachycardia, arrhythmia, profuse sweating, hypercarbia, and pyrexia.[200, 201] Autonomic dysfunction or complications may cause death despite intensive care.[202] Mild neuropathy, often asymmetric, occurs in some patients with distal weakness and sensory loss but may be apparent only after remission of the spasms.

The lack of a known wound, although uncommon, must not exclude the diagnosis. Ear infections, injections, drug abuse, foreign bodies, minor surgical procedures, or vaginal and rectal instrumentation are other possible portals of entry.[200]

Localized tetanus may be a prodrome of the generalized form or probably a consequence of partial immunity; this condition involves muscles near the site of inoculation.[198] The rigidity may be mild and persist for weeks or months, usually resolving spontaneously.[200]

A special form of localized tetanus is cephalic tetanus. Peripheral facial nerve weakness is usually the first manifestation, accompanied by trismus, dysphagia, and sometimes extraocular muscle involvement.[200, 203]

Motor and sensory nerve conduction velocities may be mildly slowed. Electrophysiologic tests show evidence of denervation and reinnervation. Continuous muscle activity, even on attempted relaxation; lack of inhibition when antagonistic muscles are activated; and absence of a silent period in the masseter following a jaw jerk are characteristic.[200]

Neonatal tetanus usually follows infection of the umbilical stump when the mother lacks immunity.[204] High mortality rates are reported, which are especially related to early age at admission, presence of fever, and risus sardonicus.[205]

The diagnosis is based on clinical features. Antitetanus antibodies may be either undetectable or above "protective" concentrations.[206] Culture is useless because it is commonly negative, and if positive it does not necessarily indicate disease.

Differential diagnoses must exclude strychnine poisoning, dystonic reactions to neuroleptic or antiemetic drugs, stiff-man syndrome, tetany due to hypocalcemia, and psychogenic disorders.[200] Trismus and visible contraction of the platysma are important clues to diagnosis, mainly in localized forms.

Respiratory support, caloric and fluid-electrolyte balance, and passive immunization are the leading aspects of treatment. Benzodiazepines, including diazepam, lorazepam, or midazolam, constitute the main symptomatic therapy by indirectly antagonizing the effect of the toxin.[200] Nasogastric delivery of benzodiazepines should be the first choice, except in patients with gastrointestinal motility impairment. Continuous infusion of midazolam may also be useful. NMJ blockade using vecuronium by continuous infusion or pancuronium by intermittent injection may be necessary in cases of benzodiazepines failure.[198] Intravenous labetalol that combines alpha- and beta-adrenergic blockade may help the control of autonomic dysfunction.[207]

Treatment of trismus with botulinum toxin A was successfully reported in a patient with cephalic tetanus in order to improve oral hygiene, aspiration, and feeding.[208] Antibiotic therapy remains controversial. The clinical course seems to be unrelated to wound débridement. Passive immunization with human tetanus immunoglobulin seems to reduce the severity and duration of the disease, but once the toxin has already been transported within the neuron it is inaccessible to antitoxin.[200] Active immunization is also necessary to prevent recurrence. Partial immunization may decrease the severity of the symptoms. A detailed management protocol is suggested by Bleck.[198]

The mortality rate is higher in severe cases, particularly in heroin addicts and neonatal tetanus,[201] and is increased with age.[209] Recovery may take several weeks.[202] Poor outcome has been correlated with respiratory failure, hemodynamic instability, hyperglycemia, hyperthermia, and anticoagulation therapy.[210]

Prophylaxis with tetanus toxoid provides almost complete immunity for at least 5 years, and routine booster injections are necessary every 10 years.[198]

Botulism

Botulism is caused by the neurotoxin from *Clostridium botulinum,* a large, usually gram-positive, strictly anaerobic bacillus,[211] which may contaminate canned foods, fish, or wounds. Botulinum toxin is structurally similar to tetanus toxin. It is also synthesized as a precursor with low toxicity, and its transport within nerve seems to be analogous. Their different clinical effects depend on different target cells.[199] Types A, B, E, and F botulinum toxins act on the peripheral NMJ and autonomic synapses, blocking acetylcholine release, producing primarily weakness and autonomic dysfunction. Recovery requires sprouting of presynaptic axon.

The clinical forms described are food-borne, wound, infant, and botulism of undetermined etiology. Food-borne botulism is easily diagnosed in outbreaks. The other forms are usually sporadic.

Food-borne botulism often begins 12–36 hours (range 6 hours to 8 days) after ingestion of contaminated food, with nausea, vomiting, dry mouth, abdominal pain, constipation, and occasionally diarrhea. Fever is present only in complications.[211]

Neurologic symptoms most commonly start with blurred vision; ptosis; and diplopia due to parasympathetic and third-, fourth-, or sixth-nerve dysfunction, followed by dysphagia, dysphonia, facial and neck weakness, and proximal upper and then lower limb muscle involvement, in a descending symmetric pattern over several days. Respiratory muscle weakness may lead to respiratory failure and is often disproportionate to limb weakness. Limb weakness and ptosis may be asymmetric. The reflexes may be normal or become hypoactive, even in cases with severe weakness. Mydriasis with poor response to light and accommodation, a hallmark of botulism, may not appear until late.[212, 213] The lateral rectus is the most commonly affected eye muscle. The triad of ptosis, medial rectus weakness, and dilated or hyporeactive pupils is thought to be predictive of respiratory failure, the main cause of death in severe cases.[214]

Autonomic dysfunction may occur with constipation, urinary retention or hesitation,[215] impairment of lacrimation and salivation, orthostatic hypotension, or hypothermia. Paresthesias without objective sensory loss, nystagmus, ataxia, and Babinski's sign may be atypical features of the disease.[213]

CSF examination may show a slight protein level elevation in some cases.[213] Electrophysiologic studies present increased numbers of myopathic units. There are often small CMAPs and motor unit potential amplitudes that suggest a lesion of the small nerve terminal branches. Decremental response at low rates of repetitive stimulation and incremental response after exercise or repetitive nerve stimulation at higher rates is also found. Electromyographic findings are not generalized and may be absent early in the disease. Single-fiber electromyography may reveal impulse blocking and increased jitter in clinically normal muscles.[216, 217] Fibrillation may be present in the recovering period. Nerve conduction velocities and terminal latencies are usually normal. F waves may be absent in cases with very low CMAP. H reflexes are usually normal, but a low-amplitude H reflex with prolonged latency or prominent H reflexes has been reported.[218] The sensitivity of electrophysiologic tests has been questioned in cases of infant botulism.[219]

Detection of botulinum toxin in the stool or serum, in the contaminated food, or in culture of *C. botulinum* is required for diagnosis. Epidemiologic data are the most important clues for diagnosis. Edrophonium may be a useful test, causing brief clinical and electrophysiologic improvement.[213]

MG, Lambert-Eaton myasthenic syndrome, tick paralysis, toxic exposure to organophosphates or heavy metals, GBS, and Miller-Fisher syndrome may be considered in the differential diagnosis.

Treatment is usually supportive.[220] Antitoxin seems to have no clear effect once neurologic symptoms have begun, but the fatality rate seems to be lower in patients treated with antitoxin even after 24 hours.[221]

The high mortality in the past has decreased with modern intensive care. Respiratory support and adequate care with the paralyzed patient allow complete recovery unless complications supervene. A detailed description of the critical care management of botulism was published by Tacket and Rogawski.[222]

Proper food management is the leading aspect of preventing botulism.

Wound botulism is rare and often associated with compound fractures or crush injuries, as well as puncture wounds and skin lesions in chronic drug abusers.[223–225] *C. botulinum* infects and produces toxin in traumatized tissue. The incubation period is longer (4–14 days), and the onset is slower. Classic signs are similar to those of food-borne botulism, except for a prodromal gastrointestinal disorder. Fever may occur due to wound infection. Wound débridement is necessary despite the good appearance of the wound,[223] and antibiotic treatment, although questioned, is frequently recommended.

Infant botulism[226] occurs most exclusively in infants receiving breast milk,[227] at a mean age of 15 weeks; it results from gut colonization with *C. botulinum* prior to toxin production.[228] Constipation is typically the first symptom, followed after 3 weeks by a weak sucking reflex, swallowing, weak cry, and generalized progressive weakness in a descending pattern. There are also decreased spontaneous movements, hypotonia, ptosis, and extraocular and facial weakness. Hyporeflexia or areflexia may occur in more than half of patients. Respiratory failure is common.[226,227] The pupillary reaction to light may be normal or reduced. Patients may also present with impaired salivation and lacrimation and with hemodynamic instability.[227] Relapses may occur. Botulinum toxin is usually found in the stool but not in the serum. Electrophysiologic features are classic but brief; small abundant motor-unit action potentials (BSAPs) are particularly common.[228]

Botulism of undetermined etiology has no known wound or ingestion of toxin and could be associated with gut colonization by *C. botulinum* after gastrointestinal surgical procedures or enteritis.[229, 230] Persistent constipation is typical besides clinical signs and symptoms of the other forms of botulism.

Acute Viral Myositis

Acute viral myositis is usually a febrile illness with myalgia as the major symptom, often accompanied by weakness, muscle tenderness, and swelling. Elevated serum CK, myoglobinuria, abnormal electromyographic and muscle biopsy results, and abnormal laboratory findings suggest a recent viral infection.[231]

This syndrome has been related mostly to influenza,[232–241] but coxsackievirus,[242, 243] adenovirus,[244] herpesvirus,[245] parainfluenza virus, Epstein-Barr virus,[246–248] echovirus,[248–250] cytomegalovirus,[251] and human immunodeficiency virus (HIV)[242, 252, 253] have also been described.

The pathophysiology of the syndrome remains unclear; viral infection, immunologic, or other indirect mechanisms are possible causes of tissue injury.[231]

Although usually benign and self-limited, acute viral myositis can be generalized and severe, particularly in adults,[233, 235, 237, 239, 241] with myoglobinuria and renal failure, sometimes leading to cardiopulmonary failure and death.[233, 235, 241] Most adults reported presented with fever, generalized myalgia, weakness, and myoglobinuria. Pulmonary congestion, pulmonary embolism, and arrhythmias were also described.[233, 235] Deaths were related to cardiopulmonary complications[233, 235] or renal failure,[241] but all dying patients had myoglobinuria.

Necrosis,[235, 236, 238, 241] regeneration,[241] and inflammatory infiltrates,[232, 235, 236] as well as normal muscle biopsy results, have been described,[233, 239] perhaps related to differences in the stage of the disease at examination or to the focal pattern of pathological changes.[235] Viral particles found by electron microscopy[236] and isolation of virus from muscle have been rarely described.[234, 235, 237]

Arbovirus, as well as dengue virus, produces an acute clinical syndrome characterized by fever, severe myalgia, and joint pain. Perivascular mononuclear infiltrates and lipid accumulation without actual myositis are the main muscle biopsy findings.[254]

Treatment is limited to symptomatic procedures. Cardiac, renal, and pulmonary complications must be promptly treated.

ACUTE INVOLVEMENT OF THE NEUROMUSCULAR SYSTEM DUE TO DRUGS, METALS, AND TOXINS

The practitioner is frequently confronted with disorders caused by accidental or willful intoxication with drugs or toxic agents. Some of these agents have widespread effects on the different cells and organs; others more specifically affect the neuromuscular system.[255] Skeletal muscle, an extremely active tissue, is very susceptible to the effects of poisons and drugs.[256] The PNs and the myoneural junctions are also susceptible to harm by drugs and toxins.

The precise incidence of toxic neuromuscular disorders in clinical practice is difficult to establish, because the association with drug therapy or toxic substance is not always recognized, and subclinical forms are probably more common than is generally appreciated.[257] The most useful diagnostic approach is a detailed occupational and social history, specifically inquiring about solvent exposure, inhalant abuse, and use of drugs. Without a precise history or a few clear physical signs, identification of a drug or toxic substance via toxicologic analysis of serum, urine, or gastric contents is more difficult but may be the only method of establishing a definitive diagnosis.[258]

The critical determinant of outcome should be the interval between intoxication and arrival at the emergency room. This assumes an ability of the physician to differentiate other forms of disease from that caused by toxic agents, recognize the patterns of dysfunction caused by different and specific agents, and promptly initiate appropriate therapy. Specific treatment, however, is rare.

This review considers acute manifestations on the neuromuscular system caused by exogenous substances.

Involvement of Peripheral Nerves

Involvement of PN trunks may occur as a complication of intramuscular injections of drugs, attributable either to direct needle trauma or to local toxic effect of the drug itself. The best-known example is the sciatic nerve damage that may occur with injections into the buttock. A more generalized involvement of PNs is related to a large variety of agents, including organic and inorganic substances, particularly metals.[259] These agents may cause sensorimotor neuropathy or pure motor or sensory neuropathy.

Most of these agents appear to produce chronic and distal axonopathy, usually after prolonged exposure. Certain agents, however, may produce acute involvement of the PNs. The mechanisms involved in the production of neuropathy are not always well understood. In general, the agents that cause peripheral neuropathy do so either by interfering with axonal or Schwann cell metabolism or through a vascular effect.

The following agents are selected because of recognized associations with acute neuropathy and distinctive features.

Pharmaceutical Agents

ISONIAZID

Isoniazid-induced polyneuropathy was common in the early 1950s,[260] when this drug was first used for the treatment of tuberculosis. Symptoms of neuropathy appeared in about 10% of patients receiving therapeutic doses of the drug, between 3 and 35 weeks after treatment was begun. The initial symptom is symmetrically painful neuropathy in the lower extremities. Severe degrees of weakness and loss of deep sensation are rare. The effect on the PN is related with the inhibition of pyridoxine phosphorylation. The daily administration of 0.2–0.65 mg/kg of pyridoxine (vitamin B_6) prevents the neuropathic disorder.[261]

PYRIDOXINE (VITAMIN B_6)

Pyridoxine is an essential, water-soluble vitamin (B_6), which is a coenzyme in many important biologic reactions. It has several medical uses, including therapy for intoxication secondary to the false morel mushroom and isoniazid treatment. Paradoxically, when pyridoxine is used in high doses and over a prolonged time, it may cause an acute, diffuse, and irreversible sensory neuropathy in experimental animals and humans.[262]

NITROFURANTOIN

Peripheral neuropathy is a relatively frequent complication of treatment with nitrofurantoin, mainly in patients with impaired renal function.[263] Symptoms usually appear within the first 45 days of treatment. The majority of patients present with distal sensory symptoms followed after a few days by pain and muscle weakness. Occasionally, predominant motor neuropathy occurs.[264] The prognosis for recovery depends on the severity of the condition.[265]

METRONIDAZOLE

Metronidazole (Flagyl), a commonly used antiprotozoal and antibacterial agent, can cause distal axonopathy related to prolonged treatment; however, occasional instances have appeared at lower doses, and one report suggests the absence of a clear dose-effect relationship.[266] Metronidazole peripheral neuropathies produce pure sensory deficits and may be reversible when the drug is discontinued. In rodent experiments, metronidazole was found to bind selectively to neuronal RNA; this may inhibit protein synthesis and cause axonal degeneration.[267]

PHENYTOIN

Long-term diphenylhydantoin administration can cause reversible neuropathy characterized by axonal shrinkage, secondary demyelination, and remyelination.[268] Acute or subacute involvement of PNs is rare, and the symptoms are easily reversible after the drug is discontinued.[269]

ANTIRHEUMATIC DRUGS

Gold therapy in rheumatoid arthritis is related to peripheral neuropathy. Motor involvement is usually prominent and may be asymmetric, and sensory signs may be inconspicuous. The onset may be abrupt and progression rapid, mimicking GBS. CSF protein has been raised in some cases.[261]

TAXOL

Taxol is a plant alkaloid used as an antineoplastic agent for solid tumors. Doses above 200 mg/m^2 are associated with sensory neuropathy.[270] Paresthesias and disesthesias in hands and feet with proximal spread begin suddenly within days of administration. Weakness is unusual. The drug binds to tubulin and promotes microtubule assembly. When taxol is injected directly into rat sciatic nerve, microtubules aggregate into unusual arrangements in both axons and Schwann cells, leading to acute demyelination and chronic loss of axoplasmic transport.[271] Electromyographic studies support the presence of both axonal degeneration and demyelination. Administration of nerve growth factor can delay the onset of neuropathy in experimental animals[272] and could have some significance for human taxol neuropathy.

VINCA ALKALOIDS

Alkaloids derived from the periwinkle plant, Vinca Rosea Linn, are useful agents for the treatment of a variety of neoplastic diseases, particularly the lymphomas, because of their effects on the mitotic spindle in proliferating cells. Vincristine and vinblastine are inhibitors of tubulin polymerization (microtubule formation) that disrupt the microtubules of the axonal cytoskeleton and cause axonal neuropathy.[273] Paresthesias of the feet or hands may occur within a few weeks of the beginning of treatment; with continued use of the drugs, a progressive, symmetric motor-sensory and reflex loss occurs. Cranial nerves are affected less frequently. Autonomic involvement with postural hypotension and constipation may be early symptoms. Recovery may occur if the drug is stopped or the dose is reduced, but mild sensory impairment and reflex depression often persist. Electrophysiologic studies have shown evidence of severe axonal damage involving both motor and sensory fibers.[274]

MELANOMA IMMUNOTHERAPY

The vaccine used in melanoma immunotherapy, prepared from the supernatant of centrifuged lysate of vaccinia killed melanoma cells from a single allogenic melanoma cell line, has been associated with inflammatory demyelinating neuropathy, acute inflammatory demyelinating polyneuropathy, and chronic inflammatory demyelinating polyneuropathy.[275]

OCCUPATIONAL, BIOLOGIC, AND ENVIRONMENTAL AGENTS

An enormous number of potentially toxic chemicals are deployed in the workplace and general environment. Many have been implicated as causes of chronic peripheral neuropathy, usually of the distal axonopathy type, whereas some of them cause acute or subacute involvement of PNs.

Inorganic Substances

HEAVY METALS

Lead

Lead neuropathy is an uncommon disorder mostly seen in children; it seldom occurs as a unique manifestation in children, in whom the poisoning usually also results in encephalopathy.[276] The characteristic feature is the predominantly motor affection, involving mainly the upper extremities, that develops over a period of a few weeks. The radial nerves are most frequently affected, producing wrist and finger drop with few or no sensory manifestations. The diagnosis depends on a high index of suspicion and on certain laboratory and clinical findings: anemia, basophilic stippling of red cell precursors in the bone marrow, lead line along the gingival margins, and increased urinary excretion of lead and coproporphyrins. Blood levels of more than 70 μg/dL are always abnormal. The treatment consists in terminating the exposure to lead and eliminating lead from the bloodstream and bones using combined chelation therapy (dimercaprol or $CaNa_2$ EDTA), penicillamine, or both.[259]

Mercury

Most of the neurologic effects of mercury are manifested by the CNS; symptomatic peripheral neuropathy is rare.[277] Nevertheless, mercury metal vapor exposure can cause subacute, diffuse, predominantly motor neuropathy, mimicking acute inflammatory demyelinating polyneuropathy.[259]

Thallium

Because thallium is odorless and tasteless, it is one of the most potentially toxic metals. Thallous salts have been widely employed in rodenticides and insecticides, and reports of intoxication come from suicidal, criminal, or accidental ingestion. Acute intoxication can cause death within 12 hours to 14 days from heart failure or brain damage. If a massive dose is ingested, acute and extremely painful ascending polyneuropathy may develop. Sensory symptoms predominate. Intoxication by other metals (arsenic, cadmium, lead, and mercury), porphyria, GBS, and botulism must be excluded.[278] The diagnosis of acute thallium neuropathy is difficult unless there is clear evidence of ingestion. Alopecia, the classic indication of thallium poisoning, is not present in the early stages of acute neuropathy.[279] Clinical suspicion of thallotoxicosis has to be confirmed by determination of thallium in the urine or blood. The treatment includes activated charcoal or Prussian blue.[280]

Arsenic

Human neurotoxicity from arsenic is usually associated with ingestion of trivalent arsenic (arsenite), an often-used substance for homicide and suicide. Pentavalent arsenic (arsenate) is less toxic. The clinical presentation of arsenic poisoning may be divided into three forms: acute massive, acute gastrointestinal, and chronic intoxication. A single large dose of arsenic can produce death within a day because of profound circulatory collapse or CNS depression.[281] Survivors may develop neuropathy within 10 days to 3 weeks following the ingestion.[282] The neuropathy progresses in an ascending fashion to involve proximal arms and legs, presenting as a GBS-like syndrome.[283] Whenever apparent Guillain-Barré neuropathy is associated with hyperpigmentation or keratosis of the skin, or is heralded by gastrointestinal symptoms, arsenic poisoning must be considered.[284] The severity of the neuropathy depends on the ingested dose. Recovery is slow and incomplete in severe cases. The diagnosis is based on the results of toxicologic analysis of urine, nails, and hair. It is suggested that arsenic may be primarily toxic to the nerve cell body, leading eventually to axonal dysfunction that produces, initially, segmental demyelination before axonal degeneration ensues.[283] Treatment involves chelation therapy with either dimercaprol or penicillamine.

Organic Substances

Organophosphorus Esters

Over 50,000 organophosphorus compounds, most of which inhibit acetylcholinesterase, can produce acetylcholinesterase side effects and a relatively uncommon form of peripheral neuropathy.[285] The most infamous organophosphate is triorthocresyl phosphate. Many instances of neuropathy have resulted from adulteration or misuse of triorthocresyl phosphate in food, drink, or cooking oil.[286, 287] Clinical symptoms may develop after a single dose or following repeated doses. Distal sensory symptoms in the limbs develop first, followed within a few days by distal limb weakness, which may progress for about a month. Recovery is often incomplete, probably because of failure of repair of coincidental CNS damage, leaving residual spasticity.

Trichloroethylene

Trichloroethylene is used in dry cleaning, in rubber production, and as a degreasing agent. Acute industrial exposure is associated with a typical neurotoxic syndrome characterized by trigeminal involvement, followed by dysfunction of the facial, oculomotor, and optic nerves. Peripheral limb nerves have not been implicated.[288]

Vacor

Vacor, N-3-pyridylmethyl-N-p-nitrophenyl urea (PNU), is a structural analog of nicotinamide. It is used as a rodenticide, and its accidental ingestion causes unusual, rapid-onset, severe, distal axonopathy with prominent autonomic involvement. The neuropathy is accompanied by acute diabetes mellitus secondary to necrosis of pancreatic beta cells.[289] Very early niacinamide therapy has a potential therapeutic benefit and may prevent PNU-induced diabetes.

Intoxication Related to Health Food and Herbal Preparations

So-called alternative, nontraditional, or unconventional medicine is practiced throughout the world. Nutritional supplements and herbal compounds are available in pharmacies, supermarkets, health food stores, and offices of ethnic herbalists. Because many of these preparations are derived from botanical species, they are considered "natural" and safe. However, these products are not well regulated by federal laws, and their efficacy and safety have not been determined. Intoxications resulting from these products are common, including involvement of PNs. Specific queries about ingestion of those products should become a routine part of the medical history and may be critical when a peripheral neuropathy of unknown origin is under consideration. Some examples of acute peripheral neuropathy related to those conditions are considered in the following sections.

Brazilian Indians. A form of acute peripheral neuropathy has been described in Brazilian Indians. Male pubertal seclusion is a cultural characteristic habit in tribes in the Alto Xingu region of central Brazil. This period, varying from several months to 3 years, is marked by many rules and taboos. Involvement of the PN is related to the use of some native plants in infusions or ointments during rites of purification.[290] The main clinical manifestations are tachycardia, sweating, and muscle weakness. A study of the PN has shown axonal degeneration.[291]

Podophyllin. Podophyllum peltatum, a source of podophyllotoxin, an antimicrotubule agent, is a constituent of herbal preparations used in some parts of the world as cathartics and in the treatment of inflammation.[292] Systemic manifestations of toxicity consist of nausea, vomiting, and diarrhea, followed by marrow suppression and hepatic failure. Neurotoxicity includes encephalopathy, sensory, motor, and autonomic neuropathy. The clinical course is sometimes fatal.[293]

Buckthorn. Accidental ingestion of the fruit from the buckthorn shrub, *Karwinskia humboldtiana* (wild cherry), found in Mexico, Texas, and New Mexico, is followed by a rapidly evolving, diffuse motor polyneuropathy that may be fatal. The clinical picture is that of progressive and symmetric polyneuropathy, starting in the lower limbs and ending with respiratory and bulbar paralysis.[294] The illness is sometimes confused with poliomyelitis; its severity is proportional to the amount ingested. If the patient survives, there is a slow and progressive improvement to almost complete functional recovery. The exact nature of the neuropathy is still uncertain.

SEAFOOD POISONING

Paralytic Shellfish Poisoning

Paralytic shellfish poisoning is an acute paralytic illness that follows ingestion of shellfish contaminated with saxitoxin, a compound similar to tetrodotoxin. Under favorable conditions, mainly associated with red tide, the toxin is concentrated in shellfish at levels sufficient to cause disease in humans. The clinical manifestations are acute bulbar and respiratory paralysis. Serial electromyography/NCV studies performed in one patient showed transitory demyelination in the PNs.[295] The main differential diagnoses to be considered are Miller-Fisher syndrome, botulism, and tick paralysis.

Ciguatera

Ciguatera poisoning is a common form of fish poisoning occurring in humans.[296] The clinical manifestations are the sudden onset of nausea, vomiting, diarrhea, and abdominal pain, followed by paresthesia, dysesthesia, myalgia, and weakness. The neurologic disturbance is usually self-limiting, resolving within 2–3 weeks, but mild symptoms may persist for months or even years. Significant slowing of sensory conduction velocity and prolongation of the absolute refractory, relative refractory, and supernormal periods have been demonstrated.[297] Ciguatera poisoning apparently produces no immunity, and the second attack may be more severe. The symptoms and signs are caused by a neurotoxin, ciguatoxin, that causes an abnormally prolonged sodium channel opening in nerve membranes. No drugs given empirically have been found to be consistently effective in this disease.[297]

Involvement of the Neuromuscular Junction

A great variety of drugs and toxins produce an MG-like syndrome, either by interfering with acetylcholine formation or its release at the synaptic terminal of the myoneural junction, or by binding with the receptor. Other drugs produce this effect by a direct influence on the postsynaptic membrane.

Antibiotics

Many antibiotics are known to interfere with neuromuscular transmission.[298] These include neomycin, streptomycin, kanamycin, gentamicin, polymyxin B, bacitracin, colistin, oxytetracycline, lincomycin, clindamycin, and imipenen.[299]

Antiarrhythmics

Quinidine and beta-adrenoceptor blockers have anticholinergic effects on neuromuscular conduction and may unmask previously unsuspected MG or aggravate a previously mild, stable case of clinical MG.[300] The use of these drugs should be avoided in MG; the use of other antiarrhythmic agents is suggested.

Organophosphorus Esters

The acute toxicity of anticholinesterase organophosphate compounds is caused by inhibition of carboxylic esterases. After proper treatment, there is complete control of the acute cholinergic crisis. Nevertheless, prolonged and later manifestations described as an intermediate syndrome have been described and related with fenthion or its analogues.[301] It has been suggested that prolonged circulation of these agents from adipose tissue might play a role. The syndrome is characterized by cholinergic symptoms emerging 24–96 hours after an apparently well-treated acute crisis that persists for weeks. The severe cases present with respiratory paresis and weakness in the territory of many motor cranial nerves and proximal limb and neck flexor muscles.

Black Widow Spider Envenomation

Black widow spider (*Latrodectus* sp) produces one of the most potent known venoms by volume. The venom acts at the NMJ by binding to glycoproteins or gangliosides on the presynaptic membrane and opening cation channels.[302] Large quantities of acetylcholine are released from the presynaptic neuron; the reuptake of choline is inhibited simultaneously. The venom also causes severe skeletal muscle pain, cramping, and autonomic disturbances. Some patients with generalized pain have elevated CK levels. Many of these patients require admission for observation and pain control, but symptoms usually resolve within 24–48 hours. The treatment includes calcium gluconate, parenteral opioids, and *Latrodectus*-specific antivenin. The latter should be restricted to patients who have severe envenomation and no allergic contraindications.[303]

Involvement of Muscle

Drugs and toxins may produce myopathic changes in several ways. They may act directly on muscle cells, and their effects can be generalized or local, as occurs when a drug is injected into a muscle. Muscle damage can also be secondary to electrolyte disturbances, to excessive energy requirements due to neural activation, or to the inadequate delivery of oxygen and nutrients due to muscle compression and ischemia. The resulting clinical syndromes vary in severity, mode of onset, and rate of progression.[256]

Intramuscular injections produce localized areas of muscle damage as a result of needle insertion and local effects of the agent injected, such as cephalothin, lidocaine, or diazepam. Some organic poisons, such as formalin, Lysol, or turpentine, may cause more severe tissue damage. Muscle fibrosis leading to progressive induration and contractures may occur in children who have undergone intramuscular injections of antibiotics[304] and in adults addicted to pethidine.[305]

Rhabdomyolysis, a necrotizing form of myopathy in which injury to skeletal muscle results in the leakage of intracellular contents from myocytes into plasma, is the most frequent myotoxic syndrome. It is characterized by acute or subacute onset of local or generalized muscle pain, tenderness and weakness, and rapid elevation of serum CK.

Myoglobinuria may complicate any skeletal muscle injury, resulting in acute renal failure.[306] Myoglobin has a nephrotoxic effect that is increased by low urine flow states and acidic urine pH values. The incidence of such renal failure has been as high as 50%. There are about 100 types of drug- and toxin-induced rhabdomyolysis and myoglobinuria.[307] Myoglobinuria has accounted for more than 8% of all cases of acute renal failure in some hospitals,[308] most of them induced by drugs or alcohol.[309]

Treatment consists of terminating exposure to the toxic agent, correcting intravascular volume depletion, and urine alkalinization to prevent acute renal failure.[306]

The main primary myopathies caused by toxins or drugs are described in the following sections.

Pharmaceutical Agents

TRYPTOPHAN

Tryptophan is an essential amino acid that has been associated to eosinophilia-myalgia syndrome. The illness is characterized by peripheral eosinophilia fatigue and myalgia. The disorder is often disabling and may become chronic. The symptoms may progress even after the ingestion of L-tryptophan has been discontinued. Muscle biopsy discloses inflammatory changes.[310] The pathological and clinical features suggest that it is an autoimmune illness in which T-lymphocytes play a major role. Immunosuppressive treatment may be beneficial in eosinophilia-myalgia syndrome.[311]

PROCAINAMIDE

Procainamide is known to induce a conditioned autoimmune response similar to systemic lupus, except that the kidneys are rarely involved.[256] Myositis is an unusual manifestation of the drug. The myopathy remits rapidly after withdrawal of the drug and a short course of azathioprine.[312]

LABETALOL

Labetalol, an antihypertensive alpha/beta blocker, may cause severe generalized myopathy that can be reversible after discontinued use of the drug.[313]

ANTIMALARIALS

Quinine and chloroquine, used in the treatment of malaria, scleroderma, and discoid erythematosus lupus, are known for their myotoxic effects.[314] The main symptom is a painless weakness. Pathologically, chloroquine is associated with vacuolar myopathy, mainly affecting type I fibers. The vacuoles in the muscle are autophagic, containing cytoplasmic degeneration products.[314]

COLCHICINE

Colchicine has been used therapeutically for more than 200 years. It affects mitosis and other microtubule-dependent functions. Muscle involvement can occur after the long-term use of colchicine at customary doses or as result of acute intoxication accompanying renal failure.[315, 316] It usually presents with proximal weakness, elevation of serum CK, and frequently mild axonal polyneuropathy. Electromyographic studies show myopathy that is marked by abnormal spontaneous activity. The myopathy is vacuolar, characterized by accumulation of lysosomes and autophagic vacuoles. The weakness remits within 3–4 weeks after the drug is discontinued. The axonal neuropathy resolves slowly.

VINCRISTINE

Vincristine, an oncolytic alkaloid widely used in the treatment of leukemia, has been known to produce mild sensorimotor polyneuropathy. However, when large doses are administered, painful proximal necrotizing and acute myopathy may occur.[317] Electron-microscopic studies have shown that the drug has a profound effect on membrane systems and causes severe autophagic degeneration of muscle fibers. Inflammation is minimal, and only rare fibers show phagocytosis. The disparity between the degree of muscle degeneration and inflammation may be explained by vincristine's action in suppressing the immune response.

EMETINE AND IPECAC

The ipecac alkaloid called emetine, which is used in the treatment of amebiasis, inhibits protein synthesis in a variety of cell types. It causes polyfocal myonecrosis of skeletal and cardiac muscle,[318] sometimes fatal.[319] Muscle weakness caused by emetine varies from moderate to complete paralysis. Resolution of the neurologic symptoms may take weeks. The myofibrillar degeneration affects mainly type I fibers and closely resembles that observed in multicore disease.[319]

Drugs Used in the Treatment of Hyperlipoproteinemias

Clofibrate (Atromid-S), lovastatin, and nicotinic acid, used clinically as a means of reducing the lipid content of the blood, have been found to occasionally induce acute myopathy with cramps, severe myalgia, weakness, tenderness of muscles, and elevation of CK.[320] The main differential diagnosis is polymyositis; muscle biopsy is an important diagnostic procedure to distinguish the two. The administration of lovastatin in combination with certain drugs increases the risk of toxic myopathy. When associated with cyclosporine, the risk of myopathy increases to 30%, and prominent rhabdomyolysis may occur.[321, 322] Lovastatin and its analogues are excreted primarily in the bile and cause cholestasis at high doses. The degree of bile acid elevation increases by more than 13 times in the presence of cyclosporine, which also undergoes biliary excretion.[323] These myopathies are usually entirely reversible within weeks to a few months after drug withdrawal.

EPSILON-AMINOCAPROIC ACID

The antifibrinolytic agent epsilon-aminocaproic acid has been associated in a number of cases with rhabdomyolysis, myoglobinuria, and myonecrosis. Usually, it has appeared after 1 or 2 weeks of therapy. Muscle symptoms begin with muscle tenderness, followed by weakness, most pronounced in the limb-girdle and axial musculature.[256]

THEOPHYLLINE

Theophylline in toxic concentrations may produce a wide spectrum of symptoms and signs. Neurologic, cardiac, and metabolic manifestations are well documented in standard texts. A rare but fatal form of theophylline poisoning with massive rhabdomyolysis has been described.[324, 325] The main clinical features are rhabdomyolysis, renal failure, and compartment syndrome, as well as the more usual features of severe theophylline poisoning. Dantrolene appeared to be useful in controlling the hypermetabolic state associated with the overdose and may have a role in the treatment.[324]

PODOPHYLLIN

Podophyllin is a resin commonly used in the topical treatment of warts and condylomata. Neurotoxic effects may involve the central and peripheral nervous system,[326] but involvement of skeletal muscle is not described. We saw a 21-year-old male who ingested podophyllin in a suicide attempt. The disorder was marked by seizures, coma, hepatic dysfunction, cardiac failure, peripheral neuropathy, and acute necrotizing myopathy (Fig. 13–3), an unusual finding. The state of coma and systemic disturbances resolved within 3 weeks. The myopathy resolved in 7 weeks, demonstrating a high capacity of muscle recuperation (Fig. 13–4). The sensorimotor peripheral neuropathy persisted until the patient's death 9 weeks after the ingestion.

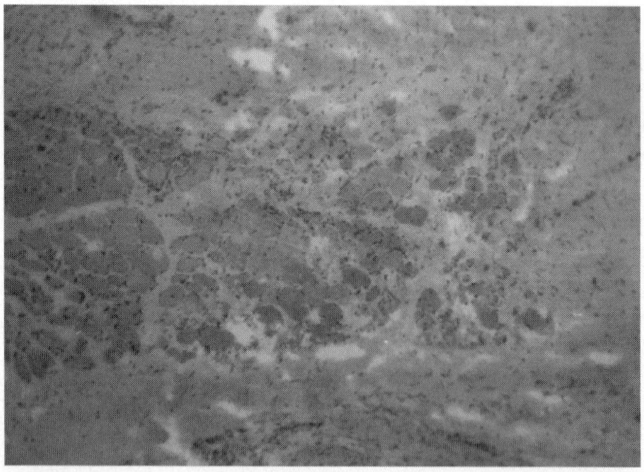

FIGURE 13–3 • Acute podophyllin myopathy. Massive necrosis of muscle fibers without inflammatory changes (H&E ×40).

ANTIBIOTICS

Myopathy rarely occurs with the use of antibiotics. Rifampicin has once been related to a severe proximal myopathy.[327]

STEROIDS

Corticosteroids have long been known to cause muscle fiber necrosis under experimental conditions.[328] The synthetic analogues, fludrocortisone and triamcinolone, are more toxic to muscle. Although usually subacute or chronic in its development, corticosteroid myopathy may also develop acutely. Several reports implicate high-dose, intravenously administered corticosteroids in the development of an acute myopathy in patients with status asthmaticus[329] and other disorders requiring corticosteroid therapy. Different from the chronic manifestation, the acute form entails muscle weakness that is more generalized, and involvement of the respiratory

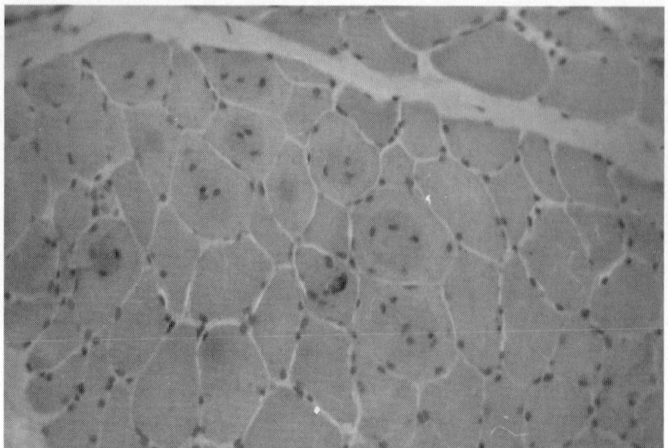

FIGURE 13–4 • Regeneration phase of podophyllin myopathy. Some fibers are still small, and others show nuclear centralization (H&E ×120).

muscles is common.[330] Steroid myopathy is associated with type II muscle fiber atrophy. Severe cases entail polyfocal myonecrosis or vacuolar degeneration of muscle.[331] The precise cause of this disorder remains uncertain. Because it occurs predominantly during the treatment of severely ill asthmatics, it is possible that the particular drugs used in this setting promote acute myopathy. Paralytic agents (pancuronium or vecuronium) or aminophylline might enhance or modify the toxic response to corticosteroid. Recovery from the myopathy is the rule within weeks to months and is usually complete.[332]

Organic Substances

ETHYL ALCOHOL

Patients who develop acute alcoholic myopathy are usually heavy drinkers. The onset is abrupt, with severe muscle cramps, pain, and swelling, following a rapidly evolving bilateral and symmetric muscle weakness. There may also be evidence of myocardial involvement. Usually, the condition is relatively benign, with recovery within 2 or 3 weeks. Alcohol may account for at least 20% of all cases of myoglobinuria secondary to rhabdomyolysis.[333] Only in the most fulminating cases is there a threat of myoglobinuria and acute renal failure. Severe muscle necrosis can occur in these situations.[334] The principal histologic change is widespread segmental necrosis of muscle fibers. Depending on the age of the lesion, one observes eosinophilic alteration of sarcoplasm, myophagocytosis, and regeneration (Fig. 13–5).

CARBON MONOXIDE

Carbon monoxide poisoning is an important cause of morbidity and mortality. Rhabdomyolysis has been well recognized as a complication.[335] Rhabdomyolysis with anuric renal failure is unfortunately not infrequent.[336] After removal from the site of intoxication, patients should receive 100% oxygen by a non-rebreathing mask. If the patient is in a coma, oxygen should be delivered via an endotracheal tube. Hyperbaric oxygen is considered in patients whose symptoms do not subside with oxygen at normal pressure.[337]

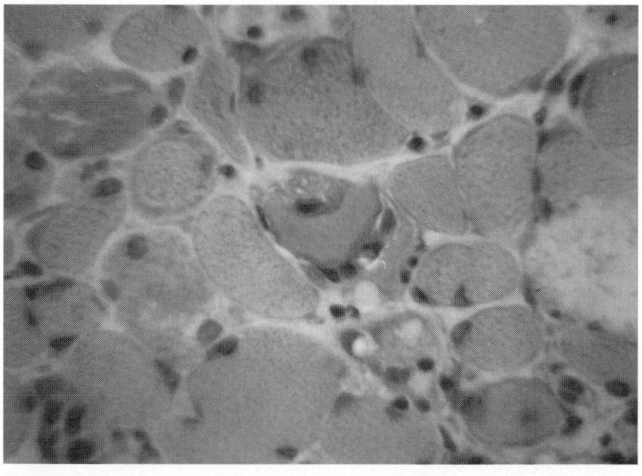

FIGURE 13-5 • Acute alcoholic myopathy. Widespread segmental necrosis of muscle fibers, eosinophilic alteration of sarcoplasm (center of photograph), phagocytosis, and regeneration (H&E ×120). (See color plate.)

GASOLINE

A patient not previously known to be MH-susceptible developed acute rhabdomyolysis after accidentally inhaling gasoline vapors. The patient recovered well from the episode.[338]

Addicting Drugs

COCAINE AND OPIOIDS

An association between cocaine and a direct effect on skeletal muscle has been described. Thirty-nine patients with acute myoglobinuria have been described after cocaine use; 13 of these patients had acute renal failure, and 6 of them died.[339]

The rapid evolution of widespread rhabdomyolysis as a complication of intravenous heroin injection has been reported.[340, 341] Rarely, heroin-induced myoglobinuria occurs in the absence of unconsciousness. The lower limbs are affected to a greater extent, and the proximal muscles are more affected than the distal. Muscle biopsy has revealed swelling and necrosis of muscle fibers, more in proximal than in distal muscles, sometimes with focal hemorrhage.

Similar lesions have been noted in patients with barbiturate intoxication and in patients on meprobamate.[256]

PHENCYCLIDINE (PCP, "ANGEL DUST")

Phencyclidine was largely used in the United States as a recreational drug in the 1970s. A related substance, ketamine, an anesthetic, is still used. The usual toxic manifestations are agitation, convulsions, and catatonic muscular rigidity. About 2% of patients with phencyclidine intoxication may develop myoglobinuria, and some of them develop acute renal failure.[342]

AMPHETAMINE, PHENFORMIN, AND FENFLURAMINE

Acute rhabdomyolysis has been observed when patients take large doses of amphetamine, phenformin, or fenfluramine over a period of months.[343, 344]

Phenformin has been used as a hypoglycemic agent in patients with diabetes mellitus, and fenfluramine, a derivative of amphetamine, has been used as a means of reducing appetite in the control of obesity.

TOLUENE

Muscle weakness is a common complaint in chronic abusers of volatile substances, especially in those who have inhaled toluene frequently. The weakness is symmetric and usually accompanied by other neurologic alterations and metabolic abnormalities caused by distal renal tubular acidosis. Once toluene is discontinued, weakness resolves within days. However, severe electrolyte abnormalities can be complicated by myoglobinuria.[345]

Poisoning Due to Bites and Stings

SNAKE BITE

Snake venoms are highly complex mixtures of proteins with a wide variety of actions. Many snake poisons are myotoxic, producing muscle fiber necrosis that is severe enough to cause myoglobinuria and acute renal failure. Necrosis of skeletal muscle is produced by two types of snake venom components: single-chain peptides consisting of 42–44 amino acid residues, and phospholipases A2. Vacuolation, lysis, and necrosis of skeletal muscle cells are the major pathological effects of these myotoxins. Although the exact mode of action of these toxins is not clear, interactions with the plasma membrane leading to permeability changes for ions and to their complete destruction is evident.[346] The South American rattlesnake, *Crotalus durissus terrificus,* has an extremely potent myotoxic venom responsible for myonecrosis and myoglobinuria, often misdiagnosed as hemoglobinuria.[347]

CENTUROIDES SCORPION STING

Centuroides scorpion envenomation in children, common in Arizona, can be dramatic and life-threatening. The sting produces symptoms ranging from local pain to severe systemic and neuromuscular symptoms characterized by extreme neuromuscular activity, tachycardia, and respiratory distress. Rhabdomyolysis occasionally occurs, probably related to excessive motor activity. Administration of anti-*Centuroides* antivenin developed in the goat is recommended in patients with severe clinical manifestations.[348]

SPIDER ENVENOMATION

Involvement of the neuromuscular system is common in latrodectism—envenomation due to the red-back spider, *Latrodectus hasselti.*[349] It includes tetanic spasms, tingling in the teeth, trismus, shooting pains in the fingers and the toes, confusion, and convulsions. Rhabdomyolysis is rare.[350]

References

1. Lehmann-Horn F, Engel AG, Ricker K, et al: The periodic paralysis and paramyotonia congenita. In Engel AG, Franzini-Armstrong C (eds): Myology, 2nd ed, vol 2, pp 1303–1334. New York, McGraw-Hill, 1994.
2. Pearson CM: The periodic paralysis: Differential features and pathological observations in permanent myopathic weakness. Brain 1964;87:341–354.
3. Johnsen T: Familial periodic paralysis with hypokalemia. Dan Med Bull 1981;281:1–22.
4. Ptacek LJ, Tawil R, Griggs RC, et al: Dihydropyridine receptor mutations cause hypokalemic periodic paralysis. Cell 1994;77:863–868.
5. Talbott JH: Periodic paralysis: A clinical syndrome. Medicine 1941;20:85–143.
6. Tengan CH, Oliveira ASB, Gabbai AA: Paralisia periodica: Analise clinica de 20 pacientes. Arq Neuropsiquiatr 1994;52:501–509 (Port).
7. Ferrebee JW, Gerity MK, Atchley DW, Loeb RF: Behavior of electrolytes in familial periodic paralysis. Arch Neurol 1940;44:830–840.
8. Weisler MJ: The electrocardiogram in periodic paralysis. Dis Chest 1961;40:217–218.
9. Minaker KL, Meneilly GS, Flier JS, et al: Insulin-mediated hypokalemia and paralysis in familial hypokalemic paralysis. Am J Med 1988;84:1001–1006.
10. Rüdel R, Lehmann-Horn F, Ricker K, et al: Hypokalemic periodic paralysis. In vitro investigation of muscle fiber membrane parameters. Muscle Nerve 1984;7:110–120.
11. Buruma OJS, Schipperheyn JJ, Bots GTAM: Heart muscle disease in familial hypokalemic periodic paralysis. Acta Neurol Scand 1981;64:12–21.
12. McArdle B: Metabolic myopathies: The glycogenoses affecting muscle, and hypo- and hyperkalemic periodic paralysis. Am J Med 1963;35:661–672.
13. Fontaine B, Khurana TS, Hoffmann EP, et al: Hyperkalemic periodic paralysis and the adult muscle sodium channel gene. Science 1990;250:1000–1002.
14. Herman RH, McDowell MK: Hyperkalemic paralysis (adynamia episodica hereditaria): Report of four cases and clinical studies. Am J Med 1963;35:749–767.
15. Gould RJ, Steeg CN, Eastwood AB, et al: Potentially fatal cardiac dysrhythmia and hyperkalemic periodic paralysis. Neurology 1985;35:1208–1212.
16. Subramony SH, Wee AS: Exercise and rest in hyperkalemic periodic paralysis. Neurology 1986;36:173–177.
17. Riggs JE, Griggs RC, Moxley RT: Acetazolamide-induced weakness in paramyotonia congenita. Ann Intern Med 1977;86:169–173.
18. McClatchey AI, McKenna-Yasek D, Cros D, et al: Novel mutations in families with unusual and variable disorders of the skeletal muscle sodium channel. Natl Genet 1992;2:148–152.
19. Hoffman EP, Lehmann-Horn F, Rüdel R: Overexcited or inactive ion channels in muscle disease. Cell 1995;80:681–686.
20. Lehmann-Horn F, Küther G, Ricker K: Adynamia episodica hereditaria with myotonia: A non-activating sodium current and the effect of extracellular pH. Muscle Nerve 1987;10:363–374.
21. Aarons JJ, Moron R, Camporesi E: General anesthesia and hyperkalemic periodic paralysis. Anesthesiology 1989;71:303–304.
22. Van Der Meulen JP, Gilbert GJ, Kane KA: Familial hyperkalemic paralysis with myotonia. N Engl J Med 1961;264:1–6.
23. Oh V, Taylor E, Yeo S, et al: Cation transport across lym-

phocyte plasma membranes in euthyroid and thyrotoxic men with and without hypokalemic periodic paralysis. Clin Sci 1990;78:199–206.

24. McFadzean AJS, Yeung R: Periodic paralysis complicating thyrotoxicosis in Chinese. Br Med J Clin Res 1967;1:451–455.
25. Bergeron L, Sternbach G: Thyrotoxic periodic paralysis. Ann Emerg Med 1988;17:843–845.
26. Conway MJ, Seibel JA, Eaton P: Thyrotoxicosis and periodic paralysis: Improvement with beta-blockade. Ann Intern Med 1974;81:332–336.
27. Shulkin D, Olson B, Levey G: Thyrotoxic periodic paralysis in a Latin-American taking acetazolamide. Am J Med Sci 1989;297:337–338.
28. Lewi Z, Bar-Khayim Y: Food-poisoning from barium carbonate. Lancet 1964;2:342–343.
29. Gallant EM: Barium-treated mammalian skeletal muscle: Similarities to hypokalemic periodic paralysis. J Physiol 1983;335:577–590.
30. Pasman J, Gabreëls F, Semmekrot B, et al: Hyperkalemic periodic paralysis in Gordon's syndrome: A possible defect in atrial natriuretic peptide function. Ann Neurol 1989;26:392–395.
31. Levinsky NG: Fluids and electrolytes. In Isselbacher KJ, Braunwald E, Wilson JD, et al (eds): Harrison's Principles of Internal Medicine, 13th ed, vol 1, pp 242–253. New York, McGraw-Hill, 1994.
32. Gronert GA: Malignant hyperthermia. In Engel AG, Franzini-Armstrong C (eds): Myology, 2nd ed, vol 2, pp 1661–1678. New York, McGraw-Hill, 1994.
33. Ellis FR, Halsall PJ, Christian AS: Clinical presentation of suspected malignant hyperthermia during anesthesia in 402 probands. Anaesthesia 1990;45:838–841.
34. Gronert GA, Mott J, Lee J: Aetiology of malignant hyperthermia. Br J Anaesth 1988;60:253–267.
35. Gillard EF, Otsu K, Fujii J, et al: A substitution of cysteine for arginine 614 in the ryanodine receptor is potentially causative of human malignant hyperthermia. Genomics 1991;11:751–755.
36. MacLennan DH, Phillips MS: Malignant hyperthermia. Science 1993;256:789–794.
37. Larach MG: Standardization of the caffeine halothane muscle contracture test. North American malignant hyperthermia group. Anesth Analg 1998;69:511–515.
38. MacKenzie AE, Allen G, Lahey D, et al: A comparison of the caffeine halothane muscle contracture test with the molecular genetic diagnosis of malignant hyperthermia. Anesthesiology 1991;75:4–8.
39. Harriman DGF: Malignant hyperthermia myopathy—A critical review. Br J Anaesth 1988;60:309–316.
40. Sethna NF, Rockoff MA, Worthen HM, et al: Anesthesia-related complications in children with Duchenne muscular dystrophy. Anesthesiology 1988;68:462–465.
41. Harrison GG: Propofol in malignant hyperthermia [Letter]. Lancet 1991;i:503.
42. McGraw TT, Keon TP: Malignant hyperthermia and the clean machine. Can J Anaesth 1989;36:530–532.
43. Ruthberg H, Hakanson E: Malignant hyperthermia: Clinical course and metabolic changes in two patients. Acta Anaesthesiol Scand 1986;30:211–214.
44. Kolb ME, Horne ML, Martz R: Dantrolene in human malignant hyperthermia: A multicenter study. Anesthesiology 1982;56:254–262.
45. Wedel DJ, Quinlam JG, Iaizzo PA: Clinical effects of intravenously administered dantrolene. Mayo Clin Proc 1995;70:241–246.
46. Desnick RJ: The porphyrias. In Isselbacher KJ, Braunwald E, Wilson JD, et al (eds): Harrison's Principles of Internal Medicine, 13th ed, vol 2, pp 2073–2079. New York, McGraw-Hill, 1994.
47. Adams RD, Victor M: Diseases of the peripheral nerves. In Adams RD, Victor M (eds): Principles of Neurology, 5th ed, pp 1117–1169. New York, McGraw-Hill, 1993.
48. Ridley A: Porphyric neuropathy. In Dyck PJ, Thomas PK, Lambert E, et al (eds): Peripheral Neuropathy, vol 2, pp 1704–1716. Philadelphia, WB Saunders, 1984.
49. Windebank AJ, Bonkovsky HL: Porphyric neuropathy. In Dyck PJ, Thomas PK, Bunge R, et al (eds): Peripheral Neuropathy, 3rd ed, vol 2, pp 1161–1168. Philadelphia, WB Saunders, 1993.
50. Goldberg A: Lead poisoning as a disorder of heme synthesis. Semin Hematol 1968;5:424–445.
51. Mustajoki P, Nordmann Y: Early administration of heme arginate for acute porphyric attacks. Ann Intern Med 1993;153:2004–2008.
52. Kauppinen R, Timonen K, Mustajoki P: Treatment of the porphyrias. Ann Med 1994;26:31–38.
53. Muthane UB, Vengamma B, Bharati KC, et al: Porphyric neuropathy: Prevention of progression using heme arginate. J Intern Med 1993;234:611–613.
54. Engel AG: Acquired autoimmune myasthenia gravis. In Engel AG, Franzini-Armstrong C (eds): Myology, 2nd ed, vol 2, pp 1769–1797. New York, McGraw-Hill, 1994.
55. Willis T: De anima brutorum, p 406. Oxford, England, Theatro Sheldoniano, 1672.
56. Jolly F: Über Myasthenia gravis pseudoparalytica. Berl Klin Wochenschr 1895;32:1–7.
57. Campbell H, Bramwell E: Myasthenia gravis. Brain 1900;23:277–336.
58. Buzzard EF: The clinical history and post-mortem examination of five cases of myasthenia gravis. Brain 1905;28:438–448.
59. Sorensen TT, Holm E-B: Myasthenia gravis in the county of Viborg, Denmark. Eur Neurol 1989;29:177–179.
60. Kurtzke JF, Kurland LT: The epidemiology of neurologic disease. In Joynt RJ (ed): Clinical Neurology, revised ed, vol 4, pp 80–88. Philadelphia, JB Lippincott, 1992.
61. Osserman KE, Genkins G: Studies in myasthenia gravis: Review of a 20 year experience in over 1200 patients. Mt Sinai J Med 1971;38:497–537.
62. Grob D, Arsura EL, Brunner NG, et al: The course of myasthenia gravis and therapies affecting outcome. Ann N Y Acad Sci 1987;505:472–479.
63. Patrick J, Lindstrom J: Autoimmune response to acetylcholine receptor. Science 1973;180:871–872.
64. Fambrough DM, Drachman DB, Satyamurti S: Neuromuscular junction in myasthenia gravis: Decreased acetylcholine receptors. Science 1973;182:293–295.
65. Pestronk A, Drachman DB, Self SG: Measurement of junctional acetylcholine receptors in myasthenia gravis: Clinical correlates. Muscle Nerve 1985;8:245–251.
66. Drachman DB: Myasthenia gravis. Review. N Engl J Med 1994;330:1797–1810.
67. Daroff RB: The office Tensilon test for ocular myasthenia gravis. Arch Neurol 1986;43:843–844.
68. Keesey JC: Electrodiagnostic approach to defects of neuromuscular transmission. Muscle Nerve 1989;12:613–626.
69. Lindstrom J: An assay for antibodies to human AchR in serum from patients with myasthenia gravis. Clin Immunol Immunopathol 1977;7:36–43.
70. Oh SJ, Kim DE, Kuruoglu R, et al: Diagnostic sensitivity of the laboratory tests in mysthenia gravis. Muscle Nerve 1992;15:720–724.
71. Kuncl RW, Pestronk A, Drachman DB, et al: The pathophysiology of penicillamine-induced myasthenia gravis. Ann Neurol 1986;20:740–744.
72. Howard JF Jr: Adverse drug effects on neuromuscular transmission. Semin Neurol 1990;10:89–102.
73. Marrs TC: Organophosphate poisoning. Pharmacol Ther 1993;58:51–66.
74. Sghirlanzoni A, Pareyson D, Benvenuti C, et al: Efficacy of intranasal administration of neostigmine in myasthenic patients. J Neurol 1992;239:165–169.
75. Keesey J, Buffkin D, Kebo D, et al: Plasma exchange alone for the therapy of myasthenia gravis. Ann N Y Acad Sci 1981;377:729–743.
76. Cosi V, Lombardi M, Piccolo G, et al: Treatment of myasthenia gravis with high-dose intravenous immunoglobulin. Acta Neurol Scand 1991;84:81–84.
77. American Medical Association: Consensus Conference: The utility of therapeutic plasmapheresis. JAMA 1986;256:1333–1337.

78. Dau PC, Lindstrom JM, Cassel CK, et al: Plasmapheresis and immunosuppressive drug therapy in myasthenia gravis. N Engl J Med 1977;297:1134–1140.
79. Evoli A, Bartoccioni E, Batocchi AP, et al: Anti-AchR-negative myasthenia gravis: Clinical and immunological features. Clin Invest Med 1989;12:104–109.
80. Arsura E: Experience with intravenous immunoglobulin in myasthenia gravis. Clin Immunol Immunopathol 1989;53(Suppl):S170–S179.
81. Sekul EA, Cupler EJ, Dalakas MC: Aseptic meningitis associated with high-dosage immunoglobulin therapy: Frequency and risk factors. Ann Intern Med 1994;121:259–262.
82. Steg RE, Lefkowitz DM: Cerebral infarction following intravenous immunoglobulin therapy for myasthenia gravis. Neurology 1994;44:1180–1181.
83. Landry O: Note sur la paralysie ascendant aigue. Gaz Hebdomadaire 1859;6:472–474.
84. Guillain G, Barré JA, Strohl A: Sur un syndrome de radiculonebrite avec hyperalbuminose du liquide cephalo-rachidien sans reaction cellulaire. Remarques sur les caracteres cliniques et graphiques des reflexes tendineux. Bull Soc Med Hop Paris 1916;40:1462.
85. Kurland LT: Descriptive epidemiology of selected neurologic and myopathic disorders with particular reference to a survey in Rochester, Minnesota. J Chron Dis 1958;8:378–418.
86. Kennedy RH, Danielson MA, Mulder DW, et al: Guillain-Barré syndrome: A 42-year epidemiologic and clinical study. Mayo Clin Proc 1978;53:93–99.
87. Hankey GJ: Guillain-Barré syndrome in Western Australia, 1980–1985. Med J Austr 1987;146:130–133.
88. Hurwitz ES, Holman RC, Nelson DB, et al: National surveillance for Guillain-Barré syndrome: January 1978–March 1979. Neurology 1983;33:150–157.
89. Leneman F: The Guillain-Barré syndrome: Definition, etiology, and review of 1100 cases. Arch Intern Med 1966;118:139–144.
90. Hart IK, Kennedy PGE: Guillain-Barré syndrome associated with cytomegalovirus infection. Q J Med 1988;67:425–430.
91. Ricker W, Blumberg A, Peters CH, et al: The association of the Guillain-Barré syndrome with infectious mononucleosis wih a report of two fatal cases. Blood 1947;2:217–226.
92. Dayan AD, Ogul E, Graveson GS: Polyneuritis and herpes zoster. J Neurol Neurosurg Psychiatry 1972;35:170–175.
93. Bernsen HJJA, Van Loon AM, Poels RFJ, et al: Herpes simplex virus specific antibody determined by immunoblotting in cerebrospinal fluid of a patient with the Guillain-Barré syndrome. J Neurol Neurosurg Psychiatry 1989;52:788–791.
94. Bosh VV, Dowling PC, Cook SD: Hepatitis A virus imunoglobulin M antibody in acute neurological disease. Ann Neurol 1983;14:685–687.
95. Berger JR, Ayyar DR, Sheremata WR: Guillain-Barré syndrome complicating acute hepatitis B (a case with electrophysiological and immunological studies). Arch Neurol 1981;38:366–368.
96. De Klippel N, Hautekeete ML, De Keyser J, et al: Guillain-Barré syndrome as the presenting manifestation of hepatitis C infection. Neurology 1993;43:2143.
97. Melnick SC, Flewett TH: Role of infection in the Guillain-Barré syndrome. J Neurol Neurosurg Psychiatry 1964;27:395–407.
98. Aguayo JM, Ramos JT, Lumbreras C: Campylobacter jejuni infection and Guillain-Barré syndrome [Letter]. N Engl J Med 1996;334:802.
99. Perez-Perez GI, Dworkin BM, Chodos JE, et al: Campylobacter pylori antibodies in humans. Ann Intern Med 1988;109:11–17.
100. Winer JB, Hughes RAC, Anderson MJ, et al: A prospective study of acute idiopathic neuropathy. II. Antecedent events. J Neurol Neurosurg Psychiatry 1988;51:613–618.
101. Langmuir AD, Bregman DJ, Kurland LT, et al: An epidemiologic and clinical evaluation of Guillain-Barré syndrome reported in association with the administration of swine influenza vaccines. Am J Epidemiol 1984;119:841–879.
102. Kinnunen E, Färkkilä M, Hovi T, et al: Incidence of Guillain-Barré syndrome during a nationwide oral poliovirus vaccine campaign. Neurology 1989;39:1034–1036.
103. Rodin A, Ferner RE, Russell R: Guillain-Barré syndrome in pregnancy and the puerperium. J Obstet Gynecol 1988;9:39–42.
104. Arnason BG, Asbury AK: Idiopathic polyneuritis after surgery. Arch Neurol 1968;18:500–507.
105. Chakraborty TK, Rudell WS: Guillain-Barré neuropathy during treatment with captopril. Postgrad Med J 1987;63:221–222.
106. Cicale MJ: Guillain-Barré syndrome after streptokinase therapy. South Med J 1987;80:1068.
107. Asbury AK, Arnason BG, Adams RD: The inflammatory lesion in idiopathic polyneuritis. Medicine 1969;48:173–215.
108. Asbury AK, Arnasn BG, Karp HR, et al: Criteria for diagnosis of Guillain-Barré syndrome. Ann Neurol 1978;3:565–566.
109. Asbury AK, Cornblath DR: Assessment of current diagnostic criteria for Guillain-Barré syndrome. Ann Neurol 1990;27(Suppl):S21–S24.
110. Feasby TE, Gilbert JJ, Brown WF, et al: An acute axonal form of Guillain-Barré polyneuropathy. Brain 1986;109:1115–1126.
111. McKhann GM, Cornblath DR, Ho TW, et al: Clinical and electrophysiological aspects of acute paralytic disease of children and young adults in northern China. Lancet 1991;338:593–597.
112. McKhann GM, Cornblath DR, Griffin JW, et al: Acute motor axonal neuropathy: A frequent cause of acute flaccid paralysis in China. Ann Neurol 1993;33:333–342.
113. Thomas PK: The Guillain-Barré syndrome: No longer a simple concept. J Neurol 1992;239:361–362.
114. Hartung HP, Hughes RAC, Taylor WA, et al: T cell activation in Guillain-Barré syndrome and in MS: Elevated serum levels of soluble IL-2 receptors. Neurology 1990;40:215–218.
115. Honavar M, Tharakan JKJ, Hughes RAC, et al: A clinicopathological study of the Guillain-Barré syndrome: Nine cases and literature review. Brain 1991;114:1245–1269.
116. Winer JB, Gray IA, Gregson NA, et al: A prospective study of acute idiopathic neuropathy. III. Immunological studies. J Neurol Neurosurg Psychiatry 1988;51:619–625.
117. Yuki N, Yoshino H, Sato S, et al: Acute axonal polyneuropathy associated with anti-GM1 antibodies following Campylobacter enteritis. Neurology 1990;40:1900–1902.
118. Winer JB, Hughes RAC, Osmond C: A prospective study of acute idiopathic neuropathy. I. Clinical features and their prognostic value. J Neurol Neurosurg Psychiatry 1988;51:605–612.
119. Kotsoris H, Schleifer L, Menken M, et al: Total locked-in state resembling brain death in polyneuropathy [Abstract]. Ann Neurol 1984;16:150.
120. Ropper AH: Unusual clinical variants and signs in Guillain-Barré syndrome. Arch Neurol 1986;43:1150–1152.
121. Dyck PJ, Lais AC, Ohta M, et al: Chronic inflammatory polyradiculoneuropathy. Mayo Clin Proc 1975;50:621–637.
122. Singh NK, Jaiswal AK, Misra S, et al: Assessment of autonomic dysfunction in Guillain-Barré syndrome and its prognostic implications. Acta Neurol Scand 1987;75:101–105.
123. Lichtenfeld P: Autonomic dysfunction in the Guillain-Barré syndrome. Am J Med 1971;50:772–780.
124. Van Zandycke M, Martin JJ, Vander Gaer J, et al: Facial myokymia in the Guillain-Barré syndrome: A clinicopathological study. Neurology 1982;32:744–748.
125. Löffel NB, Rossi LN, Mumenthaler M, et al: The Landry-Guillain-Barré syndrome: Complications, prognosis and natural history in 123 cases. J Neurol Sci 1977;33:71–79.
126. Culbertson LR: A case of Landry's disease with involvement of the eye muscles. Am J Ophthalmol 1902;19:113–114.
127. Nikoskelainen E, Riekkinen P: Retrobulbar neuritis as an

early symptom of Guillain-Barré syndrome. Report of a case. Acta Ophthalmol 1972;50:111–115.
128. Farrell K, Hill A, Chuang S: Papilledema in Guillain-Barré syndrome. A case report. Arch Neurol 1981;38:55–57.
129. Ropper AH, Marmarou A: Mechanism of pseudotumor in Guillain-Barré syndrome. Arch Neurol 1984;41:259–261.
130. Haymaker W, Kernohan JW: The Landry-Guillain-Barré syndrome: A clinicopathologic report of fifty fatal cases and a critique of the literature. Medicine 1949;28:59–141.
131. Dawson DM, Samuels MA, Morris J: Sensory form of acute polyneuritis. Neurology 1988;38:1728–1731.
132. Young RR, Asbury AK, Corbett JL, et al: Pure pan-dysautonomia with recovery. Description and discussion of diagnostic criteria. Brain 1975;98:613–636.
133. Fisher CM: An unusual variant of acute idiopathic polyneuritis (syndrome of ophthalmoplegia, ataxia and areflexia). N Engl J Med 1956;255:57–65.
134. Ropper AH, Shahani B: Proposed mechanism of ataxia in Fisher's syndrome. Arch Neurol 1983;40:537–538.
135. Phillips MS, Stewart S, Anderson JR: Neuropathological findings in Miller Fisher syndrome. J Neurol Neurosurg Psychiatry 1984;47:492–495.
136. Landau WM, Glenn C, Dust G: MRI in Miller Fisher variant of Guillain-Barré syndrome. Neurology 1987;37:1431.
137. Elizan TS, Spire JP, Andiman RM, et al: Syndrome of acute idiopathic ophthalmoplegia with ataxia and areflexia. Neurology 1971;21:281–292.
138. Fross RD, Daube JR: Neuropathy in the Miller Fisher syndrome: Clinical and electrophysiologic findings. Neurology 1987;37:1493–1498.
139. Feasby TE, Hahn AF, Brown WF, et al: Severe axonal degeneration in acute Guillain-Barré syndrome: Evidence of two different mechanisms? J Neurol Sci 1993;116:185–192.
140. Albers JW, Donofrio PD, McGonagle TK: Sequential electrodiagnostic abnormalities in acute inflammatory demyelinating polyradiculoneuropathy. Muscle Nerve 1985;8:528–539.
141. Ropper AH, Wijdicks EFM, Shahani BT: Electrodiagnostic abnormalities in 113 consecutive patients with Guillain-Barré syndrome. Arch Neurol 1990;47:881–887.
142. Brown WF, Feasby TE: Conduction block and denervation in Guillain-Barré polyneuropathy. Brain 1984;107:219–239.
143. Kimura J: Proximal versus distal slowing of motor nerve conduction velocity in the Guillain-Barré syndrome. Ann Neurol 1978;3:344–350.
144. Markand ON, Kincaid JC, Pourmand RA, et al: Electrophysiologic evaluation of diaphragm by transcutaneous phrenic nerve stimulation. Neurology 1984;34:604–614.
145. Morgan GW, Barohn RJ, Bazan C III, et al: Nerve root enhancement with magnetic resonance imaging in inflammatory demyelinating polyradiculoneuropathy. Neurology 1993;43:618–620.
146. Perry JR, Fung A, Poon P, et al: Magnetic resonance imaging of nerve inflamation in the Guillain-Barré syndrome. Neuroradiology 1994;36:139–140.
147. Cornblath DR, McArthur JC, Kennedy PGE, et al: Inflammatory demyelinating peripheral neuropathies associated with human T-cell lymphotropic virus type III infection. Ann Neurol 1987;21:32–40.
148. Halperin JJ, Little BW, Coyle PK, et al: Lyme disease: Cause of a treatable peripheral neuropathy. Neurology 1987;7:1700–1706.
149. Mancardi GL, Del Sette M, Primavera A, et al: Borrelia burgdorferi infection and Guillain-Barré syndrome. Lancet 1989;ii:485–496.
150. Bolton CF, Laverty DA, Brown JD, et al: Critically ill polyneuropathy: Electrophysiological studies and differentiation from Guillain-Barré syndrome. J Neurol Neurosurg Psychiatry 1986;49:563–573.
151. McKhann GM, Griffin JW, Cornblath DR, et al: Plasmapheresis and Guillain-Barré syndrome: Analysis of prognostic factors and the effect of plasmapheresis. Ann Neurol 1988;23:347–353.
152. van der Meché FGA, Schmitz PIM, Meulstee J, et al: Prognostic factors in the Dutch Guillain-Barré study [Abstract]. J Neurol 1992;239(Suppl 2):S52.
153. Fergusson RJ, Wright DJ, Willey RF, et al: Suxamethonium is dangerous in polyneuropathy. BMJ 1981;282:298–299.
154. Loh L: Neurological and neuromuscular disease. Br J Anaesth 1986;58:190–200.
155. Ropper AH, Kehne SM: Guillain-Barré syndrome: Management of respiratory failure. Neurology 1985;35:1662–1665.
156. Newton-John H. Prevention of pulmonary complications in severe Guillain-Barré syndrome by early assisted ventilation. Med J Aust 1985;142:444–445.
157. Consensus Conference: The utility of therapeutic plasmapheresis for neurological disorders. JAMA 1986;256:1333–1337.
158. Guillain-Barré Study Group: Plasmapheresis and acute Guillain-Barré syndrome. Neurology 1985;35:1096–1104.
159. French Cooperative Group on Plasma Exchange and Guillain-Barré syndrome: Efficiency of plasma exchange in Guillain-Barré syndrome: Role of replacement fluids. Ann Neurol 1987;22:753–761.
160. van der Merché FGA, Schmitz PIM, Dutch Guillain-Barré Study Group: A randomized trial comparing intravenous immune globulin and plasma exchange in Guillain-Barré syndrome. N Engl J Med 1992;326:1123–1129.
161. Hughes RAC, Newsom-Davis JM, Perkin GD, et al: Controlled trial of prednisolone in acute polyneuropathy. Lancet 1978;ii:750–753.
162. Hughes RAC; Ineffectiveness of high-dose intravenous methylprednisolone in Guillain-Barré syndrome. Lancet 1991;338:1142.
163. Irani DN, Cornblath DR, Chaudhry V, et al: Relapse in Guillain-Barré syndrome after treatment with human immune globulin. Neurology 1993;43:872–875.
164. Castro LHM, Ropper AH: Human immune globulin infusion in Guillain Barré syndrome: Worsening during and after treatment. Neurology 1993;43:1034–1036.
165. MacGregor RR: Corynebacterium diphtheriae. In Mandell GL, Bennett JE, Dolin R (eds): Mandell, Douglas and Bennett's Principles and Practice of Infectious Diseases, 4th ed, pp 1865–1872. New York, Churchill Livingstone, 1995.
166. Groman NB: Conversion by corynephages and its role in the natural history of diphtheria. J Hyg (Camb) 1984;93:405–417.
167. McDonald WI, Kocen RS: Diphtheritic neuropathy. In Dyck PJ, Thomas PK, Lambert EH (eds): Peripheral Neuropathy, 2nd ed, pp 2010–2017. Philadelphia, WB Saunders, 1984.
168. Scheid W: Diphtherial paralysis. An analysis of 2292 cases of diphtheria in adults, which included 174 cases of polyneuritis. J Nerv Ment Dis 1952;116:1095–1101.
169. Créange A, Meyrignac C, Roualdes B, et al: Diphtheritic neuropathy. Muscle Nerve 1995;18:1460–1463.
170. Fisher CM, Adams RD: Diphtheritic polyneuritis—A pathological study. J Neuropathol Exp Neurol 1956;15:243–268.
171. Naiditch MJ, Bower AG: Diphtheria. A study of 1433 cases observed during a ten-year period at the Los Angeles County Hospital. Am J Med 1954;17:229–245.
172. Kurdi A, Abdul-Kader M: Clinical and electrophysiological studies of diphtheritic neuritis in Jordan. J Neurol Sci 1979;42:243–250.
173. Solders G, Nennesmo I, Person A: Diphtheritic neuropathy, an analysis based on muscle and nerve biopsy and repeated neurophysiological and autonomic functions tests. J Neurol Neurosurg Psychiatry 1989;52:876–880.
174. Gothe R, Kunze K, Hoogstraal H: The mechanism of pathogenicity in the tick paralysis. J Med Entol 1979;16:357–369.
175. Wilson BB: Ticks. In Mandell GL, Bennett JE, Dolin R (eds): Mandell, Douglas and Bennett's Principles and Practice of Infectious Diseases, 4th ed, pp 2565–2567. New York, Churchill Livingstone, 1995.
176. Wright SW, Trott AT: North American tick-born disease. Ann Emerg Med 1988;17:964–972.

177. Stanbury JB, Huyck JH: Tick paralysis. A critical review. Medicine 1945;24:219–242.
178. Cherington M, Snyder RD: Tick paralysis. Neurophysiologic studies. N Engl J Med 1968;278:95–97.
179. Swift TR, Ignacio OJ: Tick paralysis. Electrophysiologic studies. Neurology 1975;25:1130–1133.
180. Finkel MF: Lyme disease and its neurologic complications. Arch Neurol 1988;45:99–104.
181. Halperin JJ, Golightly M, and the Long Island Neuroborreliosis Collaborative Study Group: Lyme borreliosis in Bell's palsy. Neurology 1992;42:1268–1270.
182. Hansen K, Lebech A-M: The clinical and epidemiological profile of Lyme neuroborreliosis in Denmark 1985–1990. Brain 1992;115:399–423.
183. Pachner AR, Steere AC: The triad of neurologic manifestations of Lyme disease: Meningitis, cranial neuritis, and radiculoneuritis. Neurology 1985;35:47–53.
183a. Debue M, Gautier P, Hackel C, et al: Detection of *Borrelia burgdorferi* in biological samples using the PCR assay. Res Microbiol 1991;142:565–572.
184. Ettestad PJ, Campbell GL, Welbel SF, et al: Biliary complications in the treatment of unsubstantiated Lyme disease. J Infect Dis 1995;17:356–361.
185. Nkowane BM, Wassilak SGF, Orenstein WA, et al: Vaccine-associated paralytic poliomyelitis. United States: 1973 through 1984. JAMA 1987;257:1335–1340.
186. Strebel PM, Sutter RW, Cochi SL, et al: Epidemiology of poliomyelitis in the United States one decade after the last reported case of indigenous wild virus-associated disease. Clin Infect Dis 1992;14:568–579.
187. Modlin JF: Poliovirus. In Mandell GL, Bennett JE, Dolin R (eds): Mandell, Douglas and Bennett's Principles and Practice of Infectious Diseases, 4th ed, pp 1613–1620. New York, Churchill Livingstone, 1995.
188. Ren R, Racaniello VR: Poliovirus spreads from muscle to the central nervous system by neural pathways. J Infect Dis 1992;166:747–752.
189. Auld PAM, Kevy SV, Eley RC: Poliomyelitis in children. Experience with 956 cases in the 1955 Massachusetts epidemic. N Engl J Med 1960;263:1093–1100.
190. Horstmann DM: Clinical aspects of acute poliomyelitis. Am J Med 1949;6:592–605.
191. Baker AB: Bulbar poliomyelitis. Am J Med 1949;6:614–619.
192. Weinstein L, Shelokov A, Seltser R, et al: A comparison of the clinical features of poliomyelitis in adults and children. N Engl J Med 1952;246:296–302.
193. Johnson EW, Guyton JD, Olsen KJ: Motor nerve conduction velocity studies in poliomyelitis. Arch Phys Med Rehabil 1960;41:185–190.
194. Openshaw H, Lieberman JS: Vaccine-related poliomyelitis [Editorial]. Arch Intern Med 1982;142:1617.
195. Ferris BG, Auld PAM, Cronkhite L, et al: Life-threatening poliomyelitis. Boston, 1955. N Engl J Med 1960;262:371–380.
196. Wright PF, Karzon DT: Minimizing the risks associated with the prevention of poliomyelitis. N Engl J Med 1995;332:529–530.
197. So YT, Olney RK: AAEM case report #23: Acute paralytic poliomyelitis. Muscle Nerve 1991;14:1159–1164.
198. Bleck TP: Clostridium Tetani. In Mandell GL, Bennett JE, Dolin R (eds): Mandell, Douglas and Bennett's Principles and Practice of Infectious Diseases, 4th ed, pp 2173–2178. New York, Churchill Livingstone, 1995.
199. Cutler D: Progress by poisoning. Nature 1992;359:773.
200. Bleck TP: Tetanus: Pathophysiology, management and prophylaxis. Dis Mon 1991;37:545–603.
201. Weinstein L: Current concepts. Tetanus. N Engl J Med 1973;289:1293–1296.
202. Edmondson RS, Flowers MW: Intensive care in tetanus: Management, complications, and mortality in 100 cases. BMJ 1979;1:1401–1404.
203. Mayo J, Berciano J: Cephalic tetanus presenting with Bell's palsy. J Neurol Neurosurg Psychiatry 1985;48:290.
204. Schofield FD, Tucker VM, Westbrook, GR: Neonatal tetanus in New Guinea. Effect of acctive immunization in pregnancy. BMJ 1961;2:785–789.
205. Gürses N, Aydin M: Factors affecting prognosis of neonatal tetanus. Scand J Infect Dis 1993;25:353–355.
206. Crone NE, Reder AT: Severe tetanus in immunized patients with high anti-tetanus titers. Neurology 1992;42:761–764.
207. Domenighetti GM, Savary G, Stricker H: Hyperadrenergic syndrome in severe tetanus: Extreme rise in catecholamines responsive to labetalol. BMJ 1984;288:1483–1484.
208. Andrade LAF, Brucki SMD: Botulinum toxin A for trismus in cephalic tetanus. Arq Neuropsiquiatr 1994;52:410–413.
209. Nollas-Salas M, Garcés-Brusés J: Severity of tetanus in patients older than 80 years: Comparative study with younger patients. Clin Infect Dis 1993;16:591–592.
210. Luisto M: Outcome and neurological sequelae of patients after tetanus. Acta Neurol Scand 1989;80:504–511.
211. Bleck TP: Clostridium botulinum. In Mandell GL, Bennett JE, Dolin R (eds): Mandell, Douglas and Bennett's Principles and Practice of Infectious Diseases, 4th ed, pp 2178–2182. New York, Churchill Livingstone, 1995.
212. Cherington M: Botulism. Ten-year experience. Arch Neurol 1974;30:432–437.
213. Hughes JM, Blumenthal JR, Merson MH, et al: Clinical features of types A and B food borne botulism. Ann Intern Med 1981;95:442–445.
214. Terranova W, Palumbo JN, Breman JG: Ocular findings in botulism type B. JAMA 1979;241:475–477.
215. Koenig MG, Spickard A, Cardella MA, et al: Clinical and laboratory observations on type E botulism in man. Medicine 1964;43:517–545.
216. Martinez AC, Anciones B, Ferrer MT, et al: Electrophysiologic study in benign human botulism type B. Muscle Nerve 1985;8:580–585.
217. Valli G, Barbieri S, Scarlato G: Neurophysiological tests in human botulism. Electromyogr Clin Neurophysiol 1983;23:3–11.
218. Tyler HR: Physiologic observations in human botulism. Arch Neurol 1963;9:661–671.
219. Graf WD, Hays RM, Astley SJ, et al: Electrodiagnosis reliability in the diagnosis of infant botulism. J Pediatr 1992;120:747–749.
220. Lecour H, Ramos MH, Almeida B, et al: Food-borne botulism. A review of 13 outbreaks. Arch Intern Med 1988;148:578.
221. Tacket CO, Mann JM, Hargrett NT, et al: Equine antitoxin use and other factors that predict outcome in type A food-borne botulism. Am J Med 1984;76:794–798.
222. Tacket CO, Rogawski MA: Botulism. In Simpson LL (ed): Botulinum Neurotoxin and Tetanus Toxin, pp 351–378. San Diego, Academic Press, 1989.
223. Swedberg J, Wendel TH, Deiss F: Wound botulism. West J Med 1987;147:335–338.
224. MacDonald KL, Rutherford GW, Friedman SM, et al: Botulism and botulism-like illness in chronic drug abusers. Ann Intern Med 1985;102:616–618.
225. Rapoport S, Watkins PB: Descending paralysis resulting from occult wound botulism. Ann Neurol 1984;16:359–361.
226. Schreiner MS, Field M, Ruddy, R: Infant botulism: A review of 12 years' experience at the Children's Hospital of Philadelphia. Pediatrics 1991;87:159–165.
227. Long SS, Gajaweski JL, Brown LW, et al: Clinical, laboratory, and environmental features of infant botulism in southeastern Pennsylvania. Pediatrics 1985;75:935–941.
228. Arnon SS, Midura TF, Clay SA, et al: Infant botulism. Epidemiological, clinical, and laboratory aspects. JAMA 1977;237:1946–1951.
229. Chia JK, Clark JB, Ryan CA, et al: Botulism in an adult associated with food-borne intestinal infection with Clostridium botulinum. N Engl J Med 1986;315:239–241.
230. Sonnabend WF, Sonnabend OA, Grundler P, et al: Intestinal toxicoinfection by Clostridium botulinum type F in an adult. Case associated with Guillain-Barré syndrome. Lancet 1987;1:357–360.

231. Hays AP, Gamboa ET: Acute viral myositis. In Engel AG, Franzini-Armstrong C (eds): Myology, Basic and Clinical, 2nd ed, pp 1399–1418. New York, McGraw-Hill, 1994.
232. Congy F, Hauw JJ, Wang A, et al: Influenzal acute myositis in the elderly. Neurology 1980;30:877–878.
233. Cunningham E, Kohli R, Venuto RC: Influenza-associated myoglobinuric renal failure. JAMA 1979;242:2428–2429.
234. Farrel MK, Partin JC, Bove KE: Epidemic influenza myopathy in Cincinnati in 1977. J Pediatr 1980;96:545–551.
235. Gamboa ET, Eastwood AB, Hays AP, et al: Isolation of influenza virus from muscle in myoglobinuric polymyositis. Neurology 1979;29:1323–1325.
236. Greco TP, Askenase PW, Kashgarian M: Postviral myositis: Myxovirus-like structures in affected muscle. Ann Intern Med 1977;86:193–194.
237. Kessler HA, Trenholme GM, Harris AA, et al: Acute myopathy associated with influenza A/Texas/1/77 infection: Isolation of virus from a muscle biopsy specimen. JAMA 1980;243:461–462.
238. Ruff RL, Secrist D: Viral studies in benign acute childhood myositis. Arch Neurol 1982;39:261–263.
239. Simon NM, Rovner RN, Berlin BS: Acute myoglobinuria associated with type A2 (Hong Kong) influenza. JAMA 1970;212:1704–1705.
240. Stang H: Acute transient myositis associated with influenza virus infection. Pediatr Infect Dis J 1989;8:257–258.
241. Zamkoff K, Rosen N: Influenza and myoglobinuria in brothers. Neurology 1979;29:340–345.
242. Beressi A, Sunheimer RL, Huish S, et al: Acute rhabdomyolysis in a human immunodeficiency virus-seropositive patient associated with rising anti-coxsackie B viral titers. Ann Clin Lab Sci 1994;24:278–281.
243. Lépine P, Desse G, Sautter V: Biopsies musculaires avec examen histologique et isolement du virus coxsackie chez l'homme atteint de myalgie épidemique (maladie de Bornholm). Bull Acad Nation Med 1952;136:66–69.
244. Wright J, Couchonnal G, Hodges GR: Adenovirus type 21 infection: Occurence with pneumonia, rhabdomyolysis, and myoglobinuria in an adult. JAMA 1979;241:2420–2421.
245. Schlesinger JJ, Gandara D, Bensch KG: Myoglobinuria associated with herpes-group viral infections. Arch Intern Med 1978;138:422–424.
246. Kantor RJ, Norden CW, Wein TP: Infectious mononucleosis associated with rhabdomyolysis and renal failure. South Med J 1978;71:346–348.
247. Friedman BI, Libby R: Epstein-Barr virus infection associated with rhabdomyolysis and acute renal failure. Clin Pediatr 1986;25:228–229.
248. Poels PJE, Ewals JAMP, Joosten EMG, et al: Rhabdomyolysis associated with simultaneous Epstein-Barr virus infection and isolation of echovirus 6 from muscle: A dual infection [Letter]. J Neurol Neurosurg Psychiatry 1989;52:412–413.
249. Josselson J, Pula T, Sadler JH: Acute rhabdomyolysis associated with an echovirus 9 infection. Arch Intern Med 1980;140:1671–1672.
250. Jehn, UW, Fink MK: Myositis, myoglobinemia, and myoglobinuria associated with enterovirus echo 9 infection. Arch Neurol 1980;37:457–458.
251. Naylor CD, Jevnikar AM, Witt NJ: Sporadic viral myositis in two adults. Can Med Assoc J 1987;137:819–821.
252. Younger DS, Hays AP, Uncini A, et al: Recurrent myoglobinuria and HIV seropositivity: Incidental or pathogenic association? Muscle Nerve 1989;12:842–843.
253. del Rio C, Soffer O, Widell JL, et al: Acute human immunodeficiency virus infection temporally associated with rhabdomyolysis, acute renal failure, and nephrosis. Rev Infect Dis 1990;12:282–285.
254. Malheiros SMF, Oliveira ASB, Schmidt B, et al: Dengue. Muscle biopsy findings in 15 patients. Arq Neuropsiquiatr 1993;51:159–164.
255. Adams RD, Victor M: Disorders of the nervous system due to drugs and other chemical agents. In Adams RD, Victor M (eds): Principles of Neurology, 5th ed, pp 922–956. New York, McGraw-Hill, 1993.
256. Victor M, Sieb JP: Myopathies due to drugs, toxins, and nutritional deficiency. In Engel AG, Franzini-Armstrong C (eds): Myology, 2nd ed, vol 2, pp 1697–1725. New York, McGraw-Hill, 1994.
257. Le Quesne PM: Neuropathy due to drugs. In Dyck PJ, Thomas PK, Lambert EH, et al (eds): Peripheral Neuropathy, 2nd ed, vol 2, pp 2162–2179. Philadelphia, WB Saunders, 1984.
258. Schaumburg HH, Spencer PS: Human toxic neuropathy due to industrial agents. In Dyck PJ, Thomas PK, Lambert EH, et al (eds): Peripheral Neuropathy, 2nd ed, vol 2, pp 2115–2132. Philadelphia, WB Saunders, 1984.
259. Windebank AJ, McCall JT, Dyck PJ: Metal Neuropathy. In Dyck PJ, Thomas PK, Lambert EH, et al (eds): Peripheral Neuropathy, 2nd ed, vol 2, pp 2133–2161. Philadelphia, WB Saunders, 1984.
260. Gammon GD, Burge FW, King G: Neural toxicity in tuberculous patients treated with isoniazid (isonicotinic acid hydrazide). Arch Neurol Psychiatry 1953;70:64–69.
261. Le Quesne PM: Iatrogenic neuropathies. In Vinken PJ, Bruyn GW (eds): Handbook of Clinical Neurology, pp 527–551. Amsterdam, North-Holland, 1970.
262. Albin RL, Albers JW, Greenberg HS, et al: Acute sensory neuropathy-neuronopathy from pyridoxine overdose. Neurology 1987;37:1729–1732.
263. Ellis FG: Acute polyneuritis after nitrofurantoin therapy. Lancet 1962;ii:1136–1138.
264. Morris JS: Nitrofurantoin and peripheral neuropathy with megaloblastic anaemia. J Neurol Neurosurg Psychiatry 1966;29:224–228.
265. Toole JF, Parrish ML: Nitrofurantoin polyneuropathy. Neurology 1973;23:554–559.
266. Duffy LF, Daum F, Fisher SE, et al: Peripheral neuropathy in Crohn's disease patients treated with metronidazole. Gastroenterology 1985;88:681–684.
267. Bradley WG, Karlson IJ, Rassol CG: Metronidazole neuropathy. BMJ 1977;3:610–611.
268. Ramirez JA, Mendell JR, Warmolts JR, et al: Phenytoin neuropathy: Structural changes in the sural nerve. Ann Neurol 1986;19:162–167.
269. Dobkin BH: Reversible subacute peripheral neuropathy induced by phenytoin. Arch Neurol 1977;34:189–190.
270. Lipton RB, Apfel SC, Dutcher JP, et al: Taxol produces a predominantly sensory neuropathy. Neurology 1989;39:368–373.
271. Roytta M, Raine CS: Taxol induced neuropathy: Chronic effects of local injection. J Neurocytol 1986;15:483–496.
272. Apfel SC, Lipton RB, Arezzo JC, et al: Nerve growth factor prevents toxic neuropathy in mice. Ann Neurol 1991;29:87–90.
273. Luduena RF: Biochemistry of tubulin. In Roberts K, Hyams JS (eds): Microtubules, pp 65–116. New York, Academic Press, 1979.
274. Casey EB, Jellife AM, Le Quesne PM, et al: Vincristine neuropathy, clinical and electrophysiological observations. Brain 1973;96:69–86.
275. Fuller GN, Spies JM, Pollard JD, et al: Demyelinating neuropathies triggered by melanoma immunotherapy. Neurology 1994;44:2404–2405.
276. Mahaffey KR: Exposure to lead in childhood. The importance of prevention. N Engl J Med 1992;327:1308–1309.
277. Clarkson TW: Mercury: An element of mystery. N Engl J Med 1990;323:1137–1139.
278. Vergauwe PL, Knockaert DC, Van Tittelboom TJ: Near fatal subacute thallium poisoning necessitating prolonged mechanical ventilation. Am J Emerg Med 1990;8:548–550.
279. Davis LE, Standefer JC, Kornfeld M, et al: Acute thallium poisoning: Toxicological and morphological studies of the nervous system. Ann Neurol 1981;10:38–44.
280. Kamerbeek HH, Raws AG, Van Heijst ANP: Prussian blue in therapy of thallotoxicosis. Acta Med Scand 1971;189:321–324.
281. Jenkins RB: Inorganic arsenic and the nervous system. Brain 1966;89:479–498.
282. LeQuesne PM, McLeod JG: Peripheral neuropathy follow-

ing a single exposure to arsenic. J Neurol Sci 1977;32:437–451.
283. Donofrio PD, Wilbourn AJ, Albers JW, et al: Acute arsenic intoxication presenting as Guillain-Barré-like syndrome. Muscle Nerve 1987;10:114–120.
284. Heyman A, Pfeiffer JB, Willett RW, et al: Peripheral neuropathy caused by arsenical intoxication: A study of 41 cases with observations on the effect of BAL (2,3 dimercaptopropanol). N Engl J Med 1956;254:401–409.
285. Stamboulis E, Psimaras A, Vassilopoulos D, et al: Neuropathy following acute intoxication with mecarban (OP ester). Acta Neurol Scand 1991;83:198–200.
286. Aring CD. The systemic nervous affinity of triorthocresyl phosphate (Jamaican ginger palsy). Brain 1942;65:34–47.
287. Senanayake N, Jeyaratnam J: Toxic polyneuropathy due to gingili oil contaminated with tri-cresyl phosphate affecting adolescent girls in Sri Lanka. Lancet 1981;1:88–89.
288. Feldman RG, Mayer RM, Taub A: Evidence for peripheral neurotoxic effect of trichlorethylene. Neurology 1970;20:599–606.
289. Pont A, Rubino JM, Bishop D, et al: Diabetes mellitus and neuropathy following vacor ingestion in man. Arch Intern Med 1979;139:185–187.
290. Pinto NRS, Baruzzi RG: Male pubertal seclusion and risk of death in indians from Alto Xingu, Central Brazil. Hum Biol 1991;63:821–834.
291. Gabbai AA, Schmidt B, Oliveira ASB, et al: An original peripheral neuropathy associated with a seclusion rite in male adolescent Brazilian Indians. Muscle Nerve 1986;5(Suppl):123.
292. Chang MH, Lin KP, Wu ZA, et al: Acute ataxic sensory neuronopathy resulting from podophyllin intoxication. Muscle Nerve 1992;15:513–514.
293. Cassidy DE, Drewry J, Fanning JP: Podophyllin toxicity: A report of a fatal case and a review of the literature. J Toxicol Clin Toxicol 1982;19:35–44.
294. Bermudez de Rocha MV, Lozano Melendez FE, Salazar Leal ME, et al: Familial poisoning with Karwinskia humboltiana. Gac Med Mex 1995;131:100–106.
295. Long RR, Sargent JC, Hammer K: Paralytic shellfish poisoning: A case report and serial electrophysiologic observations. Neurology 1990;40:1310–1312.
296. Bagnis R, Kuberski T, Laugier S: Clinical observations on 3009 cases of ciguatera (fish poisoning) in the South Pacific. Am J Trop Med Hyg 1979;28:1067–1073.
297. Cameron J, Flowers AE, Capra MF: Electrophysiological studies on ciguatera poisoning in man (Part II). J Neurol Sci 1991;101:93–97.
298. McQuillen MP, Cantor HE, O'Rourke JR: Myasthenic syndrome associated with antibiotics. Arch Neurol 1968;18:402–413.
299. O'Riordan J, Javed M, Doherty C, et al: Worsening of myasthenia gravis on treatment with imipenem/cilastatin [Letter]. J Neurol Neurosurg Psychiatry 1994;57:383.
300. Kornfeld P, Horowitz SH, Genkins G, et al: Myasthenia gravis unmasked by antiarrhythmic agents. Mt Sinai J Med 1976;43:10–14.
301. Merril DG, Mihm FG: Prolonged toxicity of organophosphate poisoning. Crit Care Med 1982;10:550–551.
302. Baba A, Cooper JR: The action of black widow spider venom on cholinergic mechanisms in synaptosomes. J Neurochem 1980;34:1369–1379.
303. Clark RF, Wethern-Kestner S, Vance MV, et al: Clinical presentation and treatment of black widow spider envenomation: A review of 163 cases. Ann Emerg Med 1992;21:782–787.
304. Hagen R: Contracture of the quadriceps muscle in children: A report of 12 cases. Acta Orthop Scand 1968;39:565–578.
305. Mastaglia FL, Gardner-Medwin D, Hudgson P: Muscle fibrosis and contractures in a pethidine addict. BMJ 1971;4:532–533.
306. Penn AS: Myoglobinuria. In Engel AG, Franzini-Armstrong C (eds): Myology, 2nd ed, vol 2, pp 1679–1696. New York, McGraw-Hill, 1994.
307. Curry SC, Chang D, Connor D: Drug and toxin induced rhabdomyolysis. Ann Emerg Med 1989;18:1068–1084.
308. Thomas MAB, Ibels LS: Rhabdomyolysis and acute renal failure. Aust N Z J Med 1985;15:623–628.
309. Knochel JP: Rhabdomyolysis and myoglobinuria. Semin Nephrol 1981;1:75–86.
310. Martin RW, Duffy J, Engel AG, et al: The clinical spectrum of the eosinophilia-myalgia syndrome associated with L-tryptophan ingestion: Clinical features in 20 patients and aspects of pathophysiology. Ann Intern Med 1990;113:124–134.
311. McKinley KL, Harati Y, Schneider LW: Chronic immune activation in the eosinophilia-myalgia syndrome. Muscle Nerve 1993;16:947–951.
312. Fontiveros ES, Cumming WJK, Hudgson P: Procainamide-induced myositis. J Neurol Sci 1980;45:143–147.
313. Willis JK, Tilton AH, Harkin JC, et al: Reversible myopathy due to labetalol. Pediatr Neurol 1990;6:275–276.
314. Rewcastle NB, Humphrey JG: Vacuolar myopathy: Clinical, histochemical, and microscopic study. Arch Neurol 1965;12:570–582.
315. Kuncl RW, Duncan G, Watson D, et al: Colchicine myopathy and neuropathy. N Engl J Med 1987;316:1562–1568.
316. Murray SS, Kramlinger KG, McMichan JC, et al: Acute toxicity after excessive ingestion of colchicine. Mayo Clin Proc 1983;58:528–532.
317. Slotwiner P, Song SK, Anderson PJ: Spheromembranous degeneration of muscle induced by vincristine. Arch Neurol 1966;15:172–176.
318. Carraccio C, Blotny K, Ringel R: Sudden onset of profound weakness in a toddler. J Pediatr 1993;122:663–667.
319. Fewings JD, Burns RJ, Kakulas BA: A case of acute emetine myopathy. In Kakulas BA (ed): Clinical Studies in Myology. Proceedings of the 2nd International Congress on Muscle Diseases, part 2, p 594. Amsterdam, Excerpta Medica, 1971.
320. Langer T, Levy RI: Acute muscular syndrome associated with administration of clofibrate. N Engl J Med 1968;279:856–858.
321. Tobert JA: Efficacy and long-term adverse effect pattern of lovastatin. Am J Cardiol 1988;62:28j–34j.
322. Corpier CL, Jones PH, Suki WN, et al: Rhabdomyolysis and renal injury with lovastatin use: Report of two cases in cardiac transplant recipients. JAMA 1988;260:239–241.
323. Smith PF, Eydelloth RS, Grossman SJ, et al: HMG-CoA reductase inhibitor-induced myopathy in the rat: Cyclosporine A interaction and mechanism studies. J Pharmcol Exp Ther 1991;257:1225–1235.
324. Parr MJA, Willatts SM: Fatal theophylline poisoning with rhabdomyolysis. Anaesthesia 1991;46:557–559.
325. Laurence AS, Wight J, Forrest ARW: Fatal theophilline poisoning with rhabdomyolysis [Letter]. Anaesthesia 1992;47:82.
326. Cassidy DE, Drewry J, Fanning JP: Podophyllin toxicity: A report of a fatal case and a review of the literature. J Toxicol Clin Toxicol 1982;19:35–44.
327. Jenkins P, Emerson PA: Myopathy induced by rifampicin. BMJ 1981;283:105–106.
328. Ellis JT: Necrosis and regeneration of skeletal muscle in cortisone-treated rabbits. Am J Pathol 1956;32:993–1013.
329. Lacomis D, Smith TW, Chad DA: Acute myopathy and neuropathy in status asthmaticus: Case report and literature review. Muscle Nerve 1993;16:84–90.
330. Williams TJ, O'Hehir RE, Czarny D, et al: Acute myopathy in severe acute asthma treated with intravenously administered corticosteroids. Am Rev Respir Dis 1988;137:460–463.
331. Rewcastle NB, Humphrey JG: Vacuolar myopathy: clinical, histochemical, and microscopic study. Arch Neurol 1965;12:570–582.
332. Hirano M, Ott BR, Raps EC, et al: Acute quadriplegic myopathy: A complication of treatment with steroids, nondepolarizing blocking agents or both. Neurology 1992;42:2082–2087.
333. Haller RG, Knochel JP: Skeletal muscle disease in alcoholism. Med Clin North Am 1984;68:91–103.

334. Ferraz ML, Gabbai AA, Oliveira ASB, et al: Estudo histoquímico do músculo esquelético no alcoolismo crônico. Arq Neuropsiquiatr 1987;47:139–149, (Port).
335. Maunter LS: Muscle necrosis associated with carbon monoxide poisoning. Arch Pathol 1955;60:136–138.
336. Florkowski CM, Rossi ML, Carey MP, et al: Rhabdomyolysis and acute renal failure following carbon monoxide poisoning: Two case reports with muscle histopathology and enzyme activities. J Toxicol Clin Toxicol 1992;30:443–454.
337. Lovejoy Jr FH, Linden CH: Acute poison and drug overdosage. In Isselbacher KJ, Braunwald E, Wilson JD, et al (eds): Harrison's Principles of Internal Medicine, 13th ed, vol 2, pp 2441–2461. New York, McGraw-Hill, 1994.
338. Anetseder M, Hartung E, Klepper S, et al: Gasoline vapors induce severe rhabdomyolysis. Neurology 1994;44:2393–2395.
339. Roth D, Alarcón FJ, Fernandez JA, et al: Acute rhabdomyolysis associated with cocaine intoxication. N Engl J Med 1988;319:673–677.
340. Penn AS, Rowland LP, Fraser DW: Drugs, coma, and myoglobinuria. Arch Neurol 1972;26:336–343.
341. Richter RW, Challenor YB, Pearson J, et al: Acute myoglobinuria associated with heroin addiction. JAMA 1971;216:1172–1176.
342. Akmal M, Valdin JR, McCarron MM, et al: Rhabdomyolysis with and without acute renal failure in patients with phencyclidine intoxication. Am J Nephrol 1981;1:91–96.
343. Lane RJM, Mastaglia FL: Drug-induced myopathies in man. Lancet 1978;2:562–566.
344. Palmucci L, Bertolotto A, Schiffer D: Acute muscle necrosis after chronic overdosage of phenformin and fenfluramine. Muscle Nerve 1978;1:245–247.
345. Streicher HZ, Gabow PA, Moss AH, et al: Syndromes of toluene sniffing in adults. Ann Intern Med 1981;94:758–762.
346. Mebs D, Ownby CL: Myotoxic components of snake venoms: Their biochemical and biological activities. Pharmacol Ther 1990;48:223–236.
347. Azevedo-Marques MM, Cupo P, Coimbra TM, et al: Myonecrosis, myoglobinuria and acute renal failure induced by South American rattlesnake (Crotalus durissus terrificus) envenomation in Brazil. Toxicon 1985;23:631–636.
348. Bond GR: Antivenin administration for centuroides scorpion sting: Risks and benefits. Ann Emerg Med 1992;21:788–791.
349. Sutherland SK, Trinca JC: Survey of 2144 cases of redback spider bites: Australia and New Zealand, 1963–1976. Med J Aust 1978;2:620–623.
350. Gala S, Katelaris CH: Rhabdomyolysis due to redback spider envenomation [Letter]. Med J Aust 1992;157:66.

14

Traumatic Disorders of the Peripheral Nervous System

Madjid Samii, M.D. • Götz Penkert, M.D.

The introduction of microsurgery in connection with the increased possibilities of application of nerve grafts during the last 30 years not only extended the indications for reconstruction of peripheral and cranial nerve lesions, but also improved the results significantly.

Although the operative microscope had been already developed for a long time, and microsurgery had been used in otosurgery and ophthalmology since 1923, they were not introduced in peripheral nerve surgery early on. The largest impact in other surgical fields was engendered by Jacobson and coworkers, who developed microsurgical techniques in small blood vessels. In 1963, Jacobson described the advantages of microsurgical techniques in the repair of peripheral nerve injuries.[1] He pointed out the two major requirements: (1) delicate handling of tissue and (2) accurate approximation of nerve ends with fascicular orientation. Both are easily fulfilled with the operating microscope.

In 1964, Smith,[2] Michon and Masse,[3] and Kurze[4] introduced microsurgical techniques in peripheral and cranial nerve surgery. Accordingly, the microsurgical possibility of preparation of the individual fascicles of a nerve trunk, along with adequate knowledge on the microtopography of the fascicular structures and their relation to the connective tissue of the nerve trunk, allowed for progress in diagnosis and ascertainment of extension and form of a nerve lesion during operation. Thus, improved results could be achieved.

PREOPERATIVE MANAGEMENT: TIMING OF OPERATION

Theoretically, we may be confronted with an extremity with open wound or even fracture, so that a primary wound control with osteosynthesis, tendon repair, and reconstruction of vessels will be indicated at once. During this procedure, immediate identification and inspection of all nerves or nerve stumps within the region of the open wound are of great importance.

In our opinion, primary repair of nerve continuity is allowed only in case of a really clean and sharp nerve transsection, without any risk of additional laceration of the involved nerve stumps, so that secondary fibrotic reactions of the epi- and perineural tissue would not occur.

If there is any doubt concerning the mechanism of nerve lesion, or if there are additional soft tissue lacerations, we postpone nerve reconstruction for an early secondary repair a few weeks after the nerve injury. Because the nerve cell response to trauma has its peak during the third week, theoretic considerations are also in favor of early secondary nerve reconstruction.

If we do not find the opportunity of a primary wound inspection, or if the patient's extremity has sustained a closed lesion, there is no available information about the continuity of the theoretically involved nerves, the degree of lesion, the question of wallerian degeneration, the tendency for fibrotic reactions within the nerve secondary to injury, or about pseudoneuroma or neuroma formation. Nerve conduction may be blocked because of segmental demyelination or wallerian degeneration. Recovery will last some weeks in the first case, but 6–9 months in case of loss of axon continuity, depending on the distance between lesion and target. Circular compressing forces of soft tissue scarring around and within the nerve may hinder nerve recovery and block some or all axon sprouts. Soft tissue proliferation within the nerve may induce a pseudoneu-

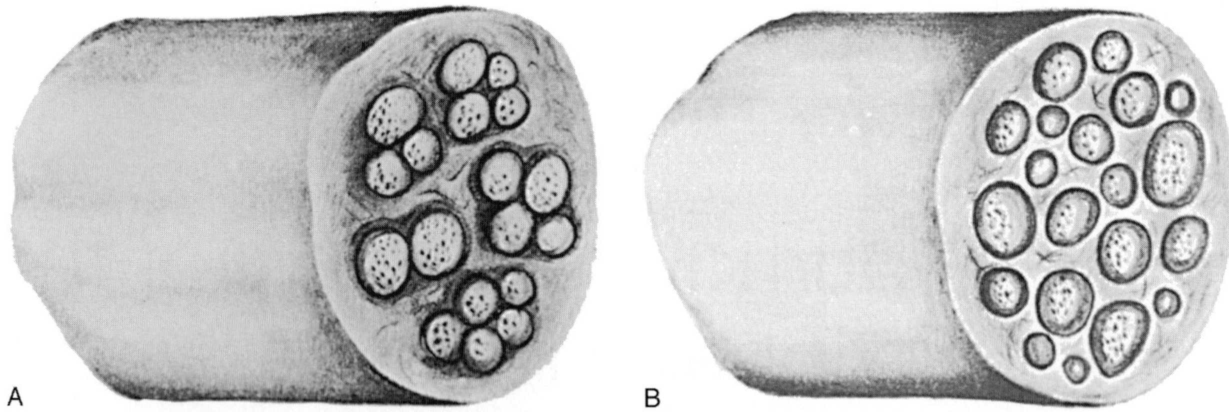

FIGURE 14-1 • *A,* Cross-section of a nerve with group arrangement (five fascicle groups). *B,* Cross-section of a polyfascicular nerve. (*A, B,* From Samii M: Fascicular peripheral nerve repair. Modern Technics in Surgery, Neurosurgery 1980;17:1–22. Futura Publishing.)

roma, or even a neuroma in continuity. Unfortunately, most patients fall into this category, with primarily unclear nerve lesions. In these cases, only repeated clinical, neurographic, and electromyographic examinations can be advised.

If, however, the above-mentioned evaluation fails to reveal any sign of nerve recovery, a late secondary exploration must be performed. Since approximately 6–7 months after injury there is a significant drop in the extent of regeneration due to degenerative processes within the muscles, timing of the so-called late secondary operation must be within half a year. In patients operated on later than that, the axon sprouts will reach their target, thus sustaining excessive irreversible atrophy. Therefore, decision making for secondary nerve repair is difficult, because several factors must be taken into account. Among those are the mechanism of injury, the patient's age, the importance of the involved nerve, its chances of recovery, and simultaneous or secondary tendon transfers, especially after longer time intervals.

NERVE LESIONS IN CONTINUITY

In order to understand the different types of nerve lesions in continuity, it is necessary to know about the anatomic composition of each individual peripheral nerve. The smallest surgical unit of a peripheral nerve is a fascicle, consisting of a great number of nerve fibers and the endoneurium. Each fascicle is enclosed by the perineurium. Often some fascicles are arranged as groups and then surrounded by the perineurium. Thus, a nerve may consist of three to five or more groups of fascicles (group arrangement [Fig. 14–1*A*]). Far peripherally, there are no more groups of fascicles, but a certain number of single fascicles within the cross-section, individually surrounded by the so-called epifascicular perineurium, and all fascicles are surrounded by connective tissue called epineurium (polyfascicular structure [Fig. 14–1*B*]).

According to studies of Sunderland, the number, size, and contribution of the fascicles are different not only in each individual nerve but also in the same nerve at different levels.[5] These fascicular structures influence microsurgical dissection, as well as the choice of operative technique.

In case of a nerve lesion in continuity, a thickened nerve segment is macrosurgically found (Fig. 14–2). However, from a microsurgical point of view (during microsurgical preparation under magnification), three types of nerve lesions in continuity can be differentiated:

Type 1. The fascicles are in continuity and surrounded by scar tissue. Fibrotically changed epineurium is mainly located in the external sheet or in the interfascicular tissues between the individual fascicles. The size and form of the fascicles can be normal or can be diminished in diameter—a pseudoneuroma (Fig. 14–3).

Regarding Seddon's classification of peripheral nerve injuries,[6] type 1 of our scale may present a neurapraxia, an axonotmesis, or both, at the same time. It is important to point out, however, that it is not easy to apportion Seddon's classification to

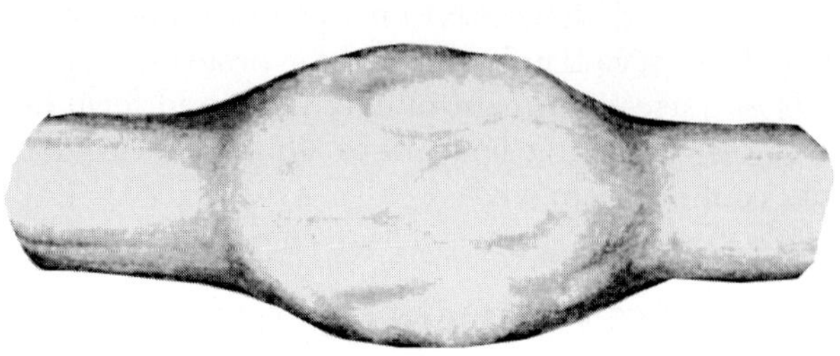

FIGURE 14-2 • Nerve lesion in continuity with thickened segment. (From Samii M: Fascicular peripheral nerve repair. Modern Technics in Surgery, Neurosurgery 1980;17:1–22. Futura Publishing.)

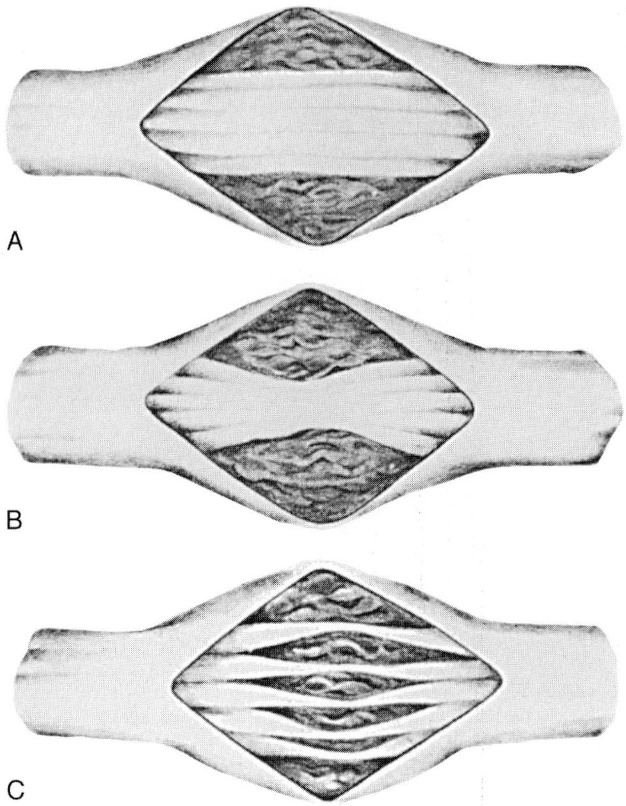

FIGURE 14–3 • *A,* Pseudoneuroma: external fibrosis, fascicles not changed and in continuity. *B,* Pseudoneuroma: external fibrosis with compressed fascicles as unit, but in continuity. *C,* Pseudoneuroma: external and interfascicular fibrosis with compressed fascicular groups in continuity. (*A–C,* From Samii M: Fascicular peripheral nerve repair. Modern Technics in Surgery, Neurosurgery 1980;17:1–22. Futura Publishing.)

each peripheral nerve injury. In case of neurapraxia, and the "temporary state" of functional deficit due to demyelinization of nerve fibers, functional restitution does not necessarily occur after 3–4 weeks. Along with creating neurapraxia, the same injury can cause fibrosis, which ultimately prevents the return of normal function.

The same holds true with *axonotmesis,* which is associated with wallerian degeneration in the distal part and regeneration in the proximal part of the injured nerve. Despite optimal regeneration of the nerve fibers after a few months, and good contact of cell body with end organ by means of axoplasm, scar strangulation can decrease or prevent electrical stimulation, if the nerve is stimulated proximal to the lesion. In contrast, stimulation of the motor branches distal to the nerve lesion leads to muscle contraction.

Type 2. The fascicles can either be interrupted with development of a neuroma or show signs of thickening of the caliber inside the perineurium. The latter is an intrafascicular neuroma. In both circumstances, the nerve fibers are completely interrupted, which, according to the Seddon's classification, constitutes *neurotmesis.* There is always extensive fibrosis of the epineurium in the lesioned region (Fig. 14–4).

Type 3. This type is a combination of the two above-described modalities occurring simultaneously, where several fascicles are in continuity while the remaining ones are interrupted (Fig. 14–5*A*).

NERVE LESIONS WITH INTERRUPTION OF CONTINUITY

The first question in cases of total interruption of nerve continuity is the indication for primary and early secondary repair (a few weeks after injury).

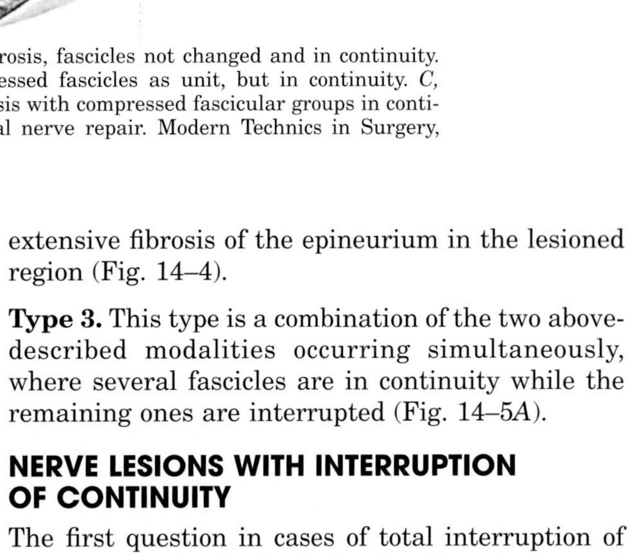

FIGURE 14–4 • Type 2 of lesion in continuity: after opening of the epineurium, some thickened and other interrupted fascicle structures—neuroma in continuity. (From Samii M: Fascicular peripheral nerve repair. Modern Technics in Surgery, Neurosurgery 1980;17:1–22. Futura Publishing.)

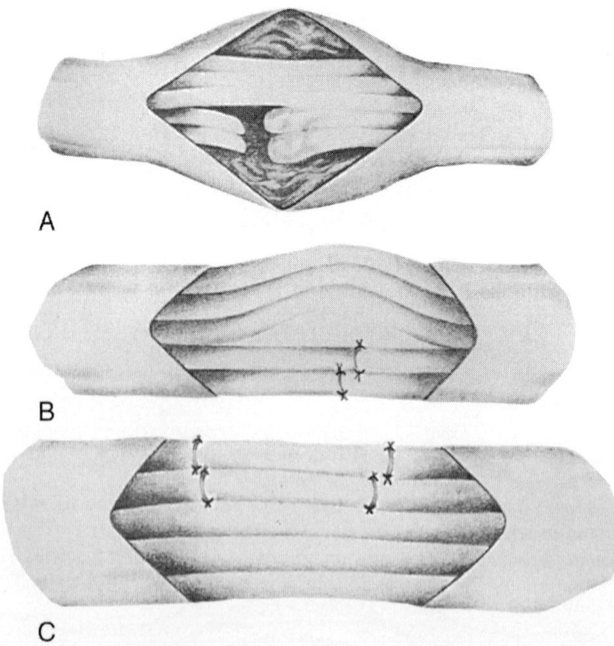

FIGURE 14-5 • *A,* Type 3 of lesion in continuity: combination of pseudoneuroma and neuroma in continuity. *B,* End-to-end suture of some fascicles within neuroma in continuity. *C,* Restoration of some fascicles within neuroma in continuity by individual grafts. (*A–C,* From Samii M: Fascicular peripheral nerve repair. Modern Technics in Surgery, Neurosurgery 1980;17:1–22. Futura Publishing.)

The extension of an open peripheral nerve lesion can be very different. The spectrum reaches from the simple superficial and clean-cut section of a nerve to amputation of the extremities.

Primary treatment is indicated only in a clean-cut wound of the nerve trunk. A coexistent vessel or tendon injury is no contraindication to primary treatment. The reconstruction of the severed nerve, however, in principle is executed after suture of vessel and tendon.

In case of contusion of soft tissues and bony damage, primary nerve treatment is not indicated, because of the following aspects:

1. The extension of a nerve lesion may be difficult to estimate at times, because of later scar tissue formation within the nerve stumps.
2. In case of nerve graft, the transplant may be strangulated by developing scar tissue and, therefore, negatively influence the axonal sprouting.
3. Necessary secondary treatment may also be of disadvantageous influence.
4. The risk of disturbance of wound healing endangering the nerve graft is increased.

The advantage of early secondary treatment, 4–6 weeks after injury, is to be seen in an already terminated sequence of wound healing. In addition, the nerve graft can be located in healthy tissue of the wound, without the risk of secondary wound healing.

An additional important decision is the choice between an end-to-end suture or application of a nerve graft. This question remained unanswered for a long time in the history of peripheral nerve repair.

The general idea was that a nerve graft, because of two suture lines, would lead to results inferior to end-to-end suture. All measures were applied to avoid nerve grafts and to render possible end-to-end suture of the nerve. These efforts focused on the important question of tension at the site of nerve suture over a period of more than 90 years.

In 1882, however, Mikulicz first tried to keep the suture line free of tension by using traction sutures.[7] Subsequently, Loebke and Kirschner recommended the use of a shortening osteotomy, in order to obtain a tension-free junction between nerve stumps.[8, 9] To reduce tension at the site of nerve suture, different manipulative procedures were recommended and used. Mobilization and transposition of nerves found general application, as did primary flexion of neighboring joints with secondary postoperative extension. The critical size of the defect and resection length, which may be closed with nerve end-to-end suture by the techniques described, have been assessed by Sanders,[10] Highet and Holmes,[11] Brooks,[12] and Seddon.[13] However, in the long run, all these manipulative procedures could not solve the problem of tension at the suture line. Although a tension-free suture can be executed and fixed by maximal flexion position of the neighboring joints, traction by later mobilization of the

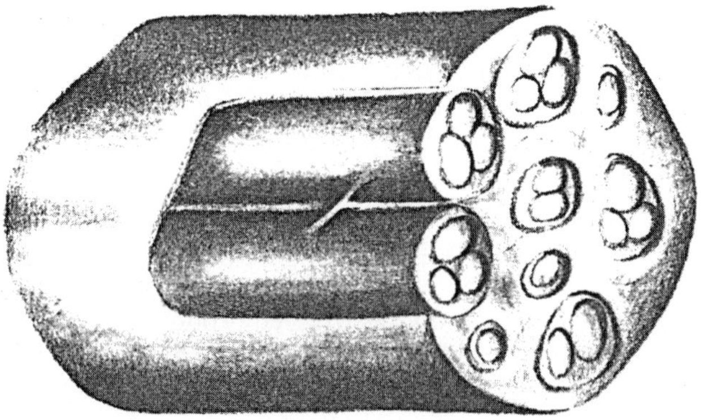

FIGURE 14–10 • Nerve with group arrangement and intercommunication between the groups. (From Samii M: Fascicular peripheral nerve repair. Modern Technics in Surgery, Neurosurgery 1980;17:1–22. Futura Publishing.)

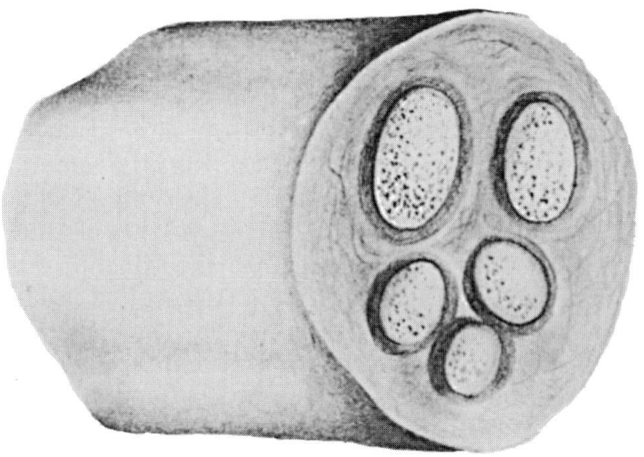

FIGURE 14–12 • Nerve with oligofascicular structure, e.g., proximal radial nerve. (From Samii M: Fascicular peripheral nerve repair. Modern Technics in Surgery, Neurosurgery 1980;17:1–22. Futura Publishing.)

topographic position and size, it is not difficult to connect the corresponding fascicles (Fig. 14–12). However, as previously mentioned, almost every peripheral nerve lesion that we have seen over the last 20 years of experience had to be reconstructed by means of nerve grafts, owing to the presence of scar tissue at the nerve stumps, and a tendency for nerve stump retraction.

Nerve Grafting

For a long period of time, the choice of a nerve graft has been characterized by the comparison of homologous and autologous nerve grafts. After the first experimental homologous nerve graft in 1870, by Philipeaux and Vulpian,[42] Albert[43] performed the first nerve graft in humans 8 years later. Since then, much experimental research on nerve grafting has been performed. After extensive, detailed experimental studies, Bielschowsky and Unger[44] showed the superiority of the autologous versus homologous nerve graft. In 1916, Foerster[45] reported on nine cases involving autologous nerve grafts, where he had used thin skin nerves for bridging the nerve defect. In two of these cases, satisfactory results were achieved. Owing to the results of their experiments and Foerster's clinical experience, Bielschowsky and Unger suggested the use of thin skin nerves as autologous nerve graft material. Because of the caliber difference between skin nerves, however, and the need for repairing the nerve stump, no further attention was paid to the use of autografts in peripheral nerve repair.

Unfortunately, the search for an ideal homologous nerve graft continued. After the negative results arising from the introduction of fresh homologous nerve grafts, due to the immunologic body reaction of the recipient, various methods were used to decrease or abolish the graft's antigenicity. Bethe[46, 47] used nerve grafts that were immersed in saline solution and refrigerated for 14 days. Bielschowsky and Unger[44] conserved the homograft in buric acid that was mixed with formalin. Huber[48, 49] used paraffin solution for graft storage purposes. Nageotte,[50] as well as Gosset and Bertrand,[51, 52] used alcohol as a fixing agent for achieving the same results. Weiss and Taylor[53] used frozen-dry homografts. Storage of homografts in petroleum was carried out by Dujarier and Francois[54] as well. Cajal[55] reported on the possibility of denaturation of nerve graft by means of chloroform, hot water, formalin, or chloral hydrate.

The use of radiation for decreasing the antigenicity of nerve grafts has been reported by Marmor,[56] Ashley,[57] Lewis and McLaurin,[58] Buch,[59] and Ducker and Hayes.[60] Nerves stored in cialit solution were used by Afanassieff.[61] Motta[62] showed the superiority of autograft over the cialit solution–stored nerves. Jacoby and associates[63] reported very good clinical results from newly developed lyophilized

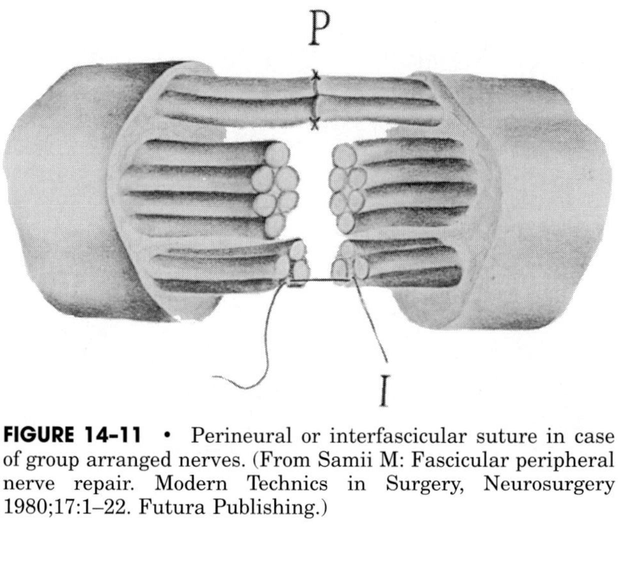

FIGURE 14–11 • Perineural or interfascicular suture in case of group arranged nerves. (From Samii M: Fascicular peripheral nerve repair. Modern Technics in Surgery, Neurosurgery 1980;17:1–22. Futura Publishing.)

homografts. These latter authors[63] suggested an additional graft wrapping with lyophilized dura, to protect the nerve regeneration from being infiltrated by connective tissue. In 1971, after extensive experimental studies, we showed that the quota of regeneration of even very short (only 5 mm) lyophilized homografts was much inferior to that of autologous nerve grafts. Our further experiments with lyophilized grafts longer than 4 cm resulted in failures.[64] An additional possibility for decreasing the antigenicity of the homografts is immunosuppressant treatment. Nigst[65] proved experimentally that the use of cortisone delayed the immune response.

It seems quite understandable that, because of the unfavorable results of homologous nerve grafting, there was a long-lasting tendency to force end-to-end nerve suture even in cases of larger defects. Exceptions were those cases in which suture could not be performed even with manipulative methods.[66] However, 16 years later, Seddon improved his own results after the Second World War in 55 cases involving nerve transplantation.[13, 67, 68] A pedicle nerve graft was attempted by Strange in 1947. This technique has mostly been used in cases of combined peripheral nerve lesions, in which one nerve was sacrificed for the benefit of the other.[69] The good results of this kind of transplantation were attributed to the good protection of the vascular supply of nerve transplant during wallerian degeneration.

The success of free autologous nerve grafts is also dependent on prompt nutrition and revascularization of the transplants. Revascularization of the nerve graft not only occurs through both nerve stumps to which the transplant is anastomosed. In fact, Hiller[70] experimentally showed that the transplant receives its blood supply mainly from the bed in which the transplant lies. We could experimentally underline this thesis and prove that sprouting vessels occur within the grafted nerve after 3 days.[29] It should be emphasized, however, that the sciatic nerve of the rabbit is of approximately the same diameter as the human sural nerve that we use for nerve graft, so that the preconditions for revascularization are the same ones.

In human nerve repair, the difficulty of free nerve transplantation lies mostly in overcoming the caliber difference between the skin nerve and the nerve stump requiring repair. Bunnell[71] attempted to build a cable from several nerve grafts in order to approach the same diameter as that of the injured nerve. In this latter work, the individual thin skin nerves were sutured together.[71] In 1947, Seddon claimed that the suture technique of a cable transplant was difficult, and therefore he preferred Young and Medawar's[72] technique of "fibrin suture." Using cable transplants, adequate revascularization could be delayed or even lead to a central necrosis.[68] After the introduction of the operating microscope, most of these technical difficulties in autologous nerve transplantation were solved. Millesi, Ganglberger, and Berger[73] recommended that attention should not be focused so much upon the nerve stump and the consequent necessary adjustment in the size of nerve grafts. Rather, the nerve stump should be divided under the microscope into fascicles or fascicular groups with the same diameter as that of the individual thin skin nerve transplant. This method has been designated as interfascicular autologous nerve grafting.[73] The subsequent microsurgical use of nerve grafts has led to clear improvement in functional results.[17, 18, 21, 74, 75]

Nerve Grafting Technique

For the performance of nerve grafting, size and distribution of the fascicular structures of the nerve stumps must be taken into consideration. From the topographic point of view, there is an exchange of nerve fibers in peripheral nerves over a short distance. Because of this feature, there is also a change in size and distribution of the fascicles within a certain distance of a nerve trunk. The longer the distance, the more the fascicle structures of one and the same nerve trunk will be changed. According to the nerve defect, there will be differences in the structures of the proximal and distal nerve stumps. Regarding the preparation of nerve stumps for nerve grafting, one must consider each nerve stump separately. Different preparation techniques can be applied to each nerve stump depending on the fascicular structures. A division of the fascicles or fascicle groups is to be recommended if:

1. There are enough interfascicular connective tissues between the individual fascicles or fascicle groups.

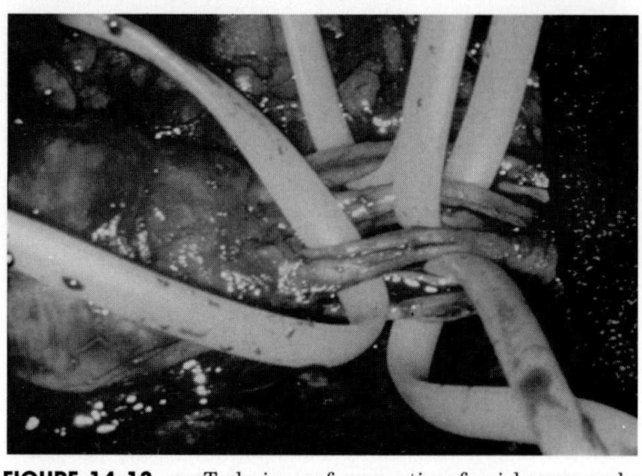

FIGURE 14–13 • Technique of separating fascicle groups beside the neuroma.

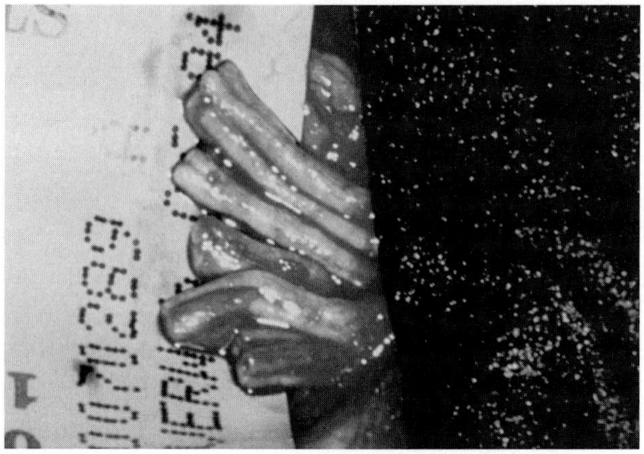

FIGURE 14–14 • The situation after transsection of the fascicle groups and removal of the neuroma.

2. No fascicular intercommunication exists in immediate proximity to the nerve ends.

In such a case, one should try to perform fascicular dissection after removal of the outer layer of the epineurum, as a means of choosing fascicle groups of about the same caliber as those of the sural nerve grafts. These fascicle groups may consist of two or more fascicles, depending on the caliber (Figs. 14–13 and 14–14).

If a fascicle is of the same diameter as the nerve graft, it can be dissected, isolated, and anastomosed with one nerve graft. A fascicle group of about double the caliber of the graft, resisting division, should be connected corresponding to the distal fascicle groups by means of two grafts (Figs. 14–15 through 14–17). In a case of polyfascicular nerve with only little interfascicular tissue, the nerve stumps may not be divided into different fascicles or fascicular groups. Several grafts of the sural nerve may be sutured side-by-side with the nerve end so that the whole surface of the nerve stump is covered up (Fig. 14–18). The same technique is used if the nerve stump consists of only one large fascicle, as in the case of brachial plexus in the supraclavicular region. The epineurium can be totally removed (Figs. 14–19 and 14–20).

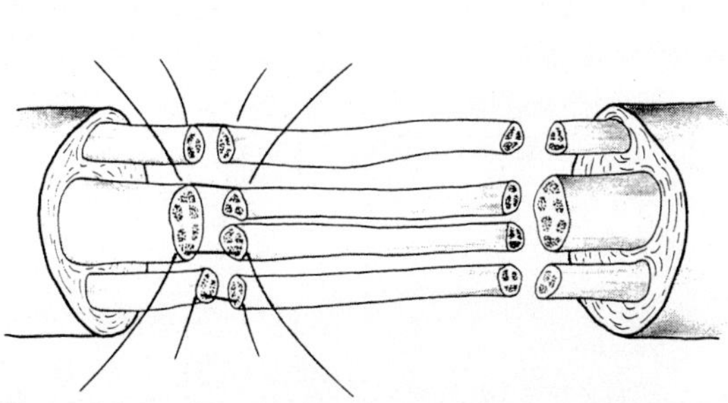

FIGURE 14–15 • Technique of nerve grafting: perineural or interfascicular stitches at the nerve stumps and epiperineural stitches at the grafts. (From Samii M: Fascicular peripheral nerve repair. Modern Technics in Surgery, Neurosurgery 1980;17:1–22. Futura Publishing.)

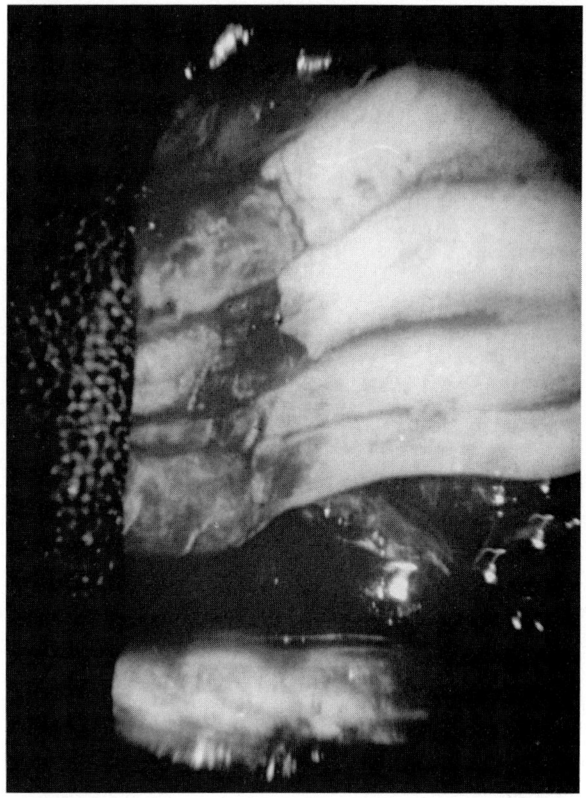

FIGURE 14–16 • Proximal suture line after grafting.

For all different techniques of nerve grafting, most attention should be paid to the graft's length, which, in any case, should be a little longer than the nerve defect, in order to avoid tension at the suture line and guarantee optimal adaptation. For adaptation and fixation of the individual graft ends at the nerve stumps, we generally place one or two sutures with 10-0 suture material. Further sutures will not be necessary because of sticking between the nerve end and nerve graft by normal fibrin clotting in a relatively short time. By the described details of the technique of nerve grafting, it becomes clear that different suture techniques can be performed. According to the circumstances, in one and the same case, either the epineural, perineural, epiperineural, or interfascicular suture technique can be applied. Nerves of thin caliber of about the same size as the sural nerve, consisting of individual fascicles, will allow for an epineural or epiperineural suture. The sural nerve should be the first choice for nerve grafts because of its length of approximately 40 cm in adults. We usually need only one sural nerve for bridging the nerve defect in most cases of single nerve lesion. In combined nerve lesions, where two or three nerves are dissected simultaneously, we remove both sural nerves.

Long sciatic nerve defects provide an exception. For bridging such a long and broad defect, we need not only both the sural nerves but also the cutane-

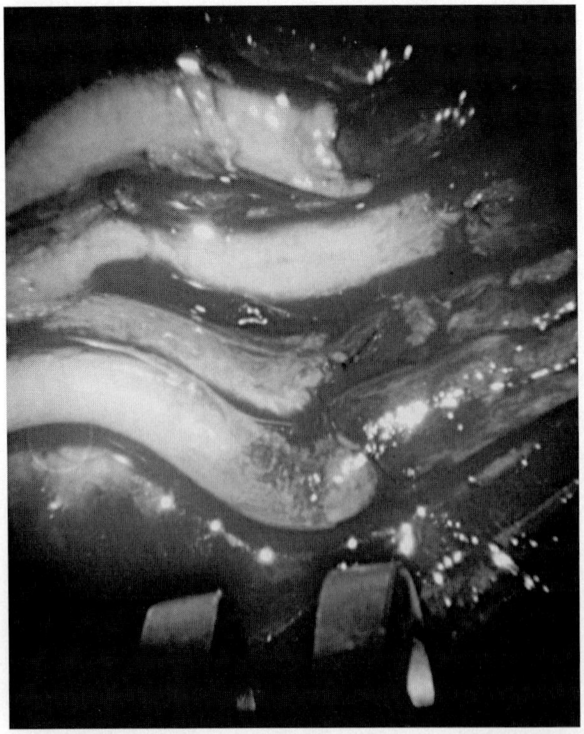

FIGURE 14-17 • Distal suture line after grafting.

ous brachei and antebrachei medialis nerves. Very seldom, the lateral femoral cutaneous nerve or the superficial branch of the radial nerve may be used as grafts. For removal, after a skin incision, the sural nerve is exposed behind the lateral malleolus, somewhat behind or beside the saphena parva vein. The nerve then has to be looped, and by slight pulling will allow for the palpation in proximal direction. After multiple short skin incisions, the sural nerve can be prepared up to the popliteal fossa and, after section, is gently extracted through the skin incision.

POSTOPERATIVE TREATMENT

In the past, it was routine to immobilize the affected extremities for some weeks with a plaster cast after

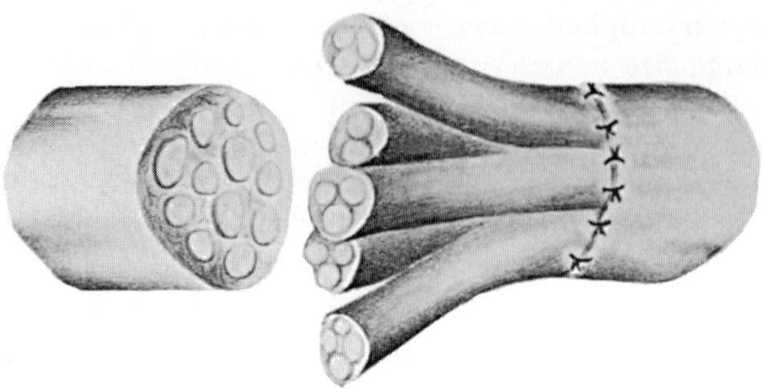

FIGURE 14-18 • Positioning of grafts at polyfascicular nerve stumps—covering the whole cross-section of the stump. (From Samii M: Fascicular peripheral nerve repair. Modern Technics in Surgery, Neurosurgery 1980;17:1–22. Futura Publishing.)

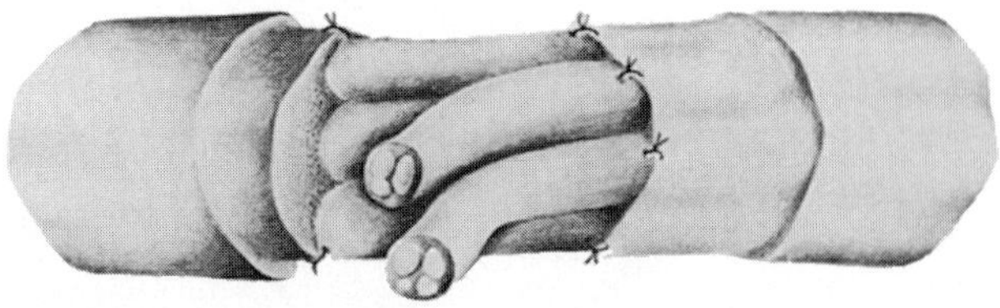

FIGURE 14-19 • Positioning of grafts at monofascicular nerve stumps, e.g., at roots of the brachial plexus. (From Samii M: Fascicular peripheral nerve repair. Modern Technics in Surgery, Neurosurgery 1980;17:1–22. Futura Publishing.)

nerve suture or nerve grafting. As the question of the effects of postoperative mobilization remained unanswered, we have attempted to gather data regarding these effects by experimental studies. We especially focused our interest on the postoperative resistance against tension forces at the suture line within 7 days. A very delicate question should be whether sutures under tension and sutures without tension would show different attachments.[76] The studies were performed on sciatic nerves of rabbits by comparison of four groups:

First group: 36 sciatic nerves were cut and merely sutured end-to-end.

Second group: 36 sciatic nerves were cut and,

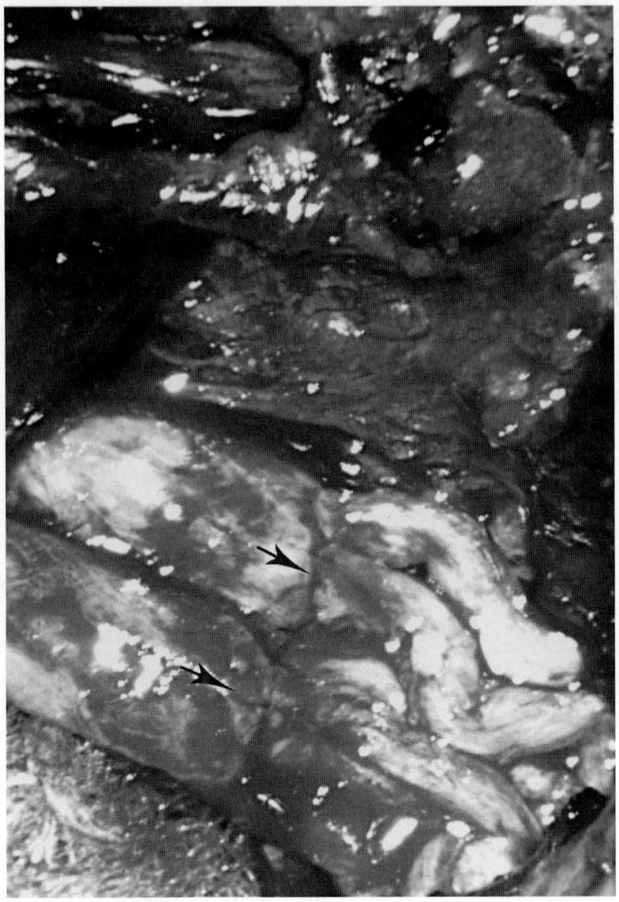

FIGURE 14-20 • Positioning of grafts at two nerve roots (arrows).

TABLE 15–1 **CAUSES OF ACUTE MYELOPATHY**

	TRAUMATIC	NONTRAUMATIC Acute	NONTRAUMATIC Subacute
Compressive	Canal encroachment Bone Disc Hematoma	Epidural hematoma	Neoplastic infiltration Spinal Epidural
	Translational deformity	Infection Epidural abscess Osteomyelitis Discitis	Infection Epidural abscess Osteomyelitis Discitis
Noncompressive	Vascular injury SCIWORA* Traction injury	Vascular Ischemia Hemorrhage Necrotizing myelitis	Inflammatory Multiple sclerosis Sarcoidosis Necrotizing myelitis

*Spinal cord injury without radiographic abnormality.

Therefore, recirculation was not related to reversibility of spinal cord function, and mechanical damage rather than ischemia was thought to be responsible for loss of neural function.

Spinal cord distraction has been studied in a dog model, using a Harrington-outrigger distraction apparatus.[19] The interstitial pressure of the spinal cord (CIP) was measured and correlated with the degree of distraction. In this model, spinal cord blood flow and somatosensory evoked potentials (SSEPs) were also measured. Baseline CIP was 6.5 mm Hg and increased to 46.5 mm Hg. At this pressure, spinal cord blood flow fell to 27% baseline and evoked potentials were abolished. CIP increased negligibly during initial elongation, and 80% CIP elevation occurred in the final 20% of elongation. Release of distraction caused a reactive hyperemia, in which spinal cord blood flow was 224% of baseline. CIP remained elevated. SSEP returned to 79% normal after 15 minutes of relaxation. Spinal cord perfusion pressure (Pperf) was defined as: Pperf = MAP − CIP, where MAP equals mean arterial pressure. Therefore, increased CIP was responsible for decreased spinal cord perfusion. Furthermore, any decrease in MAP also caused decreased spinal cord perfusion for any given CIP.

An increasing body of literature is building that indicates that following the acute injury to the spinal cord, local tissue metabolism at the site of injury is altered, which can contribute to further spinal cord injury, referred to as secondary injury. The cause of injury is not fully understood, but it appears to be multifactorial, including blood flow changes,[20] edema, hemorrhage, electrolyte abnormalities, membrane injury, and release of cytotoxic mediators and excitotoxic neurotransmitters. These factors appear to converge on a common mechanism, furthering membrane injury and alternating metabolism, resulting in progressive neural cell lysis. Such processes may be the cause of lethal injury to a cell that had initially sustained a reversible injury, thereby limiting recovery from a spinal cord injury.

A number of experimental models have been used to elucidate some of the above-mentioned factors mediating secondary injury. Decrease in blood flow during compression was proportional to the increased height in the static-load model.[21] Recovery of blood flow to baseline after decompression was also progressively prolonged with increased height and remained at a 60% baseline after 60 minutes post injury. Therefore, ischemic conditions after the primary injury may further exacerbate underlying cord injury. Microangiography after 1 minute of clip compression (51 g) revealed progressively worsened avascularity of the cord up to 24 hours.[22] In this study, progressive occlusion of the sulcal arteries also occurred up to 24 hours after compression. The anterior and posterior spinal arteries, however, remained patent. Scanning electron microscopy of vascular casts demonstrated profound lack of capillary refilling as early as 15 minutes after injury. Mild narrowing of the anterior spinal artery was noted and persisted up to 24 hours after injury. This may have represented vasospasm, which could have contributed to decreased blood flow at the injury site. Extravasation of injected resin from sulcal arteries represented severe damage of vascular walls. Progressive occlusion of sulcal arteries was also confirmed by electron microscopy.[23, 24] Experimental attempts to improve blood flow post injury have demonstrated varying results. Furthermore, reactive hyperemia has been noted immediately following spinal cord injury in some models.[16]

The disruption of energy metabolism after spinal cord injury may cause further damage and has been correlated with increasing severity of impact and reduced blood flow in rats.[25] The accumulation of metabolites measured by microdialysis after compression by static loads of increasing weight was found to be profoundly elevated. Profound elevation of lactate in the most severely injured animals correlated with continued impairment of perfusion, as well as irreversible paraplegia. Disruption of energy metabolites due to secondary ischemia parallels penumbra conditions seen in cerebral ischemic studies. Therefore, improvement of blood flow and reduction of tissue metabolic needs may improve final outcome after ASCI.

Disturbances of calcium and other electrolytes may contribute to post-traumatic ischemia. Increases of tissue calcium, sodium, and water have been observed after spinal cord injury in ischemic studies.[26] Intracellular shift of calcium activates calcium-dependent proteases and impairs mitochondrial and other intracellular functions, which contribute to cell death. Treatment with nimodipine, a calcium channel blocker, has been shown to decrease post-traumatic edema, improve blood flow, as well as improve final outcome.[27] Excitotoxic neurotransmitter release may be linked to increased intracellular calcium and worsening spinal cord damage post injury. Hemorrhage and edema also may contribute to secondary injury in spinal cord trauma. Magnetic resonance imaging (MRI) and histologic studies have been used to delineate the time course of these mechanisms.[28, 29] Hemorrhage occurs immediately after injury and resolves after 1 week. Low-impact injuries produce abnormalities in the gray matter with the relative sparing of the white matter. Hemorrhage was noted at remote sites from the area of injury in severe impact injuries and spread into the white matter. Edema was first seen 6 hours after injury and became maximal after 1 week. In clinical studies, patients with cord contusion or hematoma seen on MRI had worse neurologic outcome, and many developed post-traumatic cysts when compared with patients without demonstrable cord parenchymal abnormality on MRI.[30, 31] The patients who had only edema of the cord post injury had better outcomes. Therefore, patients with hemorrhage or contusion may be at higher risk for worsening neurologic outcome.

In summary, secondary injury following spinal cord injury can cause progressive cell lysis. Although the precise mechanisms are uncertain, the process is likely multifactorial and forms a cascade of events that accelerate the process. The direct traumatic injury, extravasated blood products, and ischemia alter the extracellular ionic environment. These changes alter membrane potentials across neural cell membranes, contributing to cell swelling and the entry of extracellular calcium into the cytocel. This process liberates proteases and lipase enzymes within the neural cell, which exacerbates cell membrane injury and liberates arachidonic acid for prostaglandin synthesis. The prostaglandins combine with oxygen free radicals to cause further intracellular organelle destruction, membrane injury, and release of liposomal enzymes. These mediators internally consume the cell structure, causing cell death. The mediators are then liberated into the extracellular fluid, which contributes to further edema, ischemia, and electrolyte disturbances propagating the destructive process.

The metabolic processes following injury form the basis of decision making regarding the management of the spinal cord injury component of the spinal injury, although current treatment modalities probably only indirectly influence the processes. A greater understanding of the metabolic derangements involved is required, along with the development of substances to act directly upon certain steps in this cascade of metabolic events to arrest the secondary process.

Current concepts regarding secondary injury to the spinal cord have been derived from experimental trauma models. The implication of such mechanisms to nontraumatic spinal cord injury is speculative.

Vertebral Injury

The osteoligamentous component of the spine has two major functions. It acts to protect the neural elements from injury by extrinsic force and functions to support the body weight for upright ambulation by enabling axial spinal movement.[32] These two functions of the spine require competing structural properties of the vertebral column—rigidity and mobility—respectively.[33] Hence, the structure of the spine is a compromise between these two properties. Pathological processes and nonphysiologic loading of the spine can affect the integrity of the osteoligamentous component of the spine, resulting in failure of the vertebral complex. Vertebral element injury or derangement of spinal motion, causing deformity or a pain syndrome, is a manifestation of such failure. The normal and abnormal properties of the vertebral column are assessed using biomechanical principles.

Spinal biomechanics is the study of spinal column structure and function as it relates to spinal movements, and its protective and mobility functions under normal and abnormal conditions. In addition to enhancing our understanding of the mechanisms of spinal injury, the study of spinal biomechanics has augmented the effectiveness of corrective procedures for spinal deformity and stability. The functional unit of the spine used for studying biomechanics is called the motion segment or functional spinal unit.[34] The motion segment consists of two adjacent vertebrae and the intervening soft tissues, including the intervertebral disc and ligaments. Except for the atlantoaxial complex, each of the cervical, thoracic, and lumbar vertebrae are composed of similar elements, although the size and configuration of the bony components vary along the length of the vertebral column. The anterior portion of the motion segment includes the vertebral body, intervertebral disc, and longitudinal ligaments. The posterior portion of the motion segment is composed of the pedicles, facets, laminae and spinous processes, and intervening ligaments, including the intraspinous, intertransverse, ligamentum flavum, and joint capsules. An understanding of basic spinal motion has been derived from studies focusing upon the above-mentioned elements of the motion segment.[35, 36] However, studies indicate that paraspinal musculature significantly contributes to spinal stability and mechanics.[32, 37, 38] Therefore, an advanced understanding of spinal biomechanics must take into consideration the paraspinal musculature.

The vertebral bodies, located in the anterior column of the spine, function predominantly to bear axial load.[33, 39] Intervertebral discs interpose between the vertebral bodies to transfer the load from one vertebra to the other and act as a fulcrum upon which the vertebrae articulate. Their elastic and deformable properties enable movement between adjacent vertebral bodies and allow dynamic load transfer between vertebrae, which varies depending upon the instantaneous configuration of the motion segment. The facets form the posterior articulations between adjacent vertebrae. The orientation of the facet joints varies along each segment of the spine. This difference in facet joint orientation determines the direction of the primary physiologic movements for a given segment of the spine. In the cervical spine, the surfaces of the facet joints are relatively horizontal, tapering both inferiorly and posteriorly (Figs. 15–1 and 15–2*A*). This shape enables the cervical spine to flex, extend, and rotate. In the thoracic spine, the facet joints are oriented almost vertically (see Fig. 15–3), with a lateral inclination. Rotation and limited forward flexion are allowed by this facet shape. The attachment of the ribs to the transverse processes and bodies of the vertebrae limits thoracic spinal motion. In the lumbar spine, the facet surfaces are aligned in a more sagittal plane, with a degree of anterior-medial inclination (see Fig. 15–4*B*). This configuration enables flexion and some degree of lateral bending, but no rotation.

The facet joint capsule fibers are generally oriented at right angles to the margins of the facet joints. This allows movement in the primary directions for a given facet joint but resists distraction or nonphysiologic primary movement of the joint.

The pedicle acts as the anchor upon which the posterior elements are based, and through which the posterior elements connect with the vertebral bodies bilaterally. The transverse and spinous processes act as attachment points for ligaments and spinal muscle tendons, thereby enabling the muscles to apply force to generate spinal motion.

Determining the stability of the spine is important in the management of a patient with a spinal abnormality. The criteria established for spinal stability have been derived from clinical and experimental studies of spinal trauma. Clinical, radiographic, and combined factors have been used to define stability.[40–45] Radiographic criteria are most important in objectively determining stability in a clinical setting, and also in determining the indication and nature of the requisite stabilization procedure. The radiographic definitions of instability are not universally applicable for all chronic deforming processes. Criteria vary depending upon the level of

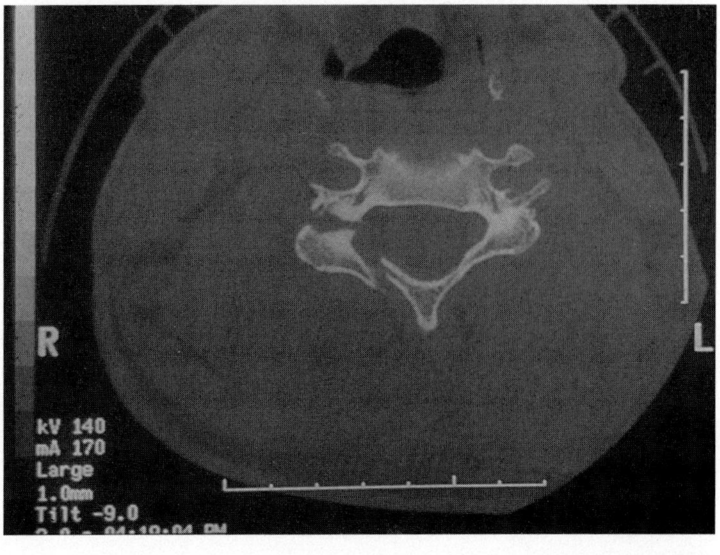

FIGURE 15–1 • An axial CT scan image of a right lateral mass fracture. The fracture runs through the posterior aspect of the pedicle and the lateral aspect of the lamina on the right. Vertebral body and left lateral mass structures are intact.

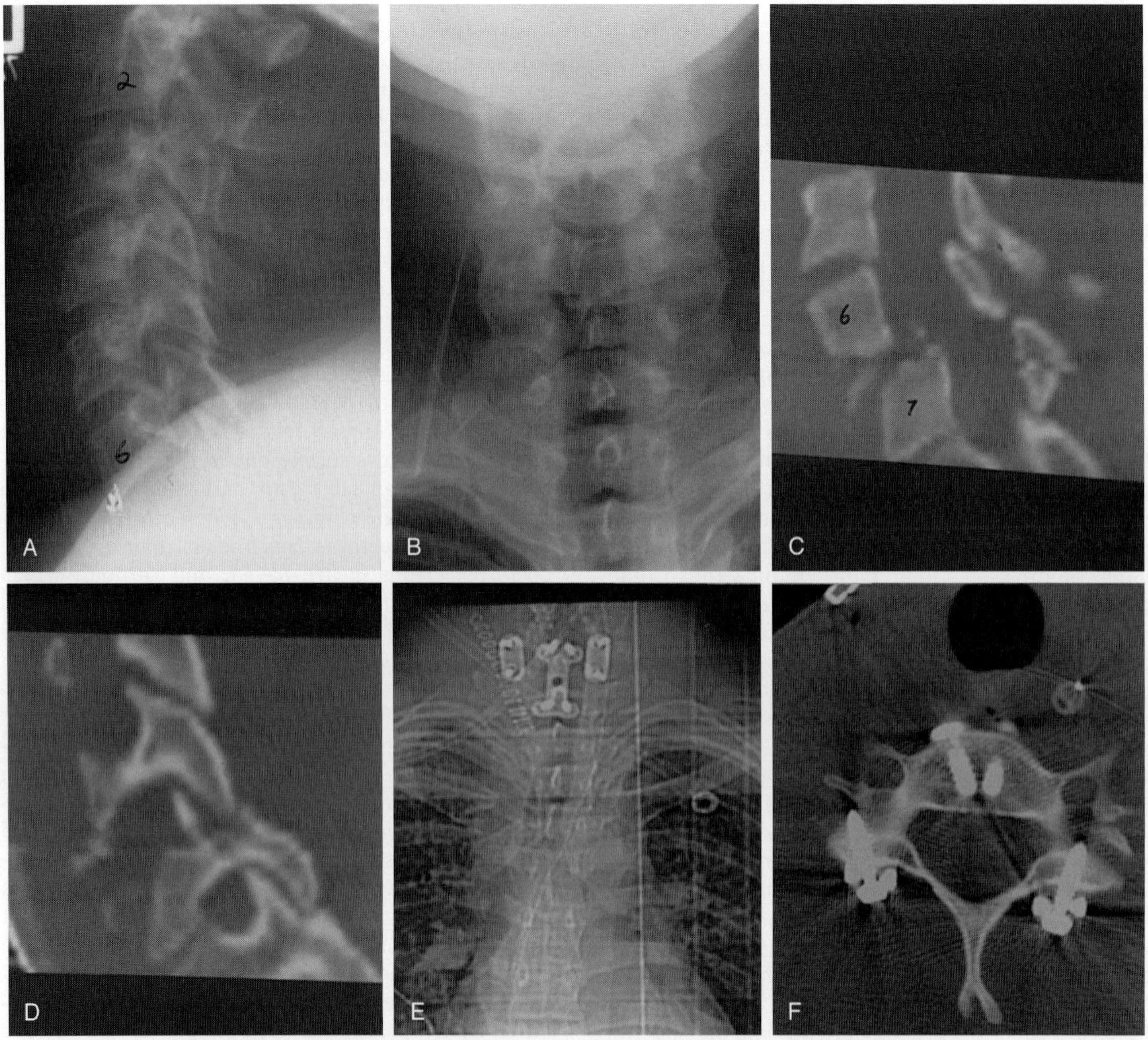

FIGURE 15–2 • Cervical fracture-subluxation. This 20-year-old patient sustained a fall from 20 feet, presenting with mild central cord syndrome. On admission, lateral *(A)* and anteroposterior *(B)* x-rays show no definite fracture-subluxations. However, the lateral view visualizes only to the inferior aspect of C6 due to obscuration by the shoulders. CT scan with sagittal reconstructions from C5 to the upper aspect of T1 was then carried out, demonstrating a severe fracture-subluxation of C6 on C7 *(C)* and the facet lock that maintained the deformity *(D)* and could not be reduced by cervical traction. Postoperative anteroposterior *(E)* and axial *(F)* views of the lower cervical region were taken following a posterior open reduction and fixation followed by a supplemental anterior fixation/fusion of the fracture. The anterior, unicortical screws are seen oriented medially. The posterior lateral mass screws are directed laterally in the axial plane to avoid the vertebral artery foramina and the intervertebral foramina *(F)*.

the spine involved. There are criteria for atlantoaxial injuries, subaxial cervical spine, and for those involving the thoracolumbar spine.[12, 46, 47] Stability has also been defined on a functional basis. The spine is considered to be unstable if, under physiologic load, the spine is unable to prevent a neurologic injury or pain.[34] The spine is considered unstable in the presence of a neurologic injury following trauma. However, exceptions to this definition exist. A central spinal cord injury due to hyperextension in the presence of cervical stenosis, unilateral facet fracture (see Fig. 15–1) presenting with radiculopathy, and spinal cord injury without radiographic abnormality (SCIWORA)[48, 49] are all examples of traumatic neurologic injury without spinal instability.

The anatomy of the atlantoaxial complex and its unique articulation necessitate different criteria to define stability than those required for the subaxial cervical spine. The major determinant of stability

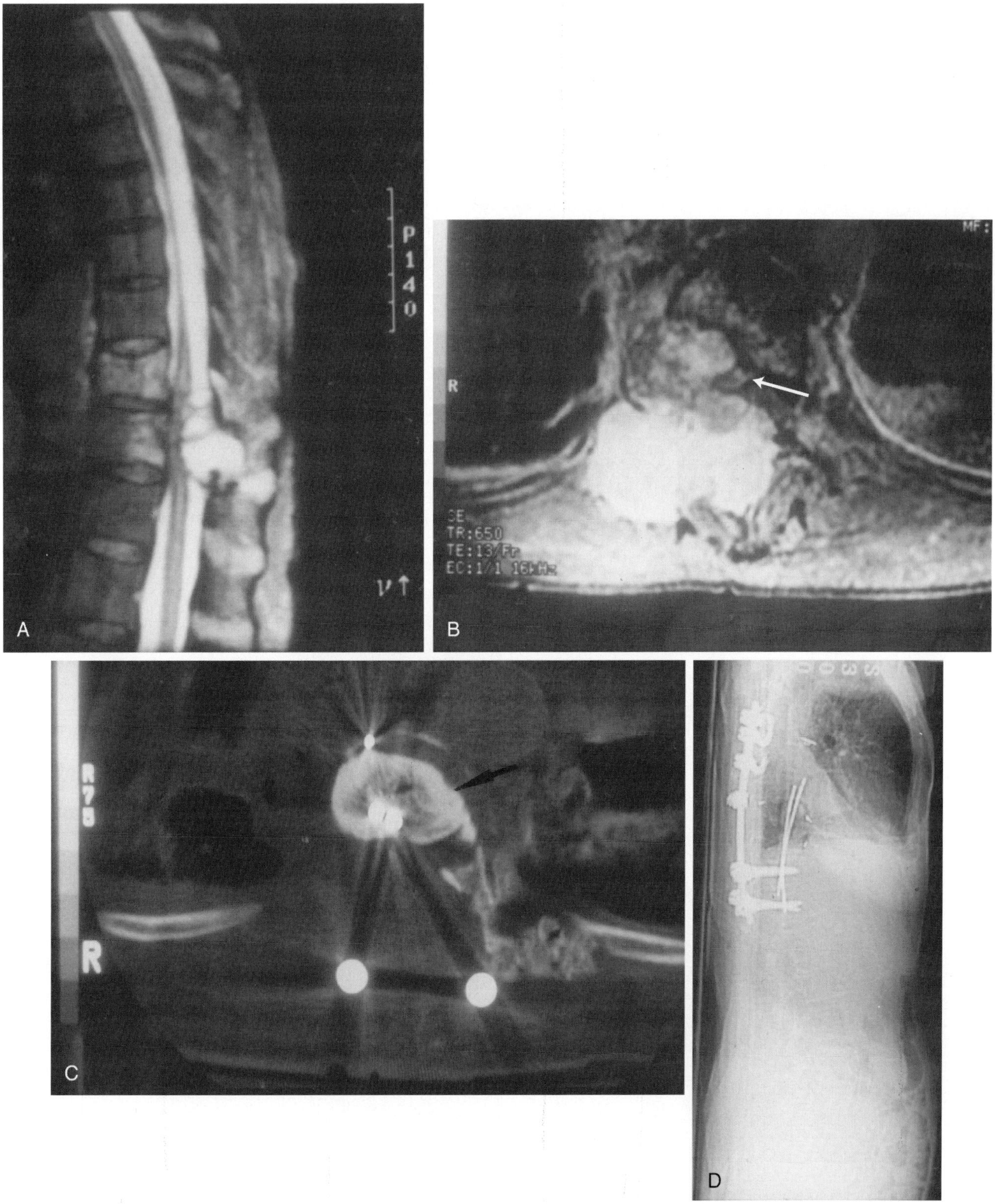

FIGURE 15–12 • Metastatic ovarian carcinoma (T9–T10). MRI with sagittal *(A)* and axial *(B)* images demonstrates involvement of the vertebral bodies of T9 and T10, indicated by the signal change within these bodies compared with the other thoracic vertebrae *(A)*. There is involvement of the posterior elements of T10. The tumor invades the spinal canal circumferentially, compressing the spinal cord. On the axial view, the compressed spinal cord is virtually imperceptible (arrow). Postoperative axial *(C)* and lateral *(D)* images of the thoracic spine demonstrate almost complete resection of the vertebrae, with only minimal residual lateral elements on the left. The vertebral body is reconstructed with stainless steel pins and methylmethacrylate (arrow). The segment of spine was fixated with a Universal system incorporating interfacet hooks superiorly and pedicle screws inferiorly *(D)*.

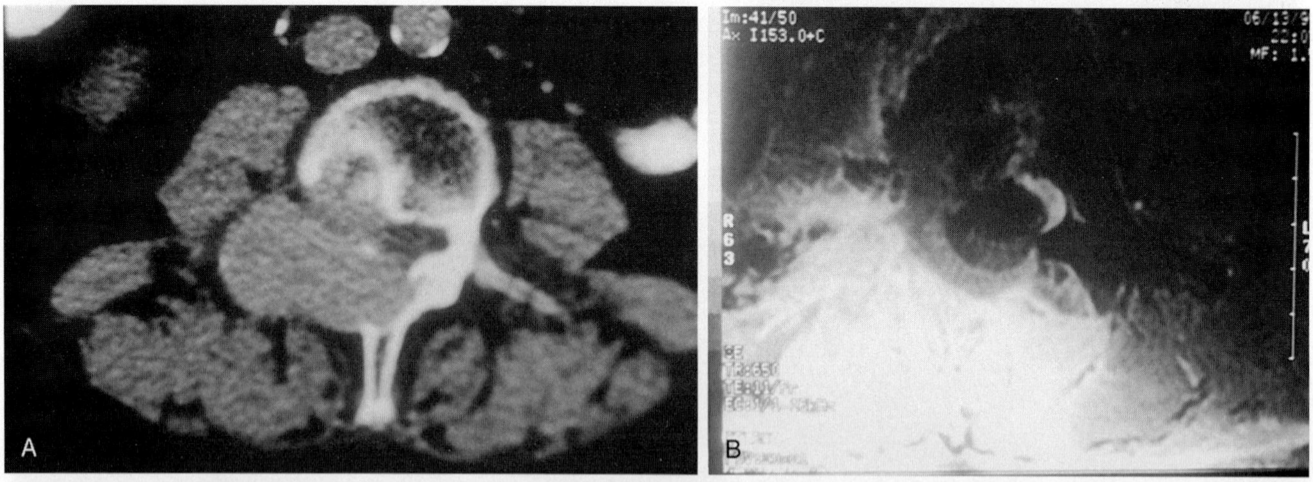

FIGURE 15–13 • An axial CT scan *(A)* of L3 demonstrating a metastasis involving the right-sided posterior elements and posterolateral vertebral body with early encroachment upon the spinal canal. The postoperative MRI with gadolinium *(B)* demonstrates radical resection of the tumor mass via laminectomy, resection of the lateral elements on the right, and the posterior aspect of the vertebral body. Residual tissue in the tumor bed represents granulation tissue. The spinal canal is widely patent.

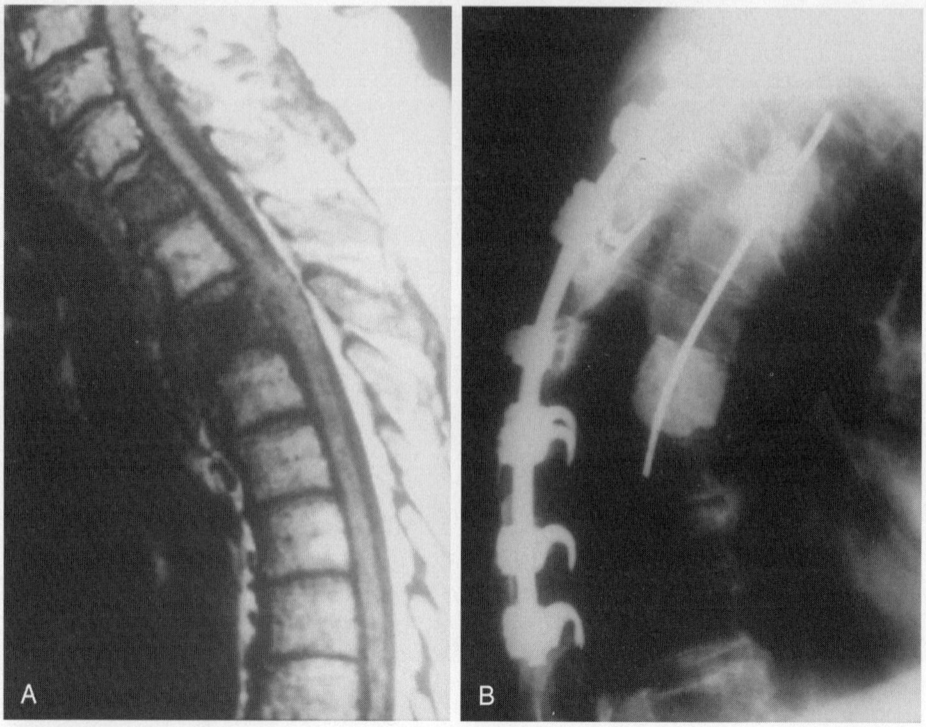

FIGURE 15–14 • Two-level thoracic metastasis. This 71-year-old man with a known primary presented with back pain and progressive myelopathy. The sagittal MRI scan *(A)* demonstrates involvement of the T5 vertebral body with extension of the tumor from the vertebral body into the epidural canal encroaching upon the spinal canal. Also, signal changes seen within the marrow of the T5 vertebral body indicate early metastatic invasion. The patient underwent transthoracic, two-level vertebrectomy *(B)*. The vertebral bodies were reconstructed with a stainless steel pin and methacrylate. The patient then underwent posterior decompression and debulking of T5 and supplementation of the anterior reconstruction by placement of a Universal hook-and-rod system.

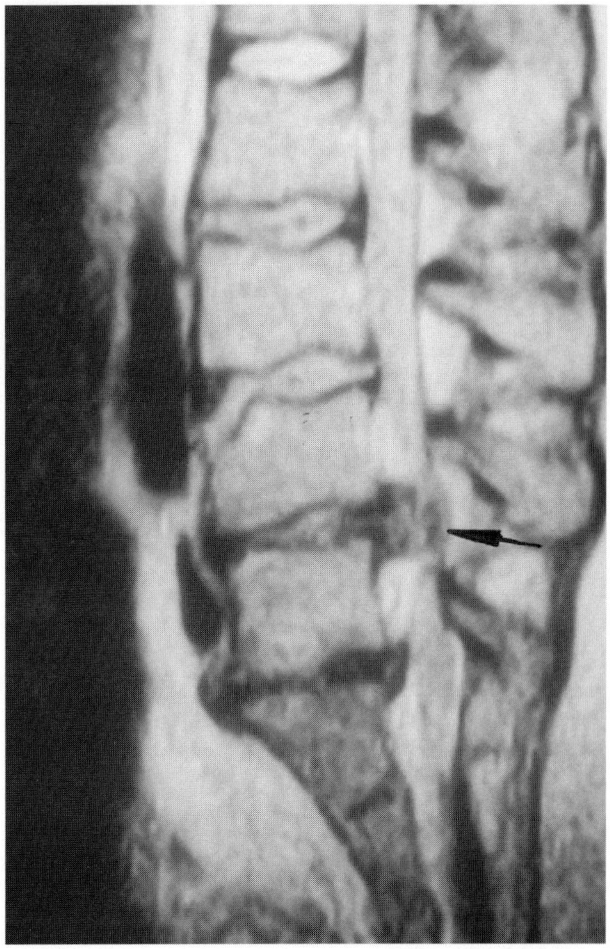

FIGURE 15–15 • Cauda equina syndrome from a lumbar disc herniation (L4–L5). This 29-year-old woman had a history of chronic low back pain. She presented with numbness involving the feet and perineum and urinary dysfunction. The MRI demonstrated a large posterolateral disc herniation at L4–L5 (arrow) filling the entire canal at this level, and a smaller midline protrusion without significant neural compression at L5–S1.

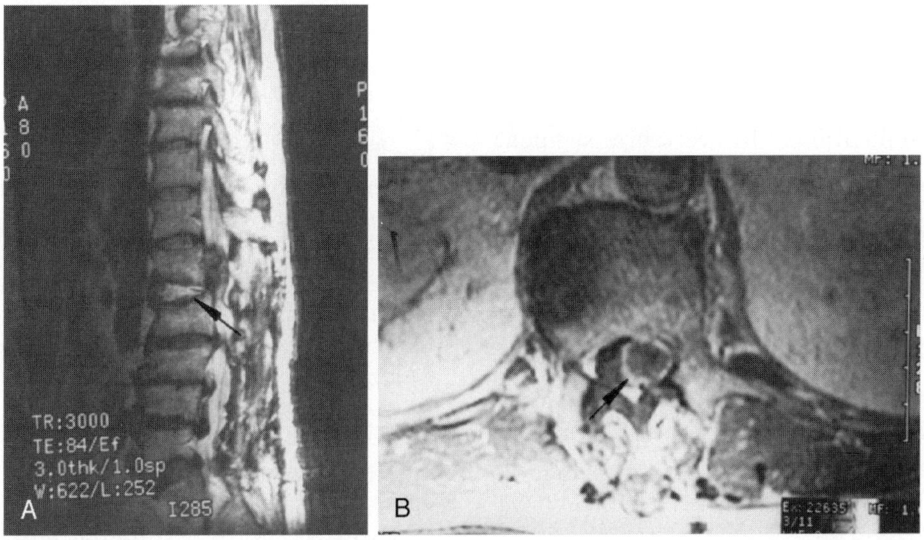

FIGURE 15–16 • Conus medullaris syndrome. This 71-year-old man presented with severe back and bilateral leg pain, progressive ataxia, and urinary retention. The sagittal MRI scan *(A)* demonstrated a large mass lesion in the spinal canal posterior to the vertebral body of L1. There were also significant degenerative changes in the disc space and end plates at L1–L2 (arrow) with high signal changes within the disc space (arrow) compared with signal characteristics of the adjacent discs. The axial view *(B)* demonstrates the mass lesion on the left side of the spinal canal (arrow) displacing the thecal sac contents to the right. The peripheral enhancing ring with the unenhancing center is characteristic of a subacute or chronic disc herniation.

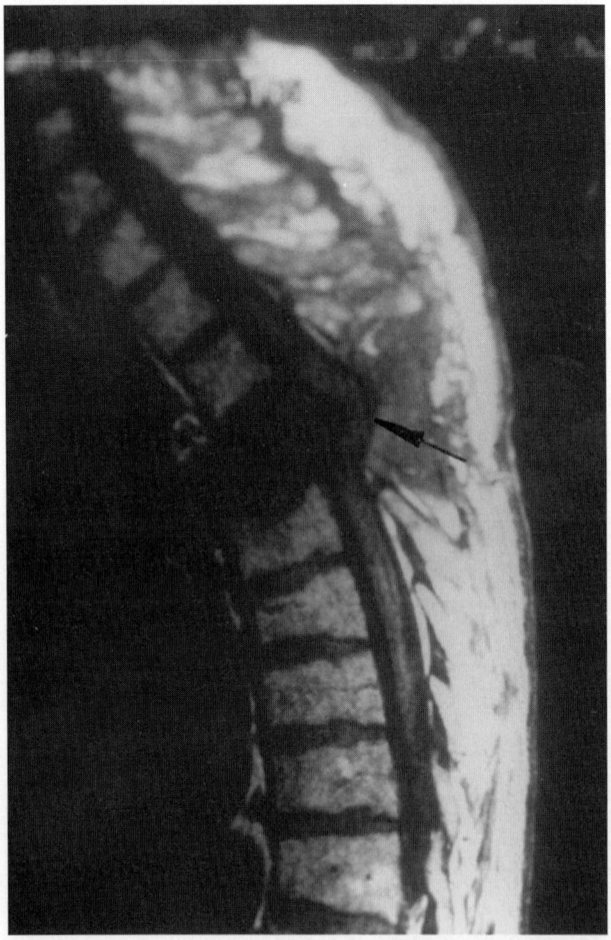

FIGURE 15–17 • Thoracic osteomyelitis/discitis. This 63-year-old man presented with thoracic back pain. MRI demonstrates signal change within the vertebral bodies of T5 and T6 and kyphotic deformity at this level and retropulsed bone and soft tissue into the spinal canal posteriorly, displacing the spinal cord (arrow). The spinous processes of T5 and T6 had been previously removed during a transpedicular vertebral body biopsy.

sive neoplastic infiltration of the vertebral segment can cause multidirectional or circumferential neural compression (see Fig. 15–12*A*, *B*). Further features of neoplastic infiltration of the spine are discussed later in the chapter.

CLINICAL ASSESSMENT

The approach to the patient with an acute spinal disorder requires the methodical process as is employed to diagnose and treat other medical conditions. The essential elements include history, physical examination, imaging studies, and other ancillary tests. However, the emphasis upon the components of the assessment varies depending upon the etiology of the disorder and the acuity of the onset of symptoms. Obviously, an otherwise young and healthy patient sustaining an acute spinal trauma with spinal cord injury does not require an extensive history to determine the etiology of neurologic deficits. His or her outcome would instead benefit from prompt imaging of the spine, followed by decompression and reduction of the vertebral injury. History is important regarding the etiology of myelopathy in a patient with nontraumatic compression and for noncompressive myelopathy.

In general, the clinical examination is intended to assess the function of the spinal cord and approximate the level of injury,[85] whereas imaging studies delineate the extent of osteoligamentous injury. Both clinical assessment and imaging contribute to the etiologic diagnosis of an acute myelopathy. The imaging studies also determine the operative approach for decompression and stabilization of the involved segment when surgery is indicated.

The goals of the neurologic assessment (history and physical examination) include determination of the extent and level of the neurologic injury; insight into possible systemic causes for the acute spinal disorder; and assessment of the patient's overall health, which may modify treatment options. Specifically, a detailed neurologic examination is required to diagnose, treat, and prognosticate in a given clinical circumstance.

The initial assessment of the patient, especially in the setting of trauma, focuses on essential functions. Airway patency and respiratory and cardiovascular function are assessed and stabilized.[3] During the evaluation of the traumatized patient, one assumes the presence of a potentially unstable cervical, thoracic, or lumbar spine injury, and precautions are taken to prevent neural injury. The patient is placed in a rigid collar, or the head is immobilized relative to the underlying backboard for cervical stabilization. Use of the backboard is common when patients are transported to the emergency room in order to prevent abnormal motion of the thoracolumbar spine.[3] It is often convenient to have the patient remain on the backboard during the initial clinical assessment and during imaging studies. It is quite effective for thoracolumbar stabilization.[3] However, in the patient who is asensate from a spinal cord injury, prolonged immobilization on the backboard can result in decubitus pressure ulcers in a matter of hours. Therefore, a backboard should be used with caution.

Secondary spinal cord injury is a relevant consideration when managing a patient with an acute spinal disorder. Hypoxia and systemic hypertension can contribute to secondary injury.[20] Therefore, these parameters must be monitored and maintained within a normal range throughout the management of the patient with a spinal injury. The presence of hypotension in the setting of trauma with or without spinal injury is not infrequent. Hypovolemia is a common cause. Sources of blood loss must quickly be identified and, if possible, con-

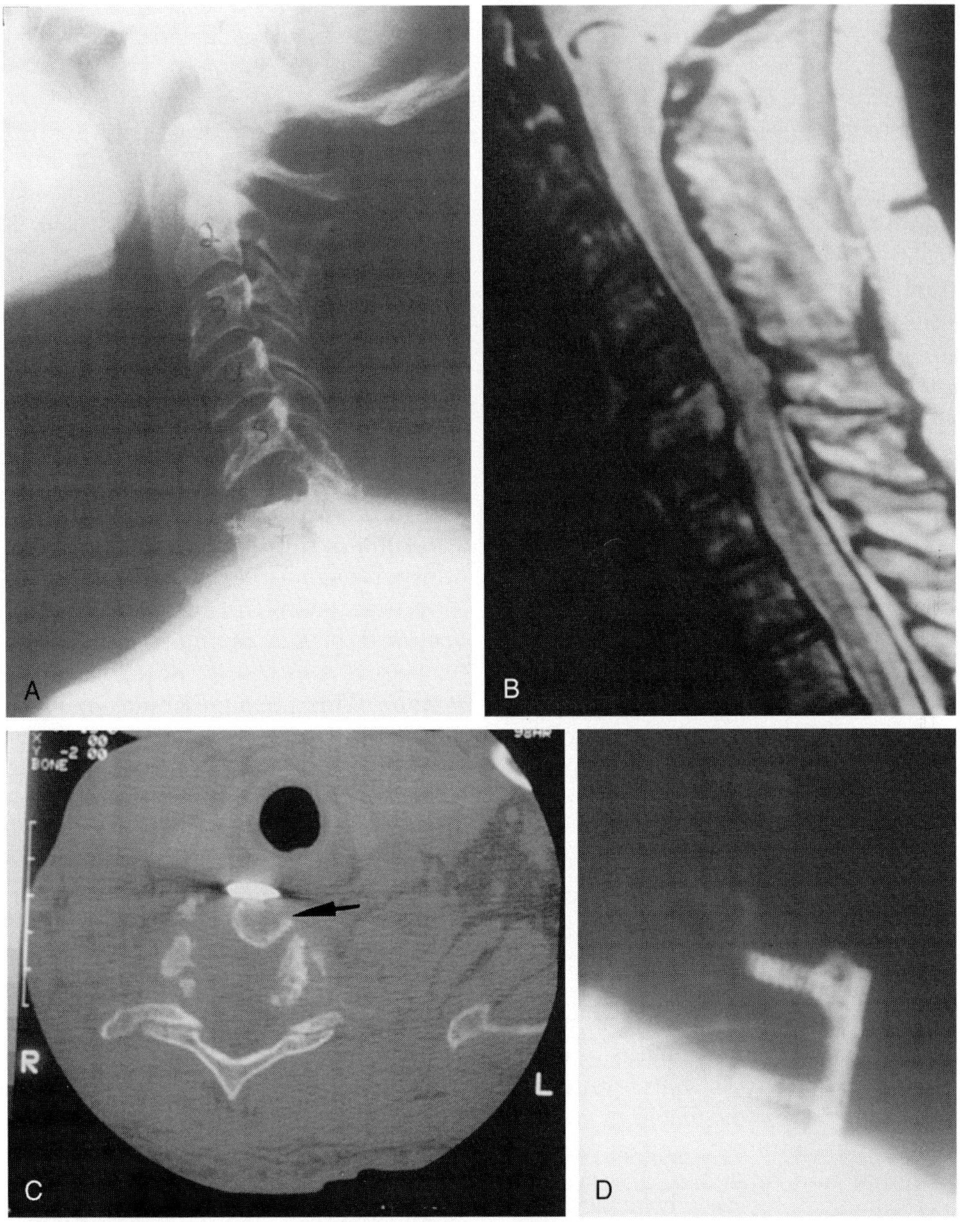

FIGURE 15-18 • Cervical metastatic tumor (C6). The lateral cervical spine x-ray *(A)* demonstrates destruction of the C6 vertebral body without significant collapse across this interval of the spine. A sagittal MRI image *(B)* outlines the vertebral body of C6 with signal change within the marrow of this vertebra. There is minimal retropulsion of bone into the canal and no significant spinal cord compression. The patient underwent radical cervical vertebrectomy and reconstruction and plating *(C, D)*. A small amount of bone around the periphery of the vertebral body remains after anterior vertebral resection *(C)*. Following the debulking of tumor, the vertebral body was reconstructed with iliac crest bone graft (arrow) and the fusion mass was stabilized with an anterior cervical plate *(C, D)*.

trolled. The abdominal and thoracic cavities can be the site(s) of significant blood loss, sufficient to destabilize a patient hemodynamically. Extensive orthopedic injury, including femoral and/or pelvic fractures, can also be a source of significant bleeding resulting in hypotension. When assessing a patient for systemic hypotension following trauma, the above-mentioned causes must always be sought. Clinical examination and imaging studies usually determine the site of significant blood loss. The differential diagnosis of nonhypovolemic hypotension includes cardiac tamponade, neurogenic shock, and agonal brain injury. Clinical and imaging criteria have been established for the diagnosis of cardiac tamponade.[86, 87] Patients with brain injury severe enough to impair cardiovascular regulation will have associated impairment of brain stem reflexes.

Neurogenic shock is a condition in which a patient has loss of blood pressure regulation following a complete spinal cord injury. The pathogenesis of the condition is the loss of sympathetic outflow to the systemic vasculature and the heart. It can occur in patients with complete spinal cord injuries above the T5 level. The clinical characteristic of neurogenic shock is hypotension with associated bradycardia. Neurogenic shock is distinct from spinal shock, although both are phenomena that can result following complete spinal cord injuries. Spinal shock is a neurologic phenomenon. It describes the loss of all neurologic function in the acute phase following a spinal cord injury.[88] Patients have no volitional movements, no sensation, and absent reflexes below the level of the spinal cord injury. Four to six weeks following the injury, the flaccid, hyporeflexic state is replaced by spastic hyper-reflexia and bilateral Babinski responses.

Following an initial general assessment of the patient, a detailed neurologic examination is required.[3] Again, the neurologic examination determines the functional status of the spinal cord and the approximate level and extent of the neurologic injury.[85] The components of the neurologic examination include mental status, motor, sensory, and reflex examinations. Emphasis is placed on motor, sensory, and reflex assessments for patients with acute neurologic events implicating the spinal cord. Assessments of mental status and cranial nerves can be made prior to the detailed peripheral neurologic assessment. In acute trauma, ascertaining cortical and brain stem function is necessary to interpret the results of the peripheral limb assessment. In nontraumatic myelopathy or neuropathy, abnormalities of mental status or cranial nerve function may indicate a systemic neurologic disorder, rather than one confined to the spinal cord and/or peripheral nerves. The spinal cord functional assessment is made by motor, sensory, and deep tendon reflex examinations. The various acute and chronic spinal cord syndromes can affect different segments of the spinal cord or certain fiber tracts and components of the cross-sectional diameter of the cord. Therefore, a full assessment is required to clearly define the extent and pattern of neurologic injury in each case. Sensory function is subserved by the spinal-thalamic tracts, which lie in the anterolateral aspect of the spinal cord, and the posterior columns, which are paramedian and posterior. The motor examination determines the integrity of the cortical-spinal tracts in the lateral aspect of the spinal cord and the gray matter at segmental levels. The reflex examination contributes to the determination of long tract functional status and at a segmental level can assist in determining the integrity of the efferent and afferent components of local reflexes. However, as outlined above, the presence of spinal shock can confound the information provided by reflex assessment in a patient with an acute spinal injury.

There are two components of the sensory examination. Spinal-thalamic tract testing is carried out by the application of noxious stimulus and, in a controlled setting, temperature sensation. Vibration and position sense testing is used to determine the integrity of the dorsal columns. The preliminary sensory assessment involves the application of noxious stimulus in the form of a pin or sharp object. A meticulous, dermatome-by-dermatome assessment from C4 to S4–S5 should be carried out bilaterally. To incorporate the lower cervical and upper thoracic dermatomes (C5–T2) and the lower lumbar dermatomes (L3–S1), the pinprick assessment must involve the proximal and distal aspects of both upper and lower limbs, respectively. The aforementioned dermatomes are exclusive to the limbs and are not represented on the anterior aspect of the torso. The cervical plexus provides innervation to the upper aspect of the thorax down to the supramammary region. This plexus includes elements from the C3, C4, and C5 nerve roots. Immediately subadjacent to this region, the T3–T4 dermatomes begin the thoracic component to anterior thoracic and abdominal sensory innervation. The inguinal region is supplied by L1, while L2 through S1 involve the lower limbs alone. Posteriorly, the perianal area represents the only cutaneous region supplied by the mid and lower sacral nerve roots. It is crucial to test for the integrity of these dermatomes in patients with a spinal cord injury. Preservation of sacral sensation alone can be the sole indication that the patient does not have a complete spinal cord injury.[13] This finding has significant prognostic implications. The potential for recovery of function is much greater for a patient with a partial spinal cord injury, as opposed to one who is complete.[3, 11–13]

Posterior column function is tested by the assessment of position and appreciation of vibration sense. Although a dermatome-by-dermatome assessment can be made, this is usually unnecessary, since the purpose of this assessment is to determine the integrity of the posterior column white matter tracts in the spinal cord. The peripheral components of proprioceptive function accompany the other sensory elements in the peripheral nerves. Hence, the peripheral integrity can be implied if pinprick sensation is intact. Therefore, the application of the tuning fork or proprioceptive sensation need only be assessed in the hands and feet of the patient.

The assessment of motor function requires detailed testing of individual muscle groups in the upper and lower limbs. As for the spinal-thalamic tract examination, cursory observation of spontaneous motor limb function can confound the interpretation of results in certain clinical settings. Patients with lower cervical spinal cord injury or a central cord syndrome can retain part or all of their proximal arm function and have severe deficits that preclude useful hand intrinsic function. In the latter example, in addition to retaining proximal limb function, patients with central cord syndrome also have good lower limb function. In such cases, the lack of a detailed motor examination may prevent the diagnosis of a partial spinal cord injury and prevent requisite acute management. A detailed lower limb examination can assist in determining the extent of a cauda equina deficit in a lumbar injury and can identify the presence of isolated radiculopathy in nontraumatic lumbar spine abnormalities. The extent and distribution of motor weakness of the lower limbs in the presence of a partial spinal cord injury are variable. Symmetric deficits of uniform severity are common in the acute setting of patients who have cervical and/or upper thoracic abnormalities. Patchy sensory and motor deficits or proximal lower limb weakness alone can be the early indicator of significant thoracic spinal cord compression.

Reflex assessment includes deep tendon and superficial reflexes. The interpretation of the reflex examination is dependent upon the acuity of the clinical setting and the severity of the spinal cord injury. In the presence of subacute or chronic cord compression, abnormal reflexes are hyperdynamic. With acute, complete spinal cord injury, deep tendon reflexes are absent as a result of spinal shock. A Babinski response (extensor plantar response) likewise is absent with acute, complete injury and may also be negative or absent in the acute phase. The Babinski response remains a sensitive indicator of an upper motor neuron lesion secondary to myelopathy or intracranial pathology.

Superficial reflexes are usually absent in the presence of a spinal cord injury. They can be of localizing value with respect to the level of the spinal injury. Upper abdominal reflexes are mediated through T6 and T9 spinal levels. Lower abdominal reflexes are subtended by T10 to T12. The presence of upper and absence of lower abdominal reflexes indicates a spinal cord injury below T9. Cremasteric reflexes are supplied by L1–L2.

The bulbocavernous reflex is tested by applying noxious stimulus to the head of the penis or manipulating the Foley catheter while feeling for contraction of the anal sphincter. Although the absence of this reflex is considered consistent with a spinal cord injury, this reflex should not be relied upon to distinguish between complete and incomplete spinal cord injuries if this is the only affirmative function present below the level of injury. It is not a highly sensitive clinical sign of retained spinal cord function.[3] Absence of rectal tone is also indicative of a complete spinal cord injury.

Based on the results of the clinical evaluation, the functional status of the spinal cord can be determined. This can be classified with respect to the extent of the spinal cord injury or the level of injury. The most basic classification of spinal cord injury is based on the severity of the injury, being complete or incomplete. The significance of this subclassification is primarily prognostic. A large percentage of patients with incomplete injury have recovery potential. Patients with retained sacral sensation only have a potential to recover spinal cord function.[13, 44] By contrast, less than 1% of patients with a complete injury recover. Partial injuries can be classified with respect to the pattern of deficit identified. The typical, partial transverse injury causes patchy or diffuse partial weakness or sensory loss below the level of the lesion.[3] Depending on the etiology of the partial myelopathy, different patterns are seen.[3, 89]

The central cord syndrome typically involves a lower cervical spine injury. Anteroposterior compressive force placed upon the cervical spine has its greatest effect upon the central portion of the spinal cord, injuring the gray matter and the deep aspects of the white matter tracts. Owing to the somatotopical organization of the white matter tracts adjacent to the gray matter, preferential involvement of fibers supplying the distal aspect of the upper extremities results. These patients have distal arm and hand intrinsic weakness, with preservation of lower limb and proximal upper limb function. Typically, this injury is seen in an older patient with significant cervical spondylosis who has sustained a hyperextension neck injury. It is less commonly seen with hyperflexion injuries in younger patients.

Pathology causing dysfunction of a lateral half of the spinal cord results in the Brown-Séquard syndrome. These patients have ipsilateral motor and posterior column deficits and contralateral pain and sensory deficits below the level of the lesion. This distribution of deficit results from the crossover of pain fibers entering the spinal cord to ascend in the contralateral spinal thalamic tract. Corticospinal and posterior column tracts remain ipsilateral in the cord and cross intracranially. Penetrating spinal cord injury or lateralized neoplasms encroaching upon the spinal canal are typical causes of this distribution of deficit.

The anterior cord syndrome is though to result from a vascular injury involving the anterior spinal artery, which supplies the anterior component of the spinal cord. These patients have severe motor deficits and loss of spinal thalamic function. There is sparing of posterior column function. This form of deficit is seen in acute trauma, peripheral vascular disease, and rarely during episodes of systemic hypotension.

The posterior cord syndrome is very rare and involves loss of posterior column function and sparing of anterior cord functions, in contradistinction to the anterior cord syndrome. Rare posteriorly placed intraspinal tumors and spinal stenosis can manifest with such deficits.

Functional classifications of spinal cord injury have also been established. The usefulness of these systems is primarily to convey the severity of an injury in a uniform manner and also for analysis of treatment protocols and prognoses. One of the first widely used classification systems was established by Frankel et al.[90] It involved five categories—A through E—depending on the severity of motor and sensory deficits. Frankel A injury represented complete motor and sensory deficits. Frankel E patients were intact neurologically. Mid-grade Frankel functional levels were thought to be too broad, thereby limiting the ability to discern functional and motor improvements in some patients.[91, 92] Based on these shortcomings, the American Spinal Injury Association (ASIA) classification and impairment scale has been established.[93, 94] The ASIA classification system involves detailed motor and sensory assessments of multiple muscle groups and dermatomes (Fig. 15–19). The ASIA impairment scale is a modification of the original Frankel grading system[90] (Table 15–2).

Following the clinical examination of the patient, which is focused on determining the functional status of the neural elements, imaging investigations are undertaken. These investigations are used to attempt to identify the etiology of the neurologic deficit if present and assess for injuries or abnormalities of the vertebral component of the spinal column. The primary consideration for both traumatic and nontraumatic causes of neurologic injury is the determination of the presence or absence of ongoing spinal cord compression. In the absence of spinal cord compression, evaluation for an intrinsic parenchymal abnormality is made. Imaging investigations are used to determine the integrity of the osteoligamentous complex and determine its stability. This is most important in the setting of acute trauma, but also is valid for infiltrative processes involving the vertebrae.

MANAGEMENT OF ACUTE SPINAL INJURY

The management principles involved in the care of the patient with an acute spinal injury are predicated on the principles outlined in the above sections. The patient must first be stable from a cardiorespiratory perspective, and other internal and peripheral injuries must be identified.[3, 83] During the initial assessment of the patient, if trauma is involved, one assumes the presence of a potentially unstable spinal injury.[95] Investigation for a spinal injury and spinal cord injury is then made, remembering that the physical examination is oriented toward the determination of spinal cord function and imaging studies determine the level, extent, and stability of the osteoligamentous injury. The goal of treatment is to prevent spinal cord injury or progression of an existing injury,[83, 92, 96] stabilize the spinal column,[12, 81, 82, 92, 97–104] and expeditiously reactivate[65, 81] and rehabilitate the patient. The pathophysiology and assessment of spinal cord injury and the criteria for determining spinal stability have been previously detailed. This section outlines the imaging investigations and treatment of the spinal-injured patient.

Imaging Techniques

The evolution of imaging techniques represents one of the most profound innovations in the management of patients with spinal injuries. Newer imaging techniques permit a detailed evaluation of the anatomy of a spinal injury and its impact on the neural elements. However, conventional radiographic studies continue to have a role in patient management.

Plain x-rays remain useful in the care of patients with an acute spinal injury. They are readily accessible in the emergency room and enable an initial survey of the entire spine. The criteria for establishing stability of the spine, especially in the cervical spine, are derived from the standard radiographs.[3] Therefore, they remain an integral part of the imaging investigation of the traumatized patient. Also, the initial plain spine views can be used as a reference for intraoperative imaging, which utilizes the same modality to identify levels and assess the

TABLE 15–2 **ASIA IMPAIRMENT SCALE**

A	**Complete:** No motor or sensory function is preserved in the sacral segments S4–S5.
B	**Incomplete:** Sensory but not motor function is preserved below the neurologic level and includes the sacral segments S4–S5.
C	**Incomplete:** Motor function is preserved below the neurologic level, and more than half of key muscles below the neurologic level have a muscle grade less than 3.
D	**Incomplete:** Motor function is preserved below the neurologic level, and at least half of key muscles below the neurologic level have a muscle grade of 3 or more.
E	**Normal:** Motor and sensory function is normal.

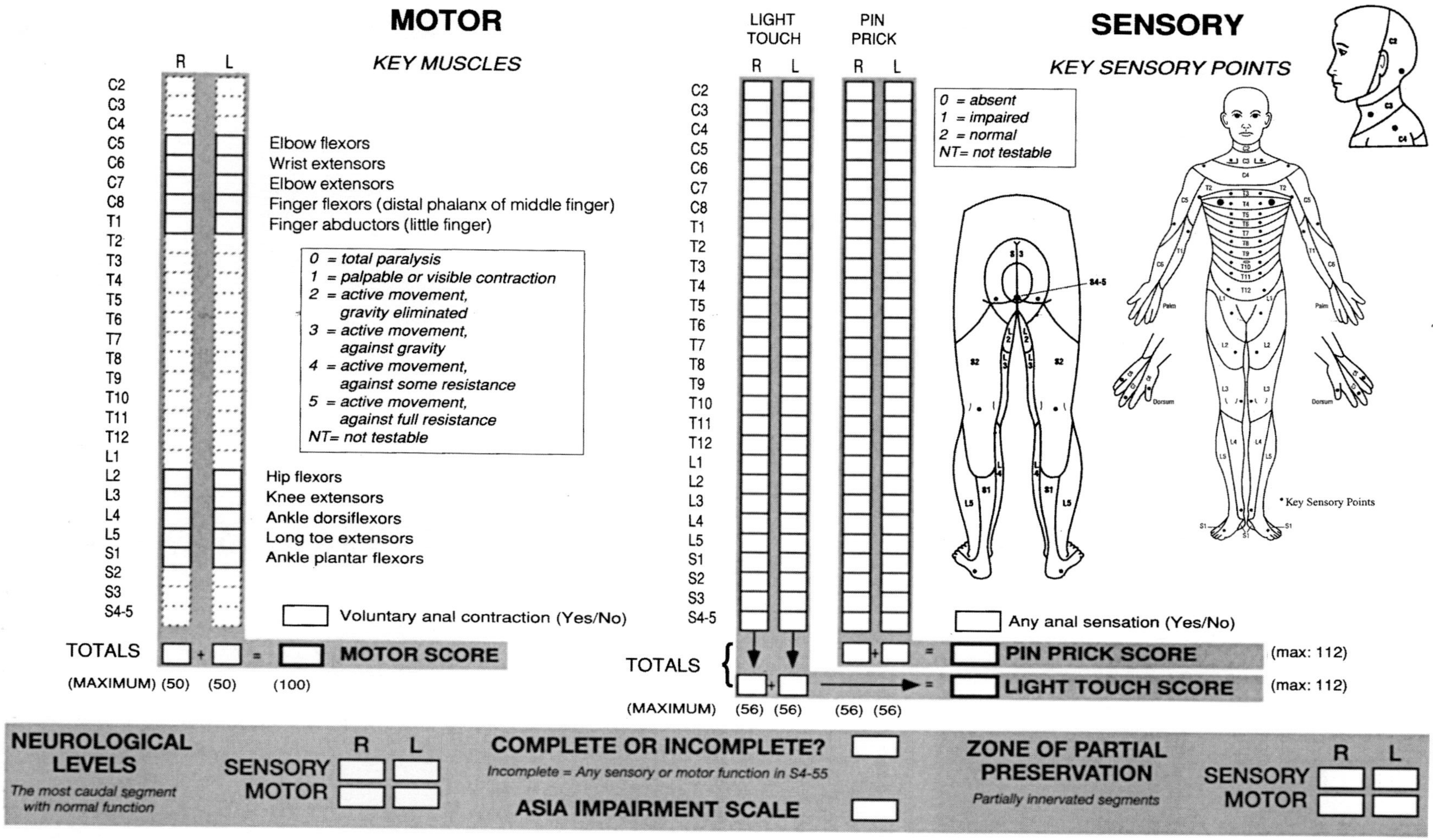

FIGURE 15-19 • ASIA motor and sensory scales. (Copyright, American Spinal Injury Association, from "International Standards for Neurological and Functional Classification of Spinal Cord Injury," revised 1996.)

degree of correction of a spinal deformity by plain film comparisons.

Computer-assisted imaging greatly enhances the detail with which bony, soft tissue, and neuroparenchymal injury can be identified. Comparisons regarding sensitivity and specificity for diagnosis of spinal disorders have been made between CT scanning and MRI scanning.[105, 106] Neither modality is universally superior for spinal imaging. The two techniques usually contribute complementary information for the diagnosis and management of patients with spinal disorders.[107] The CT scan provides superior detail of bone anatomy and pathology[64] (see Figs. 15–1, 15–5, and 15–9*B*) compared with MRI scanning.[107] High-resolution, thin-slice images with reformatting in the sagittal and coronal plains enable regional assessment of vertebral alignment (see Figs. 15–2 and 15–9). They can serve as an adjunct to plain films of the cervicothoracic junction, since this segment of the spine can be difficult to visualize with plain radiographs (see Fig. 15–2). The CT scan can be performed in an emergency setting, where images can be quickly acquired and there are no feromagnetic contraindications to proceeding with a CT scan. Neither CT scan nor MRI scan can provide dynamic imaging of the spine.

MRI provides multiplanar imaging of all the osteoligamentous[108] and neural components of the spinal column.[63, 107] Although fine detail of bony architecture and subtle fracturing are better seen on CT scan, MRI scan can detect very early signal abnormalities within the cancellous component of the vertebrae (see Figs. 15–12*A* and 15–14*A*). Bone reaction and infiltration are seen first by MRI scan, before changes are apparent on plain views or CT scans. The neural elements are seen directly by MRI (see Figs. 15–10*A*, 15–11*A*, and 15–18*B*), and in some cases, signal changes within the parenchyma of the spinal cord are identified.[109] Currently, there are no specific criteria established that firmly correlate signal abnormality within the spinal cord to the severity, extent, or prognosis of spinal cord injury[109]; clinical examination remains the most sensitive indicator of spinal cord function and injury.[85] Sagittal images usually demonstrate the relationship between the neural and osteoligamentous elements of the spinal column (see Figs. 15–10*A*, 15–11*A*, 15–12*A*, and 15–18*B*). The location and extent of the spinal canal encroachment and cord compression can be defined by this view (see Figs. 15–4, 15–11, 15–14, and 15–18). However, sagittal imaging interpretation can be hampered by coronal-oriented spinal deformities (i.e., scoliosis). MRI scans are relatively lengthy procedures, and exclusion of metal objects from the scanning room is required.[88]

Prior to computer-assisted imaging, myelography was required to image the spinal canal and its contents. Nonsoluble contrast agents were initially used but have since been discontinued because of the risk of arachnoiditis.[110, 111] Non-ionic, iodine-based contrast is now used, which augments the safety of the technique. The intracranial flow of contrast media can predispose to seizures in a susceptible population.[112, 113] In an acute setting with the possibility of an instability, lumbar injection of contrast media is impractical.[3] Positioning the patient to inject dye into the lumbar thecal sac and to pass dye superiorly is difficult in a patient with an unstable cervical injury. High cervical puncture enables introduction of contrast without manipulation of the patient and has been used in the setting of acute trauma to visualize the spinal canal.[3, 114, 115] MRI and high-resolution CT scanning enable satisfactory canal and spinal cord visualization without the inherent risks of myelography. These techniques have supplanted myelography in many clinical circumstances.[88] Myelography is used when MRI is contraindicated, or when the MRI scan resolution is limited.

Treatment

The treatment principles for acute spinal disorders are similar regardless of the underlying etiology. The primary goal of therapy is to optimize neurologic outcome by preserving or, when possible, improving neurologic function.[60] Stabilization of the osteoligamentous complex of the spine must then be achieved. Throughout treatment, monitoring for and treating potential complications resulting from the underlying condition must be continued.

Nonsurgical Treatment

There are few nonoperative treatments available for the management of acute spinal cord injury. Current guidelines regarding agents and appropriate doses have been derived from experimental and clinical trials.

Corticosteroid treatment, which has been extensively tested in animal models, is thought to reduce secondary spinal cord injury. The possible mechanisms include membrane stabilization, antioxidant effect, and action as a free-radical scavenger.[5, 6] Corticosteroids are most effective when given before, at, or shortly after the onset of the primary injury. Also, outcome in experimental animal models was improved only when very high doses of steroids were administered. The doses were much greater than those required to saturate steroid receptors on the cell membranes.[5, 6]

Based upon experimental data, multicenter clinical trials were initiated. The first study was

NASCIS I, the results of which were first published in 1984.[116, 117] This study was a prospective, randomized, double-blind trial with two treatment arms. Patients were treated for 10 days with high-dose (1000-mg bolus and 1000 mg/day) or lower dose (100-mg bolus and 100 mg/day) of methylprednisolone for 10 days. No statistically significant difference in outcome was found after 1 year of follow-up. There was also some concern about an increased complication rate associated with a 10-day course of steroids. Based upon the results of the NASCIS I trial and experimental data regarding the amount of steroids and duration of therapy for spinal cord injury, the criteria for a second trial—NASCIS II—were established.[6, 118] This was another multicenter, randomized, prospective study. The patients were randomized into three groups: placebo, methylprednisolone (30 mg/kg bolus followed by 5.4 mg/kg/hour for 23 hours), and naloxone (5.4 mg/kg bolus followed by a 23-hour infusion of 4 mg/kg/hour). At 6 months of follow-up, a statistically significant difference in the neurologic recovery (motor, pain, and light touch) was seen in the group that received the high-dose methylprednisolone. The improved outcome was experienced only in those patients who received the high-dose steroid within the first 8 hours following the injury.[6, 118] Naloxone, despite its beneficial effect in animal studies, demonstrated no benefit over placebo in the NASCIS II trial. Despite the high dose of steroid administered, the complication rate was not significantly different than that of the placebo group. Although a statistically significant difference in neurologic examination was appreciated, the changes were relatively small and did not equate to dramatic functional improvements for the patients.

Results of the third clinical steroid trial (NASCIS III) have recently been published.[118a] There were three treatment arms in this study: methylprednisolone at conventional doses (30 mg/kg bolus, 5.4 mg/kg/hour × 23 hours), methylprednisolone (30 mg/kg bolus, followed by 5.4 mg/kg for 47 hours), and tirilazad mesylate (2.5 mg/kg every 6 hours for 48 hours).[5] Tirilazad is a synthetic 21-amino steroid with potent antioxidant effect and no significant glucocorticoid receptor activity.[5] The results showed that the administration of methylprednisolone for 48 hours improved the outcome compared to patients receiving methylprednisolone for 24 hours for patients who received treatment from 3 to 8 hours following their injury. No difference in outcome was observed between the two treatment groups if steroids were administered in the first 3 hours following the injury. Tirilazad demonstrated no therapeutic advantage over methylprednisolone.[118a]

The other medication that may have some influence on outcome of spinal cord–injured patients is the ganglioside GM-1.[5, 119] A prospective study of patients randomized to placebo or treatment groups receiving GM-1 100 mg taken daily for 18–32 doses, was undertaken.[119] The first drug administration was within 72 hours of injury. Patients receiving the drug had significant Frankel and ASIA score improvements at 1-year follow up.[119] The motor improvement was based upon regaining useful motor strength in previously paralyzed muscles, as opposed to increasing strength in the previously paretic muscles. The precise mechanism of action of the gangliosides is uncertain. Unlike corticosteroids, which act as a neuroprotector against secondary injury, the gangliosides are thought to function by augmenting neuronal regeneration.[5, 119] They may possibly enhance neurite sprouting from injured axons.

In summary, progress has been made in developing medical treatment protocols for acute spinal cord injury. The beneficial effects, however, remain quite limited. Based upon the differential mechanisms of action of steroids and gangliosides, future treatment protocols may incorporate both medications given sequentially. A patient with a spinal cord injury, complete or incomplete, presenting within hours of the acute event should receive methylprednisolone 30 mg/kg bolus over the first hour, followed by a continuous infusion of 5.4 mg/kg/hour for 23 hours.

Based on the results of administering the steroid prior to or at the time of experimental spinal cord injury in animals, there appears to be a rationale for administering high-dose methylprednisolone, in doses outlined above, intraoperatively at the time of spinal surgery during procedures upon the cervical and thoracic spines, when there is a risk of spinal cord injury.[5] There are, however, no clinical data to support steroid use for this purpose. Also, in the setting of nontraumatic myelopathy, the effects of steroids on outcome is even less clear. However, the use of high-dose steroid to reduce tumor edema and cord compression is justified.[120]

Surgical Treatment

Regardless of the underlying pathology, the principles of spinal surgery include neural decompression, spinal reduction, and stabilization.[12] The advancement of our understanding of normal and abnormal spinal biomechanics, innovative approaches to decompression and fusion, and the availability of new, more versatile instrumentation systems have enabled surgeons to more successfully address various forms of spinal pathology. Current indications and techniques continue to evolve.

Neural decompression remains the first priority when addressing a surgical lesion involving the spine. Advances in spinal imaging, outlined in previous sections, have enabled the surgeon to identify the location of compressing elements. Based upon this evaluation, the optimal approach for decompression can be determined. Earlier techniques for spinal surgery usually involved posterior approaches by laminectomy. This technique enabled adequate neural decompression for some pathological entities (see Figs. 15–4, 15–11, and 15–13) but was suboptimal and sometimes risky for other conditions.[120–122] Compressive pathology, especially in the acute setting, often involves the anterior aspect of the canal[63, 84]—the vertebral body, discs, and epidural space. Access to the anterior aspect of the osteoligamentous complex must be gained to effect adequate decompression. This must be achieved without undue manipulation of the neural elements to avoid iatrogenic spinal cord or nerve root injury. The advent of direct anterior[84, 123, 124] and lateral[91, 125, 126] approaches to the vertebral column has enhanced the surgeon's ability to safely remove compressing pathology from the anterior aspect of the spine. The approach chosen in a given case is dependent upon the nature of the pathology,[120] its location within the vertebral elements, and the segment of the spine involved. For benign pathology, complete resection of the pathological tissue is unnecessary. Usually removal of the compressive component of the abnormality—a disc herniation or vertebral fracture fragment—is all that is required to relieve the reversible compressive component of the symptomatology. Adequate, safe decompression under some circumstances can be achieved by a less direct approach. Disc herniations and acute fractures can be decompressed in some circumstances by a posterolateral approach in the thoracolumbar spine (see Figs. 15–9 and 15–15). Such an approach is not feasible in the cervical spine.[120]

For other forms of pathology, such as spinal neoplasms (see Figs. 15–12 and 15–14) and infection (see Fig. 15–17), more radical excision of the abnormal tissue is required to effect decompression and to prevent local recurrence.[120, 127] Such pathology frequently requires a direct anterior approach for adequate resection, regardless of the level of the spine involved.

Reduction of a spinal deformity and re-establishment of the normal spinal alignment and curvatures are the next priority in the surgical management of an acute spinal disorder. Reduction, under some circumstances, is the means by which neural decompression is achieved. Reduction is also required to establish normal spinal biomechanics, abnormalities of which can induce pain syndromes or possibly evolve into neurologic deficit if the deformity progresses.[24, 91, 128, 129] In order to realign the spine, the deformed segment must be mobile. In the circumstance of acute trauma, destabilization induced by the injury renders a segment mobile and often readily reducible. Chronic deforming processes are often fixed. Prior to reduction, the deformed segments must be mobilized by bone resection and soft tissue release. Mobilization is sometimes achieved by spinal element removal during the decompression component of the procedure. Once mobile, force is applied to the spine by external or internal devices to effect realignment. In the cervical spine, externally applied traction is often effective to reduce a mobile spinal deformity (see Fig. 15–8). This is applied by attaching a halo ring or traction tongs to the skull and applying weight in an axial orientation. Acute, translational deformities of the spine can be corrected or improved with traction. Patients with bilateral or unilateral locked facets can often be effectively reduced with traction.[59, 60, 130]

Use of traction has been a mainstay of acute treatment for cervical translational deformity.[131] Controversy does exist regarding the amount of traction that can be safely applied, as well as the need to image the spinal canal prior to applying traction. In adults, the traditional guideline has been to begin with a weight of 10 pounds, and then increase the weight by increments of 5 pounds, up to a maximum of 5 pounds per vertebral level below C2 (maximum weight at C5–C6 would equal 10 + 5 pounds × 4 vertebrae = 30 pounds).[130] There is a broad spectrum of opinion regarding the maximum amount of weight that can be applied. Some authors would not go beyond 50–60 pounds,[3, 60, 61, 132, 133] whereas others have applied in excess of 100 pounds.[59, 60] The concern of high-weight traction is the induction of overdistraction, which could theoretically cause a traction-type injury upon the spinal cord.[134, 135] Overdistraction is defined as an increase in the height of the disc space at the injured level, relative to the disc space height at the adjacent motion segment levels (see Fig. 15–8). However, no definite correlation between neurologic deterioration and this radiographic finding has been proven. Regardless of the weight applied, the most important aspect of applying cervical traction is to closely monitor the patient clinically and obtain frequent follow-up radiographs. If the patient begins to deteriorate clinically during traction, the weight should be reduced and immediate cervical spine x-rays should be taken. If no overdistraction is identified, or if the patient undergoes reduction, the patient should have a canal study to assess the unlikely possibility of a disc herniation or hematoma as the underlying explanation for the neurologic deterioration during traction. If a patient cannot undergo reduction in traction, operative reduction should be considered[60] (see Fig. 15–2).

Most patients with cervical subluxations have sustained an injury that renders the spine unstable. Therefore, these patients will require stabilization procedures on an elective basis. Since open reduction can be accomplished relatively expeditiously and safely by either an anterior or posterior surgical approach, some proponents of moderate-weight traction would advocate proceeding with surgery for open reduction before considering high-weight traction and its theoretical risks of overdistraction, since the patient is committed to a surgical procedure at some time in the future for stabilization.

The benefits of cervical traction in the patient with a kyphotic deformity involving retropulsed bone fragments into the canal are less clear. Cervical traction under such circumstances marginally increases the anteroposterior cervical canal diameter but does not remove the retropulsed fragment from the anterior aspect of the canal.

Besides reduction, cervical traction is a very effective technique for stabilizing an injured cervical spinal segment, thereby preventing further translation, which could cause additional spinal injury. In the presence of a known, unstable spinal injury, or if the stability of the cervical spine is uncertain, a patient can be placed in traction during investigation and early management, so as to protect the spinal cord. During anesthesia, or with an uncooperative patient, applying traction to the neck can protect against spinal cord injury.

Application of cervical traction can be deleterious to a patient with an atlantoaxial injury. Injuries of the atlantoaxial complex that are unstable, including some Jefferson's fractures, type II and type III odontoid fractures, complex comminuted atlantoaxial fractures, and hangman's fractures, can all be overdistracted with injudicious use of inline traction. Many of these deformities involving the atlantoaxial complex are reducible by the application of translational force. To stabilize the reduced injury in such cases, the patient can be placed in a halo ring and vest.

The application of external distractive force upon the thoracolumbar spine is much more difficult to achieve and less efficient than cervical traction. The forces required for reduction are much greater than in the cervical spine, and the skeletal fixation points are more difficult and involved to obtain. Halo pelvic and halo femoral fixation and traction can be used as a means of external reduction for some thoracolumbar deformities.[136, 137] Many internal thoracolumbar spinal instrumentation systems are capable of applying force to effect reduction. These devices are usually required to realign the thoracolumbar spine.

The final principle of spinal surgery is to achieve stability of the involved spinal segment. Stabilization of the spine must be considered temporally in two phases. Ultimate spinal stabilization results from bone healing or incorporation of bone graft. This represents the ultimate, long-term means by which a previously destabilized segment becomes stable. Most authors agree that healing of ligamentous injury generally does not re-establish stability of an injured motion segment.[60] Bone healing and fusion are processes that can take 1–3 months, depending upon the nature of the abnormality and the segment of the spine involved. Therefore, immediate or short-term stabilization must be achieved. Postural immobilization, external fixators, and internal fixation devices represent the techniques for immediate stabilization. Despite the proliferation of spinal instrumentation for fixation, some authors continue to reduce and immobilize injured spinal segments by postural reduction and bed rest.[46, 99, 102, 138, 139] Satisfactory neurologic outcome and stability can be achieved in selected patients.[102, 139] This method is generally applicable for patients who are neurologically intact.[92, 102] The patients are immobilized in a brace for 6–8 weeks following the injury.[102, 139] Complication rates from prolonged bed rest are apparently comparable to complications following surgery for thoracolumbar instability in selected patients.[102, 139] Significant progress, however, has been made in the development of spinal instrumentation systems. The versatility and efficiency of these systems have enabled direct surgical approaches to complex spinal disorders, with limited morbidity and excellent outcomes.[92, 140]

All instrumentation systems share basic components. Each has a vertical member—a device that spans motion segments—to which individual vertebrae are attached to provide stabilization. The vertical member takes the form of a plate or rod. All systems have a fixation or anchoring device to attach the vertical member to the vertebrae. The fixation device is usually oriented at right angles to the vertical member, attaching it to the bones in the horizontal plane. Fixation components are wires, screws, or hooks. The fixation device can be linked to the vertical member directly, in a semirigid manner, by a wire passing around the rod or a screw through a hole in the plate. The attachments are considered semirigid because there can be some movement between the vertical member and the fixation device. Linkage devices are used in some systems to attach the anchoring device to the vertical member. These devices usually provide rigid coupling of the two components, thereby preventing movement of the fixator relative to the vertical member.

The purpose of instrumentation is to stabilize the spine and, in some cases with certain systems, correct spinal deformity. All systems are capable of fixating spinal segments. The strength by which this can be achieved is dependent upon the properties of the fixation device and bone quality. Devices intended for the cervical spine have less rigidity and strength than those for the thoracolumbar spine. For any given segment of the spine, in general, the strength of fixation is increased by the length of the construct and the number of points of attachment between the vertical member and the spine.

Reduction capability is provided in some systems by the ability of the vertical member to attach to points along the spine under tension. In this way, distractive, rotational, and sometimes translational force can be applied to the spine. Except for the use of pediatric thoracolumbar hook-and-rod instrumentation systems in the cervical spine, currently available cervical spine instrumentation systems are intended for fixation only.

Spinal instrumentation systems have been developed to augment the surgeon's ability to treat spinal disorders. There are many advantages to their use. Spinal instrumentation enables immediate fixation of an injured segment, which permits safe, early mobilization of the patient following trauma.[81, 82, 98, 104, 126, 141, 142] The resultant immobilization augments the rate of spinal fusion. Instrumentation also enables spinal deformity correction, which cannot be achieved effectively by fusion alone or postural reduction.[98]

There are some risks and drawbacks to the use of spinal instrumentation. Instrumentation adds time to the operation and increases operative risk. There are risks of neurologic, vascular, and visceral injury during implantation. Lengthy internal fixation constructs, required for reduction and rigid fixation, compromise the normal motion segments, thereby reducing postoperative spinal motion. Instrumentation causes artifacts on computer-assisted imaging, thereby obscuring anatomic detail (see Figs. 15–2*F* and 15–20). Despite the trend toward titanium-based instrumentation systems, imaging artifact still occurs, limiting postoperative diagnostic resolution.

Despite advances in spinal instrumentation technology and biomechanics, instrumentation systems can fail. There are a variety of reasons for these failures. Improper selection of a device for a specific pathology or location in the spine predisposes to failure. The device must be properly applied to the spine to optimize its fixation capabilities. If the patient has significant osteoporosis or involvement of bone by a pathological process, points of fixation will be inadequate and result in instrumentation pull-out. These causes of failure usually occur within weeks of the operation and represent early instrumentation failure. Long-term instrumentation failure occurs, almost exclusively, from failure to achieve a bony fusion. Despite the biomechanical properties of the devices, eventually, with repetitive

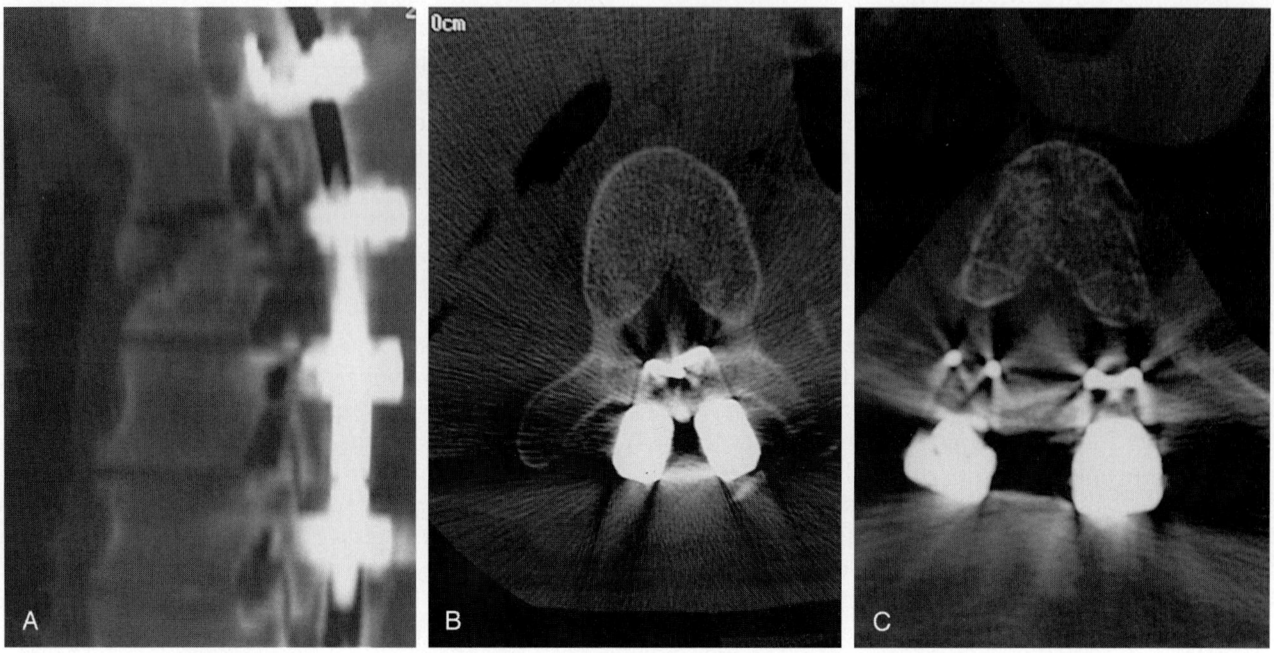

FIGURE 15–20 • Posterior reduction of a fracture-dislocation (T6). This 24-year-old male fell off a roof and sustained a complete spinal cord injury from a fracture-dislocation of T6. He underwent an open posterior reduction and fixation that realigned the midthoracic vertebrae *(A)*. The hook-and-rod device included sublaminar hooks *(B),* which are immediately superficial to the dura and spinal cord, and intrafacet *(C)* hooks, which are within the facet joints lateral to the spinal canal.

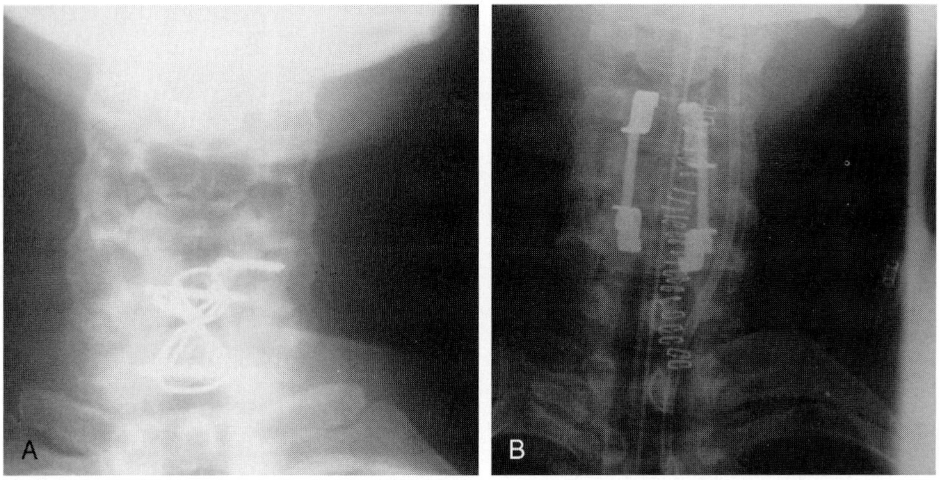

FIGURE 15–21 • Posterior cervical fixation. A posterior interspinous wire construct *(A)*. This technique re-establishes the posterior tension band between the adjacent vertebrae but has limited translational stability. Posterior clamps *(B)* help to re-establish the posterior tension band between the vertebrae but have improved translational stability compared with interspinous wiring.

loading, bone resorption at the points of fixation, or metal fatigue and breakage, will result. Instrumentation is intended to provide immediate stabilization of the spine only; long-term stabilization is provided by bone healing or bone fusion.[12]

Cervical spine instrumentation systems have continued to evolve. Initial spinous process and laminar wiring techniques have limited translational resistance (see Fig. 15–21*A*). They are best able to resist axial distractive force. Unfortunately, translational force and deformity represent the common configuration of cervical spine instability. The Halifax clamp,[143] applied to the laminar elements with a broad surface area in contact with the lamina, increased translational stability (see Fig. 15–21*B*). Facet wiring also augments translational stability by immobilizing and drawing into contact adjacent facet surfaces, thereby resisting translational movement. From these early techniques, biomechanical studies, and detailed anatomic studies of the cervical vertebrae, screw and plating systems have evolved and represent state-of-the-art fixation techniques for the cervical spine[144–149] (see Figs. 15–2*E;* 15–7*B;* 15–18*C, D*). Systems that attach to the anterior and posterior aspects of the cervical spine have been developed. Anterior plating systems are attached to the vertebral body. Available systems vary with respect to the depth of screw penetration into the vertebral body and the means by which the screws are linked to the plate. The original plating systems were semirigid, utilizing bicortical screw purchase.[144] This necessitated capture of the screw to the posterior cortex of the vertebrae, adjacent to the spinal cord. Many of the recently developed systems have rigid fixation of the screw to the plate and demand only unicortical and cancellous screw purchase within the bone[145] (see Figs. 15–2*F* and 15–7*B*).

Posterior plating systems are attached to the lateral masses of the cervical vertebrae using screws. Proper trajectory of the screws into the lateral mass is crucial to avoid complications. The vertebral artery and segmental cervical nerve roots are in close proximity to the lateral mass. There is some variation in opinion regarding the optimal trajectory of these screws within the lateral masses, although all authors agree that the screws should be oriented superiorly and laterally toward the upper anterior corner of the lateral mass from a posterior entry point in the anatomic center of the lateral mass[146–149] (see Fig. 15–2*F*).

The broad surface contact achieved between the plating systems and the vertebral body and the efficient fixation of the plate by these screws enhance translational stability of these anterior and posterior constructs. With experience and accurate determination of the anatomic landmarks, these devices can efficiently and safely be applied to the spine.

Thoracolumbar spinal instrumentation systems have been in use for 30–40 years. Both anterior and posterior devices are available. The Harrington rod was the first posterior thoracolumbar instrumentation system widely applied.[82] It was initially developed for the treatment of scoliosis but was found to be useful for trauma and other pathological conditions destabilizing the spine. Its properties enable it to be used for both fixation and deformity correction. It is a relatively simple device, with vertical rod members linked to the spine both superiorly and inferiorly by hooks (see Fig. 15–22*A*). A ratchet system enables lengthening of the construct to

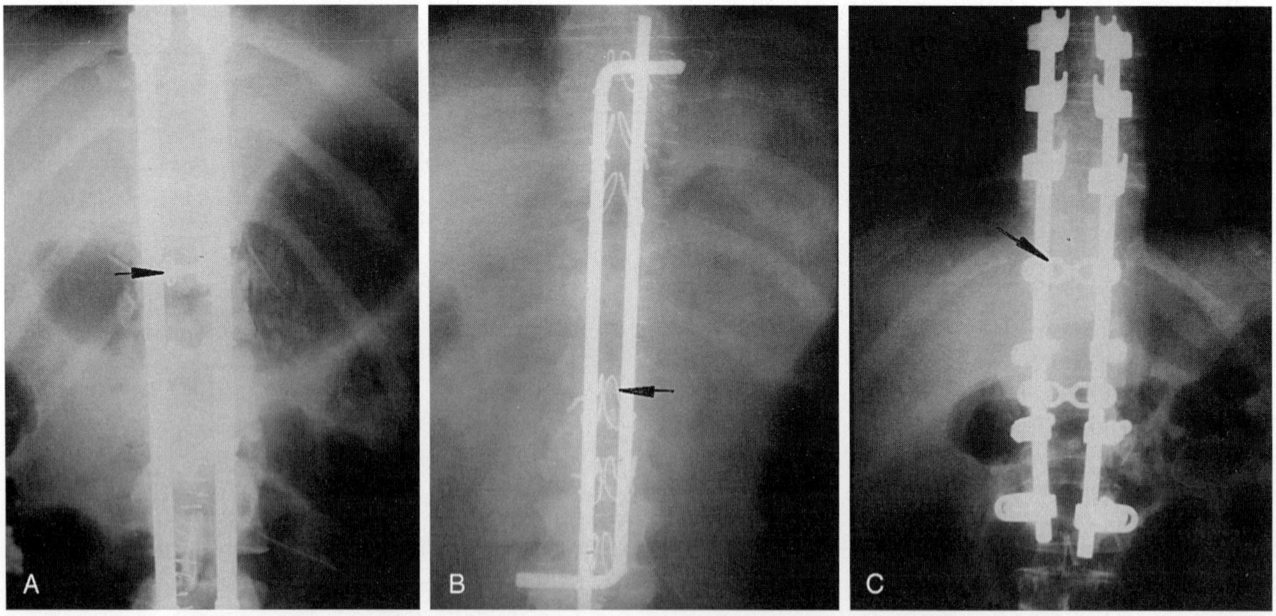

FIGURE 15–22 • Posterior thoracolumbar instrumentation. Harrington rods *(A)* are composed of parallel rods that are initially attached to the spine by superior and inferior hooks that can be placed within the facet joints, sublaminar space, or over the transverse process. To augment fixation, supplemental interspinous wiring (arrow) was placed along the mid shaft of the rod at four levels. Harrington rods have fixation and distraction capabilities. Luque *(B)* rods are primarily segmental fixators with limited translational reduction capability. They are attached to the spine at multiple levels by sublaminar wires (arrow). Universal instrumentation systems *(C)* developed from the earlier rod systems *(A, B)*. They involve parallel rods that can be attached to the spine with hooks and screws at multiple levels. These systems are quite versatile and enable multiplanar force application to the spine for deformity correction, and can rigidly fixate all segments of the thoracolumbar spine. The fixation construct shown is composed of two parallel rods attached to the spine superiorly by three interfacet hooks and inferiorly by three pedicle screws. Cross-link devices (arrow) are used to link the two rods, thereby increasing the rigidity of the fixation device.

apply corrective distracting force to the spine. The widespread use of the system enabled evaluation of its strengths and limitations,[82, 144, 150, 151] which became the basis for future system designs. One of the major shortcomings of the Harrington rod system was hook pull-out.[82, 152, 153] Supplementing the Harrington rods with sublaminar wires through intervening segments between the hooks enhanced fixation and reduced pull-out.[104, 129] The hooks could be placed within the facet joint, in the sublaminar epidural space, or over the transverse process.

The Luque rod system,[97] which utilized stainless steel L rods or a rectangular rod attached to the spine by wires,[104] was subsequently developed (see Fig. 15–22*B*). These wires could be secured to the spine through the base of the spinous process or sublaminar. The Luque system provides relatively rigid segmental fixation[97] with little translational reduction and no distraction[141] capability. The multiple points of fixation underlie the augmented stability of this device.[129]

Pedicle screw placement represents the most rigid means of spinal fixation.[144, 154] Screws are passed through the pedicles by a posterior approach into the vertebral bodies. This technique has been used throughout the thoracolumbar spine.[103] The early systems used semirigid attachment of the vertical member to the screws.[103] Modern systems have rigid coupling devices to attach the vertical member to the screw. Generally, this technique is reserved for the lumbosacral spine and the lower four thoracic vertebrae. It is ideal for fixation of the lower lumbosacral spine, since the lumbosacral lordosis can be preserved by acute contouring of the vertical member. Also, a major advantage of pedicle screws is that their fixation is independent of the presence of an intact lamina. Rigid fixation can be achieved after a patient has undergone a laminectomy for decompression.

Based upon the experience with the above-mentioned posterior thoracolumbar fixation devices, universal instrumentation systems have been developed.[44, 155, 156] These systems can combine pedicle screws and hooks in multiple configurations (see Figs. 15–9*C*, 15–14*B*, 15–20*A*, and 15–22*C*). This enables complex, multiplanar forces to be applied in the same or adjacent motion segments of the spine.[44] They can be applied to any segment of the thoracolumbar spine for any deforming or destabilizing condition.[156]

An anterior stabilization system is usually composed of a vertical member in the form of a rod or plate, although a cable system was initially introduced. The vertical member is attached to the vertebrae by screws. Early systems used a single rod, which had limited translational stability.[154] The introduction of parallel rod systems that are cross-linked by horizontal members increased translational stability.[124, 128, 154, 157] More recently, rigid plating systems have been devised (see Fig. 15–10*C–F*). Anterior plating systems have some capacity to correct the deformity, as distracting force can be applied to the screws prior to final tightening.

The properties of the anterior and posterior thoracolumbar instrumentation systems vary. Anterior systems are generally short segment fixators,[101] with a limited capacity to correct deformity by application of distractive force. The limited points of fixation and the short segment of the spine incorporated limit the strength of fixation of these systems.[100, 154] However, preservation of spinal motion by the short segment of fixation represents an advantage.[157] The posterior systems usually require incorporation of longer segments of the spine, thereby limiting the ultimate functional result. However, greater and more complex force application can be used to correct deformities with these systems. Anterior systems are difficult to apply to the upper thoracic spine[101] and lumbosacral junction due to anatomic constraints.

The choice of using the anterior versus posterior instrumentation system is dependent on the approach required for decompression and reconstruction of the spine, the location of the pathology, and the strength of fixation required to adequately stabilize the involved spinal segment. When possible, the surgeon attempts to decompress, reconstruct, and fixate the spine by using a single operative approach. Pathology involving anterior elements alone from the midthoracic to the midlumbar levels can usually be addressed by a single anterior approach for both decompression and stabilization. Extensive, three-column injury,[101] lengthy spinal deformity, or abnormalities affecting the stability of the upper thoracic or lower lumbar spines usually require posterior fixation.

SPINAL TRAUMA

Trauma is the principal cause of acute spinal injury. Most aspects of the pathophysiology, investigation, and treatment of spinal disorders of all etiologies are predicated upon the management of acute, traumatic injury. The general principles have been detailed in previous sections of this chapter. This section deals specifically with the contemporary management of acute spinal injury. As outlined in the chapter's introduction, spinal trauma affects a relatively young, male-dominated segment of the population.[2] The acute nature of the abnormality and the differences compared with the relatively older population for the other major categories of spinal disorders can influence decision making regarding therapy and have ramifications regarding morbidity and the final outcome.

The principles of assessing a traumatized patient are similar to those for other spinal disorders. However, certain aspects of the clinical assessment and imaging studies must be emphasized. The presence of other systemic injuries that can affect cardiorespiratory stability must be assessed.[3] The evaluation must be an ongoing process, since life-threatening conditions can develop following the initial survey (i.e., hypovolemia, pneumothorax, cardiac tamponade). Neurologic function must also be reassessed on an ongoing basis to identify changes caused by an intracranial expanding lesion (epidural, subdural) or progression of a spinal lesion. Until ruled out radiographically, the patient is assumed to have an unstable spinal injury.[3, 88]

Plain radiographs continue to be an important component of the imaging assessment for spinal trauma, since the criteria for stability and instability are still based upon lateral radiographs, especially in the cervical spine. Complete spinal visualization is required because there is a 5% coincidence of noncontiguous spinal fractures in trauma patients.[88, 158, 159] Active, dynamic x-ray images in the conscious, cooperative patient[160] (see Fig. 15–6), or passive radiographs under fluoroscopic control for unconscious patients, should be obtained once the patient's overall condition stabilizes to verify cervical spine stability. It is critical to image the cervicothoracic junction,[161] as this can be the site of a fracture-subluxation and is oftentimes obscured during conventional cervical spine x-rays (see Fig. 15–2*A*). Manual traction on the arms, swimmer's view,[161] and sagittal reconstructions of fine-cut CT scans of the cervicothoracic junction[162] can be used to visualize this segment (see Fig. 15–2*C*). Thoracolumbar plain films should be obtained to assess this segment of the spine. Areas of injury or questionable plain film findings should prompt computer-assisted imaging of the involved segment. There is no consensus regarding which of the two or both, MRI or CT scanning, should be performed for the assessment of trauma. In an intact patient without radiographic abnormality, MRI probably is unnecessary. A CT scan is reasonable to obtain in a patient who has a bone or ligamentous injury determined by plain films or with neurologic deficit. This study is readily obtained in emergency situations. A patient with a neurologic deficit, with or without radiographic abnormality,[48] requires a study that visualizes the spinal canal. In the patient who is both systemically and neurologically stable, high-resolution MRI scan is preferable.[88] A myelogram is also an elective option if MRI scanning is impractical or unavailable.

Controversy exists regarding the need to perform an MRI scan in a patient with significant radiographic abnormality by plain or CT scan imaging. In the vast majority of patients who have sustained a traumatic neurologic injury, translational deformity or retropulsion of bone into the canal represents the mechanism of spinal cord injury. Both of these causes of cord compression can be readily diagnosed by radiographic modalities (see Figs. 15–2*C;* 15–7*A;* and 15–9*A, B*). In the presence of a retropulsed fragment, which would be approached anteriorly, it is less necessary to perform a canal study, since the decompression will allow direct visualization of the spinal canal to assess for patency. In a patient undergoing elective fixation, especially with neurologic deficit, a canal study should be obtained.

The patient with spinal cord injury should receive high-dose corticosteroid (methylprednisolone 30 mg/kg bolus over the first hour, followed by 5.4 mg/kg/hour for 23 hours) as soon as the spinal cord injury is identified.

The role of surgical intervention for spinal trauma is somewhat controversial. Most would agree that a patient with ongoing spinal cord compression who is deteriorating clinically should undergo emergency decompressive surgery.[12, 88, 104] Such surgery would be contraindicated, however, if the patient's cardiorespiratory status is not stable.[63] Operating under such circumstances could exacerbate secondary spinal cord injury.[3] The relative indications for spinal surgery are less clear, especially the role and timing of decompressive surgery. Reduction and stabilization remain strictly elective interventions. Until surgery is carried out, there are effective means of immobilizing a patient without surgery to prevent further spinal cord injury. Decompressive surgery in a patient who is neurologically intact, followed by fixation/fusion, should be carried out under optimal circumstances to preserve cord function. Some would argue that, although it is very unlikely that decompression would be of assistance, decompressing a patient with a complete spinal cord injury represents the only treatment option available to the patient. A rationale for semiurgent decompression can be formulated on this basis alone.

A more controversial situation is a patient with a partial spinal cord injury and ongoing compression. Based upon the pathophysiology of secondary injury, the presence of cord compression may impede regional blood flow at the site of injury and promote secondary injury. Therefore, decompression may optimize the regional milieu within which the spinal cord can recover,[111, 163] and potentially counteract some of the factors involved in accelerating secondary spinal cord injury. Unfortunately, no prospective data exist.[88, 142, 163, 164] However, reports of recovery of stable neurologic deficits following delayed spinal cord decompression have been published, indicating the potential benefit of neural decompression.[91, 124, 128, 157, 165–167]

If a decompressive procedure is deemed necessary, the surgical approach is determined by the location of the pathology identified by the preoperative imaging studies.[3] As outlined earlier, spinal cord compression results from translational deformity or retropulsed material into the canal, usually bone but occasionally disc material or hematoma. Depending upon the configuration of the translational deformity and the level of the spine involved, an anterior or a posterior approach can be effective (see Figs. 15–2 and 15–7). Facet locks, which cannot be reduced with cervical traction, can be treated surgically.[60] The typical approach is posterior,[60, 133] where the facets can be unlocked under direct vision. If there is a significant disc herniation present anteriorly, an anterior approach to remove the disc followed by distraction of the spine for reduction can be considered.

In the thoracolumbar spine, translational deformities are often effectively reduced by a posterior approach (Fig. 15–20). Since the forces required to effect reduction are great, and these injuries involve the three columns, the extra leverage provided by long, multisegmental, internal fixation devices provides effective reduction and alignment maintenance.

The pathomechanics of spinal injury dictates that the spinal canal encroachment by bone, disc, or hematoma is virtually always along the anterior aspect of the spinal canal. A surgical approach to decompressing the neural elements requires access to the anterior compartments and vertebral bodies by a safe technique. Optimally, this is performed by direct anterior or anterolateral approaches (see Fig. 15–10). This is especially true in the cervical spine, where a posterior approach risks spinal cord injury due to manipulation necessary to gain adequate access anteriorly. In the thoracolumbar spine, anterior approaches are again preferable (see Fig. 15–10). However, at the level of the cauda equina and with some of the thoracic and thoracolumbar junction injuries with favorable configurations, posterolateral approaches can effect decompression (see Fig. 15–9). All of the injured anterior material does not have to be removed, as decompression alone has to be achieved, unlike malignant pathology, where radical debulking is required to prevent local recurrence.

Surgery for spinal trauma involves a population of patients who are relatively young and otherwise healthy. The patients have relatively normal anatomy, except at the focus of instability, thereby making identification of landmarks for fixator insertion easier, compared to a patient with advanced degenerative disease. The deformities, unlike chronic deforming processes, are usually readily mobile and reducible with application of relatively straightforward corrective forces. Usually a distractive force is required for reduction. With adequate fixation, site preparation, and bone grafting, these patients have a high rate of fracture union and bone fusion.

Despite the modern understanding of the pathophysiology of spinal cord injury and advanced operative techniques, the severity of the initial spinal cord injury still remains the most significant prognostic factor for acute traumatic spinal injuries. Meticulous management of these patients can optimize their neurologic recovery and augment reintegration back into society.

NONTRAUMATIC SPINAL DISORDERS

The most important features of the effective and comprehensive management of patients with acute, nontraumatic spinal cord compression are rapid but accurate assessment of the neurologic deficit, detailed radiographic determination of neural compression and vertebral column integrity, and, if possible, assessment of the natural history of the pathologic process. In general, patients who decompensate acutely require acute intervention to preserve neurologic function. In that regard, the most useful tool for assessment and initiation of treatment remains the neurologic examination. Given advances in imaging, rapid diagnostic information can, in most centers, be obtained easily, complementing clinical information and guiding surgical decision making. Finally, the expanding armamentarium provided by new surgical techniques and instrumentation systems allows a more aggressive operative approach to these difficult cases. This section outlines the physiologic basis for compression; describes common causes of acute, nontraumatic compression; and discusses some of the surgical approaches to lesions of the cervical, thoracic, and lumbar spines, with special attention to spinal metastatic lesions.

The anatomic and pathophysiologic determinants of acute, nontraumatic myelopathy may also be divided into their neural and osseous components, as one does for traumatic spinal disorders.

Neural compression can result in radicular and/or myelopathic syndromes; the level of compression determines the specific features or presentation, as outlined in the previous section. In general, spinal cord compression at any point above the conus medullaris presents in a similar fashion, with variable sensory and motor deficits below the level of the abnormality, typically hyper-reflexia and potentially bladder and bowel dysfunction. Although created and intended for use in traumatic spinal cord injury patients, the ASIA classification systems (see Table 15–2 and Fig. 15–19) outlined above can provide helpful scales by which to assess patients preoperatively and compare results postoperatively and between centers.[90]

Although more common in the setting of acute trauma, varying presentations of incomplete cord injury or compression can be seen, including anterior, posterior, central cord, and Brown-Séquard syndromes.[168] These have been previously described in this chapter.

More complex presentations occur with cervicomedullary compression or lesions at the level of the conus medullaris or cauda equina. Cervicomedullary compressive symptoms and signs reflect the onset of neural compression upon the spinal cord and lower brain stem, as well as the consequence of cerebrospinal fluid outflow obstruction and/or vascular compromise. Cervical pain, headache, cranial nerve palsy, spasticity, weakness, and a mixture of upper motor neuron findings in the upper and lower extremities are common features. In particular, the syndrome of "cruciate paralysis" may be found as a result of compression at the level of the corticospinal decussation.[169, 170] These patients have a preponderance of weakness involving the hands. It results from compression of some of the motor fibers in the corticospinal tract that supply the distal upper extremities as they cross in the anterior aspect of the cervicomedullary junction.

Thoracolumbar junction lesions are likely to cause conus medullaris syndrome. Anatomic studies, augmented by clinical and pathological correlations,[41] demonstrate that nearly all the lumbar spinal cord segments are found opposite the T12 vertebral body and the sacral segments are at the level of L1. The spinal cord terminates generally opposite the L1–L2 interspace.[171] Patients present with a combination of lower motor neuron deficits in the lower extremities, variable sensory deficits often involving the sacral region, and bladder and bowel dysfunction.

Compression below the spinal cord termination at L1–L2 leads to cauda equina syndrome. Motor fibers tend to be more susceptible to compression than sensory fibers. Asymmetric motor lesions are possible. A common cause of acute cauda equina syndrome is acute, large disc herniations or disc herniations in patients with congenital spinal stenosis. They usually occur at L4–5 and L5–S1 (see Fig. 15–15). The typical presentation is bladder and bowel dysfunction and perineal numbness. Leg function is generally spared, since the disc herniation compresses maximally on the midline sacral nerves and the laterally exiting L5 and S1 nerves are not as intimately involved with the herniation.[89, 172]

A second component of the evaluation of nontraumatic, acute spinal cord compression is the determination of the integrity of the osteoligamentous complex. Although originally devised for the classification of thoracic and lumbar fractures, the three-column scheme of Denis remains relevant to a comprehensive appreciation of spinal column integrity[42] (see Fig. 15–3). It is useful to define the extent of involvement of the pathological process in terms of the various compartments of the spine. However, the definition of instability, being based upon two columns or middle column involvement by the pathological process, may not be valid for chronic deforming or destabilizing processes. Often, with two or more columns involved by a chronic deforming process—for example, a tumor—the patient does not have gross instability as defined by conventional flexion/extension views (see Figs. 15–12, 15–14, 15–18). The inherent stability likely resides in the fact that the ligamentous components of the motion segment remain intact, preventing translation or acute angulation. Despite its limitations, there remains a rationale for defining abnormalities with regard to the three columns of the spine, since the surgical approach for radical excision or decompression of the neural elements, involving two or more columns of the spine, will often render the spine unstable, necessitating fixation/fusion (see Figs. 15–12 and 15–14).

Classification of Causes

Although there are a variety of infectious, inflammatory, vascular, and neoplastic conditions that may cause acute spinal cord dysfunction, this chapter deals with the most common causes: metastatic tumors, acute disc herniations, and infection.

In adults, the majority of spinal metastases have their origins from the breast, lung, and prostate. Renal and rectal carcinomas, as well as thyroid carcinoma, are the next most common forms of spinal metastasis, each comprising approximately 5% of all cases.[173] Up to 10% of the patients will present with neurologic deficit as the initial manifestation of their spinal metastasis.[174] Spread of tumor to the spinal neuraxis may be by direct extension, hematogenous dissemination, or lymphatic or venous spread through Batson's plexus.[173]

Breast carcinoma is the most common spinal metastasis.[173] The biologic behavior of the metastatic tumor may be different than that of the primary tumor.[173, 174] Many breast carcinomas are radiosensitive, and most with high levels of estrogen or progesterone receptors will respond to pharmacologic manipulation. The vertebral body and anterior epidural space are the most commonly affected.[175] Patients who have failed or are not responding to chemotherapy or radiation become candidates for surgical decompression and stabilization.[176, 177] Even though breast carcinoma most frequently metastasizes to the thoracic spine (because of the large number of vertebral bodies), it may nevertheless spread to any spinal level.

Lung carcinoma behaves more aggressively than breast or prostate lesions. They affect the spine through hematogenous, lymphatic, and contiguous spread from the primary lesion. Of the three histologic types (small cell, squamous cell, and adenocarcinoma), adenocarcinoma is the most common to present for surgical resection.[178] Small cell carcinomas are frequently radiosensitive, thereby not requiring surgery. Squamous cell tumors are much more radioresistant and less often a source of metastasis to the spine than adenocarcinomas. The presence of distant metastasis as well as the possibility of direct spread from the chest wall influences the choice of operation. Young patients without systemic disease are candidates for radical resection and reconstruction; those with adjacent chest wall lesions are amenable to anterior and posterior vertebral resection. Primary lung carcinomas preferentially metastasize to the thoracic spine. The reasons appear to be anatomic.[120, 178, 179]

The majority of prostate tumors that evade regional control frequently invade the spine, principally in the lumbosacral region. Most are radiosensitive or respond to hormonal therapy, and, like breast carcinoma, the bone lesions, whether lytic or blastic, may have a biologic behavior different than that of the primary lesion.[180] Most lesions have been previously treated with hormones or irradiation before they present for surgical management. Involvement is usually in the vertebral bodies, pedicles, and epidural space. Rarely are the posterior elements infiltrated. With well-differentiated lesions, even aggressive, abdominal approaches are well tolerated and permit several years of local disease-free survival.[120, 176, 177, 179]

Renal cell carcinoma (RCCA) (see Fig. 15–13) not infrequently makes its initial presentation by a spinal metastatic lesion.[181] More radioresistant than lung or prostate tumors, RCCA is a well-vascularized, aggressive tumor that can nonetheless can be quite amenable, in suitable candidates, to aggressive surgical management.[181, 182] Preoperative angiography and embolization can significantly reduce the vascularity of these lesions and reduce intraoperative blood loss.[182] RCCA most frequently metastasizes to the thoracolumbar or upper lumbar spinal levels.

Although the above-mentioned tumors are often accessible to surgery, a crucial aspect of caring for these patients is to make a proper decision regarding the appropriate indication and candidate for surgery. Unlike patients with traumatic disorders, those with metastasis are usually relatively old and may be otherwise ill and debilitated by other metastases, coexistent medical conditions, and/or medications. Such coincident conditions can significantly impact upon perioperative morbidity and mortality. No firm guidelines exist regarding the criteria for inclusion or exclusion for surgical therapy. However, some factors should be considered. The patient should have a potential survival of at least 3–6 months, relatively stable systemic disease, good potential to regain or maintain ambulation, failure of other treatment modalities, and radioresistance of the metastatic lesion. Wound healing can be a major problem with these debilitated patients. This problem is amplified if the surgical site has been previously irradiated. Therefore, it is preferable prior to initiating radiotherapy to determine whether or not a patient is a surgical candidate. If so, the use of adjunctive radiation therapy should be reserved for the postoperative period.

Disc herniations causing progressive neurologic deficit, although uncommon, do occur and, if recognized, can be treated with gratifying results.[172] While possible in the subaxial cervical spine, especially C5–6 and C6–7, as well as the mid and lower thoracic and upper lumbar spine regions (see Fig. 15–16), the most common emergent presentation of a disc herniation occurs in the lower lumbar spine (L4–L5, L5–S1) (see Fig. 15–15). The acute herniations manifest clinically with an acute cauda equina syndrome: variable motor weakness, especially distal legs; fluctuating sensory abnormalities; and, in particular, bowel, bladder, and sexual dysfunction. If dealt with expeditiously, within the first day or two of presentation, patients have the potential to recover. Delay in decompression can result in significant, permanent deficits impacting upon the patient's daily functioning.[172]

Infectious processes affecting the vertebrae and extradural spaces can be caused by bacteria, fungi, and parasitic organisms.[183–186] The principles of management are similar regardless of the inciting organism—that is, pathogen-directed therapy complemented by conservative measures such as bracing to diminish pain. Those in whom primary treatment fails can be considered for surgery.

The most common infectious processes to involve the spine are iatrogenic, pyogenic osteomyelitis and discitis. MRI is particularly useful in both situations (see Fig. 15–17). Predisposing factors for osteomyelitis include diabetes, intravenous drug use, and an immunosuppressed state. The causative organism varies according to the patient and the potential source of infection. The most common causes include *Staphylococcus* (*S. aureus* and *S. epidermidis*) and anaerobic streptococci. Gram-negative rods are more frequently seen in association with osteomyelitis and intravenous drug use (see Fig. 15–4). The ability to image the spine in detail with magnetic resonance has indicated that solitary epidural abscesses (see Fig. 15–4) are relatively rare in the absence of vertebral osteomyelitis. A focal abscess usually results from direct invasion from a contiguous infection.[185]

In the absence of progressive neurologic deficit, medical management is the cornerstone of therapy for osteomyelitis and discitis.[184, 186] Surgery is reserved, in general, for three situations: (1) when there has been severe bony destruction with resultant pain, malalignment, or instability; (2) progressive neurologic deficit; and/or (3) persistent infection despite an adequate trial of antibiotics. Pyogenic osteomyelitis, with or without epidural abscess, is a disease affecting the anterior and middle columns. Anterior and anterolateral approaches involving vertebrectomy followed by autologous fusion represent the treatment of choice. Some surgeons would proceed with grafting at the time of the decompression, without a concern for inserting an avascular graft in an infected site. In a patient without diabetes, immunocompromised state, or frank pus at the site of surgery, this is likely to be adequate and successful. However, if the above-mentioned risk factors are present, an initial decompression and débridement procedure with a subsequent spinal reconstruction operation after an adequate course of antibiotics is a therapeutic option. The use of instrumentation in the presence of osteomyelitis also requires similar considerations.

Surgical Approaches

This section explores one management philosophy for handling acute, nontraumatic surgical and spinal emergencies. It does not review the techniques of each particular approach. Discussion instead is centered on using a three-column concept model, as well as the merits and liabilities of anterior, lateral, posterior, and combined approaches to compressive and invasive pathology.[187–189]

In general, contraindications to surgical intervention, irrespective of pathology, include severe, debilitating cardiac or pulmonary disease; short life expectancy (especially <6 months); and diffuse, multilevel vertebral disease that prohibits reconstruction and stabilization.[120, 190]

More specific factors must be considered for the patient with metastatic disease. Preeminent is the presence of neurologic deficit, its duration and degree. Long-standing (>24 hours), complete deficits are unlikely to be reversed by a decompressive intervention. Other important considerations include the pathology of the tumor; the presence of local, contiguous, and distant metastases; and the radiosensitivity of the lesion. Also, life expectancy, the systemic health of the patient, the presence of spinal deformity, instability, and intractable pain influence the decision to proceed with a major operative intervention.[120, 191]

At times, when some of these questions cannot be easily settled, a less optimal posterior decompressive surgical intervention may be considered to arrest the progressive deterioration and allow for some time to complete systemic investigations.[191, 192] However, in the majority of situations in which sufficient clinical and radiographic information (high-quality MR imaging) can be obtained, most of the questions required to plan treatment can be answered. Then, a single-staged operation designed to eradicate the offending pathology, provide stability, alleviate pain, and promote independence can be undertaken primarily.

The basic principles of surgical planning involve the assessment of neurologic deficit and the assessment of the integrity of the osteoligamentous complex. Irrespective of the location along the spine, Denis' three-column assessment system can be used to guide a decompressive operative approach and subsequent stabilization.

Pathological processes that involve the vertebral body and anterior epidural space compromise the anterior and middle columns. The central canal and anterior and middle columns are best approached anteriorly or anterolaterally, depending upon the segment of the spine involved (see Fig. 15–14). Invasion of one pedicle can be addressed directly during the ipsilateral anterior or anterolateral approach. Involvement of the pedicles bilaterally requires a two-stage decompressive approach because the contralateral pedicle is difficult to access anteriorly (see Fig. 15–12). Posterolateral decompression is ideally suited for pathology that is posterior or involving the pedicle or the posterolateral aspect of the vertebral body (see Fig. 15–13). The direct posterior approach may be used for palliative treatment in a patient with extensive systemic disease with progressive paraplegia. Also, it can be effective for debulking of tumor that is strictly epidural (see Fig. 15–11).

The principles of surgical management for cancer include (1) adequately decompressing the neural elements, (2) achieving radical debulking of the tumor for local control, and (3) establishing spinal stability. Unlike trauma, a direct approach to the tumor should be obtained, whenever possible, to enable radical excision of neoplastic tissue. This generally necessitates direct anterior access by anterior or anterolateral approaches. Some have advocated bilateral posterolateral approaches, which allow greater access to the vertebral body. However, tumor that is located in the most anterior aspect of the vertebral body can be difficult to clearly identify in situ by this approach. Mediastinal vessels are in close proximity to the anterior aspect of the spine, and the normal tissue planes between these structures and the vertebrae may be obscured by the tumor, thereby increasing the risk of injury to the mediastinal vessels, which can be fatal during such an operative approach. Also, the anterior approach is best for a vertebral body reconstruction to regain stability of the spine. It is much more difficult to achieve the reconstruction by a posterolateral approach.

Radical resection for local control of spinal metastasis represents a formidable procedure. Unfortunately, patients with metastatic cancer are generally more elderly than the trauma patient and have coexistent medical conditions. Therefore, one can expect significant perioperative morbidity. These risks of surgery must therefore be weighed against the benefits of local control and overall patient longevity to determine if radical excision is appropriate.

In the subaxial cervical spine, an anterior approach for corpectomy is usually sufficient to accomplish eradication of vertebral body lesions (see Fig. 15–18). Intrapedicular extension can sometimes be addressed through this approach. However, if bipedicular or three-column involvement is present, the anterior approach must be combined with posterior debulking. Spinal reconstruction should be focused on re-establishment of the anterior two columns, since these columns are the weight-bearing component of the osteoligamentous complex. Sometimes fixation must be achieved anterior and posteriorly to adequately stabilize the involved segment.[187, 193]

A number of options exist for the management of thoracic spine lesions. The level of the spine and the extent of local involvement play a role in selecting the surgical technique. In general, there are three basic approaches: anterior or anterolateral, posterior, or posterolateral.[194–197]

In the upper thoracic spine (T1–T3), anterior cervical approaches may be combined with median sternotomy or manubrial windowing to gain direct anterior access. Transaxillary, or high transthoracic approaches, can also enable access to this region.[194, 195]

From T4 through the thoracolumbar junction, all approaches are possible to gain access to the anterior column, except the direct posterior procedure. The posterolateral approach includes costotransversectomy and pedicle resection (which has limited visualization of the anterior extent of disease and limits the ability to gain access for anterior column reconstruction). The lateral extracavitary approach limits the ability to visualize the contralateral pedicle.[125, 196] Posterior approaches include laminectomy and transpedicular decompression.[197] Anterior and anterolateral access is provided by thoracotomy (see Figs. 15–12 and 15–14); below T8, one must be cognizant of the presence of the artery of Adamkiewicz (usually found between T9 and L2, and more commonly located on the left; spinal angiography may be helpful); and, between T10 and L1, the diaphragm requires mobilization to gain direct access for decompression and reconstruction.

In the lumbar spine, anterolateral and transthoracic approaches can provide access as far down as L2.[197] Below that level, a left retroperitoneal approach is appropriate. This approach also allows access to L1 and can be extended into the lower thoracic area if required. If the pathology resides anteriorly at or below L5, a transabdominal approach is necessary. The specifics of the approaches, and merits and deficiencies of each, are well discussed in recent articles. Predominant posterior pathology can be accessed for radical tumor debulking by a posterior approach. Pedicle fixation is an efficient means of re-establishing stability in such cases.[198]

In summary, surgical intervention in acute nontraumatic spinal cord compression begins with accurate preoperative clinical assessment and high-quality, comprehensive image studies. The results of the initial assessment enable a comprehensive determination of neurologic function and osteoligamentous integrity. The primary treatment objective is neural decompression for preservation of function. The other objectives include obtaining a diagnosis, local tumor control, alleviation of pain, and re-establishing spinal stability. Improvements in critical care medicine and anesthesia, combined with less demanding, more user-friendly instrumentation systems, have made the operative and postoperative care of these patients easier, and with reducing morbidity.

Summary • Contemporary management of acute spinal disorders requires a broad understanding of the normal and abnormal anatomy and biomechanics of the spine and the principles underlying spinal cord injury. Despite the dramatic advances in spinal imaging techniques, the clinical examination remains the most sensitive indicator of neurologic function. The imaging studies provide information regarding the etiology of the acute spinal disorder and the stability of the spine, and assist in planning surgical intervention. The nonoperative treatment available for a given pathological entity can include treatment of the primary etiology and the judicious use of corticosteroids for tumor edema or to prevent secondary spinal cord injury. Surgical intervention is sometimes indicated for acute spinal disorders. The principles of surgery, regardless of the underlying etiology, include neural decompression, spinal column reduction, and stabilization. Unfortunately, despite the advances in our understanding and treatment protocols for acute spinal disorders, the ultimate neurologic prognosis often is determined by the extent of neurologic injury at the time of diagnosis.

References

1. Tator CH, Duncan EG, Edmonds VE, et al: Changes in epidemiology of acute spinal cord injury from 1947 to 1981. Surg Neurol 1993;40:207–215.
2. DiTunno JF, Formal CS: Chronic spinal cord injury. N Engl J Med 1994;330:550–556.
3. Green BA, Callahan RE, Klose JK, et al: Acute spinal cord injury: Current concepts. Clin Orthop Rel Res 1981;154:125–135.
4. Price C, Makintubee S, Herndon W, et al: Epidemiology of traumatic spinal cord injury and acute hospitalization and rehabilitation charges for spinal cord injuries in Oklahoma, 1988–1990. Am J Epidemiol 1994;139:37–47.
5. Young W: Medical treatments of acute spinal cord injury. J Neurol Neurosurg Psychiatr 1992;55:635–639.
6. Bracken MB, Shepard MJ, Collins WF: A randomized, controlled trial of methylprednisolone or naloxone in the treatment of acute spinal-cord injury. N Engl J Med 1990;322:1405–1411.
7. Ducker TB: Treatment of spinal cord injury. N Engl J Med 1990;322:1459–1461.
8. Tator CH, Duncan EG, Edmonds VE: Complications and costs of management of acute spinal cord injury. Paraplegia 1993;31:700–714.
9. Bucholz RW, Gill K: Classification of injuries to the thoracolumbar spine. Orthop Clin North Am 1986;17:67–73.
10. Bracken MB, Webb SB, Wagner FC: Classification of the severity of acute spinal cord injury: Implications for management. Paraplegia 1977–1978;15:319–326.
11. Horsley WJ, Tucker WS, Hudson AR: Experience with early anterior operation in acute injuries of the cervical spine. Paraplegia 1977–1978;15:110–122.
12. Donovan WH, Dwyer AP: An update on the early management of traumatic paraplegia (nonoperative and operative management). Clin Orthop Rel Res 1984;189:12–21.
13. Suwanwela C, Alexander E, Davis CH: Prognosis in spinal cord injury, with special reference to patients with motor paralysis and sensory preservation. J Neurosurg 1962;19:220–227.
14. Allen AR: Surgery of experimental lesions of spinal cord equivalent to crush injury of fracture/dislocation of spinal column: A preliminary report. JAMA 1911;57:878–880.
15. Iwahara T, Atsuta Y, Watakabe M, et al: Analysis of spinal cord evoked potential and locomotor function during

acute spinal cord compression in cats. Spine 1992;17:1375–1380.
16. Cain CM, Langston PG, Weston PF, et al: Assessment of spinal cord blood flow and function in sheep after anterolateral cervical interbody fusion in the presence of cord damage. Spine 1994;19:511–519.
17. Guha A, Tator CH: Acute cardiovascular effects of experimental spinal cord injury. J Trauma 1988;28:481–490.
18. Ueta T, Owen JH, Sugioka Y: Effects of compression on physiologic integrity of the spinal cord on circulation and clinical status in four different directions of compression: Posterior, anterior, circumferential and lateral. Spine 1992;17:S217–S226.
19. Jarzem PF, Quance DR, Doyle DJ, et al: Spinal cord tissue pressure during spinal cord distraction in dogs. Spine 1992;17:S227–S233.
20. Tator CH, Fehlings MG: Review of the secondary injury theory of acute spinal cord trauma with emphasis on vascular mechanisms. J Neurosurg 1991;75:15–26.
21. Holtz A, Nystrom B, Gerdin B: Spinal cord blood flow measured by 14-C iodoantipyrine autoradiography during and after graded spinal cord compression in rats. Surg Neurol 1989;31:350–360.
22. Koyanagi I, Tator CH, Theriault E: Silicone rubber microangiography of acute spinal cord injury in the rat. Neurosurgery 1993;32:260–268.
23. Koyanagi I, Tator CH, Lea PJ: Three-dimensional analysis of the vascular system in the rat spinal cord with scanning electron microscopy of vascular corrosion casts. Part I: Normal spinal cord. Neurosurgery 1993;33:277–284.
24. Koyanagi I, Tator CH, Lea PJ: Three-dimensional analysis of the vascular system in the rat spinal cord with scanning electron microscopy of vascular corrosion casts. Part II: Acute spine cord injury. Neurosurgery 1993;33:285–292.
25. Zhang Y, Hillered L, Olsson Y, et al: Time course of energy perturbation after compression trauma to the spinal cord: An experimental study in the rat using microdialysis. Surg Neurol 1993;39:297–304.
26. Chavko M, Kalincakova K, Kluchova D, et al: Blood flow and electrolytes in spinal cord ischemia. Exp Neurol 1991;112:299–303.
27. Ross IB, Tator CH, Theriault E: Effect of nimodipine or methylprednisolone on recovery from acute experimental spinal cord injury in rats. Surg Neurol 1993;40:461–470.
28. Schouman-Claeys E, Frija G, Cuenod CA, et al: MR imaging of acute spinal cord injury: Results of an experimental study in dog. Am J Neuroradiol 1990;11:959–965.
29. Fujii H, Yone K, Sakou T: Magnetic resonance imaging study of experimental acute spinal cord injury. Spine 1993;18:2030–2034.
30. Silberstein M, Tress BM, Hennessy O: Prediction of neurological outcome in acute spine cord injury: Role of CT and MR. Am J Neuroradiol 1992;13:1597–1608.
31. Silberstein M, Hennessy O: Implications of focal spinal cord lesions following trauma: Evaluation with magnetic resonance imaging. Paraplegia 1993;31:160–167.
32. Panjabi MM: The stabilizing system of the spine. Part I: Function, dysfunction, adaptation and enhancement. J Spinal Disord 1992;5:383–389.
33. Pope MH, Pflaster DS, Krag MH: Biomechanics of lumbar disc disease. AAOS Instructional Course Lecture 1992;41:187–192.
34. White AA, Panjabi MM: The problem of clinical instability in the human spine—a systematic approach. In White AA, Panjabi MM (eds): Clinical Biomechanics of the Spine, 2nd ed, pp 277–378. Philadelphia, JB Lippincott, 1990.
35. Shaffer WO, Spratt KF, Weinstein J, et al: The consistency and accuracy of roentgenograms for measuring sagittal translation in the lumbar vertebral motion segment: An experimental model. Spine 1990;15:741–750.
36. Kim YE, Goel VK: Effect of testing mode on the biomechanical response of a spinal motion segment. J Biomechanics 1990;23:289–291.
37. Stokes IA, Gardner-Morse M: Stability increase of the lumbar spine with different muscle groups: A biomechanical *in vitro* study. Spine 1995;20:2168–2178.
38. Gardner-Morse M, Stokes IA, Laible JP: Role of muscles in lumbar spine stability in maximal extension efforts. J Orthop Res 1995;13:802–808.
39. Maiman DJ, Pintar FA: Anatomy and clinical biomechanics of the thoracic spine. Clin Neurosurg 1992;38:296–324.
40. Holdsworth FW: Fractures, dislocations and fracture-dislocations of the spine. J Bone Joint Surg 1963;45B:6–20.
41. Holdworth FW: Review article: Fractures, dislocations and fracture-dislocations of the spine. J Bone Joint Surg 1970;52A:1534–1551.
42. Denis F: The three column spine and its significance in the classification of acute thoracolumbar spinal injuries. Spine 1983;8:817–831.
43. Denis F: Spinal instability as defined by the three column spine concept in acute spinal trauma. Clin Orthop Rel Res 1984;189:65–76.
44. Maiman DJ, Yoganandan N, Pintar F: Biomechanics of spinal instrumentation. In Benzel EC (ed): Neurosurgical Topics: Spinal Instrumentation. Park Ridge, IL, AANS, 1993, pp 11–29.
45. White AA, Johnson RM, Panjabi MM, et al: Biomechanical analysis of clinical stability in the cervical spine. Clin Orthop Rel Res 1975;109:85–95.
46. Gaines RW, Humphries WG: A plea for judgment in management of thoracolumbar fractures and fracture-dislocations. Clin Orthop Rel Res 1984;189:36–42.
47. Andriacchi T, Schultz A, Belytschko T, et al: A model for studies of mechanical interactions between the human spine and rib cage. J Biomechanics 1974;7:497–507.
48. Pang D, Wilberger JE: Spinal cord injury without radiographic abnormality in children. J Neurosurg 1982;57:114–129.
49. Pang D, Pollack IF: Spinal cord injury without radiographic abnormality in children—the SCIWORA syndrome. J Trauma 1989;29:654–664.
50. Fielding JW, Cochran GV, Lawsing JF, et al: Tears of the transverse ligament of the atlas. J Bone Joint Surg 1974;56A:1683–1691.
51. Jefferson G: Fracture of the atlas vertebra: Report of four cases, and a review of those previously recorded. Br J Surg 1920;7:407–422.
52. Spence KF, Decker S, Sell KW: Bursting atlantal fracture associated with rupture of the transverse ligament. J Bone Joint Surg 1970;52A:543–549.
53. Dickman CA, Mamourian A, Sonntag VK: Magnetic resonance imaging of the transverse atlantal ligament for the evaluation of atlantoaxial instability. J Neurosurg 1991: 75:221–227.
54. Anderson LD, D'Alonzo RT: Fractures of the odontoid process of the axis. J Bone Joint Surg 1974;56A:1663–1674.
55. Hadley MN, Browner C, Sonntag VK: Axis fractures: A comprehensive review of management and treatment in 107 cases. Neurosurgery 1985;17:281–290.
56. Schneider RC, Livingston KE, Cave AJ, et al: "Hangman's fracture" of the cervical spine. J Neurosurg 1965;22:141–154.
57. Levine AM, Rhyne AL: Traumatic spondylolisthesis of the axis. Semin Spinal Surg 1991;3:47–60.
58. Effendi B, Roy D, Cornish B, et al: Fractures of the ring of the axis: A classification based on the analysis of 131 cases. J Bone Joint Surg 1981;63B:319–327.
59. Star AM, Jones AA, Cotler JM, et al: Immediate closed reduction of cervical spine dislocations using traction. Spine 1990;15:1068–1072.
60. Wolf A, Levi L, Mirvis S, et al: Operative management of bilateral facet dislocation. J Neurosurg 1991;75:883–890.
61. Maiman DJ, Barolat G, Larson SJ: Management of bilateral locked facets of the cervical spine. Neurosurgery 1986;18:542–547.
62. Sturm JT, Perry JF: Injuries associated with fractures of the transverse processes of the thoracic and lumbar vertebrae. J Trauma 1984;24:597–599.
63. Blumenkopf B, Juneau PA: Magnetic resonance imaging

(MRI) of thoracolumbar fractures. J Spinal Disord 1988;1:144–150.
64. Trafton PJ, Boyd CA: Computer tomography of thoracic and lumbar spine injuries. J Trauma 1984;24:515.
65. Ferguson RL, Allen BL: A mechanistic classification of thoracolumbar spine fractures. Clin Orthop Rel Res 1984;189:77–88.
66. Schnee CL, Ansell LV: Selection criteria and outcome of operative approaches for thoracolumbar burst fractures with and without neurological deficit. J Neurosurg 1997;86:48–55.
67. Hamilton A, Webb JK: The role of anterior surgery for vertebral fractures with and without cord compression. Clin Orthop 1994;300:79–89.
68. Hollowell JP, Maiman DJ: Management of thoracic and thoracolumbar spine trauma. In Rea GL, Miller CA (eds): Spinal Trauma: Current Evaluation and Management, pp 127–156. Park Ridge, IL, AANS, 1993.
69. Kostuick JP: Anterior fixation for burst fractures of the thoracic and lumbar spine, with or without neurological involvement. Spine 1988;13:286–293.
70. Frederickson BE, Mann KA, Yuan HA, et al: Reduction of the intracanal fragment in experimental burst fractures. Spine 1988;13:267–271.
71. Benson DR: Unstable thoracolumbar fractures, with emphasis on the burst fracture. Clin Orthop Rel Res 1988;230:14–29.
72. James KS, Wenger KH, Schlegel JD, et al: Biomechanical evaluation of the stability of thoracolumbar burst fractures. Spine 1994;19:1731–1740.
73. Mumford J, Weinstein JN, Spratt KF, et al: Thoracolumbar burst fractures: The clinical efficiency and outcome of nonoperative management. Spine 1993;18:955–970.
74. Chan DP, Seng NK, Kaan KT: Nonoperative treatment in burst fractures of the lumbar spine (L2–L5) without neurologic deficit. Spine 1993;18:320–325.
75. Gertzbein SD, Offierski C: Complete fracture-dislocation of the thoracic spine without spinal cord injury: A case report. J Bone Joint Surg 1979;61A:449–451.
76. Chance GQ: Note on a type of flexion fracture of the spine. Br J Radiol 1948;21:452–453.
77. Raney EM, Bennett JT: Pediatric chance fracture. Spine 1992;17:1522–1523.
78. Green DA, Green NE, Spengler DM, et al: Flexion-distraction injuries to the lumbar spine associated with abdominal injuries. J Spinal Disord 1991;4:312–318.
79. Gertzbein SD, Court-Brown CM: Flexion-distraction injuries of the lumbar spine. Clin Orthop Rel Res 1988;227:52–60.
80. Gumley G, Taylor TK, Ryan MD: Distraction fractures of the lumbar spine. J Bone Joint Surg 1982;64B:520–525.
81. Jacobs RR, Casey MP: Surgical management of thoracolumbar spinal injuries: General principles and controversial considerations. Clin Orthop Rel Res 1984;189:22–35.
82. Dickson JH, Harrington PR, Erwin WD: Results of reduction and stabilization of the severely fractured thoracic and lumbar spine. J Bone Joint Surg 1978;60A:799–805.
83. Meyer PR, Cybulski JR, Rusin JJ, et al: Spinal cord injury. Neurol Clin 1991;9:625–661.
84. Bohlman HH, Eismont FJ: Surgical techniques of anterior decompression and fusion for spinal cord injuries. Clin Orthop Rel Res 1981;154:57–67.
85. Bondurant FJ, Cotler HB, Kulkarni MV, et al: Acute spinal cord injury: A study using physical examination and magnetic resonance imaging. Spine 1990;15:161–168.
86. Chirilo F, Totis O, Cavarzerani A, et al: Usefulness of transthoracic and transesophageal echocardiography in recognition and management of cardiovascular injuries after blunt chest trauma. Heart 1996;75:301–306.
87. Saadia R, Levy RD, DeGiannis E, et al: Penetrating cardiac injuries: Clinical classification and management strategy. Br J Surg 1994;81:1572–1575.
88. Chesnut RM, Marshall LF: Early assessment, transport and management of patients with posttraumatic spinal instability. In Cooper PE (ed): Management of Posttraumatic Spinal Instability, pp 1–17. Park Ridge, IL, AANS, 1990.
89. Tator CH: Spinal cord syndromes with physiologic and anatomic correlations. In Menezes AN, Sonntag VK (eds): Principles of Spinal Surgery, pp 785–799. New York, McGraw-Hill, 1996.
90. Frankel HL, Hyslop HG, Melzak J, et al: The value of postural reduction in the initial management of closed injuries of the spine with paraplegia and tetraplegia. Part I. Paraplegia 1969;7:179–192.
91. Maiman DJ, Larson SJ, Benzel EC: Neurological improvement associated with late decompression of the thoracolumbar spinal cord. Neurosurgery 1984;14:302–307.
92. Larson SJ: Unstable thoracic fractures: Treatment alternatives and the role of the neurosurgeon. Clin Neurosurg 1980;36:624–640.
93. Ditunno JF, Young W, Donovan WH, et al: The international standards booklet for neurological and functional classification of spinal cord injury. Paraplegia 1994;32:70–80.
94. International standards for neurological and functional classification of spinal cord injury. Revised 1996. American Spinal Injury Association, International Medical Society of Paraplegia (ASIA/IMSOP), 1996.
95. Cohn SM, Lyle WG, Linden CH, et al: Exclusion of cervical spine injury: A prospective study. J Trauma 1991;31:570–574.
96. Burney RE, Waggoner R, Maynard PM: Stabilization of spinal injury for early transfer. J Trauma 1989;29:1497–1499.
97. Luque EQ, Cassis N, Ramirez-Wiella G: Segmental spinal instrumentation in the treatment of fractures of the thoracolumbar spine. Spine 1982;7:312–317.
98. Jacobs RR, Asher MA, Snider RK: Thoracolumbar spinal injuries: A comparative study of recumbent and operative treatment in 100 patients. Spine 1980;5:463–477.
99. Weinstein JN, Collalto P, Lehmann TR: Thoracolumbar (burst) fractures treated conservatively: A long term follow up. Spine 1988;13:33–38.
100. Kostuik JP: Anterior fixation for burst fractures of the thoracic and lumbar spine with or without neurological involvement. Spine 1988;13:286–293.
101. Dunn HK: Anterior spine stabilization and decompression for thoracolumbar injuries. Orthop Clin North Am 1986;7:113–119.
102. Krompinger WJ, Fredrickson BE, Mino DE, et al: Conservative treatment of fractures of the thoracic and lumbar spine. Orthop Clin North Am 1996;17:161–170.
103. Roy-Camille R, Saillant G, Mazel C: Plating of thoracic, thoracolumbar and lumbar injuries with pedicle screw plates. Orthop Clin North Am 1996;17:147–159.
104. Sullivan JA: Sublaminar wiring of Harrington distraction rods for unstable thoracolumbar spine fractures. Clin Orthop Rel Res 1984;189:178–185.
105. Wittenberg RH, Boetel U, Beyer HK: Magnetic resonance imaging and computer tomography of acute spinal cord trauma. Clin Orthop Rel Res 1990;260:176–185.
106. Goldberg AL, Rothfus WE, Deeb ZL: The impact of magnetic resonance on the diagnostic evaluation of acute cervicothoracic spinal trauma. Skel Radiol 1988;17:89–95.
107. Tracy PT, Wright RM, Hanigan WC: Magnetic resonance imaging of spinal injury. Spine 1989;14:292–301.
108. Emery SE, Pathria MN, Wilber RG: Magnetic resonance imaging of posttraumatic spinal ligament injury. J Spinal Disord 1989;2:229–233.
109. Schaefer DM, Flanders A, Northrup BE. Magnetic resonance imaging of acute cervical spine trauma: Correlation with severity of neurologic injury. Spine 1989;14:1090–1095.
110. Skalpe IO: Adhesive arachnoiditis following lumbar myelography. Spine 1978;3:61–64.
111. Petersen HO: The hazards of myelography. Radiology 1975;115:237–239.
112. Drory VE, Neufeld MY, Avrahamy E, et al: Serial EEG recordings following intrathecal metrizamide administration. Clin EEG 1989;20:202–208.

113. Maly P, Bach-Gansmo T, Elmqvist D: Risk of seizures after myelography: Comparison of iohexol and metrizamide. Am J Neuroradiol 1988;9:879–883.
114. Harris JH: Radiographic evaluation of spinal trauma. Orthop Clin North Am 1986;17:75–86.
115. Katoh Y, Itoh T, Tsuji H, et al: Complications of lateral C1–2 puncture myelography. Spine 1990;15:1085–1087.
116. Bracken MB, Shepard MJ, Hellenbrand KG, et al: Methylprednisolone and neurological function one year after spinal cord injury: Results of the national acute spinal cord injury study. J Neurosurg 1985;63:704–713.
117. Bracken MB, Collins WF, Freeman DF, et al: Efficacy of methylprednisolone in acute spinal cord injury. JAMA 1984;251:45–52.
118. Bracken MB, Holford TR: Effects of timing of methylprednisolone or naloxone administration on recovery of segmental and long tract neurological function in NASCIS-II. J Neurosurg 1993;79:500–507.
118a. Bracken MB, Shepard MJ, Holford TR, et al: Administration of methylprednisolone for 24 or 48 hours or tirilazad mesylate for 48 hours in the treatment of acute spinal cord injury. JAMA 1977;227:1597–1604.
119. Geisler FH, Dorsey FC, Coleman WP: Recovery of motor function after spinal cord injury: A randomized placebo-controlled trial with GM1 ganglioside. N Engl J Med 1991;324:1829–1838.
120. Cybulski GR: Methods of spinal stabilization for metastatic disease of the spine. Neurosurgery 1989;25:240–252.
121. Bohlman HH: Traumatic fractures of the upper thoracic spine with paralysis. J Bone Joint Surg 1974;56A:1299.
122. Morgan TH, Wharton GW, Austin GN: The results of laminectomy in patients with incomplete spinal cord injuries. Paraplegia 1971;9:14–23.
123. Paul RL, Michael RH, Dunn JE: Anterior transthoracic surgical decompression of acute spinal cord injuries. J Neurosurg 1975;43:299–307.
124. Kostuick JP, Matsusaki H: Anterior stabilization, instrumentation, and decompression for posttraumatic kyphosis. Spine 1989;14:379–386.
125. Larson SJ, Holst RA, Hemmy DC: Lateral extracavitary approach to traumatic lesions of the thoracic and lumbar spine. J Neurosurg 1976;45:628–637.
126. Garfin SR, Mowery CA, Guerra J, et al: Confirmation of the posterolateral technique to decompress and fuse thoracolumbar spine burst fractures. Spine 1985;10:218–223.
127. Hammerberg KW: Surgical treatment of metastatic spine disease. Spine 1992;17:1148–1153.
128. Kostuik JP: Anterior Kostuik-Harrington distraction systems for the treatment of kyphotic deformities. Spine 1990;15:169–180.
129. McAfee PC, Werner FW, Glisson RR: A biomechanical analysis of spinal instrumentation systems in thoracolumbar fractures: Comparison of traditional Harrington distraction instrumentation with segmental spinal instrumentation. Spine 1985;10:204–217.
130. Crutchfield WG: Skeletal traction and treatment of injuries of the cervical spine. JAMA 1954;115:29–32.
131. Sussman BJ: Early management of spinal cord trauma. J Neurosurg 1976;44:766–767.
132. Gardner WJ: The principle of spring-loaded points for cervical traction. J Neurosurg 1973;39:543–544.
133. Hollin SA, Hayashi H, Gross SW: Management of cervical spine dislocations with locked facets. Surg Gynecol Obstet 1967;124:521–524.
134. Brieg A: Overstretching of circumscribed pathological tension in the spinal cord: A basic cause of symptoms in cord disorders. J Biomechanics 1970;3:7–9.
135. Fried LC: Cervical spinal cord injury during skull retraction. JAMA 1974;229:181–183.
136. Kostuik JP: Decision making in adult scoliosis. Spine 1970;4:521–525.
137. Bradford DS, Ahmed KB, Moe JH: The surgical management of patients with Scheuermann's disease. J Bone Joint Surg 1980;62A:705–712.
138. Davies WE, Morris JH, Hill V: An analysis of conservative (nonsurgical) management of thoracolumbar fractures and fracture-dislocations with neural damage. J Bone Joint Surg 1980;62A:1324–1327.
139. Jones RF, Snowdon E, Coan J, et al: Bracing of thoracic and lumbar spine fractures. Paraplegia 1987;25:386–393.
140. Denis F, Armstrong GW, Searls K, et al: Acute thoracolumbar burst fractures in the absence of neurologic deficit: A comparison between operative and nonoperative treatment. Clin Orthop Rel Res 1984;189:142–149.
141. Wenger DR, Carollo JJ: The mechanics of thoracolumbar fracture stabilized by segmental fixation. Clin Orthop Rel Res 1984;189:89–96.
142. Braakman R: The value of more aggressive management in traumatic paraplegia. Neurosurg Rev 1986;9:141–147.
143. Holness RO, Huestis WS, Howes WJ, et al: Posterior stabilization with an interlaminar clamp in cervical injuries: Technical note and review of the long term experience with the method. Neurosurgery 1984;14:318–322.
144. Caspar W, Barbier DD, Klara PM: Anterior cervical fusion and Caspar plate stabilization for cervical trauma. Neurosurgery 1989;25:491–502.
145. Rechtine GR, Cahill GW, Gruenberg M, et al: The Synthes cervical spine locking plate and screw system in anterior cervical fusion. Tech Orthop 1994;9:86–91.
146. Roy-Camille R, Saillant G, Mazel C: Internal fixation of the unstable cervical spine by posterior osteosynthesis with plates and screws. In Cervical Spine Research Society Editorial Committee (eds): The Cervical Spine, 2nd ed, pp 390–404. Philadelphia, JB Lippincott, 1989.
147. Haid RW, Papadopoulos SM, Sonntag VK, et al: Posterior cervical stabilization with lateral mass osteosynthetic plate technique. In Levtech technical bulletin. Jacksonville, FL, Levtech, 1991.
148. Cooper PR, Cohen A, Rosiello A, et al: Posterior stabilization of cervical spine fractures and subluxations using plates and screws. Neurosurgery 1988;23:300–306.
149. An HS, Gordon R, Renner K: Anatomic considerations for plate-screw fixation of the cervical spine. Spine 1991;16(S):548–554.
150. Swank SM, Mauri TM, Brown JC: The lumbar lordosis below Harrington instrumentation for scoliosis. Spine 1990;15:181–186.
151. Hasday CA, Passoff TL, Perry J: Gait abnormalities arising from iatrogenic loss of lumbar lordosis secondary to Harrington instrumentation in lumbar fractures. Spine 1983;8:501–511.
152. McAfee PC, Bohlman HH: Complications following Harrington instrumentation for fractures of the thoracolumbar spine. J Bone Joint Surg 1985;67A:672–686.
153. Gertzbein SD, MacMichael D, Tile M: Harrington instrumentation as a method of fixation in fractures of the spine. J Bone Joint Surg 1982;64B:526–529.
154. Krag MH: Biomechanics of thoracolumbar spinal fixation: A review. Spine 1991;16:S84–S99.
155. Cotrel Y, Dubousset J, Guillaumat M: New universal instrumentation in spinal surgery. Clin Orthop Rel Res 1988;227:10–23.
156. Gurr KR, McAfee PC: Cotrel-Dubousse instrumentation in adults: A preliminary report. Spine 1988;13:510–520.
157. Kaneda K, Abumi K, Fujiya M: Burst fractures with neurologic deficits of the thoracolumbar-lumbar spine: Results of anterior decompression and stabilization with anterior instrumentation. Spine 1984;9:788–795.
158. Calenoff L, Chessare JW, Rogers LF: Multiple-level spinal injuries. Importance of early recognition. Am J Roentgenol 1978;130:665–669.
159. Tearse DS, Keene JS, Drummond DS: Management of noncontiguous vertebral fractures. Paraplegia 1987;25:100–105.
160. Lewis LM, Doucherty M, Ruoff BE, et al: Flexion-extension views in the evaluation of cervical spine injuries. Ann Emerg Med 1991;20:117–121.
161. Davidorf J, Hoyt D, Rosen P: Distal cervical spine evaluation using swimmer's flexion-extension radiographs. J Emerg Med 1993;11:55–59.
162. Borock EC, Gabram SG, Jacobs LM: The prospective analysis of a two-year experience using computer tomography

as an adjunct for cervical spine clearance. J Trauma 1991;31:1001–1006.
163. Levi L, Wolf A, Rigamonti D, et al: Anterior decompression in cervical spine trauma: Does the timing of surgery affect the outcome? Neurosurgery 1991;29:216–222.
164. Tator CH, Duncan EG, Edmonds EH, et al: Comparison of surgical and conservative management in 208 patients with acute spinal cord injury. Can J Neurol Sci 1987;14:60–69.
165. Benzel EC, Larson SJ: Functional recovery after decompressive operation for thoracic and lumbar spine fractures. Neurosurgery 1986;19:772–778.
166. McAfee PC, Bohlman HH, Yuan HA: Anterior decompression of traumatic thoracolumbar fractures with incomplete neurological deficit using a retroperitoneal approach. J Bone Joint Surg 1985;67A:89–104.
167. Transfeldt EE, White D, Bradford DS, et al: Delayed anterior decompression in patients with spinal cord and cauda equina injuries of the thoracolumbar spine. Spine 1990;15:953–957.
168. Tator CH: Classification of spinal cord injury based on neurological presentation. In Narayan RK, Wilberger JE, Povlishock JT (eds): Neurotrauma, pp 1039–1074. New York, McGraw-Hill, 1996.
169. Bell HS: Paralysis of both arms from injury of the upper portion of the pyramidal decussation (cruciate paralysis). J Neurosurg 1970;33:376–380.
170. Menezes AH: Tumors of the craniocervical junction. In Menezes AH, Sonntag VK (eds): Principles of Spinal Surgery, pp 1335–1353. New York, McGraw-Hill, 1996.
171. Tator CH: Spine-spinal cord relationships in spinal cord trauma. Clin Neurosurg 1983;30:479–494.
172. Shapiro S: Cauda equina syndrome secondary to lumbar disc herniation. Neurosurgery 1993;32:743–747.
173. Byrne TN: Spinal cord compression from epidural metastasis. N Engl J Med 1992;327:614–619.
174. Kollmer H, Diemath HE, Strohecker J, et al: Spinal metastasis as a first manifestation. Adv Neurosurg 1984;12:44–46.
175. Harris JR, Morrow M, Norton L: Malignant tumors of the breast. In De Vita VT, Hellman S, Rosenberg SA (eds): Cancer: Principles and Practice of Oncology, pp 1557–1616. Philadelphia, Lippincott–Raven, 1997.
176. Cooper PR, Errico TJ, Martin R, et al: A systematic approach to spinal reconstruction after anterior decompression for neoplastic disease of the thoracic and lumbar spine. Neurosurgery 1993;32:1–8.
177. Sundarasan N, DiGiacinto GV, Hughes GE, et al: Treatment of neoplastic spinal cord compression: Results of a prospective study. Neurosurgery 1991;29:645–650.
178. Bach S, Agerlin N, Svensen JB, et al: Metastatic spinal cord compression secondary to lung cancer. J Clin Oncol 1992;10:1781–1787.
179. Bridwell KH, Jenny A, Sawl T, et al: Posterior segmental spinal instrumentation (PSSI) with posterolateral decompression and debulking for metastatic thoracic and lumbar spine disease: Limitations of the technique. Spine 1988;13:1383–1384.
180. Oesterling JE, Fuks Z, Lee CT, et al: Cancer of the prostate. In De Vita VT, Hellman S, Rosenberg SA (eds): Cancer: Principles and Practice of Oncology, pp 1322–1385. Philadelphia, Lippincott–Raven, 1997.
181. Sundarasan N, Scher H, DiGiacinto GV, et al: Surgical treatment of spinal cord compression in kidney cancer. J Clin Oncol 1986;4:1851–1856.
182. King GJ, Kostuik JP, McBroom RJ, et al: Surgical management of metastatic renal carcinoma of the spine. Spine 1991;16:265–271.
183. Hitchon PW, Osenbach RK, Yuh WT, et al: Spinal infections. Clin Neurosurg 1992;38:373–387.
184. Osenbach RK, Hitchon PW, Menezes H: Diagnosis and management of pyogenic osteomyelitis in adults. Surg Neurol 1990;30:266–275.
185. Sharif HS: Role of MR imaging in the management of spinal infections. Am J Radiol 1992;158:1333–1345.
186. Cahill DW: Pyogenic infections of the spine. In Menezes AH, Sonntag VK (eds): Principles of Spinal Surgery, pp 1453–1456. New York, McGraw-Hill, 1996.
187. Weinstein JN: Surgical approach to spine tumors. Orthopaedics 1989;12:897–905.
188. Frymoyer JW (ed): The Adult Spine: Principles and Practice. New York, Raven Press, 1991.
189. Menezes AH, Sonntag VK (eds): Principles of Spinal Surgery. New York, McGraw-Hill, 1996.
190. Cahill DW: Malignant tumors of the bony spine. In Menezes AH, Sonntag VK (eds): Principles of Spinal Surgery, pp 1401–1421. New York, McGraw-Hill, 1996.
191. Schnee CL, Weil RJ, Freese AW, et al: Evaluation of operative technique for thoracolumbar spinal neoplasms. Manuscript submitted.
192. Weller SJ, Rossitch E: Unilateral posterolateral decompression without stabilization for neurological palliation of symptomatic spinal metastasis in debilitated patients. J Neurosurg 1995;82:739–744.
193. Shucart WA, Borden JA. Lateral approaches to the cervical spine. In Menezes AH, Sonntag VK (eds): Principles of Spinal Surgery, pp 1325–1332. New York, McGraw-Hill, 1996.
194. Fielding JW, Stillwell WT: Anterior cervical approaches to the upper thoracic spine: A case report. Spine 1976;1:159–161.
195. Sundarasan N, Shah J, Foley KM, et al: An anterior surgical approach to the upper thoracic vertebrae. J Neurosurg 1984;61:686–692.
196. Seigel T: Current considerations in the management of neoplastic spinal cord compression. Spine 1989;14:223–228.
197. Bhojraj SY, Dantawate AV, Ramakanton R: Preoperative embolization, transpedicular decompression and posterior stabilization for metastatic disease of the thoracic spine causing paraplegia. Paraplegia 1992;30:292–299.
198. McCormick B, Mayer D, Fessler RG: Anterior approaches to the lumbar spine. In Menezes AH, Sonntag VK (eds): Principles of Spinal Surgery, pp 1293–1306. New York, McGraw-Hill, 1996.

dimensional CBF measurements (stable xenon–CT CBF technique). That study then proposed the occurrence of "global cerebral ischemia" in patients with regional compression due to acute subdural hematomas.[35] Once again, true confirmation of ischemic changes was lacking, because concomitant cerebral metabolic assessment was not carried out, as would have been required in acutely comatose patients.

In light of the clinically relevant findings addressing a major mortality reduction in patients subjected to prompt removal of acute subdural hematomas,[34] it is apparent (even though not yet demonstrated) that early hematoma removal minimizes not only the undesired effects of upper brain stem compression but also compressive supratentorial ischemia in the regions underlying the clot. Accordingly, it would appear advisable to avoid delaying surgical procedures when dealing with possible compressive cerebral ischemia.

Oligemic Cerebral Hypoxia

Since we first introduced the technique for continuous fiberoptic monitoring of cerebrovenous oxygenation,[36] the term *oligemic cerebral hypoxia* (flow-dependent hypoxia) was coined to define a condition of abnormally low cerebrovenous oxygenation in the presence of normal arterial oxygenation. We later further detailed the occurrence of oligemic cerebral hypoxia (primarily in the early postinjury hours) in relation to the outcome of patients with acute intracranial hypertension.[28] Without information about clinical outcome, however, other investigators[37] used the same technique we had previously proposed and adopted the term *ischemia* to define the same changes we had defined as oligemic hypoxia.

In fact, as mentioned earlier, we later found that initially moderately increased CEO_2, with jugular oxyhemoglobin saturation levels of approximately 45%, is more indicative of global cerebral viability than ischemia because, in the absence of profound acute anemia, this moderate increase in cerebral oxygen extraction was found to be associated with excellent outcome figures in patients with traumatic brain swelling (with or without associated hemorrhagic contusions).[28] Accordingly, the term *ischemia* appears inadequate to describe moderate cerebrovenous hypoxia without concomitant assessment of cerebral ischemic metabolites such as lactate.

It should be emphasized, however, that we have routinely attempted to therapeutically normalize increased CEO_2 values,[38, 39] just as we have also routinely attempted to normalize decreased CEO_2 levels (relative cerebral hyperperfusion) whenever they are associated with intracranial hypertension.[11, 13, 14]

Relative Cerebral Hyperperfusion

Some investigators evaluating cerebral oxygenation have primarily stressed abnormalities related to low cerebral venous oxygen levels.[37, 40] In contrast with this latter approach, we have looked at "both sides of the coin"—that is, we have evaluated and managed both increased and decreased CEO_2 values. Clinically, relative cerebral hyperperfusion (decreased CEO_2) may be a most relevant pattern of cerebral hemometabolic pathophysiology in severe acute brain trauma with associated brain swelling and intracranial hypertension.[11, 13, 14, 41]

Although relative cerebral hyperperfusion may or may not be associated with intracranial hypertension, its frequent occurrence after the first 12 hours post injury[11, 18, 41] does allow for a specific therapeutic approach, as follows.

For managing acute brain swelling and related intracranial hypertension, little can be done to promptly decrease brain mass or pericontusional edema, except for the transient effects of osmotic agents such as mannitol. This therapy, however, tends to further increase CBF[23] and cerebrovenous oxygenation,[38] which may be an undesired response in some conditions such as ongoing relative cerebral hyperperfusion. Furthermore, cumulative mannitol administration frequently leads to profound serum hyperosmolality, which indicates discontinuation of this particular therapeutic modality, at least until normal osmolality values are resumed.

In addition, there is usually little or no cerebrospinal fluid (CSF) to be removed from patients with compressed lateral ventricles in brain swelling. Another frequent component contributing to acute intracranial hypertension is subarachnoid hemorrhage, which is not promptly manageable either. Accordingly, in light of the mentioned limitations in reducing brain mass, brain edema, CSF volume, and subarachnoid blood, the most logical therapeutic approach for acute intracranial hypertension consists of reducing cerebral blood volume (and thereby CBF), but without compromising cerebral oxygen delivery relative to oxygen consumption.

Under circumstances of relative cerebral hyperperfusion, optimized hyperventilation[11–14] constitutes a most physiologic, practical, inexpensive approach to normalize intracranial hypertension while offsetting the condition of relative cerebral hyperperfusion. Furthermore, optimized hyperventilation is also capable of restoring normal coupling between cerebral oxygen and glucose extraction, thereby optimizing global cerebral aerobic metabolism as well.[13]

It should be emphasized that the condition of relative cerebral hyperperfusion does not necessarily imply cerebral hyperemia (increased CBF values, in absolute terms). In fact, as mentioned earlier, all previous studies in this area have disclosed pathologically reduced cerebral oxygen consumption, so that even normal CBF levels do represent relative cerebral hyperperfusion. Accordingly, one should not try to explain intracranial hypertension as being exclusively caused by absolute cerebral hyperemia (abnormally high CBF levels).[24] Rather, considering that many factors (besides blood volume and blood flow) may contribute to acute intracranial hypertension, the notion of manageable relative cerebral hyperperfusion (decreased CEo_2) with associated intracranial hypertension should be kept in mind, irrespective of any particular value of relative or absolute hyperemia according to CBF alone.

INITIAL EVALUATION AND MANAGEMENT

Early Patient Stabilization

In recent years, much has been improved in terms of prehospital care, as well as fast transportation to specialized trauma centers. Thus, early restoration of airway patency at the trauma scene appears to be a major contribution in itself, especially in patients with clinical signs of respiratory depression. In fact, reports from the prehospital care team have sometimes addressed restoration of pupillary reactivity and motor responses in initially unresponsive patients shortly following intubation and manual hyperventilation (unpublished observations).

An additional major contribution of the emergency care teams working at the trauma scene is their ability to rapidly administer intravenous solutions in patients found to be initially hypotensive. This approach tends to minimize potential undesired effects of ischemic brain damage in patients with defective cerebral pressure autoregulation. Because the status of pressure autoregulation is not assessable at the scene of the accident, vigorous intravenous crystalloid fluid loading would appear to be always advisable, at least until the hospital is reached and additional diagnostic procedures are undertaken.

Although the initial presence of normal pupillary signs grossly rules out life-threatening intracranial herniation, therefore allowing for "conservative" management, a major challenge in the ultra-early evaluation of these patients is the combination of arterial hypotension and pupillary enlargement. Under these circumstances, if pupillary responses are not restored by the fast intravenous administration of hypertonic mannitol alone, "semi-empirical" hyperventilation should follow, along with rapid intravenous fluid loading to compensate for the potentially dangerous hypovolemic effects of mannitol. Repetitive mannitol administration in the ultra-early stage of injury may be contraindicated by the simultaneous occurrence of arterial hypotension and unstable systemic hemodynamics.

In fact, even if restoration of adequate blood pressure can be rapidly achieved, the risk of recurrent arterial hypotension still contraindicates, at least in part, the frequent repetitive use of mannitol under these life-threatening conditions. A possible alternative to mannitol might be dihydroergotamine or indomethacin, but future research would be necessary regarding their use under such circumstances.

As a general rule, persistent and grossly abnormal pupillary signs for several minutes (despite prompt initial management) frequently constitute an ominous outcome predictor from the very early phase of management. In this respect, further therapeutic investigations are necessary, aiming at the prompt reversal of these ominous neurologic abnormalities at the trauma scene. Such an accomplishment would largely affect the initial management of what can be currently regarded as a most challenging entity in the ultra-early stage of severe acute brain trauma.

In contrast, when pupils are initially normal, profound hyperventilation would not appear logical and should be reserved for later times, after arteriojugular monitoring is implemented. This is because CBF may be initially decreased and properly coupled with reduced cerebral oxygen consumption in the very early stage of injury,[18, 28] in contrast with relative cerebral hyperperfusion (a logical indication for moderate and profound hyperventilation), which generally develops within a few hours and lasts for 3–4 days or occasionally longer.[11, 13, 18] Additional information on initial stabilization of patients with severe acute brain trauma can be found in Chapter 1.

Early Laboratory Findings

1. **Blood gases:** In light of recent advances regarding prehospital care, most patients arrive at the hospital with relatively acceptable values of arterial blood gases. The same, however, does not necessarily apply to certain geographic regions where advanced trauma life support at the scene has not yet been fully implemented. Under these circumstances, arterial hypoxemia, hypercarbia, or both are still frequently found on initial blood analyses. Further operational capabilities allowing paramedic professionals to intubate and ventilate patients would be

desirable wherever this approach has not yet become a routine.

As a general rule, initial ventilatory adjustments should allow for arterial Po_2 (Pao_2) and Pco_2 ($Paco_2$) in the approximate ranges of 150 and 30 torr (20 and 4 kPa), respectively. Acute acidosis may require therapeutic correction with sodium bicarbonate, because induced alkalotic hyperventilation may or may not be used until later times only (see Presumed Intracranial Hypertension, later).

2. **Blood hemoglobin:** Severe acute anemia is infrequent on the initial evaluation of severe acute brain trauma without associated systemic injuries (except in very small children, in whom an isolated intracranial hematoma may occasionally drop the total hemoglobin content significantly). Thus, markedly decreased initial values of total hemoglobin content (lower than 9–10 g/dL) should be promptly followed by a careful search for systemic sources of acute blood loss. Once these latter sources have been ruled out, the diagnosis of "idiopathic traumatic anemia" could then be contemplated, but only by exclusion. Red cell transfusions should always be considered when the total hemoglobin content drops below 10 g/dL. This approach minimizes the potential risks of anemic-hypoxic brain damage associated with low cerebral oxygen delivery.
3. **Serum electrolytes:** Marked and clinically relevant serum electrolyte abnormalities are not a general rule on the initial measurements, at least in relation to serum calcium, sodium, and potassium. One possibility for early hypernatremia (if associated with polyuria) is central diabetes insipidus (DI). DI may be an ominous outcome predictor if it occurs during the early postinjury hours. Hypotonic intravenous fluid replacement (milliliter per milliliter) should be considered, along with supplementary administration of aqueous vasopressin or arginine vasopressin, whenever the diagnosis of DI is confirmed by low levels of urine sodium, urine specific gravity, urine osmolality, or a combination thereof (see Supportive Measures, later).

Initially low serum magnesium levels (< 1.5 mEq/L) may be frequently found in alcoholics and may be associated with cardiac arrhythmias. Therefore, proper replacement should be considered early on. In recent years, abnormally low serum magnesium levels have also been postulated as possible contributors to brain injury severity. This notion, however, is largely based on small-animal experimentation revealing low magnesium concentrations in the traumatized brain tissue.[4, 7] Nevertheless, magnesium replacement therapy to maintain normal serum levels is indicated.

Although grossly abnormal serum electrolyte levels may not be a frequent problem on the initial measurements, they may be frequent at later times during the acute phase (see Supportive Measures, later).

4. **Blood clotting patterns:** Early acute coagulopathy is a frequent, clinically relevant finding in patients with severe acute brain trauma, whether or not associated with systemic injuries.[42, 43] Thus, early evaluation of blood clotting tests is of paramount importance. In fact, without early identification of acute hypocoagulopathic disorders, prompt treatment would not even be considered. Such lack of management could in turn severely compromise the efficacy of surgical interventions for removal of acute intracranial hematomas, wherein "excessive bleeding" might remain "unexplained." In addition, lack of early treatment might exacerbate the risk of acute or subacute intracranial bleeding or rebleeding.

In the presence of increased prothrombin time (> 15 seconds), increased activated partial thromboplastin time (> 35 seconds), and/or decreased platelet count (< 100,000/mm^3 in adults or < 150,000/mm^3 in children), *immediate* management steps should be taken. A most practical means of treating acute hypocoagulopathic disorders is by the intravenous administration of fresh frozen plasma, platelets, or both. Large amounts of fresh frozen plasma may be required to restore normal clotting tests. Once initial hypocoagulopathic disorders have been corrected, additional clotting abnormalities may still occur at later times during the acute phase, most frequently because of induced hypothermia, sepsis, or both.

5. **Toxicologic evaluation:** Acute ethanol intoxication may be a frequent finding, which may confound early outcome prediction. In fact, initially deeply comatose patients, sometimes presenting with Glasgow Coma Scale[44] (GCS) scores as low as 3, may rapidly improve over the initial 12–24 hours, irrespective of any specific management modality.

Acute cocaine intoxication is also frequent in some geographic regions. It may be responsible for nontraumatic acute intracranial bleeding (usually subarachnoid, intraparenchymal, or both),[45, 46] which may be confounded with traumatic intracranial hemorrhages in patients with severe acute brain trauma. Another frequent complication of acute cocaine intoxication is arterial hypertension, which may superimpose on the ongoing arterial hypertensive response of acute traumatic hypercatecholanemia.[47] These mixed pathophysiologic patterns might lead to potentially confusing interpretation of changes expected to occur in "standard" severe acute brain trauma alone.

Presumed Intracranial Hypertension

Empirical management of presumed intracranial hypertension should be carefully considered. This is because, although some patients may be initially deeply comatose, even with abnormal posturing, diffuse axonal injury (DAI) may be solely responsible for such dramatic neurologic changes. DAI, in turn, is not necessarily associated with brain swelling and elevated intracranial pressure (ICP), a condition known as "pure DAI." Thus, a less empirical therapeutic approach before ICP monitoring is initiated would be to combine hyperventilation ($Paco_2$ < 30 torr [< 4 kPa]) with intravenous boluses of hypertonic mannitol (500–750 mg/kg). This combined treatment step is based on previous demonstration that mannitol boluses during hyperventilation further potentiate the hypocapnic effects of lowering ICP while normalizing decreased levels of cerebrovenous oxygenation.[38] Such a synergistic response appears to be most relevant, especially when ICP and cerebrovenous oxygenation have not yet been measured.

In addition to administering mannitol and inducing hypocapnic changes, *transient* arterial hyperoxia is also of potential benefit. This is because hyperoxia not only increases arterial oxygenation but leads to cerebral vasoconstriction. This combination ultimately results in lowering presumably elevated initial ICP values while maintaining adequate cerebral oxygen delivery. Thus, 100% levels of fraction of inspired oxygen should be routinely considered until subsequent patient stabilization. High positive end-expiratory pressure should be initially avoided, especially because some patients may have occult pneumothorax, to be further evaluated and managed. Pneumothorax, in turn, could be rapidly and dangerously exacerbated by high positive end-expiratory pressure.

Acute Seizure Disorders

Anticonvulsant therapy should be considered in the presence of initial clinical signs of acute seizure disorder. However, there is currently no evidence to support the routine use of prophylactic anticonvulsant medication in severe acute brain trauma, except when focal lesions are documented on neurodiagnostic tests. For rapid anticonvulsant management, benzodiazepines, phenytoin, or both appear to be the most practical options. In refractory cases, however, fosphenytoin, barbiturate therapy, or propofol administration may be required as alternative steps (see also Chapter 4).

Confounding Factors in Early Neurologic Evaluation

In addition to frequent acute ethanol intoxication in severely brain injured patients,[48] early administration of muscle relaxants for emergency endotracheal intubation before hospital admission has resulted in a growing number of possibly inaccurate reported GCS scores of 3.[48, 49] In fact, although true GCS scores of 3 with associated pupillary abnormalities are frequently indicative of impending brain death, patients who might have been inaccurately classified as GCS 3 have been reported to experience good neurologic recovery.[48, 49]

Initial Neurodiagnostic Assessment

Since CT scans of the head became available, skull radiographs have only infrequently provided additional clinically relevant information in severe acute brain trauma. Conversely, although fast head CT can be easily performed, the same does not apply to spinal CT evaluation. Therefore, emergency assessment of associated spinal injuries still relies primarily on radiographic information. Subsequent spinal evaluation by imaging techniques such as CT and magnetic resonance imaging (MRI) would be considered after adequate physiologic stabilization of the patients. Because ICP problems may last several days, however, and because prolonged imaging tests frequently require placing the patient's head in the undesired flat position, spinal imaging procedures have been usually postponed to a subacute phase. Thus, the initial management of spinal injuries associated with traumatic intracranial hypertension has been largely based on combined clinical and radiologic judgment from plain spinal radiographs (see Associated Spinal Trauma, later).

With regard to imaging studies of the head, little or no evidence supports the routine adoption of MRI instead of CT. Not only are the MRI suites less suitable for physiologic monitoring, but the design of most MRI units precludes frequent reassessment of at least pupillary changes, which are crucial during the first hours. In contrast, CT suites do allow for more adequate clinical and physiologic monitoring under emergency conditions. Furthermore, for most acute traumatic lesion types, CT is as informative as MRI, except for rare forms of acute isodense intracranial hematomas and more "subtle" forms of DAI. The latter, however, are not manageable (at least in current days), and their confirmation would seem to be largely of prognostic interest. Thus, it appears that CT scan of the head will remain as the first imaging option for these patients, especially in the most acute stage of illness.

If CT is not available for emergency diagnostic evaluation, conventional cerebral angiography could still be regarded as a practical and informative alternative. Even with unilateral puncture of the common carotid artery, contrast injection with brief compression of the contralateral carotid frequently provides adequate bilateral anteroposterior visualization of the major supratentorial arterial territories. An additional lateral view may also be obtained to further elucidate vascular configuration.

This procedure, however, does not inform about changes such as brain swelling and small structural insults (small contusions, DAI). It does not inform about acute changes in the posterior fossa either. Nevertheless, surgically amenable lesions in the supratentorial space can be indirectly diagnosed on the basis of arterial displacement; associated vessel abnormalities can be also identified. A more time-consuming angiographic assessment would involve catheterization techniques. The latter provide additional information regarding the status of the posterior circulation, thus allowing for identification of acute traumatic lesions in the posterior fossa as well.

In contrast, near-infrared spectroscopy for bedside localization of intracranial hematomas[50] cannot reliably replace CT or angiography. This is particularly true because, for proper preoperative and intraoperative planning, adequate information regarding type (epidural, subdural, intraparenchymal), size, and location of the clot is of paramount importance. In the case of intraparenchymal hematomas, further information regarding extracapsular versus intracapsular location is important concerning indications for surgical versus nonsurgical management. Knowledge of associated vascular abnormalities may also be relevant in some cases. This broad spectrum of acute diagnostic changes, however, cannot be fine-tuned by near-infrared spectroscopy.[51]

On the basis of CT findings, the following steps apply: (1) For patients without an acute mass lesion, but whose CSF spaces are not fully preserved, placement of an ICP monitor would be indicated as soon as possible. (2) In cases of surgically amenable hematomas, time may be of the essence, and fast transfer from the CT suite to the operating room would be most appropriate; emergency preoperative mannitol administration (0.75–1 g/kg) should also be considered. (3) In patients with fully preserved CSF spaces—normal CT findings, small contusions, or pure DAI (all of these without associated regional, hemispheral, or diffuse brain swelling)—placement of an ICP monitor could be eventually disregarded in adult patients (unlike children).

The reason for this latter approach is that, unlike the pediatric population of severely brain-injured patients, in the adult population the development of clinically relevant subacute hemispheral or diffuse brain swelling is unusual if the first CT scan and a repeat test after 6–8 hours show fully preserved CSF spaces (unpublished observations). As to the development of subacute mass lesions, the second routine CT scan (within 6–8 hours from the first one, or sooner if clinical deterioration occurs) discloses new findings more frequently than what would be suspected from ICP monitoring. This situation is particularly true in intraparenchymal hematomas or extra-axial clots in the temporal fossa, which may result in life-threatening changes without relevant increases in ICP.[52–54] Additionally, the development of focal neurologic signs could also indicate the need for repeat CT scan of the head at any time throughout the acute phase.

ASSOCIATED SPINAL TRAUMA

Combined spinal and head injuries usually involve the cervical spine, occurring in approximately 6% of patients with acute head injuries but only 2.4% of those in acute coma.[55] Even though relatively infrequent, cervical spinal involvement in severe acute brain trauma may be a diagnostic and therapeutic challenge, even more than in isolated spinal injuries.

Because the acutely comatose patient is unable to cooperate for the neurologic examination, and because combined spinal cord and brain trauma may present with overlapping neurologic signs, plain anteroposterior and lateral radiographs of the entire spine are of paramount importance as soon as the patient is stabilized in the emergency room (if possible), to promptly confirm or rule out at least the most immediately manageable traumatic spinal cord injury—namely, that produced by vertebral displacement encroaching against the spinal canal. In acutely comatose patients with severe acute brain trauma, flexion-extension lateral radiographs of the cervical spine are contraindicated, and open-mouth odontoid views are frequently not obtainable. Once the patient has been stabilized from the intracranial and systemic life-threatening conditions, further evaluation of spinal injuries should be accomplished by more sophisticated neuroimaging studies, emphasizing areas that are sometimes poorly evaluated by plain radiographs, such as the cervicothoracic junction and the upper cervical levels.

In fact, in patients whose most life-threatening problems are felt to be associated with acute intracranial hypertension requiring early management, little can be done in terms of emergency surgical management of associated spinal injuries. Whenever traumatic vertebral body displacement is found on plain radiographs, emergency placement of a traction device may be a critically relevant step to possibly realign the displaced vertebral bodies nonsurgically and at least potentially increase the chances of a fair recovery. Early cervical traction can be used only in patients whose CT findings rule out the need for emergency craniotomy. Because time is of the essence when decompressing the spinal cord by traction, and the neurologic examination of comatose patients frequently precludes fine-tuned localization of a spinal cord injury, clinical neurologic assessment should be rapid and simple so as not to delay the quick placement of a traction device when indicated by abnormal radiographic findings.

In addition to the neurologic examination, gentle palpation of the entire spine is also indicated, because it may disclose additional signs of spinal injury, such as deformities ("steps"), crepitus, or indirect signs of a paraspinal hematoma. Again, because of several limitations regarding clinical assessment of spinal cord injuries in a comatose patient, somatosensory and motor evoked potentials should be considered for better evaluation of these suspected or confirmed insults.

Management of airway, breathing, and circulation (ABCs) is standard for the acutely comatose patient (see also Chapter 1), and also helps prevent secondary spinal cord insults. In the case of arterial hypotension, anticholinergic agents are advisable (besides intravenous fluid and vasopressor administration) to treat vagotonic effects, at least until a spinal cord injury has been ruled out. Endotracheal intubation should be with the head in neutral position or with limited movement of the neck whenever an associated cervical spinal injury is suspected or confirmed prior to intubation. This latter approach, however, is limited in many acutely comatose patients who require immediate intubation at the scene of the accident, before accurate neurologic examination can be performed.

In addition, whenever acute spinal cord trauma is suspected by clinical or radiographic findings, its emergency nonsurgical management currently involves early (within the first 4–6 hours) intravenous administration of high-dose methylprednisolone given during 24 hours only, starting with an intravenous bolus of 30 mg/kg (first hour) and following with continuous infusion of approximately 5.4 mg/kg per hour over the next 23 hours.

Early immobilization of the spine is of paramount importance and can be satisfactorily achieved with

TABLE 16–1 **CLINICAL SIGNS IN COMATOSE PATIENTS WITH ASSOCIATED SPINAL CORD INJURY**

1. Brown-Séquard syndrome—may be conclusive, but assessment is limited to cross-painful stimulation
2. Dissociated motor responses to pain in both upper versus lower limbs—usually conclusive
3. Arterial hypotension with associated bradycardia—usually conclusive
4. Priapism—conclusive
5. Motor response to pain limited to head and face movements—usually conclusive, but occasionally is due to the brain injury alone
6. Horner's syndrome—not necessarily conclusive (may be due to the brain injury alone)
7. Sweating level—not necessarily conclusive (may be due to the brain injury [severe diffuse axonal injury] alone, with sweating more pronounced on the head and upper trunk); lower sweating levels are more conclusive
8. Areflexia—not necessarily conclusive (may be due to the brain injury alone)
9. Paradoxical breathing patterns—not necessarily conclusive (may be due to associated chest trauma)

such measures as cervical collars, tongs and traction, halo vests, and fracture boards. Log rolling at 2-hour intervals is also important to prevent pressure sores and should be initiated as soon as possible.

Table 16–1 shows some of the clinical findings that may or may not indicate associated spinal cord injuries in acutely comatose patients with severe brain trauma. As seen, many of the clinical signs that frequently help in the combined diagnosis of head and spinal trauma in conscious patients do not apply to acutely comatose subjects. Therefore, clinical clues for diagnosing associated spinal cord injury in severe acute brain trauma are limited. Additional information on surgical and nonsurgical management of acute spinal injuries may be found in Chapter 15.

SURGICAL MANAGEMENT

On the basis of initial neurodiagnostic findings, intracranial hematomas with mass effect should be immediately evacuated. Extra-axial hematomas (epidural, subdural) located in the middle fossa, with basitemporal compression and perimesencephalic obliteration, should be surgically evacuated by a combination of partial aspiration through the first basitemporal burr hole and mini-craniectomy, followed by full visualization and removal through full craniotomy or craniectomy. This procedure would "buy time" to prevent severe and prolonged compression of upper brain stem structures. Additional steps for surgical management involve distinct features based on the type of hematoma (either supratentorial or infratentorial), as follows:

1. **Acute epidural hematoma**: Midsize craniotomies or craniectomies are usually

adequate, except for ultra-large clots requiring more generous craniotomies (Fig. 16–2). Hematoma removal and identification of the bleeding sources are usually uneventful. Epidural bleeding vessels may be easily cauterized or even clipped, whereas epidural blood oozing may be treated with topical hemostatic products. The bleeding source, however, is not necessarily found in some cases, especially when epidural bleeding develops from small arterial or venous branches, because bleeding from these small vessels may have resolved by the time of hematoma removal. Nevertheless, locating and cauterizing or clipping the bleeding vessels is relevant to prevent postoperative epidural hemorrhage. Other bleeding sources may originate from skull fractures (sometimes involving the skull base). In these cases, bleeding may be satisfactorily controlled with bone wax.

After hematoma removal, once the dura mater is fully visualized and hemostasis is accomplished, exploration of the subdural space by a small dural opening might be considered in selected cases, on the basis of either preoperative CT findings or the intraoperative suspicion of a subdural lesion. Subdural exploration would allow for documentation of cortical-subcortical contusions and possible additional bleeding sources. The latter would justify such an approach, because adequate hemostasis could represent the avoidance of postoperative subdural or intraparenchymal hematoma formation. Additional hemostasis of small bleeding sources may be required with topical hemostatic products, in case hemostasis is not feasible by cauterization.

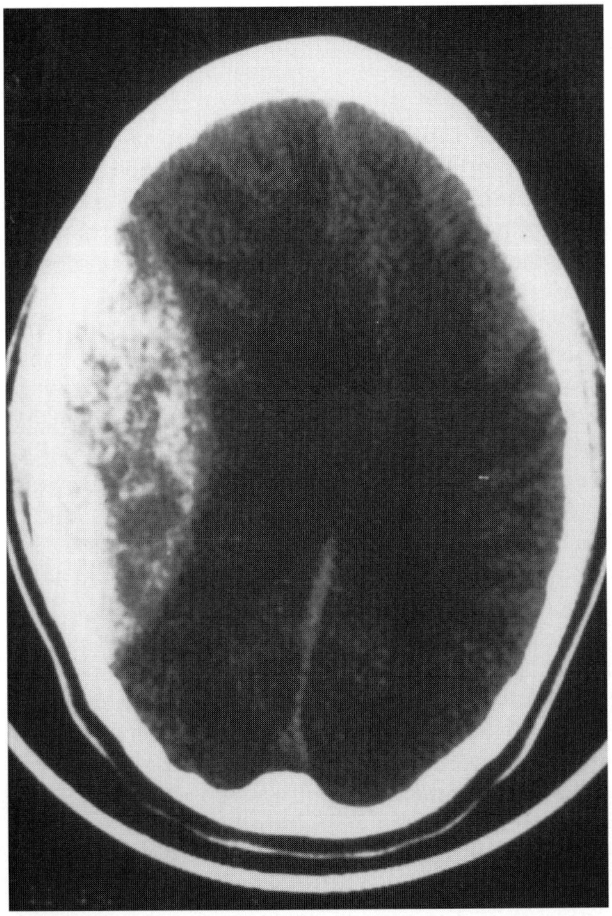

FIGURE 16–2 • Computed tomography of the head revealing a large right acute epidural hematoma, which was evacuated through a generous craniotomy.

Dural tack-up sutures are always recommended, both centrally and peripherally. This maneuver prevents epidural hematoma reaccumulation, which is particularly relevant in patients with acute hypocoagulopathic disorders or those in whom a bleeding source was missed intraoperatively because of temporary spontaneous hemostasis.

Controversy appears to surround nonsurgical management of acute epidural hematomas that are asymptomatic or nearly so. Whether this conservative approach may be contemplated for supratentorial hematomas remote from the perimesencephalic cistern, we *strongly* recommend that all acute epidural hematomas in the temporal fossa or the posterior fossa be immediately removed, even if they are small. This is because these patients may initially present relatively asymptomatic while harboring a "small" clot. The latter, however, may *rapidly* enlarge, leading to dramatic life-threatening changes within ultra-short periods.

Figure 16–3 illustrates a case wherein nonsurgical management was first sought, because the basitemporal hematoma was felt to be small (see Fig. 16–3*A*). Initially conscious and oriented, the patient rapidly became comatose, with contralateral hemiparesis and ipsilateral pupillary widening in relation to the hematoma side. Repeat CT disclosed enlargement of the acute epidural clot (see Fig. 16–3*B*), which was then evacuated. In acute intracranial hematomas, a frequently overlooked diagnostic aspect is that CT is performed over a short period and offers a steady picture of a frequently dynamic process, so that the actively bleeding lesion may further enlarge shortly after CT is done.

Despite adequate intraoperative hemostasis, hematoma reaccumulation may develop, even after rapid normalization of blood clotting tests (either therapeutic or spontaneous). Therefore, all patients with initial hypocoagulopathic disorders should undergo repeat CT immediately after surgery. If that study is unrevealing, another CT scan should be obtained within 6–8 hours.

2. **Acute subdural hematoma**: Generous

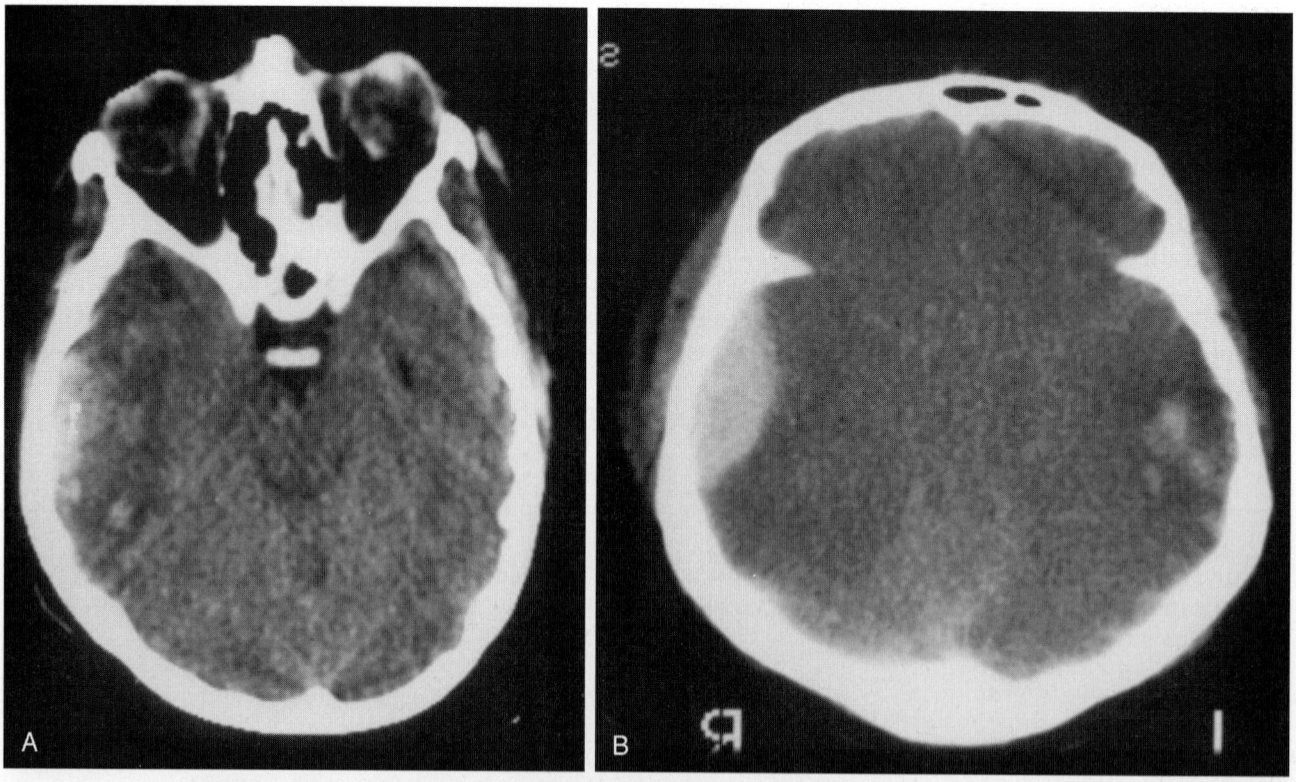

FIGURE 16–3 • The initial computed tomography of the head revealed a small right temporal acute extra-axial hematoma (*A*), which rapidly enlarged as a typical epidural hematoma (*B*) and was then evacuated. Notice the contralateral hemorrhagic contusion, as well as signs of diffuse brain swelling in *B*.

craniotomies are generally indicated because these clots frequently spread over large areas of the brain, even though they may not be always very thick (Fig. 16–4). If there is a fracture across a venous sinus, the neurosurgeon should be ready to deal with profuse sinus bleeding, which often is a challenging event, as follows: to fully visualize the sinus tear, the edge of the craniotomy may have to be expanded toward the sinus, at the same time when profuse bleeding may make it a difficult maneuver. In addition, a temporary sinus-sinus shunt may be necessary to properly repair the sinus tear without compromising sinus blood flow. Massive red cell transfusions may be required in these cases.

Sinus ligation may be performed, but our preference has been to limit this procedure to the anterior quarter of the superior sagittal sinus only while avoiding ligation involving more posterior segments of this structure.

Inverse U-shaped, as well as Y-shaped or X-shaped (cruciform) dural openings may be adopted, depending on the neurosurgeon's experience. Whether or not an associated contusion is to be removed, we do not recommend a circular dural opening with additional extended openings toward the edges of the craniotomy. Our approach is such because any one of the three mentioned types of dural opening will also expose the contusional brain while allowing for a shorter procedure than the expanded circular opening, insofar as dural closure is concerned.

Hematoma removal must be careful to minimize the chances of bleeding from previously tamponade vessels. Although small bleeding vessels may be cauterized or managed with topical hemostatic products, large cortical veins should not be definitively obliterated, unless the large venous walls have been grossly damaged and hemostasis cannot be achieved with topical hemostatic products. A major concern under these circumstances is that large venous infarction could easily develop after total obliteration of a large cortical vein, with potentially catastrophic consequences during the postoperative phase. In the presence of venous infarction, brain swelling would be expected, and a second (decompressive) operation may be required early on.

The same hemostatic features described for acute epidural hematomas would apply to acute subdural clots. Therefore, hematoma reaccumulation may occur, especially in initially hypocoagulopathic patients. As in the case of acute epidural hematoma, reoperation for acute subdural hematoma is usually easier than the initial procedure, insofar as hemo-

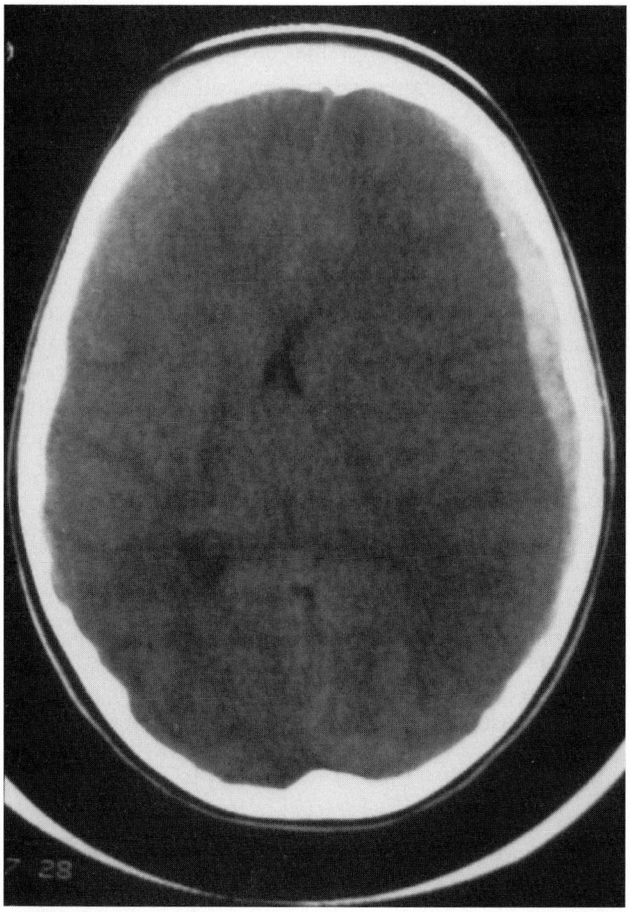

FIGURE 16–4 • Computed tomography of the head revealing a left acute subdural hematoma (which was evacuated), with associated left hemispheral swelling and midline shift out of proportion to the hematoma size.

stasis is concerned. Unlike epidural hematomas, dural tack-up sutures are optional in acute subdural hematoma surgery, because postoperative epidural bleeding is not always a concern. In hypocoagulopathic patients, however, dural tack-up sutures should be routinely performed after dural closure.

Acute subdural hematomas are more frequently associated with contusions than acute epidural hematomas. Brain swelling is also more frequent in acute subdural than epidural hematomas. Therefore, decompressive surgery may be necessary in patients harboring acute subdural clots, under the following circumstances: (1) the clot itself is not very thick but the hemorrhagic contusion is sizable, leading to mass effect (frequently compressing the basilar cisterns); (2) the clot itself is not very thick but hemispheral swelling may be pronounced, out of proportion to the hematoma size (see Fig. 16–4); and (3) the clot is large, with associated small or midsize contusions, and acute "rebound" brain swelling is found after clot removal.

These three conditions frequently require decompressive surgery. Although contemporary anesthetic techniques do allow for temporary intraoperative control of rebound brain swelling in some patients, the same is not necessarily true during postoperative care. Furthermore, in a few patients the rebound brain swelling is so pronounced that even the scalp cannot be properly closed without tension. In our experience, intraoperative management of severe brain swelling is better achieved with fast intravenous administration of high-dose 25% mannitol (approximately 1 g/kg) combined with temporary profound hyperventilation, with $Pa{CO_2}$ less than 25 torr (< 3.3 kPa) and supplemented by barbiturate therapy or propofol administration, if necessary.

Although the combination of mannitol and hyperventilation tends to simultaneously decrease brain volume and offset relative cerebral hypoperfusion,[38] prompt intravenous fluid replacement is mandatory to compensate for the rapid and massive urinary loss induced by high-dose mannitol. In addition, caution should be exercised to keep the mean arterial pressure (MAP) in the approximate ranges of 80–115 mm Hg in adults and 65–85 mm Hg in children (or lower in neonates). This latter approach is because, on one hand, lower blood pressure levels could lead to ischemic brain damage, whereas higher blood pressure values could exacerbate the brain swelling under circumstances of impaired cerebral pressure autoregulation. The latter may be, in fact, a leading cause of rebound brain swelling, even though this relationship has not yet been clearly demonstrated.

In such conditions wherein decompressive surgery could be considered, the choice for external versus internal decompression is primarily based on the magnitude of the mass effect, brain swelling, or both, as well as the involvement of eloquent areas. Because internal decompressive surgery does allow for anatomic reconstitution of the dura mater and bone flap, postoperative ICP monitoring is more reliable than in cases of external decompression, wherein the bone flap is not anatomically reconstituted. Accordingly, internal decompression by removal of the inferior temporal gyrus (extending to the midtemporal gyrus if necessary) may be regarded as an effective surgical option.

In cases of large nondominant frontal contusions, the anterior quarter of the frontal lobe could be removed for decompressive purposes. Both in temporal or frontal internal decompressive surgery, normal saline solution should be used to partially fill the cavity in which an ICP monitoring catheter could be placed. This procedure would then allow for fluid drainage (initially normal saline solution, then CSF) if elevated ICP is found postoperatively.

If external decompression is used, duraplasty is

required, sometimes using relatively large pieces of fascia lata femoris or prosthetic dura material. The main limitations of external (versus internal) decompression are in regard to: (1) the need for a cranioplastic procedure (with or without the patient's own skull) at later times; (2) the inherent risk of cortical venous infarction if severe brain swelling is still compressing cortical veins against the edges of the craniotomy; and (3) the frequent inaccuracy of ICP monitoring under circumstances of a large skull defect.

The reciprocal of intraoperative brain swelling in acute subdural hematomas is found when the underlying brain surface remains retracted, essentially nonpulsatile. Under these circumstances, visual confirmation of a poorly perfused brain indicates rapid attempts at tissue reperfusion. Because the status of cerebral pressure autoregulation is not usually assessable intraoperatively, however, caution should be exercised when iatrogenically raising the patient's blood pressure with dopamine, phenylephrine, or both in an attempt to induce re-expansion of the retracted brain. If rebound brain swelling develops, fast intravenous administration of 25% mannitol (0.75–1 g/kg) should follow, along with rapid intravenous fluid replacement. This therapeutic combination is justified, because mannitol simultaneously increases CBF and decreases brain volume.

3. **Acute intraparenchymal hematoma**: In contrast with acute epidural and subdural hematomas, acute intraparenchymal clots may be conservatively managed in a variety of circumstances, as follows: (1) intracapsular location; (2) little or no mass effect (except, perhaps, for the contribution of perihematoma edema); and (3) severe acute hypocoagulopathy. Nevertheless, subacute enlargement of initially small intraparenchymal clots is a frequent indication for surgical removal. These enlarged intraparenchymal hematomas may not cause large increases in ICP.[53, 54] Accordingly, repeat CT 6–8 hours after admission (or at any point in time if new neurologic localizing signs are found) may be a more reliable means of reevaluating these initially small lesions than changes in ICP are.

If the intraparenchymal hematoma presents with relevant mass effect on the first CT scan and is extracapsular in essence, one should consider emergency removal via corticectomy while attempting to preserve a layer of clotted blood against the walls of the hematoma cavity. The latter maneuver is to minimize the risk of clot reaccumulation from previously tamponade vessels. Accordingly, we do not recommend biopsy of the walls of these hematoma cavities for neuropathological evaluation, unless clot-free wall can be clearly seen and abnormal vasculature can be ruled out as well. Dural opening is usually less extensive than that required for acute subdural hematomas. Again, we do not recommend expanded circular dural opening, as explained earlier. Abnormal blood clotting test results may indicate the need for dural tack-up sutures.

Mixed contusional and intraparenchymal hematoma bleeding (Fig. 16–5) is a diagnostic and management challenge, because a surgical procedure may or may not reveal large-enough amounts of well-circumscribed blood to justify the operation. Nevertheless, depending on the neurosurgeon's experience, as well as on blood clotting tests, focal neurologic signs, and midline shift on CT scan of the head, early surgical evacuation of these mixed lesions may be a logical approach.

In acute intraparenchymal hematomas, we recommend routine cerebral angiography to search for vascular malformations, whose rupture may have triggered acute loss of consciousness just prior to the traumatic event. This approach is particularly relevant when the patient was the motorist or when

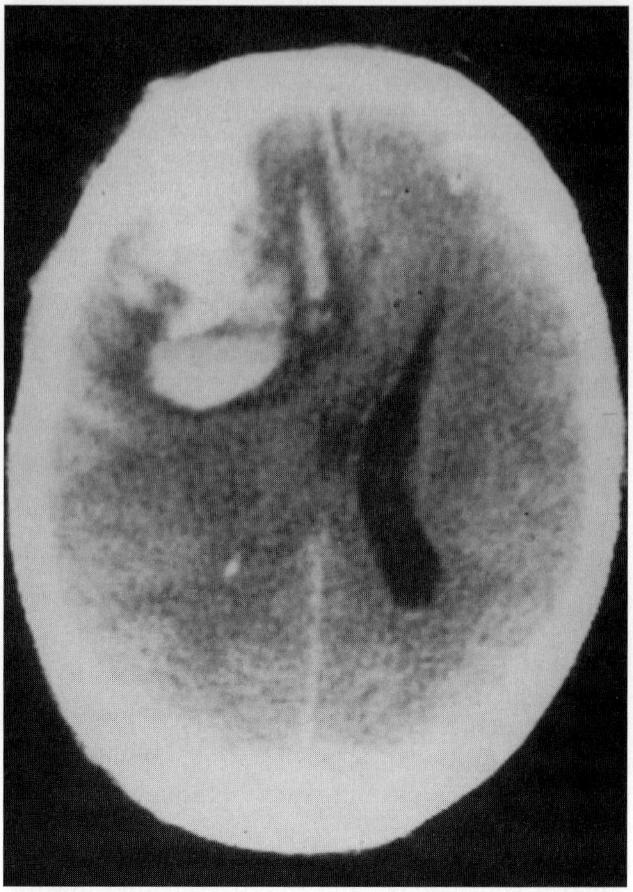

FIGURE 16–5 • Computed tomography of the head revealing large right frontal mixed hemorrhagic contusion and intraparenchymal hematoma, which was evacuated.

the mechanism of traumatic injury was a fall, both potentially associated with pretraumatic unconsciousness. Cerebral angiography should be performed preoperatively if there is no CT evidence of life-threatening mass effect; otherwise, cerebral angiography should be performed postoperatively.

For intracapsular hematomas, a nonsurgical approach has been well accepted for many years. This is because further damage to the internal capsule and surrounding structures frequently results from the surgical maneuvers. Nevertheless, in selected cases, stereotactic hematoma removal might be considered if the blood clotting test results are normal (or therapeutically normalized).

4. **Hemorrhagic contusions**: Most hemorrhagic contusions do not require surgical management, either because they are small or midsize ones or they are located away from life-threatening regions (Fig. 16–6). Accordingly, emergency surgical evacuation of these lesions is essentially limited to those in the temporal fossa, where early CT evidence of basal cisternal obliteration can be seen (even with midsize contusions). Cerebellar contusions with compression of the fourth ventricle and brain stem are also initially surgical under most circumstances. Conversely, large hemorrhagic contusions in areas remote from the basal cisterns and the brain stem may also require early removal because of substantial mass effect or refractory ICP problems.

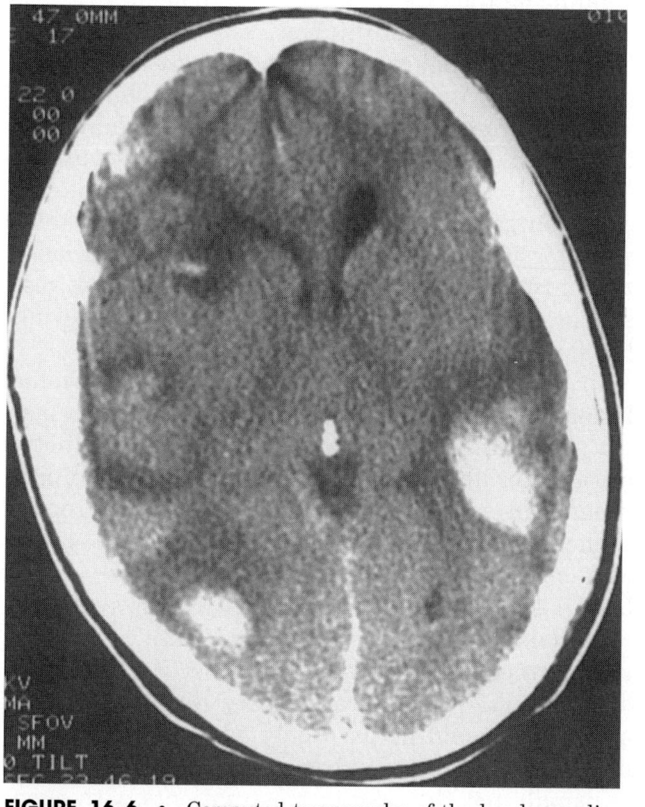

FIGURE 16–6 • Computed tomography of the head revealing bilateral small and midsize hemorrhagic contusions, which were managed nonsurgically.

Although some contusions are not initially subjected to surgical management (Fig. 16–7*A*), contusional enlargement frequently occurs (see Fig. 16–7*B*), and pericontusional edema almost invariably develops over the initial 24–48 hours, with mass effect then becoming more evident, eventually requiring surgical management. Under these sometimes challenging conditions, however, aggressive nonsurgical ICP management may have already blunted, at least in part, the primary effects of the mass on intracranial dynamics. In this case, caution should be exercised in interpreting ICP values, because even mildly increased ICP could be associated with clinical signs of neurologic deterioration. To be on a safer side, surgical indications for removal of hemorrhagic contusions should be primarily based on location and size of these lesions (also accounting for the mass effect of pericontusional edema), rather than waiting for the ICP to largely increase.

Some of the features regarding supratentorial surgical decompression were partially described earlier and are further discussed later. With regard to posterior fossa contusions, they may also be devastating, and once mass effect against the fourth ventricle or the brain stem has been identified on CT, immediate decompression should be considered, whether or not pericontusional edema has already developed. Indeed, surgical decompression of cerebellar contusions should be accomplished before clinical signs of neurologic deterioration are observed, because the nonsurgical management and reversal of such signs is usually less effective than what is observed in supratentorial contusions.

5. **Gunshot wounds to the head**: In the most severe cases, acute structural brain damage and brain swelling are the most frequent findings, whereas truly surgical clots are less frequent. Our basic approach has been to aggressively manage elevated ICP and associated changes in cerebral extraction of oxygen (see later) and to adopt surgical decompression if nonsurgical management fails to adequately maintain normalized ICP and cerebral oxygenation. The skin wounds are sutured upon the patient's admission to the emergency room or the intensive care unit (ICU) to prevent external brain exposure and infection, whereas dural closure (with duraplasty if necessary), as well as débridement of necrotic parenchyma in the operating room, may be temporarily postponed to allow for initial aggressive nonsurgical management.

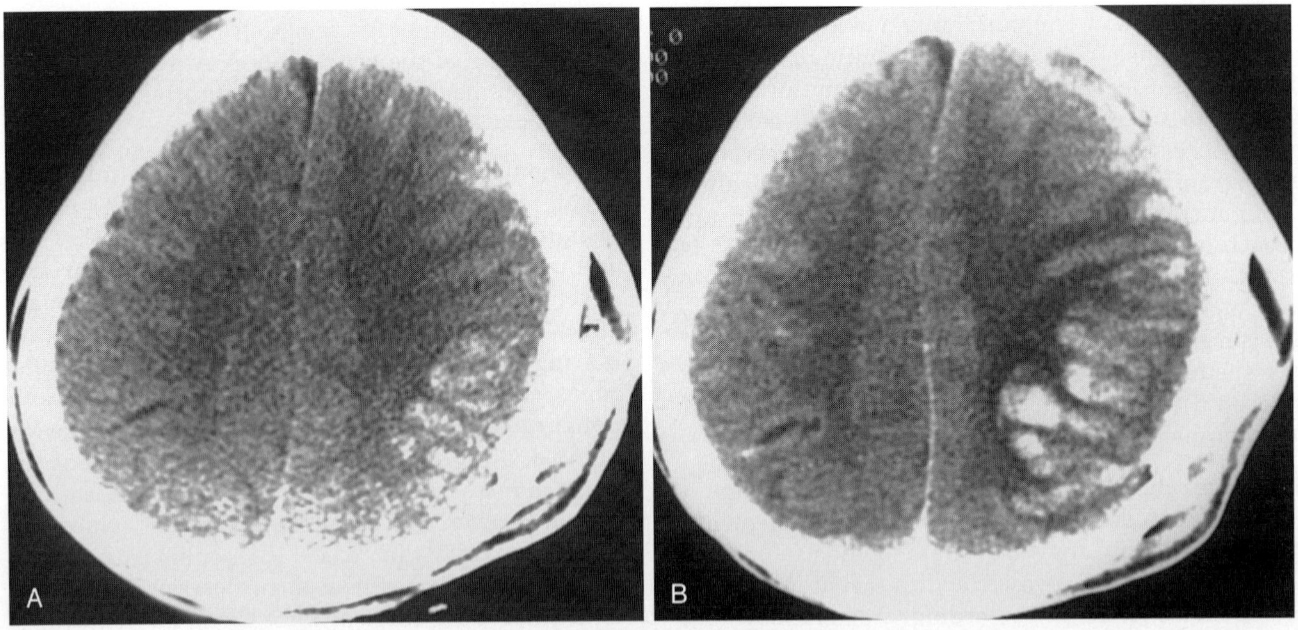

FIGURE 16–7 • Computed tomography of the head revealing a left posterior parietal "salt and pepper" type of hemorrhagic contusion (*A*), unlike the hemorrhagic contusion with associated intraparenchymal hematoma shown in Figure 16–5. *B*, Over approximately 18 hours, the lesion enlarged. Notice the development of pericontusional edema. External decompressive surgery was performed because of refractory intracranial pressure problems.

Once again, we do not recommend circular dural openings once craniotomy or craniectomy has been chosen, but one of the earlier described standard techniques. Débridement by aspiration along the bullet path may result in severe intraoperative bleeding, and therefore the use of bipolar cautery débridement appears to be safer. Generous wound irrigation with normal saline solution and bacitracin should follow, as for all open head injuries.

Duraplasty is frequently needed, and our approach has been to remove the usually irregular edges of the dural defect, which is then expanded to a square or rectangular opening. This maneuver makes the duraplasty more reliable, insofar as CSF leakage is concerned. Because the dural opening is usually small, fascia temporalis or prosthetic dura material may be used, without the need for large pieces of fascia lata femoris.

6. **Other open head injuries**: A variety of conditions may yield severe acute head injury with open scalp, skull, and dura mater unrelated to gunshot wounds. In the presence of comminuted depressed fractures or foreign bodies that are relatively superficial in relation to the brain tissue, CT alone appears to be enough for preoperative assessment. In patients whose deeper intracranial structures have been involved, however, emergency cerebral angiography should be considered. This approach is recommended because major intracranial vascular compromise may remain undiagnosed on the basis of CT alone.

Following a complete preoperative assessment, the choice of surgical technique should be based on the diagnostic findings. Accordingly, minor or major neurosurgical procedures may be required, depending on the type of lesion, as well as its location, associated vascular injuries, and other possible findings. Although resection and débridement of superficially located unviable brain tissue do not usually constitute a surgical challenge, removal of foreign bodies involving deep structures may be technically difficult. Even more challenging is the acute surgical management of major intracranial vascular injuries, which frequently allow no more than just emergently obliterating the bleeding vessels or relieving vascular compression by removing the foreign bodies.

In addition to dealing with brain and vascular lesions, duraplasty is frequently required with fascia temporalis, fascia lata femoris, or prosthetic dura material (depending on the extent of the dural repair and the neurosurgeon's option). Proper repair of the fractured skull may be either achieved on the first operation or at later times. Whenever large bone loss is observed, cranioplasty with synthetic materials such as acrylic methacrylate is a standard procedure to be adopted either early or late after injury. Acrylic cranioplasty during the first operation should be used only when there is little risk of postoperative infection. The latter, however, is usually not the case in most patients with open head injuries; thus, a second operation is frequently required for cranioplasty involving materials other than the patient's own skull. As a general rule in open head injuries, infectious prophylaxis should be always attempted by generous, repetitive wound irrigation with normal saline solution and bacitracin during surgery, along with débridement of unviable tissue.

7. **Pneumocephalus**: A relatively frequent finding in association with skull fractures, acute pneumocephalus is usually treated conservatively because of its frequently scattered distribution and small volume. In some patients, however, a large pneumocephalus may develop, most frequently occupying the frontal fossa and compressing the underlying brain (Fig. 16–8). In these cases, emergency but slow catheter drainage of the pneumocephalus through a burr hole is indicated, to lower elevated ICP and allow for re-expansion of the underlying brain. Once the brain has re-expanded satisfactorily, the choice of ICP monitoring technique depends on the size of the lateral ventricles (as well as the blood clotting tests). If a surface monitoring device is chosen, caution should be exercised not to allow communication of even small air collections with the monitoring catheter if it is fluid-filled, because air bubbles frequently dampen the ICP recordings under these circumstances. The same concern does not apply to fiberoptic subdural catheter monitoring.

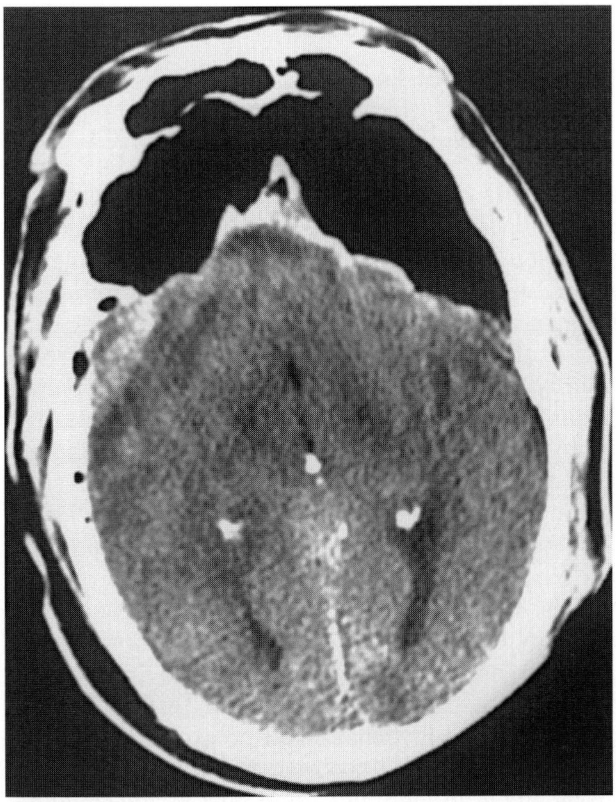

FIGURE 16–8 • Computed tomography of the head revealing a large bifrontal pneumocephalus, which required initial burr-hole drainage followed by craniotomy for repair of the dural tear.

Surgical repair of the dural tear associated with pneumocephalus formation may be performed acutely (when the pneumocephalus is first drained) or at later times, depending on other clinical or CT findings that may indicate or contraindicate acute craniotomy for dural repair. Pneumocephalus reaccumulation, however, should always be managed with dural repair, even if it is anticipated that brain swelling may make the operation more cumbersome. This is because the risks of intracranial infection and life-threatening intracranial hypertension are enhanced with pneumocephalus re-formation.

8. **Decompressive surgery**: This term refers to surgical decompressive measures other than cerebral decompression due to clot removal alone. In our experience with management of acute traumatic intracranial hypertension associated with brain swelling (whether or not in the presence of previously removed hematomas or contusions), decompressive surgery has been required in approximately 20% of the patients. The main feature regarding successful results in decompressive surgery appears to be its timing. In fact, although little or no benefit can be found when decompressive procedures are carried out after irreversible bilateral pupillary widening has developed, truly beneficial effects may be found if patients undergoing "maximum" nonsurgical management are taken to the operating room before pupillary widening is found to be irreversible by nonsurgical means.[41, 56, 57]

Conversely, "prophylactic" decompressive surgery seems inadequate before nonsurgical management of elevated ICP has been carefully maximized. The exceptions for this basic rule are lesions with mass effect located near vital structures, as mentioned earlier. In fact, waiting for the ICP to largely increase when lesions with mass effect are located in the temporal fossa appears to be inadequate, because patients may *rapidly* develop signs of brain stem dysfunction before the ICP largely increases.[56] In our experience, once a decision is made for internal decompressive surgery, generous (rather than economic) removal of noneloquent brain appears to be more effective than economic decompression, particularly because brain swelling tends to persist or even exacerbate and eventually occupy the surgical cavity. Under these circumstances, economic decompression would not allow for adequate postoperative ICP control.

In the case of eloquent areas, external decompression would be most appropriate, without removal of cerebral tissue. This is because, even when contusional tissue appears to be irreversibly damaged, viable tissue may be inadvertently removed from edematous pericontusional areas. When external decompression is carried out, a large inverse U-shaped dural opening may be necessary, supplemented by duraplasty with long strips of fascia lata femoris or prosthetic dura material, along the edges of the dural opening. This prevents CSF leakage and possible infectious complications, and it accommodates the swollen brain in the additional subdural space.

As mentioned earlier, ICP monitoring is more reliable in patients who undergo internal versus external decompressive surgery, because the former allows for anatomic dural closure and reconstitution of the bone flap, whereas the latter is performed without anatomically replacing the bone flap, thus allowing for compartmental ICP changes to influence the recordings. Another feature in favor of internal decompressive surgery is that a second (cranioplastic) procedure is not required. As mentioned earlier, however, internal decompressive surgery must not involve eloquent areas of the brain.

POSTOPERATIVE MANAGEMENT

Most features regarding postoperative care of severe acute brain trauma are described in the sections Supportive Measures and Neuromonitoring-Oriented Management. A few postoperative issues, however, may be considered separately:

1. **Surgical drains**—adequate verification of drain patency is of paramount importance, whereas early drain removal (before 24 postoperative hours) is generally contraindicated. Proper draining is particularly relevant in patients with initial hypocoagulopathic disorders.
2. **Antiseizure prophylaxis**—in patients presenting with regional (or focal) lesions, such as hematomas, contusions, or even cerebral lacerations, antiseizure prophylaxis is advisable. Phenytoin is the most widely used drug. An initial loading dose of approximately 15 mg/kg in normal saline solution is administered intravenously over 60–90 minutes. The maintenance dose is approximately 5 mg/kg/day, administered every 8 or 12 hours. Caution should be exercised not to inject the drug through a venous catheter containing dextrose (or glucose) solutions. Antiseizure prophylaxis is usually discontinued after the first week and, if patients develop seizure activity during that period or later, another anticonvulsant drug should be considered (see also Chapter 4).
3. **Infectious precautions**—in patients with open head injuries, prophylactic antibiotics may be advisable. However, even more important is local irrigation of the wound with large amounts of normal saline solution and bacitracin during the operation. In patients with closed head injuries, however, the prophylactic use of antibacterial drugs is controversial. If intracranial infection is later suspected during the acute phase, broad-spectrum antibacterial coverage is advisable (see also Chapter 5) without a diagnostic spinal tap if the patient shows compromised basilar cisterns on CT or shows elevated ICP requiring aggressive management. Once the intracranial dynamics becomes more stable, a spinal tap would be indicated for further evaluation of the infectious process.
4. **Gastrointestinal precautions**—antacid medications are advisable and administered both intravenously and via nasogastric tube. Doses vary, depending on the drugs used. In most patients the drugs may be discontinued after 2–3 weeks, once the most stressful phase of injury has subsided.

SUPPORTIVE MEASURES

Basic General Features

Accurate and frequent evaluation of vital signs stands out as a most relevant feature in the routine assessment of severely brain-injured patients. In relatively stable patients, vital signs are recorded hourly on the nursing flow sheet, or more frequently when hemodynamic or respiratory instability occurs. In addition, hourly simplified neurologic evaluation of the acutely comatose intubated patient is usually restricted to evaluation of motor responses to pain and pupillary shape, diameter, and reactivity to light (both direct and consensual), whereas confounding pupillary dilation due to direct ocular trauma must be ruled out as a potential sign of false tentorial herniation. Because these patients are frequently under the effects of sedatives and muscle relaxants, truly accurate neurologic evaluation may be hampered, except for pupillary signs.

In the normotensive patient, rapid intravenous fluid loading is not a concern, in terms of maintaining normal levels of blood pressure. In patients with acute arterial hypotension, however, *rapid* intravenous fluid loading is mandatory. The combination of normal saline solution and 5% albumin may be effective in restoring systemic volemia and arterial blood pressure, and the supplementary use of vasopressor drugs may be necessary. Vasopressor drugs, however, may cause intracranial hypertension to be triggered or exacerbated if cerebral pressure autoregulation is compromised. Although dopamine and phenylephrine appear to have clinically acceptable effects on the cerebral circulation, norepinephrine may induce cerebral vasoconstriction and at least potentially induce cerebral ischemia. Such changes have not yet been demonstrated in the emergency setting, but avoidance of norepinephrine is desirable.

In cases of severe acute brain trauma with associated severe cervical or upper thoracic spinal cord injuries (or both), arterial hypotension is better managed with anticholinergic and vasopressor drugs (rather than intravenous fluid loading), once hypovolemia has been ruled out (see Associated Spinal Trauma, earlier). If, however, there is concomitant hypovolemia, supplementary rapid intravenous fluid loading would be most appropriate.

Depending on subsequent assessment of total hemoglobin content, red cell transfusions may also be indicated. Thorough evaluation involving systemic sources of acute blood loss is of paramount importance in patients with acutely decreased total hemoglobin content. Red cell transfusions should be titrated to restore levels of total hemoglobin content in the range of 10–11 g/dL or greater.

Fluid, Electrolyte, and Nutritional Management

The approach to acute serum electrolyte abnormalities should be based on their true clinical relevance. The basic goal of fluid management is to maintain normovolemia. During the initial 48 hours, fluid management usually involves intravenous administration of normal saline solution (starting at 1.4–1.7 mL/kg per hour) with or without dextrose, depending on serum glucose levels. If patients are moderately hyperglycemic, dextrose administration should be avoided. If hyperglycemia exceeds serum glucose levels of 200–250 mg/dL, careful insulin administration should be considered. From the third day on, parenteral or enteral nutrition is started and provides much of the fluid intake (along with electrolytes and other elements). Enteral feeding is reserved for patients with active bowel movements.

In patients requiring frequent administration of hypertonic agents for ICP management, prompt intravenous fluid replacement is needed (even while enteral or parenteral nutrition is ongoing). Repetitive mannitol administration occasionally results in mild hypernatremia related to polyuria and uncorrected hypovolemia. Conversely, we have also observed hyponatremia during mannitol therapy. We believe that the mannitol-induced hyperosmolality may induce a sodium shift from the intravascular to the interstitial space. This condition should not be misinterpreted as the hyponatremia associated with the syndrome of inappropriate secretion of antidiuretic hormone (SIADH), wherein the urinary output is decreased (unlike the mannitol-induced polyuria). Attempts to normalize (increase) the serum sodium under such circumstances should be avoided because they may result in rebound hypernatremia when mannitol administration is discontinued, and because the sodium concentration in the brain is not expected to be decreased (unpublished observations).

Increased urinary output ($>$ 3 mL/kg per hour for at least 2 consecutive hours) should be evaluated for possible central DI. As mentioned earlier, early DI onset (within the first 24–48 postinjury hours) may be an ominous outcome predictor, because it may strongly suggest severe acute damage to the hypothalamus, the pituitary stalk, the neurohypophysis, or some combination thereof (as well as a possible expression of severe injury to other deep midline structures). Regardless of the time of onset, however, definitive diagnosis is important, based on the presence of high serum sodium ($>$ 150 mEq/L) as well as on low urine sodium ($\leq$ 5 mEq/L), low urine specific gravity ($\leq$ 1.005), and low urine osmolality ($<$ 150 mOsm/kg). Polyuria due to fluid overload, hyperglycemia, and therapeutic osmotic diuresis (for ICP management) must be ruled out in the differential diagnosis of central DI.

Once the diagnosis of central DI is confirmed, hypotonic intravenous fluid administration should be rapid and enough to fully replace urinary losses (milliliter per milliliter) plus approximately 10% of the most recently measured hourly diuresis. Additional steps are as follows: (1) subcutaneous antidiuretic hormone (0.03–0.07 U/kg) may be administered every 6–8 hours (dosing intervals are better adjusted according to the urinary output); (2) an alternative to the previous modality is to administer aqueous vasopressin with intravenous fluids (0.001–0.002 U/mL); (3) a second alternative is desmopressin acetate (DDAVP), which can be administered intravenously or subcutaneously (0.014–0.07 μg/kg), or intranasally (0.14–0.28 μg/kg) every 12–24 hours. These therapeutic options are usually required for adequate water retention. Frequent laboratory checks are required during management. Because central DI is frequently characterized by second and third phases of water retention and recurrent polyuria, respectively, within a span of days, careful titration of these measures is of paramount importance (see also Chapter 18).

Another clinically relevant disorder of osmoregulation is SIADH, characterized by oliguria (in the absence of hypovolemia), hyponatremia (< 135 mEq/L), and increased urine sodium (> 25 mEq/L). In severe acute brain trauma, antidiuretic hormone release may also be triggered by hypotension, hypovolemia, pain, and even stress, which should all be considered in the differential diagnosis.

In SIADH, abnormal water retention is initially associated with abnormal intravascular volume expansion, which is followed by increased urinary sodium excretion. In relatively stable patients, fluid restriction (15–20 mL/kg per day) is recommended, but this approach is frequently not feasible in patients requiring aggressive fluid replacement, such as when hypertonic agents are used for ICP management. In addition to careful (sometimes unfeasible) fluid restriction, severe hyponatremia usually responds to partial therapeutic serum sodium correction to approximately 130–135 mEq/L, which is best accomplished over 8–24 hours. Hypertonic (3%) saline solution is usually effective and may be administered in aliquots of approximately 1.5 mL/kg per hour. Frequent laboratory checks are required when managing SIADH. The cerebral salt-wasting syndrome resembles SIADH with regard to laboratory findings, but initial intravascular volume contraction is a main finding in the salt-wasting syndrome, unlike intravascular volume expansion in SIADH (see also Chapter 17).

As a general rule in managing severe acute brain trauma, in addition to maintaining normovolemia and normal serum sodium levels, electrolyte replacement should always be carried out for low serum levels of magnesium, calcium, and potassium as well. Conversely, high serum levels of those three elements is infrequent in these patients, unless complicated by systemic disorders such as acute renal failure (which may rapidly result in life-threatening hyperkalemia) or other concomitant illnesses. Regardless of concomitant systemic disorders, proper balancing of all electrolytes is important when administering parenteral or enteral nutrition.

Besides adequate caloric, fluid, electrolyte, and vitamin delivery, maintaining a neutral or positive nitrogen balance is an important additional goal of nutrition for these patients. Despite high protein delivery (2 g/kg per day), however, a positive nitrogen balance may not be achieved, especially during the most stressful phase of injury, which may extend to the first 1–3 weeks.

NEUROMONITORING-ORIENTED MANAGEMENT

Physiologic monitoring and intensive care are closely related in these patients, whether or not they initially undergo emergency surgery. As soon as the comatose patient reaches the ICU, the head should be kept partially elevated at approximately 30 degrees (except when intracranial hypertension is not suspected or confirmed), and the following monitoring modalities should be considered:

1. Continuous monitoring of electrocardioscopy
2. Continuous monitoring of arterial blood pressure, with emphasis on the MAP, keeping the pressure transducer at the level of the heart (usually at the mid-axillary line)
3. Continuous monitoring of ICP, with the pressure transducer positioned at the level of the external auditory meatus
4. Continuous monitoring of cerebral perfusion pressure (CPP, the difference between MAP and mean ICP)
5. Continuous monitoring of arterial oxygenation by pulse oximetry or alternative modalities
6. Continuous or intermittent monitoring of body temperature
7. Continuous fiberoptic[11, 14, 30, 31, 36–41, 58, 59] or even intermittent[12, 13, 28, 31, 56, 57] monitoring of SjO_2 and CEO_2
8. Continuous or intermittent monitoring of central venous pressure

Of these modalities, ICP, SjO_2, and CEO_2 monitoring may be initially disregarded in patients with fully preserved CSF spaces on the admission CT scan. If relevant changes are found on routine repeat CT after 6–8 hours (or at any point when indicated by neurologic changes), ICP, SjO_2, and CEO_2 measurements should then be initiated. As mentioned earlier, however, this is not a major concern in the adult population (unlike the case in children), in whom clinically relevant brain swelling infrequently develops if the early CT findings are associated with fully preserved CSF spaces. An exception to that rule is when patients develop early arterial hypotension, who frequently present with subacute brain swelling after initially unremarkable CT findings.

Another group of patients in whom monitoring of ICP and CEO_2 may be disregarded is that involving acute epidural hematomas without associated brain swelling. In fact, "uncomplicated" acute epidural hematomas are unlikely to present with clinically relevant changes in ICP during the postoperative period.

The basic goal of multivariate physiologic monitoring and management is to maintain normal (or therapeutically normalized) physiologic parameters, according to the following approximate ranges:

1. **ICP:** 5–19 mm Hg in adults and 0–14 mm Hg in children, or 5 mm Hg less in cases with skull defects ≥ 10 cm^2

2. **MAP:** 80–115 mm Hg in adults and 65–85 mm Hg in children
3. **CEo$_2$:** 24%–42% in adults[11] and 17%–35% (estimated) in children
4. **CPP:** 60–95 mm Hg in adults and 50–80 mm Hg in children (lower MAP and CPP in neonates)

Routine supplementary monitoring involves electroencephalographic assessment of patients undergoing barbiturate therapy for ICP management (see later). Likewise, in patients requiring more careful surveillance of systemic hemodynamics, a pulmonary artery flotation catheter should also be considered.

Near-infrared spectroscopy monitoring has been contemplated with two supratentorial probes, for possible screening of patients who develop subacute intracranial hematomas.[50] As described earlier, however, this technique essentially provides a warning on the development of a "new intracranial event" without confirmation regarding type and location of the clot.[51] Nevertheless, on the basis of a primary warning sign, indications for repeat CT might become more timely, at least with respect to supratentorial hematomas.

ICP Monitoring

Even though clinical ICP monitoring was first proposed in the early 1950s,[60] controversy still exists regarding the best monitoring modality in patients with acutely compromised CSF spaces. In fact, while some authors[61] invariably advocate ventricular catheterization for ICP monitoring and CSF drainage, our experience has demonstrated that under circumstances where the lateral ventricles are small, little help for ICP control can be obtained from draining virtually absent CSF. This limitation is particularly true during severe ICP waves, when the lateral ventricles are further compressed. Yet, these pressure waves are frequently life-threatening, and CSF drainage simply does not control the ICP satisfactorily under these circumstances.

An additional frequently overlooked contraindication for ventricular catheterization in severe acute brain trauma is the occurrence of acute hypocoagulopathic disorders. In our experience with over 700 severely brain injured patients, relevant acute hypocoagulopathic abnormalities have been found in approximately 30% of them. Yet, in acutely hypocoagulopathic patients, intraparenchymal and/or intraventricular bleeding may develop due to catheterization.

A third relevant limitation of ventricular catheterization resides on the occurrence of ventriculitis. The latter may be particularly important in an already severely injured brain, in the setting of ICU-related infectious organisms. While variable rates of severe infectious complications may be found among different units, refractory ventriculitis may be deadly.

A fourth frequently overlooked limitation of ventricular catheterization for ICP monitoring is the presence of asymmetric brain swelling (Fig. 16–9), where one of the lateral ventricles remains open and is generally used for catheterization. Under these circumstances, however, CSF drainage may induce or exacerbate a midline shift (from the most to the least swollen hemisphere), and subfalcine herniation may rapidly develop. As this latter process of enhanced midline shift progresses, even tentorial herniation may result.

From the above discussion, our preference has been to monitor the ICP from the subarachnoid or subdural spaces, except for patients in whom both lateral ventricles are open and whose blood clotting tests are normal. According to our patient selection criteria for ICP monitoring, however, open ventricles are found in a minority of cases. In fact, as mentioned above, adult patients (unlike children) whose initial CT scans show fully open lateral ven-

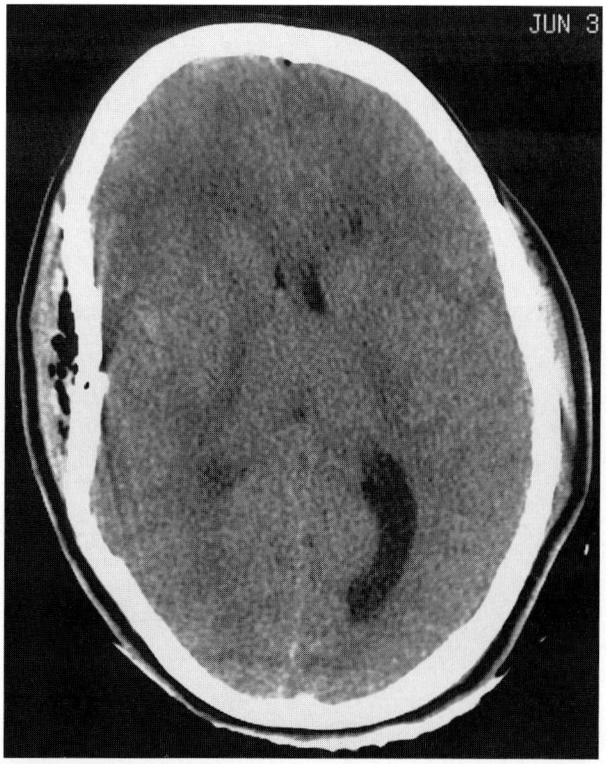

FIGURE 16–9 • Computed tomography of the head revealing right temporal depressed skull fracture and right hemispheral swelling with obliteration of the right lateral ventricle, partially sparing the left lateral ventricle (asymmetric brain swelling). This case illustrates one of the contraindications for ventricular catheterization involving intracranial pressure monitoring and management.

tricles infrequently develop severe ICP problems due to subacute hemispheral or diffuse brain swelling (except when early arterial hypotension occurs).

After the initial 5–7 days from injury, some patients may present with acute hydrocephalus, especially if traumatic subarachnoid hemorrhage is found on the initial CT scan. Under these circumstances, ventricular catheterization and CSF drainage would represent a logical even though temporary measure, whereas ventriculoperitoneal shunting may be required in several of these patients for definitive treatment.

CPP Monitoring

Because the CPP has recently been "re-visited," a proposition has been made to place both the ICP and blood pressure monitoring transducers at the level of the head.[48] Because this report addressed managing these patients with their heads flat, positioning both pressure transducers would be of little relevance. However, to the best of our knowledge, in the vast majority of head injury units patients are routinely managed with a safer positioning of the head, which is kept elevated at approximately 30 degrees (Fig. 16–10). Under these circumstances, positioning both pressure transducers at the level of the head invariably leads to artifactually low MAP (and thereby CPP) values, with all their adverse consequences regarding CPP management.

Just as is done for any other patient in the ICU without a head injury, the blood pressure transducer should be positioned at the level of the heart in brain-injured patients as well. False rather than true low MAP and CPP values are to be expected when the blood pressure transducer is positioned at the level of the head. As an obvious extension of such a technical misunderstanding, attempts to raise CBF (and cerebral blood volume) would involve unnecessary, frequently contraindicated steps such as raising the Pa_{CO_2}, the blood pressure, or both iatrogenically.

In our previously reported experience addressing simultaneous therapeutic normalization of ICP, CPP, CE_{O_2}, and cerebral extraction of glucose,[11–14] multivariate physiologic optimization was achieved with the blood pressure transducer positioned at the level of the heart (the mid-axillary line). Accordingly, had our measured CPP values been "overestimated," one would be forced to conclude that low CPP is "adequate," because not only were cerebral oxygen and glucose extraction normalized, but clinical outcome was extremely favorable as well.[11–14]

Cerebral Oxygenation Monitoring

Even though normal[19] and abnormal[23, 24] values for arteriojugular differences have been known for many years, we[36] first introduced arteriojugular oxygen monitoring and management in 1985. This methodologic and technical approach has been rapidly expanded into seven novel variables and two new concepts of cerebral hemometabolic physiology applied to patient care. The rationale for monitoring cerebrovenous oxygenation and related parameters is that, contrary to the speculation of some authors,[48] CPP monitoring and management *do not* warrant optimization of cerebral hemodynamics

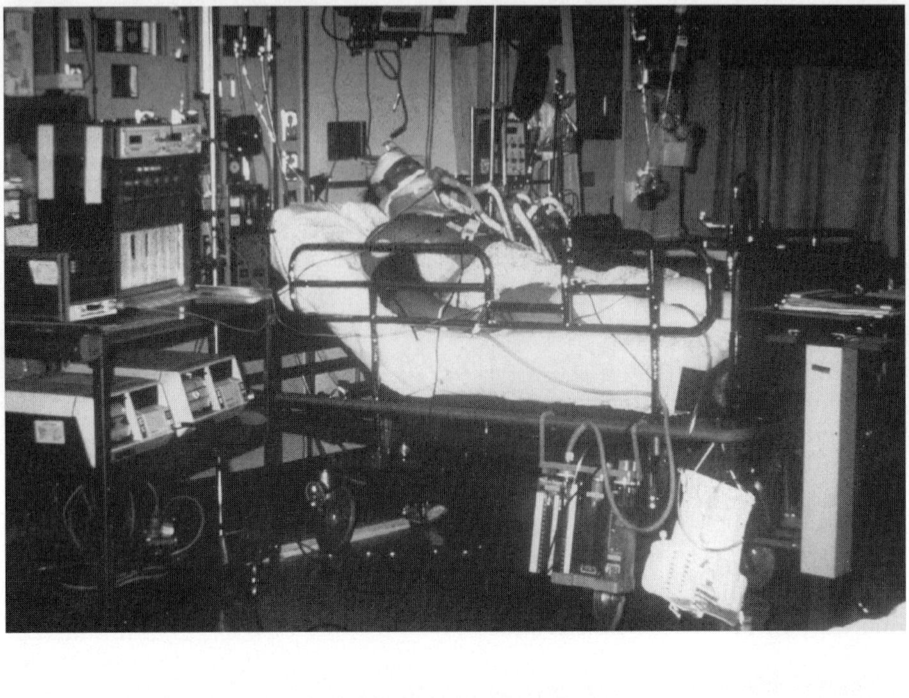

FIGURE 16–10 • A severely brain-injured patient in the intensive care unit. Notice the multiple monitoring devices for intracranial pressure, arterial blood pressure, expired carbon dioxide tension, and arterial and jugular bulb oxyhemoglobin saturation, all converged into a single recording unit. The patient's head is kept at an approximately 30-degree angle.

and oxygen metabolism once CPP is normal or high.[27, 54]

Although we have adopted jugular bulb catheterization for either frequent intermittent or continuous monitoring of global cerebrovenous oxygenation and related parameters, others have proposed monitoring of cerebral oxygenation by alternative techniques, such as focal mixed cerebral arteriolar and venular oxygenation monitoring with near-infrared spectroscopy[62] or focal monitoring of brain tissue oxygenation.[63, 64]

In our experience, global arteriojugular monitoring appears to be clinically more relevant than focal changes that may be detected by these techniques. Furthermore, from a jugular catheter, virtually any element can be measured in blood, besides oxygen. Yet, the two mentioned alternative modalities for monitoring cerebral oxygenation[62–64] do not allow for any other physiologic element to be assessed. Additional limitations should be kept in mind, as follows:

1. Acute placement of cerebral tissue probes[63, 64] may lead to focal microvascular compression, which generates artificially low tissue oxygen values. This latter feature, in turn, may have catastrophic implications regarding patient care, because many patients with compromised CSF spaces would not tolerate iatrogenic increases in cerebral blood volume and CBF, as they may rapidly develop tentorial herniation.
2. Unlike the case with normal physiology,[62] noninvasive near-infrared spectroscopy does not necessarily distinguish between arteriolar and venular oxygenation in pathological conditions. Accordingly, it may not disclose even marked changes in jugular oxygenation under clinically relevant circumstances during neuro intensive care.[40]
3. An additional limitation of near-infrared spectroscopy is its inability to "look through" layers of blood between the probe and the brain tissue. Yet subgaleal, subarachnoid, subdural, and even intraparenchymal blood is frequently found in acute brain trauma, which may be left untreated (especially subgaleal, subarachnoid, and laminar subdural blood collections).
4. Skin burns have also been associated with near-infrared spectroscopy (unpublished observations).

Jugular Bulb Catheterization

In our experience, intermittent arteriojugular monitoring requires standard intravascular catheters for periodic blood sampling, whereas continuous SjO_2 monitoring requires a fiberoptic 4 French oximetry catheter and a computerized monitor.[14]

Percutaneous placement of these catheters can be accomplished at bedside, without turning or lowering the patient's head. The right internal jugular vein is easily reached in most patients (in our experience, in over 90% of them[14]); the left internal jugular vein is an alternative when the right-sided one is not easily punctured. Just lateral to the common carotid pulse, the internal jugular vein should be initially located with a thin needle pointing cephalad, at an approximately 30-degree angle. Once the vein is located, the thin needle should be temporarily left in place to guide placement of a large-bore needle or introducer, which then replaces the thin needle.

Once the large-bore needle or introducer is properly located with its tip inside the internal jugular vein, the jugular bulb catheter is then gently threaded cephalad until resistance is felt, representing the superior wall of the jugular bulb. The catheter should then be pulled outward approximately 5 mm (to prevent endothelial damage and eventually thrombosis) and firmly stitched to the skin with a double suture involving the skin and the catheter together. A string suture involving the catheter only is interposed between the two skin-to-catheter sutures. Adequate suturing is important to prevent unintentional outward catheter mobilization during routine nursing procedures, with resulting artificially low values of cerebral oxygen extraction (from extracranial contamination of the internal jugular blood).

A plain bedside radiograph should reveal the catheter tip inside the jugular bulb. Because the suboccipital vein is a tributary of the internal jugular vein, extracranial contamination of measured SjO_2 (and CEO_2) values may be found when the catheter tip is located even at high levels of the cervical spine (atlas, axis) or lower. The catheter should then be connected to continuous slow infusion of microheparinized (1 U/mL) normal saline solution, or a heparin lock should be used, to prevent blood clotting.

In severely brain-injured patients with acutely decreased CSF spaces and ICP problems, our routine has been to maintain a cervical collar until ICP management is no longer required; neuroimaging studies are then used to evaluate the patients for more subtle spinal injuries. This approach (along with frequent sedation) is also relevant to prevent artifactual unstable recordings from the fiberoptic jugular catheter. In our experience, strict anatomic positioning of the head, neck, and shoulders (with or without cervical collars) is a basic step for preventing artifactual fiberoptic jugular catheter recordings, and the correlation between conventional laboratory and fiberoptic oximetry values is excellent in properly selected and nursed patients.[30] With proper placement and nursing, jugular bulb catheters have been used for approximately 1 week in our experience without clinically relevant complications.[14] Figure 16–11 shows a patient with a fiberoptic jugular bulb catheter in place.

ICP, CPP, and CEo_2

Our protocol for combined ICP, CPP, and CEo_2 management and normalization has been described[14, 30, 58] and consists of a cumulative treatment scheme to maintain the ICP below 20 mm Hg in adults and 15 mm Hg in children, as follows:

1. Sedation (morphine sulfate or midazolam).
2. Neuromuscular junction blockade (metocurine iodide or vecuronium bromide), which is sometimes discontinued in patients requiring aggressive pulmonary toilette and whose coughing is desirable to clear airway secretions.

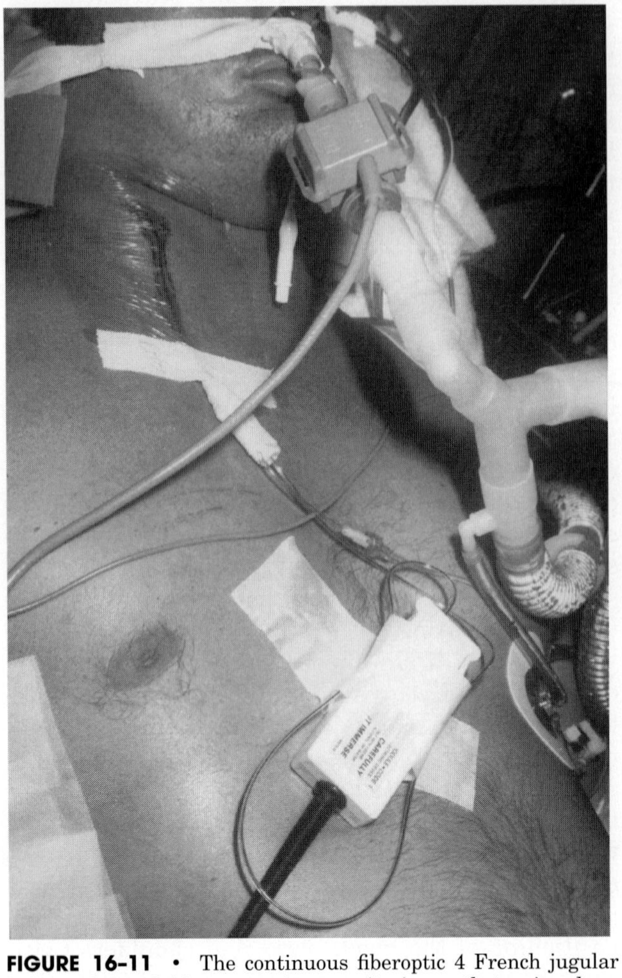

FIGURE 16–11 • The continuous fiberoptic 4 French jugular bulb oxyhemoglobin saturation monitoring catheter in place, along with the optical module (large white piece taped to the patient's chest) and the expired carbon dioxide tension monitoring sensor. The anterior portion of the cervical collar was temporarily removed for catheter placement and repositioned afterward.

3. Optimized hyperventilation,[11–14] which consists of upward or downward arterial or expired Pco_2 manipulations, aiming at the simultaneous maintenance of normalized ICP (and thereby CPP), as well as CEo_2.
4. Fast intravenous bolus injections of hypertonic mannitol (up to a serum osmolality of 315–320 mOsm/L), which are especially useful in simultaneously decreasing elevated ICP and normalizing increased CEo_2 values.[38]
5. CSF drainage (limited to patients with less challenging forms of brain swelling and open lateral ventricles).
6. Barbiturate (pentobarbital sodium) therapy, aiming at the simultaneous maintenance of normalized ICP, CPP, and CEo_2. Profound oligemic cerebral hypoxia, however, may be induced by pentobarbital bolus injections in some patients, despite apparently satisfactory CPP and ICP levels.[31] This undesired finding is presumably because cerebral pressure autoregulation is more severely compromised in some patients, and pentobarbital boluses frequently drop the systemic arterial pressure.[31]
7. Hypothermia (in carefully selected patients only, in whom infectious complications have not yet developed). In our experience (unpublished observations), this treatment modality frequently is linked to possible immunosuppressive effects, leading to unmanageable pulmonary infection and respiratory failure in some patients. Another potential complication is hypocoagulopathy, which may result in life-threatening extracranial or intracranial bleeding. Contrary to using hypothermia for all consecutively admitted comatose patients (without stratification according to different traumatic lesion types[17]), our limited need for hypothermic treatment is primarily based on managing refractory ICP. Therefore, there is no specific target for body temperature in the mild-moderate hypothermic range. Rather, low body temperature is titrated just to help maintain normal ICP. Accordingly, some patients may not require lowering their temperatures to the 32°C range.
8. Decompressive craniotomy or craniectomy (also in selected cases, before clinical signs of irreversible pupillary widening develop). Under circumstances of rapid pupillary enlargement despite ongoing "maximum" nonsurgical management, we rapidly administer mannitol irrespective of high serum osmolality to reverse pupillary widening prior to performing decompressive surgery.[41, 56]

of Monro.[89, 90] To complete the differential diagnosis, subependymal giant-cell astrocytomas in tuberous sclerosis patients, and intraventricular meningiomas arising from the choroid plexus at the trigone, may present with hydrocephalus due to local obstruction of the foramen.[86, 91]

Colloid cysts, accounting for about 1% of all brain tumors, are benign lesions usually found arising from an epithelial outpouching of the roof of the third ventricle.[85, 92] Rapid neurologic deterioration from acute obstruction of the foramen of Monro is such a well-documented phenomenon with colloid cysts that craniotomy, stereotactic drainage, and ventriculoscopic aspiration of these lesions (or a combination thereof) in asymptomatic patients is often advocated.[85, 93–95] Third-ventricular obstruction may occur with a variety of tumor types, including ependymomas, lymphomas, gliomas, and metastases. Gliomas of the hypothalamus and optic apparatus, suprasellar extension of pituitary adenomas, and up to 15% of craniopharyngiomas may present with obstruction of the third ventricle and even the foramen of Monro.[96]

Pineal region tumors almost always present with obstructive hydrocephalus at the level of the aqueduct. The incidence of hydrocephalus with these tumors is typically in the range of 90%, whereas Raimondi and Tomita[65] reported that all 21 children with pineal region masses in their series (100%) presented with some degree of hydrocephalus. In 27 of 32 patients (84%) with pineal region germ-cell tumors reported by Hoffman et al.,[97] symptoms of hydrocephalus from third-ventricular obstruction predominated. Seven of these cases were obtunded on presentation.[97]

Tumors of the mesencephalon such as gliomas can cause acute aqueductal obstruction. Acute neurologic deterioration from hydrocephalus may be the only event associated with previously undiscovered gliomas of the tectum of the midbrain.[98]

The small volume and the presence of vital structures of the posterior fossa leave little room for expanding lesions. Although these tumors rarely hemorrhage, they can be associated with either a moderate amount of mass effect or large cystic/microcystic components. Although any tumor in the infratentorial compartment can lead to obstruction, fourth-ventricular tumors are more apt to result in acute obstruction of CSF. Childhood tumors like cerebellar astrocytomas, PNETs, and ependymomas may be slow-growing but can eventually lead to obstruction. In a study of 156 pediatric patients with infratentorial tumors, 122 (78.2%) presented with hydrocephalus.[65] Of this group, 15.4% presented with impairment of consciousness, all but one of which responded to operative intervention. Because of the multitude of possible shunt complications, there is inter-observer controversy regarding the need for permanent, preoperative ventricular shunt in patients with posterior fossa tumor-related hydrocephalus.[65, 99, 100] In adults, cerebellar hemispheric tumors, such as metastases and hemangioblastomas, are more the rule, although virtually any intraparenchymal tumor, benign or malignant, can cause symptomatic obliteration of the fourth ventricle (Fig. 17–7).[101]

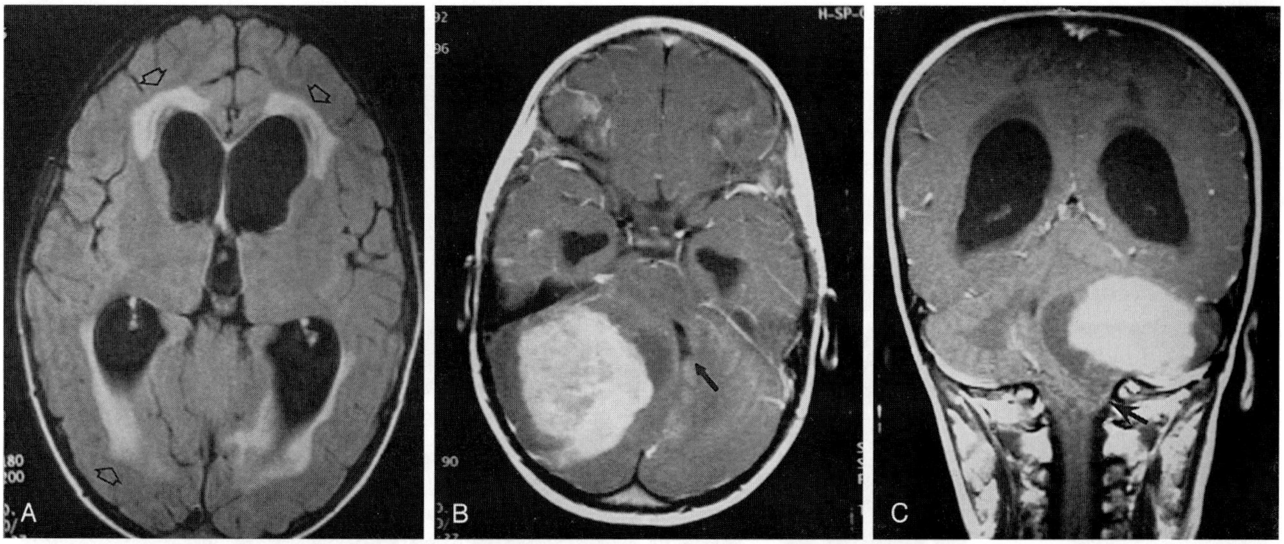

FIGURE 17-7 • *A,* Significant dilation of the ventricular system is associated with periventricular edema from transependymal flow (open arrowheads). This hydrocephalus was caused by almost complete fourth-ventricular obstruction by a right cerebellar hemispheric ependymoma noted in an axial image (*B*). Note the obliteration and marked shift of the fourth ventricle (arrow) in *B. C,* A similar tumor in the coronal view with herniation of the left cerebellar tonsil through the foramen magnum (arrow).

pression can lead to immobility. Immobility and poor nutrition may foster skin breakdown, hypoventilation, and thromboembolic disease. Concomitant radiation therapy, chemotherapy, or both may exacerbate or result in any of these factors. This all-too-common scenario paves the way for infection, often complicated by nosocomial, multidrug-resistant pathogens secondary to prolonged hospitalization. Brain tumor patients are as susceptible to these same complications as other cancer patients are. However, unique biochemical properties of brain tumors and the brain itself predisposes this subset of patients to specific intercurrent disease. These complications can be divided into two groups: those which result from a disruption of the normal physiologic milieu of the brain and those resulting from the release of tumor-specific factors.

Seizures are a common presentation for brain tumors and, depending on the tumor pathology and location, occur in 20%–90% of these patients. Compared with high-grade gliomas and metastases, patients with low-grade gliomas tend to have a higher propensity for seizures, with rates of 50%–90%.[127, 128] The majority of tumor-associated seizures are self-limited. In patients with significant mass lesions and impending herniation, one must be vigilant about therapeutic levels of antiepileptic medications. With little reserve, these patients are at particular risk for catastrophe with hypercapnia from seizures. Status epilepticus occurs rarely and should be treated via the standard medical protocols (see also Chapter 4). Investigation of the neocortex surrounding tumors has revealed both structural and neurochemical remodeling. It is thought that this neural reorganization may play a significant role in establishing epileptogenic foci in non-infiltrated, peritumoral neocortical tissue.[129]

Gastroduodenal ulceration (GDU) associated with neurologic disease is a well-described phenomenon. This brain-gut connection has been observed since the eighteenth century and documented by clinicians such as Cushing.[130] More recently, other investigators remarked on a special relationship between tumors of the fourth ventricle and massive upper gastrointestinal hemorrhage from severe GDU.[131–134] In children with posterior fossa lesions, massive hemorrhage from particularly malignant GDU seems to occur in a 7 to 10 day period post decompression.[133–135] Several of the cases reported required emergent laparotomy, vagotomy, and partial gastrectomy. At one center, the convalescence of four adult patients with a variety of posterior fossa tumors involving the fourth ventricle was complicated by massive upper gastrointestinal hemorrhage from GDU. Three of these four patients required emergent surgical intervention (unpublished data).

As noted earlier, tumor location, not tumor pathology, was the most significant factor related to the generation of GDU. This recurrent relationship between lesions involving the floor of the fourth ventricle and the development of severe GDU has led researchers to uncover specific brain stem physiologic mechanisms involved in ulcerogenesis. The dorsal motor nucleus of the vagus nerve (DMV), located just medial to the hypoglossal nucleus in the dorsomedial aspect of the medulla, is responsible for the majority of the vagal efferents to the stomach. Direct stimulation of the DMV or stimulation of the nucleus raphe obscurus, a major source of DMV innervation, results in GDU.[136–138] Stress ulcers in the neurosurgical patient are a well-described phenomenon, and prophylactic gastrointestinal protection with H_2-receptor blockade has proven efficacious in certain subgroups of neurosurgical patients, especially those with neurotrauma.[139, 140] Despite the anecdotal and scientific evidence for this relationship between tumors of the fourth ventricle and GDU, some investigators remain skeptical.[135, 141] Furthermore, controversy surrounds the method of gastric protection, pH elevation versus mucosal protection. Unlike sucralfate, prophylactic use of H_2-blockers alters the gastric pH. This may establish an environment conducive for gram-negative bacilli overgrowth and subsequent development of nosocomial pneumonia by retrograde colonization of the pharynx.[142]

Hyponatremia is an electrolyte disturbance common to both neurology and neurosurgery patients and occurs in a variety of diseases. Although a correctable condition, if left untreated it may result in seizures, coma, and life-threatening brain swelling. In neurosurgical patients, this hyponatremia with natriuresis is a result of cerebral salt-wasting syndrome, first described in 1950.[143, 144] Both CNS influences on proximal tubule sodium reabsorption and elevated plasma concentrations of atrial natriuretic factor are implicated.[145, 146] In the past, the cerebral salt-wasting syndrome has been confused with the syndrome of inappropriate secretion of antidiuretic hormone.[147, 148] Treatment of cerebral salt wasting consists of salt replacement with normal saline solution and correction of a fluid deficit, if necessary.[146, 149] Rapid correction of hyponatremia has been associated with the irreversible and catastrophic complication of central pontine myelinolysis, and correction in the acutely ill patient should not exceed 2 mmoL/L per hour.[150]

Cancer patients can have abnormalities with any of the hematologic cell lines or their related enzyme systems. In brain tumor patients, complications involving the fibrinolytic system, immunocompetence, and blood viscosity are well described. The propensity of certain brain tumors to spontaneously hem-

We reserve this latter approach for the treatment of large masses with extensive bilateral lateral extension of tumor. The use of an endoscope passed submucosally, transnasally, and trans-sphenoidally is a technique that provides a minimally invasive approach to the intrasellar space. The applicability of endoscopic treatment of the patient with apoplexy remains to be elucidated as experience with this technique grows. Postoperative radiation therapy is then employed to treat residual, surgically inaccessible tumor. Postoperative endocrinologic testing determines the type and degree of hormonal replacement therapy. Postoperative serial MRI is performed initially at 6 months then yearly to monitor for tumor recurrence and response of residual disease to adjunctive therapy. The role of focused, stereotactic radiosurgery, either as an initial or an adjunctive therapy, is under investigation.

CONCLUSION

Evaluation of the patient with life- or function-threatening pituitary disease, due to either endocrinologic or neurocompressive pathology, is extremely difficult, and diagnosis is often delayed. Patient histories and physical examinations are frequently negative or reveal only subtle evidence of pituitary pathology. Success in diagnosis and early therapeutic intervention requires a high index of suspicion during the initial work-up of the critically ill patient. If hormonal deficits are suspected, thyroid and glucocorticoid replacement therapy should be instituted immediately without waiting for confirmatory laboratory studies. When neurocompression is suggested on physical examination, radiographic confirmation with CT scan or MRI and neurosurgical evaluation should be rapidly obtained. Pituitary emergencies are potentially treatable with minimal or no sequelae when therapy is promptly instituted.

References

1. Fujisawa I, Nishimura K, Asato R, et al: Posterior lobe of the pituitary in diabetes insipidus: MR findings. J Comput Assist Tomogr 1987;11:221–225.
2. Sato N, Ishizaka H, Yagi H, et al: Posterior lobe of the pituitary in diabetes insipidus: Dynamic MR imaging. Radiology 1993;186:357–360.
3. Brooks BS, El Gammal T, Allison JD, et al: Frequency and variation of the posterior pituitary bright signal on MR images. AJNR 1989;10:943–948.
4. Elster AD: Imaging of the sella: Anatomy and pathology. Semin Ultrasound CT MRI 1993;14:182–194.
5. Davis PC, Hoffman JC, Spencer T, et al: MR imaging of pituitary adenoma: CT, clinical, and surgical correlation. AJR 1987;148:797–802.
6. Snyder PJ, Danoff BF, Schatx NJ, et al: Hypopituitarism following radiation therapy in pituitary adenomas. Am J Med 1986;81:457–463.
7. Constine LS, Woolf PD, Cann D, et al: Hypothalamic-pituitary dysfunction after radiation for brain tumors. N Engl J Med 1993;328:87–94.
8. Daniel PM, Treip CS: The pathology of the pituitary gland in head injury. In Gardner-Hill H (ed): Modern Trends in Endocrinology, 2nd ed, p 55. London, Butterworth, 1961.
9. Crompton MR: Hypothalamic and pituitary lesions. In Vinken PJ, Bruyn GN (eds): Handbook of Clinical Neurology. Injuries of the Brain and Skull, Part I, p 465. Amsterdam, North-Holland, 1975.
10. Landau H, Adin I, Spitz IM: Pituitary insufficiency following head injury. Israel J Med Sci 1978;14:785–789.
11. Edwards OM, Clark JDA: Post-traumatic hypopituitarism. Six cases and a review of the literature. Medicine 1986;65:281–290.
12. Barreca T, Perria C, Sannia A, et al: Evaluation of anterior pituitary function in patients with post-traumatic diabetes insipidus. J Clin Endocrinol Metab 1980;51:1279–1282.
13. Crompton MR: Hypothalamic lesions following closed head injury. Brain 1971;94:165–172.
14. Halimi P, Sigal R, Doyon D, et al: Post-traumatic diabetes insipidus: MR demonstration of pituitary stalk rupture. J Comput Assist Tomogr 1988;12:135–137.
15. Kornblum RN, Fisher RS: Pituitary lesions in craniocerebral injuries. Arch Pathol 1969;88:242–248.
16. Werbel SS, Ober KP: Acute adrenal insufficiency. Endocrinol Metab Clin North Am 1993;22:303–327.
17. Gaillard RC: Pituitary gland emergencies. In Burger AG, Philippe J (eds): Bailliere's Clinical Endocrinology and Metabolism, Vol VI (1), pp 57–75. London, Bailliere Tindall, 1992.
18. Baskin DS, Towsend JJ, Wilson CB: Lymphocytic adenohypophysitis of pregnancy simulating a pituitary adenoma: A distinct pathological entity. J Neurosurg 1982;56:148–153.
19. Buonocore CM, Robinson AG: The diagnosis and management of diabetes insipidus during medical emergencies. Endocrinol Metab Clin North Am 1993;22:411–424.
20. Moses AM: Clinical and laboratory observations in the adult with diabetes insipidus and related syndromes. In Czernichow P, Robinson AG (eds): Frontiers of Hormone Research. Vol 13, Diabetes Insipidus in Man, pp 156–175. Basel, S Karger, 1985.
21. Verbalis JG, Robinson AG, Moses AM: Postoperative and posttraumatic diabetes insipidus. In Czernichow P, Robinson AG (eds): Frontiers of Hormone Research. Vol 13, Diabetes Insipidus in Man, pp 247–265. Basel, S Karger, 1985.
22. Richardson DW, Robinson AG: Desmopressin. Ann Intern Med 1985;103:228–239.
23. Kimbrough RD, Cash WD, Branden LA, et al: Synthesis and biologic properties of 1-desamino-8-lysine vasopressin. J Biol Chem 1963;238:1411–1414.
24. Nicoloff JT, LoPresti JS: Myxedema coma. A form of decompensated hypothyroidism. Endocrinol Metab Clin North Am 1993;22:279–290.
25. Bonicki W, Kasperlik-Zaluska A, Koszewski W, et al: Pituitary apoplexy: Endocrine, surgical and oncological emergency. Incidence, clinical course, and treatment with reference to 799 cases of pituitary adenomas. Acta Neurochir 1993;120:118–122.
26. Cardoso ER, Peterson EW: Pituitary apoplexy: A review. Neurosurgery 1984;14:363–373.
27. Lacomis D, Johnson LN, Mamourian AC: Magnetic resonance imaging in pituitary apoplexy. Arch Ophthalmol 1988;106:207–209.
28. Kyle CA, Laster RA, Burton EM, et al: Subacute pituitary apoplexy: MR and CT appearance. J Comput Assist Tomogr 1990;14:40–44.
29. Onesti ST, Wisniewski T, Post KD: Clinical versus subclinical pituitary apoplexy: Presentation, surgical management, and outcome in 21 patients. Neurosurgery 1990;26:980–986.
30. Glick RP, Tiesi JA: Subacute pituitary apoplexy: Clinical and magnetic resonance imaging characteristics. Neurosurgery 1990;27:214–218.
31. Masago A, Ueda Y, Kanai H, et al: Pituitary apoplexy after pituitary function test: A report of two cases and review of the literature. Surg Neurol 1995;43:158–165.
32. Absalom M, Rogers KH, Moulton RJ, et al: Pituitary apo-

TABLE 19-2 **COMPARISON OF POSSIBLE ASSESSMENT FINDINGS BY SYSTEM OF SUBARACHNOID HEMORRHAGE (SAH), ALCOHOL, AND COCAINE USE**

ACUTE SAH AND HOSPITALIZATION	COCAINE	ALCOHOL
Neurologic		
Pain (headache), nuchal rigidity, photophobia Anxiety	Altered perception of pain	Agitation, hallucinations in alcohol withdrawal
Altered level of consciousness–drowsiness, agitation, unresponsiveness	Altered mood and reward behaviors	
Altered cognition–receptive, expressive aphasia, altered memory	Altered short-term memory and concentration	Cognitive disturbances due to dementing disease of alcoholism, e.g., Wernicke-Korsakoff syndrome. Decreased insight, confusion, and memory
Pulmonary		
Apnea, hypoventilation or hyperventilation Decreased airway patency and/or impaired gag/swallow Pulmonary edema Atelectasis	Decreased pulmonary function in smoked form of cocaine	Potential for esophageal varices (if patient requires intubation)
Gastrointestinal		
Decreased nutrition, dehydration, nausea	Pre-existing nutritional status may be poor	Pre-existing nutritional status may be poor, especially in alcoholic syndromes of dementia
Possible swallowing/gag reflex deficits Constipation due to bed rest, altered nutrition/hydration		Possible decreased liver function
Genitourinary / Neuroendocrine		
Bladder incontinence or retention	Possibility of exposure to sexually transmitted diseases	Urinary retention
Abnormalities of water and electrolyte conservation, e.g., diabetes insipidus Inability to void unless standing	Possibility of pregnancy due to patient population	
Immune		
Infection due to increased stress, bed rest, multiple invasive lines and procedures Possible immunosuppression due to steroid administration	Possible exposure to AIDS, hepatitis, or bacterial infection	Increased risk for infection with poor nutritional status
Psychosocial		
Separation from social support with admission to hospital	Addiction	Addiction Altered family coping
Decreased support for spouse, child, or parent Temporary or permanent unemployment for patient and family member Change in family dynamics due to illness of one member	Lack of social support	May live alone
Metabolic		
Electrolyte imbalances, hyper- or hyponatremia, hypokalemia Hyperglycemia with steroid administration		Chronic electrolyte disturbances, hyponatremia

alert the health care team of safety issues likely to be of concern in the recovery phase.

The occurrence of seizures is not uncommon with SAH or craniotomy. Some patients are placed on anticonvulsants after SAH, depending on the nature and location of the bleed and surgical manipulations. Seizures also occur in alcohol withdrawal 1–4 days after cessation of drinking. Cocaine use may cause seizures at the time of use. Prevention of seizures, especially in the first 4 or 5 days after SAH, and safety in the event of seizures are important components of care.

Partial complex seizures may occur alone, or they may be followed by more involved seizures. Partial complex seizures may be overlooked because they involve repetitive behavioral, apparently purposeful movements such as lip smacking or touching of the face or chest with one hand in a repetitive manner. Acute observation, assessment, early intervention, and communication may prevent progression to more disorganized and severe seizures.

The violent movement of a grand mal seizure may cause injury and airway compromise. The increased blood pressure involved may present the danger of confirmed by clinical examination and other neurologic testing, which vary from state to state. Upon examination, the patient exhibits fixed and dilated pupils and loss of reflexes, movement, and respiratory effort.

An apnea test may be performed. During the test, the patient's P_{CO_2} is normalized to 35–45 torr (4.7–6 kPa). The patient is respired with 100% oxygen for 10–20 minutes. In the presence of a physician, the patient is removed from mechanical ventilation for up to 10 minutes or as tolerated by the patient. Oxygen (100%) is administered via a catheter into the endotracheal tube to provide passive diffusion of O_2. The patient's chest is monitored for breathing activity. The patient's O_2 saturation, electrocardiogram readings, and blood pressure are continuously monitored. An arterial blood gas is obtained for analysis immediately prior to placing the patient back on mechanical ventilation. If the P_{CO_2} is greater than or equal to 60 torr (8 kPa) and no chest movement was noted, the apnea test has provided one measure of confirmation that the patient is brain dead.[2]

Other confirmatory tests of brain death may be an electroencephalogram showing absence of electrical activity or four-vessel arteriogram confirming absence of cerebral blood flow. These tests are especially necessary in the event that the patient's blood is positive for narcotics. Since narcotics may mimic brain death, a confirmatory test is essential in declaring brain death.

If brain death is determined, it is necessary for the physician, nurse, chaplain, social worker, or organ procurement agency representative to approach the family about their desire to donate the patient's organs. This is a very delicate subject and must be approached with great empathy and tact. It must be remembered that the family members may be confused, angry, sad, and distant due to the grieving process. A considerable amount of teaching must be provided to family members at this time. Many will have difficulty understanding that the patient is clinically and legally dead when his heart is still beating. The family may require several hours or more to accept this concept. Once understanding is reached, many families find solace and comfort in the fact that another person may find new life through the tragic death of their loved one.

When it is determined that the patient will become an organ donor, systemic hemodynamic functioning must be sustained in order to perfuse the organs. The patient may require a vasopressin infusion to counteract the excessive urine output resulting from the inability of the pituitary gland to produce antidiuretic hormone and concentrate urine. This condition is known as diabetes insipidus (DI).[2] Blood pressure and heart rate maintenance may be accomplished with cardiac and vasoactive drug infusions. Adequate oxygenation must be monitored via arterial blood gas sampling or pulse oximetry. Various laboratory and diagnostic tests may be ordered to assess the function of various organs. The blood type and tissue type must be determined in order to appropriately match the organs with recipients. The patient should be taken to the operating suite as soon as possible for organ harvesting, before systemic deterioration develops.

When the patient is not a candidate for organ donation, the nurse may participate in removal of life support systems. Any nurse involved in the decision to remove life support should be aware of both hospital and state regulations regarding the process.[2]

Psychosocial Considerations

The impact of a patient's death from head injury on the family is profound. However, the grief that is experienced by family members of the surviving patient may be as severe. Witnessing the incapacitated state of the patient may evoke feelings ranging from fear and despair to guilt, helplessness, and anger. Families must be encouraged to express their feelings as part of the coping process. Honest explanations of treatment and prognosis are necessary. Realistic goals must be set in place with input from various disciplines. Family meetings should be organized with representation by nurses, physicians, social workers, chaplains, and physical and occupational therapists. Active involvement in the acute hospitalization period prepares the family members for the in-depth care that may be required in the rehabilitation period and upon discharge.

SPINAL CORD INJURY

In the United States, spinal cord injury affects approximately 12,000 people each year. Of those individuals, 4,000 will die before reaching the hospital.[23] The survivors will require intensive care and rehabilitation to successfully reenter society. In caring for the spinal cord–injured patient, the nurse must utilize a collaborative approach, including such disciplines as physical therapy, occupational therapy, and social work. Each discipline will give the nurse insight in how to better care for the patient.

When the patient arrives at the hospital, a baseline assessment must be completed. A history of the accident will enable the nurse to predict the type of spinal cord injury, as well as the possibility of other traumatic injuries. Pre-existing medical problems will impact the patient's care and should be documented. It is important to perform a complete neurologic assessment, including strength and sensation, to provide a basis for further assessment. Documenting the patient's pulmonary status will assist the physician in determining the amount of ventilatory support, if any, that will be required. This assessment will also become more important during the early stages of treatment as the nurse assesses for ascending spinal cord dysfunction. Ascending spinal cord edema is a possible complication of spinal cord injury. Because of the structure of the spinal cord, edema may ascend the cord, causing further neurologic impairment. This may happen over the course of a few hours or less and may cause permanent damage as a result of the spinal cord's inability to tolerate compression.[24] The nurse must assess for bowel sounds and palpate the patient's bladder for distention. Absence of bowel sounds is one indicator of paralytic ileus, which may signify spinal shock.[25, 26]

When the patient arrives at the nursing unit, the nurse faces a tremendous task. She must assess the patient, plan for his or her immediate needs, and be constantly aware of the impact that nursing actions have on the patient's long-term outcome. The patient will arrive at the unit with a hard cervical collar in place if a cervical injury is suspected or confirmed.[27] This collar provides immobility to the cervical area only. It is the nurse's responsibility to maintain proper body alignment at all times. The patient's spinal column must be kept straight. This is not to say that the patient should not be turned from side to side. With the help of at least three other nurses, the patient should be log rolled. The body should be moved as a unit, with one person stabilizing the head. To keep the patient positioned on one side, the nurse may use a rolled blanket behind his back. Trochanter rolls and support for extremities in the form of blankets, towels, or specially made orthotic devices should be provided. For the patient's comfort and to decrease the work of breathing, he or she may be placed into the reverse Trendelenburg position. This position will allow the diaphragm to lower and give the patient the sensation that his or her head is up.[26]

Proper body alignment and spinal traction, if ordered, should be maintained at all times to prevent further injury. Nolan notes, "Traction is usually employed when the fractures are unstable and/or when subluxation has occurred."[27] Gardner-Wells tongs is the type of traction most frequently used. These tongs are usually placed by the physician. They consist of a "U"-shaped bar with pins at either end. The pins are secured in the patient's skull, and traction is applied using a system of weights and pulleys.[27] A halo device may be used. The latter consists of a metal or graphite halo ring, pins secured to the skull, and a vest. The vest is attached to the halo ring with bolts and upright poles.[27] It is usually the responsibility of the physician to apply and adjust the halo.

If the patient has an unstable thoracic, lumbar, or sacral injury, the nurse may consider utilizing a special bed. One such bed is a Roto Rest bed. This particular bed provides spinal immobilization while it gently rotates the patient. The bed can be set to rotate more than 300 times per day.[24] The rotation not only helps prevent pressure ulcers, but also aids in the mobilization of pulmonary secretions. The rotation of the bed may be stopped at several different positions, allowing the nurse to inspect the patient's skin. A Roto Rest bed is equipped with a scale, fan, and silent motor for the patient's comfort and the nurse's convenience. Hatches are present on the underside of the bed to allow the nurse to view the patient's skin. Urinary and fecal drainage tubing may also be tunneled through openings in the bottom of the bed. Special care should be taken when opening the cervical hatch. Another nurse should be present to hold the patient's head when this hatch is opened to prevent movement of the spine.[24]

The patient should be kept informed of all tests and procedures that are being performed. The nurse should not become so concerned with her or his duties as to neglect the patient's psychosocial needs at this crucial time.[24] Other health care disciplines, such as physical therapy, occupational therapy, social work, discharge planning, and rehabilitation medicine, should be consulted early in the patient's hospitalization to provide for his or her physical and emotional needs during the stay and after discharge.

A complete neurologic assessment should be performed at this time. In addition to the Glasgow Coma Scale, the documentation of the patient's level of sensation and his or her strength is important. To perform a sensory examination, the nurse may use a pin. The patient will be asked to close the eyes and determine whether a touch of the pin is sharp or dull, the nurse using both ends of the pin[26] (before beginning the examination, the nurse may have the patient keep the eyes open and show him which end is sharp and which is dull). Another sensory examination uses a paper clip. The nurse will again have the patient close the eyes. After opening the paper clip, the nurse will touch the patient with either one or two ends of the paper clip simultaneously, asking the patient to inform on whether he or she feels one or two ends.[24] One last sensory examination tests spatial relationships. With the patient's eyes closed, the nurse will move the patient's big toe up, down, and straight. The patient will be asked about the toe position.[24] The nurse should document a difference, if any, between the right and left sides of the patient's body in terms of strength and sensation, as a difference may indicate a Brown-Séquard injury pattern. The nurse's knowledge of the patient's level of injury will further allow prediction of the patient's strength and level of sensation. Neurologic assessment should be performed frequently during the initial phase of hospitalization.

Continued frequent neurologic assessments will enable the nurse to recognize ascending spinal cord dysfunction. This phenomenon can occur any time within the first 72 hours after injury.[24] The condition can manifest itself with worsening neurologic examinations.[24] Spinal cord ascending dysfunction can have a rapid onset—a patient who may have been breathing comfortably one half hour ago is now making a poor inspiratory effort. It is important for the nurse to detect ascending spinal cord dysfunction, owing to the potential for permanent damage.

If the patient is suffering from spinal shock, the possibility exists of regaining some of the lost function. As Hickey has noted, "When the spinal cord has been completely transsected, there is complete loss of motor, sensory, reflex, and autonomic function below the level of injury."[24] A hallmark sign of this condition is flaccid paralysis.[24]

In addition to or separate from spinal shock, the patient may suffer from neurogenic shock. This condition is manifested by a "temporary loss or dysfunction of the autonomic nervous system innervation below the level of injury, resulting in cardiovascular changes."[24] The patient may exhibit orthostatic hypotension, bradycardia, hypothermia, and/or the loss of the ability to sweat below the level of injury. The nurse should frequently assess and document the patient's cardiovascular status, including heart rate and rhythm, and blood pressure as well.

Owing to the patient's potential for prolonged bed rest, the nurse should institute measures to prevent deep venous thrombosis. The patient should have antithrombic stockings and may require pneumatic or sequential compression boots. The nurse should assess once a shift for the presence of warm or erythemic areas on the patient's calves. Because the patient may not be able to feel the pain of a deep venous thrombosis, it is vital for the nurse to perform this assessment.

Another potential hazard of prolonged bed rest is pressure ulcers. The patient should be turned and repositioned at least every 2 hours, maintaining proper body alignment, as earlier discussed. The skin should be assessed and documented every 4–8 hours for areas of redness or breakdown.[25] A pressure-reducing or alternating-pressure mattress may be useful in preventing pressure ulcers if the patient's spine is stable, but nothing takes the place of turning and repositioning the patient. If the patient's spinal cord injury is unstable, a pressure-reducing or -alternating mattress should not be used. Owing to the potential loss of vasomotor tone below the level of injury, the patient may have difficulty healing a pressure ulcer. Therefore, prevention is the key in skin care.

Another important consideration in skin care is spinal traction. If the patient is wearing a halo vest or Gardner-Wells or Crutchfield tongs, pin care must be performed every 8 hours to the insertion sites. The sites should be cleansed as per the hospital policy and assessed for signs of infection. In addition to cleansing the skin beneath the vest daily, the patient's skin should be assessed for areas of pressure from the vest. Every attempt should be made to keep the patient's skin as dry as possible beneath the vest. If the lining of the vest is removable, it should be laundered as needed.

While performing skin care and turning, the nurse also has the opportunity to perform range of motion. Although Physical Therapy may be working with the patient, it is the nurse who has the most opportunity to perform range of motion. If the patient is able, he or she may perform active range of motion to the unaffected extremities. The nurse, or a family member who has been trained by the nurse or physical therapist, should provide passive range of motion to the affected extremities at least twice daily.[28] While performing range of motion, it is important to maintain proper body alignment. Performing range of motion exercises with the patient will also allow the nurse to assess strength and skin.

The nurse can incorporate coughing and deep breathing into the range of motion routine. A patient with a cord transsection at or above the level of the seventh thoracic vertebra will need the nurse's, or a family member's, assistance to perform a quad cough. This is done by the nurse placing her or his hand between the patient's xiphoid process and umbilicus. Firm, quick pressure is then applied with the heel of the hand while the patient coughs.[24] This procedure requires practice and coordination between the patient and the nurse. If the patient is able, he or she should cough and deep breathe every 2 hours independently. It is important to maintain good hydration in the spinal cord–injured patient to produce thin secretions.

A patient with a high cervical injury (third cervical vertebra or above) is likely to require lifetime ventilation and a tracheostomy. The trach site should be cleansed every 8 hours and as needed in the acute phase with a mild soap or peroxide/saline solution according to hospital policy. This patient will need social work and rehabilitation and may require a structured living environment to re-enter society.

Patients with spinal shock exhibit atonic bladder and paralytic ileus. They will require a nasogastric tube for stomach decompression and will probably have a Foley catheter inserted in the emergency room. The nasogastric tube should remain in place and the patient should have nothing by mouth until bowel sounds return. The nurse should auscultate bowel sounds every 8 hours as part of the routine assessment. The Foley catheter, however, should be removed as soon as possible and bladder retraining begun.

Bowel and bladder retraining is a large part of a patient's rehabilitation and should be begun in the hospital. Once the Foley catheter is removed, straight catheterization should be performed every 4–8 hours, or more frequently as needed. The nurse should palpate the bladder for distention at least every 4 hours until a program has been designed to fit the patient's needs. Bowel retraining cannot be started until bowel sounds have returned. The patient may need stool softeners and/or laxatives to move the bowels and should be encouraged to eat a diet high in roughage to assist with elimination. The program should be individualized for each patient. Every 1–3 days, the patient will need to move the bowels, sitting in a comfortable position with the feet flat on the floor for elimination. Some pressure on the abdomen may be required, as well as digital stimulation, to achieve elimination.[27]

Patients with an injury at the level of the sixth thoracic vertebra and above are prone to developing autonomic dysreflexia.[24] This syndrome is triggered by a painful stimulus. The stimulus may be a distended bladder, fecal impaction, labor, ingrown toenail, or pressure ulcer.[24] The patient may exhibit paroxysmal hypertension, bradycardia, headache, and/or profuse sweating above the level of injury.[24] Treatment consists of removal of the stimulus and measures to lower the blood pressure. The nurse should raise the head of the bed, assess the bladder for distention, assess the rectum for impaction, assess the feet for ingrown toenails, and assess the skin for pressure ulcers.[24] When the stimulus is removed, the patient should return to a "normal" state.

Good nutrition is not only important for bowel function, but also necessary for healing. The nurse should assess for adequate skin turgor every 8 hours. Good hydration and adequate protein intake contribute to tissue repair. A nutrition or dietary consult may be necessary to assist the patient in meeting individual nutritional needs.

During the hospital stay, patient and family will need a tremendous amount of emotional support. They may initially experience shock and denial, but will also have many questions.[24] They will begin to ask questions when they are ready and should not be inundated with information in the early phase of hospitalization. Referrals may be made to social work, pastoral care, and psychiatric service, if the patient and family agree. It is important for the nurse to form a trusting relationship with the patient and the family, to improve the plan of care.[24]

Team conferences with all disciplines involved in the patient's care should be scheduled regularly. The patient and family should be made welcome to attend. The conference is a good time to examine the goals set for the patient, his or her attainment of those goals, and further refinement of the goals. Every patient is an individual and will progress as such. The plan of care should reflect the patient's individuality.

Upon discharge from the hospital, the patient will most likely be transferred to a rehabilitation facility and undergo intensive physical and occupational therapy, as well as learn how to successfully reenter society. Although the care of the spinal cord–injured patient is complex, with careful planning and evaluation this patient can be successfully managed. Intense and frequent nursing care will be required throughout the hospital stay. Patient and family will require a tremendous amount of support to cope with a major lifestyle change. However, with proper planning, the patient will be able to resume the lifestyle in a modified fashion. For additional information on spinal cord injuries, see Chapter 15.

BRAIN TUMORS

Nursing care of the patient with a brain tumor requires the caregiver to practice a holistic approach. The neurosurgical nurse is responsible for the physical and psychosocial needs of the patient and family and is an integral part of the planning process from the initial admission and diagnostic period through preoperative and postoperative care and rehabilitation and discharge planning.

Nursing Management During the Initial Diagnosis

The role of the nurse is crucial during all phases of a patient's hospitalization. To provide the level of care required, the nurse must be knowledgeable of the anatomy and physiology of the various types of brain tumors. Upon admission to the hospital, a thorough neurologic assessment is essential. It is on this assessment that an individualized plan of care will be developed. The patient and family's knowledge and emotional needs should be included in the initial assessment.

The patient may present with a variety of signs

and symptoms. Seizures or headaches may be the initial clue that something is astray. The location of the brain tumor may be the cause of the patient's presenting signs and symptoms. For instance, if the tumor is in the frontal region the patient may present with altered speech, mutism, personality changes, and motor function deficits. The patient and family should be reassured that the personality changes are a result of the brain tumor. If the patient is confused, all precautions should be taken to keep him or her safe and free of injury. When the patient has a motor deficit, all efforts should be made to preserve muscle tone and the affected extremity splinted and elevated. The plan of care should include range of motion exercises and slings if needed.

There are patients who present with cranial nerve dysfunction due to compression of the tumor on the nerve. If the patient presents with sensory deficits, the plan of care should include protection from injury by avoiding drastic changes in hot and cold. The patient's skin should be checked frequently and should be lubricated with lotions.

Upon the patient's admission, the nurse should recognize the deficits and institute the appropriate nursing measures. The glossopharyngeal (IX) and vagus (X) nerves innervate the swallow reflex. If the patient presents with a swallowing deficit, the role of the nurse is to prevent aspiration and to assist in controlling drooling. The patient's head should be positioned at a 45–90 degree angle to prevent aspiration, and a swallowing evaluation should be performed to assess the patient's need for a pureed or thick liquid diet. A thick liquid diet is often easier for a patient to swallow. If the swallowing reflex is absent, however, preparations may be made for an alternative method of nutrition.

The optic (II), oculomotor (III), trochlear (IV), abducens (VI), and facial (VII) nerves innervate vision, eye movement, and the opening and closing of the eyelid. If the patient is unable to completely close the eye, the nurse should instill artificial tears into the eye to prevent corneal abrasions. When the patient has diplopia or a hemianopsia, an eye patch should be placed on the affected eye and caregivers should approach the patient from the unaffected side.

It is during the initial diagnostic period that the nurse must provide information to the patient and family. The patient and family are under an extreme amount of stress trying to grasp the reality and the uncertainty of a diagnosis of brain tumor. The nurse should encourage the patient and the family to ask questions and express their concerns or worries. They should be informed of the resources available to assist them in dealing with the diagnosis. During this stressful time, there will probably be many diagnostic tests or procedures. The nurse needs to ensure that the patient and/or family is given information about these tests or procedures.

Nursing Management of the Patient Undergoing Radiation Therapy

The neuroscience nurse's role during radiation therapy is to manage the side effects of the treatment and to provide emotional support to the patient and family. The nurse should possess an in-depth knowledge of the drug to be used, including special precautions and usual side effects. If the patient suffers from nausea, vomiting, or diarrhea, the nurse should administer antiemetics and antidiarrheal agents as necessary.

The accumulation of cellular waste products in the blood, pain, sensory deprivation, alteration in sleep pattern, and the stress of coping with the disease may result in fatigue and weakness. In order to minimize these symptoms, regular rest periods should be arranged. A bedtime ritual that is consistent with the patient's usual pattern of daily living should be maintained.[29]

The nurse must continually assess the patient for signs of increased ICP. This complication can be caused by edema resulting from normal cell injury and cell breakdown. Corticosteroids are often the drugs of choice. The nurse should observe the patient for signs of gastrointestinal bleeding, often seen as a side effect of the corticosteroids.

Bone marrow depression can decrease the patient's platelet count, causing an increased risk of bleeding. The nurse should monitor the patient's blood cell count, especially the white blood cell and platelet counts, and should collaborate with the physician regarding possible discontinuation of radiation therapy if the platelet count falls below 50,000 or the white blood cell count falls below 3000 with an absolute neutrophil count less than 1000.[30]

Radiation erythema is a common side effect, causing the skin to be reddened and sensitive. Special care should be given to the area. Sunlight, powder, alcohol, and tape should be avoided. Hydrocortisone can be applied to reduce the inflammation. The skin markings that localize the radiation should not be washed off.

The neuroscience nurse should be supportive of the patient and family. She or he must continually reassure the patient and the family that the side effects will resolve once the therapy is completed.

Nursing Management of the Patient Undergoing Chemotherapy

Administration of the chemotherapeutic agent and the management of the side effects are the nursing responsibilities during chemotherapy. The nurse should assess the patient and the family's understanding of the agent used. If the patient suffers from nausea, antiemetics should be administered. Careful monitoring of intake and output is required. The physician should be informed of a discrepancy greater than 1 L. Chemotherapeutic agents should be administered as per the hospital's protocol and chemotherapeutic administration policy. The nurse should administer intravenous fluids as ordered through peripherally placed or centrally placed intravenous catheters, monitoring the site for infiltration or infection.

Upon discharge, the nurse should provide the patient and the family with information on the particular chemotherapeutic agent used. The possible side effects should be highlighted.

Preoperative Nursing Care

The two most important interventions a nurse can perform during the preoperative period are to obtain a thorough baseline neurologic assessment and ensure that the informed consent is signed. Once the consent is signed, the preoperative teaching begins. An explanation of the preparation procedure should include hair washing with pHisoHex and the subsequent hair shaving in the operating room. Following a craniotomy, the patient will probably spend at least 24 hours in the ICU. The patient and family should understand the frequent neurologic assessments, routines for vital signs, and the potential for intubation. A description of all the monitoring modalities should be provided so that the family can create a clear mental picture of how the patient will look postoperatively in the ICU. If a nasal operative approach is used, explain the use of nasal packing. It is important to assess the patient and family's understanding of the disease process and encourage them to verbalize their expected outcomes. Routine preoperative care such as instructions for deep breathing techniques should be provided, although coughing should be kept to a minimum owing to the risk of increased ICP.

Postoperative Nursing Care

The postoperative priorities of the neurosurgical nurse are to monitor the patient's level of consciousness and motor, cranial nerve, cardiac, and respiratory function. It is imperative that the nurse obtains an immediate baseline neurologic assessment upon the patient's arrival into the ICU. This assessment will be used to judge the response to therapy and should include the level of consciousness and mental status, visual disturbances, speech, and motor and sensory ability. Neurologic checks are typically performed every 15 minutes for 1 hour, progressing to every half hour for 2 hours, progressing to every 1 hour for 4 hours then every 2 hours for the remainder of the ICU stay, unless there is a change in status. This frequency of neurologic checks is essential to prevent or recognize complications of surgery that will be discussed in the following section.

The nurse must perform an ongoing assessment of the ABCs. The patient's airway is the priority. Owing to a potential for an altered level of consciousness, there is an increased chance for airway compromise. Oxygen saturation and ventilation should be monitored. The patient's vital signs should be monitored according to unit protocol.

In the postoperative period, the nurse should implement measures to reduce intracranial pressure. The patient's head of bed should be elevated 30 degrees while ensuring adequate cerebral venous return with proper neck alignment. Valsalva maneuvers should be avoided. The patient's specific gravity should be checked at least every shift and if diuresis occurs. A specific gravity of less than 1.008 should be reported as a possible sign of diabetes insipidus.

The postoperative craniotomy patient for tumor resection often receives steroids for cerebral edema. The nurse should monitor for signs of gastric irritation as a result of the steroids. Urine or blood should be monitored for excess glucose. The patient's risk for thromboembolic complications should be considered and pneumatic compression stockings applied as ordered. A headache is expected postoperatively, and pain medication will be ordered for the discomfort. The nurse should note the amount of analgesic administered when assessing the patient's neurologic status. The patient's head dressing should be assessed with the neurologic assessment and gross bleeding reported to the physician. Often the patient will have a head drain, such as a Jackson-Pratt or an external ventricular drain. The nurse should assess and document the amount and character of drainage. A strict intake and output should be maintained to monitor for fluid overload, which could lead to brain swelling.

Emotional and psychosocial support is a major element of the postoperative care for this patient population. The diagnosis may not be a pleasant one, and supportive care to both the patient and the family should be provided.

Postoperative Complications

One of the nurse's roles is to monitor the patient for postoperative complications. By performing frequent neurologic assessments, the neurosurgical nurse should be able to recognize early warning signs and possibly prevent lifelong deficits. Early identification of a CSF leak aids in the prevention of meningitis. The nurse can assess the drainage for a halo sign (white or yellow ring formation around the center of bloody fluid), which will indicate the presence of CSF. A positive glucose dipstick to confirm CSF can be performed on any clear drainage suspected to be CSF.

The nurse is responsible for the care of the lumbar drain, if one is inserted intraoperatively. Strict aseptic technique should be used when handling the lumbar drain, and nasotracheal suctioning should be avoided to prevent further infection. As a result of cranial nerve V and VII deficits, the patient may develop a corneal abrasion. The nurse should provide artificial tears and an eye shield when indicated. If a severe abrasion develops, an ophthalmologist should be consulted.

Frequent postoperative assessments make it possible for early recognition of increased ICP. This may result from insult to cerebral tissue during surgical exploration or from a hematoma forming from hemorrhage (refer to the nursing management of the patient with increased intracranial pressure).

Seizures may result postoperatively. The nurse must ensure patient safety and airway management during a seizure. Anticonvulsants should be administered as ordered by a physician.

The nurse must provide pulmonary hygiene to the patient to prevent atelectasis and infection. Proper airway alignment and patency should be ensured, especially with a decreased level of consciousness. The nurse's role is to prevent airway obstruction.

Hydrocephalus can result from surgery. The nurse should assess the patient and notify the physician of any change in status. The temporary treatment is a ventriculostomy until the decision for a permanent shunt can be made.

Tension pneumocephalus, usually associated with a sitting intraoperative position, is a postoperative complication. The trapped air can cause increased ICP leading to the signs and symptoms of intracranial hypertension. The nurse's responsibility is to observe the patient for changes and to maintain the patient's head of bed at approximately 30 degrees.

Nursing Care During the Rehabilitation Phase

Individualized care based on the neurologic deficits should be addressed during this phase. Nursing management is directed toward assisting and helping the patient maintain as optimal a health status as possible. Patients should be encouraged to participate in their care as soon as possible with minimal assistance. An altered body image may be present at this time, and the patient should be assisted in obtaining scarves, special hats, and clothing to improve his or her self-image. Every effort should be made to assist the patient to prepare for the return home. He or she should be encouraged to ambulate with the assistance of splints, braces, walkers, or canes as indicated. The nurse should ensure that the appropriate disciplines are involved to arrange for home care as needed, including physical therapy, occupational therapy, speech therapy, and social work. The patient and family need emotional support. This is a time of transition and adjustment for all involved.

Discharge Planning

The discharge process must be initiated as early as possible. Home problems should be identified and remedied as soon as possible. Community resources should be identified to assist the family. The patient should be provided with a plan that includes a follow-up appointment, a list of health problems to report, and what to do should they occur. The patient and family should thoroughly understand the medications the patient is taking and the adverse reactions to look for. The nurse should provide the patient and family with a sense of accomplishment, and they should have a phone number of the person or agency to contact if there is a problem or a question.

PEDIATRIC BRAIN TUMORS

When brain tumors occur in the pediatric population, nurses become involved in the complex care of afflicted children and their families. Nurses provide frequent reinforcement of available clinical and prognostic information as well as constant emotional support. Nurses implement plans of care, addressing issues such as alteration in body image, pain, and altered family processes as needed. Nurses should provide care to children who have brain tumors following a developmental approach. Age-appropriate care should be given to these children, who are frequently between 5 and 10 years old.

Signs and Symptoms

Thorough pediatric neurologic assessments should be performed on patients with suspected or confirmed brain tumors, with any deviations from the child's baseline noted. Clinical manifestations of pediatric brain tumors largely depend on which area of the brain is affected by the tumor. In addition, intracranial tumors can cause both general and focal effects.

General effects occur when the tumor's size leads

to increased ICP. The characteristic signs of increased ICP in infants (whose sutures have not yet completely closed) are enlarged heads and bulging fontanelles. Other general effects of brain tumors may include headaches, seizures, malaise, sleepiness, irritability, personality changes, vision changes, and isolated projectile vomiting.

Focal effects vary with the tumor's location. Cerebellar tumors can cause gait and balance problems. Pituitary tumors can cause endocrine abnormalities and vision changes. Intracranial tumor metastases to the spinal canal can cause weakness, paralysis, and bladder or bowel problems. Tumors in other intracranial locations may cause additional signs and symptoms.

Assessment

Nurses must question the patient, parents, and family members about changes in the child's health. Nurses must also assess the child's developmental level and neurologic condition.

Nurses support patients and families during diagnostic tests. The child may undergo CT scan or MRI of the brain. He or she may also undergo lumbar puncture (LP) for spinal fluid examination. Further, surgical biopsy may be performed to confirm tumor type. Questions regarding these procedures and their implications for the patient should be answered. Nursing care should be provided to the patient undergoing these tests according to established protocols.

Treatment

Complete surgical removal of the brain tumor is the treatment of choice, if possible. Perioperatively, nurses provide appropriate surgical care to these children. If performing surgery on these young patients would cause extensive residual neurologic damage, however, other treatment modalities may be implemented.

Radiation therapy, administered in high doses during approximately eight treatment periods, may be given to help reduce brain tumor size. Radiation is usually not given to children under 2 years old, because these children are at special risk for developing mental retardation after radiation therapy. Nurses can assist children undergoing radiation and their families to implement individualized plans addressing the fatigue, difficult treatment regimen, and disruption in family life that are associated with radiation therapy.

Chemotherapy is given to children who are too young to undergo radiation treatment. Chemotherapy is also used for children whose tumors were partially surgically removed or whose tumors have recurred or spread. Nurses help children undergoing chemotherapy cope with any side effects experienced, including vomiting episodes and hair loss.

Nurses provide comfort measures, emotional support, and age-appropriate nursing care to children undergoing these treatments. In addition, nurses provide parents and family members with frequent informational updates during treatment.

Follow-up Care

Nurses caring for pediatric patients with brain tumors often coordinate efforts of physicians, social workers, play therapists, occupational and physical therapists, and teachers to meet the needs of patients and family members. Nurses may also coordinate post-discharge care for these patients.

Upon discharge, nurses teach family members the importance of follow-up care. Nurses instruct family members to notify their health care providers if the child experiences any neurologic changes, including seizures and signs of increased ICP, or if the child experiences any side effects from prescribed medications. Nurses also provide information about support groups to interested patients and family members. (For additional information on brain tumors, see Chapters 17 and 18.)

SPINA BIFIDA

Spina bifida, a condition occurring when the spinal cord does not complete its normal embryonic development, is a common central nervous system developmental defect. Affecting about 1–2 of every 1000 newborn infants, it is a defect in which the posterior part of one or more vertebrae fail to fuse. The degree of defective spinal cord development caused by spina bifida depends on the type and significance of the condition.

Types

Spina bifida is classified into three types: spina bifida occulta, meningocele, and myelomeningocele. Each of the three types of spina bifida demands specialized nursing care, both acutely in the newborn and then chronically in the adult.

In spina bifida occulta, in which the spinal cord and meninges are normal and the only defect is to the vertebrae, no treatment is needed unless the patient displays neurologic symptoms. In meningocele, the infant is born with a sac containing meninges and cerebrospinal fluid protruding over the vertebrae in the lower back. Although the spinal cord itself is not affected, emergency repair and closing of the sac are indicated to prevent additional damage. In myelomeningocele, the type of spina bifida

CARE PLAN

Perioperative Nursing Care for the Infant With Spina Bifida

I. Potential for infection related to exposed area secondary to presence of meningeal sac

Nursing Goal (A): Prevent Infection

Nursing Interventions:

- Inspect myelomeningocele for any changes in appearance; possible changes could include cuts, tears, drainage, or signs of infection
- Position infant to prevent the sac from contamination by stool or urine
- Implement measures to avoid infection during sac dressing changes, including hand washing, wearing of sterile gloves and masks
- Cleanse sac with sterile saline and apply sterile dressings as ordered
- Administer antibiotics as ordered

Nursing Goal (B): Prevent Trauma to Meningeal Sac

Nursing Interventions:

- Use extreme care whenever handling infant
- Position infant on side or prone, unless otherwise contraindicated
- Utilize devices to protect sac
- Avoid dressings that could adhere to sac
- Implement care routines that decrease possible contact with sac

Nursing Goal (C): Identify Potential Complications

Nursing Interventions:

- Assess infant for signs of hydrocephalus: measure head circumference at least every day, inspect fontanelles for bulging or tenseness, note new irritability or high-pitched cry
- Assess for signs of meningeal irritation or inflammation: signs include fever, nuchal rigidity, irritability
- Check any sac drainage for glucose, which indicates a CSF leak

II. Altered family process related to infant's acute and chronic manifestation of spina bifida

Nursing Goal: Prepare Family for Patient's Discharge

Nursing Interventions:

- Implement an educational teaching plan to facilitate the family's learning about the disease process, surgery, treatment, and care regimen
- Provide family with information about the child's follow-up care needs
- Provide family with available resources and support groups
- Provide family with emotional support as needed

occurring most frequently, the external sac contains neural tissue in addition to meninges and cerebrospinal fluid. This infant requires both immediate surgical repair and vigilant nursing care and is likely to experience serious neurologic complications.

Caring for Infants

Nurses caring for an infant afflicted by spina bifida need to implement measures to both protect exposed areas of the spinal cord and prevent infection. As the infant is prepared for emergency surgery, nurses coordinate a multidisciplinary effort to keep the sac clean, moist, and intact while supporting all of the infant's body systems. A sterile, moist dressing is placed over the sac, and the infant is kept prone. After surgery, nurses assess for any neurologic changes including the onset of hydrocephalus. Nurses continually provide information and emotional support to parents and caregivers during this difficult time.

Conclusion

Nurses caring for patients with spina bifida play an instrumental role in continually assessing patients, quickly planning and coordinating treatments, competently implementing physical and educational interventions, and constantly evaluating patients' and families' responses to care.

MENINGITIS

Central nervous system infection is a serious complication of neurosurgery. Nurses in neurosurgical settings have a vital role in preventing infection, assessing for signs and symptoms of infection, and implementing treatments and supportive measures if infection has occurred.

Bacterial meningitis, the most frequently encountered neurosurgical infection, results from an invasion of bacterial organisms in the subarachnoid space. Intracranial meninges, specifically the arachnoid and the pia mater, become inflamed, causing changes in the patient's clinical status.

Organisms may invade the subarachnoid space secondary to head trauma with skull fractures, ICP monitoring, ventriculostomies, cranial surgery, lumbar punctures, facial and sinus surgery, or sepsis. The immunocompromised patient has an increased risk of developing meningitis. These patients include patients on immunosuppressive agents and people with AIDS. Most cases of meningitis are caused by specific bacterial or viral pathogens. Aseptic meningitis occurs when irritants such as blood, drugs, or contrast material cause an inflammatory reaction in the subarachnoid space.

The nurse's role in preventing meningitis includes administering ordered prophylactic antibiotic treatments. Frequent hand washing and strict aseptic technique should be maintained whenever nursing measures include contact with open neurosurgical wounds and cerebrospinal fluid.

Assessment

The classic signs and symptoms of acute meningitis in the adult are fever, headache, nuchal rigidity, photophobia, back pain, irritability, fatigue, nausea, and vomiting. Young children typically experience fever, anorexia, vomiting, diarrhea, bulging fontanelles, a high-pitched cry, and listlessness. Meningitis is not always clear-cut. Infantile cases show few typical signs, but meningitis must be suspected whenever a child is drowsy or irritable for no apparent reason.[31] In all cases of meningitis, altered levels of consciousness ranging from drowsiness to coma are common.

The nursing assessment should include monitoring for signs of meningeal irritation including headache, nuchal rigidity, irritability, Kernig's sign, and Brudzinski's sign. Nuchal rigidity (stiff neck), in which the patient resists when the neck is flexed by a clinician, is often an early sign. Kernig's sign, elicited by the clinician flexing the patient's upper leg to a 90-degree angle at the hip and then attempting to extend the knee, includes hamstring spasm and pain. Brudzinski's sign is positive when the patient flexes both of the upper legs at the hips and the lower legs at the knee in response to flexion of the neck by the physician.

Patients with meningitis may also experience increased ICP, generalized or focal seizures, cranial nerve deficits, and endocrine disorders. Increased ICP may be due to purulent drainage, cerebral swelling, or hydrocephalus. Increased ICP may lead to brain herniation. Generalized convulsions often occur secondary to cortical irritability. Focal motor seizures result from an accumulation of exudate over one cortical convexity.[32]

Cranial nerve problems often create residual neurologic dysfunction. Increased ICP causes compression of cranial nerve II. Papilledema is a frequent problem, and blindness can occur. Ocular movements are affected when there is irritation to cranial nerves III, IV, and VI. Ptosis, unequal pupils, and diplopia may also occur. If cranial nerve VIII becomes involved, the patient frequently experiences tinnitus, vertigo, and deafness (see also Chapter 5).

Endocrine disorders occasionally seen are hyponatremia and the syndrome of inappropriate secretion of antidiuretic hormone (SIADH). The resultant retention of fluid intensifies the cerebral edema in the acute inflammatory process.

Additional assessment findings in meningitis include personality changes, paresis, paralysis, decreased attention span, and photophobia. Complications to watch for are symptoms of pneumonia and endocarditis. Subdural effusions frequently complicate meningitis in children less than 4 years old. Epilepsy is particularly apt to develop in young children. The outlook is considerably worse whenever this occurs.

Intervention

Following diagnosis, the nurse's role includes administering ordered antimicrobial medications, providing general supportive measures, and assessing for further complications. Control of fever is a primary intervention. Nurses can administer antipyretic medications as ordered. Utilization of hypothermia blankets, providing cool baths, removing extra bed linens, and maintaining a cool room temperature are also effective in controlling fever. It is imperative to reduce the high fever, thereby decreasing the heart's workload and the brain's oxygen demand. The patient's vital signs must be assessed routinely, as tachypnea and tachycardia frequently accompany fever.

Febrile patients are also at risk for dehydration. An accurate measurement of intake and output (with consideration of insensible losses) is a priority. The nurse should direct close attention to excessive diaphoresis and/or oliguria. Replacement of fluid and electrolytes may be indicated if the patient has significant losses. Daily weights should also be included in the standard of care.

Maintaining adequate oxygenation is a significant goal when caring for a patient with meningitis.

Routine monitoring of the patient's respiratory status is important. The nurse should pay close attention to quality and rate of respiration, breath sounds, arterial blood gas levels, oxygen saturation values, and presence and consistency of respiratory secretions. Maintaining a patent airway is a potential clinical issue, especially if the patient has an altered level of consciousness. A bag-mask device should be kept in close proximity of the patient. Intubation equipment should also be readily accessible.

Control of back pain and headaches, nuchal rigidity, and photophobia are often challenging issues for the nurse to address. Analgesics such as acetaminophen and codeine should be administered as ordered. Elevating the patient's head to 30 degrees may also ease headache pain. Many patients are more comfortable without a pillow. A side-lying position is frequently assumed due to nuchal rigidity. It is important to establish the comfort measures each patient prefers on an individual basis.

Bed rest and a dark, quiet environment are indicated, especially if the patient is experiencing irritability, hyperalgesia, and photophobia. Patients with meningitis sometimes misinterpret stimuli, so it is necessary to create an environment they perceive as safe. A soft, calm voice and simple discussions should be used. It is best to reinforce all explanations, keeping in mind the patient may have a decreased attention span. Family members should be encouraged to participate in the patient's care but be advised to allow for frequent rest periods.

The family plays a significant role in the patient's care and recovery. Family teaching, at a minimum, should include pathophysiology, isolation protocols, medications, procedures, and details of the patient's status. Isolation practices will vary among institutions. It is common to maintain respiratory isolation for at least 24 hours after initiation of antibiotic therapy. The family may be helpful in identifying the patient's close contacts who might benefit from meningococcal vaccinations. Meningitis is a potentially fatal disease, so the family may require additional emotional support.

Seizure precautions are indicated to promote safety. If the patient presents with hydrocephalus or significant brain swelling, ICP monitoring may be indicated. Routine neurologic assessments should be completed every 1–2 hours. Assessment should consist of level of consciousness, pupillary responses, eye opening, verbal response, motor response, and cranial nerve functioning. Sensory assessment should include testing the conscious patient's response to light touch.

Further interventions should be implemented according to the patient's specific neurologic deficits. If the patient is comatose, measures should be taken to avoid complications of immobility and unresponsiveness. Cranial nerve deficits should be treated as they arise. Patient comfort and safety should be optimized as a goal of nursing intervention. Occupational therapy, physical therapy, speech therapy, and rehabilitative medicine services will play an integral role in the patient's recovery.

Rehabilitation for the patient with meningitis should focus on the specific residual deficits experienced by the patient. The type and severity of impairment will dictate the interventions that are necessary. The long-term goals are to optimize motor function, expand functional ability, and improve cognitive integration skills.

LUMBAR PUNCTURE

The nurse plays a significant role in supporting a patient throughout a lumbar puncture. During a lumbar puncture, a spinal needle is inserted into the patient's lumbar subarachnoid space and CSF is withdrawn. The CSF specimen can be evaluated for signs of hemorrhage, infection, or other disease process. A lumbar puncture is also performed to measure CSF pressure and, after proper precautions, to remove CSF to reduce that pressure. The procedure can also be utilized to administer drugs, such as antibiotics or spinal anesthesia.

Contraindications

In patients with increased ICP, the pressure changes caused by lumbar puncture can cause herniation. When increased ICP is suspected, patients should have a CT scan and a thorough baseline neurologic examination before a lumbar puncture is performed.

Patients who are following a regimen of anticoagulation therapy should not undergo a lumbar puncture. In this situation, the puncture could lead to hemorrhage. Patients who have skin infections on or around the lumbar area should not have a lumbar puncture performed. During insertion, the spinal needle could easily become contaminated, and meningitis could result.

Positioning

There are two common lumbar puncture positions: side-lying, with legs flexed and chin tucked in close to the chest (lateral recumbent position), or sitting up, bent over an overbed table or tray with the arms on a pillow.

Procedure

The lumbar area is draped and scrubbed with sterile surgical soap. Strict aseptic technique is followed as the spinal needle is inserted between the fourth and fifth (or third and fourth) lumbar vertebrae. This insertion area is below the level of the spinal cord, which ends at the first lumbar vertebral level. The specimen is collected, pressure measured, or medication may be instilled. Then the needle is removed and a sterile dressing applied. The length of the procedure varies depending on both the size of the spinal needle and how quickly the CSF drips out, but is usually about 20 minutes.

Nursing Care

Nursing care of patients undergoing a lumbar puncture is directed at prevention of complications and the reduction of any pain or anxiety related to the procedure. Continuing neurologic assessments are necessary before, during, and after the lumbar puncture, especially of the patient's level of consciousness and any unusual sensory or motor symptoms.

Anxiety due to hospitalization, procedures, or pain is common. As with all procedures, the physician and nurse are obligated to explain both the necessity for the lumbar puncture and the procedure itself. It is important to elicit the specific concerns of the patient and/or family. These concerns dictate the anxiety-relieving measures instituted.

The patient may be unable to cooperate with the procedure as a result of agitation, anxiety, altered cognition, or altered perception. If this is the case, succinct explanations, reassurance, and sedation may be necessary. If sedation is used, frequent monitoring of respiratory status is prudent.

Complications

Pain related to a lumbar puncture can be due to positioning, the puncture itself, headache, or muscle spasm. Flexing the neck forward in either the side-lying or sitting positions can be painful if nuchal rigidity is present. An analgesic, if permitted, may relieve some pain. Reassurance and gentle positioning may reduce discomfort. Asking the patient to exhale with lumbar stretching may help the patient to relax into the side-lying or sitting position. It is important to assist the patient by providing physical support and protecting against sudden involuntary movements. Patients may also experience pain and involuntary movement due to muscle spasm. Position changes and relaxation will help minimize spasm.

Removal of spinal fluid or meningeal irritation may cause mild to intense headaches. The headache can be minimized by patients lying flat for at least 8 hours after the lumbar puncture. Taking in large quantities of fluid (35–40 mL/kg) in the 24 hours following the procedure can decrease the intensity of the headache. Using the smallest possible needle for insertion further reduces patients' post–lumbar puncture headaches. Nurses should administer analgesic medications as ordered to treat patients with these headaches. The use of a pain scale will aid in the assessment, documentation, and evaluation of interventions directed at pain relief.

As with any invasive procedure, lumbar puncture increases the risk of infection because lumbar puncture penetrates the protective membranes of the central nervous system. CNS infection is a serious complication of a lumbar puncture.

Infection may be prevented by strict aseptic technique during the lumbar puncture and observation for CSF leakage afterward. CSF leaks may develop with a lumbar puncture, especially with a traumatic tap or with use of large-bore needles. If noted, CSF leakage should be reported immediately and a sterile pressure dressing applied. The dressing should be reinforced to protect against contamination. Keeping the head of the bed low or flat (if not contraindicated) reduces the pressure of CSF on the puncture site. Monitoring of vital signs and temperature periodically after the procedure can alert the clinician to changes in patient condition, such as hemorrhage or infection. The patient should be instructed to report temperature elevations after discharge to the health care provider.

When CSF sampling is completed, the color and clarity of the fluid should be noted. Typically, several tubes of CSF are analyzed for glucose, protein, cell count and differential, and culture. Bloody CSF may be due to subarachnoid hemorrhage or a traumatic lumbar puncture.

If the tap is traumatic, the bloody color should clear with successive samples. Consequently, a later and clearer tube may be designated as the tube to send for cell count and differential. If the CSF is consistently bloody or xanthochromic, subarachnoid hemorrhage may have occurred. Cloudy CSF may be due to a large number of white blood cells, protein, or microorganisms.

When increased ICP is a concern, pressure is measured using a manometer prior to, and sometimes after, fluid sampling. Pressure is dependent on body position during a lumbar puncture. In the presence of high pressure ($\geq$20 cm H_2O or 15 mm Hg), close monitoring of neurologic status is especially important.

The potential for altered neurologic status exists when lumbar puncture is performed, because of both the pressure changes created with the release of fluid from the subarachnoid space and the possibility of local trauma to spinal nerves. In order to provide safe care, it is important to obtain a baseline neurologic assessment and vital signs. Monitoring the patient's neurologic status and notation of any sensory or motor changes are possible during the procedure by talking to and eliciting responses from the patient. Afterward, a comprehensive assessment is again possible. With any change in level of consciousness, the person performing the lumbar puncture should be notified immediately. The procedure may be stopped. CT scan of the head may be ordered if the patient does not return to baseline.

Transitory urinary retention may occur after the lumbar puncture. Voiding prior to the procedure facilitates patient comfort and minimizes bladder distention. It is important to monitor intake and output for voiding pattern after the procedure, to report the inability to void (after the usual nursing interventions) for 8 or more hours to the physician, and to obtain an order to in-and-out catheterize the patient. It is also relevant to monitor for ability to void after catheterization.

MYASTHENIA GRAVIS

Myasthenia gravis (MG) is a disease of muscle weakness caused by a defect at the myoneural junction. MG is theorized as an autoimmune disease affecting the amount of acetylcholine (ACh) available at the presynaptic membrane or lack of ACh at the postsynaptic receptor sites. Although the etiology is unknown, a significant number of MG patients are diagnosed with thymoma, thymic hyperplasia, and other autoimmune disorders. The hallmark of myasthenia gravis is abnormal muscle fatigue induced by activity that is relieved by rest. The disease is chronic and progressive by nature, affecting the quality of life of those who are diagnosed with the illness.

Assessment

Diagnosis of MG is based on a history of muscle and motor weakness of certain voluntary muscle groups. Complaints of diplopia, ptosis, and ocular palsy may be the first symptoms. Weakness of fine motor movements in the hand and fingers can be early signs that cause the patient to seek medical advice. This weakness is characterized by improvement with rest, but muscle fatigue returns shortly after resumption of the activity. If facial, masticatory, speech, and neck muscles are involved, difficulty in chewing and swallowing of food, altered facial expressions, inability to hold the head upright, and changes in voice patterns occur. As the disease progresses, aspiration of food, liquids, and oral secretions can become an issue. When the intercostal muscles and diaphragm are involved, a life-threatening situation exists. Dyspnea, shortness of breath, and breathlessness are primary signs of this involvement. A neurologic emergency is apparent when the complications of respiratory failure, aspiration, myasthenic crisis, and cholinergic crisis are presented.

A comprehensive history that outlines the signs and symptoms experienced by the patient should be obtained. It is important to highlight the impact of this symptomatology on the patient's activities of daily living. If the patient is a known myasthenic, it is of paramount importance to note the anticholinesterase drugs (Table 19–3) that are taken at home, the last dose administered, the dosage, and time schedule followed. It is also very relevant to review and identify with the patient other precipitating factors of crisis (Table 19–4). The patient's and family's awareness of the disease and treatment modalities utilized is very significant in order to assess their understanding of the disease and compliance with drug therapy.

When a new diagnosis of MG is made or in the situation of myasthenic versus cholinergic crisis, the patient and family must be prepared for the testing that will identify or differentiate the diagnosis. Teaching will include information about the Tensilon (edrophonium chloride) test, electromyography (EMG), and blood tests that track serum antibodies to acetylcholine receptors.

Diagnostic Studies

Anticholinesterase Tests

The edrophonium chloride (Tensilon) test is the diagnostic test regarded as most useful and reliable in the diagnosis of MG and the differentiation of myasthenic (tolerance to or inadequate dosage of anticholinesterase drugs) versus cholinergic crisis (overdose of anticholinesterase drugs).

If symptoms improve after administration of Tensilon, the crisis is myasthenic. Conversely, if symptoms deteriorate, the crisis is cholinergic. When the Tensilon test proves inconclusive, a neostigmine test may be administered.

Laboratory Tests

ACh receptor antibody titers will be elevated in 80%–90% of patients with generalized myasthenia. MG patients will test positive with a receptor-blocking assay. A mouse transfer assay results in myasthenic symptoms in mice. Thyroid function studies are run to rule out thyroid etiology.

Nerve Conduction Studies

Repetitive nerve stimulation studies stimulate nerves electrically at various frequencies. The my-

TABLE 19–3 **DRUGS USED FOR MYASTHENIA GRAVIS**

DRUG	ACTION	DOSAGE	IMPLICATIONS
Anticholinesterases			
Neostigmine (Prostigmin)	Enhances cholinergic action by facilitating impulses across neuromuscular junction Inhibits the destruction of acetylcholine by cholinesterase enhancing	Oral (acts within 20 minutes/ peaks ~ 2.5 hours) 7.5–45 mg every 2–6 hours tailored to individual patient needs Neostigmine tablets supplied in 15 mg scored tablets	*Muscarinic type* Gastrointestinal tract: heartburn, belching, epigastric distress, abdominal cramps, increased peristalsis, diarrhea, nausea, vomiting Cardiovascular: bradycardia and hypotension, or tachycardia and hypertension Vision: blurred, constricted pupils, photophobia, myopia Respiratory tract: bronchoconstriction, increased mucus secretions, wheezing cough, chest pain and tightness Other: profuse sweating and salivation *Nicotinic type*
Pyridostigmine (Mestinon)	Inhibits destruction of cholinesterase	60–180 mg three to four times a day, orally Action is longer and smoother than neostigmine Also supplied in 180 mg time-span tablets, effective in maintaining the patient overnight	Side effects are of the muscarinic and nicotinic types Often used in combination with neostigmine for maintenance therapy, manipulated to produce maximum muscle strength with minimal side effects *Atropine* is the antidote for anticholinesterase drugs. Atropine must be available to patients receiving anticholinesterase therapy
Ambenonium (Mytelase)	Duration of action is longer than that of neostigmine or pyridostigmine, but its action is not as specific		Same as pyridostigmine Used less frequently
Corticosteroids			
ACTH and prednisone are drugs of choice	Appear to cause a remission in the severity of disease Used for those patients who do not respond well to anticholinesterase drugs	ACTH: 100–160 units daily for 10 days Prednisone: 100 mg every other day	ACTH: symptoms temporarily worsen then improve progressively after course completed Remission may last 3–6 months, requiring periodic retreatment Prednisone: current practice; symptoms worsen in first 7–10 days. Patient hospitalized for observation of respiratory problems. Concurrent administration with anticholinesterase drugs

Adapted from Alspach/Williams: Myasthenia Gravis, p 325. Philadelphia, WB Saunders, 1985; Hickey J: Guillain-Barré Syndrome, p 643. In The Clinical Practice of Neurological and Neurosurgical Nursing, 3/e. Philadelphia, JB Lippincott, 1992.

asthenic patient will demonstrate progressive decrement of muscle action potentials. EMG identifies the defect at the myoneural junction by differentiating between presynaptic and postsynaptic defects.

Other Studies

Thymoma and thymic hyperplasia may be identified by a thymus scan. Chest x-ray films or tomograms may reveal thymic abnormalities.

Treatment

The management plan for the patient with myasthenia gravis will be based on the appropriate drug therapy specific to the individual. Anticholinesterase drugs and corticosteroid therapy are the most frequently prescribed treatment modalities (see Table 19–3). Where applicable, thymectomy and plasmapheresis are approaches for a select group of patients. Thymectomy is indicated for MG related to a tumor of the thymus. Plasmapheresis is performed on those patients exhibiting severe myasthenic signs and symptoms such as imminent or actual respiratory failure.

Nursing Management

Nursing management of the patient diagnosed with myasthenia gravis involves all categories of the

TABLE 19–4 **MYASTHENIA GRAVIS: PRECIPITATING FACTORS OF CRISIS**

1. Inadequate anticholinesterase drug levels (myasthenic crisis)
2. Overdosage of anticholinesterase drugs (cholinergic crisis)
3. Influenza
4. Menstrual cycle or pregnancy (especially first trimester)
5. Certain drugs: -quinine, -mycin antibiotics, procainamide, quinidine, phenothiazines, barbiturates, tranquilizers, narcotics
6. Emotional stress and anxiety
7. Fatigue
8. Alcohol
9. Surgery

Adapted from Alspach/Williams: Myasthenia Gravis, p 323. Philadelphia, WB Saunders, 1985.

nursing process. Formulation of a comprehensive plan of care along with the appropriate teaching modalities are necessary to highlight potential or apparent problems and identify patient and family teaching needs. Hospitalization may be necessary during initial diagnosis, drug evaluation, and during periods of crisis or respiratory involvement/failure. Refer to the care plans in Tables 19–5 through 19–7 to review the nursing management of the patient diagnosed with MG, as well as Chapter 13.

GUILLAIN-BARRÉ SYNDROME

Guillain-Barré syndrome (GBS) is an acute inflammatory polyneuropathy. Although the etiology is unknown, GBS is thought to be an autoimmune response to a viral infection. Destruction of the myelin sheath surrounding spinal and cranial nerves results in edema and inflammation of the peripheral nerves secondary to the demyelination process. The hallmark of this disease process is the acute ascending paralysis caused by the demyelination that begins in distal nerves and ascends symmetrically. The paralysis may progress to quadriplegia with involvement of cranial nerves or halt at any point. Remyelination is a slow process with function returning proximally then moving distally. Complete recovery with little or no residual disability occurs in the majority of cases.

Assessment

Diagnosis of Guillain-Barré syndrome (also known as infectious polyneuritis, polyradiculoneuritis, polyneuritis, Landry-Guillain-Barré-Strohl syndrome) is based on a history of the onset of acute weakness and paralysis involving both proximal and distal limbs, recent viral infection, elevated CSF protein level with normal cell count, and EMG studies. The patient with GBS may present with complaints of extremity paresthesias, symmetric ascending weakness, dysphagia, muscle tenderness, areflexia, transient sensory loss, and varied cranial nerve (CN) involvement. CN VII involvement occurs most frequently, then VI, III, XII, V, IX, and X. GBS is classified according to four different variants, reflecting the degree of peripheral nerve involvement. These variants are ascending GBS, descending GBS, Miller-Fisher variant, and pure motor variant (see Table 19–9).

Diagnostic Studies

Clinical Presentation

Review of signs and symptoms may note acute onset of illness, motor weakness that is rapid and progressive in more than one limb, areflexia, and hypotonia without atrophy. A history of a viral infection 2–3 weeks prior to symptoms is often reported. Laboratory examination of CSF will reveal the classic finding of albuminocytologic dissociation (elevated CSF protein with a normal cell count). This increase in protein occurs in the first week after the onset of symptoms and peaks within 4–6 weeks.

Nerve Conduction Studies

Electromyography will note slowed or blocked conduction in 80% of cases and velocities that are 60% of normal in others. Abnormal EMG findings are found several weeks after onset of symptoms and are not generally used to diagnose GBS in the acute stages.

Treatment

GBS does not have a cure, and management is based on supportive care and treatment of symptoms until health is restored. Neurologic emergencies present when muscle weakness or paralysis affects breathing patterns requiring mechanical ventilation and intensive care nursing. Plasmapheresis is routinely used to remove antibodies from the bloodstream, decreasing the autoimmune response in peripheral nerves (see Table 19–7). Steroids may be prescribed for a trial period, discontinuing treatment if no response is documented after a few days.

Nursing Management

Nursing management of the patient with GBS is as challenging as it is comprehensive. This patient requires multisystem medical and nursing management, as well as psychosocial support. A plan of care that reflects both patient and family needs assessments is of paramount importance. Refer to Tables 19–7 through 19–9 to review the care plans

TABLE 19–5 **NURSING MANAGEMENT OF THE PATIENT WITH MYASTHENIA GRAVIS**

DIAGNOSIS	GOAL	INTERVENTION	EVALUATION
Ineffective breathing pattern related to weak muscles of respiration	Adequate and comfortable breathing	Assess breathing pattern noting any abnormality. Observe for weak cough, difficult swallowing, ineffective response of muscles to medication, restlessness, dyspnea Measure vital capacity every 2–4 hours. Know norm specific for patient Support inadequate breathing pattern with assisted ventilation–endotracheal intubation; tracheostomy may become necessary	Adequate pulmonary function Adequate and comfortable breathing
Risk for aspiration related to weakened muscles of swallowing	Maintenance of adequate nutrition without aspiration	Teach the patient and family to observe for signs of aspiration Encourage a soft diet, small bites, frequent swallowing Teach patient and family emergency care of aspiration May be necessary to place feeding tube during crisis	Maintains adequate nutrition Patient free of aspiration Patient and family demonstrate knowledge of emergency care of aspiration
Impaired physical mobility related to muscle weakness	Maintenance of adequate mobility and motor function to perform activities of daily living (ADL)	Assess motor function in relation to medication regimen Consult physician to adjust or reassess drug program Review daily activities with patient. Note weakest moments, scheduled periods of rest, understanding and compliance with drug program Teach patient and family the importance of maintaining a daily schedule that allows for periods of rest Teach the patient to pace activities	Patient will maintain an adequate energy level to perform ADLs, with scheduled periods of rest, and will follow prescribed drug program
Knowledge deficit related to diagnosis and hospitalization	Understanding of disease process	Teach the patient and family about the disease process, the need to alter lifestyle, and the medication program to be followed Provide verbal and written information regarding the local chapter of the Myasthenia Gravis Foundation. Medic-Alert bracelet Encourage the patient and family to lead as normal a life as possible	Demonstrates knowledge of disease process and treatment Patient and family will verbalize and demonstrate knowledge of the disease process and treatment program
Myasthenic versus cholinergic crisis	Identifying signs of crisis	Teach patient and family signs of crisis and need to seek emergent medical attention (restlessness, dyspnea, marked motor dysfunction) Inform that the Tensilon test may be used to differentiate between myasthenic and cholinergic crisis Teach the precipitating factors (see Table 19–4) of crisis Provide a written list at discharge; assess understanding, promote compliance	Patient and family demonstrate understanding of crisis and state the precipitating factors that cause crisis
Medication program Anticholinesterase Steroids Atropine	Compliance with drug program; maximum motor strength obtained	Provide verbal and written information regarding prescribed medications, their action, dosage, and side effects. Comprehensive drug cards are excellent teaching tools and reference material for patients and families Reinforce necessity to take anticholinesterase medication on schedule Teach to observe muscular response to medication, activity, etc. Suggest a diary to document response, questions	Patient and family demonstrate knowledge and understanding of prescribed medication program

TABLE 19–6 **NURSING MANAGEMENT OF THE PATIENT UNDERGOING THYMECTOMY**

DIAGNOSIS	INTERVENTION	EVALUATION
Impaired breathing pattern related to chest surgery, chest tubes, and tracheostomy	Maintain patency of airway: suction, tracheostomy care, pulmonary toilet (encourage cough, deep breathing, and perform chest physical therapy) Turn patient every 2 hours. Ensure proper positioning to maximize lung expansion and promote comfort Monitor respiratory status Institute proper care for the patient with chest tubes	Patient demonstrates adequate oxygenation and is free of pulmonary infection
Knowledge deficit related to thymectomy surgery	Anticholinesterase drugs may be discontinued prior to surgery necessitating ventilatory support. Provide all interventions necessary to care for patient on a ventilator Provide for a means of communication between patient family and members of health care team Anticholinesterase drugs and/or steroids will be reinstituted after thymectomy at low doses requiring careful assessment of motor response Remind patient and family that full effects of thymectomy may occur gradually with maximal effect noted in 1–10 years Anticholinesterase drugs and steroids will probably be required after thymectomy, although often in smaller amounts	Patient will understand reason for mechanical ventilation pre-/ post thymectomy Patient will communicate needs effectively while ventilated Patient will demonstrate understanding that medication regimens need to be followed and full effects of thymectomy may not be apparent for 1–10 years

designed for the patient with GBS, as well as Chapter 13.

HEPATIC ENCEPHALOPATHY

Hepatic encephalopathy (HE) is a complex neuropsychiatric syndrome resulting from acute or chronic hepatocellular failure. In its early stages, the syndrome is characterized by subtle behavioral, psychiatric, and cognitive changes that may be difficult for the clinician to detect. As encephalopathy progresses, intellectual abilities, motor function, and consciousness become impaired. Hepatic encephalopathy is a true neurologic emergency when fulminant hepatic failure (FHF) resulting from an acute process leads to brain swelling and coma. The nursing management of patients with FHF requires multisystem supportive care, vigilant neurologic assessment, and implementation of measures to minimize intracranial hypertension.

Etiology

FHF is defined as a sudden onset of hepatocyte necrosis and the development of encephalopathy within 8 weeks of the onset of initial symptoms.[33] The diagnosis of FHF requires adherence to the definition as well as supportive biochemical and

TABLE 19–7 **NURSING MANAGEMENT OF THE PATIENT UNDERGOING PLASMAPHERESIS**

DIAGNOSIS	INTERVENTION	EVALUATION
Impaired physical mobility related to severe myasthenia gravis (MG) Ineffective breathing pattern related to myasthenia gravis or Guillain-Barré syndrome (GBS)	Teach the patient that plasmapheresis separates blood into component parts for the purpose of removal of one or more components (MG: washes acetylcholine receptor antibodies from the plasma; GBS: removal of antibodies from bloodstream reduces autoimmune response in peripheral nerves) Explain that the exchanges take place at the bedside with a plasma separator machine For MG: (1) Procedure takes 3–5 hours depending on size of patient. (2) 3–5 exchanges every other day with improved muscle strength 24–48 hours after first exchange. (3) Albumin is used as the plasma exchanger through an antecubital shunt access. (4) Indefinite number of exchanges at 1–4 week intervals. (5) Palliates, not long-term cure For GBS: (1) 3–5 exchanges of 3–4 L each exchange. (2) Treatment must be started within 2 weeks after onset of GBS to be effective. (3) Used to decrease time on ventilator, decrease recovery time, and reduce length of hospitalization *Complications* MG: medications removed during plasmapheresis, hypotension, nausea or vomiting, transient paralysis, bleeding from anticoagulation, pulmonary emboli from venous coagulation GBS: clotting disturbances, hypocalcemia, infection, decreased serum protein, hypotension, autonomic disreflexia, phlebitis	Absence of complications post plasmapheresis

TABLE 19–8 NURSING MANAGEMENT OF THE PATIENT WITH GUILLAIN-BARRÉ SYNDROME

DIAGNOSIS	INTERVENTION	EVALUATION
Risk for ineffective breathing patterns related to neuromuscular weakness of respiratory muscles (diaphragm and intercostals)	Monitor rate and quality of respiratory pattern Monitor breath sounds throughout lung fields Monitor vital capacity and tidal volumes; be aware of normal values for patient Frequent or continuous pulse oximetric monitoring Administer oxygen as ordered Position patient to maximize lung expansion (head of bed elevated or out of bed in chair) Maintain patent airway for mechanically ventilated patient	Adequate ventilation maintained Patient is free of respiratory distress
Ineffective airway clearance related to weak cough reflex and respiratory muscles (diaphragm and intercostals)	Monitor patient's ability to manage secretions and clear airway Suction every 2 hours or as needed Monitor for effective cough reflex Position patient to facilitate maximum drainage from airway and lung expansion (turn side to side every 2 hours with postural drainage and chest physical therapy every 2–4 hours). Elevate head of bed Tracheostomy care every 4–8 hours to maintain patent airway	Patient airway maintained
Risk for disuse syndrome related to immobility secondary to paralysis and confinement to ventilator	Establish bowel program to maintain elimination pattern Meticulous skin care to prevent skin breakdown (turn every 2 hours, frequent skin assessment) Promote venous return with application of pneumatic stockings Give patient opportunity to make some decisions regarding care	Patient will demonstrate: Soft, formed stools as per bowel schedule Intact skin Absence of deep venous thrombosis Participation in decision-making activities
Impaired verbal communication related to paralysis of muscles of speech or intubation	Develop alternate communication methods (eye blinking, raising a finger, using computer board) Teach patient to communicate within physical limitations Teach family methods to communicate with patient	Communication method allows patient to convey needs Family members and other health care providers will be aware of communication system and will use it appropriately
Urinary retention related to autonomic effects on bladder	Establish bladder retraining program based on established physician protocol Maintain and monitor intake and output record Palpate suprapubic area for evidence of distention: monitor patient comfort	Bladder will be emptied every 6–8 hours When independent voiding is re-established, postvoid residuals will be less than 50 mL
Pain related to injury to the peripheral nerves	Establish character and pattern of pain Enhance comfort with frequent positioning (at least every 2 hours) Administer analgesics as ordered Teach patient imagery, relaxation, and diversional thinking techniques	Monitor patient's response to analgesics using approved pain assessment scale Patient will convey feeling of relief from peripheral pain A decrease in pain will be documented in the pain assessment scale
Knowledge deficit related to hospitalization, disease process, and changes in body function	Develop teaching plan to help patient and family understand illness, disease process, and hospital routines and equipment Answer questions and offer support to patient and family	Patient and family will demonstrate knowledge and understanding of illness, hospital routines, equipment, and what to expect
Related diagnoses Sleep pattern disturbance Risk for infection Self-care deficit Constipation Risk for aspiration Nutrition: less than body requires Impaired swallowing Sensory/perceptual deficits Fear Fatigue Anxiety Powerlessness		

Adapted from Hickey JV: Guillain-Barré Syndrome, pp 655–666, Chart 29–9. In The Clinical Practice of Neurological and Neurosurgical Nursing, 3/e. Philadelphia, JB Lippincott, 1992.

injury: Nursing concerns. J Neurosci Nurs 1988;20:217–222.
29. Kinash R: Brain tumors: Therapies and nursing interventions. AXON 1987:9:7–11.
30. Hospital of the University of Pennsylvania: Nursing management of the patient receiving radiation therapy. Clin Pract Guide Quick Ref Guide Clin 1991:4D–02–17.
31. Hickey JV: The Clinical Practice of Neurological and Neurosurgical Nursing, pp 606–614. Philadelphia, JB Lippincott, 1992.
32. Jennett B, Lindsay KW: An introduction to neurosurgery, pp 178–185. Boston, Butterworth-Heineman, 1994.
33. Trey C, Davidson C: The management of fulminant hepatic failure. In Popper H, Schaffner F (eds): Progress in Liver Disease, p 282. New York, Grune & Stratton, 1970.
34. Mathieson LR, Linglof T, Maller AM, et al: Am J Infect Dis 1979;11:303.
35. Riegler JL, Lake JR: Fulminant hepatic failure. Med Clin North Am 1993;77:1057–1083.
36. Basile AS, Jones AS, Skolnick P: The pathogenesis and treatment of hepatic encephalopathy: Evidence of the involvement of benzodiazepine receptor ligands. Pharmacol Rev 1991;43:28–71.
37. Donovan JP, Shaw BW, Langnas AN, et al: Brain water and acute liver failure: The emerging role of intracranial pressure monitoring. Hepatology 1992;16(1):267–268.
38. Munoz SJ, Robinson M, Northrup B, et al: Elevated intracranial pressure and computed tomography of the brain in fulminant hepatocellular failure. Hepatology 1991;13:209–212.
39. Williams R, Gimson AE: Intensive liver care and the management of acute hepatic failure. Dig Dis Sci 1991;36:820–826.
40. Weisner RH: Acute fulminant hepatic failure. Trans Proc 1991;23:1892–1894.
41. Walleck CA: Controversies in the management of the head-injured patient. Crit Care Nurs Clin North Am 1989;1:67–74.
42. Keith JS: Hepatic failure: Etiologies, manifestations, and management. Crit Care Nurse 1985;5(1):61–86.
43. Raabe WA: Effects of NH_4 on the function of the CNS. Adv Exp Med Biol 1990;272:99–120.
44. Kucharski SA: Fulminant hepatic failure. Crit Care Nurs Clin North Am 1993;5:141–151.
45. Manns MP: New therapeutic aspects in fulminant hepatic failure. Chest 1991;100(3 Suppl):1935–1965.
46. Sussman NL, Chong MG, Koussayer T, et al: Reversal of fulminant hepatic failure using an extracorporeal liver assist device. Hepatology 1992;16:60–65.

to the descriptive language of rehabilitation. This conceptual model distinguishes impairment, disability, and handicap. An impairment is any limitation or abnormality of psychologic, physiologic, or anatomic structure or function. Impairment encompasses those changes or losses that are associated with an underlying disease process but is not necessarily contingent on etiology. For example, while unilateral weakness may present as an impairment or a change in anatomic and physiologic function, it might also be associated with several disorders within the differential diagnosis, for example, traumatic brain injury, stroke, neuropathy, and myelopathy. Measures of impairment are organ-specific, such as pulmonary vital capacity, nerve conduction velocity, cardiac ejection fraction, renal creatinine clearance, and postvoid residual urinary volume.

A disability is any restriction or lack of ability (resulting from or associated with an impairment) to perform an activity or function in the manner and within the range considered normal for a human being. While the use of the term *function* when considering impairment is concerned with the anatomic or physiologic status of various organs, the use of the term *function* at the level of disability is concerned with the changes in performance of survival skills that one needs to negotiate through everyday life. These survival skills can be broadly categorized into three areas: (1) activities of daily living, (2) mobility, and (3) cognition/communication. Successful performance of survival skills is dependent on a relatively intact substrate of cognitive and intellectual functions, such as attention, short-term memory, visuospatial processing, language comprehension, and executive functioning. Disability involves integrated activities expected of the individual or the body as a whole. It is indicated by skills and the performance of tasks and demonstrated through behavior. For example, if a traumatic brain injury is the underlying disorder and the associated impairment is unilateral weakness, the associated disability may be an inability to ambulate up and down stairs. Walking up and down stairs successfully is dependent not only on the integrity of motor function but also on cognitive functions such as spatial processing and motor planning. The measurement of disability occurs through the process of functional assessment, which is the fundamental evaluative tool in rehabilitation.

A handicap is the result of an impairment or disability that limits or prevents an individual from fulfilling a role that is expected for that individual. Normal social roles are dependent on age, sex, social, and cultural factors and are usually described in terms of the ability to work or be economically productive or successful in an educational program. They also include fulfillment of roles within the family or more immediate social support system. Handicap is characterized by a discordance between the individual's performance and the expectations of the relevant social group. It is a socially constructed phenomenon resulting from impairment and disability. To continue the example of the traumatically brain-injured patient who presents with unilateral weakness and is unable to walk up and down stairs, the associated handicap may be defined as an inability to work or attend school, an inability to relate as a spouse because of sexual dysfunction, or an inability to participate in community activities because of physical structures that interfere with access. A handicap is measured in the broader sense through functional assessment in terms of the performance of higher-level survival skills usually required for negotiation in employment/retirement or interpersonal situations.

Basic Clinical Tools of Rehabilitation

Two fundamental tools of rehabilitation are defined. The first is the *team approach* as the basic model of service provision in rehabilitation, and the second is *functional assessment* as the basic tool of evaluation and outcome determination in response to rehabilitation and medical/surgical interventions. The rehabilitation team is discussed below. Functional assessment is discussed later in this chapter.

The Rehabilitation Team

The traditional rehabilitation team is multidisciplinary—that is, it encompasses professionals from various disciplines including the physician (specifically the physiatrist as the medical specialist in disability), physical therapist, occupational therapist, speech-language pathologist, social worker, rehabilitation nurse, psychologist, recreation therapist, and vocational counselor or special educator. The team leader is the physiatrist. A specialist known as a case manager sometimes coordinates team activities under physician direction. The team process is interdisciplinary in nature—that is, there are regular meetings in which core members of the team convene to discuss and define the plan of care and to define team goals. Further, rehabilitation team meetings serve to monitor response to the plan of care and to modify this plan and the goals accordingly. Team goals are those consensual goals that emerge from shared discipline-specific goals among different team members. These goals are articulated in terms of functional disability and handicap.

The physiatrist as team leader is responsible for orchestrating the interaction at the team meetings and then synthesizing interdisciplinary information into a realistic and specific plan of care. In inpatient settings, rehabilitation team meetings occur on a regular basis, usually weekly. In the outpatient or home care setting, more flexible approaches for team communication exist, with more dependence on telephone discussions with the physiatrist.

The team process is labor-intensive and expensive and brings about overlap of roles among various disciplines. Both rehabilitation nurses and occupational therapists, for example, have expertise and skills related to activities of daily living such as toileting. Both occupational therapy and speech therapy provide treatment in the areas of feeding and swallowing. Both social work services and counseling psychology provide supportive psychotherapies. These overlap areas, however, do not necessarily encourage duplication of services; they are utilized in a productive manner in the division of labor during team care. Discipline-specific observations are made regarding the patient's functional performance and behavior at different points in time, and this multidisciplinary approach is believed to increase the validity of clinical observations made during recovery and in response to therapies. These observations allow definition of the patient's behavioral patterns throughout the day and night. Further, conflict is considered an essential component of team process; it is utilized productively to divide rationally the labor among various personnel to serve the multiple rehabilitation needs of the patient, and it sometimes becomes an indicator of inconsistent patient behavior throughout the day. See Table 20–1 for responsibilities/roles of the neurorehabilitation team members.

The Role of the Physiatrist

Appropriate management of rehabilitation patients requires that physiatrists become "gate keepers" of rehabilitation services. Physiatrists function as both the general coordinator of rehabilitation services and the medical specialist in disability. The physiatrist provides primary medical care alone or in consultation with general medical and surgical health care providers in all rehabilitation settings, and sometimes on a continuous basis especially in the case of patients who have traumatic brain injuries and spinal cord injuries in Model Systems Programs funded by the National Institute on Disability and Rehabilitation Research. This role includes knowing when to request early and appropriate consultation from medical and surgical colleagues to prevent minor medical problems from developing into major ones, both during rehabilitation and during the community life of the person with neurologic disability.

Both inside and outside the hospital setting, the physiatrist is the best medical specialist to prescribe, monitor, and revise rehabilitation services. Therapists who practice in hospital, outpatient, and home care settings seek collegial relationships with physiatrists because these physicians have the broadest understanding of the interaction among the medical, surgical, and rehabilitation interventions.

In the acute hospital-based or skilled nursing facility subacute-based rehabilitation settings, as well as during home- or outpatient-based neurorehabilitation programs, the physiatrist must understand highly technologic state-of-the-art interventions and be prepared to respond quickly to medical emergencies. He or she integrates this knowledge by specifying medical contraindications on prescriptions during referrals to team members, and by helping these team members develop specific monitoring strategies to prevent complications. The physiatrist also coordinates medical and surgical subspecialist care and incorporates prevention, anticipation, and treatment of medical complications and emergencies into the rehabilitation process. Medical and surgical emergencies are expected and common during neurorehabilitation programs because of the high degree of comorbidity seen in neurologically injured patients, especially those who are elderly.[4]

Physiatrists serve an important consultation function to neurologists, neurosurgeons, trauma surgeons, and other medical and surgical physicians (for example, urologists and orthopedic surgeons) during the immediate acute phase after neurologic injury, and prior to entry into a neurorehabilitation program. Within 48–72 hours of injury, the physiatrist can assist with a general prediction of neurologic recovery and associated functional outcome. This can be especially helpful to family members and significant others seeking information about future functional outcome.

When the neurologically injured patient becomes relatively stable (for example, dramatic shifts in intracranial pressure have stabilized), the physiatrist can direct conservative interventions by physical, occupational, and speech/dysphagia therapists aimed at monitoring subtle changes in neural and functional recovery and prevention of anatomic and physiologic effects of inactivity. For example, passive range of motion programs are instituted to prevent soft tissue contractures. Such interventions should begin as soon as the patient is stable, while the patient still requires intensive care and monitoring. Occasionally, some patients with neurologic impairment develop dramatic increases in spasticity and may require treatments, including antispasticity medication and other modalities. Additionally, the physiatrist can make useful sugges-

TABLE 20–1 **NEUROREHABILITATION TEAM: NONMEDICAL MEMBERS AND THEIR USUAL DIVISION OF LABOR**

Physical therapist	Basic mobility skills including bed mobility, transfers, wheelchair mobility, ambulation; assistive devices for ambulation including canes, walkers, and wheelchairs; spasticity management with therapeutic exercises; sensory facilitation of motor control; gait training, including training with orthotic and prosthetic devices of the lower limb
Occupational therapist	Daily living skills including feeding, grooming, toileting, dressing, and homemaking; fine motor skills of the hand and upper limbs including splinting (orthotics) and wheelchair accessories; cognitive remediation, especially in the areas of memory and visuoperception
Speech/swallowing therapist	Cognitive remediation as it relates to meaningful communication, especially in the areas of attention, memory, language comprehension, conceptual organization, language production (including nonverbal technologies), and oral-motor articulation; swallowing evaluation and treatments, specifically regarding oral-motor and pharyngeal function, aspiration precaution, and oral feeding with different food consistencies
Cognitive remediation therapist	Cognitive remediation of basic cognitive domains (attention, memory), as well as those that are highly integrative, e.g., executive functioning; direction and tutoring of special education and vocational programs; job coaching, community re-entry
Neuropsychologist	Formal, in-depth, and quantitative evaluation of cognitive and intellectual function; translation of the cognitive and intellectual strengths and weaknesses into a behaviorally based set of strategies subsequently operationalized by therapists, nurses, family members, and other care providers
Behavioral psychologist	Explicit design of behavioral management strategies and programs (often in concert with medications) aimed at optimizing communication with patients having difficulty with self-monitoring, aggression, poor initiation, and other behaviors that disrupt rehabilitation treatments and social interactions
Counseling psychologist	Psychotherapeutic treatment (often in concert with medications) of loss reactions, depression, and other affective disorders observed during neurologic recovery and sometimes disruptive to participation in therapeutic programs
Recreation therapist	Evaluation and remediation of motor and cognitive function in both individual and group nondidactic settings while focusing on participation in leisure activities
Case manager	Orchestrates appropriate medical, surgical, rehabilitation, and social services depending on the recovery trajectory, treatment priorities, and health insurance financial resources
Social worker	Clarifies social support system, its ability to provide safe and stable emotional support, residential sites, personal care, and transportation; clarifies eligibility and coverage of health and welfare services and health insurance plans; mobilizes resources for coverage of essential health and rehabilitation services with informal and formal care providers acting in complementary roles; often defines the discharge plan; provides emotional support for patients and their social support system members
Rehabilitation nurse	Assists and supervises the patient in operationalizing cognitive and functional skills learned in therapies; patient education of medication schedule and self-monitoring of medical problems, such as diabetes, seizure disorders, skin care, bowel and bladder training programs
Nutritionist	Collaborates with physicians and therapists to establish caloric and nutritional needs during neurologic recovery, and makes recommendations for options of nutritional support depending on the most reliable means of entry of food (oral, enteral, parenteral), and dietary advancement
Prosthetist/orthotist	Assesses need for and fabricates body part replacements in amputees (prosthesis) and assesses need for and fabricates devices that facilitate motor control and conserve energy consumption during mobility (orthotics), especially of lower limbs
Vocational counselor	Assesses and provides information for vocational retraining and employment re-entry; sometimes does job coaching

tions for management of a neurogenic bowel and bladder during the acute phase of treatment and recovery.

Finally, in the consultation role on the acute medical and surgical services and in the intensive care unit, the physiatrist can provide useful advice to physician-colleagues, family members, discharge planners, and social workers about future options regarding different kinds and levels of neurorehabilitation programs, depending on the predicted recovery trajectory of the patient. The importance of early referral and involvement of the physiatrist and the rehabilitation team should not be underestimated. Such involvement will assist in the prevention of effects of inactivity, formulation of a discharge plan involving continued rehabilitation services, and progression from the acute care setting during the early phase of neural recovery after initial life-saving medical and surgical treatments.

PHYSIOLOGIC BASIS OF REHABILITATION MEDICINE AND RECOVERY OF FUNCTION AFTER NEURAL INJURY

Rehabilitation medicine is especially concerned with maximizing the functional return following neural injury and, as such, involves the integration of an understanding of physiologic processes of recovery into the treatment plan. While the acute phase of management of a neurologic emergency involves the stabilization of the patient and the limitation of irreversible neural damage, the rehabilitation phase of treatment is directed toward maximizing the functional recovery given the limitations imposed by the irreversible neural damage that has occurred. Clearly, this effort requires as comprehensive an understanding of the physiology of the recovery process as can be attained. As we will see, recovery from neural injury is a highly complicated process about which we understand remarkably little. Gains are being made on a number of fronts. Animal studies using sophisticated neurophysiologic and neuropharmacologic methods, and advancing technology for visualizing the functioning human brain, are being applied to the issue of understanding recovery from neural injury.

Residual damage to the nervous system may manifest itself clinically with a wide variety of behaviors. Rather than focusing only on the detailed description of specific behavioral deficits, the rehabilitation perspective emphasizes the residual strengths of the individual and the overriding tendency of individuals with nervous system damage to reorganize and reintegrate themselves into a reconstructed functional whole.[5] It is in the context of a holistic "systems-oriented" approach to the recovering individual that the rehabilitation perspective and the scientific orientation of rehabilitation medicine are best understood. An understanding of the physiologic bases of recovery processes in the nervous system is therefore fundamental to the rehabilitation goal of achieving maximal functional recovery.

Unfortunately, relatively little is clearly understood about how the nervous system reorganizes itself after injury. Somewhat more is understood about recovery in the peripheral nervous system than is understood about recovery in the central nervous system (CNS). The recognition that there are significant resources available within the nervous system to support recovery processes is a relatively recent observation. The metaphor of the CNS as a hard-wired "switchboard" with immutable interconnections between irreversibly committed focal brain regions and unit neurons that were assumed unable to regenerate themselves led to a widely accepted pessimism about the potential for restoring lost functions after CNS injury.

A new perspective on brain-behavior correlation and the potential for reorganization of function within the nervous system, however, appears to be emerging as the view of the nervous system as a self-organizing dynamic system begins to take shape and obtain support.[6, 7] The manner in which experience is integrated by the nervous system and how such experience influences future capacity for behavior (i.e., via memory and learning) is also being examined as new methods for looking at "neuroplasticity" are applied at different levels of organization within the nervous system. The scientific exploration ranges from distribution of neurotransmitter molecules and receptor dynamics to that of synaptic density and organization, to the manner in which different regions in the CNS link up in distributed functional networks in the context of generating recovered behaviors. A comprehensive review of this rapidly developing area within basic and applied neuroscience is beyond the scope of this chapter, but major issues relevant to rehabilitation within this area of investigation will be addressed. There is a new view of specificity within the nervous system that implies that the nervous system is a dynamic organic system that is constantly being remodeled in response to experience, primarily through the modification of synaptic distribution and the connectivity of different regions within the nervous system. How experience influences function and structure within the nervous system remains poorly understood, although some basic concepts are emerging from fundamental studies of learning-associated synaptic plasticity in simple invertebrate models[8] and studies of the capacity for reorganization of cortical maps in the monkey.[9] These studies indicate that the nervous system has well-developed mechanisms for modulating the strength of synaptic interaction based upon the detection of temporal coincidence of events that significantly impact on the survival of the organism (e.g., that allow the organism to anticipate the arrival of a noxious, threatening stimulus). Studies examining reorganization at the level of the cerebral cortex in mammals also suggest that a powerful stimulus to reorganization of cortical representations is that of correlated input bringing structured data in from the periphery.[10]

In order for this input to have an influence on the CNS, it must carry with it biologically important information, and the organism must be in a receptive state. For example, the information may be linked to a context in which it provides the subject access to a desired "reward" (e.g., food in the context of hunger). Before examining the issue of the restructuring of the organization of areas in the CNS, we will first examine how the peripheral nerves respond to injury and particularly the process involved in the recovery of strength following a partial nerve injury.

Physiologic Basis of Neural Recovery in Peripheral Nerve Injury

The response of peripheral nerve to injury is primarily a regenerative response that begins with changes in the neuronal cell body. Changes in histology and metabolism following axotomy are directed toward the reconstruction of the damaged axon. The cell body of the axotomized neuron undergoes chromatolysis and swells with displacement of the Nissl substance to the periphery of the cell. When axotomy occurs at a very proximal point close to the cell body, this can result in retrograde deterioration severe enough to lead to irreversible destruction of the cell body. But in most instances, the changes that occur in the cell body, including an increase in the rate of production of RNA, are in preparation for a reconstruction of the damaged cell appendage. When there is significant damage to the axon, the segment of the axon distal to the site of injury undergoes a process of resorption referred to as *wallerian degeneration*. The reconstructive process is supported by the transport of structural proteins along the length of the axon from the cell body to the proximal stump of the damaged axon.

The success of the regeneration process depends upon the extent of damage to axon and myelin sheath as well as the degree to which the supportive structure of the nerve has been left intact and is able to serve as a conduit for the regenerating axons. When there is severe injury with neurotmesis and significant disruption of the connective tissue investing the axons, the repair process can be set off track with the resulting formation of a disorganized swirl of axons and connective tissue frequently forming a neuroma at the site of injury. Thus when the axons and their supportive connective tissue are both significantly damaged and there is the need to reconstruct both the axons and their support structure, recovery is less likely to occur. Surgical intervention to reconstruct the nerve may eventually be necessary (see also Chapter 14).

When there is partial denervation of a muscle, there is also the possibility of restoration of muscle innervation through a process of "collateral sprouting" of the remaining distal motor fibers. Some of the denervated muscle fibers are reinnervated by "sprouts" from fibers that continue to innervate the muscle. In this manner, lost strength is restored in a partially denervated muscle through the enlargement of remaining motor units. The result of this process is the development of "giant" motor units in which the number of muscle fibers innervated by each motor fiber is much larger than that normally encountered. A larger percentage of muscle fibers can then contribute to the contraction. Because there are fewer motor units in the available pool and because each contributes a larger than normal pulse of tension to the contraction, the trade-off for the recovered strength is a loss of precision in the deployment and control of contraction forces.

Thus, in the peripheral nervous system, where the basic structure of the nerve is much simpler than the structures found within the CNS, there are two different fundamental methods available for recovery from nerve injury: (1) the regeneration of damaged axons, and (2) "sprouting" of remaining fibers when there is partial fiber loss. These recovery processes can be identified and monitored using clinical neurophysiologic techniques, in particular, electromyographic studies. Muscles that have been denervated can be assessed to determine which axons innervating the muscle have been damaged and whether or not there has been any interim "reinnervation" (i.e., re-establishment of motor units) or "sprouting" (i.e., active remodeling of existing motor units) within the affected muscles.

The regeneration and sprouting processes in the peripheral nerve remain poorly understood at the level of underlying mechanism. However, to some degree, these processes may be viewed as partial models for how recovery may take place under different circumstances following damage to the CNS. Certainly some of the general principles that can be more clearly applied to injury to the peripheral nervous system could be extended to the CNS. In less severe injuries, impairment of nerve conduction may be due to damage to the myelin only, with the axon remaining intact and in continuity. This is referred to as a "neurapraxic" injury, and, in the peripheral nervous system at least, the repair of the myelin sheath is fairly readily achieved, although it may take up to 5–6 weeks to complete.

The effects of a peripheral nerve injury are not limited to the peripheral nervous system. The significant alteration in the structure of sensory input that comes in from the periphery following a significant injury of a peripheral nerve produces transformation of central representations of the skin surface in the CNS and particularly at the level of the cerebral cortex.[9] Recovery from peripheral nerve injury therefore involves re-establishment of continuity of fibers in the periphery, but also concomitant reconstruction of sensory and motor representations within the CNS that are dynamically maintained through their direct connection to the periphery via peripheral nerve fibers. Abnormal input from the periphery induces anomalous representation in the cerebral cortex.[10] Thus, maximizing the functional recovery from peripheral nerve injury involves attention to central as well as peripheral mechanisms of recovery.

Physiologic Basis of Neural Recovery in Central Nervous System Injury

Neural recovery following CNS injury is complicated by the complex structure of neural pathways within the CNS. For the purpose of understanding the recovery process, it has been useful to view structures within the CNS with activity correlating with different forms of complex behavior as "distributed networks." From activational studies in normal human subjects, it is apparent that, for example, regions of motor cortex, premotor cortex, parietal cortex, basal ganglia, and cerebellum may all become simultaneously active when a human subject is performing a complex motor task. These zones in different parts of the nervous system appear to activate in concert as a network.[11, 12] Each element or "module" of the network may be contributing in a particular way to the support of the behavior, but the behavior emerges through a coordinated activation of all the different elements of the distributed network.[13] Within each module, there may be a representational map that is topographically organized. This is more apparent in primary sensory and motor cortical areas and is less apparent is associational regions of the cortex. Reciprocating interconnections between these modular zones may be important for maintaining temporal correlation among the activities of each of the components of the network and for ensuring a synchronized, coordinated action of the network.

Functional neuroimaging techniques can provide information on brain development and plasticity. Ontogenic changes in local cerebral metabolic rates for glucose (LCMRgl) have been described using positron emission tomography (PET) to occur over a protracted period, during which human brain is developing functionally.[14] While LCMRgl values reach adult values by the second year, they subsequently exceed adult values, reaching a plateau that extends between approximately 4 and 9 years of age, before gradually declining to adult values by the end of the second decade.[14] These changes in LCMRgl are postulated to correspond to developmental phases of overgrowth and elimination ("pruning") of neurons and their processes and synapses.[14] Emerging functional neuroimaging technology, including both PET and functional magnetic resonance imaging (fMRI) techniques, has relevance for neurorehabilitation and may provide future insights into mechanisms of recovery at different stages of the lifespan.

Recent work using PET to look at brain network activation in behaving human subjects suggests that the structure of the network may change as a new task is learned.[15] The structure of the network, particularly in terms of the localization of participating elements and the degree of symmetry of brain region activation, can change significantly in human stroke patients who have recovered hand movement following the onset of hemiparesis related to a unilateral subcortical infarct.[16–20] These studies indicate that a limb that has recovered movement following onset of hemiparesis has a very different pattern of activation associated with post-hemiparetic movement as compared with the pattern observed with movement of the opposite "non-affected" limb. While the nonaffected limb shows activation limited to discrete foci in the contralateral primary sensorimotor cortex, medial frontal cortex (supplementary motor area), and ipsilateral cerebellum, recovered hand movement of the post-hemiparetic limb is associated with more diffuse activation of nonprimary motor areas of the frontal and parietal cortices of *both* cerebral hemispheres as well as a more symmetric activation of *both* hemispheres of the cerebellum.[16, 18, 19] Furthermore, the actual pattern of activation of nonprimary motor areas of the two hemispheres associated with recovered movement varies significantly from individual to individual.[20] This suggests that the details of how the recovery occurs can vary significantly in terms of precisely how the reorganization of the functional brain network supporting hand movement is accomplished.

These studies now begin to provide information about the capacity for reorganization that exists in functional neuronal networks of the human brain to support the recovery process. What drives the reorganization process and the mechanisms through which this reorganization occurs are not well understood from a physiologic and neurochemical standpoint. Clearly, further study of such issues will have a profound impact on the manner in which rehabilitation procedures can be constructed to maximize the extent of recovery following neural trauma by supporting the naturally occurring recovery processes. Furthermore, it is clear that there is a broad distribution of the extent of recovery that occurs across affected individuals. The factors that are associated with poor versus good recovery should be more precisely understood once there is a better understanding of the necessary conditions for recovery. Certainly, these studies would suggest that the extent to which nonprimary motor regions of both damaged and unaffected hemisphere remain intact and capable of participating in a reorganizational process is a necessary condition for such recovery.

But is this a sufficient condition for optimal recovery? This is the important question for rehabilitation: to what extent does the experience of the individual during the recovery period influence the extent to which recovery occurs? And precisely what kinds of "therapeutic" experience and exactly what intensity of such experience can optimally influence the extent to which recovery of function can occur? These remain open questions that will require further investigation. However, we can speculate about some general issues based on our currently limited understanding of how experience influences reorganizational processes in the context of learning new skills in human subjects and animal models[15, 21] and in the context of the cortical response to reconstructed peripheral somatic input in an animal model.[9]

These issues have been previously reviewed in the context of examining neurophysiologic models of recovery from focal brain damage due to stroke.[22, 23] How these models may be extended to recovery from traumatic brain injury is less clear for diffuse axonal injury than it is for focal cortical contusion or secondary ischemic injury because of the significant differences in the nature of the pathology and its functional consequences. A focal lesion places a discrete "hole" in a functional brain network that necessitates a reorganization of the network to reconstitute a function without the participation of the "lost" region. The success of this process depends on the extent of redundancy within the organization of the network and the relation between the extent of redundancy and the "functional" extent of the lesion.

In contrast, diffuse axonal injury (DAI) results in a generalized disconnection of functional brain regions and therefore a more generalized disruption of brain networks. The sine qua non of DAI is loss of consciousness secondary to a disturbance of influence of the reticular activating system (RAS) projections on the cerebral cortex. Focal cerebral injury without DAI rarely produces loss of consciousness unless there is secondary involvement of the RAS projections due to edema, herniation, or concomitant brain stem injury. Focal injury, however, may be associated with remote physiologic inactivation due to secondary down-regulation of RAS systems, a process believed to underlie the phenomenon of "diaschisis" (see below). This consideration raises the issue of how the diffuse, nonthalamic cortical projections from the reticular core of the brain stem, whose cortical influence is mediated through neuromodulator-type neurotransmitters, play a critical role in the influence of recovery processes. These projections play well-established critical roles not only in controlling the sleep-wake cycle and level of consciousness but also in active attentional processes as well as influencing cortical plasticity.

It may well be disruption of these systems that is responsible for the diffuse impairment that is sometimes initially associated with focal injury and has been labelled "diaschisis." Von Monakow first introduced this concept in 1914; he argued that damage to one part of the brain deprived other intact regions remote from the site of damage of the normal afferent drive that would originate in the damaged region. This damage resulted in physiologic inactivity or "shutdown" in sites remote from that of the damage.[24, 25] The important role played by the nonthalamic cortical afferents from the reticular core in both the diaschisis phenomenon as well as the consequences of DAI has led to the development of concepts of neuropharmacologic manipulation to counteract such down-regulation of the cortical activating systems that may impede recovery.[26] There is then the emerging idea of combining neuropharmacologic therapy that activates cortical systems through neuromodulatory influence (e.g., with bromocriptine in the case of dopaminergic projections or methylphenidate in the case of noradrenergic projections) together with therapeutic training in order to maximize the influence of the training program on cortical plasticity.[27–29] This approach also recognizes that medications (e.g., haloperidol) that inhibit the cortical activating mechanisms and are frequently used as sedatives in agitated patients can have detrimental effects on recovery processes.[30] While this appears to be a useful concept supported by well-established basic studies, the clear demonstration of its effectiveness in humans using controlled clinical trial methods has not yet been published. However, there is currently work in progress examining various techniques, including single-subject designs, for developing more precise methods for documenting the effectiveness of neuropharmacologic therapy associated with rehabilitation training in a manner that is clinically accessible.[31]

In order to maximize the effect of the training, therapeutic experience must be carried out in a context in which the patient is motivated. Motivation can be defined as the extent to which the subject can focus and sustain attention on the therapeutic experience. The greater the focus of attention to task, the greater the likelihood that the experience will have lasting effects on cortical plasticity, possibly owing to the associated influence of intrinsically activated neuromodulator substances. Careful consideration may be given to enhancing the neuromodulator influence through pharmacologic means when intrinsic activation mechanisms appear to be inadequate. To whatever extent possible, the subject must be actively engaged as a participant in the activity. The actual activity itself should be on the "edge" of the subject's capability or "reach" and should ideally be carried out repetitively in a highly consistent functional context. Daily tasks (e.g., dressing, feeding, grooming) should be carried out repetitively in the context of a daily activity pattern emphasizing the functional context and the achievement of functional goals that have clear intrinsic importance to the individual. When functional "gaps" have been identified in the patient's behavioral repertoire, restorative training strategies can be employed to attempt to restore the damaged behavior, or, alternatively, compensatory strategies can be used to train the subject to substitute remaining functional abilities.

These principles in the rehabilitation of patients with neural injury remain, for the most part, empiric. However, physiologic insights into the mechanisms of functional recovery using new technologies that allow the three-dimensional visualization of patterns of brain activation in the behaving human subject, such as fMRI and PET, should provide a more solid footing for such practices and suggest more effective means for achieving the goals of a rehabilitation program.

PREDICTING OUTCOME: A REHABILITATION PERSPECTIVE

Neurosurgeons are typically more confident than rehabilitation professionals that research provides the identifiable prognostic factors that permit decision making early after an insult such as spinal cord injury or traumatic brain injury. A questionnaire survey of an international group of neurosurgeons revealed that the majority held the opinion that a prognosis could be determined within 3 days after traumatic brain injury, and that a computerized system of prognostication was as reliable as the predictions of an experienced clinician.[32]

In contrast, rehabilitation professionals remain skeptical about the clinician's ability to predict outcome, even months post injury.[33, 34] Long-range studies suggest that patients continue to improve months to years after an insult or injury to the spinal cord or brain.[35–43] On the other hand, delayed sequelae may have a deleterious effect on long-term recovery; for example, depression, psychosis, and even progressive dementia have been documented years after traumatic brain injury.[44] After any insult to the brain, including stroke, trauma, aneurysm rupture, anoxia, or tumor, an assessment of the severity of the insult is certainly important in predicting outcome but may be only one dimension to consider in prediction.[45, 46] These differences in perspective can be partly accounted for by differences in clinical approaches in the fields of rehabilitation, neurosurgery, and traumatology. While neurosurgeons and traumatologists focus on preventing mortality and responding to acute medical and surgical events, physiatrists attempt to prevent secondary complications of hospitalization and immobilization, and prepare the patient and family for the process of rehabilitation.

These differences in approach are matched by differing perspectives on studying outcome. Acute care physicians understand severity of injury to be the chief predictive factor in outcome after pathologic events; rehabilitation professionals understand the importance of premorbid factors, the availability of support systems and other environmental factors, as well as the importance of the interplay of these factors in addition to severity of injury on long-term outcome. Improvements documented during rehabilitation suggest that predictive factors that relate only to severity of injury are not always meaningful for an individual patient, who may have unique responses to the rehabilitation process or because of the interplay of a number of factors.[47, 48] Rehabilitation physicians have a perspective on outcome that is focused on long-term *recovery of function*, which may be a consequence of not only the severity of injury but also recovery processes, and of the success of rehabilitation interventions that include learned strategies that allow the individual to compensate for deficits.[49–51] Outcome measures, for example, are focused not on mortality or pathophysiologic outcome, but rather on impairment and disability.[52, 53] By definition, these rehabilitation outcome measures identify an individual in an environment and attempt to quantify the level of function. Rehabilitation professionals have stressed the need to assess the quality of life as defined by survivors rather than professionals.[54, 55] The differences in perspective may influence the content of discussions with families and patients about outcome and the confidence with which professionals communicate prognostic information.

Functional Assessment

Functional assessment is the measurement of the performance of survival skills required to negotiate through everyday life. Traditionally, rehabilitation has limited the definition of these survival skills to three broad categories that relate to physical and cognitive functioning: (1) activities of daily living (ADLs), (2) mobility, and (3) communication and/or cognition. These skills can be divided into basic and higher-level or instrumental skills. Basic survival skills are those that are generally required to live within the confines of one's home, such as eating, dressing, toileting, bathing, and household ambulation. Higher-level survival skills are those that are generally required to live in the larger community, such as paying bills, shopping, driving, ambulating on nonlevel surfaces, working, and attending school. Performance of functional skills is dependent on the integrity of cognitive and intellectual function. An understanding of the basic domains of cognition—attention, memory, language, visuospatial perception, executive function—is essential to appreciate the behaviors observed during the execution of everyday life survival skills.

Thus, functional assessment must occur with concomitant, in-depth mental status evaluation. While screening tools such as the Mini Mental Status Examination (MMSE)[56] can be useful to identify general areas of cognitive difficulty, such mental status screening tools cannot replace in-depth cognitive examination and behavioral examination.

Functional assessment can be accomplished in a medical/surgical setting in either an informal or formal manner. Both approaches require systematic thinking regarding making explicit connections between the specific interference with survival skills and the underlying disease process and related impairments. Informal functional assessment is usually carried out in the physician's office or at the bedside, and it requires that the care provider review with the patient, either as part of the history of the present illness or review of systems, the specific performance of basic and higher-level survival skills that interfere with everyday life.

Formal functional assessment utilizes specific tools that have been developed to quantify human functional performance in everyday life. These tools utilized in rehabilitation are more frequently limited to measurement of basic skills and to some degree have attempted to measure cognitive function. The Barthel Index is a prototype that is commonly used in rehabilitation settings.[57] Over the last 10 years, the Functional Independence Measure (FIM) has been developed and is now widely used in rehabilitation.[58] The FIM is reproduced in Table 20–2. A major contribution of the FIM is that it has streamlined the language describing disability such that rehabilitation professionals are now using a common terminology concerning the relative control that the patient has in everyday life along a spectrum of total dependence to complete independence. Total dependence, for example, is defined by complete assistance by the care provider and no participation by the patient. Maximal assistance is defined as 75% assistance by the helper and 25% participation in a specific survival skill by the patient. Moderate assistance is defined as 50% assistance by the helper and 50% participation by the patient. Minimal assistance is defined as 25% assistance by the helper and 75% participation by the patient. Supervision is defined as no actual physical contact between the helper and the patient, but verbal or visual cueing in the form of breaking down more complex tasks into simpler series of steps to perform a survival skill, when the patient needs it. Independence in a survival skill allows for use of those assistive devices that facilitate communication, such as computer software, and facilitate mobility, such as canes, walkers, orthoses (wrist splints, leg braces), and prostheses (artificial limbs). Functional assessment tools are used as measures of outcome assessment for neurorehabilitation programs. Outcome assessment is becoming essential for determining the design, costs, and choices of neurorehabilitation programs during this era of cost containment in health and medical care.

In pediatrics, there are developmental considerations that must be incorporated in measurement of functional outcomes. Achievement of mobility and self-care functions, for example, may be at a level that is less than fully independent, but normal for age. Functional outcome measures differ from developmental tests in that they are more likely to be consistent with goals of rehabilitative intervention and with an emphasis on independence rather than normality.[59] The FIM has been modified for children as the Functional Independence Measure for Children (Wee FIM^{SM}).[60] This instrument is a measure of disability for children ages 6 months to 7 years that includes assessment of the same domains of function assessed with the FIM for adults: ADLs, mobility, communication, mental processing, and social interaction. The Pediatric Evaluation of Disability Inventory (PEDI)[61] is another pediatric functional outcome measure for children ages 6 months to 7 years that assesses ADLs, mobility, and social

TABLE 20–2 **FUNCTIONAL INDEPENDENCE MEASURE (FIM[SM])**

L E V E L S		
	7 Complete Independence (Timely, Safely)	NO
	6 Modified Independence (Device)	HELPER
	Modified Dependence 5 Supervision 4 Minimal Assist (Subject=75%+) 3 Moderate Assist (Subject=50%+) Complete Dependence 2 Maximal Assist (Subject=25%+) 1 Total Assist (Subject=0%+)	HELPER

		ADMIT	DISCHG	FOL-UP
	Self Care			
A.	Feeding			
B.	Grooming			
C.	Bathing			
D.	Dressing– Upper Body			
E.	Dressing– Lower Body			
F.	Toileting			
	Sphincter Control			
G.	Bladder Management			
H.	Bowel Management			
	Mobility			
	Transfer:			
I.	Bed, Chair, W/Chair			
J.	Toilet			
K.	Tub, Shower			
	Locomotion			
L.	Walk/wheel Chair	w / c	w / c	w / c
M.	Stairs			
	Communication			
N.	Comprehension	a / v	a / v	a / v
O.	Expression	v / n	v / n	v / n
	Social Cognition			
P.	Social Interaction			
Q.	Problem Solving			
R.	Memory			
	TOTAL			

Note: Leave no blanks. Enter 1 if patient not testable due to risk.

Copy freely but do not change.

Reprinted with permission from Uniform Data System for Medical Rehabilitation. Functional Independence Measure (FIM), Guide for the Use of the Uniform Data Set for Medical Rehabilitation. Buffalo, Research Foundation, State University of New York at Buffalo, 1989.

function and includes separate measurement dimensions for functional skills, caregiver assistance, and modifications.

Examples of rehabilitation outcome assessment tools that have been developed for specific patient populations are discussed below. Some of these tools are global assessments of function; others are developed for evaluation of specific impairments (such as cognition) or to measure disability or handicap (such as vocational or community reintegration).

FUNCTIONAL OUTCOME IN SPECIFIC POPULATIONS

In this section, the discussion focuses on the natural course of recovery of patients after insults to the brain and spinal cord from a variety of causes: trauma, hypoxia, vascular insult, or neoplasm. For the physiatrist or other rehabilitation professionals, assessment of the patient must include determination of functional impairments associated with diagnosis of the pathologic condition. In the case of the coma-emerging or minimally responsive patient, the assessment must focus on the rudiments of function, including awareness of the environment and ability to retain information on a minute-to-minute or day-to-day basis. As the patient becomes more responsive, assessments become more complex until the patient is evaluated for levels of independence in the home, community, school, or workplace.

Included in the discussion are the following components: (1) an outline of the natural course of recovery from neurologic insult, (2) the assessment instruments employed by physiatrists and other rehabilitation professionals to assess the patient at various stages of recovery, and (3) predictive factors for various subpopulations of patients who suffer injury to the brain, brain stem, or spinal cord, from a variety of causes resulting in a medical or surgical emergency, including traumatic and vascular injury and hypoxia.

Cerebral Disorders

Coma and Post-traumatic Amnesia

After a severe insult to the brain, patients may be comatose for a period of time. During *coma*, the eyes are closed and there is no observable response to the environment except for reflexive movements. As the patient emerges from coma, eye opening occurs, but this eye opening, in association with sleep-wake cycles, may also occur in the vegetative state in the context of continued lack of awareness.[62] Patients may begin to recover after coma but have responsiveness to the environment without ongoing memory of events. More than 60 years ago, Russell[63] described the period of *post-traumatic amnesia* as a period of impaired consciousness after traumatic brain injury that often follows coma or may occur without a period of unconsciousness. More recently, post-traumatic amnesia has been described as a broader syndrome consisting of disorientation to person, place, and time, with confusion, diminished memory, and decreased capabilities to attend and respond to environmental cues. Monitoring cognitive recovery during the period of agitation is important because cognitive improvement has been shown to precede resolution of agitation.[64]

Post-traumatic Agitation

The estimated incidence of post-traumatic agitation after traumatic brain injury varies between 11% and 50%, depending on the study.[65–68] *Agitation* following brain injury was first described in the medical literature in 1945 when Denny-Brown described restlessness in patients surviving traumatic brain injuries.[69] Levin and Grossman defined post-traumatic agitation as the "thrashing of extremities, truncal rocking, dislodging intravenous tubes and catheters, yelling, combativeness, and attempts to get out of bed."[65] A similar definition was included in the Neurobehavioral Rating Scale, used to rate various behavioral disturbances in patients with head injury.[70] Reyes[66] differentiated restlessness and agitation, suggesting that restlessness was consistent activity and the patient was capable of inhibiting this behavior; agitation consisted of movement that could not be inhibited. Ommaya and Gennarelli describe a "general pattern of recovery in many patients after severe but relatively uncomplicated head injury. . . . The patient falls unconscious and remains for a while in an unresponsive, immobile coma. Emerging from his state of paralytic unconsciousness the patient successively passes through stages of stupor, confusion with or without delirium, and finally, an almost lucid phase with automatisms before becoming fully alert."[71]

Delirium is the term used by psychiatrists to describe the agitated brain-injured patient.[72] However, delirium is used to refer to both calm and agitated confusional states[73] and is considered a clinical syndrome, caused by a wide variety of metabolic, physiologic, and neurologic insults, including brain injury.[74] Another related term, which first appeared in the psychiatric literature in 1902, is akathisia, or motor restlessness.[75] Akathisia was defined as the inability to remain seated with a compulsion to move about. Akathisia occurs as a side effect of neuroleptics and has been reported after traumatic brain injury.[76]

The current edition of the *Diagnostic and Statisti-*

cal Manual of Mental Disorders (DSM-IV) defines agitation after brain injury as a cognitive disorder known as delirium that is "due to a general medical condition," i.e., an acute brain injury.[77] In contradistinction to the term agitation used by rehabilitation professionals, the criteria for delirium established by the DSM-IV are cognitive and not behavioral features of an acute confusional state. The core features of delirium as defined by the DSM-IV are impairments of consciousness that fluctuate over time, reduced attention, and other cognitive impairments. Memory deficits, disorientation, and language and perceptual disturbances are described as key associated features but not required for the diagnosis.[78] Physiatrists have recommended that post-traumatic agitation be defined as a subtype of delirium unique to survivors of a traumatic brain injury, and during which "the survivor remains in post-traumatic amnesia and the observed behaviors consist of some combination of aggression, akathisia, disinhibition or emotional lability."[78]

Assessing Coma-Emerging and Minimally Responsive Patients

The Glasgow Coma Scale (GCS) is a widely accepted, standardized, reliable procedure for assessing comatose patients. The motor score is the most predictive of outcome for patients.[79] The usefulness of the GCS ends when periods of wakefulness occur, and the clinician must determine if the patient is responsive or in a vegetative state. The Glasgow Outcome Scale (GOS)[48] includes the categories of good recovery, moderate disability, severe disability, vegetative state, and death and can be useful in identification of a patient's global outcome category. However, other scales have been developed in neurorehabilitation that are more useful in tracking recovery of responsiveness and degree of disability.

Coma recovery instruments have been developed to assess minimally responsive patients with eye opening, a situation in which the GCS is no longer a useful clinical tool. The Disability Rating Scale (DRS) provides a global score that reflects function for survivors of brain injury by combining components of the GCS and the GOS and other components ranging from cognitive and physical impairments to "employability."[80] The DRS has been found to be more sensitive to improvement in function than the GOS.[81]

The Rancho Los Amigos Level of Cognitive Functioning Scale (Rancho Scale)[82] is an eight-point scale describing Rancho level I patients with "no response" (equivalent to a GCS of 3), to Rancho level IV patients who are "confused and agitated," to Rancho level VIII patients with recovery to a stage of being essentially fully functional (Table 20–3). The Scale is widely used in clinical settings to provide "short-hand" descriptions of patients.

The Coma/Near-Coma Scale (CNCS)[83] is an instrument developed to measure small clinical changes in survivors of severe traumatic and nontraumatic brain injuries with low DRS scores. The CNCS consists of parameters such as auditory response, command responsitivity, visual response, responses to olfactory and tactile inputs and pain, and vocalization. Based on the scores, patients are classified at five levels believed to be indicative of severity of sensory, perceptual, and primitive response deficits. These levels are described as no coma, near coma, moderate coma, marked coma, and extreme coma. The instrument can be completed daily, by professionals of varied specialization and is "learned easily, and . . . completed quickly."[83] The CNCS was initially validated with a population of patients with missile injury, blunt traumatic brain injury, stroke, anoxic brain injury, and substance overdose. The instrument can be useful for assessing patients with cognitive impairments due to a variety of insults.

The Coma Recovery Scale (CRS) is an instrument for assessing subtle changes in neurologic responsiveness over time and predicting outcome in minimally responsive patients during the acute rehabilitation stage of recovery.[84] The instrument was validated in an adult population consisting of survivors of traumatic brain injury, anoxic brain injury, and vascular events, who were functioning at the equivalent of Rancho level II through IV. The CRS consists of 35 items designed to evaluate responsiveness in the areas of arousal and attention, auditory perception, visual perception, motor function, oral motor ability, communication, and initiative. The procedure requires approximately 30 minutes of administration time by clinicians of various backgrounds.[84]

The Sensory Stimulation Assessment Measure (SSAM) was designed to measure responses to a structured sensory stimulation program.[85] The instrument measures responses to standardized stimuli administered to the olfactory, gustatory, auditory, visual, and tactile senses. Responses are rated on a six-point scale that ranges from 1 (no response) to 6 (spontaneous communicative response). The procedure requires approximately 45–50 minutes of therapist time to complete both the sensory stimulation protocol and the subsequent ratings. The instrument was validated with 20 patients functioning initially at Rancho level II or Rancho level III and who survived either a blunt traumatic brain injury, or anoxic, vascular, or missile injury.[85]

The Western Neurosensory Stimulation Profile (WNSP) was designed as a measure of cognitive

TABLE 20–3 **COGNITIVE LEVELS/RANCHO LOS AMIGOS SCALE**

I. *No response:* unresponsive to any stimulus
II. *Generalized response:* limited, inconsistent, nonpurposeful responses, often to pain only
III. *Localized response:* purposeful responses; may follow simple commands; may focus on presented object
IV. *Confused, agitated:* heightened state of activity; confusion, disorientation; aggressive behavior; unable to do self-care; unaware of present events; agitation appears related to internal confusion
V. *Confused, inappropriate, nonagitated:* appears alert; responds to commands; distractible; does not concentrate on task; agitated responses to external stimuli; verbally inappropriate; does not learn new information
VI. *Confused appropriate:* good directed behavior, needs cueing; can relearn old skills as activities of daily living (ADL); serious memory problems; some awareness of self and others
VII. *Automatic appropriate:* Robot-like appropriate behavior, minimal confusion; shallow recall; poor insight into condition; initiates tasks but needs structure; poor judgment, problem-solving, and planning skills
VIII. *Purposeful appropriate:* alert, oriented; recalls and integrates past events; learns new activities and can continue without supervision; independent in home and living skills; capable of driving; defects in stress tolerance, judgment, abstract reasoning persist; many function at reduced levels in society

With permission from Rancho Los Amigos Medical Center, Downey, CA, USA, Adult Brain Injury Service.

function in survivors of severe traumatic brain injury between Rancho level II and the early stages of Rancho level V.[86] The instrument consists of 32 items that are categorized into six subscales: Arousal/Attention, Auditory Comprehension, Visual Comprehension, Visual Tracking, Object Manipulation, and Tactile/Olfactory Response. The time commitment to administer the instrument is estimated at 20–40 minutes. The total score and the Auditory Comprehension, Visual Tracking, and Arousal/Attention subscale scores all identify those brain injury survivors that improve from Rancho level II or III to level V.[86]

The scales described above require trained staff and a time commitment that may be prohibitive in this era of cost containment. However, they are useful in the evaluation of patients for determinations of responsiveness for clinical or medicolegal purposes. In many patients, a brief physician contact with the patient during bedside rounds is not sufficient to establish interaction with the environment consistent with emergence from coma. These instruments provide a more formal method of patient assessment that can be crucial in determinations of appropriate levels of care and prognosis.

Measuring Post-traumatic Amnesia

Despite the early recognition that clearing post-traumatic amnesia (PTA) represented an important milestone in the recovery continuum, the first instrument to permit an objective, prospective assessment of progress through post-traumatic amnesia appeared in the literature in 1979. The Galveston Orientation and Amnesia Test (GOAT)[87] (Table 20–4) is most appropriate for patients functioning between Rancho level IV and early Rancho level VII. The procedure can be performed at bedside, on a daily basis, in 5–10 minutes by professionals of varied background and training. The instrument evaluates temporal orientation and estimates the duration of both retrograde and anterograde amnesia. Scores range between 0 and 100, with a score of 75 or more on consecutive days being consistent with clearing post-traumatic amnesia. The GOAT was validated in a population of inpatients on an acute neurosurgical service. There is agreement with the GCS and with computed tomography scan findings as to injury severity, and the GOAT identifies spinal cord injury survivors with concurrent traumatic brain injury.[87] Although this tool requires a time commitment for administration, it provides valuable prognostic information for predicting global cognitive outcome. The Children's Orientation and Amnesia Test (COAT)[88] (Table 20–5) has been developed and demonstrated to have adequate reliability and validity as a measure of the duration of post-traumatic amnesia in children and adolescents.

The Orientation Group Monitoring System (OGMS) is a reliable method to monitor cognitive recovery through the period of clearing post-traumatic amnesia.[89] The instrument is based on behavioral ratings by a trained rater, during a daily 30-minute orientation group. Subscales include episodic recall, identity of group members and staff, associative learning, orientation to time, orientation to place, attention, and utilization of environmental cues. A weekly aggregate score is calculated, and a score greater than 2.75 correlates with clearing beyond post-traumatic amnesia. Validation of the OGMS was performed in a population of survivors of traumatic brain injury on an acute brain injury rehabilitation inpatient service.[89] Validity was supported by a 71.4% agreement with the GOAT.[90] Additionally, the OGMS was found to correlate significantly with the Mini Mental Status Examination,[64] simple reaction, and choice reaction times.[64] The OGMS was useful in documenting a decline in scores attributable to a concurrent medical etiology 93% of the time.[91] Improvement in orientation group scores preceded a decrement in agi-

TABLE 20–4 **GALVESTON ORIENTATION AND AMNESIA TEST (GOAT)**

Instructions: Error points (shown in parentheses after each question) are scored for incorrect answers and are entered in the two columns on the extreme right side of the test form. Enter the total error points accrued for the 10 items in the lower right hand corner of the test form. The GOAT score equals 100 minus the total error points. Recovery of orientation is depicted by plotting serial GOAT scores on at least a daily basis.

Name:____________________ Date of Test:____________

Age:______ Sex: M F Day of the Week: S M T W TH F S

Date of Birth:____________________ Time: AM PM

Diagnosis:____________________ Date of Injury:__________

Error Points

1. What is your name? (2)____________ When were you born? (4)____________ ______

   Where do you live? (4)____________

2. Where are you now? (5) city____________ (5) hospital____________ ______
   (unnecessary to state name of hospital)

3. On what date were you admitted to the hospital? (5)____________ ______

   How did you get here? (5)____________

4. What is the first event you can remember <u>after</u> the injury? (5)____________ ______

   Can you describe in detail (e.g., date, time, companions) the first event you can recall after the injury? (5)

   ____

5. Can you describe the last event you recall <u>before</u> the accident? (5)____________ ______

   ____________ Can you describe in detail (e.g., date, time, companion) the first event you can recall <u>before</u> the injury? (5)____________

6. What time is it now?__________(1) for each 1/2 hour removed from correct time to maximum of 5 ______

Error Points

7. What day of the week is it?__________(1) for each day removed from correct one ______

8. What day of the month is it?__________(1) for each day removed from correct date to maximum of 5 ______

9. What is the month?__________(5) for each month removed from correct one to maximum of 5 ______

10. What is the year?__________(10) for each year removed from correct one to maximum of 30 ______

Total Error Points ______

Total GOAT Score (100-total error points) ______

Courtesy of Harvey S. Levin, Ph.D., The Institute for Rehabilitation and Research, Houston, Texas.

tation,[64] and improvement in agitation was related to recovery from the period of post-traumatic amnesia.[92] Although this system of assessment is not widely used because of the organizational structure and time commitment required, it is an example of a formalized system of monitoring recovery that can be useful in rehabilitation settings.

Mental Status and Neuropsychologic Evaluations

Depending on the clinical needs or situation of the neurologically impaired patient, mental status screening tools are appropriate during the early phase of recovery, or in urgent or emergent clinical

TABLE 20–5 **CHILDREN'S ORIENTATION AND AMNESIA TEST (COAT)**

General Orientation:

1. What is your name? first (2)________________ (5) ________

   last (3)________________________

2. How old are you? (3)________ When is your birthday?

   month (1)____________ day (1)____________ (5) ________

3. Where do you live? city (3)________________

   state (2)________________________ (5) ________

4. What is your father's name? (5)________________

   What is your mother's name? (5)________________ (10) ________

5. What school do you go to? (3)________________

   What grade are you in? (2)________________ (5) ________

6. Where are you now? (5)________________ (5) ________
   (May rephrase question: Are you at home now? Are you in the hospital? If rephrased, child must correctly answer both questions to receive credit)

7. Is it daytime or night-time? (5)________________ (5) ________

General Orientation Total ________

Temporal Orientation: (administer if age 8-15)

8. What time is it now? (5)________________ (5) ________
   (correct = 5; < hr. off = 4; 1hr. off = 3; > 1 hr. off = 2; 2 hrs. off = 1)

9. What day of the week is it? (5)________________ (5) ________
   (correct = 5; 1 off = 4; 2 off = 3; 3 off = 2; 4 off = 1)

10. What day of the month is it? (5)________________ (5) ________
    (correct = 5; 1 off = 4; 2 off = 3; 3 off = 2; 4 off = 1)

11. What is the month? (10)________________ (10) ________
    (correct = 10; 1 off = 7; 2 off = 4; 3 off = 1)

12. What is the year? (15)________________ (15) ________
    (correct = 15; 1 off = 10; 2 off =5; 3 off = 1)

Temporal Orientation Total ________

TABLE 20–5 **CHILDREN'S ORIENTATION AND AMNESIA TEST (COAT)** *Continued*

Memory:

13. Say these numbers after me in the same order. (Discontinue when the child fails both series of digits at any length. Score 2 points if both digit series are correctly repeated; score 1 point if only 1 is correct.)

3	5________	35296	81493 ________		
58	42________	539418	724856________		
643	926________	8129365	4739128________	(14)	________
7216	3279________				

14. How many fingers am I holding up?

two fingers (2)______three fingers (3)______10 fingers (5)______ (10) ________

15. Who is on Sesame Street? (10)______________ (10) ________
(can substitute other major television show)

16. What is my name? (10)______________ (10) ________

Memory Total ________

OVERALL TOTAL ________

Courtesy of Harvey S. Levin, Ph.D., The Institute for Rehabilitation and Research, Houston, Texas.

situations when cognition and behavior are changing rapidly, thus requiring frequent assessment of mental status. In-depth clinical examination and extensive neuropsychologic assessment are appropriate in clinical situations in which there is a need to establish cognitive and behavioral baselines, to monitor spontaneous neural recovery, to design cognitive remediation strategies, and to monitor response to cognitive remediation and behavioral management interventions.

Mental status screening tools offer a quick and selective assessment of cognitive function. Their use is appropriate when cognition and behavior are changing rapidly. These changing behaviors often occur during the acute phase of injury and recovery, when the patient is being administered life-saving medications and surgical procedures, or in an environment that is distracting and insensitive to sleep-wake cycles. The Mini Mental Status Examination (MMSE)[56] is a widely utilized screening device that attempts to quantify cognitive function by probing several cognitive domains including orientation, verbal memory, calculation, visuoperception, and language skills including auditory comprehension, repetition, naming, and writing (Table 20–6). It also has been used as a general indicator of severity of cognitive impairment. It should not be considered predictive of future neural and functional recovery, future performance in rehabilitation, and potential ability to live safely and alone in the community.

In-depth clinical cognitive/behavioral assessment, and formal neuropsychologic assessment, during which individual patient performance is compared with established norms, is appropriate during periods of clinical stability when recovery has established a steadier course. Clinical cognitive/behavioral assessment should be performed by all rehabilitation team members. The cognitive domains evaluated will vary according to which team member is examining the patient and what areas of cognition are the focus of treatment. For example, the occupational therapist pays particular attention to visuoperception, while the speech therapist pays particular attention to language skills. As the orchestrator of rehabilitation services and as the synthesizer of information during the team process, the

TABLE 20–6 **THE MINI MENTAL STATUS EXAMINATION**

MAXIMUM SCORE = 30

Orientation	
5	What is the (year) (season) (date) (month) (day of week)?
5	Where are we (state) (country) (town/city) (hospital) (floor)?
Registration	
3	Name three objects, for example, "ball," "flag," "tree": One second to say each. Then ask the patient all three after you have said them. Give one point for each correct answer. Repeat until he learns all three. Count trials and record number of trials.
Attention and Calculation	
5	Begin with 100 and count backwards by 7 (stop after five answers). Alternatively, spell world backwards.
Recall	
3	Ask for three objects repeated above. Give one point for each correct answer.
Language	
2	Show a pencil and a watch and ask subject to name them.
1	Repeat the following: "No 'ifs,' 'ands,' or 'buts.'"
3	A three stage command, "Take a paper in your right hand; fold it in half and put it on the floor."
1	Read and obey the following: (Show subject the written item.) CLOSE YOUR EYES
1	Write a sentence
1	Copy a design

Reprinted from Folstein MF, Folstein SE, McHugh PR: The Mini Mental state: A practical guide for grading the cognitive state of patients for the clinician. J Psychiatr Res 1975;12:189. With kind permission from Elsevier Science Ireland Ltd., Bay 15K, Shannon Industrial Estate, Co., Clare, Ireland.

physiatrist, and other physicians involved in the direct care of the patient, should utilize a consistent cognitive/behavioral assessment evaluating all major cognitive domains (attention, memory, language, visuoperception, and executive function), using visual and verbal materials, requiring visual and auditory input. Such an in-depth mental status examination allows a reasonable appreciation of both preserved and impaired areas of cognition over a long recovery trajectory.

During the examination, close observation of the patient's "on-line" performance must occur; specifically, reactive or compensatory behaviors utilized by the patient to attempt to complete a specific task should be noted. It is important to observe not only whether the patient completes or does not complete a task accurately, but also what behavioral strategies are attempted or utilized that facilitate or interfere with successful task performance. Such concurrent behavioral observation provides clinical insights into behaviors that may need to be addressed later during rehabilitation. For example, a patient who consistently is distracted during task execution may require a highly structured, individualized, and quiet treatment environment. A patient who has word finding difficulties and who uses circumlocutory speech during a naming task may be encouraged to use this as a strategy for self-cueing target words during speech therapy and during interpersonal interactions.

When used by the clinician, in-depth clinical cognitive/behavioral assessment should involve a structured mental status interview applied consistently over time in order to allow direct comparison of serial examinations prospectively for each patient. The tasks presented should be practical modifications of neuropsychologic tasks established as recognized indicators and measures of each cognitive domain. The Neurobehavioral Cognitive Examination (NBCE)[93, 94] is one example of a cognitive battery used in rehabilitation patient care and research. Another approach is presented in Table 20–7. Some investigators have demonstrated that specific neuropsychologic subtests, especially measures of executive functioning such as the Trail Making Test–Part B, can be relatively predictive of future functioning in everyday life in patients with cognitive impairments.[95, 96]

In many cases, referral to the neuropsychologist for formal assessment can be useful, especially in cases of mild to moderate impairment, and in cases of diagnostic ambiguity when clinical examination demonstrates uncertainty. Formal neuropsychologic testing requires that the patient have the attentional vigilance to participate in several hours of task performance, at least during multiple testing episodes or perhaps continuously with short rest breaks. Such an approach allows comparison of each patient's performance against established norms considering age, educational background, and previous educational performance. As with in-depth cognitive assessment, concurrent behavioral observations must be made during neuropsychologic testing, and these can be important during the interpretation of task performance. Formal neuropsychologic assessment can be performed serially to follow a patient's spontaneous recovery and/or response to rehabilitation interventions. Because it involves a large investment of time, and because of practice effects, a formal assessment is not recommended more frequently than every 6 months.

Neuropsychologic evaluation should always be considered during investigational clinical trials when evaluating neuropharmacologic or behavioral interventions thought to enhance recovery. As with clinical cognitive/behavioral assessment, formal neuropsychologic testing can also be used to define cases of preserved and impaired cognitive functioning. Each patient can, subsequently, be characterized according to an individual profile of cognitive strengths and weaknesses. This information can then be used by the rehabilitation team to develop a formal cognitive and behavioral treatment program that takes the approach of treating the cognitive impairments directly, and/or enhancing the cognitive strengths and compensating with behaviors in order to bypass the cognitive weaknesses. Such an approach, in which the profile of cognitive strengths and weaknesses is translated into behavioral strategies used in rehabilitation, is becoming known as the "neuropsychologic-behavioral" approach to cognitive remediation.[97, 98]

The approach to behavioral assessment recommended here is one in which explicit behavioral descriptions, generally categorized as reactive and compensatory behaviors, must be juxtaposed with rigorous cognitive assessment. In this way, consistent patterns of "brain-behavioral" relationships can be articulated for each patient. Some neurologically injured patients may demonstrate disruptive, socially inappropriate, or aggressive behaviors, sometimes in the context of undetectable or mild neuropsychologic impairments. Many of these patients may be too difficult to assess with the usual clinical tools because of these behaviors. In these situations, the difficult behaviors and not the cognitive deficits become the target of treatment, with directed behavioral management programs.

The rehabilitation team can be especially useful in the assessment of these patients, in that different team members' observations at different times of the day and in different situations can cross-validate each other. Thus, a more focused and consistent definition of difficult behaviors that require treatment, the daily patterns of these behaviors, and the relationship of these behaviors to sensory (vision, hearing, tactile) disturbances or to situational precipitants can be articulated. Using a journal or diary over a series of days can sometimes be useful for assisting with identifying specific behavioral patterns and their precipitants, and in monitoring the efficacy of behavioral management strategies and behavior-altering medications.

Assessment of Agitation and Other Neurobehavioral Disorders

The Agitated Behavior Scale (ABS)[99] (Table 20–8) permits the objective assessment of post-traumatic agitation and provides a tool to assess the efficacy of clinical interventions. The instrument is designed to rate agitated behavior from coma through recovery from the period of post-traumatic amnesia. Ratings are based on behavioral observations after treatment sessions or after nursing shifts. Hence ratings are completed by various rehabilitation professionals. The instrument consists of 14 items or behaviors that are rated between 1 and 4.[99] Subsequent work has identified three subscales: disinhibition, aggression, and lability, but the total score remains the best overall measure of agitation.[100] The instrument was validated in a population of severe traumatic brain injury survivors on an inpatient acute traumatic brain injury rehabilitation service. The scale has been shown to be predictive of change in cognitive status.[64]

The Neurobehavioral Rating Scale (NBRS)[70] was developed as an adjunct in outcome studies and that could assist in documentation of clinical recovery. The NBRS is based on the Brief Psychiatric Rating Scale and consists of 27 scales and 7 potential rankings. The ratings yield a total score and four factor scores: cognitive/energy, metacognition, somatic/anxiety, and language. Administration requires approximately 30 minutes with subsequent ratings based on both a structured interview and behavioral observation. The instrument was initially validated with a population of 101 survivors of closed head injury that ranged from mild through severe injuries. Factor scores discriminate populations according to severity of injury and the presence of frontal lobe injury. Construct validity of NBRS is supported by the observation that scores improve with subsequent follow-up evaluations.[70]

Measuring Disability and Handicap

Until the development of the Glasgow Outcome Scale (GOS), outcome measures utilized in traumatic brain injury research consisted of determinations of mortality or simply "good" and "bad" outcome categories. The GOS is a five-point scale that measures "social outcome."[48] In some studies, the GOS is collapsed to a two-point scale, rendering it more statistically advantageous but with obvious cost.[101, 102] These broad outcome categories are useful for research purposes and for making generalizations about various predictive factors, but clinicians cannot use this information to determine outcome in individual patients. Developers of the scale voiced concern about the inappropriate use of the scale to predict individual outcome after brain injury.[48, 103] As the patient with cerebral injury recovers function, functional assessments must include evaluations of disability and handicap, which measure social and vocational reintegration and quality of life. A variety of instruments are available to clinicians and researchers and include the Craig Handicap Assessment and Reporting Technique (CHART),[104] and the Community Integration Questionnaire.[105] Both measures assess specific constructs such as the ability to live independently, to navigate the environment, and to work and maintain social relationships.

TABLE 20–7 **IN-DEPTH COGNITIVE/BEHAVIORAL ASSESSMENT**

MAJOR COGNITIVE DOMAINS	VERBAL TASKS	VISUAL TASKS
Attention/short-term memory	Auditory digit span forward and in reverse[1]	Visual pointing span forward and in reverse[1]
Long-term memory/episodic memory	Word list learning—immediately after word presentation (word span or registration), and then at set time intervals after presentation, such as 1, 5, and 10 minutes[2]	Single or complex, geometric 2-dimensional figure—recall immediately after presentation, and then at 5 and 10 minutes after presentation.[3] (See visuoperception for prototype of figure)
Remote memory	Report U.S. presidents in accurate reverse order, starting with the present leader: "Clinton, Bush, Reagan, Carter, Ford, Nixon, etc." Note if providing a cue, such as a first name. Assists with name retrieval	
Semantic memory	Category recognition task: "Is this a vegetable?" (yes or no response) "Onion, carrot, lemon, etc."[4]	Category recognition task as described under verbal tasks, but present stimuli as pictures or real objects rather than as spoken words[4]
Language	Spontaneous speech production—note accuracy of grammar, specifically the appropriate use of nouns, verbs, prepositions, and article	Visual confrontation naming of objects (real or pictured), for example, pen, shoe, button, and actions (simulated or pictured), for example, writing, saluting, hopping.[5] Note the difference in naming more and less frequently occurring word (e.g., flower vs. teepee)
	Repetition—monosyllabic and multisyllabic words and phrases (e.g. "declaration"; "opportunity"; "Declaration of Independence"; "No ifs, ands, or buts"); sentences of increasing word length and of more complex grammatical structure (e.g. "The eagle chased the hawk," "The green car was hit by the blue van")	Reading—single words that follow phonetic rules (cat, milk), and that have silent letters (bought, doubt); nonsense syllables that follow phonetic rules (bliv, dat) and that are read by analogy to real words (scatz, szine)
	Comprehension—simple comprehension (point to the window . . . point to the door, etc.), and more complex, grammatical comprehension, such as providing correct responses to probe questions about sentences with complex grammatical structures, for example, "The old gorilla was chased by the young monkey that was fast." What was chased? (gorilla) What was fast? (monkey)[6]	Writing—own name; sentence writing to dictation, e.g., "The weather is cool."; sentence writing in response to a question, e.g., "How is the weather?" (question) "It is cool." (possible response)

Predictive Factors After Cerebral Injury

TRAUMATIC BRAIN INJURY

For decades, duration of the period of coma (measured by GCS, particularly the motor score) and/or post-traumatic amnesia has been shown to correlate with severity of injury and outcome after traumatic brain injury.[63, 106] Mortality is most highly associated with subdural hematomas, severe diffuse axonal injury, or intracerebral hemorrhages with mass effect.[107] Other clinical measures of severity in traumatic brain injury have included pupillary reflexes, intracranial pressure/cerebral blood flow, evoked potentials, and cerebral spinal fluid/blood factors; static and dynamic imaging studies have also been established as useful in a number of studies and are reviewed elsewhere.[108] Factors that predict survival after severe traumatic brain injury are not necessarily also predictive of severity of disability in those who survive.[109]

For patients with mild brain injury, outcome cannot be predicted using these measures except for the period of loss of consciousness and post-traumatic amnesia (PTA); anecdotal reports highlight the difficulties of predicting outcome after mild brain injury and link functional outcome to social- and vocationally relevant deficit areas.[34]

Post-traumatic agitation may be predictive of outcome in patients with head trauma. In one study, patients with agitation after brain injury had longer periods of PTA, suggesting more severe injuries, but rehabilitation outcome did not differ in the nonagitated and agitated group, the latter treated with haloperidol.[110] Reyes and associates[66] studied pa-

TABLE 20–7 **IN-DEPTH COGNITIVE/BEHAVIORAL ASSESSMENT** *Continued*

MAJOR COGNITIVE DOMAINS	VERBAL TASKS	VISUAL TASKS
Visuoperception	Single letter or word identification (see Reading above under Language)	Visual construction of complex 2-dimensional and 3-dimensional figures[7] 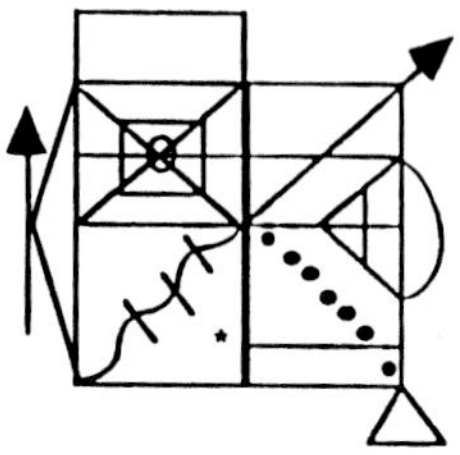 Taylor Complex Figure 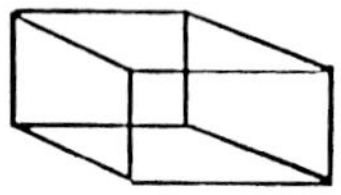 Cube Copy
Executive functioning	Verbal alternating pattern: "1–a–2–b–3–c ... 26–z"[8] Semantically guided verbal fluency[10] Phonemically guided verbal fluency[11]	Continuation of written alternation pattern[9]: 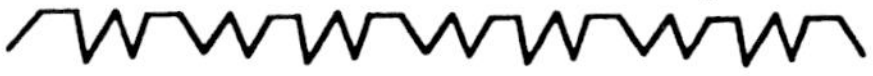 Trail-Making Test-Part B[12]: 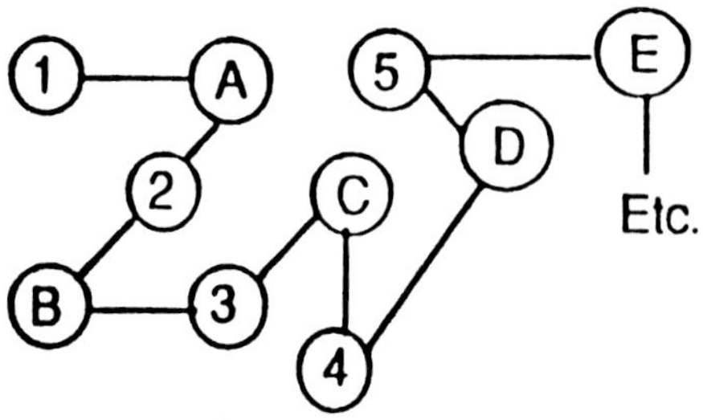

1. Adapted from Wechsler D: Wechsler Memory Scale–Revised (WMS-R). San Antonio, The Psychological Corporation, 1987. Normal auditory digit span is 6 to 7 randomly presented numbers repeated forward, and 5 to 6 numbers repeated in reverse. Normal visual pointing span is 5 to 6 forward and 4 to 5 in reverse.
2. This task can be varied depending on the patient's abilities, from 3 monosyllabic, imageable words (e.g., book, shoe, chair) or 3 non-imageable words (e.g., although, from, faith), to longer lists of imageable words varying in syllables that are not semantically related such as provided on the Rey Auditory Verbal Learning Task or RAVLT (see Lezak M: Neuropsychological Assessment. Oxford, Oxford University Press, 1983, for RAVLT).
3. Adapted from Lezak M: Neuropsychological Assessment. Oxford: Oxford University Press, 1983. The Rey-Osterreith Figure (ROF) and the Taylor Complex Figure are prototypes.
4. This task is adapted from several experimental tasks (Grossman M: Personal correspondence, Cognitive Neurology Section, University of Pennsylvania Medical Center) that probe the patient's ability to distinguish items that are from semantically related categories, such as fruits (apple, orange, etc.) and vegetables (onion, carrot, etc.). Rosch has developed a series of categories for potential use here (see Rosch E: Cognitive representation of semantic categories. J Exp Psychol–General 1975; 104:192–233.
5. Adapted from Goodglass H, Kaplan E, Weintraub S: Boston Naming Test, 1983; Obler LK, Albert M: Action Naming Task, 1986.
6. Adapted from several experimental tasks (Grossman M: Personal correspondence, Cognitive Neurology Section, University of Pennsylvania Medical Center).
7. Adapted from Lezak M: Neuropsychological Assessment. Oxford, Oxford University Press, 1983.
8. Adapted from Jones BN, Teng EI, Folstein MF: A new bedside test of cognition for patients with HIV infection. Ann Intern Med 1993; 119:1001–1004. This is a verbal version of the Trail-Making Test–Part B. Make a note of how much cueing the patient needs to continue this task, and how much time it takes to complete. It should be completed within 1 minute.
9. Adapted from Luria AR: Higher Cortical Functions in Man, 2nd ed. New York, Basic Books, 1980. Note a tendency for perseveration.
10. Adapted from the Category Fluency Test or the Set Test (Lezak M: Neuropsychological Assessment. Oxford, Oxford University Press, 1983). The patient is asked to name as many exemplars ("cat, dog, snake, fish, etc.") of a specified category (animals) during 1 minute.
11. Adapted from the Controlled Oral Word Association Test or the FAS Test (Benton A, Hamsher K: Multi-lingual Aphasia Examination. Iowa City, University of Iowa Hospital, 1978). The patient is asked to produce as many common words with a given letter ("f" or "a" or "s") during 1 minute for each letter.
12. Adapted from Reitan RM: The relation of the Trails Making Test to organic brain damage. J Consult Psychol 1955;19:393–394. The patient is instructed to alternate the sequence of numbers and letters, i.e., connect the circles, 1–A–2–B–3–C–4–etc.

tients in the rehabilitation setting, an average of 10.5 weeks post injury, and found that agitated and restless patients were "physically and mentally functioning at a higher level at the time of discharge than those exhibiting sluggishness." At long-term follow-up, approximately 4 years after discharge, 92% of restless patients were working and independent.[66]

Premorbid factors most likely influence functional outcome after a disabling injury, but few studies have addressed this issue. Estimates of premorbid intelligence may be predictive of IQ scores after traumatic brain injury[111]; on the other hand, the drop in IQ scores may be greater for patients with high premorbid IQ.[112] However, whether IQ scores predict return to work has not been established. Return to work is, of course, related to preinjury work history.[113] A history of alcohol abuse predating the brain injury worsens the chance for recovery of cognitive function.[114] Other factors such as work

TABLE 20–8 **AGITATED BEHAVIOR SCALE**

Patient: ______________________

Period of Observation:

From________am/pm ______/______/______
To__________am/pm ______/______/______

Rater: ______________________

At the end of the observation period, indicate whether each behavior was present and if so, to what degree -- slight, moderate or extreme. The degree can be based on either the frequency of the behavior or the severity of a given incident. Use the following numerical values for every behavior listed. DO NOT LEAVE BLANKS.

1 = ABSENT
2 = PRESENT TO A SLIGHT DEGREE
3 = PRESENT TO A MODERATE DEGREE
4 = PRESENT TO AN EXTREME DEGREE

______ 01. Short attention span, easy distractibility, inability to concentrate.

______ 02. Impulsive, impatient, low tolerance for pain or frustration.

______ 03. Uncooperative, resistant to care, demanding.

______ 04. Violent and/or threatening violence toward people or property.

______ 05. Explosive and/or unpredictable anger.

______ 06. Rocking, rubbing, moaning or other self-stimulating behavior.

______ 07. Pulling at tubes, restraints, etc.

______ 08. Wandering from treatment areas.

______ 09. Restlessness, pacing, excessive movement.

______ 10. Repetitive behaviors, motor and/or verbal.

______ 11. Rapid, loud or excessive talking.

______ 12. Sudden changes of mood.

______ 13. Easily initiated or excessive crying and/or laughter.

______ 14. Self-abusiveness, physical and/or verbal.

From Corrigan JD: Development of a scale for assessment of agitation following traumatic brain injury. J Clin Exp Neuropsychol 1989;11:261–277.

history, pre-existing psychiatric disorders, and socioeconomic status may affect outcome.

Age is a factor that has been linked to outcome in a number of studies, at least in regard to mortality. Mortality is highest during childhood under 2 years of age, then progressively decreases throughout childhood to a nadir at 12 years of age before steeply rising between 15 and 24 years, and continues to progressively rise from the age of 35 years.[115] To evaluate the effect of age on functional outcome, however, the data are more complex. Some studies of patients with traumatic brain injury have found age to be either not important for prediction or not useful as a single predictor.[101, 102, 116] For any severity, PTA is prolonged with advancing age, especially over age 40, and increased age and PTA in combination may be predictive of poor outcome. Patients over age 40 who were comatose over 1 hour did not achieve a good recovery at 1 year; in contrast, 50% of patients under 40 with similar durations of coma achieved a good recovery in that time frame.[117] In the pediatric age range, most studies have found worse functional outcomes in children of younger age at the time of injury.[118–121] Findings in other studies, however, have diverged, with younger age being associated either with better outcome, such as in the study by Eiben and associates[122] in which the younger children also had shorter durations of coma, or with no effect on outcome, such as in the study by Costeff and associates[123] in which duration of coma was also not associated with outcome. Adverse neurobehavioral outcome in very young children is frequently associated with intentional injury, i.e., the shaking impact syndrome of child abuse.[118, 124, 125] Interrelationships among the severity, type, and extent of brain injury, mechanism, and age complicate assessment of the effect of age on outcome in the pediatric population.

Rate of recovery may be another prognostic indicator as suggested by studies of survivors of traumatic brain injury.[84] This finding is not surprising to clinicians who care for patients in rehabilitation centers, where varying recovery rates are often subjectively appreciated by staff.

CEREBRAL ANEURYSMS AND STROKE

Increased survival rates after rupture and surgical repair of cerebral aneurysms have led to significant numbers of patients with impairments and compromised quality of life.[126] A number of outcome studies have demonstrated that cognitive and behavioral impairments are frequent sequelae of such aneurysms, even among patients who show "no neurologic impairments."[127–131] The most common site for cerebral aneurysms is the anterior portion of the circle of Willis (85%–95%).[131] The anterior communicating artery (ACoA) in the anterior portion of the circle is particularly vulnerable.[132–134]

The most consistently reported deficits and those most characteristic of the "ACoA syndrome" are memory impairments, confabulation, and "personality change."[132] Questions remain, however, as to the specific deficits and their anatomic correlates that are characteristic of this population of patients. Since memory deficits are understood to be a consequence of hippocampal injury in many other disease and injury states, the memory deficits seen after anterior communicating and anterior cerebral artery aneurysm rupture/surgery are difficult to explain, since these arteries do not supply the hippocampus. In Damasio's series,[127] the "common anatomic denominator" demonstrated by CT scans, angiography, intraoperative photographs, and single photon emission tomography (SPECT) imaging was the posterior aspect of the ventromedial sector of the frontal lobe, which includes the orbitofrontal cortex and the midline and paramedial basal forebrain, but not the medial temporal lobes. These anatomic sites have been implicated as important parts of a neural network that includes the medial temporal lobes and that is thought to mediate declarative memory.[135, 136]

As with traumatic brain injury, most neuronal recovery after stroke occurs in the first 6 months after the event.[137] Patients with cerebral hemorrhage have a higher mortality rate but a better outcome than patients with impairments from cerebral infarction.[138, 139] Approximately four of five stroke patients eventually walk, but only two of three regain self-care independence.[140]

Predictive factors after a stroke include the following: coma at onset, incontinence, cognitive impairment, especially visuoperceptual disorders, severe hemiparesis, no motor return in 1 month, previous stroke, cardiovascular disease, large and deep lesions on brain imaging; possible predictive factors include hemisensory deficit, lack of a close family member, and poor financial resources.[141–145] In a study on recovery in stroke based on a sample of over 1000 patients, however, the authors concluded that "even the most severe cases regularly experience meaningful improvement during rehabilitation."[146]

HYPOXIC-ISCHEMIC BRAIN INJURY

Patients suffering brain injury from anoxia have a poorer prognosis in general than those with traumatic injury. This poor prognosis relates to both mortality and level of function.[147–149] In a series of 169 patients, recovery of function in the small percentage of patients who regained consciousness was poor. Only one patient had a good recovery.[150, 151]

Because of the vulnerability of the hippocampus, cerebellum, and basal ganglia to anoxic or hypoxic insult, many patients who recover have profound mobility and memory deficits. Patients with traumatic brain injury may have suffered concomitant hypoxic-ischemic injury because of either hypotension or high ICP levels. Additional insults such as these presaged a poor outcome in one study.[149]

Spinal Cord Disorders

Natural Course of Recovery After Traumatic Spinal Cord Injury

There are approximately 10,000 new cases of traumatic spinal cord injury (SCI) every year in the United States.[152] With improved medical management and increased life expectancy, the prevalence of SCI is increasing and has been estimated at 906 per million population in the United States.[153] Improved emergency management has also led to an increase in the percentage of less severe injuries.[154]

Immediately following an injury to the spinal cord, all deep tendon reflexes below the lesion are absent. This finding has been ascribed to a phenomenon called spinal shock, which has been defined as the period after an acute SCI when there is motor and sensory loss accompanied by areflexia. Gradually, the reflexes return, if the lesion is upper motor neuron, and eventually become hyperactive. The anocutaneous and bulbocavernosus reflexes are often depressed only for a very short period of time and are usually the first to return. The pathophysiology and time course of spinal shock have not yet been clearly defined.[155]

Assessment Tools for SCI

The degree of recovery from SCI depends on the severity of the initial injury. The Frankel classification has been used to differentiate the severity of the neurologic impairment and is based on the degree of incompleteness of the lesion (Table 20–9).[156] Maynard and associates[157] demonstrated that only 5% of those patients who are initially Frankel A gain any lower extremity motor recovery and that none become ambulatory or fully recover. Eighty-two percent of those who are initially Frankel B regain some lower extremity recovery and 47% become ambulatory, although none fully recover. Eighty-seven percent of those who are initially Frankel C or D become ambulatory and 26% fully recover.[157] The Frankel classification is limited because of its imprecise designation of "useless" versus "useful" motor function.[158] Additionally, authors have observed an improved prognosis in patients with sacral sensory sparing.[159] Because of the limitations of the Frankel Scale, the classification system has been revised by the American Spinal Injury Association (ASIA) and is referred to as the ASIA Impairment Scale (Table 20–10).[160, 161] The neurologic level is defined as the most caudal segments which test as normal or intact for both motor and sensory function and therefore also defines which muscles are available to perform self-care and mobility tasks (Table 20–11).[160]

TABLE 20–9 FRANKEL SCALE OF FUNCTIONAL CLASSIFICATION OF NEUROLOGIC DEFICIT POST SPINAL CORD INJURY

A	Complete
B	Motor complete and sensory incomplete
C	Motor useless
D	Motor useful
E	Complete recovery

From American Spinal Injury Association: Standards for Neurological Classification of Spinal Injury Patients. Chicago, ASIA, 1990.

TABLE 20–10 ASIA IMPAIRMENT SCALE

A	Complete: No motor or sensory function is preserved in the sacral segments S4–S5.
B	Incomplete: Sensory but not motor function is preserved below the neurologic level and extends through the sacral segments S4–S5.
C	Incomplete: Motor function is preserved below the neurologic level, and the majority of key muscles below the neurologic level have a muscle grade less than 3.
D	Incomplete: Motor function is preserved below the neurologic level, and the majority of key muscles below the neurologic level have a muscle grade greater than or equal to 3.
E	Normal: Motor and sensory function is normal.

From American Spinal Injury Association: International Standards for Neurological and Functional Classification of Spinal Cord Injury, Revised 1996. Chicago, ASIA, 1996.

Other SCI Measurement Tools

There are several functional assessment scales that are used to measure self-care and mobility; how-

TABLE 20–11 KEY MUSCLES FOR MOTOR LEVEL CLASSIFICATION

C5	Elbow flexors
C6	Wrist extensors
C7	Elbow extensors
C8	Finger flexors to the middle finger
T1	Small finger abductors
L2	Hip flexors
L3	Knee extensors
L4	Ankle dorsiflexors
L5	Long toe extensors
S1	Ankle plantarflexors

From American Spinal Injury Association: International Standards for Neurological and Functional Classification of Spinal Cord Injury, Revised 1996. Chicago, ASIA, 1996.

ever, most are not designed specifically for SCI. The Modified Barthel Index and the Functional Independence Measure (FIM) have been found to be valid, reliable and sensitive assessments of function following SCI.[162, 163] ASIA endorses the use of the FIM in SCI, although it recognizes the potential difficulties in utilizing a scale that was developed for the disabled population in general.[160] The Quadriplegia Index of Function (QIF) is a functional assessment tool that was designed specifically to assess the function of quadriplegics.[164] It is composed of 10 categories: transfers, grooming, bathing, feeding, dressing, wheelchair mobility, bed activities, bladder program, bowel program, and understanding of personal care. Each category consists of several component activities, each scored separately, and each category carries a relative weight. The QIF has been found to be reliable and more sensitive than the Barthel Index in assessing functional gains in patients with quadriplegia.[164]

Other Predictive Factors

Age has an impact on both mortality[165, 166] and on the likelihood of recovery of ambulation[167, 168] after SCI. A study of the recovery of ambulation following acute traumatic central cord syndrome demonstrated that 29 of 30 patients less than 50 years of age regained ambulation, whereas only 7 of 17 patients 50 years of age or older ambulated. The greatest difference in the recovery of ambulation occurred in the Frankel C patients: all five of the younger Frankel C patients ambulated, whereas only one of seven older Frankel C patients ambulated. When the muscle strength recovery in the Frankel C patients was examined, it was noted that there was similar improvement in the lower extremity motor scores in the younger and older groups. Recovery of upper extremity strength, however, was noted to be greater for the younger patients and the one older ambulatory patient than for the nonambulatory older patients. The authors hypothesized that the difference in upper extremity recovery may be one factor that limits the ambulatory capacity of older SCI patients. They theorized that this diminished recovery of upper extremity strength may be due to a different pathophysiologic mechanism of injury that results in a greater extent of injury in the older group. They suggested that older patients may have cervical spondylosis and vertebral artery sclerosis, which result in greater injury to the anterior horn cells and lateral columns, resulting in less recovery of motor function.[167] A larger study of 105 central cord patients confirmed these findings. In this study, all ASIA D patients ambulated at time of discharge from rehabilitation, regardless of age. Among ASIA C patients, 30 of 33 patients less than 50 years of age ambulated whereas 13 of 31 patients 50 years of age or older ambulated.[168]

SCI affects sensory, motor, and autonomic functions and results in significant disability in self-care and mobility. The degree of disability generally follows the degree of motor impairment,[169] although numerous other factors, including medical complications and psychosocial factors, impact on which activities an individual patient will actually perform in the community.[170] For incomplete injuries, functional outcome is difficult to predict because the degree and timing of motor recovery is not precise.[171] The expected functional outcome of complete injuries is somewhat easier to predict and depends upon the neurologic level of injury.

Functional Outcome by Neurologic Level

Patients with complete lesions at C1 and C2 have no voluntary movement of the upper or lower extremities and no diaphragmatic function. They are dependent on a ventilator for respiration. They require a power wheelchair for mobility, often operated by chin control, with a powered recliner for pressure relief. They are dependent for all other mobility and self-care. Environmental control units (ECUs), either voice-activated or controlled by a mouthstick, may allow these patients to use a speaker phone, turn on a radio or television, and turn on and off lights.

If the phrenic nerve is not denervated, pacing of the diaphragm with an implanted phrenic nerve pacemaker may be possible.[172, 173] Pacing may not be effective in patients with lesions between C3 and C5 because some or all of the anterior horn cells or lower motor neurons of the phrenic nerve may be destroyed. Phrenic pacing is indicated in patients with SCI at or above the C3 level.[172] This would allow these patients to be ventilator-free for all or part of the day and may allow them to have their tracheostomies plugged or discontinued, if their secretions are otherwise manageable.[172, 173] This results in easier communication and may decrease the chance for respiratory infection. Additionally, the equipment required for phrenic nerve pacers is much smaller and lighter than a ventilator and allows easier transfers and mobility.[172]

Most patients at the C4 level will not require mechanical ventilation beyond the acute postinjury period; however, they will require total assistance for coughing and clearing secretions. They require a power wheelchair and may utilize pneumatic (sip and puff) or head control devices to operate their wheelchair. They may be able to drink from a cup with a long straw after set-up and may be able to do some very limited feeding with a balanced forearm orthosis that can be attached to the wheelchair.[174] They are otherwise dependent for mobility and self-care.

Patients with C5 tetraplegia have functional deltoid and biceps strength. The ability to abduct the shoulder and flex the elbow allows these patients to be independent in feeding and grooming with equipment, after set-up. An orthosis that provides wrist support and has a palm pouch that can hold an eating utensil, toothbrush, comb, or razor is needed, and the patients require assistance to don and doff such equipment. They require assistance for upper extremity dressing and are dependent for lower extremity dressing. They may be able to perform a lateral weight shift for pressure relief by hooking an elbow under the arm of their wheelchair and leaning to the side. They are independent in power wheelchair mobility with a joystick and can propel a manual wheelchair with lugs on the hand rims for short distances indoors but require assistance for transfers. They are dependent for bowel and bladder management.[175]

The ability to actively extend the wrist allows C6 tetraplegics to become independent with upper extremity dressing, bathing upper and lower extremities with equipment, and with bowel and bladder management with equipment. By actively extending the wrist, the fingers will passively flex, resulting in a tenodesis grasp, which can be used to grasp large objects, such as built-up utensils.[176] It is important to prevent finger extension contractures and to allow the finger flexors to develop some tightness in order to enhance the strength of the tenodesis grasp. Some patients will still require a universal cuff, a leather or webbing cuff that is placed on the hand and has a palm pouch, to hold utensils; wrist support is not needed. A wrist-driven flexor hinge orthosis can be utilized to provide increased pinch strength for self-catheterization and other tasks.[177] C6 tetraplegics are independent in manual wheelchair propulsion, can be independent with transfers utilizing a transfer board, and can drive a specially adapted van with a hydraulic lift and a lock-down system for the wheelchair. Although these patients do not have active elbow extensor strength, anterior deltoid and pectoralis muscles may be utilized to perform elbow extension to assist in transfers in a closed kinetic chain in both C5 and C6 tetraplegics.[178, 179]

A patient with C7 tetraplegia has active elbow extension and is independent with all manual wheelchair mobility, except stairs. A C7 tetraplegic patient can transfer independently with or without a transfer board but cannot transfer from the floor without assistance. Transfers into and driving a car with hand controls are achievable, as is independent wheelchair placement into the car. A C7 tetraplegic patient can be independent feeding without adaptive equipment, independent in grooming, bathing, and bowel and bladder management with equipment, and may be independent in upper and lower extremity dressing with equipment.[180] Upper extremity function can be improved in C6 and C7 tetraplegics by use of tendon transfer surgery. There are two main aims of tendon transfer in these patients: restoration of elbow extension and restoration of grasp.[176] It is important to wait until neurologic recovery has reached a plateau before undertaking any tendon transfer surgery. To obtain elbow extension, the posterior third of the deltoid muscle is elongated by free tendon grafts into the triceps near the olecranon. The arm is immobilized for 6 weeks, and then gradual mobilization of the elbow is begun under the supervision of a physical therapist. The force of elbow extension gained from this procedure allows patients to reach overhead, and in some lightweight patients, to assist movement in bed and transfer to a wheelchair.[176] To restore grasp in a C6 or C7 tetraplegic, flexion of the fingers and lateral key pinch of the thumb can be obtained by transfer of the extensor carpi radialis longus into the profundi and brachioradialis into the flexor pollicis longus. If wrist extension is weak, the extensor carpi radialis brevis can be reinforced by transfer of the brachioradialis. The wrist and hand are immobilized for 3–4 weeks following the surgery, and the hand cannot be used for wheelchair propulsion or transfer for at least 4 weeks after the operation.[176]

C8 tetraplegics have function of the deep finger flexors, which provide an active, although not normal, hand grip. This allows them to be independent with manual wheelchair mobility, stairs, and all transfers, including floor transfers. They are independent with all self-care and bowel and bladder management.[180]

T1 paraplegics have control of the hand intrinsic muscles and therefore have normal hand function. Function is otherwise the same as for a patient with C8 tetraplegia. Paraplegics with neurologic levels between T2 and T10 are independent with all wheelchair mobility, transfers, and self-care. Additionally, they may be able to ambulate with a "swing to" or "swing through" gait pattern with the use of bilateral knee-ankle-foot orthoses (KAFOs) with locked knees and a walker or crutches.[181] Most use a wheelchair, however, as their primary means of mobility, owing to the excessive energy cost of ambulation. Studies have demonstrated that energy consumption during wheelchair propulsion in paraplegics approximates the normal walking energy consumption.[182]

At the T12 neurologic level, there is full innervation of the abdominal muscles, including the obliques. This provides increased truncal stability as well as the ability to hip hike by use of the internal and external obliques and the latissimus dorsi muscles. With bilateral KAFOs and crutches, patients with neurologic levels between T11 and L2 can ambulate with a swing-through or a reciprocal gait indoors and can ascend and descend stairs with a railing.[181] At neurologic levels L3 and below, long leg braces are no longer necessary and the patient can ambulate independently in the community with ankle-foot orthoses and crutches or canes.[181]

Hypoxic-Ischemic Spinal Cord Injury

Prognosis for functional recovery following ischemic SCI has not been as well studied as that for traumatic SCI. Laceration of the aorta due to trauma is the most common cause of ischemic myelopathy, but other causes include cross-clamping of the aorta during surgical repair, manipulation of the aorta during intercostal artery ligation, severe hypotension associated with myocardial infarction, aortic aneurysm dissection, spinal cord vascular anomaly, aortic angiography, and possibly decompression sickness. The clinical picture produced may be complete and flaccid or incomplete and spastic, depending on the site and etiology of the injury. Ischemia due to generalized diminished perfusion preferentially damages central gray matter and results in a flaccid lower motor neuron type weakness.[183] Patients who present with complete motor loss and who are flaccid have a poor prognosis for future functional motor recovery.[183, 184]

REHABILITATION TREATMENT INTERVENTIONS

Preventive Care

Case History

VK is a 52-year-old nursing aide who was driving home after completing a late night shift when she lost control of her car, crossed a median, and hit a tree at high speed. She sustained a severe brain injury with a right temporoparietal subdural hematoma as well as multiple fractures including a left humeral head fracture, left femoral neck and femoral shaft fractures, right acetabular fracture, bilateral severely comminuted tibial fractures with knee dislocations, and a right navicular bone fracture. The subdural hematoma was evacuated, and she remained in coma for 3 weeks and then gradually emerged and was extubated and taken off the respirator. The left humeral fracture was not treated. Ender's rods were placed in the left femur to maintain alignment of the left femoral shaft fracture. The tibial fractures and ankle fracture were not treated.

Three months after her injury, she was transferred to a rehabilitation facility. At that time, she was noted to have severe bilateral equinovarus contractures of both feet, finger and wrist flexion contractures complicated by metacarpophalangeal joint contractures of both hands, an immobile and painful left shoulder, severe deformities of both knees with posterior displacement of the tibial plateau, a moderate left hemiparesis, and bilateral draining pressure sores (Grade III) on both heels. She was awake and alert and oriented to place and person and was aware of the reason for her hospitalization. She had pain in both legs and in the left shoulder but had enough voluntary control over the right arm to be able to use it to feed herself, although she could not open her grasp sufficiently to hold larger objects because of the upper limb flexion contractures. After a year of rehabilitation care and multiple orthopedic joint salvage operations (bilateral knee replacements, a left shoulder replacement, and bilateral ankle triple arthrodeses with Achilles tendon lengthening to correct severe equinovarus ankle deformities), the patient was ambulatory with a platform walker and had reached a level of minimal assistance for activities of daily living. Her mental status had improved significantly, but she remained significantly limited by residual pain in her legs and by bilateral joint flexion contractures in the hands.

The above case history illustrates the kinds of problems that are encountered in the rehabilitation phase of care when inadequate attention is paid to the potential prevention of secondary complications during the acute phase of management of the patient with neural trauma complicated by multiple musculoskeletal trauma. There are two major goals of the rehabilitation treatment program: maximizing return of function and preventing secondary complications. The prevention of secondary complications is a critical goal of the rehabilitation program that should not be delayed until many days have elapsed after the injury when the patient is ready to be transferred to a rehabilitation service.

Rehabilitation of the patient with neural injury as well as the initiation of measures to prevent secondary complications must begin *as early as possible* following the stabilization of the patient. It is not too early to begin a program of treatment to avoid skin complications, contracture, heterotopic ossification (HO), urinary tract infections, and general deconditioning (to name only a few avoidable possible complications in the neurally injured patient) in the neurointensive care unit. Early consultation and active participation of a physiatrist on the trauma team are absolutely critical in keeping the focus on preserving function and preventing complications that can place significant limitations on the recovery process. It is often the accumulation of the effects of *avoidable* secondary complications that places significant limitation on the eventual extent to which functional recovery of the patient can be maximized. It is frequently presumed that a patient with a severe traumatic brain injury along with multiple other injuries does not need to have optimal management of the associated musculoskeletal injuries, for example, since an assumption is made early on that the patient will not again become mobile or regain functional cognition. Such a patient, as that in the case study at the beginning of this section, can reach rehabilitation having started to recover significantly from the neural injury but unable to take advantage of the neural recovery to become physically mobile because of severe residual physical impairments—e.g., joint fusions due to HO, multiple contractures, limb deformities, pressure sores, etc. For example, a patient with severe traumatic brain injury whose fractures are not properly set, who is not started on prophylactic treatment for HO, whose skin is not adequately protected from pressure-related breakdown, and/or who is not initiated on a program of regular turning, sitting, and range of motion exercises can end up in the very frustrating situation in which there is a recovering nervous system in a physically incapacitated and deconditioned body. The rehabilitation team is then faced with the formidable task of attempting to assist the patient to recover mobility by "undoing" the complications that have accumulated during the acute phase of care.

In this section, we review the more common complications that are encountered in the patient who has sustained a significant neural injury. The likelihood of a patient developing such complications can be minimized. The most effective way to maximize functional recovery and avoid complications is to involve the rehabilitation team as early in the hospital course as possible. The physiatrist must be considered an integral component of the neuroemergency response team for any condition in which the patient is expected to be immobilized or require rehabilitation services during the course of recovery.

Physiologic Effects of Immobilization

One of the major results of neural damage is the loss of mobility. In severe injury to the brain and/or spinal cord, the patient may become completely immobile and essentially bedridden for extended periods of time. Prolonged immobilization has profound deleterious effect on all body systems.[186] Some of these effects are listed in Table 20–12. A complete review of preventive measures for all of these complications is beyond the scope of this chapter. General principles of prevention with a highlighting of a few of these problems will be provided.

TABLE 20–12 **EFFECTS OF PROLONGED BED REST AND INACTIVITY**

SYSTEM	EFFECTS
Musculoskeletal	Muscle weakness, atrophy, contractures, immobilization, hypercalcemia, degenerative joint disease, osteopenia/osteoporosis
Cardiovascular	Cardiovascular deconditioning, postural hypotension, thromboembolic phenomena including deep venous thrombosis and pulmonary embolism
Respiratory	Ventilatory dysfunction, upper respiratory infections, hypostatic pneumonia, aspiration pneumonia
Metabolic	Androgen, growth hormone, parathyroid, insulin, electrolyte, protein, and carbohydrate changes
Genitourinary	Stasis, urinary tract infections (especially in the presence of prolonged indwelling urinary catheter), calculi
Gastrointestinal	Constipation, loss of appetite, weight loss
Nervous	Sensory deprivation, anxiety, agitation, depression, confusion, cognitive dysfunction, incoordination, and impaired motor control
Integument	Pressure sores

Adapted from Halar EM, Bell KR: Rehabilitation's relationship to inactivity. In Kottke FJ, Lehman JF (eds): Krusen's Handbook of Physical Medicine and Rehabilitation, pp 1113–1133. Philadelphia, WB Saunders, 1990.

The accumulation of effects of prolonged immobilization can produce additional problems in patients who may already be significantly compromised by their primary injuries. It is therefore imperative that patients be actively remobilized or at least passively moved so as to change their posture and joint positions on a regular basis, and to maintain the flexibility of soft tissues. Immobilization has traditionally been viewed as a nursing issue. However, it should be viewed as a wide-reaching medical issue that should be addressed in one way or another by all the members of the treatment team so that there is a comprehensive approach to the problem of avoiding the many complications of prolonged immobilization. In remobilizing the patient, it should be recognized that passive movement without lifting the patient off the support surface can lead to shearing forces on the skin, which are the major forces involved in skin breakdown. Attention must be paid to the issue of limiting shear forces on the skin while maximizing the amount of passive joint motion that a patient experiences. To avoid muscular and joint capsule contracture, the joints should be mobilized through regular passive range of motion exercises through full available range and advanced to active assistive and active range of motion exercises as the patient recovers the ability to produce active voluntary motion at the joints. Splinting to maintain joints in a neutral position of function should also be considered as an adjunct to exercise, particularly for maintaining joint position while the patient is asleep. Splinting can also help to prevent traumatic synovitis (e.g., in the wrist) in the presence of muscle flaccidity.

Regular active lower extremity exercises may improve venous blood flow. In addition, the patient should have regular changes in truncal posture with respect to the pull of gravity, with sitting and turning to the sides in addition to the supine position, not only to avoid the development of prolonged pressure on any particular weight-bearing skin region but also to facilitate the drainage and clearance of pulmonary secretions and to avoid the development of hypostatic pneumonia. If there is any question that a patient with reduced responsiveness may be prone to aspiration of enteral feedings, various precautions should be taken to limit the possibility of precipitating an aspiration pneumonia. These would include checking of the residual volumes in the stomach regularly if a gastrostomy tube is used instead of a jejunostomy tube, elevating the trunk to at least 45 degrees during feeding, and giving enteral feeds at a slow continuous rate by pump rather than in boluses or at high administration rates. If there is any question about whether a "low-level" patient may be at major risk for aspiration, a salivagram can be performed. As soon as it is feasible, a "low-level" patient should be started on progressive weight-bearing activities on a tilt table in order to generate some gravitational axial forces on the long bones of the legs and the spine.

After sudden immobilization, urinary calcium can rise for several weeks with loss of calcium due to acceleration of osteoclastic and decreased osteoblastic activity. In young persons who are in a rapidly growing phase with normally high rates of bone turnover, the flow of calcium out of bone triggered by acute immobilization can exceed the ability of the kidneys to excrete it and serum calcium levels can rise significantly, occasionally reaching levels associated with malignant hypercalcemia (serum levels of $>$ 14 mg/100 mL). Acute treatment involves increasing the rate of urinary excretion of calcium by administering fluids with loop diuretics (e.g., furosemide). Salmon or porcine calcitonin can be used, and occasionally chelating agents are necessary for symptomatic acute hypercalcemia. Antiosteoclastic diphosphonate agents may also be effective as an adjunct for acute management.[185, 187] This condition most commonly occurs with acute onset of quadriplegia due to spinal cord injury[188] or, less commonly, Guillain-Barré syndrome[189] in young adolescents.

Heterotopic ossification (HO) can occur after traumatic brain injury or spinal cord injury, particularly in the presence of concomitant fractures involving periarticular regions.[190] This is a relatively common problem of great significance for the eventual function of the individual, since HO can essentially immobilize important large joints and can also be a source of significant musculoskeletal pain in the rehabilitation phase of care. Between 10% and 20% of patients with neural injury develop significant HO, which generally can be detected radiologically within the first 12 weeks after injury. The cause of HO following neural trauma is uncertain but may relate to neural autonomic innervation of the circulatory supply to the joints, neurohumoral factors, or direct neural influences on the rate of bone anabolic and catabolic rates. Etidronate sodium has been used for this condition after neural injury, although the long-term benefit of therapy has not been conclusively demonstrated.[191–193] Nonsteroidal anti-inflammatory medications and irradiation can also be used.[194, 195] As with the development of HO in other conditions, surgical excision should be delayed by 12–18 months to allow for maturation of the heterotopic bone in order to minimize the likelihood of recurrence. There has been one report of successful early removal of HO in patients with TBI in a small case series.[196] Bone scans can be used to identify sites at which HO has developed, and the activity of the HO process can be followed with serial measures of serum alkaline phosphatase. Clinical trials of preventive measures for neurogenic HO would be of significant value in clarifying the relative utility of different interventions.

Preservation of at-risk organ systems in the neurologically disabled individual is a key element of a successful rehabilitation program. This includes preventing additional catastrophic events for which the patient may be at risk as a result of underlying disease processes that precipitated the neurologic emergency. This is clearly important in the patient with a cerebrovascular accident where atherosclerotic involvement of the cerebral vessels increases the risk of recurrence of cerebrovascular events, or, through association with atherosclerotic disease involving other critical vascular beds, myocardial ischemia and peripheral arterial occlusion. Identification and modification of risk factors as well as the judicious selective use of antiplatelet agents and anticoagulants for preventing thromboembolic events can favorably influence the risk of vascular events in patients with established thromboembolic cerebrovascular disease.[197]

The types of medical complications that can be encountered in patients undergoing neurorehabilitation are varied and depend on the nature of the process precipitating the neurologic emergency and disease that may be associated with this causative process, the presence of pre-existing comorbid conditions, as well as the various problems that are consequential to the precipitating neurologic event including those associated with prolonged immobilization.[198, 199] Some of the more common complications are listed in Table 20–13. While preventive measures should be instituted wherever possible to minimize the risk of life-threatening complications, when they do occur, they need to be recognized quickly with early initiation of appropriate therapy. This is best accomplished in the context of a specialized neurorehabilitation unit, where such complications are most likely to be recognized earlier and managed successfully.[200]

Self-Care and Mobility Deficits

Neurorehabilitation patients experience a decline in function because of deficits in mobility secondary to primary neurologic insults and to secondary effects of immobilization. Self-care deficits may occur because of mobility deficits, awareness or cognitive deficits, or a combination of these factors. Therapists with special training and/or experience with this population of patients use a wide variety of interventions to address these impairments. These interventions may include adaptive equipment, orthotics or prosthetics, splinting, or therapeutic modalities such as range of motion, heat and cold applications, or other techniques to preserve or improve passive and active mobility. Proper positioning of the patient for feeding is essential. Appropriate assessment of swallowing by speech-language pathologists is mandatory in this population for preventing aspiration pneumonia. When patients are out of bed, proper positioning in a bedside chair or adaptive seating system is required for patients who have poor postural or head control. Restraints may be necessary to protect patients from injury in the bed or while seated out of bed. Appropriate management of survivors of brain and spinal cord disorders requires the expertise of teams of subspecialty-trained therapists and nurses.

TABLE 20–13 **COMMON MEDICAL COMPLICATIONS ENCOUNTERED DURING NEUROREHABILITATION**

Aspiration associated with dysphagia
Hypostatic pneumonia
Urinary tract infection
Acute/chronic pain syndromes
Deep venous thrombosis
Pulmonary embolism
Pressure sores
Myocardial ischemia
Congestive heart failure
Cardiac arrhythmias
Brittle diabetes mellitus
Uncontrolled hypertension

Cognitive and Behavioral Disorders

This discussion is not intended to be a comprehensive review of cognitive and behavioral management. Several principles, however, will be articulated. Several texts are available for more in-depth information in these areas.[201–205] Cognitive remediation and behavioral management will be discussed separately below, yet in practice they are highly integrated during rehabilitation of neurologically injured patients. Cognitive remediation can be viewed as the translation of information about a patient's cognitive strengths and weaknesses into a behavioral treatment plan that is operationalized by the neurorehabilitation team. This is known as the neuropsychologic-behavioral approach. The basic principles of behavior management must be heeded whether the behavioral treatments are directed toward remediating cognitive deficits or toward minimizing disturbing behaviors that interfere with social interactions occurring both within and outside of structured learning situations.

Both cognitive remediation and behavioral management can be applied concomitantly with medications that are intended to enhance neural recovery (e.g., psychostimulants, tricyclic antidepressants, dopaminergic agents) or control disturbing behaviors such as aggression (e.g., antiseizure agents, beta blockers) and abulia (e.g., psychostimulants, tricyclic antidepressants). See Table 20–14 for a summary of these medications.

Principles of Cognitive Remediation

Several principles can be articulated:

1. *A hierarchy of cognitive functions is assumed.* Among the different cognitive domains, selective attention and short-term memory can be viewed as basic domains that serve as infrastructural support for higher-level domains, i.e., language, visuoperception, and executive function, which require more complex and highly integrated processing of information. Deficits in language, visuoperception, and executive functioning thus must not only take into account impairments in fundamental processing components that interact within a neural network within each domain, but also consider whether impairments in attention and memory are contributing to the clinical presentation. Rehearsal strategies, i.e., repetition, forced usage, and practice, which are

TABLE 20–14 **COMMON MEDICATIONS USED DURING NEUROLOGIC REHABILITATION FOR ENHANCING NEURAL RECOVERY AND MANAGING DIFFICULT BEHAVIORS IN BRAIN-INJURED PATIENTS**

AGENT	POSTULATED MECHANISM OF ACTION	INDICATIONS	CAUTIONS	ADULT DOSE
Methylphenidate hydrochloride	Activates brain stem and cortical arousal network via noradrenergic and dopaminergic neurotransmitter systems	Deficits in attention and concentration; flat affect; poor initiation; depression; impulsivity	Tachycardia; hypertension; agitation; anxiety; glaucoma; lowers seizure threshold; simultaneous use with antihypertensive and pressor agents, MAO inhibitors, tricyclic antidepressants; exacerbates Tourette's syndrome; abrupt discontinuation can be unsafe, thus should be tapered	5 mg as initial test dose. Then 5 mg BID given in morning and early afternoon before therapies; increase by 5 mg every 3–5 days until desired behavioral effect to maximal dose of 20 mg BID without side effects
Bromocriptine mesylate	Activates postsynaptic dopamine receptors on neurons that modulate prolactin secretion by the anterior pituitary; modulates motor function in the basal ganglia; modulates attentional network between basal ganglia and anterior cingulate gyrus	Poor arousal; inconsistent level of alertness	Hypertension; sensitivity to ergot alkaloids; lowers seizure threshold; headache; visual disturbances; pulmonary infiltrates, pleural effusions, and thickening; delirium; hallucinations	1.75 mg BID with meals as test dose for several days Increase by 1.75–2.5 mg every 3–5 days until optimal arousal/alertness levels achieved without side effects until maximal dose 25 mg BID
Tricyclic/tetracyclic antidepressants: amitriptyline, trazodone	Amitriptyline inhibits reuptake of noradrenergic neurotransmitters presynaptically, thus increasing their availability postsynaptically; other neurotransmitter systems—serotonin, dopamine, acetylcholine, histamine—also have been implicated Trazodone may be primarily serotoninergic	Postconcussive syndrome; agitation; aggression; post-traumatic stress disorder; deficits in attention and concentration; sleep disturbance; depression; poor initiation; flat affect	Delirium, especially those with prominent anticholinergic effects; lowers seizure threshold; concurrent use with MAO inhibitors and digoxin; orthostatic hypotension; glaucoma; neurogenic bladder; cardiac disease, especially conduction block; thyroid disease; constipation; abrupt discontinuation can be unsafe, thus should be tapered	For amitriptyline, 10–25 mg at HS as test dose, then increase by 10–25 mg in single or BID dose every week to dose of 100 mg daily, at which point blood levels should be checked (amitriptyline only). Blood levels should guide gradual increase of amitriptyline over 100 mg daily to maximal dose of 200 mg daily For trazodone, start with 25 mg as first dose; increase by 25 mg every 3–5 days until desired effects without side effects to maximal dose of 300 mg daily in 2 divided doses
Beta blockers: propranolol	Nonselective blockade of beta-adrenergic receptor sites in effort to decrease noradrenergic activity	Aggression	Bronchospasm; congestive heart failure; diabetes mellitus; thyroid disease; bradycardia; depression; heart block	Start with test dose of 20 mg daily. Increase by 20 mg every 3 days to a BID schedule. Increase by 30–60 mg every 3 days if HR stays above 50, and systolic BP stays above 90 to maximal dose of 300 mg daily
Antiseizure: carbamazepine	Unknown	Aggression; disinhibition	Marrow suppression; sedation; hepatotoxicity	100 mg BID for 1 week and check CBC. Increase to 200 mg BID for 1 week and check blood level. Further increase in dose should be guided by blood levels

For a complete review of these agents, see Horn LJ: Pharmacology and brain rehabilitation. Phys Med Rehabil Clin North Am 1997;8(4).
MAO, monoamine oxidase; BID, twice daily; HR, heart rate; BP, blood pressure; CBC, cell blood count.

intended to reinforce or treat the fundamental domains of selective attention and short-term memory, are an essential component of cognitive remediation.[206]

2. *Clinical cognitive or neuropsychologic assessment is essential for developing cognitive remediation strategies.* From these assessments, an individual patient's profile of cognitive weaknesses and strengths can be defined. Fundamental deficits and strengths in attention and memory that influence performance of higher level domains also are defined. Further, basic component deficits and strengths contributing to impairment or preservation of function within each cognitive domain are defined. This information, then, can be

translated into a series of cognitive remediation strategies operationalized in different therapies as well as in interpersonal interactions. These strategies are intended either to treat the deficits directly or to bypass or compensate for these deficits by utilizing preserved or available cognitive components and cognitive strengths.[97, 207, 208]

3. *Treatment of cognitive deficits directly involves a series of replacement or substitution strategies.* These utilize external structure to provide information that cannot be processed spontaneously, or for strategies that cannot be internally generated. For example, in the amnestic patient with declarative memory deficits, a series of external aids such as memory notebooks, diaries, calendars, alarm watches, timers, and computer software can be developed to provide important "to-be-remembered" information. Rehearsal strategies are utilized to teach amnestic patients to remember to use external aids. Procedural memory strategies (see below under bypass strategies) are utilized to teach amnestic patients how to use external aids as an acquired and automatic skill or habit. As another example, in the aphasic patient with word retrieval difficulties, an external semantic or phonemic cue can be offered to induce spontaneous production of a target word or phrase. When this is not helpful, a series of choices can then be offered, giving the patient the option of a yes or no response to the possible target words.[206, 209, 210]
4. *Treatment of cognitive deficits also involves a series of bypass strategies.* These utilize available or preserved cognitive components within a larger cognitive skill or domain to bypass cognitive weaknesses, and to achieve adequate cognitive performance. For example, in the amnestic patient with declarative memory deficits, a series of procedural memory strategies, such as conditioned learning and priming, can be applied. Procedural memory strategies are thought to take advantage of preserved learning processes that require unconscious encoding of information in an effort to bypass learning that is dependent on conscious encoding of incoming information. As another example, in the aphasic patient with deficits in auditory comprehension, a series of informational input strategies that take advantage of intact visual or tactile sensory systems can be applied. These patients may have difficulty understanding acoustically presented (spoken) lexical information, but their understanding may be optimized by alternate presentation of pictorial, gestural, written, or touched stimuli.[206, 211–213]
5. *Successful cognitive remediation strategies should be internally generated by the patient.* Those strategies that are found to be successful in therapeutic or interpersonal interactions must be encouraged to become adopted by the patient as automatic or spontaneously internally generated through a series of behavioral management techniques such as "vanishing cues" and "errorless learning." The technique of "vanishing cues" involves incremental and structured removal of external cueing systems, such that the patient eventually will incorporate and demonstrate a specific strategy in response to minimal external cueing. "Errorless learning" involves provision of minimal or no feedback to patients when mistakes are made, and positive reinforcement when the appropriate strategy is used. This approach is thought to encourage the patient to learn an optimal strategy by minimizing attention to alternative or incorrect strategies.[97, 211, 212]

How cognitive remediation relates to neural recovery is not well understood. As we continue to learn more about the neural networks underpinning different cognitive domains and neural plasticity, it is hoped that the relationship between specific cognitive remediation interventions and neural recovery will be better established. Much hope is being placed on the development of physiologic imaging studies of the brain, such as PET and fMRI, to define neural networks in the brain during patient participation in a variety of cognitive assessment and remediation tasks.[206, 209]

Principles of Behavioral Management

Several principles can be articulated:

1. *The therapeutic environment must be consistent, highly structured, and goal oriented, with minimal distracting influences.* Many of the disturbing behaviors, such as distractibility, aggression, and poor initiation, that require behavioral management stem from either internally disorganized processing of incoming stimuli or an inability to monitor affective responses in specific situations. One view is that the basic cognitive deficit predisposing to such behaviors is attentional, either to the environment or to oneself. Brain-injured patients may be unable to select and prioritize incoming stimuli, leaving them relatively lost in an immediate array of environmental stimuli, processing them in no particular order, and

responding to them without purpose. Or, if incoming stimuli are processed with some degree of organization, their behavioral responses may be extreme because these patients may be unable to monitor and regulate their own responses. Thus, external structure is required in order to control the quantity and quality of incoming sensory input, to prioritize incoming stimuli, and to provide feedback as to the appropriateness of responses. This approach must be built into a therapeutic or home environment by a variety of strategies such as a structured daily schedule, and consistency of staff responses across the various rehabilitation team members and care providers.[214, 215] Finally, every effort must be made to guarantee that the patient's vision and hearing are optimized to ensure organized sensory input and processing of environmental stimuli.

2. *Target behaviors and their precipitants must be identified and then subject to reinforcement or extinction.* Most agitated and aggressive behaviors can be connected to specific environmental precipitants or antecedents that act to trigger undesirable behavioral reactions. In some situations, no one particular precipitant may trigger these behaviors, but the cumulative effect of many environmental distractions, i.e., "sensory overload," may precede them. Thus, the undesirable target behavior must clearly be identified. The environment must be explored carefully for specific precipitants or multiple distracting influences. The environment subsequently must be manipulated to remove unnecessary precipitants and/or to reduce unnecessary distractions.[214, 215]
3. *Reinforce adaptive behaviors and ignore undesirable behaviors.* All instances of desirable or adaptive behaviors should be rewarded. Undesirable behaviors should be handled with as neutral a response as possible. Reward systems that aim to encourage and reinforce adaptive behaviors range from positive verbal or facial feedback during interpersonal situations, to highly regimented, contingency-based management plans (e.g., token economy systems). Overtly negative response to, or punishment for, undesirable behaviors tends to reinforce them, thus ignoring these behaviors is preferred as an interactional technique to attempt to minimize them. With particularly obnoxious and aggressive behaviors, ignoring them is often not realistic, and more active behavioral strategies or punishment must be used to minimize changes to the patient and care providers. "Time-out," or removing the patient from a rewarding environment to an environment in which there are no possible distracting rewarding embellishments, and "overcorrection" or requiring the patient to rectify the consequences of the undesirable behaviors are examples of aggressive behavior, yet these approaches are controversial.[214, 215]
4. *Optimize self-monitoring abilities.* Lack of awareness of one's own cognitive deficits and personality changes resulting from neurologic trauma is thought to be a fundamental barrier interfering with a therapeutic response to cognitive remediation and behavioral management. Such lack of insight, self-reflection, and self-monitoring are considered to be the result of structural, physiologic disruption of the brain. This results either in basic and widespread difficulties with attentional, sensory, peripheral, and semantic processing of incoming information, or a denial of one's difficulties with other integrative cognitive domains being spared. In patients in whom there are basic and widespread impairments of input processing components, it is unlikely that they will be able to learn to generate internal compensatory strategies, and thus they will be more dependent on external systems that replace lost cognitive processing components. In patients who deny or minimize cognitive and behavioral difficulties, individual and group psychotherapies sometimes have been used to teach insightful behaviors. Self-monitoring is a target behavior that must be reinforced in any therapeutic environment requiring behavioral management.[216, 217]

Psychosocial Issues

Ask not what disease the person has, but rather what person the disease has

(attributed to) William Osler

The manifestation of a disease process is critically dependent upon the psychosocial context in which the process is expressed. This is especially true when the disease process has produced neural damage, thus affecting the organ system most directly responsible for the behavior of an individual. Premorbid personality traits, coping strategies, personal resources, individual attitudes and beliefs, availability of family supports, educational level, cultural values, socioeconomic status, and psychologic make-up all play important roles in determining how a neurologic disability will play itself out and the manner and extent to which the life of the affected person can be reconstructed. It is critically important to develop an empathic understanding of the psychosocial context of the patient in order to make the best decisions about how to set up the goals of the rehabilitation program, how best to deal with behavioral issues, and how to go about counseling the patient and significant others about what to expect and how to prepare.

It is often helpful in this regard to have the team psychologist and/or social worker perform a detailed interview of significant others as well as the patient (to the extent possible) early in the rehabilitation phase of care in order to obtain as much relevant psychosocial information as possible so that the rehabilitation program and its goals can be appropriately tailored to the psychosocial context. Discharge planning is critically constrained by the psychosocial context and the available human and economic resources. Neurologic disability reverberates through a social support system and becomes a systems problem when viewed from a psychosocial perspective.[218]

Not only must the patient adapt to new and often difficult circumstances, but also his or her entire support system must do so. This presents a stressful challenge to both the patient and those around him. For example, preinjury family functioning in families with a child with traumatic brain injury has been shown to be predictive of family functioning 1 year after injury.[219] In combination with injury severity and the child's preinjury function, preinjury family functioning has also been shown to be predictive of the child's functioning 1 year after injury.[220]

Mood disorders and particularly depression can have an important effect on functional outcome. Depression in the patient may be reactive or may have a direct organic basis in the neural damage itself. Depression can also develop among significant others when they are faced with an overwhelming burden of caring for a significantly disabled loved one. Drug abuse and alcohol abuse are frequently complicating issues particularly in young patients with spinal cord injury or traumatic brain injury where these problems are seen disproportionately and are likely to continue as a means of coping with the stress of adapting to their residual deficits.[221, 222]

Vocational and Academic Re-entry

Recent legislation in the area of education law recognizes traumatic brain injury as a specific category of disability within special education. The Education of the Handicapped Act Amendments of 1990 (PL 101–476), now titled the Individuals with Disabilities Education Act (IDEA), mandates provision, when needed, of modifications to the educational program to include a spectrum of special educational services ranging from those provided in the regular educational setting through assistance in a resource room or placement in a self-contained, special education class. In addition, physical, occupational, and/or speech-language therapies, special services for visual or hearing impairments, behavioral management, and counseling services may be provided as part of the child's individualized education program (IEP).

This legislation also mandates provision of transition services, including vocational evaluation and training, for students with disabilities to begin no later than 16 years of age. Children and adolescents with severe brain, spinal cord, or multisystem injury are at risk for abnormal vocational development and outcome. Among children with severe brain injury sustained during the preschool years and then evaluated in adulthood, half had achieved average school performance but only one fourth were able to work full-time.[120] When the onset of disability occurs during childhood or adolescence, there is risk of loss of an entire lifetime of potential productivity with enormous personal, social, and economic costs. Discharge planning with these issues in mind must take place in the acute care setting for both children and adults returning to school or work.

DEVELOPMENTAL ISSUES IN NEUROREHABILITATION

The onset of disability due to congenital and acquired conditions involving the nervous system in children occurs during the development of independence in motor, communicative, cognitive, and social function. The brain is in varying stages of development at different ages in childhood; this may result in significant age differences in types of injury, responses to injury, and outcomes.[223] Skills developing rapidly at the time of injury may be especially vulnerable, with widespread consequences in young children in whom many skills are in a rapid stage of development.[125] Acquired neurologic conditions in childhood may cause immediate loss or decline in previously accomplished age-appropriate performance in one or more domains of function relative to the pre-insult baseline. Congenital neurologic conditions may cause delayed, abnormal, or absent development of specific functions. Either congenital or acquired disability with childhood onset can have consequences on subsequent development of both the domain of function that is directly affected and other domains. For example, deficits in mobility, self-care, or communicative function may lead to secondary developmental and functional deficits in social function. Deficits may also not be apparent immediately after acquired brain injury, particularly in young children in whom higher level functions which utilize affected structures have not yet developed, and a long-term developmental perspective is required in assessing cognitive outcome and behavioral adjustment after brain injury in children.[224]

There is a paucity of information regarding the physiologic and metabolic processes associated with both acute injury and recovery in children with brain injury.[225] Brain "plasticity" and potential for recovery of function within different domains of function in children of different ages are not well understood. Functional improvement in children with traumatic brain injury can reflect the natural history of the processes of recovery, ongoing developmental changes, or the effects of rehabilitative interventions, and these are not often easy to differentiate.[122] Discriminating among natural history, developmental changes, and effectiveness of rehabilitative interventions is similarly difficult in children with other congenital or acquired insults to the nervous system. Neurorehabilitation of children and adolescents is distinguished from that of adults by the ongoing challenge of meeting special needs related to growth and development.

GERIATRIC ISSUES IN NEUROREHABILITATION

Profile of the Geriatric Neurorehabilitation Patient

Several demographic and epidemiologic observations emphasize the importance of considering the special needs of the elderly in neurorehabilitation. While absolute lifespan of humans is not being extended, more people are living to old age, and perhaps even to a healthier old age, thus increasing their risk of experiencing life events usually associated with younger age groups, such as neurologic trauma.[226–229] Normal anatomic and physiologic aging can be characterized as a linear decline in reserve capacity of different organ systems.[230] The elderly, thus, have less adaptive resilience biologically to handle stressors such as acute illnesses, traumatic events, and rehabilitation interventions. This may contribute to slower neural and functional recovery often observed in the elderly as compared to younger counterparts. Additionally, the prevalence of chronic comorbidity and associated functional disability increases with aging.[231] Further, in the United States, despite cost-containment of medical health services, older patients have not been excluded from treatment with highly technological and life-saving interventions, even though they have an increased vulnerability to the undesirable complications of these interventions.[232–234] Thus, converging evidence reinforces the observation that older and sicker people are participating in neurorehabilitation after life-saving medical and surgical interventions.

The elderly neurologically injured patient will already have entered the acute care facility with several pre-trauma chronic diseases, for example, cerebrovascular and cardiovascular diseases, and degenerative arthritides. These chronic diseases will already be associated with compromises in several daily life survival skills such as difficulty walking especially outside the household, and difficulty performing heavier household duties, for example, cleaning and gardening. If the elderly patient survives the traumatic event, the hospital course may be characterized by multiple organ system compromise.[229] Staying in the acute care facility after a neurologically traumatic event itself is associated with acquiring more functional disability.[232, 235] Thus, medical/surgical hospital stays can be disastrous for elderly patients. New areas of compromise in survival skills become manifest, for example, swallowing dysfunction during feeding associated with sedating medication leading to aspiration; urinary and bowel incontinence associated with many factors including infection, immobility, and medications. Thus, on entry into a neurorehabilitation program, an elderly patient may have progressed to a functional level far below a pre-trauma baseline because of a compromised biologic substrate (normal aging, comorbidities), the superimposed ill effects of acute trauma, side effects of life-saving treatments, and imposed but necessary immobility.

While in neurorehabilitation, it should be expected that neurologically impaired elderly patients will recover more slowly than their younger counterparts. Normal aging-related changes are irreversible, when considering rehabilitation interventions. Inactivity effects, however, are reversible. Rehabilitation interventions, especially therapeutic exercises, are directed toward reversing inactivity effects in the elderly neurologically injured patient. The positive anatomic and physiologic effects of these exercises, specifically strengthening and endurance, are well established in elderly populations.[235–242]

As the elderly, neurologically injured patient remobilizes in rehabilitation, exacerbations of underlying degenerative musculoskeletal impairments, such as degenerative arthritis, as well as previously acquired soft tissue injuries, such as rotator cuff tendinitis, are common and can impede smooth remobilization. Caution must be used by physicians, in their prescription of therapeutic exercises, and therapists, in their application of traditional modalities (for example, ultrasound, transcutaneous nerve stimulation), to treat these inflammatory and pain syndromes.[243] During rehabilitation, it should also be expected that the elderly patient's neurorehabilitation program may be interrupted by either short episodes of acute comorbid illness (for example, urinary tract infection, pneumonia, autonomic dysreflexia, deep venous thrombosis, congestive heart failure), or by minor and major surgical procedures to treat complications of neurologic trauma (for example, ventriculoperitoneal shunting to treat hydrocephalus), and to optimize neural recovery (for example, tracheostomy placement to optimize pulmonary toilet, and transabdominal parenteral feeding tube placement to optimize nutritional support and to maintain bowel integrity). An optimal level of nutrition and optimal cardiopulmonary endurance are critical for supporting their neural recovery, as well as for tolerance of ongoing surgical, medical, and rehabilitation interventions.[4, 244]

Delirium in Geriatric Patients

Acute changes in mental status, or delirium, should be expected in elderly patients during neurologic recovery and rehabilitation. Delirium can be viewed as a nonspecific clinical presentation of an acute or subacute deleterious event.[245] Delirium, as discussed above, may present as a hypoactive or hyperactive state, with or without agitation. It must be recognized and investigated aggressively by considering several precipitating factors such as the following metabolic conditions: a gradual decrease in sodium associated with a syndrome of inappropriate antidiuretic hormone secretion (SIADH); infections, for example, urinary tract infections with sepsis; aspiration pneumonitis with compromised pulmonary ventilation and hypoxemia; meningoencephalitis with abnormal glucose, protein, and cell counts on spinal fluid examination; structural abnormalities, for example, extension of cerebral hemorrhage, or cerebrovascular accident; and, importantly, psychotropic side effects of medications, for example, sedating antiseizure agents, dopaminergic agents administered to enhance neural recovery, antihypertensive agents such as beta blockers, and narcotic analgesics to treat pain.[246–252]

The elderly patient's cognitive baseline must be established by interviewing a reliable significant other. A history of premorbid changes in cognition and behavior, suggestive of an underlying cerebrovascular or neural degenerative process, must be explored, since elderly patients with dementia seem especially vulnerable to developing delirium even with minor metabolic changes, infections, or structural abnormalities.[252] Serial and consistent mental status screening must be executed in an effort to monitor changes to interventions directed at reversing the delirium and defining its resolution. Family members and therapists more often recognize subtle changes in behavior, and reports to the physician managing the neurorehabilitation program must be heeded.

In the event that no obvious explanation emerges during the investigation of delirium, an affective disorder, specifically depression, must be seriously pursued. Loss reactions, or adjustment disorders, are expected and appropriate during neurologic recovery and can present as an acute change in mental status.[253] They can progress to a full-blown clinical depression that must be treated psychotherapeutically, and with neurotransmitter-enhancing agents such as psychostimulants, tricyclic antidepressant agents, or serotonin uptake blocking agents. A diagnosis of depression can be difficult in a neurologically recovering elderly patient, given the array of precipitants of delirium, and especially if the patient displays poor initiation, a labile or flat affect, or abulic or amotivational behavior as part of his or her neurologic cognitive-behavioral presentation. Making such a diagnosis may require consultation with experienced geriatric psychiatrists or behavioral neurologists with a thorough review of all diagnostic studies, especially structural imaging, and close monitoring of behavior to establish sleep-wake cycles and affective consistency during various therapeutic interventions with different team members. If medications are necessary to treat depression, extremely low doses should be initiated, and increases in dose should be performed slowly.[254, 255]

Behavioral strategies must be considered when treating delirium, especially when there are disturbing or socially inappropriate behaviors. The importance of a structured environment including consistent daily care providers and therapeutic program, and courteous, reality-oriented interactions must be emphasized. Physical restraints sometimes are necessary to prevent potentially harmful behaviors, but these should be used as a last resort. Mildly sedating medications such as chloral hydrate or short-acting benzodiazepines may be necessary in an effort to regulate sleep-wake cycles. Ensuring that the elderly patient has optimal use of his or her special sensory systems, specifically vision and hearing, with glasses and hearing aids will assist in facilitating presentation of organized environmental information for the delirious elderly patient.[4]

The Effect of Aging on Learning in Neurorehabilitation

Normal aging is associated with changes in cognitive and intellectual function, and subsequently how we continue to learn successfully. These issues are important to consider as an elderly patient recovers and is exposed to rehabilitation interventions that demand learning of new skills and information, or relearning previously habitual or automatic skills.

Learning capacity during normal aging has been characterized as a decline in "fluid" intelligence, or the ability to learn noncontextual new information and skills, especially when time constrained and performance based. Moreover, there is maintenance or improvement in "crystallized" intelligence, or the ability to learn experientially or contextually relevant information and skills, especially when not time constrained and verbally based.[256, 257] Thus, all information must be presented to an elderly neurologically recovering patient by explicitly making connections to the individual's life experiences and relevant frames of reference. Other aging-related cognitive changes, including decrease in visuoperception, and increasing difficulty selectively attending in distracting environments, can influence or delay the elderly patient's neurologic recovery in response to rehabilitation. Thus, task deconstruction and rehearsal become essential strategies during rehabilitation. Sensory stimuli must be presented in a singular and organized manner during therapeutic and informal interactions. Communication strategies that compensate for compromises in vision and hearing include using monosyllabic words within short, grammatically simple sentences; lowering vocal pitch to compensate for high-frequency sensorineural hearing loss; and the use of controlled prosodic, gestural, and facial embellishments, and tactile hand-to-hand contact during one-to-one interactions.[4]

The Social Support System

The population of elderly patients being treated in the late twentieth and early twenty-first century has had a cohort experience of several world wars, a major economic depression, and sometimes immigration from their countries of birth. Consequently, they hold high the value of independence as operationalized by control of everyday life survival skills. After neurologic injury, compromise in such control may be inevitable. Dependence on others for personal care may be necessary. Such loss must be handled carefully during rehabilitation. The rehabilitation team members must engage the older patient in a negotiation that defines, from the patient's point of view, a hierarchy of survival skills to be improved, prioritizing those that the patient chooses actively to control and perform. These skills inevitably become the focus in skilled therapy sessions. Other survival skills will become less important and may require ongoing assistance from personal care providers. The patient's social support system may be recruited to assist the elderly patient with various survival skills as "informal" care providers. Sometimes shared residential arrangements with family members must be made, or physical architectural changes to their own residence to improve access are necessary.

The relationship between the elderly disabled patient and the social support system, and the insurance and financial resources available to both parties, can be viewed as the major determining factors for continued life in the community after neurorehabilitation. Gerontologic data suggest that older disabled patients are not inclined to share households with younger adult relatives, but they do want to live close by and remain in regular personal or telephone contact with adult children. Spouses may have died or may be disabled themselves, and thus are not readily available to provide personal care. Thus, adult children, especially women, traditionally are asked to become home-based caregivers.[257–259]

"Formal" home providers such as visiting nurses, homemakers, home health aides, and therapists continue to be available in most communities. For elderly disabled patients who have "skilled" needs, which justify receiving ongoing personal care services, insurance reimbursement (usually Medicare) for these services is limited. Realistically, formal home care services must be viewed as complementary and incomplete vis-à-vis services provided by significant others in community-based residential sites. At times, patients and their families use private financial resources and their life savings to purchase home care services not reimbursed by health insurance. When functional recovery is incomplete and personal services required by the elderly patient cannot be met by formal, reimbursable home care services and by those provided by the social support system, the option of long-term residential institutionalization must be considered. This option continues to be difficult for most elderly patients and their families, but may increasingly be necessary as the elderly population expands and American families become more disrupted by geographic mobility.

Specific Adaptation of the Neurorehabilitation Process for the Elderly Patient

Neurologic and associated functional recovery takes longer in the elderly. This observation must be considered when planning rehabilitation programs for elderly patients. Referral and entry of elderly patients into aggressive, acute hospital-based programs may set them up for failure. Aggressive acute hospital-based programs may be inconsiderate of individualized neurologic recovery trajectories. However, acute hospital-based programs for medically complex patients with high comorbidity may be appropriate for aggressive management of comorbid medical conditions during participation in a conservative rehabilitation program. Less aggressive neurorehabilitation programs, or subacute rehabilitation programs, have become increasingly available in most communities, usually based in skilled nursing facilities. These subacute rehabilitation programs are not intended to commit the slowly recovering elderly patient to long-term institutional life. They are intended to provide a program that is more appropriately paced, with ultimate return to community life.

In treating the older neurologically impaired patient, the rehabilitation team is asked to take an incremental approach to setting program goals. Global functional end points of treatment must be deconstructed into a series of units of behavior that eventually reconstruct to a functional optimum as the patient is treated and recovers. Such a goal-setting strategy is more conducive to documenting neural and functional recovery, and better guarantees insurance reimbursement for these programs.

BENEFITS OF FORMAL REHABILITATION PROGRAMS

The benefits of early medical and surgical intervention and coordination of trauma care are well established. Aggressive surgical management of patients with severe head injuries, including evacuation of epidural, subdural, and intracerebral hemorrhages and attempts to reduce intracranial pressure or increase cerebral blood flow, are among the list of successful interventions. Likewise, rehabilitation interventions that prevent complications, such as decubiti or contractures, are effective in reducing morbidity and costs associated with injury. Identification of medical problems such as hydrocephalus in the rehabilitation setting can decrease morbidity and potentially improve function.[198, 260] Early mobilization prevents complications and may shorten length of stay for a variety of disorders, for example, traumatic brain injury.[261, 262]

The question of the efficacy of various types of rehabilitation programs has been addressed by a number of studies. In one such study, a group of patients receiving inpatient rehabilitation after traumatic brain injury had better outcomes than a control group of patients discharged to home, even though those in the rehabilitation group had more severe injuries as determined by the length of post-traumatic amnesia.[263] Other studies have demonstrated improved outcomes in groups of brain-injured survivors treated in postacute programs.[45, 46, 49, 50, 57, 264] Several factors that have been shown to be associated with the occurrence of traumatic brain injury and/or its outcome are independent of rehabilitative interventions. These include pre-existing factors, injury-related factors, variables related to acute management, and factors operative after injury in the post-rehabilitation environment.[265] Some of these factors can potentially confound the results of studies attempting to evaluate the efficacy of rehabilitative interventions.[265] The methodologic issues involved in studies of rehabilitation effectiveness have undoubtedly contributed to the paucity of studies in this area.

With the initiation of capitated managed care systems of reimbursement, some speculation must be allowed regarding the distribution of resources during neurorehabilitation programs. It is expected that most rehabilitation services will be offered during the initial 3–6 months after moderate or severe neurologic insult or injury, especially to serve the immediate purposes of establishing medical/surgical stability; to document baseline neural and functional performance levels; and to establish the ability of the social support system to provide home-based treatments under the supervision of the rehabilitation team.

There may be an effort, reinforced by capitated reimbursement, to move the rehabilitation program into a setting where the "hotel costs" can be minimized, for example, in the patient's or family members' homes. Various members of the social support system may be recruited to serve as home-based agents of treatment under scheduled and intermittent supervision of various members of the rehabilitation team available in the community. Thus, various therapists may be working with the older patient and their family care providers within a more loosely organized team process. These programs may be more selective as to when specific therapy interventions are considered appropriate and necessary, at different points in the recovery trajectory during and beyond the initial year of neurologic injury. The role of the physiatrist as team leader emerges as extremely important under the proposed managed care capitated model. The physiatrist has the best overview of the range of rehabilitation services and is best trained to negotiate, within a capitated system, the best entry and exit of various rehabilitation services. Thus, the physiatrist plays an instrumental role to assist capitated reimbursement systems with the expedient rationing of services during recovery of the patient with a neurologic or neurosurgical injury or disease.

CONCLUSIONS

This chapter outlines the scientific basis of rehabilitation medicine and argues for the involvement of physiatrists (rehabilitation medicine physicians) in the early care of patients with neurologic and neurosurgical emergencies. Physiatrists must work with neurologists and neurosurgeons in the acute care setting to evaluate and treat the patient's cognitive, behavioral, self-care, and mobility impairments; implement early mobilization to prevent the complications associated with bed rest; identify rehabilitation services required during various stages of recovery; and organize appropriate discharge planning. Specialists in geriatric and pediatric rehabilitation can provide additional consultative services for these populations with special needs.

References

1. Siebens H: Deconditioning. In Kemp B, Brummel-Smith K, Ransdell, JW (eds): Geriatric Rehabilitation, pp 177–191. Boston, Little, Brown, 1990.
2. DeLisa JA, Martin GM, Currie DM: Rehabilitation medicine: Past, present and future. In DeLisa JA (ed): Rehabilitation Medicine: Principles and Practice, 2nd ed, pp 3–27. Philadelphia, JB Lippincott, 1993.
3. World Health Organization (WHO): International Classification of Impairments, Disabilities, and Handicaps. Geneva, World Health Organization, 1976.
4. Robinson KM, Siegler EL, Streim JE: Medical emergencies in rehabilitation. In DeLisa JA (ed): Rehabilitation Medicine: Principles and Practice, 2nd ed, pp 783–797. Philadelphia, JB Lippincott, 1993.
5. Goldstein K: The Organism. A Holistic Approach to Biology Derived from Pathological Data in Man. New York, Zone Books, 1995.
6. Edelman GM: Neural Darwinism. The Theory of Neuronal Group Selection. New York, Basic Books, 1987.
7. Kelso JAS: Dynamic Patterns. The Self-Organization of Brain and Behavior. Cambridge, MA, MIT Press, 1995.
8. Hawkins RD, Kandel ER, Siegelbaum SA: Learning to modulate transmitter release: Themes and variations in synaptic plasticity. Annu Rev Neurosci 1993;16:625–665.
9. Merzenich MM, Jenkins WM: Reorganization of cortical representations of the hand following alteration of skin inputs induced by nerve injury, skin island transfers, and experience. J Hand Ther 1993;6:89–104.
10. Allard T, Clark SA, Jenkins WM, et al: Reorganization of somatosensory area 3b representations in adult owl monkeys after digital syndactyly. J Neurophysiol 1991;66:1048–1058.
11. Colebatch JG, Deiber M-P, Passingham RE, et al: Regional cerebral blood flow during voluntary arm and hand movements in human subjects. J Neurophysiol 1991;65:1392–1401.
12. Grafton ST, Mazziotta JC, Woods RP, et al: Human functional anatomy of visually-guided finger movements. Brain 1992;115:565–587.
13. Posner MI, Raichle ME: Images of Mind. New York, WH Freeman, 1994.
14. Chugani HT: Functional brain imaging in pediatrics. Pediatr Clin North Am 1992;39:777–799.
15. Raichle ME, Fiez JA, Videen TO, et al: Practice-related changes in human brain functional anatomy during non-motor learning. Cerebral Cortex 1994;4:8–26.
16. Chollet F, DiPiero V, Wise RJS, et al: The functional anatomy of motor recovery after stroke in humans: A study with positron emission tomography. Ann Neurol 1991;29:63–71.
17. Frackowiak RSJ, Weiller C, Chollet F: The functional anatomy of recovery from brain injury. In Chadwick DJ, Whelan J (eds): Exploring Brain Functional Anatomy with Positron Tomography (CIBA Foundation Symposium 163), pp 235–249. New York, John Wiley, 1991.
18. DiPiero V, Chollet FM, MacCarthy P, et al: Motor recovery after acute ischaemic stroke: A metabolic study. J Neurol Neurosurg Psychiatr 1992;55:990–996.
19. Weiller C, Chollet F, Friston KJ, et al: Functional reorganization of the brain in recovery from striatocapsular infarction in man. Ann Neurol 1992;31:463–472.
20. Weiller C, Ramsay SC, Wise RJS, et al: Individual patterns of functional reorganization in the human cerebral cortex after capsular infarction. Ann Neurol 1993;33:181–189.
21. Jenkins WM, Merzenich MM, Ochs MT, et al: Functional reorganization of primary somatosensory cortex in adult owl monkeys after behaviorally controlled tactile stimulation. J Neurophysiol 1990;63:82–104.
22. Jenkins WM, Merzenich MM: Reorganization of neocortical representations after brain injury. A neurophysiological model of the bases of recovery from stroke. Prog Brain Res 1987;71:249–266.
23. Goldberg G: Neurophysiologic models of recovery in stroke. Phys Med Rehabil Clin North Am 1991;2:599–614.
24. von Monakow C: Diaschisis (original 1914 article, Harris G [trans]). In Pribram KH (ed): Brain and Behavior. I: Mood States and Mind, pp 27–36. Baltimore, Penguin, 1969.
25. Feeney DM, Baron JC: Diaschisis. Stroke 1986;17:817–830.
26. Boyeson MG, Harmon RL: Acute and postacute drug-induced effects on rate of behavioral recovery after brain injury. J Head Trauma Rehabil 1994;9:78–90.
27. Feeney DM, Gonzalez A, Law WA: Amphetamine, haloperidol, and experience interact to affect rate of recovery after motor and cortex injury. Science 1982;127:855–857.
28. Cope N: An integration of psychopharmacological and rehabilitation approaches to traumatic brain injury rehabilitation. J Head Trauma Rehabil 1994;9:1–18.
29. Wroblewski BA, Glenn MB: Pharmacological treatment of arousal and cognitive deficits. J Head Trauma Rehabil 1994;9:19–42.
30. Goldstein LB, Matchar DB, Morganlander JC, et al: Influence of drugs on the recovery of sensory-motor function after stroke. J Neurol Rehab 1990;4:137–144.
31. Whyte J: Toward rational psychopharmacological treatment: Integrating research and clinical practice. J Head Trauma Rehabil 1994;9:91–103.
32. Barlow P, Teasdale G: Prediction of outcome and the management of severe head injuries: The attitude of neurosurgeons. Neurosurgery 1986;19:989–991.
33. Johnson EW: Outcome measures . . . a chimera? Am J Phys Med Rehabil 1992;71:201.
34. Sandel ME: Outcome measures and prognosis in traumatic brain injury. J Neurol Rehab 1995;9:111–115.
35. Brooks DN, Campsie L, Symington C, et al: The five year outcome of severe blunt head injury: A relative's view. J Neurol Neurosurg Psychiatry 1986;49:764–760.
36. Thomsen IV: Late outcome of very severe blunt head trauma: A 10–15 year follow-up. J Neurol Neurosurg Psychiatr 1984;47:260–268.
37. Oddy M, Coughlan T, Tyerman A, et al: Social adjustment after closed head injury: A further follow-up seven years after injury. J Neurol Neurosurg Psychiatr 1985;48:564–568.
38. Rappaport M, Herrero-Bock C, Rappaport MI, et al: Head injury outcome up to ten years later. Arch Phys Med Rehabil 1989;70:885–892.
39. Vogenthaler DR, Smith KR, Goldfader P: Head injury, an empirical study: Describing long-term productivity and independent living outcome. Brain Injury 1989;3:355–368.
40. Kriel RL, Krach LE, Sheehan M: Pediatric closed head injury: Outcome following prolonged unconsciousness. Arch Phys Med Rehabil 1988;69:678–681.
41. Jacobs HE: The Los Angeles Head Injury Survey: Procedures and initial findings. Arch Phys Med Rehabil 1988;69:425–431.
42. Ditunno JF, Stover SL, Freed MM, et al: Motor recovery

of the upper extremities in traumatic quadriplegia: A multicenter study. Arch Phys Med Rehabil 1992;73:431–436.
43. Piepmeier JM, Jenkins NR: Neurological changes following traumatic spinal cord injury. J Neurosurg 1988;69:399–402.
44. Gualtieri T, Cox DR: The delayed neurobehavioral sequelae of traumatic brain injury. Brain Injury 1991;5:219–232.
45. Johnston MV, Lewis FD: Outcomes of community re-entry programmes for brain injury survivors. Part I: Independent living and productive activities. Brain Injury 1991;5:141–154.
46. Johnston MV: Outcomes of community re-entry programmes for brain injury survivors: Part II: Further investigations. Brain Injury 1991;5:155–168.
47. Katz DI, Alexander MP, Roberts MB: Functional outcome after closed head injury: The effects of multiple neuropathologies. Arch Phys Med Rehabil 1993;74:661–662.
48. Jennett B, Teasdale G, Braakman R, et al: Predicting outcome in individual patients after severe head injury. Lancet 1976;i:1031–1034.
49. Fryer J, Haffey WJ: Cognitive rehabilitation and community readaptation: Outcomes from two program models. J Head Trauma Rehabil 1987;2:51–63.
50. Cope ND, Cole JR, Hall KM, et al: Brain injury: Analysis of outcome in a post-acute rehabilitation system. Part I: General analysis. Brain Injury 1991;5:111–126.
51. Cope ND, Cole JR, Hall KM, et al: Brain injury: Analysis of outcome in a post-acute rehabilitation system. Part II: Subanalysis. Brain Injury 1991;5:127–140.
52. Johnston MV, Keith RA, Hinderer S: Measurement standards for interdisciplinary medical rehabilitation. Arch Phys Med Rehabil 1992;73:Suppl 12:6S–23S.
53. Johnston MV, Findley TW, DeLuca J, et al: Research in physical medicine and rehabilitation: Measurement tools with application to brain injury. Am J Med Rehabil 1991;70:S114–S130.
54. Condeluci A, Ferris LL, Bogdan A, et al: Outcome and value: The survivor perspective. J Head Trauma Rehabil 1992;7:37–45.
55. Evans RW, Ruff RM: Outcome and value: A perspective on rehabilitation outcomes achieved in acquired brain injury. J Head Trauma Rehabil 1992;7:24–36.
56. Folstein MF, Folstein SE, McHugh PR: The Mini Mental state: A practical guide for grading the cognitive state of patients for the clinician. J Psychiatr Res 1975;12:189.
57. Mahoney FI, Barthel DW: Functional evaluation: The Barthel Index. Maryland State Med J 1965;14:61.
58. Uniform Data System for Medical Rehabilitation. Functional Independence Measure (FIM), Guide for the Use of the Uniform Data Set for Medical Rehabilitation. Buffalo, Research Foundation, State University of New York at Buffalo, 1989.
59. Haley SM, Coster WJ, Ludlow LH: Pediatric functional outcome measures. Phys Med Rehabil Clin North Am 1991;2:689–723.
60. Guide for the Uniform Data Set for Medical Rehabilitation for Children (WeeFIM[SM]), Version 4.0. Buffalo, State University of New York at Buffalo, 1993.
61. Haley SM, Coster WJ, Ludlow LH, et al: Pediatric Evaluation of Disability Inventory (PEDI), Version 1.0. Boston, New England Medical Center, 1992.
62. Jennett B, Plum F: Persistent vegetative state: A syndrome in search of a name. Lancet 1972;i:734–737.
63. Russell WR: Cerebral involvement in head injury. Brain 1932;55:549–605.
64. Corrigan JD, Mysiw WJ: Agitation following traumatic head injury: Equivocal evidence for a discrete stage of cognitive recovery. Arch Phys Med Rehabil 1988;69:487–92.
65. Levin HS, Grossman RG: Behavioral sequelae of closed head injury: A quantitative study. Arch Neurol 1978;35:720–727.
66. Reyes RL, Bhattacharyya AK, Heller D: Traumatic head injury: Restlessness and agitation as prognosticators of physical and psychologic improvement in patients. Arch Phys Med Rehabil 1981;62:20–23.
67. Brooke MM, Questad KA, Patterson DR, et al: Agitation and restlessness after closed head injury: A prospective study of 100 consecutive admissions. Arch Phys Med Rehabil 1992;73:320–323.
68. Brooke MM, Patterson DR, Questad KA: The treatment of agitation during initial hospitalization after traumatic brain injury. Arch Phys Med Rehabil 1992;73:917–921.
69. Denny-Brown D: Disability arising from closed head injury. JAMA 1945;127:429–436.
70. Levin HS, High WM, Goethe KE, et al: The neurobehavioural rating scale: Assessment of the behavioural sequelae of head injury by the clinician. J Neurol Neurosurg Psychiatry 1987;50:183–193.
71. Ommaya AK, Gennarelli TA: Cerebral concussion and traumatic unconsciousness: Correlation of experimental and clinical observations on blunt head injuries. Brain 1974;97:633–654.
72. Grant I, Alves W: Psychiatric and psychosocial disturbances in head injury. In Levin HS, Grafman J, Eisenberg HM (eds): Neurobehavioral Recovery from Head Injury, pp 232–261. Oxford University Press, 1987.
73. Taylor D, Lewis S: Delirium. J Neurol Neurosurg Psychiatry 1993;56:742–751.
74. Lipowski ZJ: Delirium: Acute Confusional States. New York, Oxford University Press, 1990.
75. Haskovec L: Akathisie. Arch Bohemes Med Clin 1902;3:193–200.
76. Stewart JT: Akathisia following traumatic brain injury: Treatment with bromocriptine. J Neurol Neurosurg Psychiatry 1989;52:1200–1201.
77. Diagnostic and Statistical Manual of Mental Disorders, 4th ed. Washington, D.C., American Psychiatric Association, 1994.
78. Sandel ME, Mysiw WJ: The agitated brain injured patient. Part I: Differential diagnosis and assessment. Arch Phys Med Rehabil 1996;77:617–623.
79. Teasdale G, Jennett B: Assessment of coma and impaired consciousness. Lancet 1974;ii:81–84.
80. Rappaport M, Hall KM, Hopkins K, et al: Disability Rating Scale for severe head trauma: Coma to community. Arch Phys Med Rehabil 1982;63:118–123.
81. Hall KM, Cope DN, Rappaport M: Glasgow Outcome Scale and Disability Rating Scale: Comparative usefulness in following recovery in traumatic head injury. Arch Phys Med Rehabil 1985;66:35–37.
82. Hagen C, Malkmus D, Durham P: Levels of cognitive functioning. Read at the 3rd Annual Post-Graduate Course on Rehabilitation of Traumatic Brain-Injured Adult, Williamsburg, VA, June 14–16, 1979.
83. Rappaport M, Dougherty AM, Kelting DL: Evaluation of coma and vegetative states. Arch Phys Med Rehabil 1992;73:628–634.
84. Giacino JT, Kermarsky MA, DeLuca J, et al: Monitoring rate of recovery to predict outcome in minimally responsive patients. Arch Phys Med Rehabil 1991;72:897–901.
85. Rader MA, Alston JB, Ellis DW: Sensory stimulation of severely brain injured patients. Brain Injury 1989;3:141–147.
86. Ansell BJ, Keenan JE: The Western Neurosensory Stimulation Profile: A tool for assessing slow-to-recover patients. Arch Phys Med Rehabil 1989;70:104–108.
87. Levin HS, O'Donnell VM, Grossman RG: The Galveston orientation and amnesia test: A practical scale to assess cognition after head injury. J Nerv Ment Dis 1979;167:675–84.
88. Ewing-Cobbs L, Levin HS, Fletcher JM, et al: The Children's Orientation and Amnesia Test: Relationship to severity of acute head injury and to recovery of memory. Neurosurgery 1990;27:683–691.
89. Corrigan JD, Arnett JA, Houck LJ, et al: Reality orientation for brain injured patients: Group treatment

Index

Note: Page numbers in *italics* indicate illustrations; those followed by t indicate tables.

ISBN 0-7216-6105-X

90038

9 780721 661056